Clinical Reproductive Endocrinology

Clinical Reproductive Endocrinology

Edited by

Rodney P. Shearman

MD FRCOG FRACOG

Professor of Obstetrics and Gynaecology, University of Sydney; Head,
Division of Obstetrics and Gynaecology King George V Memorial
Hospital, Royal Prince Alfred Hospital Sydney, Australia

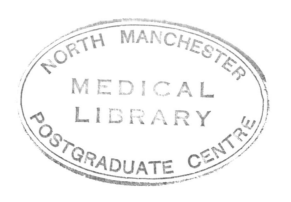

CHURCHILL LIVINGSTONE
EDINBURGH LONDON MELBOURNE AND NEW YORK 1985

CHURCHILL LIVINGSTONE
Medical Division of Longman Group Limited

Distributed in the United States of America by Churchill Livingstone
Inc., 1560 Broadway, New York, N.Y. 10036, and by associated
companies, branches and representatives throughout the world.

First published 1985

ISBN 0 443 02645 9

British Library Cataloguing in Publication Data
Clinical reproductive endocrinology.
    1. Generative organs—Diseases
    2. Endocrine glands
    I. Shearman, Rodney P.
    612'.6   RC877

Library of Congress Cataloging in Publication Data
Main entry under title:

Clinical reproductive endocrinology.

    1. Human reproduction—Endocrine aspects.
2. Generative organs—Diseases—Endocrine aspects.
3. Clinical endocrinology. I. Shearman, Rodney P.
[DNLM: 1. Endocrinology. 2. Genital Diseases, Female.
3. Genital Diseases, Male. 4. Reproduction. WQ 205
C6413]
QP252. C55   1984   612'.6   84-12156

Produced by Longman Group (FE) Limited
Printed in Hong Kong

Preface

It is not so very long ago that gynaecologists were almost exclusively surgeons and the specialties of andrology, perinatology and oncology did not exist. In the 1980s rigid and often artificial barriers between medical disciplines have largely disappeared. It is often a matter of chance, or the habit of referral patterns, whether an adolescent with, say, delayed puberty is seen and investigated by a paediatrician, a gynaecologist or an endocrinologist or a hirsute woman is referred to a dermatologist, a gynaecologist or a physician.

Reproductive endocrinology is relevant to huge areas of medicine — general practice, gynaecology, obstetrics, urology, paediatrics, endocrinology, oncology, genetics and general medicine. This book had its genesis in the publisher's belief that there was a need for a comprehensive text covering all aspects of reproductive endocrinology — not just the female, but also the male. We also felt it desirable to include significant sections dealing with endocrinology of breast cancer and neoplasia of the genital tract in men and women. This is a large text aimed at all of the groups mentioned above as a primary reference for those clinical problems with which they may not be intimately familiar but which cross their clinical horizons from time to time.

I am deeply indebted to the many contributors, each one distinguished in his own field, without whose help this book would not have been produced. No one man or small group can hope to encompass the skills and knowledge in all areas covered. I am also very conscious of my own responsibility to the contributors for delays in completion of the book. But with so many authors, there are always, unfortunately, one or two who fail to meet their previously agreed deadlines, resulting in deferments for all involved.

Throughout this long task the publishers have been extraordinarily helpful, even inspired. I am particularly grateful to them.

Sydney, 1985   Rodney P. Shearman

Contributors

J. Blankstein MD
Lecturer in Obstetrics and Gynecology, Sackler School of Medicine, Tel-Aviv University; Chief, University Clinic, Chaim Sheba Medical Centre, Tel-Hashomer, Israel

Ulf Borell MD
Professor at the Karolinska Institute; Head of the Department of Obstetrics and Gynecology, Karolinska Hospital, Stockholm, Sweden

Maxine Briggs MB ChB DPH DOH FRACMA
The Geelong Hospital, Australia

M. H. Briggs DSc PhD FRSC FI Biol FRC Path
Dean of Sciences, Deakin University, Australia

M. W. Brinsmead MB BS PhD MRCOG FRACOG
Senior Lecturer in Reproductive Medicine, The University of Newcastle, Australia

James B. Brown MSc (NZ and Melb) PhD (Edin) DSc (Edin) FRACOG
Professor, Royal Women's Hospital, Melbourne; Department of Obstetrics and Gynaecology, University of Melbourne, Australia

H. G. Burger MD FRACP
Director, Medical Research Centre, Prince Henry's Hospital; Professor of Medicine, Monash University, Melbourne, Australia

Marc Bygdeman MD
Professor and Vice-Chairman, Department of Obstetrics and Gynecology, Karolinska Hospital, Stockholm, Sweden

T. Chard MD FRCOG
Professor, Joint Academic Unit of Obstetrics, Gynaecology and Reproductive Physiology, St Bartholomews Hospital Medical College and The London Hospital Medical College, London, United Kingdom

I. D. Cooke MB BS DGO FRCOG
Professor of Obstetrics and Gynaecology, University of Sheffield; Honorary Consultant Obstetrician and Gynaecologist, Sheffield Health Authority, Jessop Hospital for Women, United Kingdom

M. Yusoff Dawood MD ChB M Med MRCOG FACOG
Professor and Director, Division of Reproductive Endocrinology; Department of Obstetrics and Gynecology, University of Illinois College of Medicine, Chicago, USA

D. M. de Kretser MD FRACP
Professor of Anatomy, Monash University, Melbourne, Australia

Sir John Dewhurst FRCS (Ed), FRCOG, Hon.FACOG
Professor of Obstetrics and Gynaecology at Queen Charlotte's Hospital for Women, London, United Kingdom

Gere S. diZerega MD
Department of Obstetrics and Gynecology, University of Southern California, Los Angeles, USA

James H. Evans MD BS FRCP (Edin) FRCOG FRACOG
Senior Endocrinologist, Royal Women's Hospital, Melbourne, Australia

C. C. Fisher FRCOG FRACGP FRACOG
Director, Fetal Intensive Care Unit, Royal Hospital for Women, Sydney, Australia

Ian S. Fraser BSc MB ChB MRCOG FRACOG
Associate Professor, Obstetrics and Gynaecology, University of Sydney; Honorary Obstetrician and Gynaecologist, King George V Memorial Hospital, Sydney, Australia

Joseph W. Goldzieher MD
Professor and Director Endocrine/Metabolic Research, Department of Obstetrics and Gynecology, Baylor College of Medicine, Houston, USA

Krister Gréen MD
Department of Clinical Chemistry, Karolinska Hospital, Stockholm, Sweden

Michael J. Gronow MB BS MRCOG MRACOG
Senior Registrar, Reproductive Biology Unit, Royal Women's Hospital, Carlton, Victoria, Australia

J. G. Grudzinskas BSc MD FRCAOG
Senior Lecturer and Honorary Visiting Medical Officer in Obstetrics and Gynaecology, University of Sydney, Royal North Shore Hospital of Sydney, St Margaret's Hospital for Women, Sydney, Australia*

Charles B. Hammond MD
E. C. Hamblen Professor and Chairman, Department of Obstetrics and Gynecology, Duke University Medical Center, Durham, USA

Joseph J. Hoet MD
Professor in Medicine, Department of Medicine, Unit of Endocrinology and Nutrition, Catholic University of Louvain, Clinique Saint-Luc, Brussels, Belgium

* Present address: Professor, Joint Academic Unit of Obstetrics, Gynaecology and Reproductive Physiology, The London Hospital Medical College and St Bartholomew's Hospital Medical College, London, United Kingdom

B. Hudson MD PhD FRACP

Associate Director, Howard Florey Institute of Experimental Physiology and Medicine, University of Melbourne, Melbourne, Australia

Elisabeth Johannisson MD PhD

Department of Obstetrics and Gynecology, Basle, Switzerland

Firyal S. Khan-Dawood PhD

Assistant Professor, Division of Reproductive Endocrinology, Department of Obstetrics and Gynecology, University of Illinois College of Medicine, Chicago, USA

Arnold Klopper MD PhD FRCOG

Professor of Reproductive Endocrinology, Department of Obstetrics and Gynaecology, University of Aberdeen, United Kingdom

Robert P. S. Jansen BSc MB BS FRACP MRCOG FRACOG

Visiting Obstetrician and Gynaecologist, King George V Memorial Hospital, Sydney; Clinical Lecturer, Department of Obstetrics and Gynaecology, University of Sydney

Ian Johnston MB BS MGO FRCOG FRACOG

Gynaecologist in Charge, Reproductive Biology Unit, Royal Women's Hospital, Melbourne, Australia

Howard W. Jones Jr MD

Professor Emeritus, Gynecology and Obstetrics, John Hopkins University School of Medicine, Baltimore, Maryland; Professor of Obstetrics and Gynecology, Eastern Virginia Medical School, Norfolk, USA

Stephen Judd MD FRACP

Department of Medicine, Flinders Medical Centre and Centre for Neuroscience, Flinders University of South Australia, Australia

Georgeanna Jones Klingensmith MD

Assistant Professor of Pediatrics, University of Colorado, Denver, USA

Gabor T. Kovacs MB BS MRCOG FRACOG

Medical Research Centre, Prince Henry's Hospital, Melbourne, Australia

Britt-Marie Landgren MD

Reproductive Endocrinology Research Unit, Karolinska Hospital, Stockholm, Sweden

P. H. Lange MD

Chief, Section of Urology, Veterans Administration Hospital, Minneapolis; Professor, Department of Urologic Surgery, University of Minnesota, Minneapolis, USA

Elizabeth A. Lenton BSc PhD

Lecturer in Reproductive Endocrinology, Department of Obstetrics and Gynaecology, University of Sheffield, United Kingdom

Derek Llewellyn-Jones OBE MD FRCOG FRACOG

Associate Professor of Obstetrics and Gynaecology, University of Sydney, Australia

Viveca Lundström MD

Associate Professor, Department of Obstetrics and Gynecology, Karolinska Hospital, Stockholm, Sweden

B. Lunenfeld MD FRCOG

Professor of Endocrinology, Bar Ilan University, Ramat-Gan; Director, Institute of Endocrinology, Chaim Sheba Medical Centre, Tel-Hashomer, Israel

Paul G. McDonough MD

Professor of Obstetrics and Gynecology; Chief, Reproductive Endocrine Division, Medical College of Georgia, Augusta, USA

William L. McGuire MD

Professor and Chief of the Division of Medical Oncology, University of Texas Health Science Center, San Antonio, USA

F. I. R. Martin MD FRACP

Professorial Associate, Department of Medicine, University of Melbourne; Physician in Charge, Department of Diabetes and Endocrinology, Royal Melbourne Hospital; Physician to Diabetes Clinic, Royal Women's Hospital, Melbourne, Australia

S. Mashiach MD

Associate Professor, Obstetrics and Gynecology, Sackler School of Medicine, Tel-Aviv University; Director, Department of Obstetrics and Gynecology, Chaim Sheba Medical Centre, Tel-Hashomer, Israel

D. R. Mishell Jnr MD

Professor and Chairman, Department of Obstetrics and Gynecology, University of Southern California School of Medicine, Women's Hospital, Los Angeles, USA

P. M. S. O'Brien MD MRCOG

Lecturer, Department of Obstetrics and Gynaecology, The Royal Free Hospital, London, United Kingdom

Colm O'Herlihy MB BCh MD (Melb) BAO DCH MRACOG MRACP (1)

Senior Registrar, National Maternity Hospital, Dublin, Ireland

Steven J. Ory MD

Assistant Professor, Division of Reproductive Endocrinology and Infertility, Department of Obstetrics and Gynecology, Duke University Medical Centre, Durham, USA★

Roger J. Pepperell MD MGO FRACP FRCOG FRACOG

Professor of Obstetrics and Gynaecology, University of Melbourne, Australia

Bengt Persson MD

Associate Professor, Karolinska Institute, Department of Pediatrics, St Goran's Hospital, Stockholm, Sweden

Derek Raghavan MB BS FRACP

Staff Specialist in Medical Oncology, Royal Prince Alfred Hospital; Honorary Consultant, Ludwig Institute for Cancer Research, Sydney, Australia

J. S. Robinson BSc MB BCh BAO MRCOG FRACOG

Professor of Reproductive Medicine, The University of Newcastle, Australia

Franz Michael Schroeder MD

Department of Radiology, Royal Prince Alfred Hospital, Sydney, Australia

Rodney P. Shearman MD FRCOG FRACOG

Professor of Obstetrics and Gynaecology, University of Sydney; Head, Division of Obstetrics and Gynaecology, King George V Memorial Hospital, Sydney, Australia

George W. Sledge MD

Staff Oncologist, Division of Medical Oncology, University of Taxas Health Science Center, San Antonia, USA

E. M. Symonds MD FRCOG

Professor of Obstetrics and Gynaecology, University Hospital, Nottingham, United Kingdom

★ Present address: Director of Reproductive Endocrinology and Infertility Clinics, Department of Obstetrics and Gynecology, Northwestern University, Chicago, USA

Pincus Taft MD FRACP
Associate Professor, Department of Medicine and Biochemistry, Monash University, Melbourne; Consultant Physician, Ewen Downie Metabolic Unit, Alfred Hospital, Melbourne; Visiting Endocrinologist, St Vincent's Hospital, Melbourne, Australia

Selwyn Taylor DM MCh FRCS
Dean Emeritus, Royal Postgraduate Medical School, Hammersmith Hospital, London, United Kingdom

B. Teisner MD
Associate Professor, Institute of Medical Microbiology, University of Odense, Odense, Denmark

Sandra P. T. Tho MD
Assistant Clinical Professor, Department of Obstetrics and Gynecology, Reproductive Endocrine Division, Medical College of Georgia, Augusta, USA

Alan O. Trounson MSc PhD
Department of Obstetrics and Gynaecology, Monash University, Queen Victoria Medical Centre, Melbourne, Australia

Frans Andre Van Assche MD PhD
Professor of Obstetrics and Gynaecology, University Hospital, Gasthuisberg, Leuven, Belgium

T. G. Williams MA MChir FRCS
Senior Surgical Registrar, St Thomas' Hospital, London, United Kingdom

Carl Wood CBE MB BS FRCS FRCOG FRACOG
Chairman and Professor, Department of Obstetrics and Gynaecology, Monash University, Queen Victoria Medical Centre, Melbourne, Australia

Contents

The neuroendocrinology of reproduction

INTRODUCTION

The relationship between the gonad and the development of secondary sexual characteristics and reproductive capacity in the human has been known for many centuries, since eunuchs first guarded harems; however, the recognition that function of the gonad depends on central stimulation is a relatively recent discovery. Over the last 80 years, since Frohlich's description of adiposogenital dystrophy, we have seen the birth and rapid maturation of the science of neuroendocrinology and with it the realisation that the pituitary, the hypothalamus and higher centres in the brain are essential for the normal function of the gonad. This chapter considers these central elements; their structure, function, and integration. It will also consider the clinical problems of reproduction which result from abnormalities in the central component of this system.

GONADOTROPHIN RELEASING HORMONE (GnRH)

A major advance in our understanding of the neuroendocrinology of reproduction was the recognition that a humoral agent in the hypothalamus, gonadotrophin releasing hormone (GnRH), stimulates the release of luteinising hormone (LH) and follicle stimulatory hormone (FSH). The peptide nature of this substance was demonstrated when bovine GnRH was found to be inactivated by pepsin (McCann & Ramirez, 1964). In rapid succession, porcine (Schally et al, 1971) and ovine (Amoss et al, 1971) GnRH were isolated, purified and sequenced and were found to be an identical linear decapeptide (Fig. 1.1).

The next step of this classic model of endocrine research was to develop antibodies to synthetic GnRH and then, using the techniques of immunohistofluorescence and radioimmunoassay, to localise the site of production and secretion of GnRH in the brain.

Gonadotropin releasing hormone

pyro Glu - His - Trp - Ser - Tyr - Gly - Leu - Arg - Pro - Gly - NH_2

Met enkephalin

Tyr - Gly - Gly - Phe - Met

Leu enkephalin

Tyr - Gly - Gly - Phe - Leu

Endorphins

Tyr[61] - Gly - Gly - Phe - Met - Thr - Ser - Glu - Lys - Ser - Gln -
Val - Ile - Ala - Aln - Lys - Phe - Leu[77] - Thr[76] - Val - Leu - Pro - Thr -
Lys - Asn - Ala - His[87] - Lys - Lys - Gly - Gln[91]

Fig. 1.1 The amino-acid structure of gonadotropin releasing hormone (GnRH), the enkephalins and the endorphins

Localisation of GnRH in the brain

The major concentration of GnRH in the mammalian brain, whether measured by radioimmunoassay or demonstrated by immunohistofluorescent staining, is found in the lateral pallisade zone of the external layer of the median eminence. In this area GnRH is found within nerve terminals, contained in granules 75–90 nm in diameter. These nerve endings are in close proximity to the portal capillaries through which they influence gonadotrophin secretion from the pituitary (Barry, 1976).

GnRH cell bodies are fusiform in shape measuring 12–20 μ in diameter with an eccentric cell nucleus and a single axon projection. There are two main sites of concentration of these cell bodies. The major group arises from the lateral portion of the arcuate nucleus and adjacent periventricular area and a second group is sited more rostrally in the anterior hypothalamus in the medial preoptic area (MPOA) and the interstitial nucleus of the striae terminalis (Fig. 1.2). Axon projections from these cell bodies have been difficult to trace over any distance, largely because they run a rather diffuse course rather than being in discrete bundles. It is thought that some of the axons from the MPOA find their way to the median eminence but others terminate in a second area more close

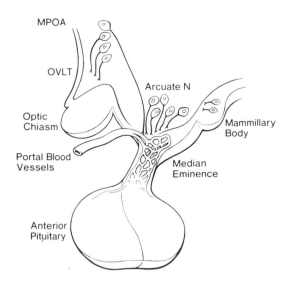

Fig. 1.2 The distribution of GnRH neurons in the human brain. The major group has its cell bodies in the arcuate nucleus and its nerve terminals in the median eminence. Some median eminence terminals may originate in the medial preoptic area (MPOA). The organ vasculosum of the lamina terminalis (OVLT) also contains a portal circulation.

by, the organ vasculosum lamina terminalis (OVLT), which also contains a systemic portal circulation.

Evidence has also been presented to suggest that some GnRH reaches the portal blood, supplying the pituitary by means of specialised ependymal cells (tanycytes) which line the third ventricle (Koyabashi, et al, 1970). These cells are congregated in the infundibular process of the third ventricle and on one side send long filamentous projections

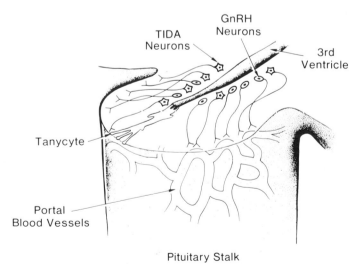

Fig. 1.3 Morphological connections between dopamine and GnRH neurons and tanycytes in the hypothalamus. GnRH and tuberoinfundibular dopamine (TIDA) cell bodies arise in the arcuate nucleus and their nerve terminals intermingle in the lateral pallisade zone of the external layer of the median eminence. Tanycytes connect the third ventricle to the portal blood vessels. Dopamine nerve terminals also end close to the tanycytes

into the lumen of the ventricle; from the other side, an irregular cytoplasmic process extends through the width of the median eminence to end close to portal capillaries (Fig. 1.3). These cytoplasmic processes contain mitochondria and microtubules arranged parallel to the long axis in an orientation which suggests that they might also be involved in transport of substances between the CSF and portal blood. Radioactive protein, including GnRH, injected into the CSF can be located in tanycytes (Ondo et al, 1972; Scott et al, 1974) and immunoreactive GnRH material has been located in tanycytes of mice but not other species (Zimmerman et al, 1974a). Moreover, tanycytes undergo structural changes when exposed to changing levels of ovarian steroids or catecholamines. However, the exact role of the tanycytes in the physiological transport of GnRH to the portal capillaries is still not established and it seems more likely that the tanycytes are of secondary importance to axoplasmic transport of GnRH in nerve cells.

Biosynthesis of GnRH

Immunofluorescent studies have established that GnRH is localised within neuronal structures in the hypothalamus and it is now accepted that GnRH is one of an increasing number of neuropeptides which are synthesised in neuronal cell bodies. From basic principles of peptide synthesis elsewhere in the body and by analogy with the neurohypophyseal hormone, vasopressin, (Sachs et al, 1969) it would be expected that the biosynthesis of GnRH requires transcription and translation of messenger RNA in the sophisticated biomachinery of the endoplasmic reticulum in the neuronal cell body. This would necessitate axonal transport of GnRH (or a more complex prohormone) to the nerve terminals for processing, storage and eventual release (Fig. 1.4). The occurrence of a genetic abnormality (with autosomal recessive inheritance) resulting in reduced GnRH synthesis and hypogonadism in both mice and humans (Cattanach et al, 1977) tends to support this concept because of the well established link between gene abnormality and nuclear protein synthesis. Moreover colchicine, which inhibits axonal transport of proteins, leads to accumulation of GnRH immunofluorescence in the nerve cell body (Barry et al, 1974) and immunoelectron-microscopic studies of the cell body and nerve axon have shown dense core vesicles of GnRH indicating that this is the most likely site of hormone synthesis (Krisch, 1978).

There is some evidence to support the existence of a precursor or prohormone for GnRH in the hypothalamus. Barnea & Porter (1975) isolated a large molecular weight protein (60 000 daltons) which cross-reacted with some, but not all antibodies to GnRH. This could be either a prohormone or GnRH associated with a binding protein, analogous to the association of neurophysin and vasopressin. If a prohormone form does exist, it would require

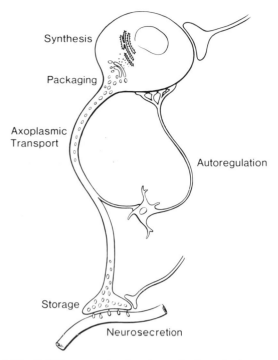

Fig. 1.4 The GnRH neuron showing the synthesis packaging, transport, storage and secretion of GnRH. Neurons containing other neurotransmitters influence the GnRH neuron either at its cell body or its nerve terminal

a final processing step to form the active decapeptide, and this would probably occur in the axon terminals.

Neurosecretion

Secretion of GnRH is directly linked to the activity of the GnRH neuron which, in turn, depends on the input from a variety of peptidergic and monoaminergic neurons making contact by axo-somatic, axo-dendritic, or axo-axonic connections (Fig. 1 4) Depolarisation of the cell body causes a rapid increase in the permeability of a voltage-dependent calcium channel which results in a rise of intracellular calcium content (Kelly et al, 1979). This initiates a series of intracellular events which results in exocytosis of vesicles containing GnRH (Rasmussen & Goodman, 1977). The concentration of intracellular calcium ions determines the amplitude of GnRH secretion (Drouva et al, 1981).

Metabolism

Although GnRH is relatively stable when incubated *in vitro* with blood or urine, it has a short half-life in the serum (first phase disappearance of 4 minutes). This is the result of widespread distribution of peptidases in liver, kidney, lung, and skeletal muscle which degrade GnRH rapidly and specifically (Swift & Crighton, 1979). Local inactivation of GnRH in the hypothalamus and pituitary is physiologically more important. Several peptidases may be involved. A neutral endopeptidase which splits Gly^6–Leu^7, is present in the cytoplasm of both the hypothalamus and the pituitary and is an important, initial, inactivation step (Koch, et al, 1974). Other peptidases cleave the C terminal Gly -NH_2 and Tyr^5-Gly^6. These enzymes may have physiological importance since their activity is influenced by castration, treatment with gonadal steroids (Griffiths et al, 1974) and dopamine (Marcano De Cotte et al, 1980).

The physiology of GnRH secretion

It is now clearly established that GnRH release into the portal venous blood is characterised by intermittent pulses superimposed on a lower level of continuous secretion. Evidence for this is derived from various sources.

1. Electrical recordings of neuronal activity by electrodes positioned in the medial basal hypothalamus of ovariectomised rhesus monkeys show intermittent electrical activity at hourly intervals which correlates well with the pulsatility of LH in the peripheral circulation (Knobil, 1981).

2. Studies with push-pull cannulae inserted into the median eminence of ovariectomised sheep show pulsatile release of GnRH every 40 minutes, with peak levels of 1–6 pg per 10 minute sample (Levine & Ramirez, 1980).

3. Finally, using a method of collecting portal vein blood which does not require anaesthesia or section of the pituitary stalk, Clarke & Cummins (1982) found portal blood concentrations of GnRH ranging between 5–30 pg/ml in ovariectomised sheep. This elegant techinique does not significantly alter pituitary function and contemporaneous measurement of peripheral blood LH showed that all pulses of LH are preceded by an increase in portal blood GnRH (Fig. 1.5).

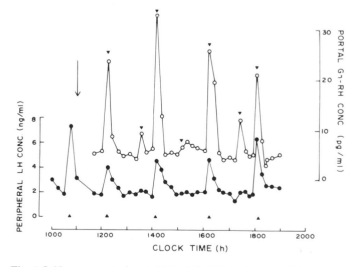

Fig. 1.5 Measurement of portal blood GnRH (o-o) and peripheral blood LH (●–●) in the undisturbed, conscious, ovariectomised sheep. GnRH secretion is pulsatile and each pulse of LH is preceeded by a substantial secretion of GnRH. Reproduced with permission from Clarke & Cummins (1982)

The site of origin of pulsatile secretion of GnRH appears, in the monkey at least, to reside in the hypothalamic island containing the arcuate nucleus, the median eminence, part of the ventromedial nucleus, the premamillary area, and the mamillary bodies (Krey et al, 1975), although a wider area of the hypothalamus may be involved with pulsatile secretion of LH in the rat (Gallo, 1981). Moreover, in the monkey relatively discrete lesions of the arcuate nucleus abolish the pulsatile pattern of LH secretion while lesions sparing the arcuate have a less devastating effect (Plant et al, 1978).

The frequency of GnRH secretion is determined by the firing rate of the neuron, a function which is likely to originate in the perikaryon. The amplitude of the GnRH pulses is determined not only by stimuli acting at the cell body but also by those affecting the nerve terminals in the median eminence. Moreover, the LH response to this pulse is dependent on the sensitivity of the pituitary gonadotrope to GnRH stimulation.

Many different approaches have been used to study the effect of different neurotransmitters on the GnRH neuron. Until recently, factors that influence the *magnitude* of LH have received most attention, but the critical importance of the *frequency* of GnRH secretion to ovulation has now been established and these will be considered independently.

Factors modulating the frequency of GnRH secretion

The frequency of LH secretion in women varies at different times of the menstrual cycle (Fig. 1.6). LH pulses occur every 1–2 hours in the early follicular phase with increasing amplitude until preovulation. Recent studies have suggested that there is an increase in frequency, as well as amplitude, in the preovulatory phase in both the human (Backstrom et al, 1982) and the rat (Gallo, 1981).

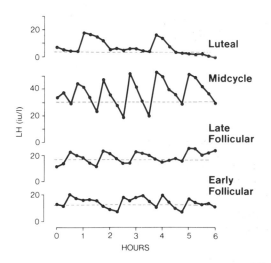

Fig. 1.6 The pattern of LH secretion in a normal woman at different times of the menstrual cycle showing the variation of amplitude and frequency of LH pulses. Modified from Yen et al (1974b)

It is possible that oestrogen modulates the frequency of GnRH secretion at this time, but this remains to be established.

During the luteal phase, there is a remarkable reduction in LH pulsatility to one pulse every 4 hours. This change is probably related to the increase in serum progesterone which characterises the luteal phase. In the ovariectomised ewe, chronic administration of progesterone in doses equivalent to those normally found in the luteal phase, causes a reduction in LH pulsatility (Fig. 1.7). A similar effect in

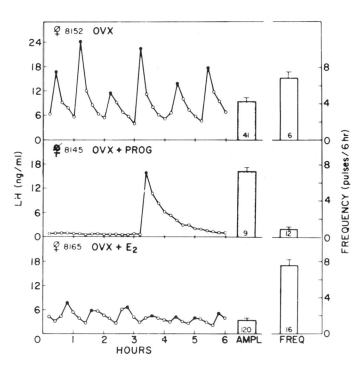

Fig. 1.7 The influence of 17 β oestradiol (E₂) and progesterone (Prog) on the frequency and amplitude of LH secretion in the ovariectomised sheep. Progesterone reduced the frequency but not the amplitude whereas oestradiol reduces amplitude but not frequency. Reproduced with permission from Goodman & Karsch (1980)

progesterone has also been described in the ovariectomised woman (Yen, 1978). Progesterone is known to have anaesthetic properties and to alter electroencephalographic recordings in the human which, combined with the demonstration of progesterone receptors in the brain, indicate that it *may* have a direct effect on brain neurons. However, its action on the firing rate of GnRH neurons appears to be mediated indirectly by increasing the activity of opioid peptide neurons in the brain. This is suggested by the observation that naloxone, an opiate antagonist, increases the frequency of LH pulses in normal women in the luteal but not the early follicular phase (Ropert et al, 1981) (Fig. 1.8) and also with the studies that show that naloxone increases the frequency of LH secretion in ovariectomised rats treated with oestrogen and progesterone but not oestrogen alone (Sylvester et al, 1982).

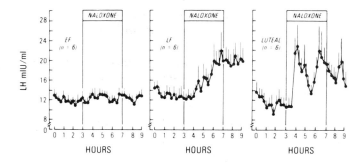

Fig. 1.8 The effect of naloxone on serum LH levels in 6 women in the early follicular (EF), late follicular (LF) and the luteal phase of the menstrual cycle. Naloxone increases serum LH in the late follicular phase without changing the frequency of secretion. In the luteal phase, naloxone increases the frequency of LH secretion from its normal rate of one pulse per 4 hours. Reproduced with permission from Quigley & Yen (1980) Journal of Clinical Endocrinology and Metabolism 51: 179–181

Endogenous opioids

The discovery of endogenous opioid peptides in the brain resulted from the observation that the brain contained specific receptors for morphine. The pentapeptides, leu and met-enkephalin (Fig. 1.1) were the first 'endorphins' to be isolated (Hughes et al, 1975); this was followed by the observation that fragments 61–76, 61–77, 61–87, and 61–91 of the pituitary hormone lipotropin (subsequently named α, γ, δ, and β endorphin respectively) had opiate activity (Guillemin et al, 1976) (Fig. 1.1)

Enkephalin cell bodies are widely distributed through the central nervous system, including the arcuate, ventro-medial, premamillary, and paraventricular nuclei of the hypothalamus (Hokfelt et al, 1978); met-enkephalin is present in three times the concentration of leu-enkephalin. Although the greatest concentration of β endorphin is found in the pituitary, significant concentrations are also found in the arcuate nucleus. Nerve endings containing enkephalins are found throughout the central nervous system including the external layer of the median eminence (Hokfelt et al, 1978). Nerve fibres containing β endorphin are distributed from the arcuate nucleus cell bodies to various areas of the brain including the locus coeruleus, an important area containing noradrenaline cell bodies (Adler, 1980). Hence, there is a great potential for interaction between opiate peptide and GnRH neurons either directly or via monoaminergic intermediates.

A third opioid compound, humoral endorphin (H-endorphin) has been described which is apparently distinct from the enkephalins and endorphin (Sarne et al, 1978). This material is similar in structure to leu-enkephalin since it crossreacts with the same antibody, but it differs by having a larger molecular size, being more stable in blood and CSF than the enkephalins and by having different pharmacological effects (Sarne et al, 1980). H-endorphin has a similar distribution in the brain to the enkephalins

although the proportion varies in different areas. The physiological role of this peptide remains to be determined.

Several studies have indicated an important role for the endogenous opioid peptides in the control of GnRH secretion. The earliest indication of this was the report that morphine prevents ovulation in rats when injected during the critical phase of proestrus (Barraclough & Sawyer, 1955); this was later shown to be due to an inhibition of the proestrus LH surge (Pang et al, 1977). Chronic anovulation in the human is a common association of morphine addiction (Gaulden et al, 1964) although it has not been established whether this is a specific effect of morphine. Met-enkephalin and β endorphin both decrease serum LH in the rat (Van Vugt & Meites, 1980) and the enkephalin analogue, DAMME, reduces serum LH in the human (Grossman et al, 1981). Conversely, increases in serum LH occur after administration of the opiate antagonist, naloxone, in the late follicular or luteal phases of the cycle (Fig. 1.8), indicating that the endogenous opioid peptides exert a tonic inhibiting action on the GnRH neurons at these times. *In vitro* studies, have shown that this inhibitory action of opioid peptides occurs in the medial basal hypothalamus (Wilkes & Yen, 1981) although a role of the amygdala in mediating the opioid peptide inhibition of GnRH neurons, as suggested by Lakoski & Gebhart (1981) cannot be excluded by these *in vitro* studies.

More detailed studies have shown that the reduction in serum LH seen after administration of opiates is the result of a reduced frequency of pulsatility rather than to a reduced amplitude of each individual secretory pulse (Sylvester et al, 1982). This role of the endogenous opioid peptides in modulating the frequency of GnRH secretion may have an important physiological role in the human, particularly with respect to the luteal phase and puberty. It is now realised that the gonadotrope responds optimally to a narrow range of frequency signals and that variation in this frequency profoundly affects the ratio of secretion of LH relative to FSH (Hausler et al, 1979). The reduced frequency of GnRH secretion in the luteal phase may be important in resting ovarian follicles between cycles or providing an optimal ratio of FSH to LH for new follicle development.

Factors affecting the magnitude of GnRH secretion

A wide range of studies using different approaches indicate the importance of various monaminergic brain neurotransmitters in the control of GnRH neuronal activity and hence the magnitude of GnRH secretion. To date, it has not been possible to monitor the electrical activity of a functionally homologous group of monoaminergic neurons and then to correlate this with minute to minute fluctuation of GnRH secretion in an undisturbed animal. Hence less direct methods have, by necessity, been used.

The wide range of approaches and models have made this important, though complex, area difficult to elucidate. However certain generalisations can be made about the role of individual neurotransmitters.

(a) *Noradrenaline.* Noradrenaline nerve terminals are present in the areas of the brain which contain GnRH cell bodies (Fuxe et al, 1978), and are generally considered to have a *facilitatory* action on the GnRH cell body. This may be a direct effect on the cell body or it may act more indirectly by reducing the activity of an inhibitory neurotransmitter affecting GnRH neurons.

Numerous models have been established to examine the relationship between noradrenaline activity in the brain and GnRH secretion. Early studies revealed that generalised depletion of brain catecholamines blocked ovulation in the rat, presumably by inhibiting the midcycle surge of LH (Barraclough & Sawyer, 1955; Coppola et al, 1966); drugs which specifically depleted only peripheral catecholamines were without effect (Coppola, 1968). More selective depletion of noradrenaline with diethyldithiocarbamate reduced the surge of LH induced by progesterone treatment of the oestrogen-primed castrate rat (Kalra et al, 1972). Castration was found to increase the concentration of noradrenaline in pooled blocks of the anterior hypothalamus (Donoso & Stefano, 1967) and oestrogen replacement reduced noradrenaline concentration. More recently, Selmanoff and others showed that noradrenaline concentration increased sharply in discrete hypothalamic nuclei at the time of the pre-ovulatory surge of LH (Selmanoff et al, 1976).

In an attempt to obtain a more dynamic assessment of noradrenaline activity in the brain, other groups have measured the turnover rate of noradrenaline in areas of the brain and have found it is increased at the time of the pre-ovulatory LH surge (Löfström, 1977). In other studies, intracerebroventricular injections of noradrenaline were found to increase serum LH and to induce ovulation while α adrenergic blockers, e.g. phenoxybenzamine, reduce serum levels of LH in the monkey (Bhattacharya et al, 1972) though not in the human (Santen & Bardin, 1973).

(b) *Dopamine.* Histofluorescent studies show an accumulation of both GnRH and dopamine nerve endings in the lateral pallisade zone of the external layer of the median eminence (Löfström et al, 1976) (Fig. 1.3). Electron microscopic examination of this area show numerous granules, some of which are undoubtedly catecholamines and others which are probably releasing factors (Kobayashi et al, 1970). These granules are closely related but do not coexist in the same axon since destruction of dopamine terminals does not change the local concentration of GnRH (Kizer et al, 1975). Moreover, numerous 'synaptoid' contacts have been described between nerve axons containing dopamine and cytoplasmic processes of tanycytes (Guldner & Wolff, 1973). In addition, dopamine nerve terminals of the incerto-hypothalamic tract supply and hence may influence the medial preoptic area containing GnRH cell bodies.

Hence, there are numerous sites at which dopamine could influence GnRH secretion. At the nerve terminal level, local release of dopamine may alter release of GnRH from adjacent nerve terminals by changing nerve membrane activity or the process of exocytosis; also, high local concentration of dopamine may alter the local degradation of GnRH after release from nerve terminals (Marcano De Cotte et al, 1980). If tanycytes are involved in the transport or storage of GnRH then the synaptoid contact demonstrated between dopamine neurons and tanycyte processes may be physiologically relevant. On the basis of electron microscopic changes, it has also been suggested that tanycytes may be structurally altered by local dopamine release and that this forces GnRH nerve terminals further away from portal capillaries and hence reduces portal blood concentration of GnRH (Hokfelt et al, 1978).

The role of dopamine in the control of GnRH is more controversial than that of noradrenaline though most recent studies suggest that dopamine is an inhibitory neurotransmitter acting chiefly at the GnRH nerve terminal. In early studies, McCann and his colleagues showed that dopamine had no effect on the pituitary; however, when hypothalamic tissue was co-incubated with the pituitary, dopamine *stimulated* the release of LH and FSH (Schneider & McCann, 1969; Kamberi et al, 1969). A subsequent report from the same group was unable to confirm these findings (Quijada et al, 1973) and in a similar *in vitro* experiment, dopamine was found to *inhibit* LH secretion from the pituitary left attached to the median eminence (Miyachi et al, 1973).

Injection of both dopamine and noradrenaline into the third ventricle stimulated LH, FSH and bioassayable GnRH from the brain (Kamberi et al, 1971). In contrast, relatively large doses of dopamine were without effect in another study although noradrenaline caused an ovulatory LH surge (Sawyer et al, 1974). This apparent paradox may be explained by rapid uptake and conversion of dopamine to noradrenaline after injection into the CSF, or perhaps oxidation and inactivation of dopamine (Takahara et al, 1974). A further technical factor raised as a possible explanation of these findings is that gonadotrophin secretion can be induced in some models by non-specific mechanical stretching of the ventricle (Porter et al, 1972.).

Local injection of dopamine into the arcuate nucleus inhibits ovulation in rats (Craven & McDonald, 1973) and implantation of dopamine into the median eminence also inhibits LH secretion (Uemura & Kobayashi, 1971). In detailed studies of ovariectomised rats given large intraperitoneal or subcutaneous injections of the dopamine agonists apomorphine and peribedil, several groups have reported that LH secretion is inhibited (Gnodde & Schuilling, 1976; Mueller et al, 1976; Drouva & Gallo,

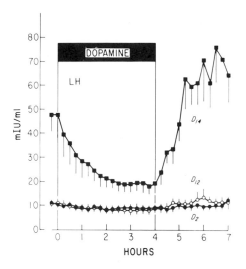

Fig. 1.9 The influence of dopamine (4 μg/kg/min) infusion on serum levels of LH in six normal women in the early follicular phase (D_2), late follicular phase (D_{12}) and preovulatory phase (D_{14}) of the menstrual cycle. Dopamine causes an inhibition of serum LH, particularly in the pre-ovulatory phase. Reproduced with permission from Judd et al (1979)

1977). However, systemic injections of dopamine antagonists do not increase serum LH which suggests that endogenous dopamine does not exert a tonic effect on GnRH secretion in rats (Drouva & Gallo, 1977).

In human studies, systemic infusion of dopamine causes a consistent reduction in circulatory LH without altering the frequency of LH pulsatility. Moreover, this effect of dopamine is influenced by the prevailing concentration of oestrogen (Fig. 1.9). Since dopamine delivered systemically does not cross the blood brain barrier and since cessation of dopamine is followed by a rebound increase in serum LH, it is likely that dopamine directly inhibits the release of GnRH by an action on GnRH nerve terminals. This does not exclude a different action at another site, e.g. the GnRH cell body. Indeed, if dopamine does exert a stimulatory action at the GnRH cell body, then the recent report that GnRH inhibits the biosynthesis of dopamine (Wang et al, 1982) raises the possibility that dopamine neurons may be important in the autoregulation of GnRH neurons (Fig. 1.4).

(c) *Serotonin*. Most of the serotonin-containing neurons in the hypothalamus are derived from the dorsal raphe nucleus in the midbrain and high concentrations of nerve terminals are found in the median eminence (Mulder & Snyder, 1976), and in the suprachiasmatic and arcuate nuclei (Palkovits et al, 1974). Elegant studies by Gallo have suggested that serotonin is an inhibitory neurotransmitter which acts at the GnRH cell bodies in the arcuate nucleus. Hence, stimulation of the dorsal raphe nucleus inhibits the secretion of LH but this effect is abolished if serotonin synthesis is blocked (Gallo & Moberg, 1977). Direct stimulation of the arcuate nucleus suppresses serum LH levels since serotonin neurons are stimulated and these inhibit

GnRH secretion. However, when serotonin synthesis is blocked, arcuate stimulation produces an unrestrained secretion of GnRH and hence the serum LH response is increased (Gallo, 1980). In other studies, intraventricular injection of the serotonin neurotoxin 5,7 dihydroxytryptamine which destroys serotonin neurons caused a *decrease* in serum LH levels (Wuttke et al, 1978) which supports an earlier view that serotonin is *excitatory* for GnRH secretion (Hery et al, 1976). Hence the precise role of serotonin remains to be established.

(d) *Other potential neurotransmitters*. Early work implicated acetylcholine as a stimulatory neurotransmitter on the basis of release of LH after intraventricular injection of acetylcholine and inhibition of the pre-ovulatory surge after intra-ventricular atropine (Ojeda and McCann, 1978). However, these effects were only seen with very high doses of the drugs and a physiological role of acetylcholine is doubtful. The same can be said of histamine which, in high doses, also causes LH release (Libertun & McCann, 1976).

The amino acids gamma amino butyric acid (GABA) and glycine are present in large amounts in the hypothalamus. GABA releases LH in anaesthetised rats (Ondo, 1974), but not in unanaesthetised rats (Pass & Ondo, 1977). Moreover, the GABA antagonist, bicuculline, had no effect on serum LH (Ojeda & McCann, 1978).

Alpha melanocyte stimulating hormone (α MSH) has the same sequence as the first 13 amino acids of ACTH. α MSH is found in high concentrations in the neuro-intermediate lobe but also in the arcuate nucleus and the zone inserta, an area richly supplied with dopamine neurons (Eskay et al, 1979; Watson & Akil, 1980). Menstrual bleeding occurred after injection of α MSH into amenorrhoeic women (Kastin et al, 1968), raising the possibility that α MSH may influence LH secretion. However, more detailed studies failed to show any effect on normal women at different times during the menstrual cycle (Runnebaum et at, 1976), although it does stimulate LH secretion in the normal male (Reid et al, 1981). It is possible that αMSH modulates the effect of monoaminergic neurons on GnRH secretion.

THE GONADOTROPE

GnRH stimulates secretion of LH and FSH from the pituitary gonadotrope, a medium sized pituitary cell scattered throughout the anterior lobe of the pituitary. The gonadotrope contains two different types of secretory granules and is thought to have the capacity, at least, of secreting both LH and FSH (Phifer et al, 1973).

The gonadotropins

LH and FSH are glycoproteins composed of two polypeptide chains linked by non-covalent bonds. Part of their sequence (the α subunit) is common to both hormones and to the other glycoproteins, human chorionic gonadotrophin (hCG) and thyrotrophin (TSH). The remainder (the β subunit) is distinct for each of the glycoproteins. Attached to the polypeptide chains, at different locations for each hormone, is a carbohydrate moiety containing various monsaccharides including their N acetyl derivatives. One of these amino sugars is sialic acid which has an important role in determining the rate of catabolism of the various glycoproteins in the liver. Thus, the circulatory half life of FSH (which contains 5% sialic acid) is 4 hours compared to 20 minutes for LH (which contains 2 per cent sialic acid). α and β subunits of the glycoproteins are translated on the ribosomes from two separate messenger RNA's. In the case of TSH, β subunit synthesis is the rate limiting step. Glycosylation takes place on the microsomal membrane, after conjugation of the α and β subunits, by attachment of preformed oligosaccharide chains to asparagine residues. Gonadotrophins are largely metabolised in the liver which removes the sialic acid residues although 10–15 per cent are excreted unchanged in the urine (Coble et al, 1969; Raiti et al, 1975).

The GnRH receptor

GnRH exerts its effects on the gonadotrope by stimulating a specific receptor on the cell membrane. Using radiolabelled GnRH agonists which resist metabolic degradation, studies have shown that the pituitary contains a single class of saturable, high affinity receptors (Ka 3×10^{-9}M) scattered over the surface of selected pituitary cells (Clayton & Catt, 1980; Naor et al, 1981). Calculations suggest that each gonadotrope contains 10 000–15 000 receptor sites and that only a small fraction needs to be occupied to produce maximum cellular response.

The number of GnRH receptors is increased in the preovulatory phase of the cycle and in the gonadectomised animal; oestrogen and testosterone treatment reverses the increase produced by gonadectomy (Clayton & Catt, 1981). GnRH receptor number is reduced in the prepubertal and postpartum state, when endogenous GnRH levels are low. There is convincing evidence which links the *number* of GnRH receptors on the gonadotrope to the *activity* of GnRH neurons and the *magnitude* of GnRH secretion. Thus, the proestrus rise of GnRH receptors is obliterated if the LH (and GnRH) surge is blocked by barbiturates (Clayton & Catt, 1981); the post castration rise in GnRH receptors is prevented by prior destruction of GnRH neurons in the median eminence, by GnRH receptor antagonists or by GnRH antiserum (Frager et al, 1981; Clayton & Catt, 1981). These studies indicate that there is an increase in the secretion of endogenous GnRH after gonadectomy and in the preovulatory phase of the cycle and suggest that in these situations endogenous GnRH 'up regulates' the number of GnRH receptors.

In other situations, however, when GnRH is administered in pharmacological doses or in a non-physiological way (i.e. by continuous infusion or by very frequent pulses), the response of the pituitary gland decreases as a result of 'down regulation' of GnRH receptors (Belchetz et al, 1978; Heber & Swerdloff, 1981). These receptor studies have provided considerable information about the normal physiology of GnRH secretion and have also given rise to new therapeutic interest in GnRH and its long acting analogues. Pulsatile delivery of small doses of GnRH have been used to treat various forms of chronic anovulation associated with endogenous deficiency of GnRH (Leyendecker et al, 1980; see also Chapter 21) and it has also proved a useful alternative for the treatment of cryptorchidism (Keogh et al, 1982b) and male hypogonadotropic hypogonadism (Keogh et al, 1982a). Conversely, administration of long acting GnRH *agonists* has been used to 'down regulate' pituitary GnRH receptors and to reverse precocious puberty (Comite et al, 1981).

The biochemistry of the gonadotrope

Within 20 minutes of interaction of GnRH with its receptor, there is aggregation of receptor-GnRH complexes and by 30 minutes these complexes are internalised into the cell (Hazum et al, 1980). Here, presumably they are degraded by lysosomes, or possibly, recirculated. Activation of the gonadotrope occurs well before GnRH is internalised and studies using GnRH analogues in conditions where internalisation does not occur, show that the intracellular activity of the gonadotrope is triggered by interaction of GnRH with the cell membrane receptor rather than by some effect of the GnRH-receptor complex within the cell (Conn et al, 1981a).

The biochemistry of gonadotrophin synthesis and release has not been studied in as much detail as that of insulin but, by analogy, the amino acid sequence is assembled in the rough endoplasmic reticulum of the cytoplasm; packaging of LH and FSH into microvesicles then occurs in the Golgi apparatus and these microvesicles are then guided by the microtubule/microfilament system to the cell membrane where secretion occurs by exocytosis (Fig. 1.10) (Lambert, 1976). This formulation, although still unproven, provides a setting which explains the response of the gonadotrope to GnRH. Interaction of GnRH with the membrane bound receptor stimulates immediate secretion of pre-packaged LH and FSH in vesicles which are contained within the microtubule/microfilament system, close to the cell membrane.

It is likely that calcium ions play a central role in mediating this effect of GnRH (Conn et al, 1981b). Elegant studies have shown that interaction of GnRH with its receptors results in rapid movement of calcium ions from extracellular fluid through specific calcium channels into the cytosol of the gonadotrope. Once into the cell, calcium

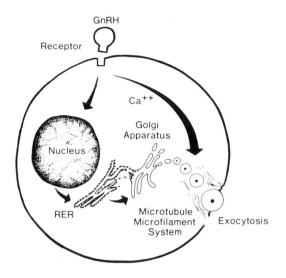

Fig. 1.10 The synthesis and secretion of gonadotropins in the gonadotrope. GnRH interaction with its receptor results in an activation of new gonadotropin synthesis and (by alteration of intracellular calcium concentration) acute secretion of gonadotropins

The dynamics of gonadotropin secretion

The response of the gonadotrope, in terms of the increase in serum levels of LH and FSH, is determined by the input of GnRH and the prevailing concentration of circulating gonadal steroids, particularly oestrogen. The relationship between these variables is complicated and depends not only on the magnitude but also on the duration of exposure of the gonadrotrope to GnRH and oestrogen.

The effect of GnRH

In the normal early follicular phase in women serum LH and FSH respond to exogenous GnRH in a dose dependent way with a maximum response being seen after 100 mg given intravenously. Serum levels of LH reach a maximum at 15–30 minutes and return to baseline levels at 2 hours. Serum FSH increases less dramatically and its level is maintained for longer because of its longer half-life (Fig. 1.11).

ions bind to calmodulin and this complex (or calcium ions *per se*) acts on the microtubule/microfilament system to transport and release stored LH (Khar et al, 1979). The importance of calcium ions to secretion of gonadotrophins (as it is to insulin) is strongly supported by the close correlation between induced increases in cytosol calcium ion concentration (by bacterial ionophores or calcium specific liposomes) and the rapid release of LH, even in the absence of GnRH (Conn et al, 1979).

In addition to stimulating the release of LH and FSH from the acute storage pool within the gonadotrope, GnRH also activates an increase in new synthesis of gonadotrophins in the rough endoplasmic reticulum. In this way, GnRH activates a larger reserve of gonadotrophins than that which. is immediately available for secretion. The second, larger, pool of gonadotrophins is dependent on new protein synthesis and is blocked by inhibitors of protein synthesis but not by inhibitors of DNA replication or RNA polymerase II (Pickering & Fink, 1976, 1977). It does not appear that calcium ions, *per se*, mediate the activation of this second pool (Fink & Geffen, 1978) but it is known that the calcium-calmodulin complex activates a number of important intracellular enzymes, including adenyl cyclase, phosphylase kinase and adenosine triphosphatase, which suggests that calcium may have a more indirect action on new protein synthesis (Means & Dedman, 1980; Cheung, 1980).

Cyclic AMP may be involved in new biosynthesis of gonadotropins but, contrary to earlier opinion, it is unlikely that it is involved in the acute secretion of LH from the gonadotrope (Conn et al, 1981a).

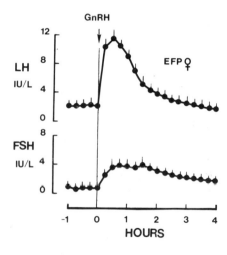

Fig. 1.11 The effect of GnRH (10 μg i.v.) on serum LH and FSH secretion in six women in the early follicular phase (EFP) of the normal menstrual cycle

Submaximal doses of GnRH infused at a rate of 0.2 μg/minute show a separation of the LH response into two components (Fig. 1.12). The early phase secretion probably reflects release of stored hormone and is influenced by the magnitude of the GnRH stimulus, the number of GnRH receptors, the efficiency of intracellular generation of calcium ions and the quantity of preformed gonadotrophins stored in vesicles on the microfilament/microtubule system. The second larger phase is dependent on a longer duration of exposure to GnRH and is thought to represent new gonadotrophin synthesis and its distribution to the golgi and microtubule system for subsequent release. With very low rates of GnRH infusion (0.5 μg/h), it is possible to selectively

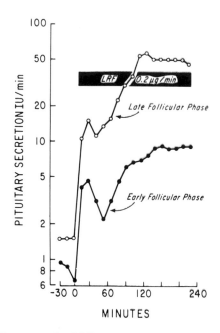

Fig. 1.12 The two pools of LH release from the pituitary in response to low dose infusion (0.2 μg/min) of GnRH (LRF) in normal women in the early follicular and late follicular phases of the cycle. Reproduced with permission from Yen (1978)

increase the size of the acute releasable pool without influencing the basal rate of LH secretion (Hoff et al, 1979). This suggests that redistribution of LH within the gonadotrope, as opposed to acute secretion, is favoured by prolonged exposure to GnRH at a low dose, this provides a rationale for the *in vivo* situation of a continuous low amplitude secretion of GnRH as well as the intermittent, higher amplitude pulses.

The negative feedback effect of oestrogen

Administration of oestrogen inhibits the greatly increased synthesis and secretion of LH and FSH induced by gonadectomy — known as the negative feedback effect of oestrogen. Deafferentation experiments clearly show that this effect of oestrogen is exerted within the mediobasal hypothalamus — pituitary complex (Blake et al, 1974) but the exact site of action is still controversial.

Tritiated oestradiol, administered systemically, is localised in different areas of the hypothalamus including the medial preoptic area and the amygdala (Pfaff & Keiner, 1973). Local injection of oestrogen into the mediobasal hypothalamus reduces serum LH concentration (Ferin et al, 1974; Weick, 1981) but these studies do not exclude the possibility that some oestrogen diffuses into the portal blood and hence influences the pituitary. Technical difficulties have hampered interpretation of portal blood levels of GnRH but more recent studies indicate that the amplitude of GnRH secretory pulses *is* increased after ovariectomy (Sherwood & Fink, 1980) and GnRH content of the hypothalamus is reduced in orchidectomised rats after

oestrogen treatment (Rudenstein et al, 1979; Kalra & Kalra, 1980). The oestrogen induced decrease in pituitary GnRH receptors in the castrated animal and its dependence on endogenous GnRH (Frager et al, 1981) is further support for a hypothalamic action of oestrogen.

There are several mechanisms by which oestrogen could, potentially, reduce GnRH release in the hypothalamus.

1. Oestrogen increases the activity of the peptidase which metabolises GnRH (Tate & Swift, 1981).

2. Oestrogen increases the turnover of dopamine in the hypothalamus and this is closely correlated, in time, to the fall in serum LH (Löfström et al, 1977).

3. The hypothalamus metabolises oestrogen to catechol oestrogens and this conversion is increased in ovariectomised animals (Fishman, 1973). Catechol oestrogens have a higher affinity for catechol-o-methyl transferase than the catecholamines themselves and hence function as competitive inhibitors. In this way oestrogen could augment the inhibitory action of dopamine (Fishman, 1976; Schinfeld et al, 1980).

On the other hand, oestrogen receptors are also found in the pituitary and local injection of oestrogen into the pituitary of ovariectomised animals causes reduction of serum LH and FSH (Ramirez et al, 1964). Studies of the effect of oestrogen on the pituitary *in vitro* have produced conflicting results probably as a result of the variety of protocols used, particularly with respect to the duration of exposure to oestrogen and the dose used. Inhibition of GnRH induced release of LH by oestrogen was reported *in vitro* after short term (4–6 h) exposure to oestrogen (Tang & Spies, 1975) but not after exposure for 40 hours (Drouin et al, 1976). In stalk sectioned, gonadectomised rats, oestrogen did not inhibit the LH response to GnRH. However, in rhesus monkeys in whom the arcuate nucleus had been destroyed, and endogenous GnRH secretion ablated, oestrogen inhibited the effect of hourly pulses of GnRH (Nakai et al, 1978). At the present time, there appears to be evidence to support both a hypothalamic and pituitary site of action for the negative feedback effect of oestrogen on gonadrotropins; it is not clear which of these sites of action is the more important.

The positive feedback effect of oestrogen

Although the initial effect of oestrogen is to inhibit secretion of LH from the pituitary, exposure to oestrogen for a longer duration produces a paradoxical increase in serum LH — the positive feedback effect of oestrogen. This phenomenon is seen in both the rat and the primate but whilst it occurs at an early age in lower animals, positive feedback does not occur until late puberty in the primate (Dierschke et al, 1974). Moreover, there are more critical requirements for induction of the positive feedback in primates; whereas a single injection of oestrogen causes an

LH surge in rats and sheep, prolonged exposure to concentrations of oestradiol in excess of 150 pg/ml for a duration not less than 36 hours are needed in the monkey (Karsch et al, 1973).

In the rat, the medial preoptic area seems to be the site of major importance for the production of the LH surge by oestrogen (Goodman, 1978) although the limbic system connection with the preoptic area may also be important (Kawakami et al, 1978). In the primate, only the mediobasal hypothalamus (excluding the medial preoptic area) and the pituitary gland are necessary for oestrogen induced LH secretion (Goodman & Knobil, 1981). Indeed, Knobil's elegant studies have shown that the LH surge can be induced by an increasing serum oestrogen concentration in the presence of a *constant* input of GnRH, suggesting that the pituitary may be the major site of positive oestrogen feedback. This would be in keeping with the known biphasic effect of oestrogen and its ability to increase the sensitivity of the pituitary to stimulation by GnRH (Drouin et al, 1976).

However, *in vivo* increased concentrations of GnRH have been described in portal blood after oestradiol administration, at a time when peripheral blood concentration of LH was increasing (Neill et al, 1977). Moreover, the preovulatory LH surge, which is dependent on the positive feedback effect of oestrogen, is associated with an increase of portal blood GnRH and a GnRH dependent increase in pituitary GnRH receptors. Overall, it would seem that although the positive feedback effect of oestrogen *can* be induced by an action on the pituitary gland, it is probably also associated with an increased secretion of endogenous GnRH.

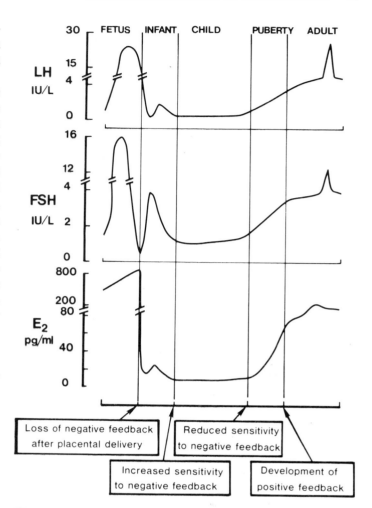

Fig. 1.13 Diagrammatic representation of the changes in the hypothalamic-pituitary-gonadal axis during life. Modified from Winter et al (1976)

MATURATION OF THE HYPOTHALAMIC — PITUITARY — GONADAL AXIS (Fig. 1.13)

(a) Fetus.

GnRH is first detectable in the fetus at 11 weeks of development and continues to increase until 24 weeks (Kaplan et al, 1976). It is not clear whether there is a sex difference in the hypothalamic secretion of GnRH but serum levels of LH and FSH are higher in female fetuses than male. It is possible that testosterone may play a role in reducing GnRH secretion in the male fetus (Rosenfield, 1982). In late gestation, serum levels of gonadotrophins decline partly as a result of increasing feto-placental sex steroids and partly because of maturation of hypothalamic inhibitory connections with the GnRH neuron.

(b) Childhood

After delivery, serum gonadotrophins rapidly increase as the negative feedback effect of placental steroids is lost. In boys, FSH levels reach a peak level at 1–12 weeks of life and decrease after this to prepubertal levels. The FSH rise in girls is higher and more sustained than in boys reaching a peak level at 6 months and declining to a nadir after 4 years of age.

By 6 years of age, both serum LH and FSH are low, despite low levels of circulating oestrogen, and the response to GnRH is minimal. This situation is thought to result from an increasing sensitivity of the hypothalamic — pituitary axis to negative feedback by oestrogen (Steel & Weisz, 1974). This concept has received some experimental support from studies showing an increased number of hypothalamic oestrogen receptors in the prepubertal, compared to the adult, rat (Rosenfield, 1977). However, low levels of LH and FSH are seen even in agonadal children in whom there are undetectable levels of oestrogen. This indicates that increased sensitivity to oestrogen is not the only factor operating to suppress the activity of the GnRH neuron at this time; presumably, some other brain mechanism, independent of oestrogen, causes activation of neurons which are inhibitory to GnRH secretion. Despite low levels of gonadotrophins between the ages of 4 and 6 years, it *is* possible to detect gonadotrophic activity in urine specimens and even intermittent bursts of increased LH excretion.

Urinary FSH excretion doubles between the ages of 5 and 9 years and there is a steady, though less obvious, increase in urinary LH. This results from an increase in GnRH neuronal activity and is accompanied by a rapid growth of ovarian follicles to the antral stage of development, although these later undergo atresia (Peter et al, 1978; Bourginon et al, 1979).

(c) Puberty

The factors which initiate puberty are not well delineated. Evidence suggests that the state of nutrition, energy expenditure and weight are all critical for the onset of puberty but the means by which these influence GnRH secretion is not known (Frisch, 1974; Warren, 1980). It seems likely that the changes in gonadotrophin secretion that occur during puberty are the end result of a cascade of events which collectively depend on an increase in activity of the GnRH neuron; this is currently attributed to a 'maturation of the gonadostat' which results in a reduced sensitivity to negative feedback by gonadal steroids (Rosenfield & Fang, 1974).

According to the proposals of Hausler et al (1979), the changing pattern of gonadotrophin secretion seen at different phases of puberty can be explained on the basis of a gradual increase in the firing rate of GnRH neurons, perhaps as a result of attenuation of the inhibiting action of opioid neurons on GnRH secretion (Wilkinson & Bhanot, 1982). At low pulse frequency (one pulse every 3 hours), there is a preferential increase of FSH compared to LH as a result of the longer circulating half-life of FSH and its accumulation between pulses. As puberty advances, the firing rate of GnRH neurons increases; initially this increased frequency is entrained to a sleep related rhythm (Fig. 1.14) and serum LH rises during non-REM sleep (Boyar et al, 1972). Eventually, the increase in GnRH firing rate (one pulse every 1–2 hours) allows LH, which is more sensitive to GnRH, to increase proportionally more than FSH (Fig. 1.15).

Late puberty in the female is characterised by increasing amplitude of gonadotrophin secretion, increasing levels of gonadal steroids and the appearance of the positive feedback effect of oestrogen (Reiter et al 1974). Eventually, follicular maturation and gonadotrophin surges are coordinated and regular menstrual cycles are established.

If a changing frequency of GnRH secretion is the most important factor influencing the pattern of gonadotrophin secretion in puberty, puberty may be induced by a decrease in opiate activity in the brain. This would certainly be in keeping with the concept that opioid peptidergic activity mediates the negative feedback action of gonadal steroids in the rat (Cicero et al, 1979; Van Vugt et al, 1982). The observation that naloxone is more effective at increasing serum LH levels in prepubertal rats than in adult animals (Blank et al, 1979), is an indication that the increased sensitivity of the gonadostat before puberty may be due to an increased opioid peptide activity at this time.

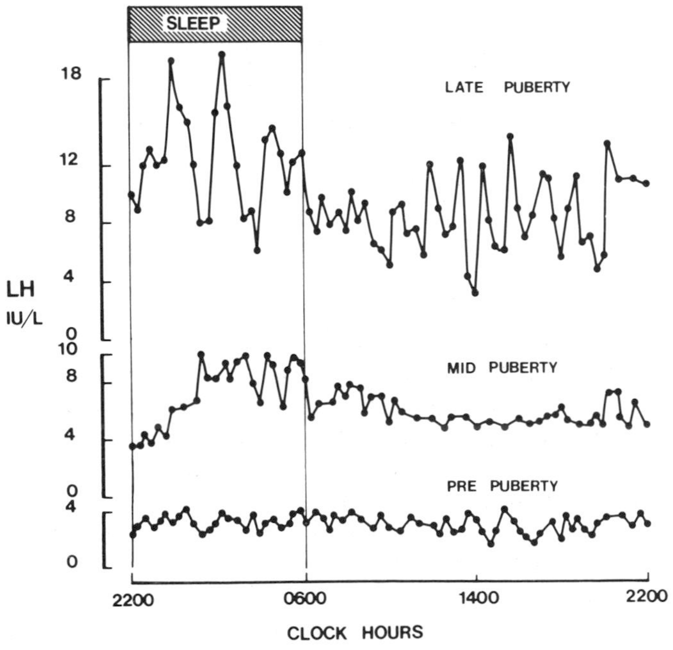

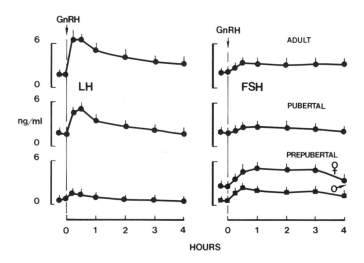

Fig. 1.14 The pattern of LH secretion during puberty showing the increasing amplitude of LH pulsatility and the nocturnal episodic secretion which develops, transiently, during mid and late puberty. Modified from Katz et al (1976)

Fig. 1.15 The effect of GnRH on LH and FSH secretion at different phases of puberty. Before puberty FSH secretion exceeds that of LH, particularly in females. As puberty progresses, LH secretion exceeds that of FSH. Modified from Grumbach et al (1974)

CHANGES IN GONADOTROPIN SECRETION THROUGHOUT THE MENSTRUAL CYCLE

The alterations in gonadotropin secretion which climax in the preovulatory mid-cycle surge of LH and FSH are the result of a highly integrated sequence of events. The current knowledge about this process is discussed in detail in Chapter 2 and is summarised here.

(a) Early follicular phase (Fig. 1.16a)

This part of the cycle is characterised by low amplitude secretion of GnRH at a frequency of one pulse every 1 to 2 hours. The gonadotrophe has a low rate of new gonadotrophin synthesis and small quantities of gondotrophins available for acute release. Relative to other times of the cycle, the ratio FSH:LH is high. The pattern of LH secretion is pulsatile but of low amplitude. Under the influence of FSH and LH, a number of ovarian follicles become activated and begin to produce increasing amounts of 17 β oestradiol. By day 6 of the cycle, a dominant follicle has been selected as the one producing most oestrogen and this will progress to full development at the time of ovulation.

(b) Mid follicular phase

Under the influence of increasing circulating oestradiol and a continuing pulsatile input of GnRH, the synthesis and storage of gonadotrophins increases. Pulsatile secretion of LH becomes more obvious and the ratio of FSH : LH decreases.

(c) Late follicular phase (Fig. 1.16b)

As the ovarian follicle matures, there is a rapid increase in circulating 17 β oestradiol commencing about 4 days before the mid-cycle surge of gonadotrophins. The rate of synthesis and storage of gonadotrophins is further increased until the day before the mid-cycle surge when oestradiol concentration reaches its peak and begins to decline. Around this time, there is an acceleration in the rate of secretion of GnRH and an increase in the number of GnRH receptors on the gonadotrope. Each pulse of LH increases in magnitude as the gonadotropes, now with maximum stores of gondotrophins, also develop an increase in sensitivity. At this stage, it is likely that the magnitude and frequency of GnRH pulses is also transiently increased, perhaps as a result of oestrogen altering the activity of brain neurotransmitter neurons which, in turn, activate GnRH neurons; an increase in noradrenaline and a decrease in dopamine activity at this time seems best documented. The net result is a major increase in circulating gonadotrophins (the mid-cycle surge) which is followed 28–36 hours later by ovulation and formation of the corpus luteum.

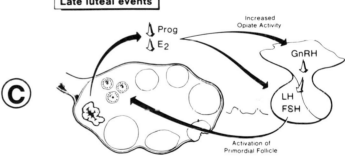

Fig. 1.16 The hypothalamic–pituitary–gonadal events of the menstrual cycle. For details see text

(d) The luteal phase (Fig. 1.16c)

The mid-cycle surge is limited in duration perhaps by the increase in serum progesterone which is secreted in vast amounts by the corpus luteum. Under the influence of progesterone, opioid activity is increased and there is a slowing of the frequency of LH pulses, although the amplitude remains high. During this phase, new follicular development is inhibited until 1–2 days before menses when the function of the corpus luteum begins to fail, serum FSH and LH increase and a new cycle of follicle development is initiated. The function of the luteal phase is critically dependent on the level of FSH in the early follicular phase of the cycle. Reduction of early follicular phase FSH levels by inhibin impairs function of the subsequent corpus luteum (Stouffer & Hodgen, 1980). A normal tonic level of LH is also a necessity (Vande Wiele et al, 1970).

PROLACTIN

The observation that pituitary tumours could be associated with pathological lactation was recognised in 1896 and reviewed in a classic work by Krestin (1932). Animal work extended these clinical observations by demonstrating that pituitary extracts had lactogenic activity (Gruter & Stricker, 1929). In 1931, the pigeon crop sac bioassay was developed to measure lactogenic activity in a variety of animal species including humans (Riddle et al, 1932). For some time in the human there was confusion as to whether growth hormone alone could explain the lactogenic activity of the pituitary, but this was finally resolved by the purification of human prolactin and the development of a radioimmunoassay (Hwang et al, 1971).

In lower animal forms, prolactin has been found to be responsible for a variety of actions including nesting behaviour, growth promotion, fluid and electrolyte balance and maintenance of the corpus luteum (Nicoll, 1974). Some of the actions may yet be found to apply to the human but, to date, the single function for human prolactin that is beyond question is the initiation and maintenance of lactation.

The control of prolactin secretion

Prolactin inhibitory factor

A case report of galactorrhoea associated with post enkephalitic Parkinson's disease in 1928 (Riese, 1928) correctly attributed these clinical features to damage in the hypothalamus and the extrapyramidal system, respectively. In retrospect, this is the first indication that the hypothalamus exerts an inhibitory control over prolactin secretion and that dopamine may be an important neurotransmitter controlling its release (as it is in Parkinson's disease). However, it remained until 1954 for this to be firmly established when it was discovered that pseudopregnancy in the rat (known to be due to 'lactogenic hormone') occurred when the pituitary was removed and transplanted under the renal capsule away from the influence of the hypothalamus (Everett, 1954).

The tonic inhibitory influence of the hypothalamus is confirmed by observations that damage to the hypothalamus, interruption of the pituitary stalk or culture of the pituitary *in vitro* results in increased prolactin secretion and that extracts of the hypothalamus inhibit this. It is now generally accepted that the hypothalamic factor of major importance in controlling prolactin secretion is dopamine itself, although there is still some support for a non-catecholamine, possible peptide, prolactin-inhibitory factor (Greibrokk et al, 1975; Enjalbert et al, 1977). Other studies

have isolated a different, non-peptide, inhibitory factor, which was later shown to be gamma aminobutyric acid (GABA) but it seems that this is unlikely to be of physiological importance (Schally et al, 1977; Locatelli et al, 1979).

Dopamine

Early studies showed that dopamine is a potent inhibitor of prolactin secretion both *in vivo* and *in vitro* (MacLeod et al, 1970; Lu & Meites, 1972). The prolactin inhibiting activity of hypothalamic extracts is proportional to its catecholamine content (Takahara et al, 1974) and is reduced by removal of catecholamines with monoamine oxidase or aluminium oxide (Shaar & Clemens, 1974). Increased serum concentrations of prolactin are seen after inhibition of catecholamine synthesis with α methyl tyrosine, after depletion of catecholamine stores with reserpine or by dopamine receptor blockade, all of which reduce the action of dopamine Lu et al, 1970; (Donoso et al, 1971; Judd, et al, 1976).

Dopamine concentration in the portal blood vessels is higher than in the systemic circulation and is sufficient to inhibit prolactin secretion (Gibbs & Neill, 1978) although the suppression is incomplete. Using an electrochemical probe to study changes in median eminence of dopamine concentration, the same workers found that dopamine declined by 70% for 1–3 minutes after mammary nerve stimulation and that this was associated with a contemporaneous decrease in concentration of portal blood dopamine and an increase in serum prolactin (Plotsky & Neill, 1982), providing further support for the physiological role of dopamine in the control of prolactin secretion.

Although most studies have assumed that dopamine in the portal blood is derived from nerve terminals in the median eminence, tuberoinfundibular dopamine neurons also pass directly to the posterior lobe of the pituitary (Bjorklund et al, 1973). The demonstration of a rich network of capillaries connecting the anterior and posterior lobes of the pituitary (Bergland & Page, 1979) has raised the possibility that dopamine may reach the anterior pituitary via the posterior lobe (Fig. 1.17) and indeed this has received some support from the observation that selective removal of the posterior lobe is associated with an increase in prolactin secretion (Peters et al, 1981) and that synthesis of dopamine in the posterior lobe of the pituitary is increased in suckling rats compared to those whose pups have been removed (Ben-Jonathon, 1982).

Prolactin releasing factor (PRF)

Although it is possible that an increase in prolactin secretion may merely be the result of reduced dopamine inhibition, it seems likely that the hypothalamus also contains a factor which, in certain circumstances at least, directly stimulates the pituitary to release prolactin. This was first indicated by studies showing that prolactin is stimulated by ether stress in rats whose dopamine stores had been depleted by reserpine (Valverde et al, 1973) or whose dopamine activity had been blocked with receptor antagonists (Shin, 1979b).

Hypothalamic extracts are known to contain substances which stimulate prolactin secretion *in vitro* (Boyd et al, 1976). An early candidate was thytotropin releasing hormone (TRH) which was found to increase prolactin as well as thyrotropin (TSH) secretion from a tumour cell line in rats (Tashjian et al, 1971). However, in most situations prolactin and TSH secretion do not increase in parallel; suckling, for example, is associated with prolactin but not TSH secretion (Gautvik et al, 1974) and although decreases in serum prolactin occur after administering TRH anti-serum, it is generally agreed that TRH is not a physiological prolactin releasing factor.

More recently, vasoactive intestinal polypeptide (VIP) has been suggested as a more likely alternative. VIP is contained in nerve terminals of the medial basal hypothalamus and is present in the portal blood in high concentration (Said & Porter, 1979). Unlike many other brain peptides which only stimulate prolactin secretion *in vivo*, VIP is also effective in very low concentrations and in a dose dependent way *in vitro* (Ruberg et al, 1979) even when dopamine is administered concurrently (Frawley & Neill, 1981). Although its role as prolactin releasing factor is not yet established, VIP does fulfil the essential requirements.

Neurotransmitters and prolactin secretion.

The tuberinfundibular dopamine (TIDA) neurons and the putative PRF secreting neurons provide a final common pathway through which stimuli can be channelled to bring about prolactin secretion. TIDA neurons provide tonic inhibitory control of prolactin secretion while PRF mediates rhythmic stimulation and acute release (Fig. 1.17). A number of neurotransmitter substances are known to influence the secretion of dopamine or PRF and hence to alter prolactin release (Weiner & Bethea, 1981).

Serotonin There is considerable evidence which suggests that serotonin neurons increase prolactin secretion by increasing PRF release (Clemens et al, 1978). An increase in serotonergic activity in the brain induced by drugs which increase serotonin synthesis such as the serotonin precursors, L tryptophan or 5-hydroxytrytophan, cause an increase in serum prolactin (Kato et al, 1974). Similarly, serum prolactin is elevated by fluoxetine which blocks re-uptake of serotonin by neurons and by quipazine which acts on serotonin receptors (Meltzer et al, 1976; Krulich et al, 1979). Moreover, these increases in serotonergic neurotransmission are associated with raised PRF activity in the serum (Garthwaite & Hagen, 1979) and an increase in VIP secretion into the portal blood (Shimatsu

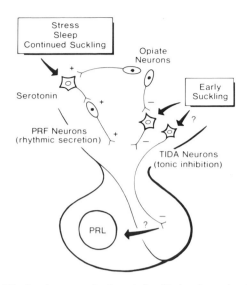

Fig. 1.17 The involvement of tubero-infundibular dopamine (TIDA), serotonin, opiate and prolactin releasing factor (PRF) neurons in the control of prolactin secretion. TIDA neurons provide tonic inhibition while PRL neurons cause rhythmic secretion

et al, 1982). On the other hand, serotonin antagonists or destruction of serotonergic neurons are *not* associated with a change in the *tonic secretion* of prolactin which is in keeping with the concept that serotonin has its effect on PRF and not TIDA neurons which provide tonic inhibitory control (Gallo et al, 1975) (Fig. 1.17).

Endogenous opioid peptides. The opioid peptides increase serum prolactin, probably by decreasing the activity of TIDA neurons. Prolactin secretion is stimulated in rats by morphine, β endorphin and met-enkaphalin (Meites et al, 1979) and in the human by the enkephalin analogue, D-ala, MePhe, Met (0)-ol enkephalin (DAMME), as well as morphine (Stubbs et al, 1978; Hemmings et al, 1982). The effect of these opiates is blocked by naloxone but, by itself, naloxone does not influence the basal secretion of prolactin (Quigley et al, 1980a). The evidence for an action of opiate peptides on TIDA neurons is based on the observation that dopamine turnover in the hypothalamus and the portal blood concentration of dopamine are reduced by administration of opiates (Gudelsky & Porter, 1979; Van Loon et al, 1980).

In addition, opioid peptides may also exert an action on PRF neurons by stimulating serotonergic activity since destruction of serotonin neurons in the brain or administration of serotonin antagonists inhibit the prolactin stimulating effect of morphine (Koenig et al, 1979; Spampinato et al, 1979).

Finally, although opiates have no direct action *per se* on the pituitary, they do interfere with the inhibition of prolactin by dopamine *in vitro* (Enjalbert et al, 1979). This raised the possibility that opiates may behave as dopamine receptor antagonists (Lal et al, 1977), in part supported by behavioural studies, but this possibility has been specifically excluded by *in vitro* experiments (Caron et al, 1978).

Other potential neurotransmitters. In early *in vitro* studies, *noradrenaline* was found to inhibit prolactin secretion (MacLeod, 1969) but only in supraphysiological doses which probably also affect dopamine receptors (Cronin et al, 1978). Furthermore, most noradrenaline terminals are found in the internal layer of the median eminence, removed from the portal capillaries, and portal blood concentration of noradrenaline is not different from that of the peripheral circulation (Ben-Jonathon et al, 1977). Administration of adrenergic agonists and antagonists have not been associated with any change in prolactin secretion and, with the possible exception of the oestrogen induced prolactin surge observed in rats, noradrenaline does not seem to be of major importance as a neurotransmitter involved in prolactin secretion (Weiner & Berthea, 1981).

In the rat and the human, *histamine* appears to stimulate prolactin secretion possibly by reducing dopamine concentration in portal blood (Pontiroli & Pozza, 1978; Gibbs et al, 1979). However, histamine antagonists also increase serum prolactin (Bateson et al, 1977; Donoso & Banzan, 1980) which complicates this conclusion. Similarly, no definite conclusions can be made about the role of *acetylcholine*. *In vitro*, inhibition of prolactin secretion has been shown after treatment with high doses of acetylcholine or cholinergic agonists which can be reversed by atropine (Snyder et al, 1980). However, treatment of rats with either nicotinic or muscarinic antagonists does not alter the basal secretion of prolactin (Lawson & Gala, 1975).

Autoregulation of prolactin secretion

Although mastectomy is associated with an increase in serum prolactin in the human (Herman & Kalk, 1980), this is probably due to chronic stimulation of nerves involved in the suckling reflex rather than to a removal of end organ inhibition. In this regard, prolactin differs from that of other pituitary hormones which are regulated mainly by negative feedback by a hormone secreted from a target organ. Control of prolactin secretion is exerted by a short loop feedback whereby prolactin increases the activity of tuberoinfundibular dopamine neurons (Fig. 1.18).

This 'autoregulation' of prolactin has been demonstrated by a number of studies which have shown an increase in hypothalamic dopamine turnover and portal vein dopamine concentrations after pharmacological or physiological elevation of serum prolactin concentration (Fuxe et al, 1969; Eikenberg et al, 1977; Cramer et al, 1979b). Autoregulation is produced by local implants of prolactin into the hypothalamus and even in animals with complete deafferentation of the hypothalamus, indicating that the site of this action of prolactin is in the mediobasal hypothalamus (Voogt & Meites, 1973; Gudelsky et al, 1978). *In vitro* studies, which show that prolactin enhances the synthesis and release of dopamine from incubated mediobasal hypothalamic fragments, indicate that this is a

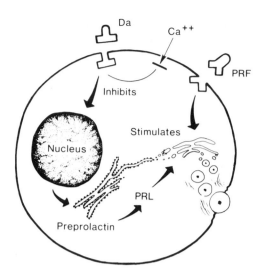

Fig. 1.18 The effects of dopamine (DA) and prolactin releasing factor (PRF) on the lactotrope. DA inhibits new synthesis of prolactin by a mechanism involving a reduced influx of calcium ions. PRF stimulates acute release of performed stores of prolactin

direct effect of prolactin and not one that requires an intermediary (Perkins & Westfall, 1978; Perkins et al, 1979). Finally, it would seem that there is a lag period of between 1 and 4 hours before prolactin induces this increase in the synthesis of dopamine (Advis et al, 1977; Perkins et al, 1979).

The lactotrope

Having been released into the portal circulation, PRF and dopamine are carried to the anterior pituitary where they have their effect on the lactotrope. The structure of the lactotrope remained uncertain for many years even though it had been recognised that pregnancy is associated with the appearance of a specific pituitary cell type, thought to be involved in lactation (Erdheim & Stumme, 1909). These cells stained erythrosinophilic with tetrachromic stains (Pasteels, 1963) or carmoisinophilic with Brook's stain (Goluboff & Ezrin, 1969) but could only be identified in the pituitaries of women dying during pregnancy or in the puerperium. It remained until the introduction of the immunocytochemical staining technique for prolactin-containing cells to be identified in the pituitaries of non-pregnant adults and for the recognition that these cells undergo hypertrophy and hyperplasia during gestation (Pasteels et al, 1972; Zimmerman et al, 1974b). Using this technique, lactotropes of varying size and shape have been identified (Baker & Yu, 1977). One type has a small perikaryon with long cytoplasmic processes extending towards neighbouring capillaries; this type is chiefly located in the posterolateral zones of the anterior pituitary. A second type has a larger perikaryon with short cytoplasmic processes; these are fewer in number and are mainly located in the anteromedian zone. Lactotropes have been identified in 14-week-old fetuses with a marked increase around 23 weeks of development. The number of lactotropes is only slightly greater in adult females compared to males and both sexes show regression of lactotropes with age (Baker & Yu, 1977).

The dopamine receptor

Like GnRH, labelled dopamine has proved to be an unstable ligand for use in pituitary receptor studies and more sensitive techniques have been devised using radiolabelled neuroleptics, which function as dopamine receptor antagonists, or [3H]-dihydroergocryptine, a potent dopamine agonist. Initial studies revealed binding sites with two affinities but recently, using [3H]-domperidone and preparations of dispersed bovine anterior pituitary cells comprising 25 per cent lactotropes, a single class of high affinity receptors (Kd = $9.1 \pm 1.0 \times 10^{-10}$M) were identified (Ramsdell et al, 1982). They found approximately 50 000 binding sites per cell with effective displacement of ligand by dopamine ($K_1 = 298 \pm 74 \times 10^{-9}$M) and in this system biologically active butaclamol was 1000 times more effective at displacing [3H]-domperidone than the inactive isomer 1-butaclamol. Other studies, using [3H]-dihydroergocryptine have shown the affinity of various agonists and antagonists for displacement of radioligand correlates well with their ability to modulate prolactin secretion in vitro (Labrie et al, 1978).

Dopamine receptors are located at the plasma membrane of the lactotrope and it is likely that dopamine exerts its major inhibitory action on the lactotrope through a mechanism which is triggered by this initial interaction. However, some studies have shown that the dopamine-receptor complex, like that of other hormones, is internalised into the cell (Goldsmith et al, 1978). Although this has been seen as a mechanism to conserve and recycle hormone receptors, it is interesting that once inside the lactotrope, dopamine appears to become associated with secretory granules containing prolactin and may even be present with prolactin in the same granule (Nansel et al, 1979; Ajika et al, 1982). These observations have raised the possibility that dopamine may also have an intracellular action in regulating the synthesis or secretion of prolactin.

It is now established that there are at least two distinct dopamine receptors which are different in terms of their location in various parts of the body, in the selectivity of their response to different agonists and antagonists and in the mediation, or otherwise, of their action by cyclic AMP (Iverson, 1978; Costall & Naylor, 1981). It seems that the lactotrope dopamine receptor is of the D2 (or alpha) type which dose not require cyclic AMP for its action. It is selectively antagonised by domperidone, metoclopramide or sulpiride and is stimulated, probably selectively, by bromocriptine (and other ergolines) and piribedil.

There is good evidence that dopamine receptors on the lactotrope mediate their response by way of changes in calcium ion flux rather than using cyclic AMP as a second messenger. Electrophysiological studies of normal pituitary cells and cultured prolactin secreting cells show that the lactotrope has a membrane potential which is stimulated by TRH and inhibited by dopamine (Taraskevich & Douglas, 1977; Dufy et al, 1979). These action potentials are produced by movement of calcium ion into the cytosol; once into the cytoplasm, calcium binds to calmodulin and thereafter activates various intracellular enzymes which cause prolactin secretion. The inhibition of prolactin secretion is prevented if calcium ion flux is maintained by calcium ionophores (Thorner & MacLeod, 1980). Conversely agents which block calcium channels (manganese or verapamil) or the interaction of calcium with calmodulin (neuroleptics in high dose) inhibit lactotrope action potentials (Dufy et al, 1980) and secretion of prolactin, even in the absence of dopamine (Thorner & MacLeod, 1980).

The number of dopamine receptors varies at different times of the oestrus cycle in the rat, being maximal on the afternoon of pre-oestrus at the time of the prolactin surge (Herman & Ben-Jonathon, 1982). The number of dopamine receptors is also profoundly influenced by the level of dopamine activity at the receptor level; at times of high dopamine secretion, dopamine receptors become 'down regulated' and reduced in number, whilst rats with electrolytic lesions of the median eminence and reduced dopamine secretion show an increase in the number of dopamine binding sites without a change in binding affinity (Cheung & Weiner, 1978; Libertun et al, 1980).

The biochemistry of the lactotrope (Fig. 1.18).

Rapid developments in the fields of gene structure and function are gradually unravelling the mechanism of the synthesis of peptide hormones. In view of the close structural homology of prolactin, growth hormone and placental lactogen and their presumed evolution from a common genome, it is thought that the three genes for these hormones are situated close together, perhaps on one chromosome (Gorski, 1981). The sequences of nucleotides which make up the gene for prolactin probably contain more information than is required for synthesis of the hormone and, if it follows the example of other proteins, transcription of the DNA into RNA is followed by cleavage and splicing before the final messenger RNA is produced.

The mRNA is used by ribosomes on the rough endoplasmic reticulum to synthesise pre-prolactin which, in the rat, is prolactin with an additional 29 amino acid sequence (Maurer & McKean, 1978). This additional sequence confers a hydrophobic aminoterminal which aids in the extrusion of the peptide sequence across the membrane of the rough endoplasmic reticulum (Blobel & Dobberstein, 1975). Having been partly extruded, the additional sequence is removed by a highly specific protease (McKean

& Maurer, 1978) and the completed prolactin sequence is passed on through the smooth endoplasmic reticulum into the Golgi apparatus where it is packaged, possibly with dopamine, into a secretory granule. Some of these granules fuse with lysosomes present in the lactotrope and prolactin is then destroyed before it can be released; other granules fuse with the cell membrane and, after exocytosis, prolactin enters the blood stream. It has been reported that dopamine increases the lysosomal enzyme activity of the lactotrope and, by increasing the intra-lactotrope degradation of prolactin, this may provide another means whereby dopamine inhibits prolactin secretion (Nansel et al, 1981).

The dynamics of prolactin secretion have been studied in depth in the lactating rat (Grosvenor et al, 1979). According to these authors, soon after the suckling stimulus is applied, there is a rapid 'apparent depletion' of prolactin within the lactotrope and transformation into a form which is made available for secretion; this phase, in the resting state, is inhibited by dopamine (Fig. 1.18). Once transformation has occurred, secretion is greatly accelerated by more prolonged suckling, ether stress or TRH, factors which are thought to be associated with, or to simulate, secretion of prolactin releasing factor. This theory had considerable experimental support and provides a framework in which both dopamine and prolactin releasing factor (?VIP) play important and complementary roles (Fig. 1.17).

Oestrogen and prolactin secretion

The effect of oestrogen on prolactin secretion has been widely studied. Women respond to many stimuli with an increased secretion of prolactin compared to men (Judd et al, 1976). Moreover, physiological changes in oestrogen concentration alter the prolactin response to stimulation (Yen et al, 1974a). This effect of oestrogen is apparently due to an action at various sites. In the hypothalamus, oestrogen decreases activity of TIDA neurons (Cramer et al, 1979a) and, in high doses, this may even result in permanent damage to the arcuate dopamine cell bodies (Brawer & Sonnenschein, 1976). At the pituitary level, oestrogen blocks the inhibition of lactotrope action potentials induced by dopamine agonists and stimulates prolactin secretion (Labrie et al, 1978); these actions suggest an effect at the receptor level. In addition, oestrogen reduces the capacity of lactotropes to incorporate dopamine into the prolactin secretory granule either by reducing the uptake of dopamine or accelerating its intracellular degradation (Gudelsky et al, 1981).

Oestrogen also has an important effect on cell replication and increases the number and the activity of lactotropes (Maurer, 1979; Gorski, 1981). DNA synthesis is greatly accelerated and, in particular, the mRNA for pre-prolactin synthesis (Vician et al, 1979). This action of oestrogen on lactotrope proliferation is of considerable clinical import-

ance because of the potential for pituitary enlargement during pregnancy and particularly in those patients who are harbouring a prolactin secreting tumour. It is of some interest that this action of oestrogen is rapidly reversed by the dopamine agonist, bromocriptine; this effect seems to be due to an action at the level of the cell nucleus (Lloyd et al, 1975) and possibly involves competition with oestrogen receptors (Nagy et al, 1979).

Circulating prolactin

Human prolactin, as measured by radioimmunoassay, is shown on chromatography of serum to be in three forms. In the basal state, a normal adult has about 60% in the monomeric form ('little prolactin'; mol. wt. 22 000); another 18 per cent elutes with a mol. wt. of 50 000 ('big prolactin'), thought to be a mixture of prolactin dimeric and trimeric forms; a third form ('big, big prolactin'; mol. wt. around 100 000) elutes with the void volume (Farkough et al, 1979). The ratio of these forms is altered in favour of 'little prolactin' when the pituitary is stimulated with TRH (Farkough et al, 1979) or is in a state of increased activity (Suh & Frantz, 1974). It seems likely that the pituitary secretes only monomeric prolactin and that the additional forms are produced during circulation in the plasma by formation of disulphide bonds (Benveniste et al, 1979). Moreover, 'big prolactin' and 'big, big prolactin' have reduced biological activity as judged by radio receptor assay although they are freely measured in the radioimmunoassay (Farkough et al, 1979). This may be the explanation for the absence of pathological effects in some patients with apparent high levels of serum prolactin (Whittaker et al, 1979).

Depending on the assay procedure and the preparation used as a standard, serum prolactin measured by radioimmunoassay ranges between 2–30 μg/l. The normal adult pituitary gland contains about 100 μg of prolactin and the volume of distribution for prolactin is close to that of extracellular fluid. The half-life of circulating prolactin is between 20 and 30 minutes with metabolism occurring mainly in the liver and kidney.

Rhythms of prolactin secretion

A variety of rhythms governs the secretion of prolaction into the circulation and these vary for different animal species. In the rat, circadian, oestrus and seasonal rhythms as well as random brief secretion are all well characterised (Willoughby, 1980). In the human, the variety is no less varied. In the basal state, particularly in the luteal phase of the cycle, serum prolactin increases contemporaneously with luteinising hormone (Fig. 1.19). Although this raises the possibility that there is a common dopaminergic pathway controlling GnRH and prolactin secretion, this is

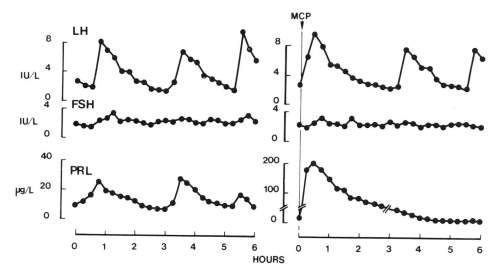

Fig. 1.19 The pattern of LH, FSH and PRL secretion in a normal luteal phase woman before and after metoclopramide (MCP). The pulsatile secretion of LH is associated with synchronous release of PRL. Blockade of dopamine receptors increases PRL and abolishes its synchrony with LH but pulsatility of LH is unaffected. From Braund et al (1984)

unlikely in view of the dichotomy in response of LH and prolactin after metoclopramide (Fig. 1.19) (Braund et al, 1984). This concurrence is over-ridden by other physiological stimuli affecting prolactin secretion, including secretion in relation to food intake (Quigley et al, 1981b), and stress. Recent studies suggest that this synchrony is due to the lactotrope responding to a paracrine secretion produced by the gonadotrope in response to GnRH (Denef & Andries, 1983).

In the early hours of the morning, there is a marked increase in prolactin secretion (Fig. 1.20) which requires but is not dependent on any particular phase of sleep

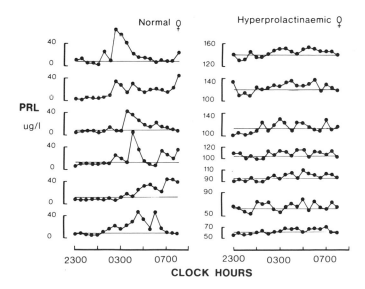

Fig. 1.20 The pattern of PRL secretion during sleep in six normal women and seven women with hyperprolactinaemia. Note the nocturnal rise of PRL in normal women which is not present in hyperprolactinaemic women. From Judd (unpublished data)

(Parker et al, 1974; Van Cauter et al, 1982). Episodic secretion of prolactin, including that occurring in sleep, are mediated by serotonin stimulated PRF release (Mendelson et al, 1975).

Small increases of prolactin occur in the preovulatory and luteal phases of the cycle in women, and this is thought to be due to increases of circulating oestrogen seen at these times (Vekemans et al, 1977).

Physiological stimuli of prolactin secretion (Table 1.1)

Increases in serum prolactin occur in response to a number of physiological stimuli (Table 1.1; Figure 1.17).

Pregnancy. During pregnancy, there is a steady increase in serum prolactin to a maximum level of ten times that of the non-pregnant state, at full term (Rigg & Yen, 1977). It is likely that this rise is a result of increased circulating oestrogen, derived from the placenta, acting at both the hypothalamus and the pituitary. Despite these increased basal levels of prolactin during pregnancy, sleep related

Table 1.1 Stimuli of prolactin secretion

1. Physiological
   — Normal rhythms (Sleep, circhoral etc)
   — Suckling
   — Pregnancy
   — Stress
2. Pharmacological
   — Dopamine antagonists (anti emetics, neuroleptics etc.)
   — Insulin hypoglycaemia
   — Thyrotropin releasing hormone
   — Oestogen
3. Pathological
   — Reduced clearance (Hypothyroidism, Renal failure)
   — Hypothalamic damage (Trauma, tumour, infiltration)
   — Pituitary tumour (chromophobe, Acromegaly, Cushings)
   — 'Primary' hyperprolactinaemia

secretion still persists (Boyar et al, 1975) although, at the time of delivery, stimulation of prolactin secretion by stress is impaired (Rigg & Yen, 1977). The amniotic fluid contains large amounts of prolactin derived from the decidua-chorion (Healy et al, 1977). In this situation, prolactin may play a role in osmoregulation and the maintenance of amniotic fluid and sodium ion content. This is supported by clinical studies showing elevated amniotic fluid prolactin levels in patients with oligohydramnios (Josimovich, 1977), and by *in vivo* and *in vitro* studies showing that prolactin influences fluid transport in human amnion (Leontic & Tyson, 1977; Josimovich et al, 1977).

Lactation. Suckling induces an increase in serum prolactin within a few minutes with a maximum response being apparent at 30 minutes. The effectiveness of suckling as a stimulus for prolactin secretion is time dependent; it is most effective between 2 and 16 weeks after delivery when peak responses may be ten times the basal level. Thereafter, the prolactin response to suckling is less consistent and of a smaller magnitude (Tyson et al, 1972), possibly due to a decreasing sensitivity of the nipple to stimulation by suckling (Robinson & Short, 1977). Although milk let down can occur during preparation for suckling without actual stimulation of the breast, prolactin increase only occurs after stimulation of the nipple (Noel et al, 1974). The neural pathway involved in this reflex includes the spino-thalamic sensory projection, the dorsal longitudinal fasciculus, the median forebrain bundle and the lateral and medial pre-optic areas (Tindall & Knaggs, 1977). Denervation or local anaesthesia of the nipple (Findlay, 1968) or interruption of this neural pathway abolishes the prolactin response to suckling. Serotonergic pathways (and hence PRF) play an important role in mediating continued prolactin secretion in response to suckling. This is shown by inhibition of the prolactin rise after suckling by disruption or blockade of serotonergic pathways in the medial forebrain bundle (Gallo et al, 1975; Delitala et al, 1977) and is in keeping with the observed increase in serotonin turnover in the hypothalamus during suckling (Mena et al, 1976).

According to the hypothesis proposed by Mena & Grosvenor (1980), within 5 minutes after the initiation of suckling there is a rapid depletion of prolactin from the rough endoplasmic reticulum and a transfer to the Golgi apparatus; this is mediated by an initial decrease in dopamine inhibition. More prolonged suckling activates serotonin pathways and PRF secretion, which in turn, causes prolonged prolactin secretion (Fig. 1.18). Continued prolactin secretion is terminated by an increase in TIDA neuron activity by the normal process of autoregulation (Mena et al, 1976).

There is debate concerning whether the amount of milk secretion is dependent on the prolactin response to suckling. Some have found an impaired prolactin response to suckling in women who have problems establishing lactation (Aono et al, 1977) and have suggested that drugs which stimulate prolactin may improve lactational performance. Others have found no such correlation between the prolactin response to suckling and the quantity of milk produced (Howie et al, 1980).

Stress. Prolactin secretion is increased by physical and emotional stress, though the degree is variable. Surgery and anaesthesia are relatively constant stimuli but stressful exercise and venesection produce more variable increases (Noel et al, 1972). Psychological stress is less well documented as a stimulus of prolactin secretion but can be demonstrated to occur in normal parachute jumpers (Noel et al, 1976) and in neurotic women subjected to psychological testing (Miyabo et al, 1977). As with most other stimuli of prolactin secretion, the effect is more pronounced in females. It is likely that these stimuli which arise in higher brain centres are carried in projections of the limbic system to the hypothalamus (Willoughby, 1980). Stress release of prolactin in rats can be induced by restraint, short exposure to ether or to a novel environment; this release is inhibited by serotonin antagonists suggesting that serotonergic-PRF releasing pathways are involved (Goodman et al, 1976; Shin, 1979b).

Pharmacological stimuli of prolactin secretion. Pharmacological stimuli increase prolactin concentration in the circulation by reducing the effective activity of dopamine at lactotrope receptors, by activating the release of PRF or by simulating the action of PRF on the pituitary gland (Table 1.1).

Drugs which reduce the inhibitory action of dopamine may do so by reducing the synthesis or release of dopamine or by blocking the dopamine receptor on the lactotrope. Acute blockade of dopamine receptors by metoclopramide causes a rapid rise in serum prolactin which is maximal by 30 minutes and which is prolonged for up to 8 hours. As

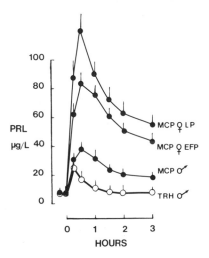

Fig. 1.21 The effect of metoclopramide (MCP 2.5 mg i.v.) on prolactin secretion in men and women in the early follicular phase (EFP) and the luteal phase (LP) of the cycle compared with the effect of thyrotropin releasing hormone (TRH 200 μg i.v.) in men

is the case with most stimuli for prolactin secretion, the response is augmented by endogenous oestradiol concentration and hence is higher in women than men, and higher in the luteal phase than in the follicular phase (Fig. 1.21).

Direct stimulation of the pituitary by thyrotropin releasing hormone also results in prompt prolactin secretion but the magnitude and duration of the response is reduced compared to dopamine blockade (Fig. 1.21). Insulin induced hypoglycaemia is a less reliable stimulus of prolactin, particularly in men but after substantial hypoglycaemia, there is a clear rise in serum prolactin (Noel et al, 1972); it is likely that the effect of insulin on prolactin secretion is mediated by increase in serotoninergic activity in the brain (Whitaker et al, 1980).

Pathological hyperprolactinaemia

Although uncommon, hyperprolactinaemia may be caused by damage to or infiltration of the hypothalamus, particularly if it involves the tuberoinfundibular dopamine neurons. Decreased metabolic clearance of prolactin is an important factor causing hyperprolactinaemia in hypothyroidism and chronic renal failure.

Hyperprolactinaemia may also reflect excessive secretion from a pituitary tumour which may greatly enlarge the pituitary fossa (macroadenoma) or which may cause subtle or no change in its normal configuration (microadenoma). Macroadenomas may secrete only prolactin and be largely asymptomatic or excessive prolactin secretion may only be one of several pituitary hormones secreted in excess (Heitz, 1979). Hyperprolactinaemia without major radiological change in the pituitary fossa is more common and in many of these a discrete microadenoma can be identified (Robert & Hardy, 1975). These tumours are less than 10 mm in diameter, and are generally located in the postero-lateral aspects of the gland. Electron microscopy of these lesions show a scarcity of secretory granules, well developed rough endoplasmic reticulum and prominent Golgi areas, all suggesting increased secretory activity. Frequently, exocytosis of secretory granules occurs through the lateral membranes of the lactotrope into adjacent tumour cells rather than into the perivascular space. This 'misplaced exocytosis' (Horvath & Kovacs, 1974) is apparently the result of increased secretory activity combined with a relative reduction of cell membranes in contact with perivascular spaces.

In some situations, hyperprolactinaemia is associated with generalised lactotrope hyperplasia, without discrete tumour formation. This is most clearly seen in the state of pregnancy (Baker & Yu, 1977) but is also recognised in association with end organ failure of the thyroid or testis. It is not clear whether all women with persistent hyperprolactinaemia do harbour microadenomas or whether some may have generalised hyperplasia. Unfortunately, no radiological technique is sensitive enough, at this time, to

be definitive about the frequency of microadenoma in primary hyperprolactinaemia and with the increasing reliance on medical treatment of primary hyperprolactinaemia, it is unlikely that a series of unselected patients will be referred for surgical exploration of the pituitary to enable this question to be answered.

CHRONIC ANOVULATION DUE TO NEURO-ENDOCRINE ABNORMALITIES

Chronic anovulation due to primary disorders of the ovary are considered in other chapters of this book and, clearly, for ovulation to occur there must be an ovary containing primordial follicles capable of being stimulated by gonadotrophins. Abnormalities of the end organ are characterised by low levels of gonadal steroids, increased serum gonadotrophins (particularly FSH) and an increased pituitary response to GnRH.

Chronic anovulation may be due to a loss of pituitary gonadotropes as a result of pituitary tumour, pituitary surgery or irradiation. These disorders are characterised by low serum levels of gonadotropins, despite low levels of oestradiol, and a reduced response to exogenous GnRH.

Chronic anovulation due to a hypothalamic abnormality results from a disturbance in the function of GnRH neurons. This may take the form of complete absence of neurons or be due to a functional abnormality of a variable degree (Table 1.2).

Table 1.2 Neuroendocrine causes of chronic anovulation
1. Absence of Pituitary Gonadotropins
   — Pituitary tumour
   — Pituitary surgery
   — Pituitary irradiation
2. Absence or Global loss of GnRH neuron function
   — Congenital (Kallman's Prader-Willi)
   — Infiltrative (Craniopharyngioma, histiocytosis X)
   — Functional (Anorexia, Delayed Puberty)
3. Moderate or Selective dysfunction of GnRH neurons
   — Hyperprolactinaemic chronic anovulation
   — Normoprolactinaemic hypothalamic chronic anovulation
   — Luteal phase dysfunction
   — Failure of positive feedback
4. Inappropriate or Extra-ovarian oestrogen secretion
   — Increased precurssor availability (androgen excess syndromes)
   — Excessive aromatase activity (obesity)
   — Non-ovarian production of oestrogen (Pregnancy, Oral oestrogen)

Conditions associated with an absence or global disturbance of the GnRH neuron

In the complete absence of GnRH neuron activity, serum levels of gonadotrophins, and gonadal steroids are very low, there is no measurable pulsatility of LH and the ovaries are infantile in appearance with greatly reduced growth of follicles to the antral stage and virtual absence of Graafian follicles (Goldenberg, 1976); in male patients,

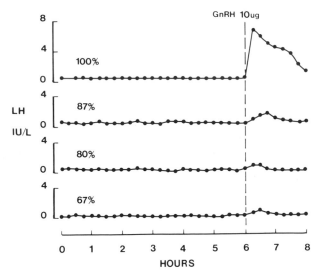

Fig. 1.22 Serum LH before and after GnRH (10 μg i.v.) in four women with anorexia nervosa of varying severity (ideal body weight 67–100%). There is a low mean basal level of LH with absent pulsatility. The responses to GnRH range from minimal (IBW 67%) to normal (IBM 100%). From Russell & Judd (unpublished data)

testicular biopsy shows immature seminferous tubules with undifferentiated germinal epithelium (Bardin & Paulsen, 1981). Depending on the degree of GnRH deficiency, individual patients will respond suboptimally, or not at all, to an initial dose of exogenous GnRH (Fig. 1.22). However, continued exposure to GnRH, particularly if delivered in a physiological manner, leads to an increasing gondotropin response and steady rise in gonadal steroids. Moreover, if GnRH is continued, normal ovulatory menstrual cycles in women and spermatogenesis in men are established, indicating that the abnormality is indeed hypothalamic. Disorders of the hypothalamus which result in isolated hypofunction of the GnRH neuron can be congenital, infiltrative or functional.

Congenital causes

Kallman's syndrome (Fig. 1.23). In this disorder, hypogonadism is associated with varying degrees of anosmia. This is related to hypoplasia or agenesis of the olfactory apparatus as well as incomplete development in mammillary bodies and parts of the anterior hypothalamus (Steinberger, 1979). It may be associated with colour-blindness, midline facial defects, unilateral renal agenesis, cryptorchidism or short metacarpals (Sparkes et al, 1968). The inheritance is variable, being variously reported as an autosomal dominant, an autosomal recessive and a sex-linked dominant disorder.

A form of hypogonadotropic hypogonadism which is not associated with any of the added features of Kallman's syndrome also exists and this is transmitted as an autosomal recessive disorder. This disorder usually manifests itself as delay in the onset of puberty and is difficult to

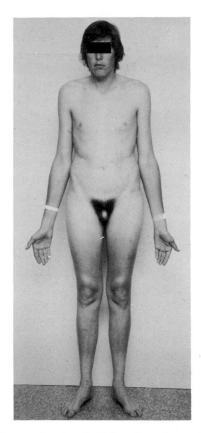

Fig. 1.23 A 23-year-old male with Kallman's syndrome. Note the eunuchoid stature and poorly developed genitalia. Pubic hair appeared after treatment with human chorionic gonadotropin at the age of 16

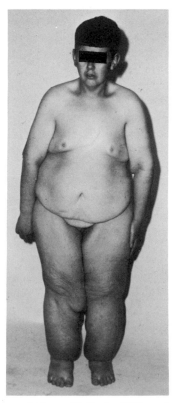

Fig. 1.24 An 18-year-old boy with Prader-Willi syndrome

distinguish from the functional, self limiting form of delayed puberty. However, in the latter group, puberty can be initiated by treatment with testosterone or human chorionic gonadotrophin in the male, or oestrogen in the female, and if pubertal changes continue after this, then an organic deficiency of GnRH is excluded.

Prader-Willi syndrome (Fig. 1.24). This disorder is characterised by neonatal and infantile hypotonia, mental retardation of a variable degree, massive obesity associated with glucose intolerance, short stature and hypogonadism. The condition is usually sporadic and is not associated with any major morphological hypothalamic abnormality. These patients usually have low levels of gonadotrophins with absent pubertal changes but onset of puberty has been described after weight reduction and after clomiphene administration (Hamilton et al, 1972) suggesting a functional disorder of the hypothalamus rather than complete absence of the GnRH neuron.

Infiltrative hypothalamic lesions

Tumours or infections which infiltrate the hypothalamus usually cause marked hypothalamic damage and secondary deficiency of a number of pituitary hormones. When the secretion of growth hormone is affected as well as the gona-

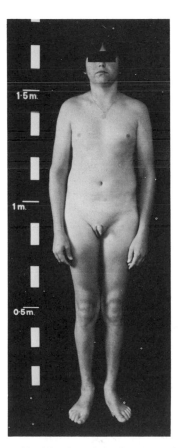

Fig. 1.25 A 21-year-old with a hypothalamic tumour showing hypogonadism without an eunuchoid stature

dotrophins, then hypogonadism is not associated with the usual eunochoid stature (Fig. 1.25). Occasionally, hypogonadism with or without hyperprolactinaemia may be the only clinical feature of an infiltrative lesion of the hypothalamus.

Craniopharyngioma (Fig. 1.25). This tumour arises from remnants of Rathke's pouch and is usually situated anterior and superior to the pituitary fossa although it may be confined to the sella turcica. It frequently causes visual disturbance because of its close proximity to the optic chiasm and optic tracts. It may be associated with diabetes insipidus or other dysfunctions of the hypothalamus including polyphagia, somnolence and loss of thirst sensation, although this more commonly occurs as a result of post-operative surgical trauma. The tumour may be solid or cystic with a high concentration of cholesterol. Skull X-ray or CAT scanning of the head commonly shows calcification within the tumour. Other tumourous infiltrations of the hypothalamus include dysgerminomas arising in the anterior or posterior parts of the third ventricle which may involve the medio-basal hypothalamus, optic gliomas, occuring as a complication of von Ricklinghausen's disease or as an isolated anomaly, and meningiomas arising from the sphenoid ridge.

Other causes of hypothalamic damage or infiltration. Histiocytosis X is a generalised malignant disease characterised by infiltration of many body tissues, including the hypothalamus, with lipid-laden histiocytic cells. This is usually associated with diabetes insipidus, hypogonadism and growth failure; skeletal X-rays show multiple cystic lesions in the skull, ribs and long bones.

Rapid deceleration of the brain during accidental head injury commonly leads to pituitary stalk and hypothalamic damage; in 106 patients dying of traumatic head injury, hypothalamic lesions were found in 45 patients (42.5 per cent) (Crompton, 1971). Radiotherapy given for non hypothalamic brain tumours or for leukaemia in children is also associated with hypothalamic damage and variable pituitary dysfunction, including gonadotrophin deficiency. Although rare, tuberculosis or bacterial meningitis may also be associated with impaired hypothalamic function.

Functional disorders

Anorexia nervosa. This disorder occurs most frequently in girls and is characterised by severe weight loss associated with a distorted body image and a pathological fear of gaining weight. Patients tend to be obsessional, intelligent 'achievers' and in those severely affected there may be defective temperature regulation, bradycardia, hypokalaemia and carotenaemia.

Fasting is associated with a number of changes in hormone metabolism including preferential conversion of thyroxine to reverse triiodothyronine (rT_3) at the expense of normal triiodothyronine (Moshang et al, 1975), increased conversion of androgens to etiocholanolone instead of androsterone (Bradlow et al, 1976) and increased conversion of oestradiol to catechol oestrogens rather than oestriol (Fishman et al 1975). The metabolic clearance rate of cortisol is reduced, apparently as a result of the reduction of circulating triiodothyronine (Boyar et al, 1977).

The degree of suppression of GnRH neuron activity seems closely related to the amount of weight loss. When body weight is less than 70 per cent of that which is ideal for height, response to exogenous GnRH is imperceptible. With increasing weight gain, response to GnRH increases (Fig. 1.26) and the dynamics of gonadotropin secretion within the gonadotrope becomes more normal (Abraham et al, 1977). Continued administration of pulsatile GnRH, given in physiological doses, causes an increase in FSH which is initially rapid but which reaches a plateau level after 2 days; this is followed by a gradual fall in serum FSH despite continued GnRH administration. Conversely, serum LH is more slow to rise but continues to increase while GnRH is given and there is also a steady rise in 17β oestradiol (Marshall & Kelch, 1979). These alterations in LH:FSH ratios are the same as those which occur during the course of normal puberty and which follow pulsatile GnRH administration in the rhesus monkey with lesions of the arcuate nucleus (Hausler et al, 1979).

The nature of the functional impairment of the GnRH neuron has been widely speculated upon. On a theoretical basis, Barry & Klawans (1976) proposed that excessive

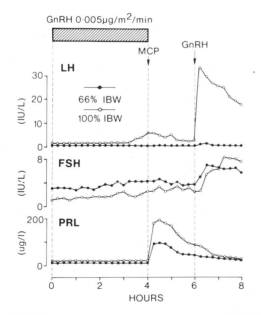

Fig. 1.26 LH, FSH and PRL responses to metoclopramide (MCP 10 mg i.v.) and GnRH (10 μ i.v.) after priming with GnRH in two women with anorexia nervosa. In the patient most severely affected (ideal body weight 66% ●-●, neither MCP nor GnRH increases serum LH or FSH. In a less severely affected patient with normal body weight but continuing amenorrhoea (o–o), the last 30 minutes of the infusion of GnRH is associated with an increase in serum LH and GnRH causes a substantial increase in both LH and FSH; there is no response to MCP. From Russell & Judd (unpublished data)

dopaminergic activity in the brain and hypothalamus could explain the psychiatric and neuroendocrine manifestations of the disorder. Excessive dopamine activity might well cause suppression of GnRH secretion but acute administration of metoclopramide does not cause any increase in serum LH in anorexic women, even when the gonadotrope has been primed with GnRH to increase its sensitivity to endogenous GnRH (Fig. 1.26). However, in another study, longer treatment with metoclopramide led to an increase in pituitary responsiveness to GnRH which could be explained by a blockade of dopamine neurons inhibiting endogenous GnRH secretion (Larsen, 1981). It seems likely that severe weight loss causes a regression to a prepubertal pattern of GnRH secretion by a mechanism which is not well understood but which probably involves brain neurotransmitters. This may be the result of an increase in activity of inhibitory neurons such as dopamine or the brain opiates or to an impairment in function of stimulatory neurons such as noradrenaline.

Severe systemic illness. Chronic anovulation associated with reduced gonadotrophin secretion may occur in adolescents with chronic debilitating diseases and malnutrition. These conditions are usually associated with a delay in skeletal growth and maturation; they include chronic renal disease, chronic, poorly controlled diabetes with ketosis, and chronic anaemias.

Functional delayed puberty. This diagnosis is one of exclusion and is, to some extent, retrospective since it depends on the spontaneous appearance of puberty at future date. Chronic illness and anorexia are usually easy to exclude but idiopathic hypogonadotrophic hypogonadism may be very difficult, particularly in the teenage years. A family history of delayed puberty is sometimes helpful and complete absence of sexual development by the age of 18 in females is rarely a functional problem. The appearance of early signs of puberty is an encouraging sign; this will be followed, in time, by the characteristic changes in LH secretion (Figs 1.14 and 1.15). The development of nocturnal secretion of LH is a clear indication that puberty is preceding normally but by this time, the clinical situation is usually clear.

Management

Chronic anovulation due to these conditions does not respond to clomiphene and the most appropriate treatment, if indicated, is for replacement treatment with pulsatile administration of GnRH or by direct stimulation of the ovaries with exogenous gonadotrophins (Chapters 26, 27).

Conditions associated with moderate impairment or selective dysfunction of the GnRH neuron

This group of disorders is characterised by normal basal levels of LH but an absent or reduced frequency of LH pulsatility. This is associated, in some, with an inability to respond to the positive feedback effect of oestrogen with a preovulatory surge of gonadotrophins. Serum FSH levels are either normal or slightly increased and the response of both LH and FSH to GnRH is not impaired. Serum oestradiol levels are variable but usually not greater than those found in the normal early follicular phase; however, stimulation of the ovary by LH and FSH induced by pulsatile GnRH administration leads to a normal ovarian response and an increase in oestradiol. This type of GnRH neuron abnormality is seen in women with chronic anovulation due to hyperprolactinaemia or 'hypothalamic amenorrhoea' and may also apply in the condition of 'luteal phase dysfunction'.

Chronic anovulation and hyperprolactinaemia

In addition to elevated levels of PRL, hyperprolactinaemic women have a disturbed pattern of PRL secretion. Episodic secretion of PRL continues but the physiological increase seen during sleep, after eating and during suckling is abolished or greatly diminished (Judd, 1982; Fig. 1.27).

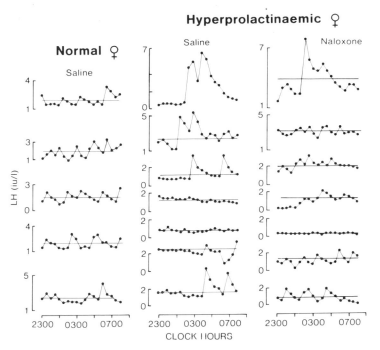

Fig. 1.28 The frequency of LH secretion in seven hyperprolactinaemic women (middle panel) and five normal women (left panel) during saline infusion showing the reduced rate of LH pulsatility (with normal mean levels of LH) in the hyperprolactinaemic women. After infusion of naloxone, there is an increase in the frequency of LH pulsatility in the hyperprolactinaemic women (right panel) suggesting that in hyperprolactinaemia there is an increase in opiate activity operative on the GnRH neuron. From Judd & Roeger (unpublished data)

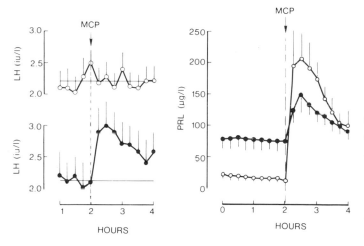

Fig. 1.27 The effect of metoclopramide (MCP; 10 mg i.v.) on serum LH and PRL in six normal women in the early follicular phase (o-o) and ten hyperprolactinaemic women (o-o). MCP causes an increase in serum LH, but only in the hyperprolactinaemic women; the pattern of this increase is similar to that seen after GnRH administration. The increase in serum PRL after MCP is reduced in hyperprolactinaemic women. Reproduced with permission from Judd (1982)

In some patients, the pulsatile pattern of LH secretion is lost, even though the mean basal level of LH is no different from that seen in early follicular phase women; others show a pulsatile pattern of LH secretion but with a reduced frequency of LH pulses (Fig. 1.28). The positive feedback effect of oestrogen, as judged by the LH response to clomiphene or 1 mg of 17 β oestradiol intramuscularly, is lost (Glass et al, 1975; Kandeel et al, 1979).

The pathophysiology of chronic anovulation has been studied in some detail in hyperprolactinaemic women (Quigley et al, 1979, 1980a; Judd, 1982). There is evidence of *increased* dopamine activity at the level of the GnRH nerve terminals in the median eminence which inhibits the secretion of GnRH and hence disturbs gonadotrophin release. Hence, the dopamine antagonist, metoclopramide, causes an increase in the secretion of serum LH (probably as a result of blockade of GnRH inhibition by dopamine) in hyperprolactinaemic women (Fig. 1.27) but not normal or anovulatory women with normoprolactinaemia (Judd, 1980). In keeping with this, infusion of dopamine is less effective at inhibiting LH secretion in hyperprolactinaemic women than normal women (Quigley et al, 1980b). Conversely, at the level of the lactotrope, there is evidence of *decreased* dopamine activity as suggested by the impaired PRL response to metoclopramide (Fig. 1.27) and the excessive suppression of PRL by dopamine in hyperprolactinaemic women compared to normal (Quigley et al, 1980a).

On the basis of these findings, it has been proposed that in hyperprolactinaemic anovulation the afferent arm of the normal feedback control system of prolactin is intact but that there is an abnormality in the efferent arm so that the increase in tuberoinfundibular dopamine activity is not reflected at the level of the lactotrope (Fig. 1.29; Judd,

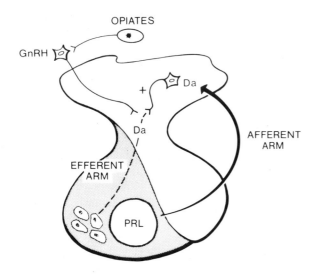

Fig. 1.29 Proposed pathophysiology of hyperprolactinaemic chronic anovulation. Excessive secretion of PRL is associated with an increase in TIDA activity, i.e. the afferent arm of the short loop feedback is intact. Increased dopamine activity at the level of the GnRH nerve terminal inhibits secretion of GnRH. The efferent arm of the short loop feedback is abnormal (see text) which maintains excessive prolactin secretion. In addition, there is increased opiate activity affecting the GnRH neuron, causing a reduced rate of GnRH and hence LH secretion

1982). Two fundamentally different mechanisms can be proposed to explain this paradox. Firstly, it is possible that a separate group of TIDA neurons control PRL secretion and GnRH secretion and there is a selective abnormality in the group controlling PRL secretion. This would be in keeping with the work of Fine & Frohman (1978) and Van Loon (1978) who have found evidence of a defect in TIDA neurons in hyperprolactinaemic women and also with pathological studies that suggest that the lactotropes outside prolactin secreting tumours are hyperplastic (Halmi & Duello, 1976; Kovacs et al, 1978; Heitz, 1979). However, this hypothesis does not explain the apparent cure of some patients after selective removal of a microadenoma, with return to normal of the prolactin response to metoclopramide (Barbarino et al, 1978).

The alternative hypothesis is that a group of lactotropes become autonomous as a result of isolation from the influence of portal vein dopamine (Porter et al, 1978) or because they possess abnormal dopamine receptors (Malarkey et al, 1977) or because they have a greater capacity for local inactivation of dopamine. These uninhibited lactotropes cause hypersecretion of PRL, the short loop feedback remains intact and the non-adenomatous lactotropes and thyrotropes are exposed to increased concentration of dopamine in the portal blood (Scanlon et al, 1980). This provides a satisfactory explanation for the return of normal lactotrope and thyrotrope function after selective microadenectomy but does not explain why some hyperprolactinaemic women show a negliglible increase in PRL, even after chronic exposure to metoclopramide (Judd, 1982).

The final solution to the nature of the abnormality in the efferent arm of the feedback system, therefore, remains to be determined.

The dopamine hypothesis does not explain the pathophysiology in those hyperprolactinaemic women whose major abnormality is a reduced frequency of LH secretion since dopamine does not influence the frequency of LH pulsatility. In these women, infusion of naloxone restores the frequency of LH pulsatility to normal (Fig. 1.28) suggesting that, in addition to increased dopamine activity, there is also an increase in the activity of opiate neurons in the brain affecting GnRH neurons (Fig. 1.29). Whether this increase in opiate activity is due to hyperprolactinaemia *per se* or as a secondary effect of the increase in dopamine activity, remains to be determined.

It is intriguing to speculate that a change in frequency of GnRH secretion may so profoundly affect the frequency of LH pulsatility (or the ratio LH : FSH) that stimulation of ovarian follicles is inhibited. This would be in keeping with the absence of folliculogenesis during the luteal phase of the normal menstrual cycle and with the induction of ovulation in hyperprolacinaemic women who have their normal LH pulsatility restored with intermittent GnRH injections at a frequency of one pulse every 90 minutes (Leyendecker at al, 1980). Moreover, one of the effects of reducing prolactin levels to normal with bromocriptine is to restore the normal frequency of LH secretion (Moult et al, 1982).

Normoprolactinaemic hypothalamic chronic anovulation

This is a rather heterogenous syndrome and includes a wide range of women with persisting anovulation but normoprolactinaemia. These women are characterised by the normal onset of secondary sexual characteristics but with amenorrhoea developing after menarche. This group includes those women who undertake vigorous physical exercise ('athletes amenorrhoea') and those women who are less than ideal body weight and who are overly preoccupied with their diet although not to the same pathological extent as women with anorexia ('low weight amenorrhoea'). Frequently, depression or stressful life events can be identified at the onset of amenorrhoea ('psychological amenorrhoea') even such factors as removal from a familiar, emotionally comfortable environment ('boarding-school amenorrhoea').

Despite its heterogeny, the fundamental abnormality appears to be a functional, usually reversible, abnormality of the GnRH neuron resulting in normal basal levels of LH, variable loss of LH pulsatility, retention of response to exogenous GnRH, a prolonged negative feedback suppression by oestradiol and a failure of the positive feedback effect of oestrogen. Numerous attempts have been made to differentiate this group on the basis of their response to clomiphene (Vaitukaites et al, 1974), oestrogen, progesterone or GnRH (Keller et al, 1975 Santen et al, 1978; Rakoff et al, 1978); however, to date, this has not led to a more specific classification of this disorder (Lachelin & Yen, 1978).

Since the condition is largely reversible, it can be assumed that its aetiology lies in an alteration in the normal activity of stimulatory or inhibitory neurons affecting GnRH activity. These alterations might be triggered by a change in energy balance, reduced body fat ratio or weight (Frisch & McArthur, 1974) or the primary abnormality may arise centrally as a result of stress.

The concept of increased inhibitory activity on the GnRH neuron imposed by dopamine and opiate neuron has been strongly suggested by the work of Quigley et al (1980c). These authors showed that serum LH was increased by metoclopramide in some patients with hypothalamic chronic anovulation and, in the same patients, naloxone stimulated an increase in both frequency of pulsatility and amplitude of secretion. Other women with hypothalamic chronic anovulation did not respond to either metoclopramide or naloxone. These could be distinguished from the responsive group by a lower basal serum LH level, but there was no difference in their basal serum PRL, oestradiol or their gonadotrophin response to GnRH. In another study, metoclopramide was given to women with hypothalamic chronic anovulation and was found to increase significantly the subsequent response to GnRH; this improved response was also attributed to an increase in endogenous GnRH induced by dopamine blockade in these women (Larsen, 1981). These neuroendocrine studies have provided important insights into the mechanisms of this condition and although, our understanding of the pathophysiology of hypothalamic chronic anovulation is still incomplete, careful clinical neuroendocrine studies can be expected to add much more in the next few years.

Management. Specific treatment with the long acting dopamine agonist, bromocriptine, is highly effective in lowering serum prolactin in hyperprolactinaemic women and in restoring the normal frequency of LH ssecretion and ovulation (Ch. 26). Despite some reports suggesting a therapeutic role for bromocriptine in normoprolactinaemic hypothalamic chronic anovulation (Seppala et al, 1976; Corenblum & Taylor, 1980), most studies have not found bromocriptine to be valuable in these situation and the preferred form of treatment is clomiphene (Ch. 26). Pulsatile administration of exogenous GnRH is a valuable addition to the treatment of these conditions.

Luteal phase dysfunction

This condition was first characterised by Jones (1949) on the basis of a study of endometrial biopsies. She proposed that the abnormality was due to a decreased progesterone production from the corpus luteum or a result of a local endometrial resistance to progesterone action. Since then,

this abnormality has been described in a number of clincal situations including hyperprolactinaemia (Del Pozo et al, 1979), stressful exercise programmes and ovulation induction with clomiphene (Van Hall & Mastboom, 1969). It is likely that luteal phase dysfunction represents part of the continuum of impaired GnRH function rather than a separate entity of its own.

Detailed study of women with luteal phase dysfunction has confirmed that both serum FSH and LH are low in the early follicular phase of the cycle and, in particular, the FSH : LH ratio is low (Strott et al, 1970). Others have described an absence of the mid-cycle surge of FSH (Aksel, 1980). Significant progress has been made in understanding this condition since the development of an elegant animal model (Di Zerega & Hodgen, 1981a,b). These authors found that administration of porcine follicular fluid caused a selective fall in serum FSH (probably due to its Inhibin activity) and that this was followed by a reduced rise of oestrogen during the follicular phase, a reduced preovulatory rise of serum FSH and LH and a low luteal phase level of oestradiol and progesterone. Moreover, in later studies these authors demonstrated that these abnormalities induced by porcine follicular fluid could be partly overcome by administration of FSH during the early follicular phase (Di Zerega & Hodgen, 1981c).

To date, it is not clear why the serum FSH : LH ratio is altered in those conditions that give rise to luteal phase dysfunction but it is tempting to speculate that there is a selective dysfunction in the GnRH neuron — perhaps an alteration in the frequency of its secretion. It naturally follows that the appropriate treatment of this abnormality is to restore the normal early follicular phase hormone pattern with bromocriptine (in hyperprolactinaemia) or exogenous FSH, perhaps by a pulsatile mode of delivery.

Failed positive feedback effect of oestrogen

In some patients with apparently regular menstrual cycles and normal increase in oestradiol during the follicular phase, ovulation does not occur because of a failure of the mid-cycle gonadotrophin surge (Van Look, 1976). This may occur in hyperprolactinaemia and in women undergoing ovulation induction or it may occur as an isolated event (Fraser et al, 1973). In this latter situation it is often associated with dysfunctional uterine bleeding and particularly in the perimenarchial or perimenopausal woman. Detailed studies of these women to show the frequency of pulsatile LH secretion and the FSH:LH ratio have not been performed although one study has shown a lower mean basal level of serum LH and FSH and an elevated level of oestradiol (Fraser et al, 1973). It is not possible therefore to decide whether this condition is due to a primary abnormality in the GnRH neuron leading to an absence of midcycle GnRH secretion only, or if it really represents, like luteal phase dysfunction, a more basic defect in early follicular phase secretion of GnRH. In some patients, ovulation and fertility can apparently be restored by properly timed replacement of the endogenous LH surge with human chorionic gonadotropin.

Conditions associated with inappropriate or extraovarian oestrogen secretion.

In the normal, premenopausal, fertile female, the ovary is the major source of oestrogen (in the form of 17β oestradiol). However, some oestrogen is produced by peripheral conversion of androgens, resulting from the action of aromatase. This enzyme is found in skin, muscle, peripheral fat tissue and in the hypothalamus. It actively converts androstenedione and testosterone (derived from the ovary and the adrenal) to oestrone and oestradiol, repectively. Approximately 40 μg of oestrone each day is produced from androstenedione in the premenopausal woman but this amount is greatly increased in obese women and with advancing age. Oestrone is, therefore, the major oestrogen after the menopause. As long as the ovary produces an increasing amount of oestradiol during the follicular phase, the hypothalamus and the pituitary are able to receive the correct feedback signals to allow for the appropriate timing of the positive feedback response and the preovulatory discharge of gonadotrophins. However, if a substantial proportion of oestrogen is derived from tissues other than the ovary, then the normal feedback system is interrupted and a continuous, low grade positive feedback effect occurs (Fig. 1.30). This leads to a high basal level of LH with increased frequency of LH secretion and an augmented LH response to exogenous GnRH; conversely, serum FSH is often suppressed and acyclical because of its greater sensitivity to the negative feedback action of oestrogen (Yen et al, 1970; Baird, 1976).

This pathophysiology contributes, to a varying extent, to a number of conditions. These include those disorders in which there is increased precursor availability (androgen excess syndromes),where there is increased aromatase activity (obesity) or when there is an extraovarian source of oestrogens (oral oestrogen administration, pregnancy and oestrogen producing adrenal tumours). Moreover, in the rat it is possible that oestrone and oestradiol have different sites of action in the hypothalamus which may contribute to the abnormal function of GnRH neurons (Kawakami et al, 1978). However this has not been investigated in the primate.

Polycystic ovary syndrome

This is a heterogenous syndrome but is characterised clinically by a normal age of menarche with menstrual cycles becoming increasingly irregular. Patients commonly are overweight and hirsute even from the time of menarche (Yen et al, 1976). Basal levels of serum LH are elevated and the frequency of LH pulsatility is increased to one pulse every hour (Fig. 1.31); the normal negative feedback response to oestrogen is retained (Rebar et al, 1976) as is the positive feedback response to clomiphene and oestradiol (Baird et al, 1975; Shaw et al, 1975; Rebar et al, 1976); the LH response to exogenous GnRH is exaggerated. All these features are consistent with an increased sensitivity of the gonadotrope, perhaps associated with an increased activity of GnRH neurons. In keeping with the speculation that GnRH activity is increased, (a well as pituitary sensitivity to GnRH) is the observation that serum LH is more sensitive to the inhibitory actions of dopamine in women with polycystic ovary disease than in normal or agonadal women (Judd et al, 1977; Quigley et al, 1981a).

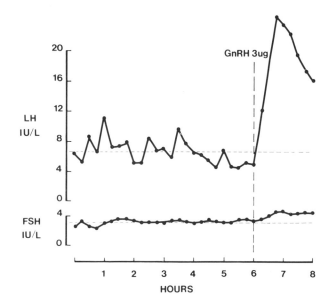

Fig. 1.31 The pattern of gonadotropin secretion in a 29-year-old woman with polycystic ovary disease showing the increase in mean basal level of serum LH, the increased frequency of LH secretion and the increased LH sensitivity to GnRH

Inappropriate oestrogen feedback

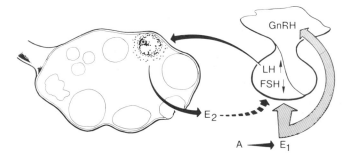

Fig. 1.30 Chronic anovulation associated with inappropriate oestrogen feedback. In conditions of inappropriate feedback of oestrogen, there is excessive production of oestrogens (often oestrone) from tissues other than the ovary. This process interrupts the normal feedback signals from the ovarian follicle and produces, at the same time, excessive secretion of LH and decreased FSH (see text for details)

Under the influence of increased circulating levels of LH, the theca interna is stimulated to produce more testosterone which interferes with the maturation of follicles in the ovary. High intraovarian concentration of androgens are maintained by a deficiency of granulosa cell aromatase (secondary to FSH deficiency). The ovary remains acutely sensitive to FSH, both *in vitro* and *in vivo*, and addition of FSH causes a marked increase in ovarian oestrogen production (Erikson et al, 1979). Increased circulating testosterone is responsible for hirsutism and, by increasing precursor availability, for maintaining increased extra-ovarian oestrogen production (Fig. 1.32).

Management. In all the conditions associated with inappropriate or extraovarian oestrogen secretion, the logical method of treatment is to treat the cause where possible (e.g. weight reduction or adrenal androgen suppression with glucocorticoids in congenital adrenal hyperplasia). Clomiphene is a useful adjunct competing, as it does, for oestrogen receptors in the hypothalamus and pituitary.

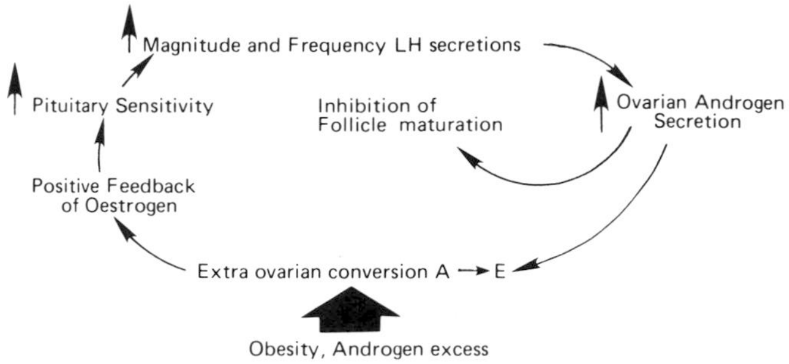

Fig. 1.32 The proposed pathophysiology of polycystic ovary disease (and other conditions of inappropriate oestrogen feedback). Modified from Yen et al (1976)

Pulsatile GnRH administration is neither logical or effective. The possibility of reducing excessive endogenous GnRH effect (by dopamine infusion or GnRH antagonists) or selectively blocking peripheral aromatase activity has not been explored.

REFERENCES

Abraham S F, Beumont P J V, Argall W J, Turtle J H 1977 LH and FSH responses to a 4 hour infusion of luteinising hormone-releasing hormone (LHRH) in patients with anorexia nervosa. Abstract 3 2oth Annual Meeting Endocrine Society Australia, Melbourne

Adler M W 1980 Opioid peptides. Life Sciences 26: 497–510

Advis J P, Hall T R, Hudson C A, Mueller G P, Meites J 1977 Temporal relationship and role of dopamine in 'short loop' feedback of Prolactin. Proceedings of the Society for Experimental Biology and Medicine 155: 567–570

Advis J P, Krause J E, McKelry J F 1980 Evidence that endopeptidase-catalysed LHRH cleavage contributes to the regulation of median eminence LHRH levels during positive feedback. Abstract 10.1 10th Annual Meeting Society for Neuroscience, Cincinnati, Ohio

Ajika K, Arai K, Okinaga S 1982 Localisation of dopamine in the prolactin cell of the rat anterior pituitary gland — a fluorescence and immunoelectron microscopical study. Abstract 367 64th Annual Meeting Endocrine Society San Francisco

Aksel S 1980 Sporadic and recurrent luteal phase defects in cyclic women: comparison with normal cycles. Fertility and Sterility 33: 372–377

Amoss M, Burgus R, Blackwell R, et al 1971 Purification, amino acid composition and N terminus of the hypothalamic luteinising hormone releasing factor (LRF) of ovine origin. Biochemical and Biophysical Research Communication 4: 205–210

Aono T, Shioji T, Shoda T, Kurachi K 1977 The initiation of human lactation and prolactin response to suckling . Journal of Clinical Endocrinology and Metabolism 44: 1101–1106

Backstrom C T, McNeilly A S, Liask R M, Baird D T 1982 Pulsatile secretion of LH, FSH, Prolactin, oestradiol and progesterone during the human menstrual cycle. Clinical Endocrinology 16: 29–42

Baird D T 1976 Disturbance in the negative feedback loops of the pituitary-ovarian axis. Clinics in Obstetrics and Gynaecology 3: 535–554

Baird D T, Corker C S, Fraser I S, Hunter W M, Michie E A, Van Look P F A 1975 Pituitary-ovarian relationships in polycystic ovarian disease. Journal of Endocrinology 64: 53–54

Baker B L, Yu Y Y 1977 An immunocytochemical study of human pituitary mammotropes from fetal life to old age. American Journal of Anatomy 148: 217–234

Barbarino A, De Marinis L, Maira G, Menini E, Anile C 1979 serum prolactin response to thyrotropin-releasing hormone and metoclopramide in patients with prolactin secreting tumours before

and after trans sphenoidal surgery. Journal of Clinical Endocrinology and Metabolism 47: 1148–1151

Bardin C W, Paulsen C A 1981 The testes. In: Williams R H (ed) Endocrinology, Ch 6, pp 293–354. W B Saunders, Philadelphia

Barnea A, Porter J 1975 Demonstration of macromolecule cross reacting with antibodies to luteinising hormone releasing hormone and its tissue distribution. Biochemical and Biophysical Research Communications 67: 1346–1352

Barraclough C A, Sawyer C H 1955 Blockade of the release of pituitary ovulating hormone in the rat by chlorpromazine and reserpine: possible mechanism of action. Endocrinology 61: 341–351

Barry J 1976 Characteristics and topography of LH-RH neurons in the human brain. Neuroscience Letters 3: 287–291

Barry V C, Klawans H L 1976 On the role of dopamine in the pathophysiology of anorexia nervosa. Journal of Neural Transmission 38: 107–122

Barry J, Dubois M P, Carette B 1974 Immunofluorescence study of the preoptico-infundibular LRF neurosecretory pathway in the normal, castrated or testosterone treated male guinea pig. Endocrinology 95: 1416–1423

Bateson M C, Browning M C K, Maconnachie A 1977 Galactorrhoea with cimetidine. Lancet ii: 247–248

Belchetz P E, Plant T M, Nakai Y, Keogh E J, Knobil E 1978 Hypophysial responses to continuous and intermittent delivery of hypothalamic gonadotropin releasing hormone. Science 202: 631–633

Ben-Jonathon N 1982 Dopamine synthesis by the posterior pituitary: alteration during lactation. Abstract 854, 64th Annual Meeting Endocrine Society San Francisco

Ben-Jonathon N, Oliver C, Weiner H J, Mical R, Porter J 1977 Dopamine in hypophysial portal blood of the rat during the estrus cycle and throughout pregnancy. Endocrinology 100: 452–458

Benveniste R, Helman J O, Orth D N, McKenna T J, Nicholson W E, Rabinowitz D 1979 Circulating big hPRL: conversion to smaller hPRL by reduction of disulphide bonds. Journal of Clinical Endocrinology and Metabolism 48: 883–886

Bergland R M, Page R B 1979 Pituitary-brain vascular relations — a new paradigm. Science 204: 18–24

Bhattacharya A, Dierschke D I, Yamagi T, Knobil E 1972 Pharmacologic blockade of the circhoral mode of LH secretion in the ovariectomised rhesus monkey. Endocrinology 90: 778–786

Bjorklund A, Moore R Y, Nobin A, Stenevi U 1973 The organisation of tubero-hypophyseal and reticulo-infundibular catecholamine neuron systems in rat brain. Brain Research 51: 171–191

Blake C A, Norman R L, Sawyer C H 1974 Localisation of the
inhibitory actions of estrogen and nicotine on release of luteinising
hormone in rats. Neuroendocrinology 16: 22–35

Blank M S, Panerai A C, Friesen H G 1979 Opioid peptides modulate
luteinising hormone secretion during sexual maturation. Science
203: 1129–1131

Blobel G, Dobberstein B 1975 Transfer of protein across membranes. I.
Presence of proteolytically processed and unprocessed nascent
immunoglobulin light chains on membrane-bound ribosomes of
murine myeloma. Journal of Cell Biology 67: 835–851

Bourginon J-P, Hayoux C, Reuter A, Franchimont P 1979 Urinary
excretion of immunoreactive luteinising hormone releasing hormone-
like material and gonadotropins at different stages of life. Journal of
Clinical Endocrinology and Metabolism 48: 78–84

Boyar R M, Finkelstein J, Roffwarg H, Kapen S, Weitzman E,
Hellman L 1972 Synchronisation of augmented luteinising hormone
secretion with sleep during puberty. New England Journal of
Medicine 287: 582–586

Boyar R M, Finkelstein J W, Kapen S, Hellman L 1975 Twenty-four
hour prolactin secretory pattern during pregnancy. Journal of
Clinical Endocrinology and Metabolism 40: 1117–1120

Boyar R M, Hellman L D, Roffwarg H, Katz J, Zumoff B, O'Connor
J, Bradlow H L, Fukushima D K 1977 Cortisol secretion and
metabolism in anorexia nervosa. New England Journal of Medicine
296: 190–193

Boyd A E, Spencer E, Jackson I, Reichlin S 1976 Prolactin-releasing
factor (PRF) in porcine hypothalamic extract distinct from TRH.
Endocrinology 99: 861–871

Bradlow H L, Boyar R M, O'Connor J, Zumoff B, Hellman L 1976
Hypothyroid-like alterations in testosterone metabolism in anorexia
nervosa. Journal of Clinical Endocrinology and Metabolism
43: 571–574

Braund W, Roeger D C and Judd S J 1984 Synchronous secretion of
luteinising hormone and prolactin in the human luteal phase:
neuroendocrine mechanisms. Journal of Clinical Endocrinology and
Metabolism. 58: 293–298

Brawer J R, Sonnenschein C 1976 Cytopathological effects of estradiol
on the arcuate nucleus of the female rat. A possible mechanism for
pituitary tumorigenesis. American Journal of Anatomy 144: 57–88

Caron M G, Beaulieu M, Raymond V, Gagne B, Drouin J, Lefkowitz
J, Labrie F 1978 Dopaminergic receptors in the anterior pituitary
gland. Journal of Biological Chemistry 253: 2224–2253

Cattanach B M, Iddon C A, Charlton H M, Chiappa S M, Fink G 1977
Gonadotrophin-releasing hormone deficiency in a mutant mouse
with hypogonadism. Nature 269: 338–340

Cheung W Y 1980 Calmodulin plays a pivotal role in cellular
regulation. Science 207: 19–27

Cheung C Y, Weiner R I 1978 In vitro supersensitivity of the anterior
pituitary to dopamine inhibition of prolactin secretion.
Endocrinology 102: 1614–1620

Cicero T J, Schainker B A, Meyer E R 1979 Endogenous opioids
participate in the regulation of the hypothalamic-pituitary-luteinising
hormone axis and testosterone's negative feedback control of
luteinising hormone. Endocrinology 104: 1286–1291

Clarke I J, Cummins J T 1982 The temporal relationship between
gonadotropin releasing hormone (GnRH) and luteinising hormone
(LH) secretion in ovariectomised ewes. Endocrinology 111: 1737–
1739

Clayton R N, Catt K J 1980 Receptor binding affinity of gonadotropin-
releasing hormone analogues; analyses by radioligand receptor assay.
Endocrinology 106: 1154–1159

Clayton R N, Catt K J 1981 Gonadotropin-releasing hormone receptors:
characterisation, physiological regulation and relationship to
reproductive function. Endocrine Reviews 2: 180–209

Clemens J A, Roush M E, Fuller R W 1978 Evidence that serotonin
neurons stimulate secretion of prolactin releasing factor. Life
Sciences 22: 2209–2214

Coble Y D, Kohler P O, Cargille C M, Ross G T 1969 Production rates
and metabolic clearance rates of human follicle-stimulating hormone
in premenopausal and postmenopausal women. Journal of Clinical
Investigation 48: 359–363

Comite F, Cutler G B, Rivier J, Vale W W, Loriaux D L, Crowley Jr
W F 1981 Short term treatment of idiopathic precocious puberty

with a long acting analogue of luteinising hormone-releasing
hormone. New England Journal of Medicine 305: 1546–1550

Conn P M, Rogers D C, Sandham F S 1979 Alteration of the
intracellular calcium level stimulates gonadotropin release from
cultured rat anterior pituitary cells. Endocrinology 105: 1122–1127

Conn P M, Smith R G, Rogers D C 1981a Stimulation of pituitary
gonadotropin release does not require internalisation of gonadotropin
releasing hormone. Journal of Biological Chemistry 256: 1098–1100

Conn P M, Marian J, MacMillan M, Stern J, Rogers D, Hamby M,
Penna A, Grant E 1981b Gonadotropin-releasing hormone action in
the pituitary: a three step mechanism. Endocrine Reviews 2: 17–185

Coppola J A, Leonardi W, Lippman W 1966 Ovulatory failure in rats
after treatment with brain norepinephrine depletors. Endocrinology
78: 225–228

Coppola J A 1968 The apparent involvement of the sympathetic
nervous system in the gonadotrophin secretion of female rats.
Journal of Reproduction and Fertility Suppl. 4: 35–45

Corenblum B, Taylor P J 1980 A rationale for the use of bromocriptine
in patients with amenorrhoea and normoprolactinaemia. Fertility
and Sterility 34: 239–241

Costall B, Naylor R J 1981 The hypothesis of different dopamine
receptor mechanisms. Life Sciences 28: 215–229

Cramer O M, Parker C R, Porter J C 1979a Estrogen inhibition of
dopamine release into hypophysial portal blood. Endocrinology
104: 419–422

Cramer O M, Parker C R, Porter J C 1979b Secretion of dopamine into
hypophysial portal blood by rats bearing prolactin-secreting tumours
or ectopic pituitary glands. Endocrinology 105: 636–640

Craven R R, McDonald P G 1973 The effect of intrahypothalamic
infusions of dopamine and noradrenaline on ovulation in reserpine
treated rats. Journal of Endocrinology 58: 319–326

Crompton M R 1971 Hypothalamic lesions following closed head
injury. Brain 94: 165–172

Cronin M J, Roberts J M, Weiner R I 1978 Dopamine and
dihydroergocryptine binding to the anterior pituitary and other
brain areas of the rat and sheep. Endocrinology 103: 302–309

Del Pozo E, Wyss H, Toles G, Alcaniz J, Campana A, Naftolin F 1979
Prolactin and deficient luteal function. Obstetrics and Gynaecology
53: 282–286

Delitala G, Lodico G, Masala S, Alagna S, Devilla C 1977 Action of
metergoline in suppressing prolactin release induced by mechanical
breast emptying. Journal of Clinical Endocrinology and Metabolism
44: 763–765

Denef C, Andries M 1983 Evidence for paracrine interaction between
gonadotrophs and lactotrophs in pituitary cell aggregates.
Endocrinology 112: 813–823

Dierschke D J, Weiss G. Knobil E 1974 Sexual maturation in the
female rhesus monkey and the development of estrogen-induced
gonadotropic hormone release. Endocrinology 94: 198–206

Di Zerega G S, Hodgen G D 1981a Luteal phase dysfunction infertility:
a sequel to aberrant folliculogenesis. Fertility and Sterility
35: 89–499

Di Zerega G S, Hodgen G D 1981b Folliculogenesis in the primate
ovarian cycle. Endocrine Reviews 2: 27–50

Di Zerega G E, Hodgen G D 1981c Follicular phase treatment of luteal
phase dysfunction. Fertility and Sterility 35: 428–432

Donoso A O, Stefano F J E 1967 Sex hormones and concentration of
noradrenalin and dopamine in the anterior hypothalamus of
castrated rats. Experientia 23: 665–666

Donoso A O, Bishop W, Fawcett W, Krulich C P, McCann S M 1971
Effects of drugs that modify brain monoamine concentrations or
plasma gonadotrophin and prolactin levels in the rat. Endocrinology
89: 774–784

Donoso A O, Banzan A M 1980 H and H histamine receptor
antagonists and induced release of prolactin in male rats.
Neuroendocrinology 30: 11–14

Drouin J, Lagace L, Labrie F 1976 Estradiol-induced increase of the
LH responsiveness to LH releasing hormone (LHRH) in rat
anterior pituitary cells in culture. Endocrinology 99: 1477–1481

Drouva S V, Gallo R V 1977 Further evidence for inhibition of
episodic luteinising hormone release in ovariectomised rats by
stimulation of dopamine receptors. Endocrinology 100: 792–798

Drouva S V, Epelbaum S, Itery M, Tapia-Arancibia L, Laplante E,

Kordon C 1981 Ionic channels involved in the LHRH and SRIF release from rat medio basal hypothalamus. Neuroendocrinology 32: 155–162

Dufy B, Vincent J-D, Fleury H, Du Pasquier P, Gourdji D, Tixier-Vidal A 1979 Dopamine inhibition of action potentials in a prolactin secreting cell line is modulated by oestrogen. Nature 282: 855–857

Dufy B, Vincent J-D, Gourdji D, Tixier-Vidal A 1980 Electrophysiological study of prolactin-secreting pituitary cells in culture. In: L'Hermite, Judd (ed) Advances in Prolactin, pp 31–43 Karger, Basel

Eikenburg D C, Ravitz A J, Gudelsky G A, Moore K E 1977 Effects of estrogen on prolacin and tuberoinfundibular dopaminergic neurons. Journal of Neural Transmission 40: 235–244

Enjalbert A, Priam A, Kordon C 1977 Evidence in favour of the existence of a dopamine-free prolactin-inhibiting factor (PIF) in rat hypothalamic extracts. European Journal of Pharmacology 41: 243–244

Enjalbert A, Ruberg M, Aranciba S, Priam M, KordonC 1979 Endogenous opiates block dopamine inhibition of prolactin secretion in vitro. Nature 280: 595–597

Erdheim J,·Stumme E 1909 Uber die Schwangershafts veranderung der hypophyse. Beitraege zue Pathologischen Anatomie und Allgemeinen 46: 1–132

Erickson G F, Hsuch A J W, Quigley M E, Rebar R W, Yen S S C 1979 Functional studies of aromatase activity in human granulosa cells from normal and polycystic ovaries. Journal of Clinical Endocrinology and Metabolism 49: 514–519

Eskay R I., Girand P, Oliver C, Brownstein M J 1979 Distribution of α melanocyte stimulating hormone in the rat brain: evidence that αMSH-containing cells in the arcuate region send projections to extra hypothalamic regions. Brain Research 178: 55–67

Everett J 1954 Luteotrophic function of autografts of the rat hypophysis. Endocrinology 54: 685–690

Farkough N H, Packer M G, Frantz A G 1979 Large molecular size prolactin with reduced receptor activity in human serum: high proportion in basal state and reduction after thyrotropin-releasing hormone. Journal of Clinical Endocrinology and Metabolism 48: 1026–1032

Ferin M, Carmel P W, Zimmerman E A, Warren M, Perez R, Vande Wiele R L 1974 Location of intrahypothalamic estrogen responsive sites influencing LH secretion in the female rhesus monkey. Endocrinology 95: 1059–1068

Findlay A I R 1968 The effect of teat anaesthesia on the mild ejection reflex in the rabbit. Journal of Endocrinology 40: 127–128

Fine S A, Frohman L A 1978 Loss of central nervous system component of dopaminergic inhibition of prolactin secretion in patients with prolactin-secreting pituitary tumours. Journal of Clinical Investigation 61: 973–980

Fink G, Geffen L B 1978 The hypothalamus-hypophysial system: Model for central peptidergic and monoaminergic transmission. In: Porter R (ed) International Review of Physiology, Neurophysiology III, Vol III, pp 1–48. University Park Press, Baltimore

Fishman J 1973 Catechol oestrogen formation by the rat hypothalamus. Abstract 39 Endocrine Society Meeting

Fishman J 1976 The catechol estrogens. Neuroendocrinology 22: 363–374

Fishman J, Boyar R M, Hellman L 1975 Influence of body weight on estrogen metabolism in young women. Journal of Clinical Endocrinology and Metabolism 41: 989–991

Frager M S, Pieper D R, Tonetta S A, Duncan J A, Marshall J C 1981 Pituitary gonadotropin-releasing-hormone receptors effects of castration, steroid replacement, and the role of gonadotropin-releasing hormone in modulating receptors in the rat. Journal of Clinical Investigation 67: 615–623

Fraser I S, Michie E A, Wide L, Baird D T 1973 Pituitary gonadotropins and ovarian function in adolescent dysfunctional uterine bleeding. Journal of Clinical Endocrinology and Metabolism. 37: 407–414

Frawley L S, Neill J D 1981 Stimulation of prolactin secretion in rhesus monkeys by vasoactive intestinal polypeptide. Neuroendocrinology 33: 79–83

Frisch R E 1974 Critical weight at menarche, initiation of the adolescent growth spurt and control of puberty. In: Grumbach

M M, Grave G D, Mayer F E (Ed) The Control of the Onset of Puberty. John Wiley and Sons, New York

Frisch R E, McArthur J W 1974 Menstrual cycles: fatness as a determinant of minimum weight for height necessary for their maintenance or onset. Science 185: 949–951

Fuxe K, Hokfelt T, Nilsson O 1960 Factors involved in the control of the activity of the tubero-infundibular dopamine neurons during pregnancy and lactation. Neuroendocrinology 5: 257–270

Fuxe K, Hökfelt T, Nilsson O 1969 Castration, sex hormones and tubero-infundibular dopamine neurons. Neuroendocrinology 5: 107–120

Fuxe K, Ferland L, Andersson K, Eneroth P, Gustafsson J A, Skett J P 1978 On the functional role of hypothalamic catecholamine neurons in control of the secretion of hormones from the anterior pituitary, particularly the control of LH and PRL. In: Scott O E (ed) Brain-Endocrine Interaction III, pp 172–198. Karger, Basel

Gallo R V 1980 Neuroendocrine regulation of pulsatile luteinising hormone release in the rat. Neuroendocrinology 30: 122–131

Gallo R V 1981 Pulsatile LH release during the ovulatory LH surge on pro-estrus in the rat. Biology of Reproduction 24: 100–104

Gallo R V, Moberg G P 1977 Serotonin mediated inhibition of episodic luteinising hormone release during electrical stimulation of the arcuate nucleus in ovariectomised rats. Endocrinology 100: 945–954

Gallo R V, Moberg G P 1977 Serotonin mediated inhibition of episodic luteinising hormone release during electrical stimulation of the arcuate nucleus in ovariectomised rats. Endocrinology 100: 945–954

Garthwaite T L, Hagen T C 1979 Evidence that serotonin stimulates a prolactin-releasing factor in the rat. Neuroendocrinology 29: 215–220

Gaulden E C, Littlefield D C, Sutoff U E, Sievert A L 1964 Menstrual abnormalities associated with heroin addiction. American Journal of Obstetrics and Gynaecology 90: 155–160

Gautvik K M, Tashjian A H, Kourides I A, Weintraub B D, Graeber C T, Maloof F, Suzuki K. Zuckerman J E 1974 Thyrotropin-releasing hormone is not the sole physiologic mediator of prolactin release during suckling. New England Journal of Medicine 290: 112–1165

Gibbs D M, Neill J D 1978 Dopamine levels in hypophysial stalk blood are sufficient to inhibit prolactin secretion in vivo. Endocrinology 102: 1895–1900

Gibbs D M, Plotsky P M, de Greef W S, Neill J D 1979 Effect of histamine and acetylcholine on hypophysial stalk plasma dopamine and peripheral plasma prolactin levels. Life Sciences 24: 2063–2070

Glass M R, Shaw R W, Butt W R, Logan Edwards R, London D R 1975 An abnormality of oestrogen feedback in amenorrhoea — galactorrhoea. British Medical Journal ii: 274–275

Gnodde H P, Schuilling G A 1976 Involvement of catecholaminergic and cholinergic mechanisms in the pulsatile release of LH in the long-term ovariectomised rat. Neuroendocrinology 20: 212–223

Goldenberg R L, Powell R D, Rosen S W, Marshall J R, Ross G T 1976 Ovarian morphology in women with anosmia and hypogonadotropic hypogonadism. American Journal of Obstetrics and Gynaecology 126: 91–94

Goldsmith P C, Cronin M J, Rubin R J, Weiner R I 1978 Immunocytochemical staining of dopamine receptors on mammotrophs. Abstract 1098, Fifth Annual Meeting Society for Neuroscience, St Louis

Goluboff L G, Ezrin C 1969 Effect of pregnancy on the somatotroph and the prolactin cell of the human adenohypophysis. Journal of Clinical Endocrinology and Metabolism 29: 1533–1538

Goodman R L 1978 The site of positive feedback action of estradiol in the rat. Endocrinology 102: 151–159

Goodman W 1, Karsch J R 1980 Pulsatile secretion of luteinising hormone: differential suppression by ovarian steroids. Endocrinology 107: 1286–1290

Goodman R L, Knobil E 1981 The sites of action of ovarian steroids in the regulation of LH secretion. Neuroendocrinology 32: 57–63

Goodman G, Lawson D M, Gala R R 1976 The effects of neurotransmitter receptor antagonists on ether-induced prolactin release in ovariectomised oestrogen-treated rats. Proceedings of the Society for Experimental Biology and Medicine 153: 225–229

Gorski J 1981 Prolactin biosynthesis and its regulation by oestrogens. In: Jaffe R B (Ed) Prolactin, pp 57–83. Elsevier, New York

Greibrokk T, Hansen J, Knudsen R. Lam Y-K, Folkers K 1975 On the isolation of a prolactin inhibiting factor (hormone). Biochemical Biophysical Research Communications 67: 338–344

Griffiths E C, Hopper K C, Jeffcoate S L, Holland D T 1974 The presence of peptidases in the rat hypothalamus inactivating luteinising hormone releasing hormone (LHRH). Acta Endocrinologia 77: 435–442

Grossman A, Moult P J A, Gaillard R C, Delitalia G, Toff W D, Rees L H, Besser G M 1981 The opioid control of LH and FSH release: effects of a met-enkephalin analogue and naloxone. Clinical Endocrinology 14: 41–48

Grosvenor C E, Mena F, Whitworth N S 1979 Ether releases large amounts of prolactin from rat pituitaries previously 'depleted' by short term suckling. Endocrinology 105: 884–887

Grumbach M M, Roth J C, Kaplan S L, Kelch R P 1974 Hypothalamic-pituitary regulation of puberty in man: evidence and concepts derived from clinical research. In: Control of the Onset of Puberty. John Wiley, New York

Grüter F, Stricker P 1929 Über die Wirkung eines Hypophysenvorderlappenhormons und die Auslösung der Milchsekretion. Klinische Wochenschrift 8: 2322–2323

Gudelsky G A, Porter J C 1979 Morphine and opioid peptede-induced inhibition of the release of dopamine from tuberoinfundibular neurons. Life Sciences 25: 1697–1702

Gudelsky G A, Annunziato L, Moore K E 1978 Localisation of the site of the haloperidol-induced, prolactin-mediated increase of dopamine turnover in the median eminence: studies in rats with complete hypothalamic deafferentations. Journal of Neural Transmission 42: 181–192

Gudelsky G A, Nansel D D, Porter J C 1981 Role of estrogen in the dopaminergic control of prolactin secretion. Endocrinology 108: 440–444

Guillemin R, Ling N, Burgus R 1976 Endorphines, peptides, d'origine hypothalamique et neurohypophysaire a activite morphinomimetique. Isolement et structure moleculaire de 1' β-endorphine. C R Academie Science 282: 783–785

Guldner F H, Wolff J R 1973 Neurono-glial synaptoid contacts in the median eminence of the rat: ultrastructure, staining properties and distribution of tanocytes. Brain Research 61: 217–234

Halmi N S, Duello T 1976 'Acidophilic' pituitary tumours. A reappraisal with differential staining and immunocytochemical techniques. Archives Pathology and Laboratory Medicine 100: 346–351

Hamilton C R, Scully R E, Kliman B 1972 Hypogonadotropinism in Prader-Willi syndrome. American Journal of Medicine 52: 322–329

Hausler A, Wildt L, Marshall G, Plant T M, Belchetz P E, Knobil E 1979 Modulation of pituitary gonadotropin secretion by frequency of GnRH input. Federation Proceedings 38: 1107

Hazum E, Cuatrecases P, Manan J, Conn P M 1980 Receptor mediated internalisation of fluorescent gonadotropin-releasing hormone by pituitary gonadotropes. Proceedings of the National Academy of Science, USA 77: 6692–6695

Healy D L, Muller H K, Burger H G 1977 Immunofluorescence shows localisation of prolactin to human amnion. Nature 265: 642–643

Heber D, Swerdloff R S 1981 Down-regulation of pituitary gonadotropin secretion in post menopausal females by continuous gonadotropin-releasing hormone administration. Journal of Clinical Endocrinology and Metabolism 52: 171–172

Herman M L, Ben Jonathon N 1982 Dopamine receptors in the rat anterior pituitary change during the estrous cycle. Endocrinology 111: 37–41

Heitz P V 1979 Multihormonal pituitary adenomas. Hormone Research 10: 1–13

Hemmings R, Fox F, Tolis G 1982 Effect of morphine on the hypothalamic-pituitary axis in postmenopausal women. Fertility and Sterility 37: 389–391

Herman V S, Kalk W S 1980 Neurogenic Prolactin release: effects of mastectomy and thoracotomy. In: Progress in Reproductive Biology, Advances in Prolactin. Karger, Basel

Hery M, Laplante E, Kordon C 1976 Participation of serotonin in the phasic release of LH (1) Evidence from pharmacological experiments. Endocrinology 99: 496–503

Hoff J D, Lasley B L, Yen S S C 1979 The functional relationship between priming and releasing actions of luteinising hormone-releasing hormone. Journal of Clinical Endocrinology and Metabolism 49: 8–11

Hokfelt T, Elde R, Fuxe K, Johansson O, Ljungdahl A. Goldstein M, et al 1978 Aminergic and peptidergic pathways in the nervous system with special reference to the hypothalamus. In: Reichlin S, Baldessarini R J, Martin J B (ed) The Hypothalamus. Raven Press, New York

Horvath E, Kovacs k 1974 Misplaced exocytosis- distinct ultrastructural feature in some pituitary adenomas. Archives of Pathology 97: 221–224

Howie P W, McNeilly A S, McArdle T, Smart L, Houstin M 1980 The relationship between suckling-induced prolactin response and lactogenesis. Journal of Clinical Endocrinology and Metabolism 50: 670–673

Hughes J, Smith T W, Kosterlitz H W, Fothergill L A, Morgan B A, Morris H R 1975 Identification of two related pentapeptides from the brain with potent opiate agonist activity. Nature 258: 577–579

Hwang P, Guyda H, Friesen H 1971 A radioimmunoassay for human prolactin. Proceedings National Academy of Science, USA 68: 1902

Iverson L L 1978 More than one type of dopamine receptor in brain? Trends in Neuroscience November V

Jones G S 1949 Some newer aspects of the management of infertility. Journal of the American Medical Association 141: 1123–1127

Josimovich J B 1977 The role of pituitary prolactin in fetal and amniotic fluid and water and salt balance. In: Crosignani P G, Robyn C (ed) Prolactin and Human Reproduction, p 27. Academic Press, London

Josimovich J B, Merisko K, Buccella L 1977 Amniotic prolactin control over amniotic and fetal extracellular fluid water and electrolytes in the rhesus monkey. Endocrinology 100: 564–570

Judd S J 1980 Autoregulation of prolactin secretion. In: L'Hermite M, Judd S J (eds) Progress in Reproductive Biology, Advances in Prolactin, pp 87–91. Karger, Basel

Judd S J 1982 Primary hyperprolactinaemia and chronic anovulation: pathophysiology and management. Clinical Reproduction and Fertility 1: 95–116

Judd S J, Lazarus L, Smythe G 1976 Prolactin secretion by metoclopramide in man. Journal of Clinical Endocrinology and Metabolism 43: 313–317

Judd S J, Rakoff J S, Rigg L A, Yen S S C 1977 Dopamine suppression of pituitary release of LH and prolactin — effects of gonadal steroids. Endocrinology 100: 157

Judd S J, Rakoff J S, Yen S S C 1978 Inhibition of gonadotropin and prolactin release by dopamine: effect of endogenous estradiol levels. Journal of Clinical Endocrinology and Metabolism 47: 494–498

Judd S J, Rigg L A, Yen S S C 1979 The effect of ovariectomy and oestrogen treatment on the dopamine inhibition of gonadotropin and prolactin release. Journal of Clinical Endocrinology and Metabolism 49: 182–184

Kalra P S, Kalra S P, Krulich L, Fawcett C P, McCann S M 1972 Involvement of norepinephrine in transmission of the stimulatory influence of progesterone on gonadotropin release. Endocrinology 90: 1168–1176

Kalra P S, Kalra S P 1980 Modulation of hypothalamic luteinising hormone-releasing hormone levels by intracranial and subcutaneous implants of gonadal steroids in castrated rats: effects of androgen and oestrogen antagonists. Endocrinology 106: 390–397

Kamberi I A, Mical R S, Porter J C 1969 Luteinising hormone releasing activity in hypophysial stalk blood and elevation by dopamine. Science 166: 388–390

Kamberi I A, Mical R S, Porter J C 1971 Hypophysial portal vessel infusion: in vivo demonstration of LRF, FRF and PIF in pituitary stalk plasma. Endocrinology 88: 1012–1020

Kandeel F R, Butt W R, Rudd B T, Lynch S S, London D R, Logan Edwards R 1979 Oestrogen modulation of gonadotropin and prolactin release in women with anovulation and their responses to clomiphene. Clinical Endocrinology 10: 619–635

Kaplan S L, Grumbach M M, Aubert M L 1976 The ontogenesis of pituitary hormones and hypothalamic factors in the human fetus. Recent Progress in Hormone Research 32: 161–243

Karsch F J, Weick R F, Butler W R, Dierschke D J, Krey L C, Weiss G et al 1973 Induced LH surges in the rhesus monkey: strength-duration characteristics of the estrogen stimulus. Endocrinology 92: 1740–1747

Kastin A J, Kullander S, Borglin N E, Dahlberg B, Dyster-Aas K, Krakau C E T et al 1968 Extra pigmentary effects of melanocyte stimulating hormone in amenorrhoeic women. Lancet i: 1007–1010

Kato Y, Nakai Y, Imura H, Chihara K, Ohgo S 1974 Effects of 5-hydroxytryptophan (5HTP) on plasma prolactin levels in man. Journal of Clinical Endocrinology and Metabolism 38: 695–697

Katz J L, Boyar R M, Weiner H, Gorzynski G, Roffwarg H, Hellman L 1976 Towards an elucidation of the psychoendocrinology of anorexia nervosa. In: Sachar E J (ed) Hormones Behaviour and Psychopathology, pp 263–283. Raven Press, New York

Kawakami M, Yoshioka E, Konda N, Arita J, Visessuran S 1978 Data on the sites of stimulatory feedback action of gonadal steroids indispensable for luteinising hormone release in the rat. Endocrinology 102: 791–798

Keller E, Dahlen H G, Friedrich E, Bohnet H G, Richter R, Joel E W, et al 1975 Human pituitary index I Standardised LRH test criteria for evaluation of functional amenorrhoea. Journal of Clinical Endocrinology and Metabolism 40: 959–964

Kelly R B, Deutsch J W, Carlson S S, Wagner J A 1979 Biochemistry of neurotransmitter release. Annual Review of Neuroscience 2: 299–446

Keogh E J, Dunn A, Mallal S, Somerville C, McColm S, Marshall T, et al 1982a Induction of spermatogenesis by pulsatile administration of GnRH. Abstract 37 25th Annual Meeting Endocrine Society of Australia

Keogh T, Somerville C, Lawson-Smith C, MacKillar A, Mallal S, Marshall T, Altikouzel J 1982b Treatment of cryptorchidism with pulsatile gonadotrophin releasing hormone (GnRH). Abstract 38 25th Annual Meeting of the Endocrine Society of Australia

Khar A, Kunnert-Radek J, Jutisz M 1979 Involvement of the microtubule and microfilament system in the GnRH induced release of gonadotropin by rat pituitary cells in culture. FEBS Letters 104: 410–414

Kizer J S, Arimura A, Schally A V, Brownstein M J 1975 Absence of luteinising hormone-releasing hormone (LH–RH) from catecholaminergic neurons. Endocrinology 96: 523–525

Knobil E 1981 Patterns of hypophysiotropic signals and gonadotropin secretion in the rhesus monkey. Biology of Reproduction 24: 44–49

Kobayashi H, Matsui T, Ishii S 1970 Functional electron microscopy of the hypothalamic median eminence. International Review of Cytology 29: 281 381

Koch Y, Baram T, Chobsieng P 1974 Enzyme degradation of luteinising hormone releasing hormone (LHRH) by hypothalamic tissue. Biochemical and Biophysical Research Communications 61: 95–103

Koenig J I, Mayfield M A, McCann S M, Krulich L 1979 Stimulation of prolactin secretion by morphine: role of the central serotonergic system. Life Sciences 25: 853–864

Kovacs K, Ryan N, Horvath E, Ezrin C, Penz G 1978 Prolactin cell adenomas of the human pituitary. Morphologic features of prolactin cells in nontumorous portions of the anterior lobe. Hormone and Metabolic Research 10: 409–412

Krestin D 1932 Spontaneous lactation associated with enlargement of the pituitary. Lancet i: 928–932

Krey L C, Butler W R, Knobil E 1975 Surgical disconnection of the medial basal hypothalamus and pituitary function in the rhesus monkey. I Gonadotropin secretion Endocrinology 96: 1073–1087

Krisch B 1978 The distribution of LHRH in the hypothalamus of the thirsty rat. A light and electron microscopic immunocytochemical study. Cell and Tissue Research 186: 135–148

Krulich L, Vijayan E, Cappings R J, Giachetti A, McCann J M, Mayfield M A 1979 On the role of the central serotoninergic system in the regulation of the secretion of thyrotropin and prolactin: thyrotropin-inhibiting and prolactin releasing effects of 5 hydroxytryptamine and quipazine in the male rat. Endocrinology 105: 276–283

Labrie F, Beaulieu M, Caron M C, Raymond V 1978 The adenohypophysial dopamine receptor: specificity and modulation of its activity by estradiol. In: Robyn C, Harter M (eds) Progress in Prolactin Physiology and Pathology, pp 121–136. Elsevier, North Holland.

Lachelin G C L, Yen S S C 1978 Hypothalamic chronic anovulation. American Journal of Obstetrics and Gynaecology 130: 825–831

Lakoski J M, Gebhart G F 1981 Attenuation of morphine's depression of serum luteinising hormone by lesions in the amygdala. Neuroendocrinology 33: 105–111

Lal H, Brown W, Drawbaugh R, Hynes M, Brown G 1977 Enhanced Prolactin Inhibition following chronic treatment with haloperidol and morphine. Life Science 20: 101–106

Lambert A E 1976 The regulation of insulin secretion. Review of Physiology, Biochemistry and Pharmacology 75: 97–115

Larsen S 1981 Responses of luteinising hormone, follicle stimulating hormone and prolactin to prolonged administration of a dopamine antagonist in normal women and women with low-weight amenorrhoea. Fertility and Sterility 35: 642–646

Lawson D M, Gala R R 1975 The influence of adrenergic, dopaminergic, cholinergic and serotonergic drugs on plasma prolactin levels in ovariectomised, estrogen treated rats. Endocrinology 96: 313–318

Leontic E A, Tyson J E 1977 Prolactin and fetal osmoregulation: water transport across isolated human amnion. American Journal of Physiology 232: 124–127

Levine J E, Ramirez V D 1980 In vivo release of luteinising hormone releasing hormone estimated with push-pull cannulae from the medio-basal hypothalami of overiectomised steroid primed rats. Endocrinology 107: 1782–1790

Leyendecker G, Struve T, Plotz E J 1980 Induction of ovulation with chronic intermittent (pulsatile) administration of LHRH in women with hypothalamic and hypoprolactinaemic amenorrhoea. Archives of Gynaecology 229: 177–190

Libertun C, McCann S M 1976 The possible role of histamine in the control of prolactin and gonadotropin release. Neuroendocrinology 20: 110–120

Libertun C, Larrea G A, Vacas M I, Cardinali D P 1980 [³H] Dihydroergocryptine binding in anterior pituitary and prolactin secretion: further evidence of brain regulation of adenohypophyseal receptors. Endocrinology 107: 1905–1909

Lloyd H M, Meares J D, Jacobi J 1975 Effects of oestrogen and bromocriptine on in vivo secretion and mitosis in prolactin cells. Nature (London) 255: 497–498

Locatelli V, Cocchi D, Frigerio C, Betti R, Krogsgaard-Larsen P, Racagni G, Muller E 1979 Dual γ amino butyric acid control of prolactin secretion in the rat. Endocrinology 105: 778–785

Löfström A 1977 Catecholamine turnover alterations in discrete areas of the median eminence in the 4 and 5 day cyclic rat. Brain Research 120: 113–131

Löfström A, Jonsson G, Fuxe K 1976 Microfluorimetric quantitation of catecholamine fluorescence in rat median eminence. I Aspects on the distribution of dopamine and noradrenaline nerve terminals. Journal of Histochemistry and Cytochemistry 24: 415–429

Löfström A, Eneroth P, Gustafsson J A, Skett P 1977 Effects of estradiol benzoate on catecholamine levels and turnover in discrete areas of the median eminence and the limbic forebrain and on plasma LH, FSH and prolactin concentrations in the ovariectomised female rat. Endocrinology 101: 1559–1569

Lu K H, Amenomori Y, Chen C L, Meites J 1970 Effects of central acting drugs on serum and pituitary prolactin levels in rats. Endocrinology 87: 667–672

Lu K H, Meites J 1972 Effects of L dopa on serum prolactin and PIF in intact and hypophysectomised pituitary-grafted rats. Endocrinology 91: 868–972

Malarkey W B, Groshong J C, Milo G E 1977 Defective dopaminergic regulation of prolactin secretion in a rat pituitary tumour cell line. Nature 266: 640–641

Marcano De Cotte D, De Menezes C E, Bennett G W, Edwardson J A 1980 Dopamine stimulates the degradation of gonadotropin releasing hormone by rat synaptosomes. Nature 283: 487

Marshall J C, Kelch R P 1979 Low dose pulsatile gonadotropin-releasing hormone in anorexia nervosa: a model of human pubertal development. Journal of Clinical Endocrinology and Metabolism 49: 712–718

Maurer R A 1979 Estrogen-induced prolactin and DNA synthesis in immature female rat pituitaries. Molecular and Cellular Endocrinology 13: 291–300

Maurer R A, McKean D J 1978 Synthesis of preprolactin and conversion to prolactin in intact cells and a cell free system. Journal of Biological Chemistry 253: 6315–6318

Means A R, Dedman J R 1980 Calmodulin: an intracellular calcium receptor. Nature 285: 73–77

Meites J, Bruni J R, Van Vugt D A, Smith A F 1979 Relation of endogenous opioid peptides and morphine to neuroendocrine functions. Life Sciences 24: 1325–1336

Meltzer H Y, Fang V S, Paul B M, Kalusker R 1976 Effect of quipazine on rat plasma prolactin levels. Life Sciences 19: 1073–1078

Mena F, Enjalbert A, Carbonell L, Priam M, Kordon C 1976 Effect of suckling on plasma prolactin and hypothalamic monoamine levels in the rat. Endocrinology 99: 445–451

Mena F, Grosvenor C E 1980 New concepts concerning the release of prolactin induced by suckling. In: Cumming I A, Funder J W, Mendelsohn F A O (eds) Endocrinology, 1980, pp 194–198. Australian Academy of Science, Canberra.

Mendelson W B, Jacobs L S, Reichman J D, Othner E, Cryer P E, Trivedi B, Daughaday W H 1975 Methysergide suppression of sleep-related prolactin secretion and enhancement of sleep-related growth hormone secretion. Journal of Clinical Investigation 57: 690–697

Miyachi Y, Mecklenberg R S, Lipsett M B 1973 In vitro studies of pituitary-median eminence unit. Endocrinology 93: 492–503

Miyabo S, Asato T, Mizushima N 1977 Prolactin and growth hormone responses to psychological stress in normal and neurotic subjects. Journal of Clinical Endocrinology and Metabolism 44: 947–951

Moshang T, Parks J S, Baker L, Vaidya V, Utiger R D, Bongiovanni A M, Snyder P J 1975 Low serum triiodothyronine in patients with anorexia nervosa. Journal of Clinical Endocrinology and Metabolism 40: 470–473

Moult P J A, Rees L H, Besser G M 1982 Pulsatile gonadotropin secretion in hyperprolactinaemic amenorrhoea and the response to bromocriptine therapy. Clinical Endocrinology 16: 153–162

Mueller G P, Simpkins J, Meites J, Moore K J 1976 Differential effects of dopamine agonists and haloperidol on release of prolactin, thyroid stimulating hormone, growth hormone and luteinising hormone in rats. Neuroendocrinology 20: 121–135

Mulder A H, Snyder S 1976 Putative central neurotransmitters. In: Gispen W H (ed) Molecular and Functional Neurobiology, pp 161–191. Elsevier Scientific, Amsterdam

McCann S, Ramirez V 1964 The neuroendocrine regulation of luteinising hormone releasing hormone secretion. Recent Progress in Hormone Research 20: 131–181

McKean D J, Maurer R A 1978 Complete amino-acid sequence of the precursor region of rat prolactin. Biochemistry 17: 5215–5219

MacLeod R M 1969 Influence of norepinephrine and catecholamine-depleting agents on the synthesis and release of prolactin and growth hormone. Endocrinology 85: 916–923

MacLeod R M, Fontham E H, Lehmeyer J E 1970 Prolactin and growth hormone production as influenced by catecholamines and agents that affect brain catecholamines. Neuroendocrinology 6: 283–294

Nagy I, Valdenegro C A, Login I S, Snyder F A, MacLeod R M 1979 Oestradiol and anti-estrogens in pituitary hormone production, metabolism and pituitary toumour growth. In: Jacobelli (ed) 1st International Congress on Hormones and Cancer, Rome. Raven Press, New York

Nakai Y, Plant T M, Hess D L, Keogh E J, Knobil E 1978 On the sites of the negative and positive feedback actions of estradiol in the control of gonadotropin secretion in the rhesus monkey. Endocrinology 102: 1008–1014

Nansel D D, Gudelsky G A, Porter J C 1979 Subcellular localisation of dopamine in the anterior pituitary gland of the rat: apparent association of dopamine with prolactin secretory granules. Endocrinology 105: 1073–1077

Nansel D D, Gudelsky G A, Raymond M J, Neaves W B, Porter J C 1981 A possible role for lysosomes in the inhibitory action of dopamine on prolactin release. Endocrinology 108: 896–902

Naor Z, Atlas D, Clayton R N, Forman D S, Amsterdam A, Catt K J 1981 Fluorescent derivative of gonadotropin-releasing hormone:

visualisation of hormone-receptor interaction in cultured pituitary cells. Journal of Biological Chemistry 256: 3049–3052

Neill J D, Patton J M, Dailey R A, Tsou R C, Tindall G T 1977 Luteinising hormone releasing hormone (LHRH) in pituitary stalk blood of rhesus monkeys. Relationship to level of LH release. Endocrinology 101: 430–434

Nicholl C S 1974 Physiological actions of prolactin. In: Knobil E, Sawyer W H (ed) Handbook of Physiology Section F, Vol IV, Part 2, pp 253–292. American Physiological Society, Bethesda

Noel G L, Suh H K, Stone G J, Frantz A G 1972 Human prolactin and growth hormone release during surgery and other conditions of stress. Journal of Clinical Endocrinology and Metabolism 35: 840–851

Noel G L, Suh H K, Frantz A G 1974 Prolactin release during nursing and breast stimulation in postpartum and non-postpartum subjects. Journal of Clinical Endocrinology and Metabolism 38: 413–420

Noel G L, Dimond R C, Earll J M et al 1976 Prolactin, thyrotropin and growth hormone release during stress associated with parachute jumping. Aviation and Space Environmental Medicine 47: 534–537

Ojeda S R, McCann S M 1978 Control of LH and FSH release by LHRH: Influence of putative neurotransmitters. Clinics in Obstetrics and Gynaecology 5: 283–303

Ondo J G 1974 Gamma-aminobutyric acid effects on pituitary gonadotropin secretion. Science 186: 738–739

Ondo S R, Mical R, Porter R J 1972 Passage of radioactive substances from CSF to hypophysial portal blood. Endocrinology 91: 1239–1246

Palkovits M, Brownstein M, Saavedra J M 1974 Serotonin content of the brain stem nuclei in the rat. Brain Research 80: 237–249

Pang C N, Zimmerman E, Sawyer C H 1977 Morphine inhibition of the preovulatory surges of plasma luteinising hormone and follicle stimulating hormone in the rat. Endocrinology 101: 1726–1732

Parker D C, Rossman L G, Vanderlaan E F 1974 Relation of sleep-entrained human prolactin release to REM-non REM cycles. Journal of Clinical Endocrinology and Metabolism 38: 646–651

Pass K A, Ondo J G 1977 The effects of γ aminobutyric acid on prolactin and gonadotropin secretion in the unanaesthetised rat. Endocrinology 100: 1437–1442

Pasteels J L 1963 Recherches morphologiques et experimentales sur la secretion de prolactine. Archives de Biologie 74: 439–553

Pasteels J L, Gausset P. Danguy A, Ectors F, Nicoll C S, Varavudha P 1972 Morphology of the lactotropes and somatotropes of man and rhesus monkeys. Journal of Clinical Endocrinology and Metabolism 34: 959–967

Perkins N A, Westfall T C 1978 The effect of prolactin on dopamine release from rat striatum and medial basal hypothalamus. Neuroscience 3: 59–63

Perkins N A, Westfall T C, Paul C V, MacLeod R, Rogol A D 1979 Effect of prolactin on dopamine synthesis in medial basal hypothalamus: evidence for a short loop feedback. Brain Research 160: 431

Peters H, Byskov A G, Grinsted J 1978 Follicular growth in fetal and prepubertal ovaries in humans and other primates. Clinics in Endocrinology and Metabolism 7: 469–485

Peters L H, Hoeffer M T, Ben-Jonathon N 1981 The posterior pituitary: regulation of anterior pituitary prolactin secretion. 1. Science 213: 659–661

Pfaff D W, Keiner M 1973 Atlas of oestradiol-concentrating cells in the central nervous system of the female rat. Journal of Comparative Neurology 151: 121–158

Phifer R G, Midgley A R, Spicer S S 1973 Immunohistologic and histologic evidence that follicle stimulating hormone and luteinising hormone are present in the same cell type in the human pars distalis. Journal of Clinical Endocrinology and Metabolism 36: 125–141

Pickering A J M C, Fink G 1976 Priming effect of luteinising hormone releasing factor: in vivo and in vitro evidence consistent with its dependence upon protein and RNA synthesis. Journal of Endocrinology 69: 373–379

Pickering A J M C, Fink G 1977 A priming effect of luteinising hormone releasing factor with respect to release of follicle-stimulating hormone in vitro and in vivo. Journal of Endocrinology 75: 155–159

Plant T M, Moossy J, Hess D L, Nakai Y, McCormack J T, Knobil 1978 The arcuate nucleus and the control of gonadotropin and prolactin secretion in the female rhesus monkey (Macaca mulatta). Endocrinology 102: 52–62

Plotsky P M, Neill J D 1982 The decrease in hypothalamic dopamine secretion induced by suckling: comparison of voltametric and radioisotopic methods of measurement. Endocrinology 110: 691–696

Pontiroli A E, Pozza G 1978 Histamine stimulates prolactin release in normal men. Acta Endocrinologica 88: 23–28

Porter J C, Mical R S, Cramer O M 1972 Effect of serotonin and other indoles on the release of LH, FSH and Prolactin. Gynaecological Investigation 2: 13–22

Porter J C, Barnes A, Cramer O M, Parker C R 1978 Hypothalamic peptide and catecholamine secretion: roles for portal and retrograde blood flow in the pituitary stalk in the release of hypothalamic dopamine and pituitary prolactin and LH. Clinics in Obstetrics and Gynaecology 5: 271–282

Quijada M, Illner P, Krulich L, McCann S M 1973 The effect of catecholamines on hormone release from anterior pituitaries and ventral hypothalami incubated in vitro. Neuroendocrinology 13: 151–163

Quigley M E, Judd S J, Gilliland G B, Yen S S C 1979 Effect of a dopamine antagonist on the release of gonadotropin and prolactin in normal women and women with hyperprolactinaemic anovulation. Journal of Clinical Endocrinology and Metabolism 48: 718–720

Quigley M E, Sheehan K L, Casper R R, Yen S S C 1980a Evidence for an increased opioid inhibition of luteinising hormone secretion in hyperprolactinaemic patients with pituitary microadenoma. Journal of Clinical Endocrinology and Metabolism 50: 427–430

Quigley M E, Judd S J, Gilliland G B, Yen S S C 1980b Functional studies of dopamine control of prolactin secretion in normal women and women with hyperprolactinaemia pituitary microadenomas. of Clinical Endocrinology and Metabolism 50: 994–998

Quigley M E, Sheehan K L, Casper R F, Yen S S C 1980c Evidence for increased dopaminergic and opioid activity in patients with hypothalamic hypogonadotropic amenorrhoea. Journal of Endocrinology and Metabolism 50: 949–954

Quigley M E, Rakoff J S, Yen S S C 1981a Increased luteinising hormone sensitivity to dopamine inhibition in polycystic ovary syndrome. Journal of Clinical Endocrinology and Metabolism 52: 231–234

Quigley M E, Robert J F, Yen S S C 1981b Acute prolactin release triggered by feeding. Journal of Clinical Endocrinology and Metabolism 52: 1043–1045

Quigley M E, Yen S S C 1981 The role of endogenous opiates on LH secretion during the menstrual cycle. Journal of Clinical Endocrinology and Metabolism 51: 179–181

Raiti S, Foley T P, Penny R 1975 Measurement of the production rate of human luteinising hormone using the urinary excretion technique. Metabolism 24: 937–941

Rakoff J S, Rigg L A, Yen S S C 1978 The impairment of progesterone-induced pituitary release of prolactin and gonadotropin in patients with hypothalamic chronic anovulation. American Journal of Obstetrics and Gynaecology 130: 807–812

Ramsdell J S, Monnet F, Weiner R I 1982 Dopamine receptors on dispersed bovine anterior pituitary cells. Abstract 856 64th Annual Meeting of the Endocrine Society, San Francisco

Ramirez V D, Abrams R M, McCann S M 1964 Effect of estradiol implants in the hypothalamo-hypophysial region of the rat on the secretion of luteinising hormone. Endocrinology 75: 243–248

Rasmussen H, Goodman D B P 1977 Relationships between calcium and cyclic nucleotides in cell activation. Pharmacological Review 57: 421–509

Rebar R, Judd H L, Yen S S C, Rakoff J, Vanden Berg G, Naftolin F 1976 Characterisation of the inappropriate gonadotropin secretion in polycystic ovary syndrome. Journal of Clinical Investigation 57: 1320–1329

Reid R L, Ling N, Yen S S C 1981 Melanocyte stimulating hormone induces gonadotropin release. Journal of Clinical Endocrinology and Metabolism 52: 159–161

Reiter E O, Kulin H E, Hamwood S M 1974 The absence of positive feedback between estrogen and luteinising hormone in sexually immature girls. Paediatric Research 8: 740–745

Riddle O, Bates R W, Dykshorn S W 1932 A new hormone of the anterior pituitary. Proceedings of the Society for Experimental Biology and Medicine 29: 1211–1215

Riese W 1928 Milchsekretion and zwischenhirn. Klinisch Wochenschrift 41: 1954–1955

Rigg L A, Yen S S C 1977 Multiphasic prolactin secretion during partuition in human subjects. American Journal of Obstetrics and Gynaecology 128: 215–217

Robert F, Hardy J 1975 Prolactin-secreting adenomas. Archives of Pathology 99: 625–633

Robinson J E, Short R V 1977 Changes in breast sensitivity at puberty, during the menstrual cycle and at partuition. British Medical Journal i: 1188–1191

Ropert J F, Quigley M E, Yen S S C 1981 Endogenous opiates modulate pulsatile luteinising hormone release in humans. Journal of Clinical Endocrinology and Metabolism 52: 583–585

Rosenfield R L 1977 Hormonal events and disorders of puberty. In: Gynaecologic Endocrinology Year Book, Year Book Medical Publishers

Rosenfield R L 1982 The ovary and female sexual maturation. In: Kaplan S A (ed) Clinical Paediatric Adolescent Endocrinology, pp 217–268, W B, Saunders, Philadelphia

Rosenfield R L, Fang V S 1974 The effects of prolonged physiologic estradiol therapy on the maturation of hypogonadal teenagers. Journal of Paediatrics 85: 830–837

Ruberg M, Rotsztejn W H, Arancibia S, Besson J, Enjalbert A 1978 Stimulation of prolactin release by vasoactive intestinal peptide (VIP). European Journal of Pharmacology 51: 319–320

Rudenstein R S, Bidgcli II, McDonald M H, Snyder P J 1979 Administration of gonadal steroids to the castrated male rat prevents a decrease in the release of gonadotropin releasing hormone from the incubated hypothalamus. Journal of Clinical Investigation 63: 262–267

Runnebaum B, Heep J, Geiger W, Vecsei P, Andor J 1976 Effect of α MSH on plasma levels of LH, FSH, progesterone and cortisol during the corpus luteum phase of the menstrual cycle. Acta Endocrinologia 81: 243–251

Said S I, Porter S C 1979 Vasoactive intestinal polypeptide release into hypophysial portal blood. Life Sciences 24: 227–230

Sachs H, Fawcett P, Takabatake Y, Portanova R 1969 Biosynthesis and release of vasopressin and neurophysin. Recent Progress in Hormone Research 25: 447–491

Santen R J, Bardin C W 1973 Episodic luteinising hormone secretion in man. Pulse analysis, clinical interpretation, physiologic mechanisms. Journal of Clinical Investigation 52: 2617–2628

Santen R J, Friend J N, Trojanowski D, Davis B, Samojlik E, Bardin C W 1978 Prolonged negative feedback suppression after estradiol administration. Proposed mechanism of eugonadal secondary amenorrhoea. Journal of Clinical Endocrinology and Metabolism 47: 1220–1229

Sarne Y, Azov R, Weissman B A 1978 A stable enkephalin-like immunoreactive substance in human CSF. Brain Research 151: 339–403

Sarne Y, Keren O, Dalith M, Weissman B A 1980 Heterogeneity of endogenous opiates: H-endorphin is not correlated with enkelaphin or with β endorphin. Life Sciencer 27: 2167–2173

Sawyer C H, Hilliard J, Kanematsu S, Scaramuzzi R, Blake C A 1974 Effects of intraventricular infusions of norepinephrine and dopamine on LH release and ovulation in the rabbit. Neuroendocrinology 15: 328–337

Scanlon M F, Rodriguez-Arnao M D, McGregor A M, Weightman D, Lewis M, Cook D B, et al 1980 Altered dopaminergic regulation of thyrotropin release in patients with prolactinomas: comparison with other tests of hypothalamic-pituitary function. Clinical Endocrinology 14: 133–143

Schally A V, Kasten A J, Arimura A 1971 Hypothalamic follicle-stimulating hormone (FSH) and luteinising hormone (LH) — regulating hormone: structure, physiology and clinical studies. Fertility and Sterility 22: 703–721

Schally A V, Redding T W, Arimura A, Dupont A, Linthicum G L 1977 Isolation of gamma-amino butyric acid from pig hypothalami and demonstration of its prolactin release-inhibiting (PIF) activity in vivo and in vitro. Endocrinology 100: 681–691

Schinfield J S, Tulchinsky D, Schiff I, Fishman J 1980 Suppression of prolactin and gonadotropin secretion in post menopausal women by 2 hydroxyestrone. Journal of Clinical Endocrinology and Metabolism 50: 408–410

Schneider H P G, McCann S M 1969 Possible role of dopamine as transmitter to promote discharge of LH-releasing factor. Endocrinology 85: 121–132

Scott D E, Dudley G K, Knigge K M, Koztowski G P 1974 In vitro analysis of the cellular localisation of luteinising hormone-releasing factor (LRF) in the basal hypothalamus of the rat. Cell and Tissue Research 149: 371–378

Selmanoff M K, Pramik-Holdaway M J, Weiner R I 1976 Concentrations of dopamine and norepinephrine in discrete hypothalamic nuclei during the rat estrous cycle. Endocrinology 99: 326–329

Seppala M, Hirvonen E, Ranta T 1976 Bromocriptine treatment of secondary amenorrhoea. Lancet i: 1154–1156

Shaar C J, Clemens J A 1974 The role of catecholamines in the release of anterior pituitary prolactin in vitro. Endocrinology 95: 1202–1212

Shaw R A, Duignan N M, Butt W R, Logan Edwards R, London D R 1975 Hypothalamic-pituitary relationships in the polycystic ovary syndrome. Serum gonadotropin levels following injection of oestradiol benzoate. British Journal of Obstetrics and Gynaecology 82: 952–957

Sherwood N M, Fink G 1980 Effect of ovariectomy and adrenalectomy on luteinising hormone-releasing hormone in pituitary stalk blood from female rats. Endocrinology 106: 363–367

Shimatsu A, Kato Y, Matsushita N, Katakami H, Yanaihara N 1982 Stimulation by serotonin of vasoactive intestinal polypeptide release into rat hypophysial portal blood. Abstract 13 64th Annual Meeting Endocrine Society, San Francisco

Shin S H 1979a Pulsatile secretion of prolactin in the male rat after pimozide administration is not due to pulsatile inhibition of PIF secretion. Life Sciences 24: 1751–1756

Shin S H 1979b Prolactin secretion in acute stress is controlled by prolactin releasing factor. Life Sciences 25: 1829–1836

Snyder G, Mukherjee A, McCann S M 1980 Properties of muscarine receptors on intact anterior pituitary cells. Federation Proceedings 39: 488

Spampinato S, Locatelle V, Cocchi D, Vincentini L, Bajusz S, Ferri S, Muller E E 1979 Involvement of brain serotonin in the prolactin-releasing effect of opioid peptides. Endocrinology 105: 163–170

Sparkes R S, Simpson R W, Paulsen C A 1968 Familial hypogonadism with anosmia. Archives of Internal Medicine 121: 534–538

Steele R E, Weisz J 1974 Changes in sensitivity of the estradiol-LH feedback system with puberty in the female rat. Endocrinology 95: 513–520

Steinberger E 1978 Disorders of testicular function (male hypogonadism). In: De Groot L J (ed) Endocrinology, Ch 124, pp 1549–1565. Grune and Stratton, New York.

Stouffer R L, Hodgen G D 1980 Induction of luteal phase defects in rhesus monkeys by follicular fluid administration at the onset of the menstrual cycle. Journal of Clinical Endocrinology and Metabolism 51: 669–671

Strott C A, Cargilli C M, Ross G T, Lipsett M B 1970 The short luteal phase. Journal of Clinical Endocrinology and Metabolism 30: 246–251

Stubbs W A, Jones A, Edwards C R W, Delitalia G, Jeffcoate W S, Ralter S J, et al 1978 Hormonal and metabolic responses to an enkephalin analogue in normal man. Lancet ii: 1225–1227

Suh H K, Frantz A G 1974 Size heterogeneity of human prolactin in plasma and pituitary extracts. Journal of Clinical Endocrinology and Metabolism 39: 928–935

Swift A D, Crighton D B 1979 Relative activity, plasma elimination and tissue degradation of synthetic luteinising hormone releasing hormone and certain of its analogues. Journal of Endocrinology 80: 141–152

Sylvester P W, Van Vugt D A, Aylsworth C A, Hanson E A, Meites J 1982 Effects of morphine and naloxone on inhibition by ovarian hormones of pulsatile release of LH in ovariectomised rats. Neuroendocrinology 34: 269–273

Takahara J, Arimura A, Schally A J 1974 Suppression of prolactin release by a purified porcine PIF preparation and catecholamines infused into rat hypophysial portal vessels. Endocrinology 95: 462–465

Tang L K L, Spies H G 1975 Effects of gonadal steroids on the basal and LRF-induced gonadotropin secretion by cultures of rat pituitary. Endocrinology 96: 349–356

Taraskevitch P S, Douglas W W 1977 Action potentials occur in cells of the normal anterior pituitary gland and are stimulated by the hypophysiotropic peptide thyrotropin releasing hormone. Proceedings of the National Academy of Sciences, U.S.A. 74: 4064–4067

Tashjian A, Barowsky N, Jensen D 1971 Thyrotropin releasing hormone: Direct evidence for stimulation of prolactin production by pituitary cells on culture. Biochemical and Biophysical Research Communications 43: 516–523

Tate A C, Swift A O 1981 The effects of sex steroids on the degradation of LRH by hypothalamic homogenates. Acta Endocrinologica 98: 321–325

Thorner M O, MacLeod R M 1980 The lactotrope — regulation of its activity. In: L'Hermite, Judd (ed) Advances in Prolactin, pp 1–23 Karger, Basel

Tindall J S, Knaggs G S 1977 Pathways in the forebrain of the rat concerned with the release of prolactin. Brain Research 119: 211–221

Tyson J E, Friesen H G, Anderson M S 1972 Human lactational and ovarian respose to endogenous prolactin release. Science 177: 897–900

Uemura H, Kobayashi H 1971 Effects of dopamine implanted in the median eminence on the estrous cycle of the rat. Endocrinology Japonica 18: 91–100

Vaitukaites J, Becker R, Hansen J, Mecklenburg R 1974 Altered LRF responsiveness in amenorrhoeic women. Journal of Clinical Endocrinology and Metabolism 39: 1005–1011

Valverde R C, Chieffo V, Reichlin S 1973 Failure of reserpine to block ether induced release of prolactin: physiological evidence that stress induced prolactin release is not caused by acute inhibition of PIF secretion. Life Sciences 12: 327–335

Van Cauter E, Desir D, Refetoff S, Spire J -P, Noel P, L'Hermite M, et al 1982 The relationship etween episodic variations of plasma prolactin and REM — non REM cyclicity is an artifact. Journal of Clinical Endocrinology and Metabolism 54: 70–76

Vande Wiele R L, Bogumil J, Dyenfurth I, Ferin M, Jewelewicz R, Warren M, et al 1970 Mechanisms regulating the menstrual cycle in women. Recent Progress in Hormone Research 26: 63–87

Van Hall E V, Mastboom J L 1969 Luteal phase insufficiency in patients treated with clomiphene. American Journal of Obstetrics and Gynaecology 103: 165–171

Van Look P F A 1976 Failure of positive feedback. Clinics in Obstetrics and Gynaecology 3: 555–578

Van Loon G R 1978 A defect in catecholamine neurons in patients with prolactin secreting adenomas. Lancet ii: 868–869

Van Loon G R, Ho D, Kim C 1980 β endorphin-induced decrease in hypothalamic dopamine turnover. Endocrinology 106: 76–80

Van Vugt D A, Meites J 1980 Influence of endogenous opiates on anterior pituitary function. Federation Proceedings 39: 2533–2538

Van Vugt D A, Sylvester P W, Aylsworth C F, Meites J 1982 Counteraction of gonadal steroid inhibition of luteinising hormone release by naloxone. Neuroendocrinology 34: 274–278

Vekemans M, Delvoyi P, L'Hermite M, Robyn C 1977 Serum prolactin levels during the menstrual cycle. Journal of Clinical Endocrinology and Metabolism 44: 989–993

Vician L, Shupnik M A, Gorski J 1979 Effects of estrogen on primary ovine pituitary cell cultures: stimulation of prolactin secretion, synthesis and preparation messenger ribonucleic acid activity. Endocrinology 104: 736–743

Voogt J L, Meites J 1973 Suppression of proestrus and suckling-induced increase in serum prolactin by hypothalamic implant of prolactin. Proceedings of the Society for Experimental Biology and Medicine 142: 1056–1058

Wang W -K, Jeng L S, Chiang Y, Chien N K 1982 Inhibition of dopamine biosynthesis by gonadotropin-releasing hormone in the rat. Nature 296: 354

Warren M P 1980 The effects of exercise on pubertal progression and reproductive function in girls. Journal of Clinical Endocrinology and Metabolism 51: 1150–1157

Watson S J, Akil H 1980 α MSH in rat brain: occurrence within and outside of β endorphin neurons. Brain Research 182: 217–223

Weick R F 1981 Induction of luteinising hormone surge by intrahypothalamic application of estrogen in the rhesus monkey. Biology of Reproduction 24: 415–422

Weiner R I, Bethea C L 1981 Hypothalamic control of prolactin secretion. In: Jaffe R B (ed) Prolactin, pp 19–43. Elsevier, North Holland

Whitaker M D, Corenblum B, Taylor P J, Harasym P H 1980 Control of the hypoglycemic release of prolactin. In: L'Hermite M, Judd S J (ed) Advances in Prolactin, pp 77–82. Karger, Basel

Whittaker P G, Wilcox T, Lend T 1981 Maintained fertility in a patient with hyperprolactinaemia due to big, big prolactin. Journal of Clinical Endocrinology and Metabolism 53: 863–866

Wilkes M M, Yen S S C 1981 Augmentation by naloxone of efflux of LRF from superfused medial basal hypothalamus. Life Sciences 28: 2355–2359

Wilkinson M, Bhanot R 1982 A puberty-related attenuation of opiate peptide-induced inhibition of LH secretion. Endocrinology 110: 1046–1048

Willoughby J O 1980 Prolactin: questions without answers. In: L'Hermite, Judd (ed) Advances in Prolactin, pp 142–165. Karger, Basel

Winter J S D, Hughes I A, Reyes F I, Faiman C 1976 Pituitary gonadal relations in infancy. 2. Patterns of serum gonadal steroid concentrations in man from birth to two years of age. Journal of Clinical Endocrinology and Metabolism 42: 679–686

Wuttke W, Hancke J L, Hohn K G, Baumgarten H G 1978 Effect of intraventricular injection of 5, dihydroxytryptamine on serum gonadotropins and prolactin. Annals of New York Academy of Science 305: 423–436

Yen S S C 1978 The human menstrual cycle. In: Yen S S C, Jaffe R B (ed) Reproductive endocrinology. Physiology, pathophysiology and management, pp 126–151. W B Saunders, Philadelphia

Yen S S C, Vela P, Rankin J 1970 Inappropriate secretion of follicle-stimulating hormone and luteinising hormone in polycystic ovarian disease. Journal of Clinical Endocrinology and Metabolism 30: 435–442

Yen S S C, Ehara Y, Siler T 1974a Augmentation of prolactin secretion by estogen in hypogonadal women. Journal of Clinical Investigation 53: 652–655

Yen S S C, Vandenberg G, Tsai C C, Parker D C 1974b Ultradian fluctuations of gonadotropins. In Ferin M et al (ed) Biorhythms and Human Reproduction, pp 203–219. John Wiley and Sons, New York

Yen S S C, Chaney C, Judd H L 1976 Functional aberrations of the hypothalamic-pituitary system in polycystic ovarian syndrome. A consideration of the pathogenesis. In: James V H T, Serio M, Guisti G (ed) The endocrine function of the human ovary, pp 373–385. Academic Press, New York

Zimmerman E A, Hsu K C, Ferin M, Kozlowski G P 1974a Localisation of gonadotropin releasing hormone (GnRH) in the hypothalamus of the mouse by immunoperoxidase technique. Endocrinology 95: 1–8

Zimmerman E A, Defendini R, Frantz A G 1974b Prolactin and growth hormone in patients with pituitary adenomas. A correlative study of hormone in tumor and plasma by immunoperoxidase and radioimmunoassay. Journal of Clinical Endocrinology and Metabolism 38: 577–585

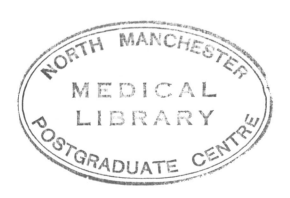

The physiology of puberty in the female

Puberty may be defined in a narrow or a wide sense. In the narrow sense it may simply be taken to indicate the achievement of the state of being functionally capable of procreation in which sense it is defined by the Oxford English Dictionary; in the wider sense it may be taken to encompass those years during which secondary sexual characteristics are being developed, menstruation starts and the psychosexual outlook of the patient changes. It is in this wider sense that it will be considered here.

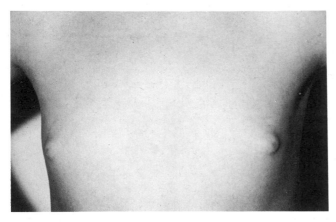

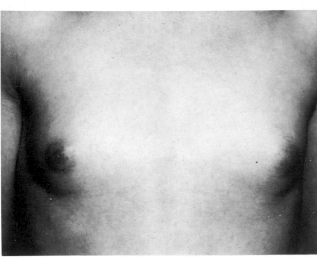

THE PHYSICAL CHANGES OF PUBERTY

Six physical changes of puberty will be discussed. They are breast growth, pubic hair growth, axillary hair growth, growth in height, menstruation and ovulation.

A generalisation must first be made about the relationship of these physical features to each other. There is variation from one girl to another in the age at which they appear for the first time; similarly there is variation in the time taken from their onset to full development whilst the order in which they make their appearance is, at least to some extent, variable. For these reasons a clinican should never expect puberty changes to conform to too definite a pattern. Very wide limits of variation exist — so wide that in two girls of the same age one may show no sign of puberty whilst the other may be already menstruating and both could be normal.

Breast growth

Breast growth has been divided into five stages by Tanner (1962) (Fig. 2.1).

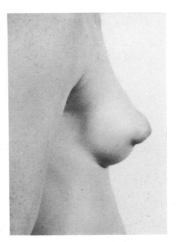 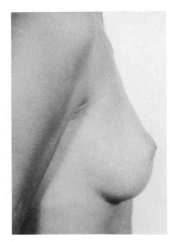

Fig. 2.1 (a) Showing Stage 2 of normal breast development. (b) Showing Stage 3 of normal breast development. (c) Showing Stage 4 (left) and 5 (right) of normal breast development

Stage 1. This is the prepubertal stage when there is no development whatever.

Stage 2. There is development of the breast bud as a very small mound beneath the nipple.

Stage 3. The breast and areolar are now both enlarged to a greater extent and resemble a small adult breast with a continuous rounded contour.

Stage 4. Here the nipple and areolar enlarge disproportionately so as to produce a secondary projection above the contour of the remainder of the breast.

Stage 5. The breast has now attained its normal adult size and shape with smooth rounded contours, the secondary mound of Stage 4 having been absorbed into the whole breast form.

Some children pass directly from breast Stage 3 to breast Stage 5 without passing through Stage 4 at all. By contrast, other girls may show persistence of Stage 4 until they have had their first child or perhaps even later. Figure 2.2 shows the variation which occurs in the time of appearance of these different stages. It is clear from this figure that there is considerable variation. As a generalisation it may be said that breast development may be evident for the first time from the age of 8½–9 onwards and it is rare for there to be no breast development at all by the age of 13 years. It may be seen too that one girl might not have mature breasts until she is 19 or 20 years of age, whilst another might show full breast development as early as 12 years old. It is worthy of mention that during breast growth inequality in size is not uncommon. One breast appears to enlarge more quickly than the other and, for a period of time, this inequality in size may persist until towards maturity the breasts become equal. What is particularly important about this inequality is that if one breast begins to develop significantly before the other, and perhaps at a rather early age, it may be taken to be an abnormality and biopsy may be unwisely attempted with the result that much or all of the breast bud on one side might be removed (Capraro & Dewhurst, 1975). Some of these features are considered more fully by Dewhurst, (1981).

Growth of pubic hair

Like breast development, pubic hair development is also described in five stages (Fig. 2.3).

Stage 1. This is the prepubertal stage where there is no true pubic hair at all.

Stage 2. There is a small amount of sparse, pigmented hair which is first noticeable on the labia and then in the midline on the mons pubis.

Stage 3. There is slightly greater spread over the symphysis pubis, the hair forming a narrow triangle with the base upwards.

Stage 4. The triangle of hair is now much broader and resembles the appearance in the adult but does not cover the entire area normally covered in the adult. In particular, the lateral corners of the triangle remain deficient.

Stage 5. This is the normal adult stage with its typical triangular distribution. There may be hair on the medial aspects of the thighs also.

From Fig. 2.2 it will be evident that pubic hair growth shows similar variation to breast growth. The ages at which pubic hair makes its first appearance and passes through its various stages are similar, in general terms, to those for

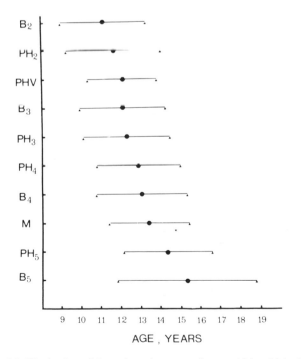

Fig. 2.2 The horizontal bars show the range of ages within which the stages of breast and pubic hair development are reached in 95 per cent of English girls. The mean age is indicated by the dark dot. Based on data from Marshall & Tanner (1969)

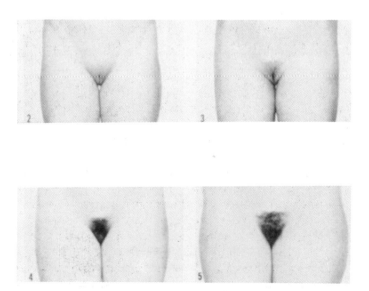

Fig. 2.3 Stages 2 to 5 of pubic hair development (By kind permission of J. M. Tanner and W. B. Saunders Co.)

breast development, although as we will see, there is considerable variation from one girl to another.

Axillary hair growth

The growth of axillary hair is described in only three stages.

Stage 1: being the infantile stage

Stage 2: being when there is a little hair present, but growth is not complete and

Stage 3: full development

Growth in height

The general pattern of growth during childhood and through puberty is illustrated in Figs. 2.4 and 2.5 (Marshall, 1974). It is, of course, common knowledge that children grow at different rates and attain different final heights. They also grow at different rates at different times so that if a child's growth is measured accurately during the years of childhood, it will be evident that, initially, growth is rapid for a period of perhaps 1 or 2 years after which the rate of growth becomes more stable until puberty is approached. Then the growth spurt makes it appearance. This is a period of much more rapid growth during which a girl may be growing almost twice as fast as she was prior to that time. When the child is growing fastest of all she has attained what is called 'peak height velocity' and thereafter the rate of growth falls off rapidly and stops. These growth effects are seen much more satis-

factorily if the velocity of growth in centimeters per year is plotted against age as is shown in Fig. 2.5.

Like the other features we have been discussing, the growth spurt occurs in different children at different times and may lead to considerable differences in size which are apt to cause a good deal of parental anxiety and perhaps anxiety in the child herself as well. Thus if a girl undergoes an adolescent growth spurt at an early age she will, temporarily, be much taller than other girls in her class. However, she is likely to stop growing sooner, as her epiphyses fuse, and those who experience a growth spurt at a later time will eventually catch her up. However if one girl has achieved peak height velocity and another has not started her growth spurt, the difference in height at that time may be considerable. Marshall & Tanner (1969), whose work in this field has been pre-eminent, showed that the majority of adolescent girls achieved the maximum growth rate between their tenth and fourteenth birthdays, although a few did so outside these limits; 12.14 years was the mean age for attaining peak height velocity.

Menstruation

Some 95 per cent of girls in Britain and in Western European countries will achieve the menarche between the ages of 11 and 15 years (Marshall, 1974) and the same is true for the USA and other countries with similar living standards.

There are a number of interesting relationships between the menarche and other features which are evident about the time of puberty. For example, the menarche generally occurs after a girl has reached peak height velocity and her growth is slowing down. There are exceptions to this rule, but they are rather few. It is an important consideration for those girls who have experienced a growth spurt at an

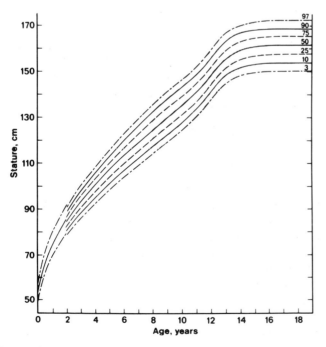

Fig. 2.4 Centiles for stature in British girls based on data from Tanner et al, 1966 (By kind permission of Dr. W. A. Marshall and W. B. Saunders Co.)

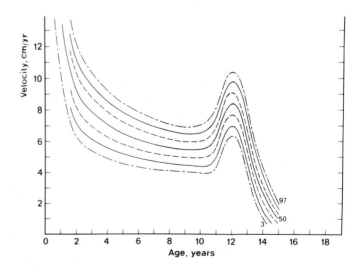

Fig. 2.5 Centile charts for growth velocity in British girls. Based on data from Tanner et al, 1966. (By kind permission of Dr. W. A. Marshall and W. B. Saunders Co.)

early age and fear that they are going to be very tall since once menstruation begins it is unlikely that they will grow significantly thereafter.

It was at one time believed that there was a comparatively close relationship between the menarche and body weight. Frisch & Revelle (1969, 1970) reported the mean body weight at the menarche to be 47 kg. It was suggested that this weight did not differ significantly in early or late maturing girls. Others have disputed this view (Johnston et al, 1975; Faust, 1977; Marshall, 1978) and it now seems less likely that the menarche is initiated by the patient achieving a particular body weight. Many clinicians who see adolescent patients with weight-related secondary amenorrhoea may, however, be reluctant to accept that there is no relationship here whatever.

The majority of girls menstruate when their breasts are in Stage 4. Perhaps 25 per cent or so may begin to menstruate sooner during breast Stage 3 and a small number may not menstruate until full breast development has been achieved.

Menstruation bears a very interesting relationship to bone age, although the earlier signs of puberty do not show the same close relationship. The majority of girls will experience the menarche between bone ages 13 and 14 and most of the remainder between bone ages $12\frac{1}{2}$ and $14\frac{1}{2}$ (Marshall, 1981). Such bone age may be estimated by taking radiographs of the wrist and hand and comparing the appearances with the atlas compiled by Greulich & Pyle (1959). Tanner et al (1975) use a somewhat more precise method in which a score is given to each bone in the hand and wrist, but confirm the relationship.

Genetic and environmental factors also influence the age of menarche. Tisserand-Perrier (1953) showed a difference in the menarcheal age of identical twins of only 2 months; the menarcheal age difference between non-identical twin sisters was 8 months, whilst sisters from different pregnancies may show an age difference of over a year and unrelated women an average difference of $1\frac{1}{2}$ years.

In general however, environmental influences on the age of the menarche are more important. In most populations the age of the menarche has been declining over the last 100 years or so, although it now appears that in the United Kingdom and Norway (Tanner, 1973) and Japan (Matsumoto, 1981, personal communication) this decline may have come to an end. The reason for the decline is generally held to be improvements in environmental conditions and standards of living. Better nutrition has often been regarded as the most important factor here and although this seems likely to be true, it is perhaps not the only one concerned. It is even possible in some communities to demonstrate an alteration in the age of the menarche in relation to social class. Thus in the Netherlands the daughters of upper class parents showed a mean menarcheal age of 13.5 years whilst those of lower or middle class parents had a mean age of 13.8 years (De Wijn, 1966). In Turkey

the difference is more striking being 12.4 years for the upper social groups and 13.2 for the lowest ones (Neyzi et al, 1975). Demonstrable differences of this kind are not apparent in the United Kingdom or in the United States of America.

Other interesting influences on menarcheal age include altitude, urban or rural dwelling, obesity, diabetes and blindness. Girls living at high altitudes tend to commence menstruation later than those living at low ones, whilst the menarche is generally earlier in urban than in rural areas (Marshall, 1981); this latter effect may reflect social class differences, not necessarily merely geographical ones. Obesity, within limits (Zacharias et al, 1970), diabetes and blindness (Hafez & Peluso, 1976) may be associated with an earlier puberty.

Relationship between puberty changes

These various changes of puberty follow a somewhat loose pattern to which there are many exceptions. In perhaps 50 per cent of girls breast development will appear first and this will coincide closely with the onset of the growth spurt. Pubic hair development is likely to appear soon afterwards, followed by axillary hair development and then by menstruation. The remaining 50 per cent will show one or other variation such as the appearance of pubic hair before breast development or menstruation before axillary hair development (Dewhurst, 1969). The rarest exception of all is the appearance of menstruation before there is any other sign of secondary sexual development; I have seen this on only three or four occasions, but am satisfied that it must be regarded as a very uncommon variant of the norm.

Whatever the pattern it must be stressed that there is much variation from one girl to another in the time taken to pass through all these stages, which may be as little as 1 year or more than 5 years. Marshall & Tanner (1969) found the average time from the beginning of breast development to the menarche to be 2.3 years.

Early menstrual cycles

The early menstrual cycles which a girl has shortly after her menarche are likely to be much more irregular than those which will characterise her later life. In the minority of girls a fair degree of regularity is achieved quickly, but most take a number of months, or even a year or two, before this regularity is evident. Zacharias et al (1970), gathering data from almost 5000 normal girls in the United States showed regular menstruation to occur a little more than a year after the menarche. Dewhurst et al (1971) showed that it was not uncommon for girls to have intervals between periods of 4, 5 or even 6 months during their first five cycles, these intervals becoming shorter and less frequent as time went by, although regularlity took more than a year to be achieved in many girls. Matsumoto (1981, personal communication) confirms very similar findings in Japanese girls. The duration of the period itself is much less variable than the cycle length. Ovulation too, is probably infrequent during early cycle and Zacharias et al (1970) found that on average 2 years elapsed before painful menses, and therefore presumably ovulation, began. The occurence of the occasional precocious pregnancy before a patient has had a menstrual period at all shows that rarely even the first cycle may be ovulatory. It is not easy to obtain precise data on this point. Matsumoto (1981, personal communication) simply states that most of the early cycles after the menarche are anovulatory whilst Vollman (1977) gives 55 per cent of cycles as anovulatory at gynaecological age 1–2 (i.e. 1–2 years from the menarche) decreasing to 3 per cent at gynaecological age 11–12. It is interesting too, that once ovulation does begin the luteal phase is unusually short for a time. Vollman (1977) comments that during the first 5 years after the menarche the median length of the premenstrual phase is about 9 days; it then begins to rise until the length is 12 days at gynaecological age 14. Matsumoto et al (1981) report similar data.

THE ENDOCRINOLOGY OF PUBERTY

The physical changes that we have been discussing result, of course, from hormonal activity, but it should be remembered that before there is any secondary sexual development at all the different sex hormones are produced if only in very small amounts. The pattern of events is similar in different studies although for various technical reasons a precise comparison between the results obtained in different laboratories around the world is not possible. The subject has been well reviewed by Pennington (1974), Faiman & Winter (1974) and Tanner (1981).

Gonadotrophic hormones

The pattern of serum FSH and LH during childhood and puberty is extremely interesting. Soon after birth both FSH and LH rise to pubertal levels reaching a peak during the first 3 months of life (Grumbach et al, 1975). In girls this elevated FSH persists for between 2 and 4 years although the LH levels usually fall 4–6 months after birth. Plasma levels of both these hormones then remain low until the end of the prepubertal stage; their actual levels are perhaps fractionally higher in the older girls than in somewhat younger ones (Penny et al, 1974) so a slight gradient may be perceived. As puberty changes become evident FSH levels rise and appear to reach a peak about the time of the menarche. LH levels do not rise until mid-puberty, nor do they reach their peak until some time after the menarche. It is interesting to note that during the time

when these puberty changes are taking place FSH and LH are released mainly at night, but with advancing puberty greater daytime release occurs until levels become equal (Lee et al, 1978). A comparison between the serum values of FSH and LH from pre-adolescence through the menarche and into the post-menarcheal period is illustrated in Fig. 2.6. It will be evident that during puberty considerable variation exists from day to day so single readings are of limited value.

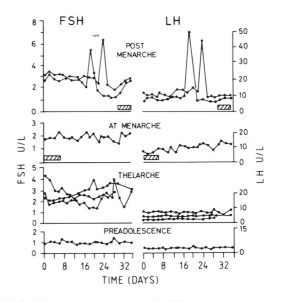

Fig. 2.6 Serial serum concentrations of FSH and LH in 7 perimenarcheal girls. The menstrual periods are denoted by the hatched bars. Adapted from Faiman & Winter (1974)

LHRH stimulation

After LHRH injection there is a different pattern of response for FSH and LH whilst each varies with the stage of puberty.

At breast Stage 1 there is a small response in FSH maximal about 60 minutes after the bolus injection and persisting for more than $1\frac{1}{2}$ hours. At breast Stage 2, however, the FSH response is much increased and is greater than at any other puberty stage. Stages 3, 4 and 5 show a smaller degree of response than at breast Stage 2 but remain considerably above the prepubertal figure (Fig. 2.7) (Apter et al, 1979; Tanner, 1981).

The LH response is quite different. That at breast stage 1 is similar to the response of FSH but is maximal somewhat earlier, about 30 minutes. Thereafter, there is a progressive increase in response all becoming maximal about the same time and declining somewhat more rapidly than FSH values (Fig. 2.8 Dickerman et al, 1976).

The pattern at the end of puberty therefore is similar to the response in the adult with the LH response being the more pronounced.

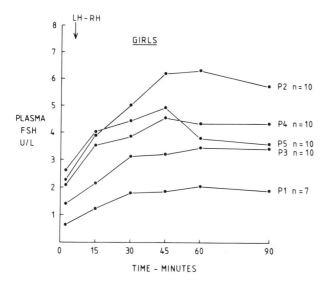

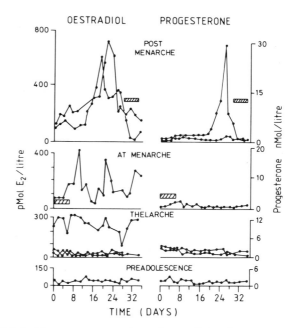

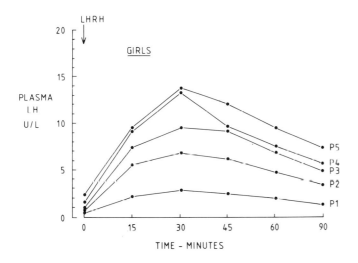

Fig. 2.7 Plasma FSH response to a single bolus injection (50 μg/m² iv) of LH-RH in girls before puberty (P1) and at various puberty stages (P2–5). (Adapted from Dickerman, et al, 1976)

Fig. 2.8 Plasma LH response to a single bolus injection (50 μ/m² iv) of LH-RH in girls before before puberty (P1) and at various puberty stages (P2–5). (Adapted from Dickerman, et al, 1976)

Fig. 2.9 Serial serum concentrations of oestradiol and progesterone in the seven perimenarcheal girls illustrated in Fig. 2.6; the menses are indicated by hatched bars. (Adapted from Faiman & Winter, 1974)

Oestrogens

Comparatively little change in plasma oestrogen levels occur during the prepubertal years although coincident with breast Stage 2 oestradiol levels begin to rise. The rate of rise increases until breast Stage 4 and the highest levels of all are associated with ovulation, a variable time after the menarche. To what extent there may be increases in plasma oestradiol during the years prior to the onset of puberty changes is a matter of debate. Pennington (1974) and Radfar et al (1976) suggest a slow rise might take place, although others (Ducharme et al, 1976; Lee et al, 1976) could not confirm this.

Although adult cycling becomes evident around the time of menarche or soon afterwards, the smooth, rhythmic pattern, characteristic of ovulation does not appear until some time later. The graphic representation of these oestrogen changes may be seen in Fig. 2.9.

Progesterone

It will also be evident from Fig. 2.9 that there is scarcely any alteration in serum porgesterone until some time after the menarche. This is in keeping with the delay in ovulation which does not usually make its appearance as a regular event until some time after the menarche. The pattern of early menstrual cycles has already been shown to be a variable one, the great majority of these early cycles being anovulatory.

Prolactin

Prolactin values remain low in the prepubertal state and during the early stages of puberty. They appear to rise either at breast Stage 3 or breast Stage 4 and by the time of the menarche adult values have been attained. The increased pattern of prolactin secretion during sleep which is evident in adults is also evident in both prepubertal and pubertal subjects.

Androgens

The relationship between androgen production and the early changes of puberty is most interesting. It has been known for some years that a rise in adrenal androgens occurs in both sexes from about the age of 7 or 8 (Migeon et al, 1957). By the time early puberty signs become evident androgen levels have reached about one-third of those in the adult. Throughout the rest of puberty into adolescence this rise continues: some describe the rise as progressive (Tanner, 1981), but others (Apter et al, 1979) have found a plateau formation occurring about bone age 12.5–15.5 years with continuous increase thereafter.

The existence of the increase before any puberty signs are apparent has given rise to much speculation as to its possible purpose. One suggestion which has much to commend it is that the androgens are concerned with the initiation of puberty, perhaps by reducing the hypothalamic sensitivity to low levels of oestrogens which have been sufficient to suppress it earlier in childhood, as will be described in the next section on the initiation of puberty.

THE INITIATION OF PUBERTY

Despite a large amount of work in recent years, we still do not know precisely what initiates puberty. It was at one time thought that puberty began when the pituitary became capable of function. Harris & Jacobsohn (1952), however, demonstrated this to be false by implanting the pituitaries of newborn rats beneath the hypothalami of their mothers who had been hypophysectomised; once vascular connections had been re-established the implanted pituitaries began to function: clearly then, the pituitary was capable of function long before it actually began to do so. The hypothalamus also appears to be capable of function earlier than the normal age of puberty. This cannot easily be shown in the human but it can be demonstrated in the rat that releasing hormone is present in the hypothalamus in considerable quantities well before the end point of puberty which, in that rodent, is vaginal opening. Despite this the hormone is released into the pituitary portal system in only tiny quantities which appear to be sufficient to cause the production of small amounts of FSH and LH which, in turn, lead to the production, by the ovary, of a small amount of oestrogen, charateristic of the prepubertal period.

There has, therefore, been much speculation upon the reason for delay in effective hypothalamic/pituitary function when both these structures are clearly capable of

working at an earlier age. What stimulates their activity; alternatively what keeps it in abeyance?

It seems likely that the most significant fact here is the very low setting of the hypothalamic rheostat. Suppression of the hypothalamus is possible by the relatively small amounts of oestrogen which the child's ovaries produce; gradually as puberty approaches the degree of sensitivity seems to lessen leading ultimately to stimulation of sufficient ovarian activity to bring about the physical changes of puberty. The evidence of this effect occurs in two contrasting forms. It has been shown that in children with 45X gonadal dysgenesis, where the gonads produce literally no oestrogens, there is much greater production of FSH and LH than in normal children, suggesting that the lack of even the small amounts of oestrogen which a normal child produces are sufficient to release the hypothalamus from inhibition (Conte et al, 1972; Kelch et al, 1972). Just the opposite effect can be shown by giving tiny quantities of oestrogens to prepubertal children when significant reduction in levels of FSH and LH were achieved by using as little as 2 μg daily of ethinyl oestradiol for 5 days (Grumbach et al, 1974); as puberty approaches larger doses of oestrogen (5–10 μg) are necessary to bring about this inhibition and by the time mid-puberty is reached these are inadequate. It has already been suggested that one reason for the diminution in the sensitivity of the hypothalamus to small doses of oestrogen may be the rising levels of adrenal androgens which are evident from the age of 7 or 8 onwards. It must be mentioned also that the higher centres may modify hypothalamic activity during the years of childhood. In particular the pineal body and the limbic system may have some involvement. Experimental work in the rat suggests that in the prepubertal animal there may be a degree of inhibition exerted on the hypothalamus by the limbic system (the amygdala, the cingulate gyrus and the hippocampus) and the pineal. Precocious puberty changes are evident in most species following pineal destruction whilst, in the human similar precocity is associated with pineal tumours which, as a rule, destroy the function of the gland. The pineal is a neuro-endocrine transducer. It receives afferent stimuli from the eye and perhaps the nose through the sense of smell; its effects are transmitted to the hypothalamus through specific indoles and appear to be inhibitory to FSH and LH (Shearman, 1981). It must be admitted however that our understanding of the real importance of these higher centres in the physiology of normal puberty is only elementary.

REFERENCES

Apter D, Pakarinen A, Hammond G L, et al 1979 Adrenocortical function in Puberty. Acta Paediatrica Scandinavia 68:599

Capraro V J, Dewhurst C J 1975 Breast Disorders in Childhood and Adolescence. Clinical Obstetrics and Gynaecology 18: 25

Conte F, Grumbach M M, Kaplan S L 1972 Variations in plasma LH and FSH with age in 35 patients with XO gonadal dysgenesis. Pediatric Research 6: 353

Dewhurst C J 1969 Variations in physical signs in pubertal girls. Journal of Obstetrics and Gynaecology of the British Commonwealth 76: 831

Dewhurst J 1981 Breast disorders in children and adolescents. Pediatric Clinics of North America 28: 287

Dewhurst C J, Cowell C A, Barrie L C 1971 The regularity of early menstrual cycles. Journal of Obstetrics and Gynaecology of the British Commonwealth 78: 1093

De Wijn J F 1966 Estimation of age at menarche in population. In: Van der Werff ten Bosch J J, Haak A (eds) Somatic Growth of the Child, p 16. Stenfert-Kroese, Leiden

Dickerman Z, Prager-Lewin R, Laron Z 1976 Response of plasma LH and FSH to synthetic LH-RH in children at various pubertal stages. American Journal of the Disabled Child 130: 634

Faiman C, Winter J S D 1974 Gonadotrophins and sex hormone patterns in puberty, clinical data. In: Grumbach M M, Grave G D, Mayer F E (eds) The Control of the Onset of Puberty, Ch 2, p 32. Wiley, New York

Faust M S 1977 Somatic development of adolescent girls. Monographs of the Society for Research in Child Development 42: 1

Frisch R E, Revelle R 1969 Variation in body weights and the age of adolescent growth spurt among Latin American and Asian populations in relation to calorie supplies. Human Biology, 71: 185

Frisch R E, Revelle R 1970 Height and weight at menarche and a hypothesis of critical body weights and adolescent events. Science 169: 397

Greulich W W, Pyle S I 1959 Radiographic Atlas of Skeletal Development of the Hand and Wrist, 2nd edn. Stanford University Press, Stanford, California

Grumbach M M, Grave G D, Mayer F E (eds) 1974 The Control of the Onset of Puberty. Wiley, New York

Grumbach M M, Roth J C, Kaplan S L, Kelch R P 1975 Hypothalamic-pituitary regulation of puberty in man: evidence and concepts derived from clinical research. In: Grumbach M M, Grave G D, Mayer F E (eds) The Control of the Onset of Puberty, Ch 6, p 115. Wiley, New York

Hafez E S E, Peluso J J (eds) 1976 Sexual Maturity: Physiological and Clinical Parameters, Vol 3. Ann Arbor Science, Michigan

Harris G W, Jacobsohn D 1952 Functional grafts of the anterior pituitary gland. Proceedings of the Royal Society of London (Biology) 139: 263

Johnston F E, Roche A F, Schell L M, et al 1975 Critical weight at menarche: critique of a hypothesis. American Journal of Diseases of Children 129: 19

Kelch R P, Conte F A, Kaplan S L, Grumbach M M 1972 Evidence for the episodic secretion of L H and decreasing sensitivity of the hypothalamic-pituitary 'gonadostat' in adolescent patients with gonadal dysgenesis. Pediatric Research 6: 349

Lee P A, Plotnick L P, Migeon C J, et al 1978 Integrated concentrations of follicle stimulating hormone and puberty. Journal of Clinical Endocrinology and Metabolism 46: 488

Marshall W A, Tanner J M 1969 Variation in the pattern of pubertal changes in girls. Archives of Disease in Childhood 44: 291

Marshall W A 1974 Growth and secondary sexual development and related abnormalities. Clinics in Obstetrics and Gynaecology 1: 593

Marshall W A 1978 The relationship of puberty to other maturity indicators and body composition in man. Journal of Reproduction and Fertility 52: 437

Marshall W A 1981 Normal Puberty. In: Brook C G D (ed) Clinical Paediatric Endocrinology, Ch 11, p 193. Blackwell Scientific Publications, Oxford

Matsumoto S, Ishizuka N, Takenaka Y 1981 Basal Body Temperature Findings of girls aged 18 and 19 years old. Japanese Journal of Adolescent Medicine 4: 17

Migeon C J, Keller A R, Lawrence B, et al 1957 Dehydrepiandrosterone and androsterone levels in human plasma. Effects of age and sex: day to day and diurnal variations. Journal of Clinical Endocrinology and Metabolism 17: 1051

Neyzi O, Alp H, Orhon A 1975 Sexual maturation in Turkish girls. Annals of Human Biology 2: 49

Pennington G W 1974 The reproductive endocrinology of childhood and adolescence. Clinics in Obstetrics and Gynecology 1: 509

Penny R, Olambiwonna N, Frasier S D 1974 Serum gonado-trophin concentrations during the first four years of life. Journal of Clinical Endocrinology and Metabolism 38: 320

Radfar N, Ansusingha K, Kenny F M 1976 circulating bound and free estradiol and estrone during normal growth and development and in premature thelarche and isosexual precocity. Journal of Pediatrics 89: 719

Shearman R P 1981 Control of Ovarian Function. In: Dewhurst Sir John (ed) Integrated Obstetrics and Gynaecology, 3rd edn, Ch 3, p 29. Blackwell Scientific Publications, Oxford

Tanner J M 1962 Growth at Adolescence. Blackwell Scientific Publications, Oxford

Tanner J M 1973 Trend towards earlier menarche in London, Oslo, Copenhagen, the Netherlands and Hungary. Nature 243: 95

Tanner J M 1981 Endocrinology of Puberty. In: Brook C G D (ed) Clinical Paediatric Endocrinology, Ch 12, p 207. Blackwell Scientific Publications, Oxford

Tanner J M, Whitehouse R H, Marshall W A, et al 1975 Assessment of Skeletal Maturity and Prediction of Adult Height (TW2 Method). Academic Press, London

Tisserand-Perrier M 1953 Etudes comparatives de certains processus de croissance chez les jumeaux. Journal Genetique Humaine 2: 87

Vollman R F 1977 The Menstrual Cycle. In: Major Problems in Obstetrics and Gynaecology, Vol 7. W B Saunders, Philadelphia

Zacharias L, Wurtman R J, Schatzoff M 1970 Sexual maturation in contemporary American girls. American Journal of Obstetrics and Gynecology 108: 833

Virility and fertility

GONADOTROPHIN SECRETION AND FEEDBACK CONTROL

Methods for the assessment of gonadotrophin secretion

Present concepts of gonadotrophin secretion are based on sensitive and specific radioimmunoassays for FSH and LH, which were developed from about 1965 onwards (Franchimont & Burger, 1975), and have been applied widely to characterise the regulation of male reproductive function from fetal life to old age. Evidence, which has accumulated over the past decade, has indicated that the ratio of biological to immunological gonadotrophin activity (B/I ratio) in blood may vary in different reproductive states; for example, the B/I ratio of LH varied from 0.7 to 2.1 during the normal menstrual cycle (Dufau et al, 1976). Sensitive bioassays have not been used extensively to examine circulating gonadotrophin levels in adult men but the possibility that immunoassayable hormone concentrations may not reflect circulating biological activity must be borne in mind.

A further caution with regard to gonadotrophin immunoassays is that investigators have used a range of different antisera and different gonadotrophin standards in their assays (Burger, 1972); thus, the absolute values obtained from different laboratories cannot be compared and interpretation requires a knowledge of the normal ranges for the individual laboratory. This is of particular importance in assessing the significance of reported hormone concentrations in evaluating individual patients — in addition to the attention that must be given to the patient's age, and the presence of other diseases (see below).

Assays of urinary gonadotrophins have not been used frequently in measurement in adult men, but have achieved some popularity in paediatric endocrinology (Kulin et al, 1975).

Patterns of basal gonadotrophin secretion

Fetal levels

Levels of both gonadotrophins are low or undetectable prior to 12 weeks' gestation. Fetal serum LH rises 3–4 weeks after the onset of testosterone secretion, and reaches peak levels at 12–16 weeks (Clements et al, 1976), while FSH levels peak between 13 and 30 weeks. Concentrations of both gonadotrophins reach those found in adult life, but decline to low levels in the latter stages of fetal life (Faiman et al, 1981).

Levels in the first two years of life

Although gonadotrophin and testosterone levels are low at birth, there is a temporary activation of the pituitary-testicular axis between 2 and 6 months of age, with a transient rise and fall in the levels of FSH, LH and testosterone, the peak concentration reaching the lower level of the adult normal range (Forest et el, 1976). This has been attributed to immaturity of the gonadostat, a concept which refers to the mechanisms regulating hypothalamic-pituitary secretion and their sensitivity to feedback control (Kaplan et al, 1976). The biological significance of this activation is unknown.

Levels from infancy to puberty

Gonadotrophin levels remain low but usually detectable from the age of 1–2 years up to 9–10 years, and during this period, the hypothalamo-pituitary unit is highly sensitive to the feedback effects of sex steroids. The phenomenon probably depends on central nervous system inhibition of the release of LH-releasing hormone (LHRH) (Styne & Grumbach, 1978).

The importance of central inhibition is reflected in the frequent finding of normal or only minimally elevated gonadotrophin levels in prepubertal children with primary gonadal failure, e.g. anorchia, Klinefelter's syndrome or ovarian dysgenesis (Conte et al, 1975) although the levels may be elevated (Winter & Faiman, 1972).

Levels during pubertal development

Starting from the age of 9–10 years, rises in LH and FSH

are best correlated with sexual development, LH levels increasing progressively during gonadal maturation, whilst FSH levels rise until mid-puberty and subsequently plateau (Franchimont & Burger, 1975). Plasma levels in adults are two to four fold greater than those in children, although if urinary measurements are compared, after correction for body size, adults excrete eight times as much LH and three times as much FSH as prepubertal boys (Santen & Kulin, 1981).

Episodic LH secretion is observable prepubertally (Penny et al, 1977). An early event in pubertal development is the occurrence of increased nocturnal secretion of LH and testosterone (Boyar et al, 1974), the LH increase resulting from an increase in both nadir and peak levels of the LH pulses (Santen & Bardin, 1973). A circadian rhythm of LH secretion has also been observed before puberty (Kulin et al, 1976). The increased nocturnal testosterone secretion may give rise to the first visible changes of puberty, including the stimulation of testicular enlargement in synergism with FSH.

Levels in adult men

Wide ranges of normal values for serum FSH and LH have been reported (Franchimont & Burger, 1975). The major characteristic of LH secretion is its pulsatile nature (Santen & Bardin, 1973), which in turn reflects the pulsatile nature of LHRH release from the hypothalamus into the hypophyseal portal blood (Clarke & Cummins, 1982). Pulses are characterised by a rapid upswing over 10–15 minutes, followed by a slower decline with a half-time of about 50 minutes. Nadir to peak increment averages 100–300 per cent, and pulses occur every 1–2 hours. FSH secretion is also pulsatile, but the amplitude of pulses is much less, 10–15 per cent, due largely to a longer half-time of disappearance (LH 34–60 minutes, FSH 2.4–3 hours) (Franchimont & Burger, 1975).

There has been extensive controversy regarding the existence of a circadian rhythm of LH and FSH secretion, but the current consensus of opinion would hold that there is no significant diurnal rhythm in adult men, whereas a rhythm for plasma testosterone is demonstrable in many studies. Plasma gonadotrophin levels show little fluctuation from day to day in normal men. Most studies indicate that the levels of both increase over 50–60 years of age, an observation interpreted as being due to a progressive failure of the spermatogenic and endocrine functions of the testis (Franchimont & Burger, 1975).

Although the pulsatile nature of LH secretion must be taken into account in any detailed clinical study of the pituitary-testicular axis, single plasma samples are usually adequate to allow characterisation of gonadotrophic status for routine clinical purposes. The measurement of serum FSH is of particular importance in the indirect assessment of the integrity of the seminiferous epithelium; the constancy of serum FSH makes single sampling adequate for this purpose.

LHRH and feedback control of gonadotrophin secretion

The secretion of the pituitary gonadotrophins can be considered to be the result of the interaction of three basic phenomena:

  (i) The basal secretory activity of pituitary gonadotrophs.
  (ii) The stimulatory activity of hypothalamic LHRH.
  (iii) The feedback effects of hormones of gonadal origin.

Basal secretory activity of the gonadotroph

Experimentally induced LHRH deficiency using arcuate nucleus-median eminence ablation in the castrated rhesus monkey or sheep leads to a fall of gonadotrophins to undetectable levels, suggesting that the basal secretory activity of the gonadotroph is low, although dispersed cultured anterior pituitary cells continue to secrete gonadotrophins for several days despite the absence of LHRH and feedback suppression.

In man, hypophyseal portal LHRH levels cannot be studied: inferences must be drawn from indirect studies of the frequency and amplitude of LH pulses, and from studies in experimental animals where access to stalk blood can be gained (Clarke & Cummins, 1982). Inferences can also be drawn from the results of exogenous LHRH administration, but must be interpreted with caution, as responsiveness is determined by the degree of prior exposure of the gonadotrophs to LHRH, as well as to feedback factors.

Gonadotrophin responses to LHRH

Most investigators have used single intravenous bolus injections of varying doses of LHRH to assess pituitary responses. These result in brisk releases of both LH and FSH, the LH response being quantitatively greater than FSH under virtually all circumstances in the male. Responsiveness to LHRH is demonstrable during fetal life (Takagi et al, 1977). Before puberty, low doses of LHRH (e.g. 25 µg) reproducibly lead to LH release, with the FSH response being more variable; at higher doses, both gonadotrophins respond (Franchimont & Burger, 1975). With achievement of stage 2 pubertal development, there is a marked increase in LH responsiveness to the same LHRH dose, while there is some controversy about changes in FSH responses, with reports indicating either no change (Roth et al, 1973) or an increase (Beck & Wuttke, 1980) as puberty progresses. In the adult male, responses of both gonadotrophins are linearly related to LHRH dose over the range 1–3000 µg (Wollesen et al, 1976). The LH response is proportional to the basal level in normal males, but is relatively attenuated (as demonstrable by repeated measures analysis of variance) in men with delayed puberty or hypogonadism secondary to hypothalamic-pituitary disease (Harman et al, 1982).

In contrast with the abrupt rise and fall of LH in response to a bolus injection of LHRH, the response to a 4-hour continuous LHRH infusion is biphasic, with an initial peak about 45 minutes after the start of the infusion, and a second prolonged response phase (de Kretser et al, 1975). The biphasic response is generally absent before puberty, and in patients with hypothalamic-pituitary disease (Burger et al, 1981a). In women with anorexia nervosa or severe hypothalamic amenorrhoea, LH responses are also low and monophasic; an increased and biphasic response can be restored by repetitive LHRH administration (Burger et al, 1981a). Taken together with the changes observed at puberty, and the postulate that there is a relative deficiency of LHRH secretion prior to puberty, in anorexia nervosa and in hypothalamic disease, it can be inferred that pituitary responsiveness to LHRH is in fact determined by its prior exposure to LHRH. Responsiveness is also influenced by gonadal feedback factors.

Feedback control of gonadotrophin secretion

The testis exerts a negative feedback effect on gonadotrophin secretion, mediated by steroidal and non-steroidal hormones, which may act at hypothalamic and/or pituitary levels. Orchidectomy in men is followed by relatively slow increases in FSH and LH levels to values found also in post-menopausal women. Administration of testosterone to normal men leads to suppression of LH, whilst variable effects on FSH have been reported (Franchimont & Burger, 1975). Oestrogen administration suppresses the levels of both gonadotrophins, though when given for relatively short periods (e.g. 40 μg ethinyl oestradiol daily for 4 days), selective suppresion of FSH is observed (Legros et al, 1972). It has been proposed that testosterone may exert some or all of its effects on the central nervous system (and hence some of its effect on the gonadotrophins) through aromatisation to oestradiol (Naftolin et at, 1972), but non-aromatisable androgens (such as dihydrotestosterone, DHT) are capable of suppressing gonadotrophin levels (Santen, 1975). Infusion of physiological amounts of testosterone and oestradiol into normal men leads to similar suppression of LH levels. Testosterone increases the amplitude but decreases the frequency of LH pulses, without any change in pituitary responsiveness to LHRH, while oestradiol decreases pulse amplitude and the pituitary response to LHRH, but does not alter pulse frequency (Santen, 1975). It can be inferred that testosterone is acting particularly on hypothalamic LHRH secretion, whilst the effect of oestradiol is predominantly on the pituitary.

There is a large body of evidence that the secretion of FSH is under the control of a non-steriodal gonadal hormone, inhibin, produced by the Sertoli cell and providing a feedback factor reflecting the state of the seminiferous epithelium (Baker et al, 1976). Deficiency of inhibin production is postulated to account for the selective elevation of serum FSH that is observed in a number of conditions causing damage to the seminiferous epithelium; this is supported indirectly by the demonstration that inhibin levels in the seminal plasma of normal men and men with various forms of infertility are inversely related to serum FSH (Scott & Burger, 1981).

TESTICULAR FUNCTION

The function of the testis is divisible into sperm production and steroidogenesis which results in the secretion of the principal androgen, testosterone. Spermatogenesis occurs within the seminiferous tubules of the testis and testosterone production is the province of the interstitial or Leydig cells which are distributed as clumps in the intertubular tissue. It has been traditional to consider the two units of the testis as being functionally separate but there is increasing evidence to indicate that there are important links between the two compartments. In this section the seminiferous tubules and intertubular compartments are considered separately and the functional links are described subsequently.

Seminiferous tubules

These structures are lined by the seminiferous epithelium which is composed of germ cells undergoing the steps involved in spermatogenesis, supported by the radially distributed Sertoli cells (Fig. 3.1). The formation of spermatozoa from the stem cells called spermatogonia is termed the process of spermatogenesis which is divisible into several steps:

(i) the division and renewal of spermatogonia by mitosis;

(ii) the meiotic process;

(iii) spermiogenesis — the metamorphosis of conventional cells, the early spermatids, to mature spermatozoa.

The spermatogonial population consists of at least three types in the human testis (Clermont, 1963) and by the process of mitosis the stem cell population is renewed. For unknown reasons groups of spermatogonia lose their connection with the basement membrane of the tubule to become pre-leptotene spermatocytes. This stage represents the earliest phase of the meiotic process in which the chromosomal number is reduced from the diploid to the haploid number. During the first prophase, the primary spermatocytes pass through the leptotene, zygotene, pachytene, diplotene and diakinetic stages each identifiable by their chromosomal configurations (Clermont, 1963). The primary spermatocytes then divide to give rise to the secondary spermatocytes which have a short lifespan before

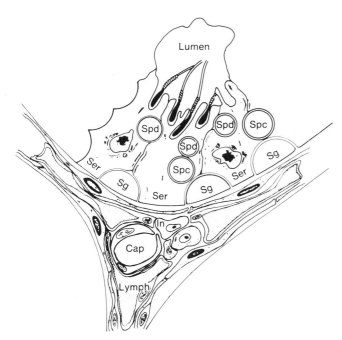

Fig. 3.1 The relationship between germ cells, Sertoli cells and Leydig cells is diagramatically illustrated. Abbreviations used :Ser = Sertoli cell; Sg = Spermatogonia; Spc = Spermatocytes' Spd = Spermatids; In – Interstitial or Leydig cells; Cap = Capillary (Reproduced with permission from Burger et al 1976 In: Hafez E S E (ed) Human Semen and Fertility Regulation in Men pp 3–16 C V Mosby, St Louis

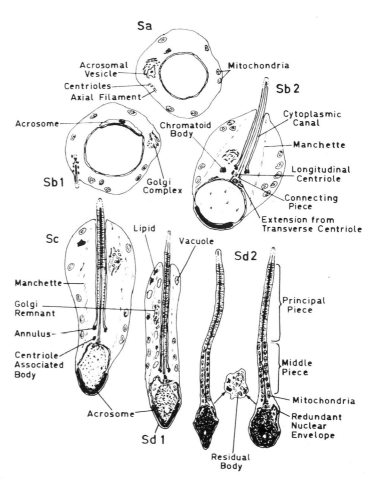

Fig. 3.2 The cytological features in human spermiogenesis are illustrated using Clermont's classification of spermatid stages (Reproduced with permission from de Kretser D M 1969 Z. Zellforsch 98: 477–5–5

dividing to form the spermatids, thereby completing the meiotic process.

The metamorphosis of the spermatids to spermatozoa, termed spermiogenesis, does not involve further cell division but is the result of a complex sequence of changes in the cell organelles. The details of these changes in the human testis have been described (de Kretser, 1969) but can be summarised as follows (Fig. 3.2): (i) The volume of the nucleus decreases, chromatin condensation occurs and the nucleus takes up an eccentric position. (ii) The Golgi complex gives rise to a cap-like structure, the acrosome, which is apposed over the half of the nucleus adjacent to the cell membrane of the spermatid. (iii) Development of the sperm tail from one of the pair of centrioles which lie adjacent to the Golgi complex; the developing tail migrates and lodges in a facet at the abacrosomal pole of the nucleus. (iv) Caudal migration of the cytoplasm and organisation of the mitochondria into a helix which surrounds the proximal portion of the tail. (v) As the mature spermatid is released from the epithelium the excess cytoplasm is shed and phagocytosed by the Sertoli cell as the residual body. The release of sperm from the epithelium is termed spermiation and the sperm are moved down the tubules by the contraction of the network of peritubular myoid cells and secretion of fluid by the Sertoli cells.

The time taken to produce spermatozoa from spermatogonia has been shown in man to be 70 ± 4 days (Heller & Clermont, 1964). This time span is a biological constant in that germ cells progress through the process at predetermined rates or they degenerate. Additionally the rate of spermatogenesis varies between species but in each, the time taken for the process cannot be altered (Clermont, 1972). Consequently, a patient with an arrest of spermatogenesis at the spermatogonial stage cannot be expected to show a response in sperm output to a therapeutic agent for at least 70 days. We know very little of the mechanisms which govern the time taken for this process. Additionally, the spermatogenic process is so organised that the epithelium in the tubules undergoes a series of sequential cellular associations which have been termed stages of the seminiferous cycle. Thus in man any specific region of the seminiferous epithelium cyclically passes through the defined six cell associations prior to the reappearance of the first one. In other species the organisation surpasses that seen in man, such that in the rat fourteen stages have been identified (Le Blond & Clermont, 1952).

The last decade has seen a considerable increase in our understanding of the functions of the Sertoli cells. These cells extend from the basement membrane of the seminiferous tubule in a radial direction towards the lumen. Their nuclei are large, indented, basally placed and contain a prominent nucleolus. However the centrally placed boundaries of the cell are indistinguishable by light microscopy since the cytoplasm forms an arborising network of processes which surround germ cells other than spermatogonia (Fawcett, 1975). Specialised cell junctions are present where the lateral boundaries of adjacent Sertoli cells come into contact. They effectively obliterate the inter-cellular space between adjacent Sertoli cells and isolate the centrally-placed germ cells from the extratubular environment dividing the epithelium into luminal and adluminal compartments (Dym & Fawcett, 1970). Since these junctions occur at the junction of the basal one-third and luminal two-thirds of the epithelium, transport of substances to the germ cells other than spermatogonia, must involve the Sertoli cells. It is generally agreed that in most mammalian testes, these inter-Sertoli cell junctions form the morphological basis for the blood-testis barrier.

The existence of the blood-testis barrier emphasises the importance of the Sertoli cells in the normal function of the seminiferous epithelium. Several studies have demonstrated that the production of seminiferous tubule fluid is a function of the Sertoli cell (Setchell, 1969) and is dependent on the integrity of the blood-testis barrier and the inter-Sertoli cell junctions (Vitale et al, 1973). Fluid production can be measured experimentally by the technique of efferent duct ligation and is a useful index of Sertoli cell function (Jegou et al, 1982).

The discovery that in some mammalian species the Sertoli cells produce an androgen binding protein (ABP), distinct from their androgen receptors provided another useful biochemical index of the function of these cells (Ritzen et al, 1973; Rich & de Kretser, 1977). No definitive experiments have been performed to delineate the role of ABP, but many investigators believe that this protein acts as a transport mechanism for testosterone from Leydig cells to the seminiferous epithelium. Furthermore since ABP is secreted into seminiferous tubule fluid, the bound testosterone is available to spermatozoa contained within the fluid and to the androgen-dependent cells of the caput epididymis wherein a large proportion of the ABP is absorbed and degraded (Hansson et al, 1975).

Sertoli cells in the immature rat are the site of aromatase enzyme activity converting androgens such as testosterone and androstenedione to oestradiol (Dorrington & Armstrong, 1975). However this activity is lost as the animal matures; in the adult aromatase activity appears to be confined to Leydig cells (Pomerantz, 1979). Other proteins and enzymes are also produced by the Sertoli cell, namely plasminogen activator (Lacroix et al, 1977) 5α-reductase (Welsh & Weibe, 1976) and inhibin (Steinberger & Steinberger, 1976; Le Gac & de Kretser, 1982).

There is accumulating evidence to show that the structure and function of the Sertoli cells vary with the stage of the seminiferous cycle (Kerr & de Kretser, 1975). Under transillumination it is possible to dissect segments of rat seminiferous tubules at various stages of the seminiferous cycle and to assess their function (Parvinen et al, 1980). In addition to inducing its own receptors FSH induces cyclic AMP formation, ABP production, RNA synthesis and the production of an aromatase inhibitor all of which vary cyclically according to the stage of the seminiferous cycle (Parvinen et al, 1980; Ritzen et al, 1980; Boitani et al, 1981; Davies & Lawrence, 1981). These results indicate that the heterogeneity in function must be taken into account when the response of the testis as a whole is assessed since the stages of the seminiferous cycle are not represented equally due to the differing times taken to pass through each stage.

Control of seminiferous tubule function

The dependence of spermatogenesis on the function of the hypothalamo-hypophyseal unit has been well recognised since the studies of Smith (1930) in which he hypophysectomised mammals and showed that the testis atrophied. There is a consensus view that during pubertal maturation FSH is required to initiate spermatogenesis and receptors for FSH have been demonstrated on Sertoli cells and spermatogonia (for reviews see Steinberger, 1971; Hodgson et al, 1982; Orth & Christensen, 1978). This action is completed by testosterone being secreted in response to rising LH levels and acting through androgen receptors in Sertoli cells (Tindall et al, 1977).

It is also generally agreed that testosterone is required for the maintenance of spermatogenesis in the adult but there is considerable argument concerning the role of FSH in the adult. The fact that following hypophysectomy in the rat, high doses of testosterone, if commenced immediately, can maintain spermatogenesis (Clermont & Harvey, 1965) has been supplemented by additional data questioning the requirement for FSH in the adult rat. Passive immunisation with antisera specific for FSH did not alter the spermatogenic process (Dym et al, 1979). However in adult male primates the use of antisera specific to FSH resulted in a decline in sperm count and fertility (Murty et al, 1979; Nieschlag et al, 1980), raising the possibility of species differences in the requirements for FSH.

Several other factors have added to the confusion. Studies on whole testis preparations have shown that the immature Sertoli cell is FSH responsive but in the adult FSH produces no response in the same parameters. However the evidence that the FSH responsiveness of Sertoli cells varies with the stage of the seminiferous cycle must now raise questions as to the interpretation of these studies. Studies in man by Bremner et al (1981) raise important questions. They showed that in men whose sperm counts had been suppressed with testosterone, the addition of hCG injections to the regime restored spermatogenesis, i.e. in the presence of unmeasureable FSH levels hCG, by raising intratesticular testosterone levels, could restore spermatogenesis. Thus a convincing case could be made that FSH was not required for spermatogenesis in adult men. However in additional experiments using a similar design, they showed that administration of FSH to men whose sperm counts were suppressed by testosterone, could also restore spermatogenesis (Matsumoto et al, 1982). They were unable to determine the mechanism by which this occurred since peripheral testosterone levels were considerably lower than those in the men treated with hCG in addition to testosterone.

As discussed before, the duration of spermatogenesis cannot be modified by hormones and the mechanisms by which hormones exert their effects on spermatogenesis are still unclear. There is evidence that FSH can decrease the proportion of germ cells that degenerate during spermatogenesis thereby increasing the throughput (Means & Huckins, 1974).

The intertubular compartment

This compartment of the testis contains the blood vessels, lymphatics and Leydig cells together with the sheath of myoid cells that surrounds the seminiferous tubules. The arrangement of the intertubular tissue varies between species particularly with respect to the volume of Leydig cells and the organisation of the lymphatics (Fawcett et al, 1973). Depending on this organisation, the Leydig cells discharge their products into the lymphatic sinusoids or the capillaries.

There is considerable variation in the size and microscopic features of the Leydig cells in man and these cells must be distinguished from the macrophages which are also found in the intertubular tissue. The Leydig cells have an ovoid nucleus, a prominent nucleolus and the cytoplasm, sometimes vacuolated, frequently contains the rod-shaped crystals of Reinke (de Kretser, 1967). In man, external to the peritubular sheath of myoid cells, elongated spindle-shaped cells are present and these have termed mesenchymal cells or immature Leydig cells. These cells are present in the prepubertal testis and thought to be responsible for testosterone production when the immature testis is stimulated by hCG.

The Leydig cells are responsible for testosterone and 30–50 per cent of oestradiol production, the remainder being derived from peripheral conversion of circulating androgens (Kelch et al, 1972). The subcellular organelles responsible are the the abundant smooth endoplasmic reticulum, mitochondria and tubular cristae, the lipid droplets probably representing stored substrate (de Kretser et al, 1982).

Control of the intertubular compartment

It is well recognised that the Leydig cells are stimulated by LH or hCG and a common receptor for these hormones has been demonstrated on the cell membranes of Leydig cells (de Kretser et al, 1971; Catt & Dufau, 1976). These high affinity, low capacity receptors were originally identified in the rat testis but have subsequently been shown to exist in human and subhuman testes (Hsu et al, 1978; Davies et al, 1979). Stimulation by LH/hCG results in cyclic AMP production and through a protein kinase mechanism in testosterone secretion (Dufau et al, 1978). In addition to initiating the secretion of testosterone, both LH and hCG are trophic to the Leydig cell stimulating enlargement and hyperplasia of the cells (Christensen & Peacock, 1980; de Kretser & Hodgson, 1982).

Several interesting features have emerged from recent studies of the Leydig cell's response to stimulation. Dufau et al (1978) have shown that there is a rapid internalisation of LH receptors following large stimulatory doses of hCG. Accompanying this loss of receptors, it was noted both *in vitro* and *in vivo* that the testes were refractory to further stimulation with hCG (Sharpe 1976; Haour & Saez, 1977). The two phenomena are not causally related since the use of cycloheximide, an inhibitor of protein synthesis, prevents the receptor loss but does not alter the refractoriness to further stimulation (Haour et al, 1978). The refractoriness is associated with an inhibitor of the 17α-hydroxylase and 17–20 lyase enzymes and can last for 48–72 hours after the hCG injection. Repeated injections of hCG over the initial 3 days have no additional stimulatory effects on testosterone secretion; however, if continued for 7 days, it can overcome the block and lead to high plasma testosterone levels and hyperresponsiveness to hCG stimulation *in vitro* (Risbridger et al, 1982). This finding suggests that the refractoriness noted to the initial stimulation is a temporary phenomenon and is not seen with subsequent injections.

The refractoriness to the initial injection results in an unusual plasma testosterone response (Fig. 3.3) since the levels rise acutely and then decline, rising again 48–72 hours later (Saez & Forest, 1979; Padron et al, 1980). This biphasic response results from the prolonged half-life of hCG since the second peak represents restimulation of the Leydig cells as they recover from their refractory period. LH which has a much shorter half-life does not produce the second testosterone peak (Hodgson & de Kretser, 1982). The prolonged response of the human testis to large doses of hCG has important clinical applications since injections of hCG do not have to be administered every 48 hours as has been practised but can be spaced at weekly intervals.

There is evidence that prolactin can modify Leydig cell function, and receptors for this hormone have been shown on these cells (Rajaniemi et al, 1974; Aragona & Friesen,

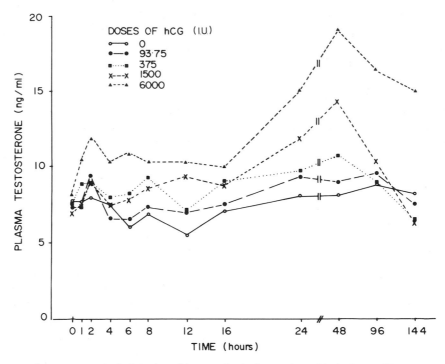

Fig. 3.3 The plasma testosterone 6 response to single injection of human chorionic gonadotrophin is shown. Data represents the mean levels from five normal men given the range of doses of hCG in random order, each dose being separated by at least a 2 week interval (Reproduced with permission from Padron et al, 1980 Journal of Clinical Endocrinology and Metabolism 50: 1100–1104

1975). However, the mechanism of its action is still unclear. There is evidence to suggest that prolactin can enhance LH binding to the testis and increase the gonadal stores of cholesterol esters, thereby augmenting the gonadal response to LH. Opposite effects have been found in clinical states where hyperprolactinaemia depresses testosterone levels resulting in hypogonadism (Thorner et al, 1977).

FSH has also been shown to modify Leydig cell function since Johnson & Ewing (1971) showed that FSH increased testosterone secretion by perfused rabbit testes exposed to LH. Furthermore, Odell et al (1973), from their experiments, suggested that during pubertal maturation FSH induced sensitivity of the testis to LH. However, to date no receptors for FSH have been found on Leydig cells but the evidence described in the next section may provide an alternative mechanism, namely FSH may influence Leydig cell function by modifying the function of Sertoli cells.

Tubule-intertubular relationships

As described earlier, it is accepted that the Leydig cells maintain a high intratesticular concentration of testosterone which stimulates spermatogenesis via receptors in the Sertoli cell. However, the concept that the Sertoli cell may influence Leydig cells is novel, and has arisen from our studies and those of Aoki & Fawcett (1978). During experiments which induced spermatogenic damage we noted that

Sertoli cell function was also rapidly impaired as measured by ABP and fluid production (Rich & de Kretser, 1977; Jegou et al, 1982). This was accompanied by elevated FSH levels, which was expected, but we also found a two to three fold elevation of LH. Investigations of Leydig cell function *in vivo* revealed an impaired testosterone response to low doses of hCG but when higher doses were administered, the damaged testes responded to a greater degree than controls (Risbridger et al, 1981a). This pattern would be consistent with a decline in blood flow to the damaged testes, as has been shown in cryptorchidism by Damber et al (1978), since our *in vitro* studies demonstrated that the damaged testis is hyperresponsive to hCG. The Leydig cells in the damaged testes were shown to be hypertrophied and to contain a lower number of LH receptors (Kerr et al, 1979; Rich et al, 1979; de Kretser et al, 1979). During further studies in which unilateral testicular damage was induced either by cryptorchidism or efferent duct ligation, the Leydig cell changes were confined to the damaged testis only (Risbridger et al, 1981b, c). This evidence was consistent with the hypothesis that the seminiferous tubules produce a signal which modulates Leydig cell function and that following spermatogenic damage, this inhibition is removed resulting in Leydig cell hypertrophy. The study by Bergh (1982) adds further support since he has shown that the size of Leydig cells changes according to the stage of the seminiferous cycle in the surrounding tubules. The nature of the factor(s) produced by the tubule which influences the Leydig cells remains unknown.

TESTICULAR STEROIDS IN BLOOD

The principal steroid secreted by the Leydig cell is testosterone which is quantitatively the most important androgen in blood. Several other steroids, which are intermediates in testosterone biosynthesis, are also secreted by the testis. These include: progesterone, 17α-hydroxyprogesterone, pregnenolone, 17α-hydroxypregnenolone, androstenedione, DHEA, dihydrotestosterone, oestradiol and small amounts of DHEA and testosterone sulphates. Some of these steroids are also secreted by the adrenal cortex. Steroids secreted by the Leydig cell enter the blood mainly by way of the spermatic vein; only a small amount is conveyed by testicular lymphatics (Eik-Nes, 1970).

More than 95 per cent of testosterone is directly secreted; this is between 15 and 25 μmol/day (~ 4.5–7 mg) in the young adult and falls with age (Kent & Acone, 1966; Baker et al, 1977). The plasma concentration of testosterone ranges between 10 and 35 nmol/l (~ 2.9–10 ng/ml). The most significant regulator of Leydig cell function is LH. Like LH testosterone is secreted episodically, the secretory pulses of LH being of greater amplitude than those of testosterone which are not completely entrained to those of LH. Plasma concentrations of testosterone show relatively small circadian fluctuations with a peak in the early morning, related possibly to the sleep-associated rise in LH that occurs during puberty; this rhythm is lost with age (Baker et al, 1975).

In blood 98 per cent of testosterone is protein bound, about 40 per cent to albumin, 42 per cent to a β-globulin, sex hormone binding globulin (SHBG) with 16 per cent bound to transcortin and acid α_1-glycoprotein. Between 1 and 2 per cent is free or unbound. SHBG is a glycoprotein made in the liver with a molecular weight of 84 000 daltons; it has 34 per cent carbohydrate and has one binding site per mole for testosterone and dihydrotestosterone (Vermeulen et al, 1969). SHBG is a high affinity binding protein (K_A: $1.6 \times 10^9 M^{-1}$) with a low capacity (~ $3 \times 10^{-8}M$). The concentration of SHBG is lower in men than women, lower in normal men than in hypogonadal men, greatly increased following treatment with oestrogens, and reduced in women treated with testosterone. Patients with hyperthyroidism have higher levels of SHBG than normal, while the converse is true for hypothyroid subjects. It is increased in patients with cirrhosis. Because the capacity for albumin to bind testosterone is virtually unlimited, and the binding affinity is relatively low (K_A: $3–4 \times 10^4M^{-1}$) the value of measuring fractions or concentrations of unbound testosterone in plasma has been questioned. Since a large amount of testosterone is loosely bound to and dissociates easily from albumin, any reduction in the local concentration of unbound testosterone is quickly replaced by dissociation from albumin. Whatever the theoretical objections may be to the measurement of free testosterone, there is enough experience to support the measurement of

non-SHBG bound testosterone as an index of biological activity (Vermeulen et al, 1971; Rosenfield, 1971; Hammond et al, 1980), rather than total testosterone concentrations. For instance, plasma concentrations of testosterone are frequently increased in women during pregnancy or with thyrotoxicosis, but plasma free testosterone concentrations are normal and masculinisation is not found. The implication of these observations — that only the free steroid is available for metabolism — is supported by the finding of an inverse relationship between the degree of protein binding and the metabolic clearance rate (MCR). Thus in women the MCR of testosterone is lower and the protein binding higher than in men (Verneulen et al, 1969; Baird et al, 1969). Similar relationships exist following oestrogen treatment or in patients with hyperthyroidism or myxoedema.

We may only speculate about the biological role of SHBG. It is suggested that binding protects steroids from degradation, and damps down fluctuations in concentrations of unbound steroids. Burke & Anderson (1972) have suggested that SHBG may be an oestrogen amplifier (for review on SHBG, see Anderson, 1974). It seems that whatever the action of SHBG it is not essential for androgen action since there are several species in which this binding protein is absent (Corvol & Bardin, 1973).

The other steroids of testicular origin and of known biological significance are dihydrotestosterone and oestradiol. Although the testis secretes both these steroids, less than 10 per cent of dihydrotestosterone and 50 per cent of oestradiol production are derived from direct testicular secretion. Dihydrotestosterone and oestradiol are derived by peripheral interconversion from secreted testosterone. Testosterone must thus be regarded as a hormone and prohormone (Baird et al, 1969).

ACCESSORY GLAND FUNCTION

The important accessory glands are the epididymis, seminal vesicles and prostate; others include the ampulla of the vas, the bulbo-urethral and urethral glands. Each of these contributes secretions to seminal plasma and is important for the viability of sperm. It is not known with certainty how most of these secretions interact with sperm. Other functions, however, are better understood — such as sperm transport and storage in the epididymis.

The epididymis

Structure

The single coiled duct of the epididymis originates from the mesonephros and lies on the posterolateral aspect of the testis. The epididymis is formed by the union of several ciliated efferent ducts which comprise most of the head or upper pole of the epididymis where they join the epididymal duct. These several efferent ducts arise from a sinus at the posterior aspect of the testis, the rete testis, into which the seminiferous tubules empty.

The epididymal duct in man is 5–6 metres in length, coiled and lined by two major cell types, principal and basal cells. The principal cells are more numerous, line the lumen and show evidence of both resorptive and secretory activity. The subepithelial wall of the epididymis is a thin covering of poorly differentiated smooth muscle which gradually increases in thickness along the duct. At the junction of the body and tail a thicker layer of smooth muscle becomes superimposed on the subepithelial muscle fibres and ultimately merges with the thick smooth muscle fibres of the vas deferens with which the epididymal duct joins. The efferent and epididymal ducts show spontaneous contractions which transport the fluid secretions and sperm toward the vas.

Function

The epididymis has a variety of functions of which the most obvious is the transport of sperm from the testis to the vas and the storage of sperm in the cauda. In man the average transit time of sperm along the epididymal duct is 5–12 days (Rowley et al, 1970). Spermatozoa mature during their passage through the epididymis; when they enter the head of the epididymis they are either non-motile or show sluggish circular swimming movements and have no capacity to fertilise; when they reach the cauda where they are stored, they are motile and are able to fertilise. Sperm undergo a number of changes with maturation, such as the loss of the cytoplasmic remnant from the neck of the sperm, modification of their membranes as a result of changes in surface glycoproteins and changes in the shape and ultrastructure of the acrosome (Bedford, 1975). At present we do not understand the functional significance of these modifications to sperm membranes during maturation. We do know, however, that with passage through the epididymis metabolic activity of sperm increases; there is an increase in fructolysis, increased oxidation of lactate and fatty acids and an increase in intracellular cAMP, at least in bovine sperm (Hoskins et al, 1975).

These changes are the effects of the epididymal environment. There is a small number of substances that are specifically secreted or concentrated in the epididymis : glycerophosphorylcholine (GPC), sialic acid, inositol and at least one glycoprotein are secreted; the concentration of carnitine in epididymal fluid is about seven times that in blood. Carnitine may play a role in sperm motility since flagellar movement without progression can be induced in non-motile sperm from the caput epididymidis by diluting these in solutions containing carnitine and moderate concentrations of carnitine can produce sustained increases in motility (Brooks et al, 1974).

The epididymis is extremely androgen sensitive and the maturation process depends on the special environment created by the androgen dependent activity of epididymal epithelium which has cytoplasmic androgen receptors (Blaquier, 1971). The epididymis which has a limited capacity for steroid synthesis (Hamilton & Fawcett, 1970) is supplied with androgens from two sources — the seminiferous tubule fluid which is rich in androgens and supplies mainly the head, and the blood which supplies the whole organ with androgens. Regressive changes in the epididymis quickly follow removal of androgens. The principal cells have a rich endoplasmic reticulum, Golgi apparatus and pinocytic vesicles which are implicated chiefly in the synthesis of proteins, GPC, sialic acid and steroids and for the concentration and secretion of carnitine. They become completely atrophic following androgen deprivation.

The epididymis continues to remain an enigma. If we were able to understand better the mechanisms by which sperm mature, and the factors directly responsible for this maturation, the prevention of this process could be a very direct way of reducing or abolishing male fertility and thus providing a valuable form of male contraception. Also, if epididymal function were better understood it is possible we may be more effective in treating some men with infertility — particularly those who produce normal numbers of sperm but with poor sperm motility (for review, see Orgebin-Crist, 1981).

Vas deferens

The vas is a single duct, about 35 cm in length, that passes from the cauda epididymis and joins the duct of the seminal vesicle behind the bladder to form the ejaculatory duct. The final part of the vas is dilated and forms the ampulla. The vas is lined by a simple mucosa which is surrounded by a thick muscular wall, made up of two layers of longitudinal and one of circular muscle which allow a peristaltic action, which is fully developed during ejaculation.

The function of the vas is the transport of sperm, particularly at the time of ejaculation from the epididymis to the urethra. However, in between ejaculations the vas undergoes small, spontaneous peristaltic movements which transport sperm along its length to the ampulla and seminal vesicles. At the time of ejaculation sperm are moved from the cauda epididymis, all parts of the vas and the seminal vesicle to the urethra. The control of ejaculation is through sympathetic nerves and the release of noradrenaline.

Seminal vesicles

The seminal vesicles are paired lobulated glands lying symmetrically above the prostate and behind the bladder. Each seminal vesicle arises from a diverticulum of the lower part of the vas deferens. The gland is lined by a complex folded mucosa, the cells of which have a substantial secretory capacity. The mucosa is surrounded by a fibromuscular stroma. The total volume of each vesicle is between 2 and 3 ml. The vesicles are filled with a viscous proteinaceous fluid which contains unique components: fructose and prostaglandins. Fructose is the principal natural energy source of ejaculated spermatozoa. Although found in many other tissues, prostaglandins are in high concentration in the seminal vesicles and seminal plasma, but their function is not known. There is no convincing evidence of any association between abnormalities of prostaglandin synthesis and secretion and infertility. The secretions of the seminal vesicles make up more than half of the total volume of seminal plasma.

Prostate

The prostate is a fibromuscular gland lying at the neck of the bladder and surrounding the first part of the urethra into which 50 or 60 prostatic collecting ducts open. These ducts drain the glandular tissue of the prostate, most of which form the lateral lobes and lie in the fibromuscular stroma of the gland. The glandular tissue consists of compound tuboalveolar glands with secretory acini that are quite irregular in size and shape. The current view is that the glandular tissue surrounding the middle portion of the urethra, the peri-urethral glands, are morphologically distinct and embryologically different from the rest of the glandular tissue. These peri-urethral glands are derived from the Wolffian duct, while the rest of the gland arises from the urogenital sinus (McNeal, 1972). Benign prostatic hyperplasia commences in the peri-urethral glands.

The prostate has a secretory function and as such contributes to about 20 per cent of the seminal plasma — citric acid, zinc and acid phosphatase are secreted by the prostate.

Like the epididymis the seminal veisicles and prostate are androgen sensitive tissues. Cytoplasmic androgen receptors and the enzyme 5α-reductase which reduces testosterone to 5α-dihydrotestosterone are present. This latter androgen is responsible for the androgen mediated effects, and in the prostate is responsible for the growth of the prostate at puberty and for benign prostatic hyperplasia which is found in more than 50 per cent of men over the age of 50 (Wilson, 1980) (see also Ch. 38).

Seminal plasma

The complex nature of seminal plasma has led to much speculation about its role in reproduction. Although the composition of seminal plasma is well known, the physiological importance of prostaglandins, zinc, a number of carbohydrates and specific proteins — several of which undergo coagulation at the time of ejaculation — is not known. Abnormalities in the volume of seminal plasma, normally between 2–4 ml, or in some of its constituents, may give some indication about abnormalities in accessory gland function. For instance, an absence of fructose indicates an absence of the seminal vesicles, a developmental anomaly which is coupled with absence of the vasa. However, changes in other constituents are rarely so sensitive or specific in diagnosis.

MECHANISM OF ANDROGEN ACTION

The mechanism by which androgens act is similar to other steroid hormones. Androgens diffuse through cell membranes, a process which is thought to be passive, although it may be more complex than this. The rate of diffusion is limited by the concentration of non-protein bound hormone. Once in the cytoplasm of the hormone sensitive cell the hormone is bound to a high affinity receptor. As far as testosterone is concerned there is further metabolism in most androgen sensitive tissues; the enzyme responsible for this metabolism is 5α-reductase which converts testosterone to dihydrotestosterone, which in turn binds to the high affinity cytosol receptors.

Steroid receptors are proteins with molecular weights of the order of 2×10^5 daltons and are made of two subunits. The responsiveness of any tissue to a steroid is determined by the concentrations of the receptors so that those with low concentrations are fairly insensitive to hormones, while androgen sensitive tissues such as the prostate, epididymis and seminal vesicles have high concentrations of 5α-dihydrotestosterone receptors. The steroid binds to one of the receptor subunits and the hormone-receptor complex undergoes some form of activation, the nature of which is not fully understood. Once activated the steroid-receptor complex is transferred to the nucleus and interacts with specific genes and causes a biological response. The nature of these nuclear acceptor sites is not known.

Nuclear binding stimulates RNA polymerases and the transcription of new message (mRNA) which promotes ribosomal synthesis of proteins involved in these functions of the cell which are identified as androgen effects, e.g. growth of the prostate and seminal vesicles in androgen deficient animals.

DISORDERS OF PUBERTAL DEVELOPMENT

Normal puberty

The initial physical sign of puberty is testicular enlargement: this occurs at an average age of approximately 11 years in boys in Western industrialised societies, with 99 per cent showing a testicular volume of 4 ml or greater (length ≥2.5 cm) by the age of 14 years. The clinical description of puberty most usefully comprises the recording of testicular volume (with the aid of the Prader orchidometer) or testicular length, together with the stage of pubic hair development, using the rating scale of Marshall & Tanner (1970), as follows:

Stage 1: Pre-pubertal, no true pubic hair.
Stage 2: Sparse growth of long, slightly pigmented hair.
Stage 3: Hair becomes darker, coarser, and more curled and begins to spread over the pubic symphysis.
Stage 4: Hair is adult in character but not in distribution; no spread to medial surface of the thighs.
Stage 5: Hair is adult in quantity and type, distributed as an inverse triangle, with spread to the medial surface of the thighs.
Stage 6: Hair spreads up the linea alba.

Delayed puberty

From a practical clinical view-point, a testicular size less than 2.5 cm length, or 4 ml volume, in a boy aged 14–15 years, is the criterion for making the diagnosis of delayed puberty. It is important to emphasise that growth of the testes may precede other signs of puberty, such as the development of pubic hair, by 1–2 years or more: thus, testicular volume may be 8–10 ml while pubic hair is still absent.

Varieties of delayed puberty

By far the commonest reason for presentation because of apparently delayed puberty is late maturation of an otherwise normal hypothalamic-pituitary-gonadal axis — the condition known as constitutional delay in puberty, usually associated with delay in growth. Much rarer are the varieties of true hypogonadism, which may result from defects either at the hypothalamic-pituitary level (hypogonadotrophic hypogonadism) or at the testicular level (hypergonadotrophic hypogonadism).

Constitutional delay in growth and pubertal development

Characteristically, there is a history of short stature which dates back to the boy's commencement at kindergarten or primary school where he was among the shortest in the class. There is frequently a family history of pubertal delay, the father having been a 'late bloomer' who entered puberty at 15–17 years, or the mother having had a delayed menarche. The remainder of the history is usually unremarkable from the viewpoint of illness. In contrast, psychological features which may result from the delay include tension, irritability or depression, non-specific abdominal pain, feelings of inferiority often associated with compensatory aggressiveness, and/or withdrawal from social contact. Physical examination shows that height age is delayed 1–2 years behind chronological age, and height is usually around the 3rd to the 10th centile. Proportions are appropriate for height age. Testicular

volume may still be less than 4 ml, but in the 15–16 year old boy presenting because of failure of development of the secondary sexual characteristics, testicular volume is usually more than 4 ml. The latter finding is indicative of an excellent prognosis for normal spontaneous pubertal development and growth, although ultimate stature may be somewhat less than normal. Provided that testicular volume is in the pubertal range, other investigations are unnecessary, although estimation of bone age (usually delayed in proportion to the height age) is useful to allow mature height prediction and estimation of when more obvious pubertal development, including the adolescent growth spurt, may be expected (at a bone age of 13–14 years).

In many instances, positive reassurance with regard to the prognosis is sufficient management. However, if the degree of anxiety or emotional disturbance is severe, consideration can be given to a course of chorionic gonadotrophin (hCG) or androgen therapy. A suitable dosage schedule is hCG 1500–3000 iu once weekly since recent studies have shown that more frequent administration is probably unnecessary (Padron et al, 1980). Testosterone oenanthate may also be used, 200 mg by intramuscular injection every 3 weeks for an arbitrary period of 3 months (Rosenfeld et al, 1982). Treatment is then withdrawn for 3 months to allow observation of the degree of spontaneous progression. A further 3 months course may be necessary.

An associated differential diagnostic problem in such boys is the possibility of isolated growth hormone deficiency, particularly if height is below the third centile. Observation of spontaneous growth velocity, and if low, performance of a screening test for growth hormone deficiency, e.g. the hormonal response to brief, intense muscular exercise, (Franchimont & Burger, 1975), are usually sufficient either to exclude the diagnosis, or to indicate the need for further assessment.

The finding of testes of prepubertal size in boys more than 14–15 years of age, particularly in the absence of a family history of delayed but otherwise normal puberty, is an indication to undertake the investigations necessary to clarify the diagnosis, and to examine the possibility of true hypogonadism. The most difficult differential diagnosis is between constitutional delay and idiopathic isolated gonadotrophin or growth hormone deficiency: continued observation may ultimately be the only means of management. Responses of the gonadotrophins to LHRH are variable and not sufficiently discriminatory to allow a reliable diagnosis (Santen & Kulin, 1981).

Measurement of serum gonadotrophin and testosterone concentrations provides the basis for further consideration of aetiology.

Hypogonadotrophic hypogonadism

This disorder may be idiopathic or organic, and may result

Table 3.1 Causes of hypogonadotrophic hypogonadism

Functional
    Constitutional delay of growth and puberty
Chronic illness
Idiopathic
    Isolated gonadotrophin deficiency
    Multiple pituitary hormone deficiencies
Organic
    Hypothalamic-pituitary tumour
    Granulomas, histiocytosis X
    Secondary to cranial irradiation
    Secondary to trauma, inflammation

from isolated deficiency of gonadotrophin secretion, or may be associated with multiple pituitary hormone defects (Table 3.1). In its most common form, known as Kallman's syndrome, isolated gonadotrophin deficiency is associated with anosmia or hyposmia in about 80 per cent of patients. Stature is normal or tall, and the proportions are usually eunuchoid. Cryptorchidism and midline craniofacial defects, such as hare-lip or cleft palate, may be present. It is inherited as an autosomal dominant syndrome with relative sex limitation to males (Santen & Paulsen, 1973) although recessive variants may occur.

Evidence of multiple pituitary hormone deficiencies in particular demands the exclusion of an organic basis, notably craniopharyngioma, for which a skull X-ray or cerebral CT scan is mandatory. Partial hypogonadotrophic hypogonadism is occasionally encountered: an intermediate degree of testicular enlargement and development of secondary sex characteristics occurs at puberty, but gonadotrophin levels remain at or below the lower limit for adult men, while testosterone is low.

A rarer form of hypogonadotrophic hypogonadism is the Laurence-Moon-Biedl syndrome, in which additional features are retinitis pigmentosa, obesity, mental retardation and polydactyly. Partial or severe deficiency of gonadotrophin secretion is seen in the Prader-Willi-Labhart syndrome of hypotonia, obesity, mental retardation, short stature and mild type II diabetes mellitus. Chronic systemic illnesses may be sufficiently severe to cause reduced growth and delayed puberty as incidental features, but do not usually create diagnostic difficulty. Pubertal delay is also seen in thalassaemia major, and is probably related to hypothalamic dysfunction (Modell, 1977).

The choice of management of true hypogonadotrophic hypogonadism is between hCG and testosterone administration. When there is associated deficiency of growth hormone, it may be convenient to combine injections of growth hormone and hCG (initially 500 iu twice weekly, increasing to 1500 iu once or twice weekly depending on the clinical and testicular androgen response) in the same subcutaneous injection. Where the gonadotrophin deficiency is isolated, or where other regular injections are not required, the use of parenteral testosterone is preferable on the grounds of convenience and efficacy. Initially, 100 mg

testosterone long-acting esters may be given every 2–4 weeks, and, depending on the adequacy of androgenisation, the dose is increased to 200–250 mg every 2–4 weeks. Although there is not an extensive literature, it appears that the induction of puberty either with hCG or with parenteral (or oral) testosterone is quite compatible with later successful induction of fertility using FSH containing preparations (Burger et al, 1981b). A practical consideration which often poses difficulty is the decision regarding the appropriate age at which to commence therapy: androgens are synergistic with growth hormone in stimulating skeletal growth, and it seems reasonable to recommend physiological levels of androgen replacement starting at the age of 13–14 when puberty would normally be underway. Similar considerations apply to isolated gonadotrophin deficiency.

In principle, hypogonadotrophic hypogonadism resulting from LHRH deficiency can be treated using pulsatile LHRH (Valk et al, 1980), though this approach is currently still under investigation and is not as practical nor as convenient as parenteral testosterone.

Hypergonadotrophic hypogonadism

The diagnosis of hypergonadotrophic hypogonadism is made by the finding of an elevated level of serum FSH in a patient with delayed puberty. A common variety is Klinefelter's syndrome, characterised by small testes (they rarely exceed 6 ml volume), eunuchoid proportions, gynaecomastia, and karyotypic evidence of an extra X chromosome. If the testes are impalpable in a boy with delayed puberty, the possibility of anorchia must be considered (Abeyaratne et al, 1969); the diagnosis is confirmed by the clinical features of a normal male phenotype, with an absent testosterone response to administered hCG (e.g. 3000 iu weekly for 3 weeks). A rare form of hypergonadotrophic hypogonadism is the Noonan syndrome in which the external genitalia are normal, the testes often undescended, and somatic features seen in Turner's syndrome are found, including webbed neck, ptosis, short stature, cubitus valgus and lymphoedema. A right-sided cardiac lesion may be present, and the karyotype is normal.

Precocious puberty

Signs of pubertal development in a boy before the age of 9 years are precocious. This development is truly precocious if all the features of pubertal development are found — in particular, bilateral testicular enlargement. In some boys the puberty is falsely precocious (or pseudoprecocious) since there is no testicular development and the physical changes result from the secretion of androgens by the adrenal (congenital adrenal hyperplasia) or from a unilateral testicular tumour. Normally the first signs of puberty appear between the ages of $9\frac{1}{2}$ and 13 years, and by the age of 14 between 90 and 95 per cent of boys have entered puberty. Sexual precocity in boys is an unusual disorder and less common than it is in girls.

True precocious puberty usually results from an intracranial lesion which activates the hypothalamus, pituitary and testes. In some boys no cause is found other than a family history of sexual precocity which is thought to be autosomal, dominant and sex linked. The lesion when found is usually an expanding one in the region of the posterior hypothalamus, most frequently a lesion of the pineal (pinealoma, hamartoma, teratoma).

The child with precocious puberty shows an accelerated physical development with the appearance of secondary sexual characteristics, a growth spurt and increased bone age. There is frequently a social problem because of aggressive behaviour and other features of androgen excess: acne, oily skin, voice changes, scrotal development and penile enlargement with the occurrence of erections, and an increase in the size of both testes. Plasma levels of testosterone are higher than normal (for that particular age) and there may be a sleep-associated secretion of LH, the release of which in response to LHRH is also increased.

To discover the cause may be difficult since the intracranial lesion is frequently very small; however, with the availability of computerised tomographic (CT) scanning there is an increased likelihood of finding a lesion, which cannot often be demonstrated by conventional methods.

Treatment is directed to the cause: irradiation or removal of the tumour — sometimes difficult to achieve. If there is no obvious cause the aim has been to block gonadotrophin secretion and the effects of androgens. In the past depot-medroxyprogesterone was given in doses of 200–400 mg every 2–4 weeks with some but not outstanding success. More recently cyproterone acetate has been used; this has two actions: first as an antiandrogen, and second as a strong progestational agent. Despite what are theoretically ideal properties, the use of this agent has not proved uniformly successful (Neumann, 1977). The use of LHRH agonists to inhibit gonadal function in precocious puberty is a new avenue of treatment of this disorder.

Patients with false or pseudo-precocious puberty have incomplete sexual development, and in some the development will be heterosexual. Isosexual development can result from excessive androgen production, usually from the adrenal but sometimes from a Leydig cell tumour. Androgen secretion can be stimulated by gonadotrophin-producing tumours which are malignant and rare chorio-epitheliomas or teratomas derived from the trophoblast. As a result of the secretion of LH-like peptides (e.g. hCG) the Leydig cells are stimulated to secrete testosterone.

The most common cause of pseudo-precocious puberty is unrecognised congenital adrenal hyperplasia. It may be unrecognised since there are no heterosexual symptoms such as are seen in girls. Adrenal androgen stimulates the development of secondary sexual characteristics but the testes remain small and soft. There is also a growth spurt and increased bone age. It is important to recognise this disorder to permit full skeletal development and prevent the possibility of infertility (See Ch. 18).

Leydig cell tumours are rare and usually benign. Sexual maturation is premature, plasma levels of testosterone are elevated but gonadotrophins are low. The diagnosis should be suspected on the hormonal profile and confirmed by the discovery of a testicular tumour which is usually small.

GYNAECOMASTIA

Gynaecomastia is defined as the presence of a discrete disc of subareolar tissue greater than 2 cm in diameter in the male. It is usually bilateral but may occasionally be unilateral. Gynaecomastia is a symptom (or sign) of a disturbance in the normal balance between androgens and oestrogens either in the blood where the concentrations can be measured or in the tissue (receptors) which can only be inferred but not measured.

The sexual dimorphism that is seen in breast development at puberty results from the effects of oestrogens. Oestrogens are responsible for the growth of the duct system of the breast while progesterone acts synergistically with oestrogens to develop the alveolar buds at the end of the ducts. These changes lead to the development of the normal female breast. The normal male breast is a remnant in which ducts can be distinguished, but the cells which line the ducts are atrophic.

Morphology

The changes found in breast tissue in men with gynaecomastia can be quite variable depending on the intensity and duration of the stimulus. Initially there is an elongation and proliferation of the duct system with an increase in the amount of stroma which surrounds the ducts. When gynaecomastia has been present for a long time all that may be left is hyalinised remnants of the ducts and fibrous tissue (Nicolis et al, 1970).

Pathogenesis

The basic defect is a disturbance in the ratio between the effects of androgens and oestrogens. This can result either from an excess of oestrogen effects or a deficiency of androgen effects or a combination of both. In some patients this imbalance can be demonstrated by measuring the concentrations of androgens and oestrogens in the blood — particularly testosterone and oestradiol. More often, however, it is not possible to demonstrate these effects either because single blood samples cannot detect minor changes which may only be revealed by repeated blood samples over a 24 h period (Large & Anderson, 1979) or because androgen receptors become occupied by drugs which are not androgenic and thus leave the actions of oestrogens unopposed. Subtle changes in oestrogen/androgen ratios apply particularly to the gynaecomastia that occurs in adolescents and young men. With the restoration of a normal androgen/oestrogen ratio the gynaecomastia disappears.

Clinical features

The common clinical setting for gynaecomastia is an adolescent proceeding through puberty who may complain of breast enlargement or soreness which is commonly bilateral but may be unilateral. In older men breast enlargement may only be found on physical examination. Most commonly it is possible to feel a 3–7 cm disk or button of breast tissue beneath the areola, but in some men the breasts may attain female proportions. In many young men the gynaecomastia is transient. Galactorrhoea is unusual.

The incidence of gynaecomastia in otherwise normal males is quite high. Nuttall (1979) who examined 306 normal men between the ages of 17 and 58 found palpable breast tissue (> 2 cm) in 36 per cent, in 98 per cent of whom it was bilateral. Gynaecomastia is also a common finding in adolescents. In one study in which 1855 boys were examined, gynaecomastia was found in 39 per cent (Nydick et al, 1961).

Classification of causes

Physiological gynaecomastia

This is the most common form and is seen particularly in three age groups: (a) neonatal; (b) adolescent; (c) elderly.

Neonatal breast enlargement is probably the result of placental oestrogens. It is harmless and disappears within a few weeks.

Adolescents with gynaecomastia most commonly present because of the embarrassment they experience when with their peers: sometimes the breasts may be tender. Examination usually shows that the boy has entered puberty but is otherwise normal. Unless the symptom is severe, sudden and persistent there is no requirement for elaborate or expensive investigations. The treatment is expectant in the hope the breast enlargement will regress. If the problem is long-standing and the stress is sufficiently serious, surgical removal of the breast tissue is indicated.

Gynaecomastia in the elderly is also fairly common, being found in about 40 per cent of men over the age of 50 (Williams, 1963). In this study no account was taken of the many possible causes of gynaecomastia, such as drugs or liver disease, so that 40 per cent may be an overestimate. It is therefore essential in dealing with an older man with gynaecomastia to exclude a pathological cause for the disorder.

Pathological gynaecomastia

This may occur in any disorder in which there is an excess of oestrogenic over androgenic activity. Such an excess can result from an increase in the production of oestrogens either by direct secretion, which is rare, or by increased conversion from precursors, particularly the weak androgen, androstenedione. Decreased secretion of androgens, particularly testosterone, from primary or secondary testicular failure may lead to hypogonadism of which gynaecomastia is one component, e.g. Klinefelter's syndrome. Competition for occupation of androgen receptors will, in effect, increase the effective ratio of oestrogens to androgens; for example, the drugs, spironolactone, cyproterone and cimetidine.

It is important to grasp the concept that gynaecomastia is the result of a disturbance of androgen/oestrogen dynamics; this makes it possible to draw up a rational aetiological classification (Wilson et al, 1980):

1. Deficient *production* of testosterone
   Primary testicular failure: anorchia, Klinefelter's syndrome
   Deficits in testosterone synthesis
   Secondary testicular failure: renal failure, cytotoxic drugs (Sherins et al, 1978; Trump et al, 1982)
   Deficient *action* of testosterone
   Androgen resistance syndromes
   Drugs which occupy androgen receptors — spironolactone, digitalis, cimetidine
2. Increased oestrogen production
   Increased secretion
   Increased substrate for peripheral aromatization
   Increased peripheral aromatase
   Administered oestrogen
   Chorionic gonadotrophin

There are still a few patients who develop gynaecomastia for which no reason is apparent, e.g. tricyclic antidepressants, methyldopa.

In this classification most of the causes of gynaecomastia can be appreciated. Attention can be drawn to some specific instances.

Klinefelter's syndrome

About 40 per cent of patients with Klinefelter's syndrome develop gynaecomastia at puberty, and this usually persists into adulthood. Diminished testosterone and increased oestradiol secretion are the major mechanisms for gynaecomastia in these patients. Increased oestradiol secretion may result from the high concentrations of gonadotrophin (LH).

Renal failure

Between 40 and 50 per cent of men with end stage renal

disease on haemodialysis develop gynaecomastia. This probably results from deficient testosterone secretion, although there has been no comprehensive exploration of androgen/oestrogen dynamics in these patients.

Testicular tumours

Many of these tumours produce hCG which stimulates the secretion of both testosterone and oestradiol. This is the reason why gynaecomastia occurs in patients with hCG producing tumours or in the course of treatment with hCG.

Adrenal tumours

While some tumours may secrete oestrogens directly these are unusual. Most frequently the gynaecomastia results from the substantial increases in the secretion of androstenedione which is an important substrate for the conversion to oestrogens in peripheral tissues, particularly adipose tissue.

MALE INFERTILITY

In an infertile couple it is sometimes difficult to decide whether the male is the infertile partner, but probably between 30 and 40 per cent of all marriages which are involuntarily infertile result from male factor infertility.

Men with persistent azoospermia, complete sperm immotility or total teratospermia are clearly infertile. All other men who have motile sperm in their ejaculates are potentially fertile. The point is: what is the potential? We take the view that for each couple, provided there is tubal patency, normal ovulation and no deleterious sperm-mucus interactions, a successful outcome for pregnancy can only be envisaged on a probability basis. The probability is high if the ejaculate always contains more than 20 million sperm/ml, at least 50 per cent of which show good forward active motility, and at least 60 per cent of which have normal morphology. By contrast, the probability is low if the sperm concentrations are rarely greater than 5 million/ml and show low motility (30 per cent or less) and a large number of abnormal forms (more than 50 per cent). In adopting this approach we do not take into account any form of treatment that might be possible, since there are very few treatments that are known to increase fertility in men.

Classification of male infertility

Infertile men can be classified on an aetiological basis, but because there is a large majority of men in whom the cause cannot be defined, we have found it more practical to classify them according to the therapeutic group into which they fall. There are three such groups: (a) specific therapy

possible; (b) no treatment available; (c) treatment unproven or empirical.

The relative proportions of men who fall into these different groups are shown in Table 3.2 and are based on a group of 1100 men whom we have studied over the past 8 years.

Table 3.2 Classification of infertile men according to therapeutic possibilities (N = 1440)

Prevalence of Classes	%
Specific treatment possible	7.7
No treatment possible	14.6
Treatment unproven or empirical	77.7

Recognition of male infertility

In practice the infertile couple usually present to their family physician or gynaecologist. Whoever is the physician of first contact should arrange for at least two semen analyses, which should be carried out in a laboratory with recognized expertise and which undertakes such examinations on a regular basis. Two samples should be requested because of the known variability in semen quality. If both are quite normal, then it is appropriate to direct management toward the female. This decision, however, begs a question.

The normal semen sample

Which semen sample is normal? This question cannot be answered clearly or unequivocally since there is no uniform agreement about the lower limits of normal, as with many other biological indices. Also, it is not possible to be certain that a semen sample, presumed to be normal, is also fertile since at present there is no simple *in vitro* method by which the *in vivo* fertilising capacity of sperm can be reliably measured.

There are, however, several studies from which it is possible to draw some conclusions about the normal semen sample. These conclusions are based on examination of several hundred semen samples from men whose wives were pregnant at the time, or from men of known fertility at the time of vasectomy, and the comparison of these with men presumed to be infertile (MacLeod & Gold 1951a, b, c; Eliasson, 1971; Rehan et al, 1975; Smith et al, 1977). What is clear from these studies is that there is a significant overlap between the sperm concentrations and the total sperm numbers from men known to be fertile and those presumed to be infertile. In MacLeod's study about 5 per cent of men whose wives were pregnant had sperm concentrations of less than 20 million/ml. Most studies agree that sperm motility is the single most important parameter of semen quality and could compensate for reduced sperm numbers. Notwithstanding this opinion, we believe it necessary to assess the collective characteristics of a semen sample. These include:

General appearance. Freshly ejaculated semen is liquid for a brief period and then coagulates. After 20 or 30 minutes the sample becomes liquid again but is quite viscous. Very occasionally liquefaction may not occur and the sperm are unable to achieve normal motility. Abnormalities of viscosity — too liquid or too viscous — may indicate abnormalities of accessory gland function.

Semen volume. This is between 1 and 4 ml in more than 80 per cent of fertile men. Lower or higher volumes may indicate abnormal accessory gland function; lower volumes may also be found in men who are androgen deficient or who have a congenital absence of the vasa and seminal vesicles but may also indicate an incomplete collection, one cause of which may be retrograde ejaculation.

Sperm concentration. This is measured in millions/ml and the lower limit of normal is probably between 15 and 20 million/ml. This figure was put at 100 million/ml nearly 50 years ago. Men with sperm concentrations of 15–20 million/ml are known to take longer to affect conception than men with high sperm counts, but they are not infertile. Low normal sperm concentrations become suspect when accompanied by abnormalities of motility or morphology.

Sperm motility. Although this is a qualitative or semi-quantitative measurement, the assessment of forward progression remains an important characteristic of the semen analysis. There are several ways of assessing motility, but one which is commonly accepted is to assign numerical gradings to motility (no forward progression = 0; poor or weak forward progression = 1; moderate forward progression = 2; excellent forward progression – 3). Normally more than 50 per cent of sperm should show a good or excellent forward progression. This estimate should be based on the assessment of at least 100 sperm in ten randomly selected microscopic fields. If 60 per cent of sperm show good or excellent motility, this should be reported as '60 per cent motility'. We would stress that the report should record as precisely as possible the quality and abnormalities of sperm motility.

The semen sample can be regarded as normal if more than 60 per cent of cells show good or excellent forward progressive motility, and as abnormal if this figure is less than 40 per cent. Intermediate values must be interpreted in conjunction with the sperm concentration and morphology. An ejaculate which has been collected properly and contains only immotile sperm should make the diagnosis of a cilial defect highly likely (Afzelius, 1976).

Sperm morphology. In the stained smear of the ejaculate the normal sperm have oval heads and a single tail piece. Abnormalities of sperm morphology may be found in the head or tail. Sperm heads may be larger or smaller than normal, tapering, amorphous or pyriform. The tail may be coiled, double or fragmented. The ejaculate may contain immature germ cells, spermatocytes or spermatids, leuco-cytes or epithelial cells. The morphological and staining characteristics of all these cells are very clearly presented in a WHO Monograph (Belsey et al, 1980). In fertile men the average proportion of normal sperm is 65–70 per cent, but this number may vary from as low as 50 to as high as 80 per cent. We would regard a sample which contains at least 60 per cent of normal oval forms as being within normal limits. The same man usually shows very little morphological variations between samples, although his sperm may show temporary changes in morphology with intercurrent illness. Normal oval sperm are reduced in number and replaced by tapering or amorphous forms (MacLeod, 1964). Some laboratories have difficulty in distinguishing between spermatids and peroxidase positive leucocytes which are normally less than 1×10^6/ml of ejaculate. The use of the Bryan/Leishman stain is probably the most useful for seminal fluid morphology (Couture et al, 1976).

Sperm Viability. The number of live spermatozoa can be determined by supravital staining. This technique makes it possible to distinguish between immotile but live sperm and those which are dead, and at the same time provides a check on the accuracy of the estimate of motility.

Accessory gland function.

The measurement of fructose in seminal plasma is used to assess seminal vesicle function. The normal range is large: 5–25 mmol/l. A low or absent fructose level indicates either an absence of the seminal vesicles (the vasa are also absent) or obstruction of the seminal vesicle ducts.

Acid phosphatase and zinc in seminal plasma are indices of prostatic function. We do not measure these routinely, and are unaware of evidence that would compel us to do this. At present the rewards in terms of understanding the cause or promoting a cure for infertile men by measuring seminal plasma constituents are not great.

Microbiology

The role of asymptomatic genital tract infection in reducing male fertility has been repeatedly postulated. Several studies have found that fertile males have significantly less non-specific infections than subfertile males (McGowan, 1981; Toth & Lesser, 1981). The presence of bacteria in seminal plasma is an inadequate criterion for the diagnosis of infection since bacteriospermia may be falsely positive due to contamination from the skin or urethra, or it may be falsely negative due to the existence of isolated micro-abscesses. Comhaire et al (1980) have drawn up a list of criteria which in their opinion should be established before the diagnosis of infection is made. It remains to be seen whether these criteria are proven to be reliable indices of infection.

Physical examination

This should be general, but particular attention should be paid to:

1. features of hypogonadism: complete or partial; pubertal development; secondary sexual characteristics; eunuchoid habitus;

2. optic fundi and visual fields;

3. gynaecomastia;

4. penile abnormalities: micropenis, hypospadias or phimosis are not commonly found in patients who present with infertility;

5. testicular size which should be measured objectively with an orchidometer (Prader, 1965). In the normal adult testicular volume should exceed 15 ml. Attention should also be paid to testicular location and consistency;

6. vasa and epididymides. These structures should be examined carefully. Nodularity or irregularities in the epididymides suggest previous infection or congenital cystic changes and raise the question of epididymal duct obstruction or an impairment of the process of sperm maturation. In some men the vasa (and seminal vesicles) may be congenitally absent and this can be detected by careful examination;

7. varicocele. Between 30 and 40 per cent of our patients referred with infertility have a varicocele. The significance of a varicocele is discussed later. A varicocele, which is much more common on the left side, is often not visible and may only be detected as a cough impulse or following a Valsalva manoeuvre when the patient is standing;

8. prostate. This is small in patients with prepubertal androgen deficiency, and may be abnormal in chronic genital tract infection when it can be enlarged, soft and sometimes tender.

Hormonal measurements

The main hormones which have been measured are:
1. Gonadotrophins — FSH and LH.
2. Testosterone.
3. Prolactin.

We had hoped when we were first able to measure these hormones that we may have discovered abnormalities in their concentrations or patterns of secretion which would, when corrected, lead to a restoration of fertility. Although this hope has not been realised, we have come to understand much better the relationship between the seminiferous epithelium, Leydig cells, anterior pituitary and hypothalamus (de Kretser et al, 1972, 1974; Franchimont et al, 1972; van Thiel et al, 1972; Baker et al, 1976).

An important finding is that serum concentrations of FSH are commonly raised in men with disorders of spermatogenesis. In some patients without apparent clinical androgen deficiency, testosterone concentrations may be low and LH levels higher than normal, suggesting that the disorder affects the Leydig cells as well as the seminiferous epithelium. While hyperprolactinaemia is a fairly common cause of infertility in women (Ch. 25) this abnormality is not frequently encountered in men.

FSH

An estimate of serum concentrations of FSH should be made in all men with azoospermia. A high level means that severe testicular damage is the cause of the azoospermia whereas a normal level indicates that obstruction is the likely cause. Low or undetectable levels are found in men with hypopituitarism. The finding of an elevated level of FSH in the serum of a patient with oligospermia indicates

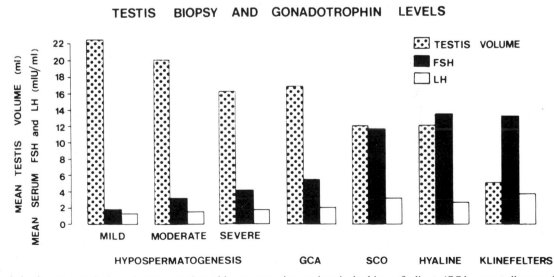

Fig. 3.4 Correlation between testicular volumes, gonadotrophin concentrations and testicular biopsy findings. (GCA: germ cell arrest; SCO : Sertoli cell only; hyaline: tubule hyalinisation)

that the seminiferous epithelium is damaged and the prognosis is poor. However, the concentrations of FSH may be normal in many men with moderate to severe hypospermatogenesis and oligospermia. In a group of infertile men from which those with obstructive azoospermia have been excluded, the levels of FSH are negatively correlated with the degree of damage to the seminiferous epithelium and testicular size (Fig. 3.4).

LH and testosterone

Not much diagnostic help is given by the measurement of these hormones in infertile men. Low values of both hormones may be found in patients with pituitary or hypothalamic disorders; high values for LH and low values for testosterone are seen in Klinefelter's syndrome and in approximately 50 per cent of patients with Sertoli cell only syndrome while high values for both LH and testosterone may be an indication of androgen resistance. The finding of a low value for LH and an increase in testosterone and other androgens would suggest congenital adrenal hyperplasia. The finding of a low value of testosterone is an indication for testosterone replacement.

Prolactin

High levels of prolactin in blood interfere with gonadal function and have been reported to cause moderate to severe oligospermia. Some men have diminished libido and potency as a result of hyperprolactinaemia. In our experience hyperprolactinaemia is an uncommon cause of infertility in men.

Cytogenetic studies

A karyotype should be obtained in all men with azoospermia or severe oligospermia and testicular atrophy. The most common cytogenetic abnormality is the presence of an additional X chromosome in patients with Klinefelter's syndrome. Sometimes more than one additional X chromosome or mosaicism is found. Chromosomal abnormalities are found in between 2 and 3 per cent of infertile men which is approximately five times the frequency found in men presenting with other disorders not associated with infertility (Chandley et al, 1975).

Testicular biopsy

This has been an important diagnostic procedure in the investigation of men with suspected disorders of spermatogenesis. However, with the advent of relatively simple hormone assays, and of the now well known correlation between hormone levels and disorders of spermatogenesis, we now undertake this procedure much less frequently. We believe it should be reserved for patients in whom

obstruction is thought to be present; that is, those men with persistent azoospermia or severe oligospermia with normal testicular size and normal hormonal levels. If surgical relief of obstruction is to be attempted, it is essential to show that spermatogenesis is normal.

Immunological factors

In the evaluation of the infertile couple, consideration must be given to the possible role of antisperm antibodies. The precise indications for undertaking investigations for the presence of such antibodies are not universally agreed. A pragmatic approach currently adopted by the authors is to screen all male partners, and all couples with unexplained (idiopathic) infertility; a useful lead can be provided by a persistently abnormal post-coital test in such couples.

Tests of antisperm antibodies. These may be found in the serum and/or genital tract secretions of both male and female partners (semen or cervical mucus, uterine, oviductal or follicular fluids) and may belong to the IgG, IgA, IgM or the secretory IgA classes (Jones, 1980). The initial screening test may be undertaken on seminal fluid or male serum (Editorial, 1981). For the former, the mixed antiglobulin reaction (Jager et al, 1978) is based on the attachment or not of motile spermatozoa to sensitised sheep red blood cells mixed with semen and antihuman IgG antiserum. The test is over 90 per cent accurate in detecting antisperm antibodies (Hendry & Stedronska, 1980). For the screening of serum, two tests are used by the authors to assess the presence of sperm immobilizins (Isojima et al, 1968, 1972) and of agglutinating antibodies (Friberg, 1974). The more significant of these two is the presence of immobilizins, which are usually accompanied by significant agglutinating antibody titres. The significance of the presence of serum immobilizins or high titre agglutinins can be assessed by the ability of the male partner's sperm to penetrate ovulatory cervical mucus; at the same time, the presence of antibodies in the female can be checked, by using a crossed mucus penetration test, in which both the male partner's and a donor's sperm are tested against the female partner's and a donor's mucus (Morgan et al, 1977). It has been shown that there is a strong negative correlation between antisperm antibody concentrations and the ability of sperm to penetrate mucus, and a good correlation between this ability and fertility (Fjallbrandt, 1968). Refinements to the technique of testing for antibodies to sperm have been described (Haas et al, 1980).

Androgen resistance

Some men with idiopathic oligospermia have been shown to have reduced numbers of androgen receptors in genital skin fibroblasts (Aiman et al, 1979). This is not yet a routine measurement that can easily be made on all men with unexplained oligospermia, so that the prevalence of androgen resistance is not yet known. This disorder is discussed in more detail in Chapter 17.

Fertilising capacity of sperm

A persistent problem in the investigation of infertile men is not having a model in which the fertilising capacity of sperm can be tested. Overstreet et al (1976) have described the use of hamster ova from which the zona pellucida has been removed as a model for testing the fertilising capacity of human sperm *in vitro*. In some hands this test is found to have good specificity and high sensitivity (Stenchever et al, 1982). It is a procedure, however, which is not available in every laboratory or indeed in every country.

The development of procedures for human *in vitro* fertilisation has now provided such a model in which the capacity of human sperm to fertilise human ova can be tested. In preliminary studies, Trounson and his colleagues (personal communication) have shown that sperm from oligospermic men have a lesser capacity to fertilise than sperm from normal men. At present this information is preliminary, but with a more widespread development of *in vitro* fertilisation procedures, we may be able to make better correlations between semen quality and the capacity of human sperm to fertilise *in vitro*.

Management

If male factor infertility is suspected on the basis of one semen sample this must be confirmed by requesting at least another two semen samples taken 3 or 4 weeks apart. This is done because of the known variability in semen quality (Fig. 3.5) and the possibility that a lowered sperm concentration may have resulted from an intercurrent pyrexial illness.

When a man is referred with infertility it is our custom to request that his wife be present at the interview, even though he will be the subject of examination. Infertility, whatever the cause, is the problem of the couple, and we feel that discussing the issues with the couple makes for a better understanding of any treatment that may be involved, and of the possible outcome. It is important to remember that this type of consultation can be quite threatening for a male, who may erroneously perceive that his virility is being questioned. At the initial consultation we try to assess the tension that may exist (frequently because of infertility), other anxieties or sexual difficulties. It is also important to establish the frequency and timing of sexual intercourse, since not all couples are well informed about the timing or recognition of ovulation. We find it helpful to instruct couples about the significance of changes in the secretion of cervical mucus as an indication of ovulation (Billings et al, 1972).

Treatable causes of infertility

In this group of patients specific treatment can be employed with a reasonable chance of producing a normal semen sample. These patients account for between 7 and 8 per cent of all men presenting with infertility.

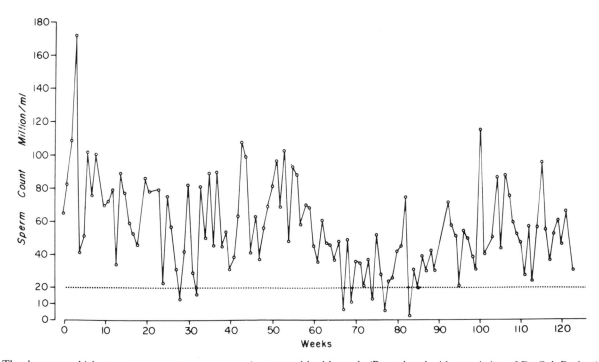

Fig. 3.5 The degree to which sperm concentrations may vary in a normal healthy male (Reproduced with permission of Dr C A Paulsen)

Gonadotrophin deficiency

The classical patient with congenital gonadotrophin deficiency is hypogonadal and eunuchoid and may have a reduced or absent sense of smell — Kallman's syndrome. He may have other congenital anomalies, such as hare lip, cleft palate or cranio-facial asymmetry. These men have a history of delayed puberty for which they may have been treated with testosterone or hCG. This may confuse the diagnosis because the treatment may have resulted in the development of secondary sexual characteristics, and have promoted normal libido and potency — particularly if the treatment is being continued. However, the testicular size is small (less than 4 ml) and the ejaculate contains no sperm.

Gonadotrophin deficiency may also be acquired. This can result from any disorder which destroys anterior pituitary function, most commonly a pituitary or suprasellar tumour or surgery for the removal of such tumours. These patients do not as a rule present with infertility, but if infertility becomes a problem, the diagnosis is usually straightforward; in addition to hypogonadism with impaired libido or potency and testicular atrophy (which varies with the degree of gonadotrophin deficiency), there may be evidence of hypothyroidism or adrenal insufficiency. Azoospermia is usually present.

Treatment is possible in men with hypogonadotrophic hypogonadism; for this reason it is crucial that the condition not be overlooked. Treatment is with gonadotrophins for those patients with pituitary lesions; GnRH may be used for those patients with Kallman's syndrome whose disorder results from a deficiency of LHRH secretion.

There is no standard therapeutic regimen for the use of gonadotrophins. Most patients require treatment with LH and FSH. It is usual to start treatment with LH, given as hCG for about three months in doses of 1500–3000 iu once or twice weekly. This phase of the treatment promotes the development of secondary sexual characteristics, increases testicular size, improves libido and potency and increases the volume of the ejaculate which usually remains azoospermic. The treatment is monitored by attention to these clinical changes as well as by measuring plasma testosterone concentration at 72–96 h after a dose of hCG. If the clinical response is inadequate or the plasma testosterone fails to reach normal levels the dose of hCG should be increased.

Many patients require FSH in addition to hCG to promote complete spermatogenesis. The common FSH preparation is derived from post-menopausal urine; it also contains some LH. The conventional dose is between 75 and 100 iu of FSH three times weekly by intramuscular injection; while this is given hCG is continued. There is frequently a variation between individual responses so that treatment should be monitored by semen analyses at approximately monthly intervals. There is no standard duration of treatment; sperm may appear in the ejaculate within 4–5 months but sometimes this may take up to 18 months.

It is now possible to use LHRH for the treatment of Kallman's syndrome. When it first became available, LHRH was given by intramuscular injection 2 or 3 times each day, and the results were disappointing. The important discovery about this hormone is that it must be given every $1-1\frac{1}{2}$ h in order to increase and maintain gonadotrophin levels. This is best achieved by the use of an infusion pump programmed to deliver the hormone over a 5–10 min period every $1-1\frac{1}{2}$ h. The dose of LHRH required for full stimulation of gonadotrophin secretion is between 5 and 10 μg per dose. Such as system of treatment thus mimics the normal episodic secretion of GnRH.

Since the accumulated experience with this form of treatment is still small, it is not possible to say whether it will be universally successful. One potential problem is the development of antibodies to LHRH; another is the need to wear the infusion pump and indwelling subcutaneous needles.

Obstruction

Patients with obstruction to sperm transport present classically with azoospermia, normal testicular size and normal levels of FSH. The obstruction can be incomplete, in which case there may be severe oligospermia, but normal levels of FSH which, in combination with normal testicular size, may indicate normal spermatogenesis. This is obstructive azoospermia and usually results from obstruction within the epididymides. The lesion is usually bilateral and congenital, with cystic changes in the upper two-thirds of the epididymides; sometimes there may be a history of epididymo-orchitis which may result from gonorrhoea, urinary tract sepsis or occasionally tuberculosis. Some patients with obstructive azoospermia may have congenital absence of the vasa and seminal vesicles. Absence of the vas, seminal vesicles and part of the epididymis is a frequent finding in patients with cystic fibrosis. Between 40 and 50 per cent of patients with obstructive azoospermia have a history of chronic sino-pulmonary disease, including bronchiectasis (Holsclaw, 1969; Eliasson et al, 1977).

The diagnostic criteria for obstructive azoospermia have been mentioned. In about half these patients there is nothing in the history to indicate a cause. In patients with epididymal obstruction the heads of the epididymides may be enlarged or nodular, and on occasions tender. Congenital absence of the vasa should be recognised on clinical examination and confirmed by the absence of fructose in the semen.

The classical operative procedure is to bypass the obstruction by vasoepididymostomy in which the vas and epididymis are anastomosed side to side. The advent of microsurgical techniques has enabled end to end rather than side to side anastomoses to be performed, but it is too early to evaluate whether such techniques will improve the success rates which have generally been poor. Although postoperative patency (sperm in the ejaculate) has been reported in up to 75 per cent of patients, the overall success rate (pregnancy) has been much lower — probably in the order of 5 to 10 per cent. For this reason the results of treatment of men with obstructive azoospermia must be regarded as discouraging and patients should be advised accordingly.

Other hormonal abnormalities

These are quite unusual, but if recognised, infertility may be successfully treated.

Hyperprolactinaemia

While this condition is a well recognised cause of secondary amenorrhoea, anovulation and infertility in women (Ch. 25) it is not in our experience a common cause of infertility in men. From a cohort of more than 100 infertile men with unexplained oligospermia we found marginally raised concentrations of prolactin in two. In none was there the gross elevation of prolactin that is frequently found in hyperprolactinaemic women. Treatment of men with marginal elevations of prolactin concentration with bromocriptine did not produce significant improvements in semen quality. We are thus unable to confirm the results described by Segal et al (1976) and Saidi et al (1977).

Congenital adrenal hyperplasia

Boys with this condition are usually recognized and treated in early childhood. Most of those in whom the disease is mild or unrecognized enter puberty and become fertile; there is, however, a small group in whom adrenal androgen production suppresses pituitary gonadotrophin secretion and thus inhibits development of the seminiferous epithelium and Leydig cells. These patients are normally virilised, may be short and stocky in build, have small underdeveloped testes, normal or high levels of testosterone and low gonadotrophins. Plasma levels of 17α-hydroxyprogesterone are high. Treatment with corticosteroids can suppress adrenal androgen production and allow normal testicular development (Urban et al, 1978; Wischusen et al, 1980).

Irreversible semen abnormalities

About 15 per cent of our patients have disorders of spermatogenesis for which no treatment is possible. In many patients the immediate cause of the disorder is unknown, while in others an association can be recognised, e.g. cryptorchidism or cytotoxic drugs. Patients who present with

irreversible disorders may in addition be androgen deficient; if this is the case replacement therapy is indicated. All couples will require counselling as to other alternatives which may exist in particular, artificial insemination or adoption.

Klinefelter's syndrome

These men may present either because of infertility or with an abnormality of sexual development or function which may be incomplete pubertal development, gynaecomastia, poor libido or reduced potency. Commonly the patient has eunuchoidal proportions and is poorly virilised with a feminine distribution of body hair, gynaecomastia and underdeveloped genitalia. Many patients with Klinefelter's syndrome are subnormal in intelligence, sometimes overtly mentally disturbed. The testes are firm and small, usually less than 6 ml in volume. By no means all patients with Klinefelter's syndrome show obvious signs of androgen deficiency and for this reason may not always be recognised. We would stress that any patient who presents with azoospermia and small testes should be suspected of having Klinefelter's syndrome; this may be confirmed by finding high levels of FSH and LH in blood and an additional X-chromosome in the karyotype. Levels of testosterone are usually lower than normal (Paulsen et al, 1968; Wang et al, 1975). Testicular biopsy, which is not required for diagnosis, shows hyalinised tubules surrounded by fibrous tissue and Leydig cells which have the appearance of hyperplasia, although their total volume is normal or subnormal.

Patients with Klinefelter's syndrome may present atypical features; in some the phenotype is close to normal. Sperm have been found in the ejaculates of some patients which is consistent with the finding of the preservation of occasional tubules. These findings probably reflect the degrees of mosaicism which may be found, such as 46XY/47XXY and do not alter the hopeless outlook for fertility in these patients (for review, see Skakkebaek, 1981).

No treatment is available to restore fertility in these patients. If the patient has symptoms of androgen deficiency, he should be given treatment with androgens. We usually use testosterone enanthate in doses of 200–250 mg by intramuscular injection every 2 or 3 weeks. The size and frequency of the dose will vary from patient to patient, and are best determined by the response in the individual patient.

Other chromosomal abnormalities

Infertility may result from other chromosomal abnormalities. Some men with an additional Y chromosome have been shown to have abnormal spermatogenesis. These men have normal sexual function, normal secondary sex characteristics and normal or slightly reduced testicular size. There are no characteristic histological changes but arrest of spermatogenesis at the primary spermatocyte stage or tubules that contain only Sertoli cells have been found. In some patients the semen sample is normal but in others there is mild to severe oligospermia or azoospermia with elevated serum levels of FSH. These patients are not androgen deficient.

Men with autosomal translocations may have abnormal spermatogenesis, reduced sperm quality and infertility. Kjessler (1973) and Chandley et al (1975) have shown that men with these abnormalities are found more commonly in an infertile population. However, these abnormalities are not common causes of infertility. Abnormalities in meiotic chromosomes have also been found in men with severe oligospermia, but most evidence suggests that meiotic chromosome abnormalities are not common, and in patients with a normal karyotype are not important factors in their infertility.

We do not believe that detailed chromosomal studies are warranted in all men with severe oligo- or azoospermia. From a strictly practical point of view, there is nothing that can be achieved therapeutically when abnormalities are found.

Germ cell aplasia

In this disorder the germ cells are not developed and the tubule is lined with Sertoli cells. This can result from irradiation or treatment with cytotoxic drugs, but in most patients there is no such history and the cause is unknown. The semen sample shows azoospermia. The testes are usually less than 15 ml in volume and the serum levels of FSH are elevated.

Germ cell arrest

The development of the germinal epithelium is arrested at a particular stage of development, e.g. at the primary spermatocyte or late spermatid stage. The cause is unknown. The semen sample may show profound oligospermia with increased numbers of abnormal (immature) forms. Some degree of testicular atrophy is the rule and serum FSH levels may be increased. Sometimes patients with germ cell arrest have normal or near normal testicular size, azoospermia and normal levels of FSH and may not be easily distinguished from those with obstructive azoospermia.

The testicular histology, in addition to the characteristic changes in the germ cells, may show some hyalinisation of tubules, and a reduction in tubule diameter. Although the Leydig cells appear normal in many patients with germ cell aplasia the plasma levels of testosterone are lower than normal and the response to hCG is also blunted. It is not possible to say whether impaired Leydig cell function is a cause or effect of these lesions, but is probably the latter.

Some of these patients may be examples of androgen resistance syndromes.

There is no treatment to restore fertility in this group of patients. Because the disorder of spermatogenesis is not uniformly distributed throughout all tubules, particularly in patients with germ cell arrest, spermatogenesis may be progressing in some and pregnancy may be achieved in a few couples. For this reason one should be hesitant in describing the prognosis for fertility as 'hopeless' or 'impossible', but the greatly lessened chances of pregnancy should be made clear to the couple.

Androgen receptor deficiency

A severe deficiency of androgen receptors leads to the syndrome of complete or incomplete testicular feminisation in which genotypic (46XY) males differentiate as females. Partial defects are associated with less severe abnormalities, such as Reifenstein's syndrome. It is only recently that androgen receptor deficiency has been recognised as a cause of male infertility (Aiman et al, 1979).

The disorder was first demonstrated in three unrelated men who presented with idiopathic infertility; two were azoospermic and one had severe oligospermia. None had any genital abnormality. The disorder appears to have been suspected because all men had higher than normal levels of testosterone while high levels of LH were found in two of them. Androgen insensitivity was demonstrated in genital skin fibroblasts in which specific high affinity binding capacity for dihydrotestosterone was less than a half that found in normal men, and comparable to that found in patients with Reifenstein's syndrome.

Following this initial report, Aiman & Griffin (1982) have investigated the frequency of androgen insensitivity as a cause of male infertility by measuring androgen receptor binding in genital skin fibroblasts in a group of men with azoospermia or oligospermia (1–17 million sperm/ml) for which there was no known cause and compared these values with those of a similar sized group of men either with azoospermia or oligospermia for which the cause was known. They showed that about two-thirds of the men with idiopathic azoospermia and one-quarter of those with oligospermia had significantly reduced dihydrotestosterone binding. Thus, the overall prevalence of androgen receptor deficiency in this group is about 40 per cent. In these patients they were unable to show the significantly high levels of LH and testosterone found in the three index patients; however, when the product, testosterone × LH, was calculated this was significantly higher than normal only in some men with idiopathic azoospermia, so that this proved to be an unhelpful diagnostic criterion. As might be expected, FSH levels were higher than in normal men and thus were not of value in recognising the syndrome. Testicular biopsies were performed on five of these men with azoospermia and androgen receptor deficiency; in three the picture was that of Sertoli cell only and in the other two spermatogenesis was arrested at the spermatid stage.

Cryptorchidism

A history of an abnormality of testicular descent is present in about 10 per cent of infertile men. It is difficult to know what proportion of men with a history of testicular maldescent remain infertile. Estimates have varied between 30 and 80 per cent. Semen samples in men with a history of cryptorchidism may show azoospermia, oligospermia or may be completely normal. There is no specific treatment for those patients with poor semen quality. Usually such patients have moderate to severe oligospermia, testicular atrophy (sometimes bilateral even with a history of unilateral cryptorchidism) and an increase in the levels of serum FSH. This reflects damage to the seminiferous epithelium which may be seen as germ cell aplasia or arrest, or severe hypospermatogenesis with a reduction in tubule diameter. Sometimes there is extensive tubule hyalinisation.

It is not known whether these abnormalities can be prevented. However, it is believed that the longer the testis remains outside the scrotum the more extensive the ultimate damage will be, and for this reason procedures to correct the maldescent should be implemented at least before the age of 2 years when ultrastructural changes can be recognised in the spermatogonia of the cryptorchid testis (Hadziselimovic et al, 1975). The question is: which is the best procedure? For those whose testes are outside the normal line of descent the appropriate treatment is surgical. A non-surgical approach can be used in those children whose testes are arrested in the normal line of descent. Until recently this has been a period of treatment with hCG, extending usually over 6–10 weeks. More recently some encouraging successes have been reported using LHRH (Illig et al, 1977; Keogh et al, 1982). Those have been achieved either by the intranasal route or by pulsatile administration of LHRH in the same way as has been used in the treatment of men with gonadotrophin deficiency. On the whole the young children tolerate the infusion pump, and the intermittent infusion quite well for the 4 to 6 weeks needed to bring about testicular descent. At present we do not know whether this form of treatment will provide a better outcome for fertility than previous treatments.

Other factors which affect spermatogenesis

Varicocele

Although Tulloch is usually credited with the first description of a direct association between varicocele and infertility, prior to his report others had suggested that an improvement in semen quality and fertility potential might be expected after varicocele ligation (Macomber & Sanders 1929; Tulloch 1952 for review, see Greenberg, 1977). At present there is still debate as to whether varicocele is a factor in infertility and whether treatment (high ligation) significantly improves fertility. We believe that claims made about varicocele as a cause of infertility remain unproven. In one prospective randomised trial in which 51 men had varicocele ligation and 45 served as controls, over follow-up periods of 3 to 6 years there was no significant improvement in semen quality and the pregnancy rate was lower in the couples in which the husband had been subjected to varicocele ligation (Nilsson et al, 1979).

Varicocele is a dilatation of veins in the scrotum; nearly all, if not all, the dilated veins are tributaries of the internal spermatic vein which can communicate with the cremasteric, vasal and other veins in the region. The cause of the dilatation is valvular incompetence in the internal spermatic vein. The lesion is predominantly one of the left internal spermatic vein (80–85 per cent). Bilateral varicoceles are found in 10–15 per cent, and right sided varicoceles in less than 5 per cent of patients with varicoceles. The reason for the much higher incidence of left sided varicoceles is not known. Theories about this and the development of varicocele have been reviewed by Verstoppen & Steeno (1977).

The diagnosis of varicocele can be made by seeing or feeling the dilated veins beneath the scrotal skin and around the testes; however, not all varicoceles are so easily detected and the condition may only be excluded if there is no venous impulse after coughing or a Valsalva manoeuvre when the patient is standing. The testis on the side of the varicocele is frequently smaller. Using these criteria a varicocele can be found in up to 39 per cent of infertile men (Dubin & Amelar, 1971), although others have reported a lesser prevalence than this. Hendry found varicocele to be present in 21 per cent of infertile men (Hendry et al, 1973). Our own figures closely approximate those of Dubin & Amelar. The incidence of varicocele in the general community is between 10 and 15 per cent (Steeno et al, 1976).

If the hypothesis that a varicocele and infertility have a cause and effect relationship, it is germane to explore the question: how does varicocele cause infertility? Why should an abnormality that is predominantly unilateral cause infertility? Hypotheses such as increased testicular temperature, hypoxia, altered steroid hormone or catecholamine concentrations or the reflux of toxins down the spermatic vein have all been postulated but are unproven as a cause of varicocele (Comhaire & Vermeulen, 1974; Verstoppen & Steeno, 1977; Caldamone et al 1980). Saypol et al (1981) created varicocele models in rats and dogs which caused a dilatation of the spermatic vein. They showed that blood flow was increased in the experimental testis, the core temperature of which was cooled by 1.5–2.0°C. They also showed histological lesions in the affected testis similar to those found in men with varicocele. Cameron et al (1980) described damage to Sertoli cells leading to spermatogenic disruption and sloughing which was often bilateral. We are unaware of any description of changes following ligation. In summary, there seems to be no convincing evidence about how a varicocele causes impaired fertility.

There is a wide range of semen quality in men with varicocele; a few patients may have azoospermia while in others the semen quality may appear perfectly normal. MacLeod described what he termed the "varicocele effect" which is the triad of depressed sperm count, poor sperm motility and an increased number of abnormal sperm in the ejaculate. He applied his motility index, a figure derived from the product of the numbers of motile sperm and the quality of motility (lower limit of normal 120) to a group of patients with varicocele, and found values that were consistently below normal in 92 per cent of patients. He also found that there was a reduction in the number of normal sperm with oval heads and an increase in the numbers of sperm with tapered heads (MacLeod, 1969). Many of our patients with varicocele have reduced sperm concentration and impaired motility, but we are not convinced that there is a classical varicocele effect.

The most significant question is: does a varicocele cause infertility? Those who support the proposition rely on a series of uncontrolled trials in which they note improvements in semen quality in 50–60 per cent and pregnancy rates in between 40 and 50 per cent of patients (Dubin & Amelar, 1971; Brown, 1976; Fernando et al, 1976; McFadden & Mehan, 1978; Rodriguez-Rigau et al, 1978). These reports suffer from the defect that none are prospective or controlled trials in which patients have been randomised into treatment and non-treatment groups, and subsequent pregnancy rates compared. In analysing the results and comparing pregnancy rates or the percentage of wives pregnant, none has taken into account the extent of exposure to pregnancy. One way of doing this is by using a life table analysis and the logrank test as a measure of significance (Peto et al, 1977). We have used this approach in a retrospective analysis of a group of patients with varicocele. The results are shown in Table 3.3. In the

ligated group there appears to be a much higher pregnancy rate than in the non-ligated group. The fact that this is not significant is because the life table analysis and the logrank test take into account the duration of exposure to pregnancy, that is the length of follow-up. This study suffers in that it is retrospective, non-randomised and uncontrolled. Using the same type of analysis in a group of patients with known gradations in varicocele size we were able to compare the pregnancy rates in these groups with those in the wives of men without varicocele. Here there is a significant difference between those with and without a varicocele; further analysis of the varicocele data shows that pregnancy rates are higher in the wives of men with larger varicoceles. We interpret from these studies that an association between varicocele and infertility remains unproven. There are other studies that support this view. Thus, Uehling (1968) examined 776 healthy army reservists and found a non-significant increase in the number of pregnancies in the wives of men with varicocele. Rodriguez-Rigau et al (1978) also found no significant difference in the pregnancy rates in the wives of men with or without varicocele. We would stress that these were non-randomised and uncontrolled studies.

It seems generally agreed that if a varicocele is to be ligated, the high ligation technique described by Palomo (1949) is the most favoured procedure. At present, however, there is no evidence that this or any other surgical treatment is clearly established to restore fertility in men with varicocele.

Infection

Acute infections with epidsodes of orchitis, epididymo-orchitis, seminal vesiculitis or prostatitis can lead to infertility. Infections of this type can produce significant testicular damage or cause obstruction in the ducts along which sperm are normally transported. When a patient presents with infertility with oligo- or azoospermia and such a history the diagnosis is usually evident and treatment should be directed to curing the acute infection and preventing further infections. The outlook for fertility will depend upon the degree of damage that is already present.

Patients with such a history are not commonly encountered. More often we are concerned about the patient who may have chronic genital tract infection. At present we are uncertain about the significance of chronic genital tract infection as a cause of abnormalities of semen quality and infertility. Some claim that occult infection can be found in 40 per cent of infertile men (Eliasson, 1976) while others attribute infertility to chronic genital tract infection in less than 10 per cent. We find it difficult to resolve which of these two figures is correct but believe that Eliasson's figure is an overestimate.

The recognition of men with chronic genital tract infection is often difficult since symptoms and signs may be

Table 3.3 Logrank test of pregnancy rates in wives of men with varicocele. Patients with azoospermia, persistent anovulation or bilateral tubal obstruction were excluded. The extent of exposure to pregnancy was calculated from the number of patients followed in each month after their first visit to the clinic (non-ligated) or the start of treatment (ligated). There is no significant difference in the pregnancy rates between groups ($P > 0.2$)

Group	Number of patients	Number of pregnancies (O)	Expected pregnancies (E)	Relative pregnancy rate (O/E)
Not ligated	306	57	53.41	1.07
Ligated	227	75	78.59	0.95

absent and even when present they may be neither characteristic nor distinctive. The diagnosis must be entertained if the patient has a history of an acute infection with urethritis, prostatitis or epididymo-orchitis, or there is a history of dysuria, low back pain or pain on ejaculation. Examination of the prostate may show evidence of infection — softness, irregularity or tenderness. Expressed prostatic fluid can be examined for leucocytes and organisms but the value of this examination has not been substantiated.

Chronic genital tract infection may be suspected from the semen sample. The sperm concentration may be normal but the sperm motility may be remarkably reduced and sperm agglutination may be present. The number of leucocytes which are normally found in the semen may be increased. Peroxidase positive cells should not exceed 1 million/ml. An increased number of leucocytes particularly polymorphs points to the diagnosis of infection; however, increased numbers of leucocytes do not occur in all men with genital tract infection and are not necessarily correlated with the presence of pathogenic organisms (Ulstein et al, 1976). Examination of expressed prostatic secretions for leucocytes as advocated by Johannisson & Eliasson (1978) may contribute to the diagnosis, although we have not found it to be of assistance in detecting patients who responded to treatment (Baker et al, 1979). We also find that cultures of semen and expressed prostatic fluid to be of little help in diagnosis or in indicating treatment. We were unable to discover any relationship between the type or number of organisms, the clinical features or the outcome of treatment. Ulstein et al (1976) have reported similar conclusions.

We do not believe that full microbiological studies of mid-stream urine or expressed prostatic secretions are indicated on men with idiopathic oligospermia or with isolated motility defects. Such studies may be warranted in men who have persistently high levels of leucocytes in their semen, or who have an unequivocal history of genital tract infection. It is important to remember that undiluted seminal plasma can inhibit the growth of some bacteria (Comhaire et al, 1980).

If treatment with antibacterial drugs is to be undertaken, it is essential to use drugs which enter the secretions and tissues of the genital tract. These drugs include erythromycin, demethylchlortetracycline and trimethoprin-sulphamethoxazole combinations. Some antibacterial agents do not enter the tissues of the genital tract while others, e.g. nitrofurantoin, depress spermatogenesis.

Immunological infertility

The management of immunologically based male infertility must remain empirical. There have been several reports of the successful use of high dose corticosteroids for the treatment of men with sperm antibodies (Shulman et al, 1978; Hendry et al, 1979). As far as we are aware there have been no controlled trials — prospective, randomised and double-blind — that unequivocally demonstrate the benefits of this therapy, which is not without the risk of potentially serious side-effects.

Cytotoxic agents

Drugs used in the treatment of cancer produce a variety of toxic effects on normal cells. Most often these are on self-regenerating populations such as the bone marrow, skin or gastro-intestinal tract where the toxic effects may result in florid symptoms. Less attention has been paid to effects on the gonads because symptoms are absent or minimal and the effects are not life-threatening. In the earlier days of cancer chemotherapy the main concern was for survival and not reproductive potential, but today substantial achievements have been made in long-term survival so that future reproductive ability becomes a much more important issue.

The cellular changes found in the testes are usually independent of the agent used but related to the total dose. The basic lesion is depletion of germ cells, so that a common finding is a tubule devoid of germ cells lined only by Sertoli cells. The tubules are atrophic and there may be some peritubular fibrosis. Leydig cells usually appear normal, but some loss of Leydig cell function may be present. These changes are reflected by a decrease in testicular volume and an increase in the serum concentrations of FSH (Schilsky et al, 1980).

Precise statements cannot be made about the doses of individual or combined anticancer drugs which affect spermatogenesis since there are insufficient controlled prospective studies. Therapy with the alkylating agents chlorambucil or cyclophosphamide can lead to azoospermia which is usually reversible. Treatment with up to 400 mg of chlorambucil produces severe oligospermia; larger doses commonly lead to azoospermia which is reversible after 24–48 months. Azoospermia is common following treatment with more than 6 or 7 g of cyclophosphamide, but recovery is usual and takes place within 15–40 months of stopping treatment (Fairley et al, 1972).

Combination chemotherapy, particularly with those regimens that contain alkylating agents or procarbazine can have severe effects on spermatogenesis. About 80 per cent of men treated with mechlorethamine, vincristine, procarbazine and prednisolone (MOPP) or cyclophosphamide, vincristine and prednisolone (CVP) develop azoospermia or severe oligospermia. A longer period of infertility with azoospermia results more often with combination agents than with single agents.

At present there is only limited information about the short- and long-term effects of the newer agents such as bleomycin and cisplatin. Enough is known about them and other agents to consider storing sperm for any young man who wants children and who faces the prospect of a period of cancer chemotherapy. The success rate of subsequent artificial insemination is good and the offer of cryopreservation should be made provided the seminal quality is adequate. Abnormalities of gonadal function may be present in men with Hodgkin's disease prior to any treatment with cytotoxic agents. Vigersky et al (1982) found decreased sperm counts in 40 per cent and motility defects in 60 per cent of a group of men with Hodgkin's disease. They found a similar prevalence of motility defects in men with other cancers. A complex series of hormonal changes which suggest a combined pituitary and gonadal disorder were also present in these patients. Similar changes have been reported by Chapman et al (1981). Glode et al (1981) have reported that in mice the seminiferous epithelium can be protected from cyclophosphamide by the concurrent administration of a synthetic GnRH analogue, [D-leu^6]-des-Gly-NH$_2$^{10} ethylamide. If the same effect can be shown in man for other agents as well as cyclophosphamide this could be of potential benefit in preventing serious testicular damage.

Germ cell damage can also result in patients receiving irradiation for cancer but screening procedures should afford protection for most subjects; it is of interest to note that testicular damage can occur in patients with thyroid cancer treated with ^{131}I. The damage appears to be dose-related; with 50 mCi there is discernible testicular damage with elevation of serum FSH but at 100 mCi there may be severe but reversible impairment of spermatogenesis with oligo-or azoospermia (Handelsman & Turtle, 1982)

Alcohol

The effects of acute and chronic alcohol ingestion on virility is generally well appreciated. The onset of impotence occurs not infrequently in the context of intoxication with alcohol. The problem of impotence is discussed elsewhere in this chapter. It has not always been appreciated that infertility may also be a feature of chronic alcoholism and that alcohol is a general tissue toxin affecting not only the liver but other tissues and organs including the testes, hypothalamus and pituitary.

In 70 to 80 per cent of chronic alcoholics with testicular atrophy there is both reproductive and Leydig cell failure. Testicular histology shows atrophy of the seminiferous tubules and loss of the mature germ cells, which are reflected in the semen by reduced numbers of sperm, decreased motility and an increased number of abnormal forms.

It was once thought that the testicular atrophy, commonly seen in chronic alcoholics, was the result of the associated liver disease but recent studies have shown that alcohol can affect the testis directly. The testosterone concentration in plasma has been shown to fall to 20 per cent of control values in normal non-alcoholic male volunteers within a few hours of ingesting sufficient alcohol to cause a hangover (Ylikahri et al, 1974). None of these subjects had liver disease so we must conclude that these changes are the result of a direct effect on the testis. Van Thiel et at (1975) induced testicular damage in rats with alcohol. When rats are fed on a diet in which alcohol accounts for 36 per cent of the caloric intake there is atrophy of the germinal epithelium and of androgen sensitive tissues, and a decrease in the concentration of plasma testosterone. No changes are found in control rats which received a diet in which sugar was substituted for alcohol (for review, see Van Thiel & Lester, 1979).

The effects of alcohol on virility and fertility are not confined to the testis. There is evidence of depression of pituitary and hypothalamic function in chronic alcoholics. Thus when normal volunteers are fed alcohol there is a reduction in both the frequency and amplitude of the episodes of gonadotrophin secretion (Gordon & Southren, 1977). Another effect is probably that of oestrogens, particularly oestrone, which are produced in excess in patients with alcoholic liver disease, particularly by the interconversion of androstenedione to oestrone.

In a series of 710 men who were not sterile (that is, not azoospermic) and whose wives were considered to be normal, we found that 27 (3.8 per cent) had a history of chronic alcoholic excess. Pregnancies occurred in the wives of five of these patients while the remainder (22) were barren. We used a life table method to analyse this data which failed to show a significant effect of alcohol.

Cigarette smoking

An association between cigarette smoking and an increased number of morphological abnormalities in sperm has been suggested by at least two studies (Evans et al, 1981; Shaarawy & Mahmoud, 1982). However, there is no evidence of which we are aware that shows a direct association between cigarette smoking and infertility.

Other drugs

A number of chemicals apart from hormones, alcohol and cytotoxic drugs have been shown to affect sperm production. One drug used for the treatment of ulcerative colitis, sulphasalazine, has been reported on numerous occasions to be associated with oligospermia which disappears once the drug has been withdrawn. One report describes oligospermia in 15 out of 21 patients; in another three patients there were other abnormalities (Birnie et al, 1981; Drife, 1982). The nature of the effect is not known. Withdrawal of the drug is followed by an improvement in semen quality.

There are other drugs which are believed to cause infertility in men but there are few satisfactory studies to prove this. Nitrofurantoin, reserpine, amoebicides and antimalarials have all been incriminated, as has the agricultural nematocide 1,2-dibrom-3-chloropropane; men working in this industry have been shown to have a higher prevalence of infertility, which is reversible.

Idiopathic infertility: empirical treatments

The man who is most commonly encountered and investigated for infertility is one who has persistent oligospermia, an increased number of abnormal forms of sperm and reduced sperm motility. None of the possible causes already referred to can be found for his disorder. Over the past 40 years or more substantial numbers of empirical treatments have been proposed for these men. These treatments have included :

Testosterone 'rebound'	Antioestrogens
Gonadotrophins	Mesterolone
Corticosteroids	Scrotal cooling
Thyroxine	Bromocriptine
GnRH	Kallikrein

Each of these treatments has their staunch advocates but none has been shown to be successful by a controlled trial which we believe should be prospective, randomised and double blind. Comments may be made about a few of these treatments.

Testosterone rebound has been used for 30 years as an empirical form of treatment. The rationale is to suppress gonadotrophin secretion and allow spermatogenesis to cease so that when the treatment is stopped the return of spermatogenesis occurs with an increased sperm production (Rowley & Heller, 1972; Lamensdorf et al, 1975). We have not found this to occur nor has a controlled trial been done to show increased pregnancy rates.

Antioestrogens such as clomiphene or cis-clomiphene citrate and tamoxifen have been used to treat men with idiopathic oligospermia. These agents, by contrast with testosterone, stimulate gonadotrophin secretion. All the alleged successes with this type of therapy have been reported from uncontrolled trials (Reyes & Faiman, 1974; Paulson, 1977; Vermeulen & Comhaire, 1978).

Gonadotrophins. We had hoped that with the availability of relatively pure forms of human gonadotrophin we would be able to identify a group of men with idiopathic oligospermia who would respond to this treatment. There have been some reports that men with persistently low sperm motility benefit from treatment with human chorionic gonadotrophin (Futterweit & Sobrero, 1968; Misarule et al, 1969). These were uncontrolled trials and, as far as we are aware, have not been confirmed.

Treatment of men with idiopathic oligospermia with FSH and hCG has also been advocated. Usually the numbers of men who have been treated have been quite small, and a variety of regimens has been used (Rosemberg, 1976). On the basis of available reports we find no convincing evidence that gonadotrophins are indicated for

men with infertility other than for those who are clearly gonadotrophin deficient.

Is there any form of treatment for these patients? We believe at present that any claim made about the superiority of one form of empirical treatment over another cannot be substantiated. We have analysed the effects of some of these treatments in men with idiopathic oligospermia by life table analysis, and have used the logrank test to test significance. The results of this analysis are shown in Table 3.4.

Table 3.4 Results of medical treatment of infertile men. Logrank test of pregnancy rates in wives of men who had been treated with the drugs specified in the table or who had received no treatment. The extent of exposure to pregnancy was calculated from the number of patients followed in each month after their first visit to the clinic or the start of treatment. There is no significant difference between the treatment groups (P > 0.1)

Treatment	No. of courses	No. of pregnancies (O)	Extent of exposure to pregnancy (E)	Relative pregnancy rate (O/E)
Antibiotics	95	25	17.56	1.42
Bromocriptine	13	3	2.94	1.02
Clomiphene	50	5	9.94	0.50
hCG	10	2	2.01	1.0
Mesterolone	49	7	12.06	0.58
T Rebound	33	6	7.38	0.81
None	583	102	98.11	1.04

This analysis shows that in this particular group of patients none of the empirical treatments was more effective, as judged by a subsequent pregnancy, than another, nor more effective than no treatment. We would emphasise that this study was neither prospective nor randomised, nor was it conducted on a double blind basis, which we believe will be the only way in which a particular form of treatment can ultimately be shown to be efficacious. Unless a treatment is discovered which has a dramatic effect, trials to show efficacy of treatment will be difficult to conduct, and will need large numbers of patients. For this reason it is imperative that basic research into the causes of idiopathic infertility should proceed along with the development of drugs that can be used to treat men with idiopathic infertility successfully.

IMPOTENCE

The inability of a male to achieve and maintain an erection of adequate quality to enable successful vaginal penetration of a normal female is termed sexual impotence. It must be differentiated from premature ejaculation which in some instances is of such severity that ejaculation occurs before or immediately after vaginal penetration.

Classification

Some men have never been able to achieve and maintain an erection for satisfactory sexual intercourse and are categorised as having primary impotence. This is very much less common than secondary impotence where the erectile tissues fail after a period of successful sexual activity. An alternative classification of impotence is based on aetiology, the term organic impotence being used to denote a pathophysiological basis as opposed to the remainder who are classed as functional or psychogenic impotence. However, a psychological element is often found in those men in whom erectile failure is based on organic factors. The extent of the psychological component in such men is dependent to a degree on the personality of the man but also on the attitude, demands and understanding of his sexual partner.

Incidence

Occasional episodes of impotence are not uncommon and may be associated with tiredness, short-term illness or mental stress. They usually do not require medical help. However, if the ability to achieve an erection fails at more than 25 per cent of opportunities then the diagnosis of secondary impotence should be made and followed by investigation and treatment. There is evidence from a number of studies that the incidence of impotence increases with age such that 65 per cent of the men over 60 years are affected (Baker et al, 1976b). However, the groups of elderly men surveyed in some of these studies may not be representative of the entire population of this age group.

Physiology of erection

The physiological basis for an erection is the engorgement of the vascular spaces of the corpora cavernosa of the penis with blood. The accumulation results from arteriolar dilatation of the internal pudendal arterial system dependent on parasympathetic fibres from the sacral segments of the spinal cord (S2,3,4). The inflow exceeds the venous drainage thereby leading to vascular engorgement (for review, see Weiss, 1972). The sacral reflex is activated by local stimuli to the penis, from interoceptive input (e.g. distension of the bladder) of from higher centre inputs resulting from auditory, visual, gustatory, tactile or imaginative stimuli. The descending pathways controlling the sacral reflex probably run in the lateral columns and some outflow may occur through the thoraco-lumbar sympathetic system. Thus individuals who have local disorders involving the sacral segments may be able to obtain an erection in response to psychogenic stimuli. Alternatively lesions of the spinal cord above the sacral segments disrupt the erectile response to psychogenic stimuli but do not prevent reflex erections in response to local stimulation.

Aetiological factors

It is important that a thorough evaluation of the factors responsible for an erection should be assessed to determine if malfunction is attributable to any single factor.

Vascular

Since distension of the corpora cavernosa is dependent on blood flow, atherosclerotic disease may play a part in impotence. Erectile failure may occur in conjunction with vascular disease of the aortic or iliac system but it is as yet unclear what influence obstruction to flow in the more minor branches of this system might cause.

Neurological

Disruption of the neural connections mediating the erection reflex will result in impotence. Neuropathic degeneration of the autonomic fibres occurs in diabetes and may result in impotence in such men. Similarly, surgical destruction of the autonomic nerve plexuses following radical prostatectomy, abdomino-perineal resection of the rectum or aortico-iliac vascular surgery may result in impotence. Clearly spinal cord lesions above the sacral segments will interfere with higher centre influence on the erectile reflex area but will not prevent erections occurring as part of local reflex stimulation.

Endocrine

An adequate supply of testosterone facilitates the ability of a male to have an erection. The specific neural mechanisms which enable testosterone to potentiate arousal by erotic stimuli are still unknown but deficiency of testosterone frequently results in loss of libido and potency. Some men are able to obtain and maintain erections in the face of testosterone deficiency but impotence frequently accompanies testicular disorders associated with impaired testosterone secretion. This may result from primary lesions of the testis such as torsion, Klinefelter's syndrome or unsuccessfully treated cryptorchidism. Alternatively the androgen deficiency may be secondary to hypothalamo-hypophysial disorders causing lowered LH secretion (e.g. Kallman's syndrome) or from hyperprolactinaemia. The latter, by some unknown mechanism impairs androgen secretion by the Leydig cells (Thorner et al, 1977).

There is also evidence to indicate that the total and free testosterone levels decline with advancing age probably through testicular mechanisms since LH levels rise (Baker et al, 1976b). This may be one of the responsible mechanisms for the greater prevalence of impotence with increasing age.

Psychogenic

The erectile response of an individual to erotic stimulation depends on personality and physical state. The psychological factors that may modify an individual's response to erotic stimuli are less well-defined than the organic causes. In primary impotence the patient's upbringing, his interaction with his parents, the presence of strict religious taboos on matters concerning sexuality and any homosexual tendencies are all considered important. Difficulties during initial sexual encounters such as the inability to complete coitus with a prostitute or an incestuous relationship may cause problems in future sexual function.

The anxiety and stress induced by erectile failure in secondary impotence may be of significance since instead of becoming involved in the sexual act, the patient my remain a 'spectator' and may not be fully responsive to the pleasurable incoming erotic stimuli. The stress can be termed 'performance anxiety' and is well illustrated by a man with a history of premature ejaculation in whom over a period of years his sexual capabilities have been questioned by his sexual partner, thereby resulting in a performance oriented attitude. Such men frequently develop secondary impotence and need to be recognised early for treatment. The case history also illustrates the important part played by the attitude of his sexual partner since an aggressive, demanding and questioning attitude may accentuate or actually precipitate secondary impotence.

Local lesions

Severe hypospadias with chordee or fibrosis following priapism are important but rare causes of diminished or absent potency.

Metabolic

The ingestion of large quantities of alcohol on a relatively long-term basis is commonly associated with impotence. This may occur as a result of several mechanisms :

1. During bouts of drinking libido declines, impotence occurs which may persist for weeks or months, but libido frequently returns spontaneously provided alcohol ingestion does not recur.

2. Impotence associated with alcohol-induced organ damage such as cirrhosis of the liver (Baker et al, 1976c).

3. Life-long abnormalities of sexual function that have contributed significantly to the onset and continuation of alcoholism.

Loss of potency occurs in chronic renal failure partly as a result of the general debility but also associated with a decline of testicular function, resulting in low plasma testosterone levels accompanied usually by high levels of LH and FSH (Holdsworth et al, 1977).

Drugs

A number of drugs used in treatment are associated with impotence or ejaculatory abnormalities usually due to neurological factors. Such drugs include alpha methyldopa, bethanidine, bretylium, guanethidine, reserpine, tricyclic antidepressants, and the phenothiazines. The treatment of prostatic carcinoma with oestrogens is usually associated with impotence.

Clinical evaluation

In the assessment of an impotent male, it is of great importance to interview both the patient and his sexual partner. Furthermore, a successful outcome of therapy is more likely if the female partner is actively informed and involved from the outset. The history and physical examination should seek to establish which of the aetiological factors may be involved. The mode of onset, frequency, duration and quality of erections should be determined, as well as the occurrence of erections at times other than during sexual intercourse. The presence of early morning erections, the occurrence of masturbation and normal libido indicate that the vascular and neurological pathways which serve the erectile reflex are normal. This association with impotence usually suggests that psychogenic factors are involved. Loss of libido, loss of sexual secondary characteristics and diminished testis volume usually indicate a testicular cause or it may be secondary to pituitary lesions.

Measurements of serum testosterone, prolactin and gonadotrophins are useful screening measurements. More recently, the monitoring of nocturnal erections by measuring penile tumescence has shown that in normal men, a considerable proportion of the sleeping hours is spent with an erection usually in association with rapid eye movement sleep (Fisher et al, 1965). It has been suggested that measuring the frequency and size of penile erections during sleep is an objective way of differentiating psychogenic from organic impotence. Marshall et al (1982) point out that the validity of these measurements has yet to be established. Diabetes, liver or renal disease should be sought if suggested by clinical assessment.

Management

The identification of a specific aetiological factor should enable therapy to be focused for that disorder. However, it should be remembered that a significant degree of counselling of the couple will be required particularly if the impotence has been long-standing. Cessation or modification of drug regimens may be required as well as attempts to correct alcoholism. The cause of specific deficiencies of testosterone should be sought and treated as outlined below. If a psychogenic cause is found, counselling and sexual guidance are warranted in an attempt to reverse the defect.

Psychogenic impotence

If a specific disorder such as depression is identified this should be treated. Sexual counselling should be undertaken by those who are appropriately trained, usually in the setting of a 'sexual difficulties clinic'. One of the major problems is the necessity to allay the man's fear of erectile failure since the attendant anxiety diminishes his receptivity to the facilitatory stimuli present during sexual arousal. It is vital that both partners be involved in the sexual guidance and attempts should be made to help the couple communicate verbally and physically.

Androgen deficiency

For patients with clinical and biochemical evidence of testosterone deficiency, treatment with androgens is indicated. Care should be taken to determine if the low testosterone is secondary to a pituitary disorder which in turn will require treatment. Specifically, hyperprolactinaemia should be sought since it responds dramatically to treatment with bromocriptine which reduces prolactin levels and results in increased testosterone secretion by the testis.

In the majority of androgen deficient patients, oral androgen therapy using agents currently available, e.g. methyl testosterone, is either less effective or results in suboptimal androgenisation. Furthermore, cholestasis may occur in some individuals and several reports have suggested that long-term oral androgen therapy may be associated with peliosis hepatis and hepatoma formation. A new ester of testosterone, testosterone undecanoate is under trial and shows promise as an orally effective androgen.

Thus, effective androgen therapy utilises the long-acting esters of testosterone such as testosterone oenanthate (250 mg) given by intramuscular injection every week for the initial three injections and subsequently lengthening the interval between injections.

If the interval between injections is too long, the patient may note a decline in libido, hot flushes, irritability, tiredness or a lack of concentration so that the optimal interval should be assessed on an individual basis; in many patients with Klinefelter's syndrome the optimal interval is 7 to 10 days. Haemoglobin and haematocrit levels should be monitored during therapy as in sensitive patients, since the development of polycythaemia may require a reduction in injection frequency and venesection.

In impotent patients desirous of fertility, testosterone therapy may be contra-indicated since sperm counts are suppressed. In the small number of patients in whom FSH and LH levels are low, therapy with these agents will restore fertility and potency. In elderly patients, inquiry should be made as to their pattern of micturition to ensure that no sudden prostatic enlargement is induced by the testosterone therapy thereby causing acute retention.

The use of androgen therapy is controversial in patients with psychogenic impotence. This arises from the fact that no double-blind trials have been undertaken. If androgens are to be used in this setting, it is useful to give weekly injections of long-acting esters for 4 to 6 weeks followed by placebo injections of vehicle (peanut oil) for a similar length of time. The patients who benefit from androgen therapy rather than a placebo effect, will experience a gradual improvement with loss of this improvement in the second phase of treatment. In all instances, such therapy should be accompanied by regular counselling of the patient and his sexual partner.

REFERENCES

Abeyaratne M R, Aherne W A, Scott J E 1969 The vanishing testis. Lancet ii: 822–824

Afzelius B A 1976 A human syndrome caused by immotile cilia. Science 193: 317–319

Aiman J, Griffin J E 1982 The frequency of androgen receptor deficiency in infertile men. Journal of Clinical Endocrinology and Metabolism 54: 725–732

Aiman J, Griffin J E, Gazak J M, Wilson J D, MacDonald P C 1979 Androgen insensitivity as a cause of infertility in otherwise normal men. New England Journal of Medicine 300: 223–227

Anderson D C 1974 Sex hormone binding globulin. Clinical Endocrinology 3: 69–96

Aoki A, Fawcett D W 1978 Is there a local feedback from the seminiferous tubules affecting activity of the Leydig cells? Biology of Reproduction 19: 144–158

Aragona C, Freisen H G 1975 Specific prolactin binding sites in the prostate and testis of rats. Endocrinology 97: 677–684.

Baird D T, Horton R, Longcope C, Tait J F 1969 Steroid dynamics under steady state conditions. Recent Progress in Hormone Research 25: 611–656

Baker H W G, Bremner W J, Burger H G, de Kretser D M, Dulmanis A, Eddie L W et al 1976a Testicular control of follicle stimulating hormone secretion. Recent Progress in Hormone Research 32: 429–469

Baker H W G, Burger H G, de Kretser D M, Hudson B, O'Connor S, Wang C, Mirovics A et al 1976b Changes in the pituitary-testicular system with age. Clinical Endocrinology 5: 349–372

Baker H W G, Burger H G, de Kretser D M, Dulmanis A, Hudson B, O'Connor S et al 1976c A study of the endocrine manifestations of hepatic cirrhosis. Quarterly Journal of Medicine 177: 145–178

Baker H W G, Burger H G, de Kretser D M, Hudson B 1977 Endocrinology of aging: pituitary-testicular axis. In: James V H T (ed) Endocrinology. Excerpta Medica International Congress Series 403, pp 479–483 Excerpta Medica, Amsterdam

Baker H W G, Straffon W E, Murphy G, Davidson A, Burger H G, de Kretser D M 1979 Prostatistis and male infertility: a pilot study Possible increase in sperm motility with antibacterial chemotherapy International Journal of Andrology 2: 193–201

Beck W, Wuttke W 1980 Diurnal variations of plasma luteinizing hormone, follicle stimulating hormone and prolactin in boys and girls from birth to puberty. Journal of Clinical Endocrinology and Metabolism 50: 635–639

Bedford J M 1975 Maturation, transport and fate of spermatozoa in the epididymis. In: Greep R O, Astwood E B (eds) Handbook of Physiology, Vol 5, pp 303–317. American Physiological Society, Washington

Belsey M A, Eliasson R, Gallegos A J, Moghissi K S, Paulsen C A, Prasad M R N 1980 Laboratory manual for the examination of human semen and semen-cervical mucus interaction. WHO Press Concern, Singapore

Bergh A 1982 Local differences in Leydig cell morphology in the adult rat testis: evidence for local control of Leydig cells by adjacent seminiferous tubules. International Journal of Andrology 5: 325–330

Billings E L, Billings J J, Brown J B, Burger H G 1972 Symptoms and hormonal changes accompanying ovulation. Lancet i: 282–284

Birnie G G, McLeod T I F, Wilkinson G 1981 Incidence of sulphasalazine induced male infertility. Gut 22: 452–455

Blaquier J A 1971 Selective uptake and metabolism of androgens in the rat epididymis. The presence of a cytoplasmic receptor. Biochemical and Biophysical Research Communications 45: 1076–1082

Boitani C, Ritzen E M, Parvinen M 1981 Inhibition of rat Sertoli cell aromatase by factor(s) secreted specifically at spermatogenic stages VII and VIII. Molecular and Cellular Endocrinology 23: 11–12

Boyar R M, Rosenfeld R S, Kapen S, Finkelstein J W, Roffwarg H P, Weitzman E D, Hellman L 1974 Human puberty. Simultaneous augmented secretion of luteinizing hormone and testosterone during sleep. Journal of Clinical Investigation 54: 609–618

Bremner W J, Matsumoto A M, Sussman A M, Paulsen C A 1981 Follicle stimulating hormone and spermatogenesis. Journal of Clinical Investigation 68: 1044–1052

Brooks D E, Hamilton D W, Mallek A H 1974 Carnitine and glycerophosphorylcholine in the reproductive tract of the male rat. Journal of Reproduction and Fertility 36: 141–160

Brown J S 1976 Varicocelectomy in the subfertile male: a ten-year experience with 295 cases. Fertility and Sterility 27: 1046–1053

Burger H G 1972 Gonadotrophins — chemistry and measurement. In: Shearman R (ed) Human Reproductive Physiology, p 729. Blackwell Scientific Publications, Oxford

Burger H G, Bremner W J, de Kretser D M, Healy D L, Hudson B, Kovacs G T et al 1981a Hypogonadotrophic hypogonadism in male and female. In: Crosignani P G, Ruben B L (eds) Endocrinology of Human Infertility — New Aspects pp 185–205. Academic Press, London

Burger H G, de Kretser D M, Hudson B, Wilson J D 1981b Effects of preceding androgen therapy on testicular response to human pituitary gonadotrophin (HPG) in hypogonadotrophic hypogonadism (HH): a study of three patients. Fertility and Sterility 35: 64–68

Burke C W, Anderson D C 1972 Sex hormone binding globulin is an oestrogen amplifier. Nature 240: 38–40

Caldamone A A, Al-Juburi A, Crockett A T K 1980 The varicocele: elevated serotonin levels and infertility. Journal of Urology 123: 683–685

Cameron D F, Snydle F E, Ross M H, Drylie D M 1980 Ultrastructural alterations in the adluminal testicular compartment in men with varicocele. Fertility and Sterility 33: 526

Catt K J, Dufau M L 1976 Basic concepts of the mechanism of action of peptide hormones. Biology of Reproduction 14: 1–15

Chandley A C, Edmond P I, Christie S, Gowans L, Fletcher J, Frackiewicz A, Newton M 1975 Cytogenetics and infertility in man. Results of a five year study of men attending an infertility clinic. Part I. Karyotype and seminal analysis. Annals of Human Genetics 39: 231–254

Chapman R M, Sutcliffe S B, Malpas J S 1981 Male gonadal dysfunction in Hodgkin's disease. Journal of the American Medical Association 245: 1323–1328

Christensen A K, Peacock K C 1980 Increase in Leydig cell number in testes of adult rats treated chronically with an excess of human chorionic gonadotrophin. Biology of Reproduction 22: 383–391

Clarke I J, Cummins J T 1982 The temporal relationship between gonadotropin releasing hormone (GnRH) and luteinizing hormone (LH) secretion in ovariectomized ewes. Endocrinology

Clements J A, Reyes F I, Winter J S D, Faiman C 1976 Studies on human sexual development: III. Fetal pituitary, serum and amniotic fluid concentrations of LH, CG and FSH. Journal of Clinical Endocrinology and Metabolism 40: 9–19

Clermont Y 1963 The cycle of the seminiferous epithelium in man. American Journal of Anatomy 112: 35–51

Clermont Y 1972 Kinetics of spermatogenesis in mammals; seminiferous epithelium cycle and spermatogonial renewal. Physiological Reviews 52: 198–236

Clermont Y, Harvey S G 1965 Duration of the cycle of the seminiferous epithelium of normal hypophysectomized and hypophysectomized-hormone treated albino rats. Endocrinology 76: 80–89

Comhaire F, Varshraegen G, Vermeulen L 1980 Diagnosis of accessory gland infection and its possible role in male infertility. International Journal of Andrology 3: 32–45

Comhaire F, Vermeulen A 1974 Varicocele sterility: cortisol and catecholamines. Fertility and Sterility 25: 88–95

Conte F A, Grumbach M M, Caplan S L 1975 A diphasic pattern of gonadotropin secretion in patients with the syndrome of gonadal dysgenesis. Journal of Clinical Endocrinology and Metabolism 40: 670–674

Corvol P, Bardin C W 1973 Species distribution of testosterone binding globulin. Biology of Reproduction 8: 277–282

Couture M, Ulstein M, Leonard J M, Paulsen C A 1976 Improved staining methods for differentiating immature germ cells from white cells in human semen. Andrologia 8: 61–66

Damber J E, Bergh A, Janson P O 1978 Testicular blood flow and testosterone concentrations in the spermatic venous blood in rats with experimental cryptorchidism. Acta Endocrinologica 88: 611–681

Davies A G, Lawrence N R 1981 Timing and localization of the stimulatory effect of follicle stimulating hormone or uridine incorporation in the mouse testis in vivo. Journal of Endocrinology 88: 443–499

Davies T F, Walsh P C, Hodgen G D, Dufau M L, Catt K J 1979 Characterization of primate luteinizing hormone receptor in testis homogenates and Leydig cells. Journal of Clinical Endocrinology and Metabolism 48: 680–685

de Kretser D M 1967 The fine structure of the testicular intestitial cells in men of normal androgenic status. Z. Zellforsch 80: 594–609

de Kretser D M 1969 Ultrastructural features of human spermiogenesis. Z. zellforsch 98: 477–505

de Kretser D M, Catt K J, Paulsen C A 1971 Studies on the in vitro testicular binding of iodinated luteinizing hormone in rats. Endocrinology 88: 332–337

de Kretser D M, Hodgson Y M 1982 Studies on the Leydig cell response to hCG. In: Mancini Fabris F (ed) Proceedings of the meeting "Therapy in Andrology". Excerpta Medica, Amsterdam

de Kretser D M, Burger H G, Fortune D, Hudson B, Long A K, Paulsen C A et al 1972a Hormonal, histological and chromosomal studies in adult males with testicular disorders. Journal of Clinical Endocrinology and Metabolism 35: 392–401

de Kretser D M, Burger H G, Hudson B, Paulsen C A 1972b Correlations between hormonal and histological parameters in male infertility. In: Scow R (ed) Endocrinology, ICS No. 273, pp 963–969. Excerpta Medica, Amsterdam

de Kretser D M, Burger H G, Hudson B 1974 The relationship between germinal cells and serum FSH levels in men with infertility. Journal of Clinical Endocrinology and Metabolism 38: 787–793

de Kretser D M, Burger H G, Dumpys R 1975 Serum LH and FSH responses in 4-hour infusions of luteinizing hormone releasing hormone (LH-RH) in normal men, Sertoli cell only syndrome and Klinefelter's syndrome. Journal of Clinical Endocrinology and Metabolism 41: 876–886

de Kretser D M, Sharpe R M, Swanston I A 1979 Alterations in steroidogenesis and human chorionic gonadotropin binding in the cryptorchid rat testis. Endocrinology 105: 135–138

de Kretser D M, Temple-Smith P D, Kerr J B 1982 Anatomical and functional aspects of the male reproductive organs. In: Bandhauer K, Frick J (eds) Handbuch der Urologie Vol XVI, pp 1–131. Springer Verlag, Berlin

Dorrington J H, Armstrong D T 1975 Follicle stimulating hormone stimulates estradiol-17β synthesis in cultured Sertoli cells. Proceedings of the National Academy of Science 72: 2677–2281

Drife J D 1982 Drugs and sperm. British Medical Journal 284: 844–845

Dubin L and Amelar R D 1971 Etiologic factors in 1924 consecutive cases of male infertility. Fertility and Sterility 22: 469–474

Dufau M L, Pock R, Neubauer A, Catt K J 1976 In vitro bioassay of LH in human serum: the rat interstitial cell testosterone (RICT) assay. Journal of Clinical Endocrinology and Metabolism 42: 958–969

Dufau M L, Hsueh A J, Cigorraga S, Baukal A J, Catt K J 1978 Inhibition of Leydig cell function through hormonal regulatory mechanisms. International Journal of Andrology Suppl. 2: 193–239

Dym M, Fawcett D W 1970 The blood-testis barrier in the rat and the physiological compartmentation of the seminiferous epithelium. Biology of Reproduction 3: 308–326

Dym M, Raj H G M, Lin Y C, Chemes H E, Kotite N J, Nayfeh S N et al 1979 Is FSH required for maintenance of spermatogenesis in adult rats. Journal of Reproduction and Fertility Suppl. 26: 175–181

Editorial 1981 Antisperm antibodies and fertility. Lancet i: 136–138

Eik-Nes K B 1970 Synthesis and secretion of androstenedione and testosterone. In: Eik-Nes K B (ed) The Androgens of the Testis, pp 1–47. Marcel Dekker, New York

Eliasson R 1971 Standards for investigation of human semen. Andrologia 3: 49–64

Eliasson R 197 Clinical examination of infertile men. In: Hafez E S E (ed) Human Semen and Fertility Regulation, pp 321–331. C V Mosby, St. Louis

Eliasson R, Mossberg B, Camner P, Afzelius B A 1977 The immotile-cilia syndrome. A congenital ciliary abnormality as an etiologic factor in chronic airway infections and male sterility. New England Journal of Medicine 297: 1–6

Evans H J, Fletcher J, Torrance M, Hargreave T B 1981 Sperm abnormalities and cigarette smoking. Lancet i: 627–629

Faiman C, Winter J S D, Reyes F I 1981 Endocrinology of the fetal testis. In: Burger H G, de Kretser D M (eds), The Testis, pp 81–105. Raven Press, New York

Fairley K F, Barrie J, Johnson W 1972 Sterility and testicular atrophy related to cyclophosphamide therapy. Lancet i: 568–569

Fawcett D W 1975 Ultrastructure and function of the Sertoli cell. In: Greep R O, Hamilton D W (eds) Handbook of Physiology, Section 7, Vol 5, pp 21–55. Williams and Wilkins, Baltimore

Fawcett D W, Neaves W B, Flores M N 1973 Comparative observations on intertubular lymphatics and the organization of the interstitial tissue of the mammalian testis. Biology of Reproduction 9: 500–532

Fernando N, Leonard J M, Paulsen C A 1976 The role of variocele in male fertility. Andrologia 8: 1–9

Fisher C, Gross J, Zuch J 1965 A cycle of penile erection synchronous with dreaming (REM) sleep. Archives of General Psychiatry 12: 29–45

Fjallbrandt B 1968 Interrelation between high levels of sperm antibodies, reduced penetration of cervical mucus by spermatozoa and sterility in men. Acta Obstetrica et Gynaecologica Scandinavica 47: 102–117

Forest M G, de Peretti E, Bertrand J 1976 Hypothalamic-pituitary-gonadal relationships in man from birth to puberty. Clinical Endocrinology 5: 551–569

Franchimont P, Millet D, Venderly E, Letawe J, Legros J J, Nettler A 1972 Relationship between spermatogenesis and serum gonadotropin levels in azoospermia and oligospermia. Journal of Clinical Endocrinology and Metabolism 34: 1003–1008

Franchimont P, Burger H 1975 Human Growth Hormone and Gonadotrophins in Health and Disease, North Holland/American Elsevier, pp 1–494 Amsterdam, New York

Friberg J 1974 A simple and sensitive micro method for demonstration of sperm agglutinating antibodies in serum from infertile men and women. Acta Obstetrica et Gynaecologica Scandinavica (Supplement) 36: 21–29

Futterweit N, Sobrero A J 1968 Treatment of normogonadotropic oligospermia with large doses of chorionic gonadotropin. Fertility and Sterility 19: 971–976

Glode L M, Robinson J, Gould S F 1981 Protection from cyclophosphamide-induced testicular damage with an analogue of gonadotropin-releasing hormone. Lancet i: 1132–1134

Gordon G G, Southren A L 1972 Metabolic effects of alcohol on the endocrine system. In: Lieber C S (ed) Metabolic Aspects of Alcoholism, p 249. University Park Press, Baltimore

Greenberg S H 1977 Varicocele and male fertility. Fertility and Sterility 28: 699–706

Haas G G, Cines D B, Schreiber A D 1980 Immunologic infertility: identification of patients with antisperm antibody. New England Journal of Medicine 303: 722–726

Hadziselimovic F, Herzog B, Seguchi H 1975 Surgical correction of cryptorchidism at two years: electron microscopic and morphometric investigations. Journal of Pediatric Surgery 10: 19–26

Hamilton D W, Fawcett D W 1970 In vitro synthesis of cholesterol and testosterone from acetate by rat epididymis and vas deferens. Proceedings of the Society of Experimental Biology and Medicine 133: 693–695

Hammond G L, Nisker J A, Jones L A, Siiteri P K 1980 Estimation of the percentage of free steroid in undiluted serum by centrifugal ultrafiltration dialysis. Journal of Biological Chemistry 255: 5023–5026

Handelsman D J, Turtle J R 1982 Testicular damage after radioactive iodine (^{131}I) for thyroid cancer. Clinical Endocrinology

Hansson V, Ritzen E M, French F S, Nayfeh S 1975 Androgen transport and receptor mechanisms in testis and epididymis. In: Hamilton D W, Greep R O (eds) Handbook of Physiology Section 7, Vol. 5, pp 173–201. Williams and Wilkins, Baltimore

Haour F, Saez J M 1977 hCG-dependent regulation of gonadotropin receptor sites: negative control in testicular Leydig cells. Molecular and Cellular Endocrinology 7: 17–24

Haour F P, Sanchez P, Cathiard A M, Saez J M 1978 Gonadotropin receptor regulation in hypophysectomized rat Leydig cells. Biochemical and Biophysical Research Communications 81: 547–51

Harman S M, Tsitouras P D, Costa P T, Loriaux D L, Sherins R J 1982 Evaluation of pituitary gonadotropic function in men: value of luteinizing hormone-releasing hormone response versus basal luteinizing hormone level for discrimination of diagnosis. Journal of Clinical Endocrinology and Metabolism 54: 196–200

Heller C G, Clermont Y 1964 Kinetics of the germinal epithelium in man. Recent Progress in Hormone Research 20: 545–575

Hendry W F, Stedronska J 1980 Mixed erythrocyte-spermatozoa antiglobulin reaction (MAR test) for the detection of antibodies against spermatozoa in infertile males. Journal of Obstetrics and Gynaecology 1: 59–62

Hendry W F, Sommerville I F, Hall R R, Pugh R C B 1973 Investigation and treatment of the infertile male. British Journal of Urology 45: 684–692

Hendry W F 1975 Male infertility. The Practitioner 214: 60–69

Hendry W F, Knight R K, Whitfield H N, Stansfield A G, Pryse-Davies J, Ryder T A et al 1978 Obstructive azoospermia: respiratory function tests, electronmicroscopy and the results of surgery. British Journal of Urology 50: 598–604

Hendry W F, Stedronska, J, Hughes, L, Cameron K M, Pugh R C B 1979 Steroid treatment of male subfertility caused by antisperm antibodies. Lancet ii: 498–500

Hodgson Y M, de Kretser D M 1982 Serum testosterone response to single injection of hCG, ovine-LH and LHRH in male rats. International Journal of Andrology 5: 81–91

Hodgson Y M, Robertson D M, de Kretser D M 1982 The regulation of testicular function. In: Greep R O (ed) Reproductive Physiology IV. University Park Press, Baltimore

Holdsworth S, Atkins R C, de Kretser D M 1977 The pituitary-testicular axis in men with chronic renal failure. New England Journal of Medicine 296: 1245–1249

Hoskins D D, Hall M L, Munsterman D 1975 Production of motility in immature bovine spermatozoa by cyclic AMP phosphodiesterase inhibitors and seminal plasma. Biology of Reproduction 13: 168–176

Holsclaw D S 1969 Cystic fibrosis and fertility. British Medical Journal iii: 356

Hsu A, Stratico D, Hosana M 1978 Studies of the human testis: X. Properties of human chorionic gonadotropin receptor in adult testis and relation to intratesticular testosterone concentration. Journal of Clinical Endocrinology and Metabolism 47: 529–536

Isojima S, Li T S, Ashitaka Y 1968 Immunologic analysis of sperm-immobilizing factor in sera of women with unexplained sterility.

American Journal of Obstetrics and Gynecology 101: 677–683

Isojima S, Tuchiya K, Koyama K, Tanaka C, Naka O, Adachi H 1972 Further studies on sperm-immobilizing antibody found in sera of unexplained cases of sterility in women. American Journal of Obstetrics and Gynecology 112: 199–207

Jager S, Kremer J, Van Slochteren-Draaisma T 1978 A simple method of screening for antisperm antibodies in the human male. International Journal of Fertility 23: 12–21

Jegou B, Risbridger G P, de Kretser D M 1982 Effects of experimental cryptorchidism on testicular function in adult rats. Journal of Andrology

Johannisson E, Eliasson R 1978 Cytological studies of prostatic fluids from men with and without abnormal palpatory findings of the prostate. I. Methodological aspects. International Journal of Andrology 1: 201–212

Johnson B H, Ewing L L 1971 Follicle stimulating hormone and the regulation of testosterone secretion in rabbit testes. Science 173: 635–637

Jones W R 1980 Immunological factors in infertility. In: Pepperell R J, Hudson B, Wood C (eds) The Infertile Couple, pp 126–146. Churchill Livingstone, Edinburgh

Kaplan S L, Grumbach M M, Aubert M L 1976 Fetal pituitary and hypothalamic hormones. Recent Progress in Hormone Research 32: 161–

Kelch R P, Jenner M R, Weinstein R, Kaplan S L, Grumbach M M 1972 Estradiol and testosterone secretion by human simian and canine testes in males with hypogonadism and in male pseudohermaphrodites with the feminizing testes syndrome. Journal of Clinical Investigation 51: 824–830

Kent J R, Acone A B 1966 Plasma testosterone and aging in males. In: Vermeulen A, Exley D (eds) Androgens in Normal and Pathological Conditions. International Congress Series 101, pp 31–35. Excerpta Medica Foundation, Amsterdam

Keogh E J, MacKellar A, Mallal S A, Dunn A G, McColm S C, somerville C P et al 1982 Treatment of cryptorchidism with pulsatile luteinizing hormone releasing hormone (LHRH). Journal of Pediatric Surgery

Kerr J B, de Kretser D M 1975 Cyclic variations in Sertoli cell lipid content throughout the spermatogenic cycle in the rat. Journal of Reproduction and Fertility 43: 1–8

Kerr J B, Rich K A, de Kretser D M 1979 Alterations of the fine structure and androgen secretion of the interstitial cells in the experimentally cryptorchid rat testis. Biology of Reproduction 20: 409–422

Kjessler B 1973 Genic and chromosomal factors in male infertility. In: Scow R G (ed) Endocrinology. International Congress Series 273, pp 956–962. Excerpta Medica Foundation, Amsterdam

Kulin H E, Bell P M, Santen R J, Ferber A J 1975 Integration of pulsatile gonadotropin secretion by timed urinary measurements: an accurate and sensitive three hour test. Journal of Clinical Endocrinology and Metabolism 40: 783–789

Kulin H E, Muller R G, Santen R J 1976 Circadian rhythms in gonadotropin excretion in prepubertal children and pubertal children. Journal of Clinical Endocrinology and Metabolism 42: 770–773

Lacroix M, Smith F E, Fritz I B 1977 Secretion of plasminogen activator by Sertoli cell enriched cultures. Molecular and Cellular Endocrinology 9: 227–236

Lamensdorf H, Compere D, Begley G 1975 Testosterone rebound therapy in the treatment of male infertility. Fertility and Sterility 24: 469–472

Large D M, Anderson D C 1979 Twenty four hour profiles of circulating androgens and oestrogens in male puberty with and without gynaecomastia. Clinical Endocrinology 11: 505–521

Le Blond C P, Clermont Y 1952 Definition of the stages of the cycle of the seminiferous epithelium in the rat. Annals of the New York Academy of Science 55: 548–573

LeGoc F, de Kretser D M 1982 Inhibin production by Sertoli cell cultures. Molecular and Cellular Endocrinology

Legros J J, Demoulin A, Burger H G, Franchimont P 1974 Influence d'une dose faible d'ethinyl oestradiol sur la liberation pulsatile des gonadotrophines et sur leur liberation hypophysaire sous l'influence du LHRH chez l'homme normale. Compte Rendus des Seances de la Societe de Biologie, Extrait du Tome, 168, nos 10–11–12. p 1432

McFadden M R, Mehan D J 1978 Testicular biopsies in 101 cases of varicocele. Journal of Urology 119: 372–374

McGowan M P, Burger H G, Baker H W G, de Kretser D M, Kovacs G T 1981 The incidence of non-specific infection in the semen in fertile and sub-fertile males. International Journal of Andrology 4: 657–668

MacLeod J 1964 Human seminal cytology as a sensitive indicator of the germinal epithelium. International Journal of Fertility 9: 281–295

MacLeod J 1969 Further observations on the role of varicocele in human male infertility. Fertility and Sterility 20: 545–563

MacLeod J, Gold R Z 1951a The male factor in fertility and infertility. II. Spermatozoon counts in 1000 men of known fertility and in 1000 cases of infertile marriage. Journal of Urology 65: 436–449

MacLeod J, Gold R Z 1951b The male factor in fertility and infertility. III. An analysis of motile activity in the spermatozoa of 1000 fertile men and 1000 men in infertile marriage. Fertility and Sterility 2: 187–204

MacLeod J, Gold R Z 1951c The male factor in fertility and infertility. IV. Sperm morphology in fertile and infertile marriage. Fertility and Sterility 2: 394–414

MacLeod J, Gold R Z 1953 The male factor in fertility and infertility. VI. Semen quality and certain other factors in relation to ease of conception. Fertility and Sterility 4: 10–33

McNeal J E 1972 The prostate and prostatic urethra: a morphologic synthesis. Journal of Urology 107: 1008–1016

Macomber D, Sanders M B 1929 The spermatozoa count: its value in diagnosis, prognosis and treatment of sterility. New England Journal of Medicine 200: 981–984

Marshall P, Morales A, Surridge D 1982 Diagnostic significance of penile erections during sleep. Urology 20: 1–6

Marshall W A, Tanner J M 1970 Variations in the pattern of pubertal changes in boys. Archives of Diseases in Childhood 45: 13–23

Matsumoto A M, Karpas A E, Paulsen C A, Bremner W J 1982 Human follicle stimulating hormone (hFSH) reinitiates spermatogenesis in gonadotropin-suppressed normal men. Clinical Research

Means A R, Huckins C 1974 Coupled events in the early biochemical actions of FSH on the Sertoli cell of the testis. In: Dufau M L, Means A R (eds) Hormone Binding and Target Cell Activation in the Testis, pp 145–165 Plenum Press, New York

Misarule F, Cognazzo G, Storace A 1969 Asthenospermia and its treatment with HCG. Fertility and Sterility 20: 650–653

Modell B 1977 Total management of thalassaemia major. Archives of Diseases in Childhood 52: 489–500

Morgan H, Stedronska J, Hendry W F, Chamberlain G V P, Dewhurst C J 1977 Sperm/cervical mucus crossed hostility testing and antisperm antibodies in the husband. Lancet i: 1228–1230

Murty G S R C, Sheela Rani C S, Moudgal N R, Prasad M R N 1979 Effect of passive immunization with specific antiserum to FSH on the spermatogenic process and fertility of adult male bonnet monkeys (Macaca radiata). Journal of Reproduction and Fertility (Suppl.) 26: 147–163

Naftolin F, Ryan K J, Petro Z 1972 Aromatization of androstenedione by the anterior hypothalamus of adult male and female rats. Endocrinology 90: 295–298

Neumann F 1977 Pharmacology and potential use of cyproterone acetate. Hormone and Metabolic Research 9: 1–13

Nicolis G L, Modlinger R S, Gabrilove J L 1971 A study of the histopathology of gynecomastia. Journal of Clinical Endocrinology and Metabolism 32: 173–178

Nieschlag E, Wickings E J, Usadel K N, Dathe G 1980 Impairment of spermaotgenesis in adult rhesus monkeys by active immunization against FSH. Proceedings VIth International Congress of Endocrinology, p 492

Nilsson S, Edvinsson A, Nilsson B 1979 Improvement of semen and pregnancy rate after ligation and division of the internal spermatic vein: fact or fiction? British Journal of Urology 51: 591–596

Nuttall F Q 1979 Gynecomastia as a physical finding in normal men. Journal of Clinical Endocrinology and Metabolism 48: 338–340

Nydick M, Bustos J, Dale J H, Rawson R W 1961 Gynecomastia in adolescent boys. Journal of the American Medical Association 178: 449–454

Odell W D, Swerdloff R S, Jacobs H S, Hescox M A 1973 FSH induction of sensitivity to LH: one cause of sexual maturation in the male rat. Endocrinology 92: 160–166

Orgebin-Crist M-C 1981 Epididymal physiology and sperm maturation. In: Bollack C V, Clarnt A (eds) Epididymis and Fertility: Biology and Pathology, pp 80–89 S. Karger, Basel

Orth J, Christensen A K 1978 Autoradiographic localization of specifically bound ^{125}I-labelled follicle stimulating hormone on spermatogonia of the rat testis. Endocrinology 103: 1944–1951

Overstreet J W, Yanagamachi R, Katz D, Heyeshi R, Hanson F W 1980 Penetration of human spermatozoa into the human zona pellucida and the zona free hamster egg: a study of fertile donors and infertile patients. Fertility and Sterility 33: 535–542

Padron R S, Wischusen J, Hudson B, Burger H G, de Kretser D M 1980 Prolonged biphasic response of plasma testosterone to single intramuscular injections of human chorionic gonadotrophin. Journal of Clinical Endocrinology and Metabolism 50: 1100–1104

Palomo A 1949 Radical cure of varicocele by a new technique: preliminary report. Journal of Urology 61: 604–607

Parvinen M, Marana R, Robertson D M, Hansson V, Ritzen E M 1980 Functional cycle of rat Sertoli cells: differential binding and action of follicle stimulating hormone at various stages of the spermatogenic cycle. In: Steinberger E, Steinberger A (eds) Testicular Development, Structure and Function. pp 425–432 Raven Press, New York

Paulsen C A, Gordon D L, Carpenter R W, Gandy H M, Drucker W D 1968 Klinefelter's syndrome and its variants: a hormonal and chromosomal study. Recent Progress in Hormone Research 24: 321–63

Paulson D F 1979 Cortisone acetate versus clomiphene citrate in pre-germinal idiopathic oligospermia. Journal of Urology 121: 432–434

Penny R, Olambiwonnu N O, Frasier S D 1977 Episodic fluctuations of serum gonadotropins in pre- and post-pubertal girls and boys. Journal of Clinical Endocrinology and Metabolism 45: 307–311

Peto R et al 1977 Design and analysis of randomized clinical trials requiring prolonged observation of each patient. British Journal of Cancer 35: 1–39

Pomerantz D K 1979 Effects of in vivo gonadotropin treatment on estrogen levels in the testis of the immaure rat. Biology of Reproduction 21: 1247–1255

Prader A 1966 Testicular size: assessment and clinical importance. Triangle 7: 240–243

Rajaniemi H J, Oksanen A, Vanha-Perttula T 1974 Distribution of ^{125}I prolactin in mice and rats. Studies on whole-body and microautoradiography. Hormone Research 5: 6–20

Rehan N-E, Sobrero A J, Fertig J W 1975 The semen of fertile men: statistical analysis of 1300 men. Fertility and Sterility 26: 492–502

Reyes F I, Faiman C 1974 Long-term therapy with low-dose cisclomiphene in male infertility: effects on semen, serum FSH, LH, testosterone and estradiol and carbohydrate tolerance. International Journal of Fertility 19: 49–55

Rich K A, de Kretser D M 1977 Effect of differing degrees of destruction of the rat seminiferous epithelium on levels of serum FSH and androgen binding protein. Endocrinology 101: 959–968

Rich K A, Kerr J B, de Kretser D M 1979 Evidence for Leydig cell dysfunction in rats with seminiferous tubule damage. Molecular and Cellular Endocrinology 13: 123–135

Risbridger G P, Kerr J B, Peake R, Rich K A, de Kretser D M 1981a Temporal changes in rat Leydig cell function after the induction of bilateral cryptorchidism. Journal of Reproduction and Fertility 63: 415–423

Risbridger G P, Kerr J B, de Kretser D M 1981b An evaluation of Leydig cell function and gonadotropin binding in unilateral and bilateral cryptorchidism. Evidence for localcontrol of Leydig cell function by the seminiferous tubule. Biology of Reproduction 24: 534–540

Risbridger G P, Kerr J B, Peake R A, de Kretser D M 1981c An assessment of Leydig cell function after bilateral or unilateral efferent duct ligation. Further evidence for local control of Leydig cell function. Endocrinology 109: 1234–1241

Risbridger G P, Robertson D M, de Kretser D M 1982 The effects of chronic human chorionic gonadotropin treatment on Leydig cell function. Endocrinology 110: 138–145

Ritzen E M, Dobbins M C, Tindall D J, French F S, Nayfeh S N 1973 Characterization of androgen-binding protein (ABP) in rat testis and epididymis. Steroids 21: 593–607

Ritzen E M, Parvinen M, Hansson V, French F S, Feldman M 1980 Role of Sertoli cell in spermatogenesis. In: Cumming J A, Funder J W, Mendelsohn F A O (eds) Endocrinology, pp 159–161. Australian Academy of Science, Canberra.

Rodriguez-Rigau L J, Smith K D, Steinberger E 1978 Relationship of varicocele to sperm output and fertility of male partners in infertile couples. Journal of Urology 120: 691–694

Rosemberg E 1976 Gonadotropin therapy of male infertility. In: Hafez E S E (ed) Human Semen and Fertility Regulation in Men, pp 465–475. C V Mosby Co, St Louis

Rosenfeld R G, Northcraft G B, Hintz R L 1982 A prospective, randomized study of testosterone treatment of constitutional delay of growth and development in male adolescents. Pediatrics 69: 681–687

Rosenfield R L 1971 Plasma testosterone binding globulin and indexes of the concentration of unbound plasma androgens in normal and hirsute subjects. Journal of Clinical Endocrinology and Metabolism 32: 717–728

Roth J C, Grumbach M M, Kaplan S L 1973 Effect of synthetic luteinizing hormone-releasing factor on serum testosterone and gonadotropins in prepubertal, pubertal and adult males. Journal of Clinical Endocrinology and Metabolism 37: 680–668

Rowley M J, Heller C G 1972 Testosterone rebound phenomenon in the treatment of male infertility. Fertility and Sterility 23: 498–504

Rowley M J, Teshima F, Heller C G 1970 Duration of transit of spermatozoa through the human male ductular system. Fertility and Sterility 21: 390–395

Saez J M, Forest M G 1979 Kinetics of human chorionic gonadotropin-induced steroidogenic response of the human testis. I. Plasma testosterone: implications for human chorionic gonadotropin stimulation test. Journal of Clinical Endocrinology and Metabolism 49: 278–283

Saidi K, Wenn R V, Sharif F 1977 Bromocriptine for male infertility. Lancet i: 250–251

Santen R J 1975 Is aromatization of testosterone to estradiol required for inhibition of luteinizing hormone secretion in men? Journal of Clinical Investigation 56: 1555–1563

Santen R J, Bardin C W 1973 Episodic LH secretion in man: pulse analysis, clinical interpretation, physiologic mechanisms. Journal of Clinical Investigation 52: 2617–2628

Santen R J, Paulsen C A 1973 Hypogonadotrophic eunuchoidism. 1. Clinical study of the mode of inheritance. Journal of Clinical Endocrinology and Metabolism 36: 47–54

Santen R J, Kulin H E 1981 Hypogonadotrophic hypogonadism and delayed puberty. In: Burger H, de Kretser D (eds) The Testis, pp 329–356. Raven Press, New York

Saypol D C, Howards S S, Turner T T, Miller E D 1981 Influence of surgically induced varicocele on testicular blood flow, temperature and histology in adult rats and dogs. Journal of Clinical Investigation 68: 39–45

Schilsky R L, Lewis B J, Sherins R J, Young R C 1980 Gonadal dysfunction in patients receiving chemotherapy for cancer. Annals of Internal Medicine 93: 109–114

Scott R S, Burger H G 1981 An inverse relationship exists between seminal plasma inhibin and serum FSH in man. Journal of Clinical Endocrinology and Metabolism 52: 796–803

Segal S, Polishuk C, Ben David M 1976 Hyperprolactinemic male infertility. Fertility and Sterility 27: 1425–1427

Setchell B P 1969 Do Sertoli cells secrete the rete testis fluid? Journal of Reproduction and Fertility 19: 391–392

Shaarawy M, Mahmoud K Z 1982 Endocrine profile and semen characteristics in male smokers. Fertility and Sterility 38: 255–257

Sharpe R M 1976 hCG-induced decrease in availability of rat testis receptors. Nature 264: 644–646

Sherins R J, Olweny C L M, Ziegler J L 1978 Gynecomastia and gonadal dysfunction in adolescent boys treated with combination chemotherapy for Hodgkin's disease. New England Journal of Medicine 299: 12–16

Shulman S, Harlin B, Davis P, Reniak J V 1978 Immune infertility and new approaches to treatment. Lancet 29: 309–313

Skakkebaek N G 1981 Cytogenics in male hypogonadism. In: Burger

H G, de Kretser D M (eds) The Testes, pp 401–417. Raven Press, New York

Smith P E 1930 Hypophysectomy and replacement therapy in the rat. American Journal of Anatomy 45: 205–256

Smith K D, Rodriguez-Rigau L J, Steinberger E 1977 Relation between indices of semen analysis and pregnancy rate in infertile couples. Fertility and Sterility 28: 1314–1319

Steeno O, Knops J, Declerck L, Adimdelja A, Van De Voorde H 1976 Prevention of fertility disorders by detection and treatment of varicocele at school and college age. Andrologia 8: 47–53

Steinberger E 1971 Hormonal control of mammalian spermatogenesis. Physiological Reviews 51: 1–22

Steinberger A, Steinberger E 1976 Secretion of an FSH-inhibiting factor by cultured Sertoli cells. Endocrinology 99: 918–921

Stenchever M A, Spadoni L R, Smith W D, Karp L E, Shy K S, Moore D E et al 1982 Benefits of the sperm (hamster ova) penetration assay in the evaluation of the infertile couple. American Journal of Obstetrics and Gynecology 143: 91–95

Styne D M, Grumbach M M 1978 Puberty in the male and female: its physiology and disorders. In: Yen S S C, Jaffe R B (eds) Reproductive Endocrinology, p 189. W B Saunders, Philadelphia

Takagi S, Yoshida T, Tsubata K, Ozaki H, Fujii T K, Nomuray Y et al 1977 Sex differences in fetal gonadotropins and androgens. Journal of Steroid Biochemistry 8: 609–620

Thorner M D, Edwards C R W, Hanker J P, Abraham G, Besser G M 1977 Prolactin and gonadotropin interactions in the male. In: Troen P, Nankin H R (eds) The Testis in Normal and Infertile Men, pp 351–366. Raven Press, New York

Tindall J J, Miller D A, Means A R 1977 Characterization of androgen receptor in Sertoli cell-enriched testis. Endocrinology 101: 13–23

Toth A, Lesser M L 1981 Asymptomatic bacteriospermia in fertile and infertile men. Fertility and Sterility 36: 88–91

Trump D L, Pavy M D, Staal S 1982 Gynecomastia in men following antineoplastic therapy. Archives of Internal Medicine 142: 511–513

Tulloch W S 1952 Consideration of sterility; subfertility in the male. Edinburgh Medical Journal 59: 29–34

Uehling D T 1968 Fertility in men with varicocele. International Journal of Fertility 13: 58–60

Ulstein M, Capell P, Holmes K K, Paulsen C A 1976 Nonsymptomatic genital tract infection and male infertility. In: Hafez E S E (ed) Human Semen and Fertility Regulation in Men, pp 355–362 C V Mosby, St. Louis

Urban M D, Lee P A, Migeon C J 1978 Adult height and fertility in men with congenital adrenal hyperplasia. New England Journal of Medicine 199: 1392–1396

Valk T W, Corley K P, Kelch R P, Marshall J C 1980 Hypogonadotropic hypogonadism: hormonal responses to low dose pulsatile administration of gonadotropin-releasing hormone. Journal of Clinical Endocrinology and Metabolism 51: 730–739

Van Thiel D H, Lester R 1979 The effect of chronic alcohol abuse on sexual function. Clinics in Endocrinology and Metabolism 8: 499–510

Van Thiel D H, Gavaler J S, Lester R, Goodman M D 1975 Alcohol induced testicular atrophy: an experimental model for hypogonadism occurring in chronic alcoholic men. Gastroenterology 69: 326–332

Van Thiel D H, Sherins R J, Myers G H, De Vita V T 1972 Evidence for a specific seminiferous tubule factor affecting FSH secretion in man. Journal of Clinical Investigation 51: 1009–1019

Vermeulen A, Stoica T, Verdonck L 1971 The apparent free testosterone concentration, an index of androgenicity. Journal of Clinical Endocrinology and Metabolism 33: 759–767

Vermeulen A, Verdonck, L, Van Den Straten M, Odrie N 1969 Capacity of testosterone binding globulin in human plasma and influence of specific binding of testosterone on its metabolic clearance rate. Journal of Clinical Endocrinology and Metabolism 29: 1470–1480

Verstoppen G R, Steeno O P 1977 Varocotele and the pathogenesis of the associated subfertility. A review of the various theories. 1: Varicocelogenesis. Andrologia 9: 133–140

Vigersky R A, Chapman R M, Berenberg J, Glass A R 1982 Testicular dysfunction in untreated Hodgkin's disease. American Journal of Medicine 73: 482–486

Vitale R, Fawcett D W, Dym M 1973 The normal development of the blood-testis barrier and the effects of clomiphene and estrogen treatment. Anatomical Record 176: 333–344

Wang C, Baker H W G, Burger H G, de Kretser D M, Hudson B 1975 Hormonal studies in Klinefelter's syndrome. Clinical Endocrinology 4: 399–411

Wiss H D 1972 The physiology of human penile erection. Annals of Internal Medicine 76: 793–799

Welsh M J, Wiebe J P 1976 Sertoli cells from immature rats: in vitro stimulation of steroid metabolism. Biochemical and Biophysical Research Communications 69: 936–941

Williams M J 1963 Gynecomastia: its incidence recognition and host characterization in 447 autopsy cases. American Journal of Medicine 34: 103–112

Wilson J D 1980 Benign prostatic hyperplasia. American Journal of Medicine 68: 745–756

Wilson J D, Aiman J, Macdonald P C 1980 The pathogenesis of gynecomastia. In: Stollerman G H (ed) Advances in Internal Medicine, Vol 25, pp 1–32

Winter J S D, Faiman C 1972 Serum gonadotropin concentrations in agonadal children and adults. Journal of Clinical Endocrinology and Metabolism 35: 562–564

Wischusen J, Baker H W G, Hudson B 1981 Reversible male infertility due to congenital adrenal hyperplasia. Clinical Endocrinology 14: 571–577

Wollesen F, Swerdloff R S, Odell W D 1976 LH and FSH responses to luteinizing-releasing hormone in normal adult human males. Metabolism 25: 845–863

Ylikahri R, Huttunen M, Harkonen M, Seuderling U, Onikki S, Karonen S-L et al 1974 Low plasma testosterone values in men during hangover. Journal of Steroid Biochemistry 5: 655–658

Young D 1970 Surgical treatment of male infertility. Journal of Reproduction and Fertility 23: 541–542

The normal menstrual cycle

The endocrine profiles of the major reproductive hormones during the menstrual cycle have been extensively reviewed (Diczfalusy & Landgren, 1977, 1981; Landgren et al, 1982). It is not our intention here to reiterate those studies but rather to consider the philosophical approach in establishing the endocrinology of the 'normal' cycle and then to evaluate the limitations imposed by our current technology and practice in achieving this objective.

THE NORMAL CYCLE

Over the past decade many authors have described the endocrine profiles of LH, FSH, oestradiol, progesterone and 17-hydroxyprogesterone during the 'normal' menstrual cycle (Neil et al, 1967; Midgley & Jaffe, 1968; Saxena et al, 1968; Taymor et al, 1968; Cargille et al, 1969; Ross et al, 1970; Yen et al, 1970; Abraham et al, 1971; Johansson et al, 1971; Mishell et al, 1971; Thorneycroft et al, 1971; Abraham et al, 1972; Briggs & Briggs, 1972; Edqvist & Johansson, 1972; Holmdahl & Johansson, 1972; Moghissi et al, 1972; Nocke & Leyendecker, 1972; Odell et al, 1973; Perez-Palacios et al, 1973; Shaaban & Klopper, 1973; Spona, 1973; Wide et al, 1973; Dyrenfurth et al, 1974; Jones et al, 1974; Saxena et al, 1974; Dodson et al, 1975; Franchimont & Burger, 1975; Kletzky et al, 1975; Leyendecker et al, 1975; Pizarro, 1975; Roger et al, 1975; Aedo et al, 1976; Frölich et al, 1976; Guerrero et al, 1976; Lehmann et al, 1976; Salmon et al, 1976; Wide, 1976; Milewich et al, 1977; Lenton et al, 1978; Schulz et al, 1978; Shumin et al, 1983).

Unfortunately the criteria used for selecting either the cycles as 'normal' or the subjects in whom the cycles occurred as 'normal', have differed significantly. The problem is partly one of experimental research expediency and partly one of imprecise definition — are we defining the characteristics of the menstrual cycle in a 'normal' woman or are we defining the caracteristics of a 'normal' cycle irrespective of the subject in whom it occurred?

If we are discussing the 'normal' woman then 'normal' could mean that she has no known gynaecological complaint, no known medical complaint and is not taking any drugs (e.g. oral contraception) which might affect her cycle. We could extend these selection criteria by excluding women above or below certain (arbitrary) age limits, or whose ponderal index (weight/height^2) is outside a defined range, or whose menstrual rhythm is irregular, or perhaps those women whose cycles although regular, are either longer or shorter than prescribed limits. This list could be continued indefinitely by imposing more and more rigid criteria on the selection of subjects in whom to study the 'normal' menstrual cycle. Just as an example of how far it might be necessary to go — should we consider excluding women who are experiencing some form of stressful life event (family illness, bereavement, examinations or even attending an artificial insemination clinic)?

Since it is commonly accepted that a 'normal' woman may not always have a 'normal' cycle, attempts have been made to impose further pre-conditions on the actual cycles themselves.

It has been suggested that certain criteria — for example, the presence of a surge of luteinising hormone (LH) or of cyclical changes in oestradiol (E_2) and progesterone (P) concentrations or both — are necessary requirements for a 'normal' cycle. Since neither of these preconditions is sufficient to define ovulation (follicular rupture and release of ovum) it is difficult to see what 'normal' means under these circumstances. Again the problem is how far to go — should cycles with short luteal phases be excluded? Should cycles with virtually no luteal progesterone secretion (aluteal cycles) be excluded? How should the limits of these parameters be defined?

The difficulty with the majority of the selection criteria outlined above is firstly that they are hypothetical and secondly that they are restrictive — subjects cannot be recruited, data must be rejected, all in an effort to reach a consensus on the endocrine limits of a normal menstrual cycle and, despite this prodigious effort, the central question 'are these cycles normal with respect to ovulation and/or normal with respect to fertility?', remains unanswered.

As has been stated before (Lenton et al, 1982b) the only (and simplest) selection criterion for establishing not only whether ovulation has occurred but also whether the cycle is fertile, is the requirement that the subject should conceive during the study cycle. Provided that the pregnancy progresses normally then it does not matter whether the subject previously had regular cycles, was overweight or was even attending for infertility investigations. The only condition is that the conception should have occurred spontaneously and not during treatment designed to induce ovulation in an otherwise abnormal subject. There are of course limitations in the use of conception cycles to define the endocrine requirements of the 'normal' non-conception cycle. Firstly, the influence of the implanting embryo is apparent from about the third week of the cycle (Lenton et al, 1982a) and so data from this stage onwards in a conception cycle are no longer comparable with the non-pregnant cycle. It is also possible that the pre-implantation embryo may influence maternal steroid levels from the time of ovulation/fertilisation, although at the present time there is no evidence to substantiate this suggestion. Nevertheless data on endocrine profiles in conception cycles and on growth of the follicle up until the time of follicular rupture should be directly comparable with the 'normal non-pregnant but potentially fertile' menstrual cycle. The second practical limitation in using conception cycles as the 'standard', is that they are much more difficult to obtain in large numbers. For this reason we propose that conception cycles should be used as the primary and most exacting standard, against which to define a group of closely comparable but non-pregnant cycles (the secondary standard). Once this has been achieved the influence of all other factors (e.g. subject age, ponderal index, cycle length) can be evaluated systematically.

Apart from the physiological goal of understanding the endocrine requirements and regulation of the normal menstrual cycle, the greatest value of information on the 'normal' cycle will be for assessing the pharmacodynamic effect of a variety of fertility regulating agents and diagnosing and understanding certain types of infertility. One of the major infertility problems constituting over 50 per cent of all infertility referrals (World Health Organisation multi-centre survey of more than 5000 couples) is the couple with unexplained infertility. In these couples, the woman has regular menstrual cycles, a normal pelvis and bilateral tubal patency, and the male will have had two or more normal semen analyses. Currently there are no adequate explanations for the prolonged inability of these couples to conceive.

Although as stated above many studies have been reported which describe circulating levels of LH, follicle stimulating hormone (FSH), prolactin (Prl), oestradiol and progesterone during the menstrual cycle of apparently normal women, very few of the studies were either directly comparable with each other (with respect to subject selection criteria, or radioimmunoassay reagents) or contained large numbers of subjects in whom most of the main reproductive hormones were measured simultaneously. Other problems with some of these older reported studies, such as the validity of the mathematical methods used to analyse the data, will be alluded to later.

Over the years detailed endocrine studies in human subjects have been carried out both in the Reproductive Endocrinology Research Unit of the Karolinska Institute, Stockholm and simultaneously in the University Department of Obstetrics and Gynaecology, Sheffield. Our two groups, although pursuing different goals, have been using similar techniques (daily blood sampling and multiple hormone analyses using radioimmunoassays) and on a number of occasions have independently reached similar conclusions.

The only completely published major series of menstrual cycle data containing information on all four main reproductive hormones is the study by Landgren et al (1980) on 68 regularly menstruating Swedish women. A similar but unpublished series of comparable endocrine data in regularly menstruating British women exists (Lenton E. A, unpublished observations). There are also a number of other similar experimental studies which have been performed by our two groups, and these all add information about the normal menstrual cycle. In this chapter we plan to draw heavily on these studies in order to compare and contrast our separate findings and to show how a concept of the 'normal' cycle is emerging.

Unfortunately space does not permit circulating concentrations of more than the four major reproductive hormones — namely LH, FSH, oestradiol and progesterone — to be reviewed. For details of the patterns of secretion of 17-hydroxy-progesterone and the other ovarian and adrenal steroids, the reader should refer to Strott & Lipsett, (1968), Abraham et al, (1974), Wu et al, (1974), Guerrero et al (1976), Diczfalusy & Landgren (1977) and Shumin et al, (1983). The range and consistency of prolactin concentrations in a group of normal cycles will be considered briefly in a later section, but no attempt will be made to consider the concentration profiles of any of the reproductive hormones in urine or other body fluids, nor to consider the effects of sampling at frequencies greater than once every 24 h. It is known that when blood samples are taken at 3 h (Aedo et al, 1977), 1 h (Lenton & Hendy-Ibbs, unpublished observations), 15 min (e.g. Yen et al, 1974) and 5 min (Lenton & Hendy-Ibbs, unpublished observations), a number of short term or ultradian rhythms can be demonstrated. Depending on the sampling frequency, it is possible to show a rapid (circhoral) pulse with a 1 h frequency within a slower (approximately 6 h) rhythm. These rhythms are not only superimposed one upon the other but may in turn be affected by circadian (diurnal) rhythms (especially those steroids with an appreciable adrenal component; Landgren et al, 1977) sleep (e.g. prolactin; Parker et al, 1973) and of course cyclical ovarian changes associated with the reproductive cycle (the so-called circatrigintan or 28 day rhythm). Clearly then the subject of 'episodic or pulsatile' hormone secretion is a complex one and beyond the scope of this review. Nonetheless it is important not to loose sight of the fact that endocrine profiles based on 24 h intermittent sampling can only give a simplified picture of the actual changes in hormone concentration and it is likely that these short-term fluctuations constitute an important part of the feedback component regulating the menstrual cycle.

Background to the present studies

The two main Swedish studies which will be referred to in this text are described in detail below. The data for the first, that of the normally menstruating women, have been subjected to identical mathematical manipulations using the same computer as has been used for the British studies (1906S, University of Sheffield Computer Services).

1. Sixty-five normally menstruating Swedish women (see Landgren et al, 1980). Originally 75 apparently healthy women with a history of regular cycles (of 25–36 days) during the previous 3 months, were recruited. They were all volunteers and none had had an abortion during the last 6 months or a delivery within 1 year. None had used steroidal contraceptives or intra-uterine devices for a minimum of 3 months prior to admission to the study and none was attempting to conceive. Their ages ranged from 18 to 39 years. Blood samples were obtained by venepuncture daily between 09.00 and 11.00 h throughout one menstrual cycle. Seventy-two women completed the study but seven cycles were later excluded from the present analysis because either cycle length or luteal phase length were outside the limits >40 days or <12 days respectively, Forty-six of the women were parous. Horomone concentrations were determined by radioimmunoassay (Aso et al, 1975 Robertson & Diczfalusy, 1977). Essential features of peptide assays were the use of the First International Reference Preparation for human pituitary gonadotrophins for bioassay (code number 69/104, Table 4.1) and the anti-

sera for LH (Kabi Diagnostica, Sweden) and for FSH (Batch #3, National Institutes of Health, Bethesda, USA). In the original analysis (Landgren et al, 1980) data from 68 women were included. This has been reduced here to 65 by specific exclusion of some cycles with short luteal phases. This group will be referred to as the Swedish control (as opposed to 'normal') group.

2. Fourteen normally menstruating women (See Diczfalusy & Landgren, 1981; Landgren et al, 1982). In this study a total of five cycles from each of 14 normally menstruating volunteers was collected. A recovery period of two cycles was allowed between each study cycle. All of these subjects were of proven fertility and a number have again conceived following the study. Hormone assays were performed as for Study No. 1 with the exception of LH concentrations which were measured using an *in vitro* bioassay (van Damme et al, 1974 as modified by Romani et al, 1977; Rajalkshmi et al, 1979). The standard preparation was 69/104 as above.

The British studies consisted of selected cycles from a data bank of 550 fully documented menstrual cycles obtained from 245 individuals. All the data are filed on a central computer (see above) and so are readily available for the retrieval of specific sub-groups of cycles.

3. Sixty-two normally menstruating British Women (unpublished). In order to match the Swedish Control group (Study No. 1) an equivalent sized group of normally menstruating British women was selected from our data bank. The basic selection requirements were age (<40 years), cycle length (<40 days) and luteal phase length (>12 days). There were only 23 cycles fulfilling these requirements which had been collected from normal volunteers directly comparable with the Swedish subjects (i.e. whose fertility was unknown and who were not attempting to conceive at that time). A further 17 cycles were added, which were obtained from women with tubal occlusion (awaiting tubal surgery, n = 10) or with azoospermic partners (awaiting AID, n = 7). Finally 22 cycles were added which were obtained from women attempting to conceive but who failed to do so in the study cycle. All these women conceived spontaneously within a maximum of 6 months (mean 2.2 months) following the study cycle. Hormone concentrations were measured by radioimmu-

Table 4.1 Details of the three standard gonadotrophin preparations* which have been used in the radioimmunoassay of human gonadotrophins

	Code No	Recommended for	Designated LH	Units/Ampoule FSH
2nd International Reference Preparations of Human Menopausal Gonadotrophin	2IRP–hMG	Bioassay	40	40
1st International Reference Preparation of Human Pituitary Gonadotrophin	69/104	Bioassay	25	10
1st International Reference Preparation of Human Pituitary LH	68/40	Immunoassay	77	0.9

* All preparations were issued through the MRC Unit for Biological Standards and Control, London. The 2nd IRP–HMG and 69/104 are both obsolete. They have been replaced for radioimmunoassay by 68/40 (LH) and 78/549 (FSH). This new FSH standard is however derived from and numerically equivalent to the old 69/104 preparation.

noassay (Lenton et al, 1978 1982b.) Essential features of the peptide assays were the use of the Second International Reference Preparation for human menopausal gonadotrophin for bioassay (code 21RP-HMG, Table 4.1), and the antisera for LH (Batch #2, National Institute of Health, Bethesda, USA) and for FSH (M91, courtesy of Dr W Butt, Birmingham, England). This group will be referred to as the British Control Group.

4. Twenty-two conception cycles in British women (see Lenton et al, 1982b). In this study 22 conception cycles were obtained. Twenty of these cycles have been described previously in a study containing 26 such cycles. The six cycles which have been omitted from present analysis were ones where ovulation had been induced with clomiphene (Clomid, Richardson-Merrell Ltd, Slough, UK). Hormone assays were as described for Study No. 3 above.

5. Seventeen normally menstruating British women (see Lenton et al, 1983a). This group is reasonably comparable with the Swedish group of 14 women (Study No. 2). Two cycles were collected from each of 17 women but unlike the Swedish study the interval between the cycles was variable and ranged from 1 month to 5.5 years. Seventy per cent of these women were attending an Infertility Clinic. Hormone assays again were as above.

6. Three normally menstruating British women (see Lenton et al, 1983a). Five cycles were obtained from each of three volunteers. The intervals between the first and last cycle ranged from 3 to 6 years. Subject A conceived twice during the study period and once again following the last cycle. Despite eventually having three pregnancies, this subject had had a history of infertility and had taken more than 5 years to achieve her first pregnancy. Subject B conceived for the first time during the fourth study cycle and she has now had a second successful pregnancy. Subject C has not yet attempted to become pregnant. These cycles were analysed for LH and progesterone only.

7. 186 normally menstruating British women (unpublished). For these studies endocrine data from 186 menstrual cycles were used. All of these 186 subjects were women with regular menstrual cycles but who were complaining of infertility (failure to conceive within 2 years). The endocrine data was part of the British cycle data bank (see above). The objective of this study was to look for associations between hormones. In order to do this, small sub-groups of the cycles containing representatively high or low concentrations of one hormone were selected, and then the concentration profiles for the remaining reproductive hormones were compared. In this way the effect of, for example, high or low follicular LH, on oestradiol and progesterone concentrations could be examined. Each sub-group consisted of about 20 cycles representing 10 per cent of the whole population. This procedure was repeated in turn for oestradiol, progesterone and prolactin.

8. Twenty normally menstruating British women. As in previous studies, normally menstruating women were recruited but this time in addition to serial blood samples, these women also underwent serial ultrasound scanning of their ovaries using the full bladder technique (Hackeloer et al, 1979). The ultrasound equipment was a Roche Superscan 50 and all scans were performed by one of two technicians. Follicle diameter (in cm) was recorded as the mean of six measurements made in three planes and follicular volume (ml) was calculated from mean follicle diameter. Photographs were generally taken and qualitative observations on the appearance of the follicle were also recorded. The blood samples were analysed for LH, oestradiol and progesterone by the methods given above. These subjects all showed clear evidence of follicular rupture on LH+1 (15 subjects) or LH+2 (five subjects) and progesterone indices were within the fertile range (see later).

9. Twelve normally menstruating British women (unpublished). The subjects in this group also underwent serial ultrasonic scanning as well as giving daily blood samples, but this study differed from Study No. 8 in that evidence of follicular rupture was not always clear and progesterone indices were not all within the normal range. Further in this group each subject gave two cycles with a maximum interval between cycles of 6 months.

Methods of hormone assay

The simplest and most widely available method of measuring hormone concentrations is the radioimmunoassay. Radioimmunoassays differ slightly from laboratory to laboratory but in practice these differences are, or should be, trivial; any major differences in results can generally be attributed to the use of different antisera or standards. In a good laboratory it should be possible to control adequately all the other factors such as reliability, precision, accuracy by careful assessment and processing of data (Cekan, 1976) and by the use of comprehensive internal and external quality controls.

The principles of radioimunoassay dictate that the hormone whose concentration is being determined should compete with a labelled variant (usually isotopically labelled) for a limited number of binding sites on an antibody. The antibody (or antiserum) is produced by immunising animals with the hormone under investigation. One advantage of the use of 'artifically produced' antisera is that they may have great sensitivity but unfortunately they may also lack specificity and be inherently variable. The antiserum may be unable to distinguish between closely related molecules (for example, free steroids and their metabolic conjugates), or in the case of peptide hormones, biologically active and inactive molecular species. Thus an antiserum that binds both biologically active and inactive hormone molecules will *overestimate* the relevant biological concentrations by the amount of biologically inactive hormone present. Although this problem can affect all radioimmunoassays whether measuring steroid or peptide hormones, the latter group is also subject to another related technical problem, that of impure standard preparations. Most of the reference preparations for the peptide hormones are impure — this means they may contain large amounts of biologically inactive hormone. When these preparations were initially calibrated using *in vivo* bioassays, the content of biologically inactive or altered hormone did not matter since this was not capable of eliciting a biological response. Unfortunately when these same standard preparations are used in an immunoassay, the antiserum is likely to recognise and bind both molecular moieties. Thus in an immunological assay system the standard preparation would appear to contain much more 'hormone' than it did in the biological assay system. Since however the standard is calibrated with respect to the bioassay, the net effect is an apparent *underestimation* of the relevant biological hormone concentration. It is likely that different antisera will 'recognise' different ratios of biological to immunological activity even in the same partially purified extract of the hormone. When plasma or serum samples are introduced into the radioimmunoassay, it is not surprising that different antisera may be further affected with the result that the true biological hormone concentration may be even more *over* or *underestimated*.

One solution to these problems is to develop *in vitro* bioassays which like *in vivo* bioassays have the ability to recognise only biologically active hormone but which compare with radioimmunoassays in terms of sensitivity and economy. In practice this goal has proved difficult to achieve — an *in vivo* bioassay for LH has been developed (van Damme et al, 1974) and modified (Romani et al, 1977; Rajalakshmi et al, 1979) and used to measure circulating LH concentrations. A comparable system for measuring FSH (Martin Ritzen et al, 1982) unfortunately lacks sensitivity and is subject to non-specific interference by plasma samples. The differences in LH concentrations when samples are measured by an *in vivo* bioassay or in two radioimmunoassays using different standards preparations are shown in Fig. 4.1. In general, results obtained by *in vivo* bioassay are higher than their equivalent radioimmunoassay concentrations.

An alternative solution to the problem of biological versus immunological measurement is to improve the hormone reference preparations. By implication adequate purification and removal of biologically inactive but immunologically active contaminants should produce the ideal standard preparations for use in radioimmunoassays. In practice these ideals too are difficult to attain (Storring et al, 1981, 1982) and even when ideal reference preparations do become available, problems due to idiosyncracies in the antisera will still remain. The search for a perfect antibody is a goal that may take a great many years to realise and in the meantime it is necessary to compromise — continuing to make use of the observation obtained by

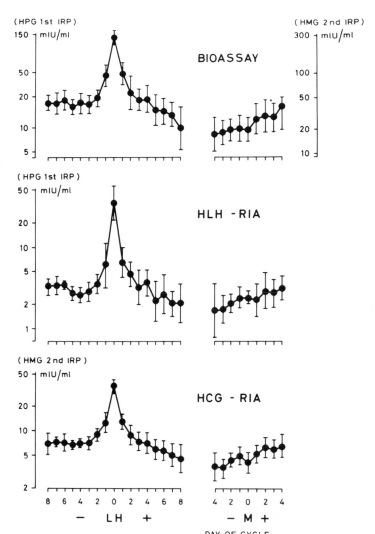

Fig. 4.1 Biological and immunological LH activities in plasma throughout the menstrual cycle. Geometric mean values and 95 per cent confidence limits. Biological activity from 12 cycles is presented both in terms of the HMG (2nd IRP) and HPG (human pituitary gonadotrophin, 1st IRP) standards. HLH–RIA represents the values obtained by a radioimmunoassay system, using a human luteinising hormone preparation (eight cycles) and HCG–RIA indicates the values obtained by a radioimmunoassay utilising an HCG preparation. (According to Romani et al, 1977)

radioimmunoassay but at the same time acknowledging the limitations of the methodology.

The currently recommended reference preparations are 68/40 (for LH) and 69/104 (for FSH) although this is gradually being phased out in favour of a new FSH reference preparation 78/549 (Table 4.1). Although 68/40 is reasonably pure, the standard 69/104, originally developed for bioassay, is very impure (containing large amounts of biologically inactive but immunologically active material) and consequently FSH concentrations determined relative to this standard are seriously *underestimated*. Just what this means in practice is shown by a recent experiment where the FSH content in ampoules of Pergonal (hMG), and

Metrodin (pure FSH, Serono Laboratories Ltd), were measured in a standard FSH radioimmunoassay. Each of these ampoules contained 70 to 75 iu of FSH calibrated against the reference preparation 69/104 using an *in vivo* bioassay. However, using a radioimmunoassay and the same standard, FSH concentrations were recorded as 16 and 11 iu/ampoule respectively. Clearly if the biological content of partially purified ampoules of FSH can be underestimated by nearly 80 per cent, then it is likely that circulating plasma levels of FSH are also being seriously underestimated. At this level of imprecision any small but possibly extremely significant alterations in circulating, biologically active FSH concentrations during the menstrual cycle are unlikely to be detected. Certainly the subcutaneous injection of 25 iu of pure FSH in a number of subjects produced no discernible alteration in circulating FSH levels over the subsequent three hours.

Without wishing to labour the point, we feel that it is important that the limitations of radioimmunoassay data are fully appreciated. If despite apparent sensitivity, the methodology is insufficiently precise to show up small but possibly important biological differences then it would be fallacious to attempt to look for such differences. Conversely because current methodology fails to show significant differences between groups of cycles (see for example, FSH concentrations between conception and non-conception cycles, Fig. 4.3 and 4.4), it may be erroneous to conclude that there are no biologically important differences.

Methods of hormone analysis

In 1945 Professor J. H. Gaddum observed that 'A large part of statistical theory is based on the assumption that measurements are distributed in normal probability curves and that the variance is constant. The mathematical conditions for normality have been firmly established but the best evidence that these conditions are fulfilled in any particular case is still the observation that the distribution is actually normal. In some cases the normal curve gives a very close approximation to the observed facts. These cases are the exception rather than the rule; but it is usually possible to transform the distribution by means of some function of the actual observations which is normally distributed' and he goes on to say that provided the distribution is normal (or can be transformed in order to make it normal) and that the variance of the distribution is constant (or varies in some predictable way) then it is relatively easy to calculate the significance of differences, regression lines, correlation coefficients, the analysis of variance and so on; but if the distribution is not normal then it is unjustifiable to assume that the arithmetic mean is the best estimate of a quantity that can be derived from a set of measurements of it. Recent developments in statis-

tical technique have thus greatly increased the importance of methods for normalising distributions by some suitable device such as taking logarithms. This is particularly important when the standard deviation is large compared with the mean. When it is small, all ordinary transformations of this kind have less effect, and in the extreme case when it is very small such transformations do not have any effect.

The example given is that of a population of men of different weight. The existence of men of more than double the average weight implies the existence of other men with negative weight. This illustration has an obvious parallel with certain biological and in particular endocrinological measurements, as is shown by the following example. The arithmetic mean of a series of prolactin measurements was found to be 343 mu/l with a standard deviation of 228 mu/l. Taking these figures at face value we obtain the limits 115 to 571 mu/l and −113 to 799 mu/l for the 68 per cent and the 95 per cent confidence ranges respectively. Now, not only is it biologically impossible to obtain a *negative* prolactin concentration, but in this case, the minimum sensitivity of the radioimmunoassay was approximately 50 mu/l and the lowest *recorded* value in the distributation was actually 69 mu/l. The difficulty arises because an arithmetic mean has been used to describe a distribution that was not normal or Gaussian. To extend these calculations by comparing prolactin concentrations between individuals using a *t*-test or performing any other mathematical manoeuvres such as those described above is clearly meaningless. [Despite the obviousness of these comments and specific Instructions to Authors, Journal of Endocrinology (1974), a glance through recent editions of most of the endocrine journals will reveal that many authors persist in quoting arithmetic means and standard deviations without regard to the distributions of their data].

Gaddum recommended testing all distributions and finding by trial and error a method of transformation that most successfully 'normalised' the distribution. Where this was not possible then he said it was 'theoretically better' to use the transformation:

$$X = \log x$$

(where the logarithms could be natural or to the base 10), than to use no transformation at all. In the example of prolactin concentrations given above, transforming all the data to logarithms (base 10) before calculating means and standard deviations in the usual way gives log 2.44 ± 0.29 mu/l. In practice these log-concentrations are unfamiliar and so it is usual to convert them back to a linear scale (by taking anti-logs). However it is necessary first to calculate the values of the 'mean plus one standard deviation' etc and then to anti-log these computed figures. Assuming a log-normal distribution, the mean prolactin concentration will become 277 mu/l, with 68 per cent and 95 per cent confidence limits of 143–537 mu/l and 74–1040 mu/l respectively. These values are much more in accord with direct observations on the data and are within the sensitivity limits of the methodology.

Testing the distribution

Standard statistical methods such as the calculation of goodness of fit will confirm whether a distribution is normal but simple graphical methods of applying transformations are more informative when attempting to find the best method of normalising the data (see Mortimer & Lenton, 1983). This technique is known as probability analysis and has been described previously (Kletzky et al, 1975; Lenton et al, 1979). In simple terms, the individual data are ranked, suitable increments known as the class interval chosen and a frequency histogram constructed. A typical skewed frequency distribution is shown in Fig. 4.2. The frequency should be expressed as a percentage, and the class (or class interval) can be individual points or groups of data depending on the numbers and range of the original observations. The approximate positions of the mode, median and mean have been indicated. The *mode* is defined as the class interval with the greatest number of observations, the *median* is the class value which occurs at a cumulative frequency of 50 per cent (i.e. at the mid-point of the ranking); the *mean* is of course the sum of all classes divided by the number of observations. Only in a special case of a normal or Gaussian distribution will the *mode*, *median* and *mean* coincide. To construct a probability plot cumulative percentage frequency values are obtained by sequentially summating percentage frequencies for each class interval. These values may be converted to probits using probability tables (Fisher & Yates, 1963) and plotted against class interval. Alternatively probability graph paper can be used directly. Any regular tendency for the plotted points to diverge from a straight line shows that the distribution was not normal (Mortimer & Lenton, 1983), and indicates that some form of transformation will be

required. Types of transformations that may be appropriate are $X = \log x$; $X = \sqrt{x}$; $X = \sqrt[3]{x}$ (Mortimer & Lenton, 1983); or $X = \log (x + x_0)$ (Gaddum, 1945). The original data are first ttransformed, then appropriate class intervals are chosen and the technique of probability analysis reapplied. The transformation which best produces a straight line is the method which will normalise the data most successfully.

The median (or 50 per cent cumulative frequency value) is given by the value probit = 5. The median should stay constant irrespective of any transformation applied to the data. In fact the median can be obtained merely from ranking the data, but probability plots yield additional information about transformation methods which will normalise the distribution (to aid later statistical analysis) and permit the confidence limits to be defined directly. For this purpose the 95 per cent confidence range corresponds with probits 3 to 7 (actually 3.04 to 6.96) and the 68 per cent confidence range corresponds approximately with probits 4 to 6. Thus confidence limits can be obtained by direct inspection of the probability plots irrespective of whether these are normal (straight line) or curvi-linear. In the special case of a normal distribution or one that has been successfully normalised the median will coincide with the mean and the probits 4 to 6 and 3 to 7 will cover the range of ± 1 s.d. and ± 2 s.d respectively.

In conclusion, the value of probability analysis is that it permits calculation of the median and ranges of the confidence limits without requiring any assumptions about the nature of the distribution. The medians and ranges provide precise information about the location and dispersion of the original data. Further probability plots can be used to check methods of transforming the data in order to normalise its distribution. Ultimately transforming the data before calculating means and confidence limits in the usual way is quicker than obtaining the same information graphically using probability plots, and it allows other statistical techniques to be applied in a valid way.

In the absence of sufficient data to describe a distribution accurately it is preferable to *assume* a log-normal distribution (Gaddum, 1945) and to quote means and confidence limits either in log-units or after transformation back to the arithmetic scale — in which case the mean is referred to as the geometric mean (Instructions to Authors, Journal of Endocrinology, 1974).

Normal ranges of reproductive hormones

When attempting to establish the normal range of any endocrine parameter, two requirements should be satisfied. Firstly the study group (more correctly the 'study population') should be homogeneous with respect to the selection criteria, and secondly there should be a sufficiently large number of observations so that addition of further data would not be expected to alter either the mean or the

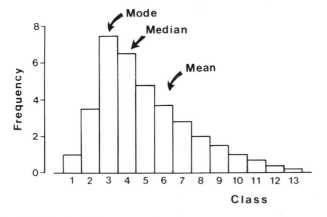

Fig. 4.2 Hypothetical example of a type of skewed frequency distribution such as is frequently seen when endocrine data are analysed. The approximate position of the *mode*, *median*, and *mean* (see text) are indicated

95 per cent confidence limits. Unfortunately there is only one published study which contains sufficient numbers of cycles to satisfy this requirement and that is the study of 68 normally menstruating Swedish women (Landgren et al, 1980). Because it is important that information of this kind be obtained in more than one laboratory (to avoid distortions due to laboratory bias) we propose to compare this Swedish control group (Study No. 1) with similar but previously unpublished data from Sheffield (the 'British control group' Study No. 3).

Results

Comparisons of the plasma profiles of LH, FSH, oestradiol and progesterone in each of the two studies are shown in Fig. 4.3. The mean profiles of the steroids, oestradiol and progesterone are virtually superimposable and the only detectable differences between the groups are slightly larger standard deviations in the Swedish group. Possible reasons for this will be discussed below. The gonadotrophin profiles were also very similar in shape (although of course numerically quite different because of the different

standards). Standard deviations were again slightly larger in the Swedish group and the magnitude of the LH and FSH peaks was greater. This is possibly a reflection of the differences in antisera.

Apart from the unavoidable numerical differences, similarities between the two control groups are remarkable. The steroid profiles where there are no problems with impure reference preparations are virtually identical and show the same features such as an oestradiol maximum on LH − 1, an oestradiol minimum following the LH peak on LH + 2, and luteal oestradiol levels which start to decline towards the end of the cycle from LH + 10 onwards. Progesterone profiles too are very similar and show the same features such as a small rise in progesterone over LH − 1 to LH + 1 with a more rapid rise from LH + 2 through to LH + 6. Maximum mean luteal progesterone concentrations were attained on LH + 6, LH + 7 (Swedish group) and on LH + 7, LH + 8 (British group). Luteal progesterone levels start to decline from about LH + 8 in both groups.

The essential features of the gonadotrophin profiles were the early follicular FSH rise (LH − 13 to LH − 6) after which concentrations decreased to a nadir on LH − 3 before rising once more at the start of the mid cycle peak. During the luteal phase mean FSH concentrations fell steadily until LH+9 when they once again began rising as the luteal phase came to an end. LH concentrations did not show an early follicular phase peak but concentrations started increasing towards the mid-cycle peak from LH − 3 (in synchrony with FSH concentrations). During the luteal phase LH levels fell slowly to reach a nadir around LH + 9 to LH + 11 again matching changes in the FSH profile.

No attempt will be made to define the 95 per cent confidence limits for specific hormones on specific days of the cycle because this has already been done (Landgren et al, 1980; Tables 4.4–4.6, and 4.9). In any case the current data merely indicate the 68 per cent confidence limits of a potentially *normal* population but not necessarily one that is potentially *fertile*. For this we need to compare the above profiles from non-pregnant women with cycles from women who actually conceived during sampling (Study No. 4).

Conception cycles are of course cycles of proven fertility and as such are a highly selected sub-group of the control population (i.e. only these control women whose cycles were actually fertile could be represented by the conception cycle group). Accordingly one would expect to find smaller confidence limits in the conception cycle group.

In Fig. 4.4 are shown the geometric mean profiles of LH, FSH, oestradiol and progesterone in 22 conception cycles from British women. The profiles of LH, FSH and oestradiol in these cycles are very similar to those of the non-conception cycles up until LH+9 when the influence of the embryo becomes apparent, but as has been reported

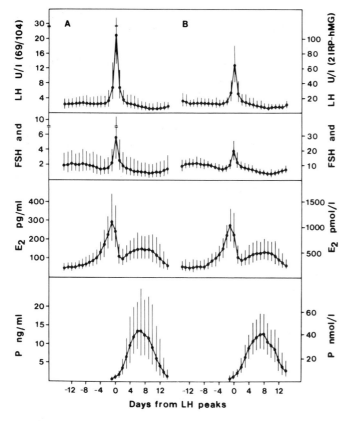

Fig. 4.3 Geometric mean (with 68 per cent confidence limits) of circulating plasma concentrations of LH, FSH, oestradiol and progesterone in (A) 65 Swedish control cycles and (B) 62 British control cycles. For details of the composition of the study populations, refer to Studies No. 1 and 3 in the text. The gonadotrophin standards employed were 69/104 (Swedish Study) and 2IRP–HMG (British Study) respectively

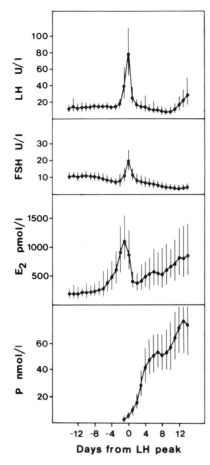

Fig. 4.4 Geometric mean levels (with 68 per cent confidence limits) of circulating plasma concentrations of LH, FSH, oestradiol and progesterone in 22 British conception cycles. The profiles of the majority of these cycles have been published before (Lenton et al, 1982) but here they have been recalculated after exclusion of six cycles where ovulation was induced with clomiphene (Study No. 4, see text). The apparent increase in LH concentrations from LH + 10 onwards is due to cross-reaction in the LH radioimmunoassay by HCG from the implanting embryo. Similarly the increases in progesterone and oestradiol concentrations from LH + 9 denotes 'rescue' of the corpus luteum. The assay reagents were identical with those used for the British Control group shown in Fig. 4.3

be to obtain evidence showing (i) that there is no pre-implantation maternal response and (ii) that pregnancies do not occur at progesterone levels below this range. At the present time there are no known embryonic signals capable of elevating luteal progesterone concentrations from day LH + 2 onwards. Moreover this signal would need to be specific for progesterone secretion since there are no detectable differences in oestradiol concentration at this early stage in the pregnancy. Since it seems improbable that such a signal exists, we must conclude for the present that these higher progesterone levels are necessary for a cycle to be fertile.

The progesterone index

It has been shown that progesterone secretion during the day is not stable, there may be diurnal rhythms (Younglai et al, 1975; but see also Runnebaum et al, 1972; Landgren et al, 1977) and other ultradian rhythms as shown in Fig. 4.5 (West et al, 1973; Pizarro, 1975). Thus single samples may not be particularly accurate or representative of the individual. Where they are used diagnostically/prognostically then difficulties over 'borderline' values may be appreciable.

In the past we have advocated the use of a progesterone index (PI) with which we have defined as the arithmetic mean progesterone concentration over the days LH + 5, +6, +7 and +8 (Lenton & Cooke, 1981). By taking an average of four samples we hoped to reduce the error associated with random episodic fluctuations. This interval was chosen merely because it represents the maximum luteal progesterone concentrations approaching the time when implantation probably occurs. It is also a time when progesterone levels are relatively stable and this too contributes towards the accuracy of the PI estimate (see also Abraham et al, 1974; Coutts et al, 1982). Clinically the major disadvantage of a PI is correctly timing the samples

before (Lenton et al, 1982b), progesterone concentrations are somewhat higher in the conception cycles. However it should be noted that the upper ranges of the 68 per cent confidence limits are very similar to the upper ranges of both the control groups (Fig. 4.3), it is only the lower range that differs.

Clearly for the hormones LH, FSH and oestradiol (as measured by radioimmunoassay) the requirements for fertility are indistinguishable from those same parameters measured in non-conception cycles up to the time of implantation. The clear differences in early luteal progesterone concentrations suggest that progesterone levels of this magnitude may be a specific requirement for pregnancy. Alternatively it is possible that they may be part of the maternal response to the presence of a pre-implantated embryo. The only way of resolving this dilemma will

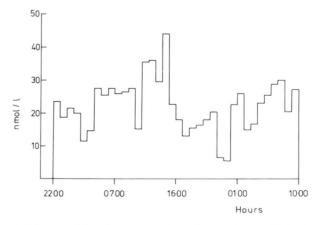

Fig. 4.5 Integrated hourly concentrations of progesterone obtained using a constant *exfusion* system, over a 36 h period during the mid-luteal phase of the cycle (see Lenton & Cooke, 1982)

relative to the LH peak. In practice the effects of slightly mis-timing the PI days are likely to be small, and eventually when salivary steroid assays become established as routine it may be better to document the whole of the luteal phase.

We have calculated PI (+5 to +8) values for all 149 cycles shown in Fig. 4.3 and 4.4 and obtained geometric means (and 95 per cent confidence limits,) using probability plots, thus avoiding any assumptions about the nature of the distributions (Table 4.2). The actual differ-

Table 4.2 Median progesterone indices (and 68 per cent and 96 per cent confidence limits) in cycles from three groups of potentially normal women. The progesterone index values were obtained from probability plots* (see text)

| Subject group | N | Progesterone index +5 to +8 (nmol/1)[†] | | | | |
		−48%	−34%	Median	+34%	+48%
British Control Cycles	62	16	28	40	53	62
Swedish Control Cycles	65	16	31	46	62	(76)**
British Conception Cycles‡	22	31	38	47	59	73

* For the control (non-conception) cycles, progesterone index values appeared normally distributed while for the conception cycles the distribution was log-normal.

† To convert to ng/ml, multiply by 0.314

** The graphical method used to determine the confidence limits was not precise at this level.

‡ The *lowest* recorded PI value in a spontaneous conception cycle in this series was 35.7 nmol/1.

ences in the distributions of the two control cycle PI (+5 to +8) values and the conception cycle values are clearly illustrated. Although the upper limits for all three distributions were very close and even the medians not markedly different, there were quite clear differences between the lower confidence limits. Incidentally inclusion of the six conception cycles where ovulation was induced by clomiphene (Lenton et al, 1982b) would not have changed the conception cycle mean and confidence limits. Thus it was obvious that whilst both control groups had PI (+5 to +8) values that were normally distributed, the data for the conception cycle group were approximately log-normally distributed.* This was interesting because it indicated that whilst the PI (+5 to +8) values in the non-pregnant cycles were distributed equally above and below their median, the PI (+5 to +8) values for the conception cycles were clustered towards the lower end of their range which was somewhat higher than the non-pregnant range (Table 4.2). The implication is that there is a specific biological 'cut-off'

* Despite the fact that non-conception PI values tended towards a normal distribution, analysing these data by taking geometric means (as was done for Fig. 4.3 and 4.4) would not effect the estimate of central tendency (Gaddum, 1945) and the results are prefectly valid.

point in a group of conception cycles associated with certain minimum progesterone concentrations. In the prolactin example quoted earlier the biological 'cut-off' point was zero hormone concentration and this absolute minimum value had the effect of 'pulling in' the distribution more rapidly towards the low hormone concentration end of the range. There is no such limiting factor at the upper end of the prolactin concentration range and so the result is a skewed distribution. In the case of conception cycle PI (+5 to +8) values, the biological 'cut-off' limit is not, of course, zero hormone concentration since progesterone levels are maximal during this part of the mid-luteal phase but could be a biological 'restraint' resulting from some inherent property of conception cycles. Again this observation does not show whether the altered PI (+5 to +8) distribution is a requirement or a consequence of the conception.

What information can be obtained from Table 4.2? Firstly it is possible to state that in a spontaneous conception cycle it is unlikely that the PI (+5 to +8) will be less than 30 nmol/1 and it is much more likely to be greater than 40 nmol/1. Further it is possible to identify the 12 per cent of Swedish and 21 per cent of British cycles that have PI (+5 to +8) values *below* the 95 per cent confidence limits of the conception group. Similarly 25 per cent and 29 per cent of the non-pregnant cycles show PI (+5 to +8) values below the 68 per cent confidence limit (i.e. 38 nmol/1) for the conception cycle group. Consequently we can postulate that about 25 per cent of cycles from normally menstruating women such as the ones described here, would not be sufficiently optimal with respect to progesterone secretion for pregnancy to occur (assuming adequate coital exposure). The small differences in the numbers of potentially fertile Swedish and British cycles probably reflects different subject selection criteria (see details of Study Nos 1 and 3).

How valuable is the PI? The only point in developing the concept of PI (+5 to +8) and in attempting to distinguish fertile cycles from control cycles is to use this information to diagnose possible endocrine defects in patients who are persistently infertile. In a series of 105 women presenting with unexplained infertility, PI (+5 to +8) values ranged from 15.9 to 49.4 nmol/1 with a median of 32.7 nmol/1. Thus in a group of regularly cycling infertile women nearly 50 per cent of the cycles showed mid-luteal progesterone concentrations that are below the 95 per cent confidence interval for conception cycles, or that are below the 68 per cent confidence limits for 'control' cycles. This suggests that a number of these infertile women may indeed have cycles with unacceptably poor luteal function. Of course this is not the same thing as saying that they fail to conceive because their progesterone concentrations are low but rather that there may be a specific functional defect resulting in poor luteal function which is associated with an inability to become pregnant.

Consistency of hormone profiles between cycles

In the foregoing section we have shown that conception is unlikely to occur in a particular cycle unless that cycle has more than a minimum progesterone concentration during the mid-luteal phase. But without some knowledge of the degree of variation in progesterone secretion between successive cycles in the *same* individual, it is impossible to use information obtained in one cycle to predict hormone concentrations in another. The primary objective in defining the endocrine parameters of a normal cycle was to provide a base against which to compare infertile cycles but such an exercise would be useless without some expression of the degree of confidence with which a study cycle can be expected to compare with subsequent cycles from the same individual.

There are three separate studies which have been carried out by the Swedish and British groups which give information on the consistency of hormonal variables *between* cycles but *within* individuals. Although study designs differ (mostly in the type of subjects selected and the number of cycles analysed) the conclusions are similar.

In the study of 17 normally menstruating women (Study No. 5) it was found that the majority of the reproductive hormones were significantly more variable *between* individuals than they were *between* cycles from the same individual when two cycles separated by intervals ranging from 1 month to 5.5 years were examined. One-way analysis of variance was used to compare representative sections of the cycles and as can be seen from Table 4.3, most of the

hormones and intervals were more significantly correlated *between* cycles than *between* individuals. In particular the LH and FSH surges, the mid-follicular phase FSH concentration and the luteal progesterone concentration (over the interval LH + 2 to LH + 8) were highly significantly ($P < 0.001$) correlated from cycle to cycle. These results are corroborated by similar observations obtained by the Swedish group (using data from the 14 regularly menstruating women Study No. 2) and two-way analysis of variance (Table 4.3). The only noteworthy difference is in the highly significant correlation in maximum pre-ovulatory concentrations in Swedish women with apparently no correlation in British women when total oestradiol over the intervals LH − 5 to LH − 0 are compared. The main conclusion to be drawn from all of these significant correlations is that it is the subjects who differ from each other whilst their cycles remain relatively constant.

Since progesterone seems to be quantitatively the most important of the four hormones under consideration (Lenton et al, 1982b) cycle to cycle variability in progesterone will be discussed in more detail. In the Swedish study (Study No. 2) five cycles were collected from each of 14 women. Identification of the maximum progesterone concentration (P_{max}) in each cycle and calculation of geometric means (and 95 per cent confidence limits) gave the results shown in Fig. 4.6. Each of the 14 individual subjects showed a range of P_{max} values within her five cycles that was less variable than that of the population overall, thus those subjects with higher P_{max} values always tended to have high values and *vice versa*. Although many of subjects showed considerable overlap there was no overlap at either end of the mean concentration range.

Results of a comparable British study (Study No. 6) are shown in Table 4.4 Here PI (+5 to +8) values were calculated for five cycles from each of three subjects. It is obvious from Table 4.4 that within subject progesterone concentrations were fairly similar. In fact the *within*-subject variance was highly significantly ($P < 0.0001$) less than the *between*-subject variance. Although both Subject A and

Table 4.3 Analyses of the variance (and the significance) of individual hormone concentrations *between* cycles (*within* individuals) and *between* individuals. The British data were obtained from 17 subjects contributing two cycles each (Study No. 5, using one-way analysis of variance) and the Swedish data were obtained from 14 subjects contributing five cycles each (Study No. 2, using two-way analysis of variance).

Hormone	Cycle interval	F-Value	Significance
British subjects			
LH	−10 to −5	1.43	ns
	−1 to +1	5.91	$P < 0.001$
	+2 to +8	2.55	$P < 0.05$
FSH	−10 to −5	4.97	$P < 0.001$
	−1 to +1	5.02	$P < 0.001$
	+2 to +8	3.26	$P < 0.01$
E_2	−10 to −5	2.59	$P < 0.05$
	−5 to 0	1.76	ns
	+2 to +8	2.78	$P < 0.05$
P	−1 to +1	1.78	ns
	+2 to +8	4.58	$P < 0.001$
Swedish subjects			
LH pre-ovulatory maximum		7.22	$P < 0.001$
E_2 pre-ovulatory maximum		12.47	$P < 0.001$
E_2 luteal maximum		4.06	$P < 0.05$
P luteal maximum		12.60	$P < 0.001$

ns = not significant

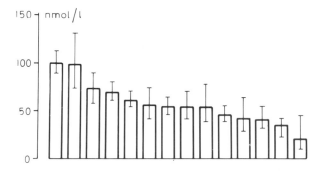

Fig. 4.6 Geometric mean levels (with 95 per cent confidence limits) of the maximum luteal progesterone concentration in five cycles in each of 14 normally menstruating women (Study No. 2, see text; unpublished data)

Table 4.4 Progesterone index concentrations in nmol/l over the interval LH + 5 to LH + 8 in five cycles from three British subjects. The intervals between the first and last cycles were 6, 5 and 3 years respectively (Study No. 6, see text)

Cycle No	1	2	3	4	5	Mean
Subject A	27.4	29.5	31.5	23.5	34.7	29.3
Subject B	42.5	44.4	38.2	49.4*	39.3	42.7
Subject C	42.8	57.0	47.9	50.4	46.5	48.9

* This was a spontaneous conception cycle.

Subject B were of proven fertility it was interesting that Subject A with the lowest PI values of the three, had previously experienced difficulty in conceiving and from Table 4.4 it was obvious that only two of her five monitored cycles fell within the conception cycle range (see Table 4.2). Even then progesterone indices were lower than the lowest recorded spontaneous conception cycle PI in the above series. These observations may offer some explanation for the length of time (in excess of 5 years) taken by this subject to conceive initially.

The use of progesterone indices has shown that women with unexplained infertility tend to have lower progesterone concentrations than normal women although some of these women do eventually conceive (Lenton & Cooke, 1981). However questions such as whether luteal function is always defective in these women and what degree of variation in progesterone secretion exists between successive cycles, needs to be answered. Although none of the present studies were designed with these objectives in mind, we felt it was worth recalculating the data (particularly of the Swedish Study No. 2) to see if it were possible to quantify cycle to cycle variability in luteal progesterone secretion within an individual.

The standard technique for quantifying variability in radioimmunoassay data is to calculate the coefficent of variation in the concentration of a single sample analysed repeatedly in successive assays. A good radioimmunoassay might give a coefficient of variation as low as 5 per cent whilst for a poor assay it could reach values of 15–20 per cent. Applying this technique to the data shown in Table 4.4 gave coefficients of variation on 10.5, 10.8 and 14.3 per cent. These values are seen to be extraordinarily low when it is considered that the coefficient of variation of the progesterone assay used to determine these data was 8.8 per cent (Lenton et al, 1982b). Similar calculations were performed on the progesterone data from the Swedish Study No. 2. Data from two subjects were not available and one subject was omitted because of occasional anovulatory cycles (PI < 7 nmol/l) but results for 11 of the 14 women are shown in Table 4.5. Individual mean progesterone index concentrations ranged from 27 to 80 nmol/l similar to but slightly lower than the mean P_{max} values for the same women shown in Fig. 4.6. Only one woman has a *mean* PI (+5 to +8) below the 95 per cent confidence limit for conception cycles (Table 4.2) and only 5/54 indi-

Table 4.5 Progesterone index concentrations in nmol/l over the interval LH + 5 to LH + 8 in five cycles from each of 11 Swedish women (Study No. 2, see text). The interval between each of the study cycles was 2 months

Cycle No	1	2	3	4	5	Mean	Coefficient of variation. (%)*
Subject 1	72	84	88	76	77	80	8.4
2	64	[103]	66	52	57	68	29.4
3	61	50	64	47	60	56	13.0
4	55	58	50	[30]	48	48	22.4
5	[36]	48	62	[38]	55	48	23.3
6	48	34	48	43	—	44	15.1
7	40	54	45	41	37	43	15.0
8	53	38	38	42	42	43	12.7
9	39	25	33	35	35	33	15.3
10	33	25	[18]	39	42	31	31.9
11	18	[40]	28	24	26	27	29.6

* Coefficients of variation calculated using all available data. When the 6 atypical cycles (indicated by the boxes) were omitted, coefficients of variation for Subjects 2, 4, 5, 10 and 11 reduced to 10.7, 8.7, 12.7, 21.5 and 17.9 per cent respectively.

vidual cycles (11.1 per cent) were below the same limit. This figure agrees closely with the 12 per cent incidence of single 'poor' quality cycles observed in the larger Swedish study (No. 1). It is noteworthy however that all of the 'poor' cycles were observed in the three subjects with lowest mean PI (+5 to +8) values. In fact most of the women were remarkably consistent throughout their five cycles, with coefficients of variation ranging from 8.4 to 31.9 per cent. A small number (approximately 11 per cent) of cycles were thought to be somewhat atypical. These cycles have been indicated in Table 4.5. They were scattered throughout the progesterone concentration range and in some cases were higher (Subjects 1 and 11) and in other cases lower (Subjects 4, 5 and 10) than the individual norm. Coefficients of variation were of course greater in the women with atypical cycles (22.4–31.9 per cent) although these reduced to 8.7 to 21.5 per cent, comparable with the remainder of the group when the atypical cycles were excluded from the calculation. Women with lower mean progesterone concentrations showed slightly greater cycle to cycle variability than women with consistently high PI (+5 to +8) values and all of the women showed one or more cycle that was within the conception cycle range and all of them were parous. Unfortunately it is not known whether Subjects 10 and 11 took longer to conceive than Subjects 1 and 2.

Attempts have been made to quantify individual variation in progesterone profiles because we feel that progesterone secretion is probably the most important indicator of the fertility potential of a cycle but the same approach could be used to show that similar individual-specific secre-

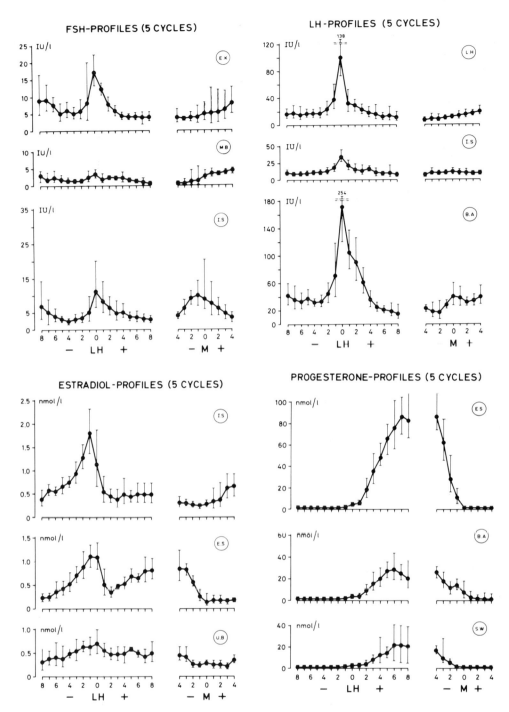

Fig. 4.7 Typical individual FSH, LH, oestradiol and progesterone profiles in the peripheral blood of normally menstruating women (Study No. 2, see text). Geometric mean levels (with 95 per cent confidence limits) have been calculated from the data of five cycles analysed in each subject. The values are synchronised around the day of the LH surge (LH) and around the day of menstruation (M) respectively. The LH results were obtained using an *in vitro* bioassay (see text), the FSH results using a conventional radioimmunoassay. The standard used in both cases was the First International Reference Preparation of human gonadotrophins for bioassay (69/104) (reprinted with permission from Landgren et al, 1982)

tion patterns exist for the other reproductive hormones. This point has already been demonstrated statistically using analyses of variance (Table 4.3) but it can also be illustrated graphically (Fig. 4.7). These examples, obtained from women in Study No. 2, clearly show both the differences in the absolute mean hormone concentrations between individuals and the differences in the shapes of the

profiles which are in turn linked to ovarian events. For example Subject IS regularly has cycles with short follicular phases (mean 10.5 day including LH – 0) and long luteal phases (mean 15.6 days). Not suprisingly we find that the normal early follicular phase rise in FSH occurs in this subject before the start of menstrual bleeding. A corresponding increase in oestradiol secretion is seen by M +

2 or M + 3. Subject MB whose cycles have longer follicular phases does not show such an early follicular rise in FSH. The vertical bars give a measure of the variability from cycle to cycle *within* the individual and it is quite obvious that the FSH profiles of IS are always different from the profiles of MB. Each woman clearly has her own specific pattern of endocrine changes which vary only slightly from cycle to cycle. Further since all the women in this study were parous (although 3/14 had not experienced a full-term pregnancy) then we must conclude that these individual patterns of hormone secretion are all compatible with fertility even though follicular growth and luteal function may not have been optimal in every cycle.

Associations between hormones within cycles

One of the obvious questions that arises from the data shown in Fig. 4.7 is whether the cycles with high progesterone concentrations are also the cycles with high preovulatory oestradiol concentrations? Is there any association between the magnitude of the LH peak and the subsequent luteal phase? (see examples in Fig. 4.8 and 4.9). Taking progesterone secretion and looking for other hormonal parameters that may correlate with it, gave the preliminary results (obtained by testing a limited number of combinations of hormones and phases of the cycle), shown in Table 4.6. It appears that there is a slight ($P < 0.05$) positive correlation between follicular oestradiol and luteal progesterone concentrations. There is a significant negative correlation ($P < 0.01$) between follicular phase LH and progesterone and a highly significant ($P < 0.001$) negative correlation between luteal phase LH and luteal phase progesterone secretion. The only directly comparable calculations which have been carried out for the British group of 17 normally menstruating women (Study No. 5) showed that the magnitude of the LH peak correlated significantly with the magnitude of the FSH peak (r = 0.49, $P < 0.01$) in 17 pairs of cycles (Lenton et al, 1983a). No other correlations between hormones have

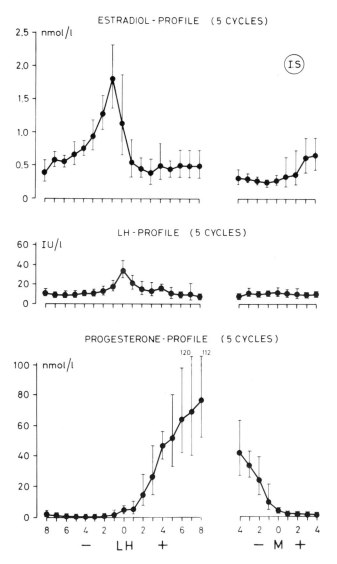

Fig. 4.8 Geometric mean of oestradiol, LH and progesterone profiles (with 95 per cent confidence limits) estimated during five cycles in a woman of proven fertility (Study No. 2, see text). The sign LH indicates the day of the LH surge and M the day of the onset of menstruation (published with permission from Diczfalusy & Landgren, 1981)

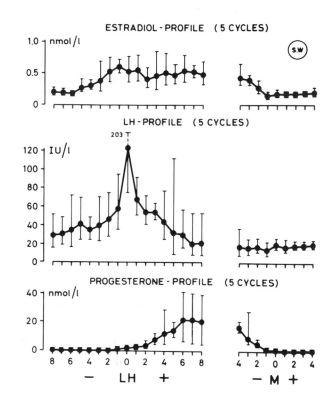

Fig. 4.9 Geometric mean of oestradiol, LH and progesterone profiles (with 95 per cent confidence limits) estimated during five cycles in a woman of proven fertility (Study No. 2, see text). The sign LH indicates the day of the LH surge and M the day of the onset of menstruation (published with permission from Diczfalusy & Landgren, 1981)

Table 4.6 Correlation coefficients between progesterone (expressed as luteal phase maximum concentration or luteal phase mean concentration) and either oestradiol or LH concentrations over selected intervals of five cycles from 14 normally menstruating women (Study No. 2)

Progesterone	Luteal maximum	Luteal phase mean
Oestradiol		
Follicular phase mean	nt	0.64*
Preovulatory maximum	0.56*	nt
Luteal phase mean	nt	0.05
LH		
Follicular phase mean	nt	−0.68†
Preovulatory maximum	−0.38	0.41
Luteal phase mean	nt	−0.79**

nt = not tested.
* $P < 0.05$; † $P < 0.01$; ** $P < 0.001$.

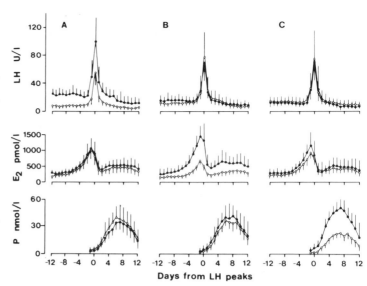

Fig. 4.10 Geometric mean levels (with 68 per cent confidence limits) of LH, oestradiol and progesterone throughout the cycle of six groups of normally menstruating women (Study No. 7, see text). The groups were selected from a data bank of 186 fully documented spontaneous cycles on the basis of specific features such as (A) a 'high' or 'low' follicular phase LH concentration (over the interval LH − 12 to LH − 5); (B) a 'high' or 'low' pre-ovulatory oestradiol concentration (over the interval LH − 5 to LH − 0) or (C) a 'high' or 'low' luteal progesterone concentration (this time over the interval LH+2 to LH+8). The number of subjects (and therefore cycles) in each group ranged from 21 to 23, and very few of the subjects appeared in more than one group. The group with 'high' concentrations are shown by the closed circles and the group with 'low' concentrations by the open circles (unpublished data)

been performed in this particular group, but there is another British study in which the question of associations between hormones was investigated (Study No. 7). The approach in this study was quite different from the Swedish study and consisted essentially of taking a large series of 186 cycles from normally menstruating women and discarding 80 per cent of the data. By selecting out 20 per cent of cycles with either the lowest or highest concentration of the hormone being tested and excluding the remaining 80 per cent of cycles which fell between these two extremes it was possible to look visually at the effects of high or low concentrations of one specific hormone on all the other reproductive hormones. The results of this procedure are shown in Fig. 4.10 for the extremes of follicular phase LH (using the mean LH per cycle over the interval LH−12 to LH−5), for oestradiol (using the interval LH−5 to LH−0) and for progesterone (using the interval LH+2 to LH+8).

Careful examination of Fig. 4.10A reveals that the group of cycles with high follicular phase LH, tend to have slightly lower luteal progesterone levels than a similar sized group of cycles with low follicular LH. There is no difference however in oestradiol concentrations between the two groups. Thus there would appear to be a negative relationship between follicular phase LH and luteal progesterone but this is obviously not of the same significance as was observed within individuals (Table 4.6). Similarly for the high and low oestradiol groups, (Fig. 4.10B) the weakly significant correlations observed in the Swedish individuals (Table 4.6) between mean follicular phase oestradiol and mean luteal phase progesterone, or between pre-ovulatory oestradiol and maximum luteal progesterone, are just discernible. The converse of this situation, namely selection of the groups with high or low progesterone levels (Fig. 4.10C), also supports the weak positive relationship between pre-ovulatory oestradiol concentrations and mid-luteal progestterone despite no detectable difference in peripheral LH concentrations.

It should be noted that hormone concentrations tend to be consistent not only between cycles from the same individual but also within the same cycle. Subjects with 'high' LH levels in the follicular phase continue to show higher levels during the remainder of the cycle than either a 'normal' LH group or the 'low' LH group. Yet absolute differences are not uniform (which they would be if their observations were merely due to fluctuations in the stability of the radioimmunoassays) and so subjects with 'high' LH shown a greater degree of LH suppression during the luteal phase than subjects with 'low' LH. Similarly for subjects with 'high' and 'low' oestradiol concentrations, early follicular (LH−12 to LH−10) concentrations were similar, but the 'high' oestradiol group show an earlier and more prolonged pre-ovulatory rise, lasting 10 days instead of only 5 days in the 'low' oestradiol group. Similar observations can be made for the 'high' and 'low' progesterone groups where the rise in mean progesterone concentrations is approximately linear over the interval LH+1 to LH+5 in both groups but the *rates* of progesterone rise are dramatically different. All of these cycles were obtained from normally menstruating women although it should be stressed that many of these women may not have been normally fertile.

At first sight it is difficult to reconcile the visual impression given by Fig. 4.8 and 4.9 where five cycles/subject were illustrated, with the large groups of 20+ cycles/20+ subjects shown in Fig. 4.10. In the individual examples it appears that cycles with high pre-ovulatory oestradiol do indeed 'correlate' with high progesterone concentrations and *vice versa*. Moreover it would also appear that there is an inverse relationship between the magnitude of the LH peak and the subsequent luteal phase. Unfortunately when the whole group of 14 subjects were analysed, these associations, although present, were not highly significant (Table 4.6). Finally when groups containing large numbers of single cycles/subject were examined (Fig. 4.10) these associations virtually disappeared. Thus these data demonstrate clearly the latent danger in using small subject numbers and selecting individual examples for illustrative purposes. In fact another of the Swedish women (Fig. 4.11) shows that a relatively poor pre-ovulatory oestradiol peak can coexist with a normal LH surge and normal luteal progesterone secretion.

Clearly then, although individual hormone concentrations within the menstrual cycle are characteristic of the woman and will show significantly less variation between cycles than between subjects, there are really no good associations between hormones. As we have said this means that a subject with low LH and high progesterone concentrations is very likely to show this same endocrine pattern in successive cycles and in this particular subject, low LH may appear to be associated with high progesterone concentrations. However there will be other subjects where high LH concentrations coexist with low progesterone concentrations and so between subjects, these associations are difficult to substantiate.

The picture that is emerging is that the 'normal' menstrual cycle results from a composite pattern of endocrine signals that allow the development of a potentially fertile reproductive state in that individual. Each woman will demonstrate a different set of endocrine values which may be characteristic of her but which may not be characteristic of other individuals. Whether or not some 'hormone-prints' are potentially more fertile than others remains an important and as yet unanswered question.

Seasonal variation in endocrine profiles

The original objective in studying five cycles from each of 14 normally menstruating women (Study No. 2) was to see if there was any seasonal variation in endocrine profiles. Since it has already been shown that there is a very strong association between successive cycles within an individual, but a lot of variability between individuals, this has to be taken into account when looking for seasonal trends. The approach used was to calculate the variance between subjects (using two-way analysis of variance) and to subtract this from the variance between seasons. No seasonal variation was found in either the LH, oestradiol or progesterone maximum values nor in the lengths of the follicular and luteal phases or in total cycle length.

Normal cycle length

In 1977 Vollman examined the basal body temperature records of 691 women and reported that the median duration of the human menstrual cycle was 27.5 days. However due to the non-Gaussian frequency distribution (McIntosh et al, 1980) the mode was 28 days and the mean 29.5 days. The observations supported the findings of older epidemiological studies (Treloar et al, 1967; Chiazze et al, 1968).

Although determination of cycle length (defined as the interval in days between the onset of menstruation) is relatively easy, the only uncertainty being the exact time of the start of menstrual bleeding, for example where this commences overnight, determination of follicular and luteal phase lengths is more difficult. Generally the follicular phase is taken as the interval (in days) from menstruation until ovulation or rupture of the follicle; from this point until the onset of the succeeding menstruation, is defined as the luteal phase. These divisions are of course only loosely related to physiological function (Hodgen,

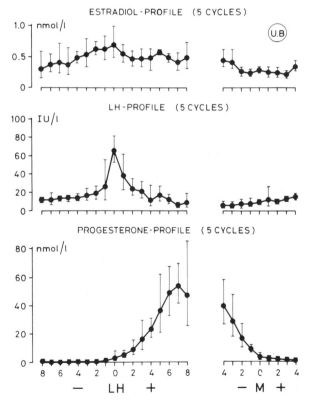

Fig. 4.11 Geometric mean of oestradiol, LH and progesterone profiles (with 95 per cent confidence limits) estimated during five cycles in a woman of proven fertility (Study No. 2, see text). The sign LH indicates the day of the LH surge and M the day of the onset of menstruation (published with permission from Diczfalusy & Landgren, 1981)

1982) and the terms proliferative and secretory phases have been preferred by some authors. In practice both systems tend to be used interchangeably. The problem of determining objectively the duration of each phase of the cycle whichever system is used, is one of imprecision in the definitions. A follicle does not instantly become a corpus luteum, ovulation cannot be measured directly (except possibly by ultrasound) and proliferative endometrium only gradually changes to a secretory pattern in response to changes in circulating steroid concentrations associated with ovulatory events. Attempts to classify the lengths of the follicular phase using the indices-thermal shift on basal body temperature recordings, intermenstrual pain or cervical mucorrhoea give poor agreement (15.7, 13.0 and 11.1 days respectively; Vollman, 1977).

If blood samples have been obtained then an endocrine signal such as the LH peak can be used to signify the change from follicular to luteal phase. This approach has the advantage of being more objective (the day of the LH maximum is readily discernible in the majority of cycles) but the disadvantage in that the LH peak may not be precisely related to ovulation (WHO Study, 1980; Brosens et al, 1978).

Other problems in determining normal follicular and luteal phase length are firstly selecting cycles that are 'normal' and secondly selecting a mathematical method that will give valid means and confidence limits.

Although spontaneous conception cycles could be used to define normal follicular phase length, they are of course, of no value in determining normal luteal phase length. The definition could be extended to include all potentially fertile cycles, i.e. those with endocrine parameters within certain limits or extended further to include all cycles from regularly (cycle length 24–35 days) menstruating women.

Using this latter definition the ranges of follicular and luteal phase length in 237 menstrual cycles were determined (Lenton et al, 1983b, 1983c). Seventy two cycles were from Swedish women (see 65 normally menstruating women, Study No. 1) and the remainder were from British women. Of these, 34 cycles were collected from volunteers (fertility unknown), 32 cycles from women aged 40–50 years and 189 cycles from regularly menstruating women attending an Infertility Clinic. The ages of the Swedish women and the younger British women were comparable and ranged from 18 to 39 years.

The first day of menstrual bleeding was defined as Day 1 and the last day of that cycle was taken as the day *before* the next menstrual period. The follicular phase was defined as the number of days up to, but *not* including the day of maximum LH concentrations and the luteal phase was defined as the number of days following but *not* including the day of maximum LH concentrations, up until the last day of the cycle.

Cycle length (and follicular phase length) have been shown to decrease with age (Sherman & Korenman, 1975;

Treloar et al, 1967; Chiazze et al, 1968) and chi-square analysis of the follicular phase data presented here confirmed that follicular phase length was significantly shorter (P < 0.0005) in the women aged 40 years and over. There were no age related changes in luteal phase length. For this reason only the 295 cycles obtained from women younger than 40 years were used to define normal follicular phase duration, but all 327 cycles were used to define normal luteal phase duration.

No assumptions were made about the normality of the distributions (McIntosh et al, 1980) and as before, probability plots were used to find the 50 per cent frequency values (medians) and to give an indication of the confidence limits of the observations.

The frequency distribution of follicular phase length was skewed and the probability plot was curvi-linear. Taking logarithms effectively normalised the distribution (straight line probability plot) as shown in Fig. 4.12. Median follicular phase duration was 12.94 days with a 95 per cent confidence range of 8.2–20.5 days.

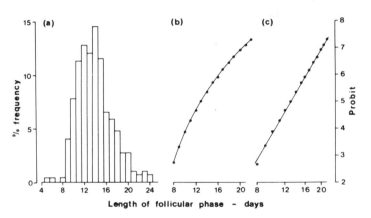

Fig. 4.12 The frequency distribution (a), and linear (b) and logarithmic (c) probability plots of follicular phase length in 295 cycles from normally menstruating women aged 18–39 years (Lenton et al, 1983b). The follicular phase was defined as the interval in days from the first day of menstruation up to but not including the day of the LH peak (Reprinted with permission from the British Journal of Obstetrics and Gynaecology)

Similarly the frequency distribution for luteal phase length was estimated and subjected to probability analysis (Fig. 4.13). On this occasion the probability plot approximated to two straight lines. This suggested that although the majority of the data followed a normal distribution, the overall group was not homogeneous and contained a small sub-population of shorter cycles. A normal frequency distribution which approximated to the majority of the data gave a mean luteal phase duration of 14.15 days, with 95 per cent confidence limits of 11.5–16.8 days respectively. From this it was concluded that any cycle with a luteal phase of 12 or more days could be considered normal. This observation supports the hypothetical limits designated by Abraham et al (1972) and Strott et al (1970).

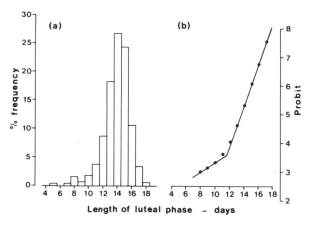

Fig. 4.13 The frequency distribution (a) and the linear probability plot (b) of luteal phase length in 327 cycles from normally menstruating women aged between 18 and 50 years (Lenton et al, 1983c). The luteal phase was defined as the interval in days following but not including the day of the LH peak until the day preceding next menstruation (Reprinted with permission from the British Journal of Obstetrics and Gynaecology)

In conclusion, normal follicular phase duration may range from 8 to 20 days and luteal phase duration from 12 to 17 days. This gives a theoretical total cycle length range of 21–38 days. In practice it is unlikely that cycles with a long follicular phase will also have a long luteal phase and in fact the reverse situation (see below) is more probable. None of the 327 cycles in this study were shorter than 24 days nor longer than 35 days.

Cycles from women over the age of 40 are likely to be abnormally short (due to decreased follicular phase duration) and cycles with luteal phases lasting less than 12 days are also probably abnormal.

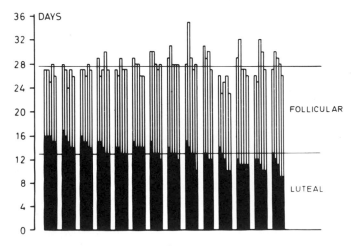

Fig. 4.14 The lengths of follicular and luteal phases in five cycles in each of 14 normally menstruating women (Study No. 2, see text). The follicular phase here was defined as the interval between the first day of menstruation up to and including the day of the LH peak. The luteal phase was defined as stated in the legend for Fig. 4.13 (with permission from Diczfalusy & Landgren, 1981)

Variability in cycle length

Again we need to consider variability *within* and *between* individuals in cycle phase length. The data from the Swedish study of 14 normally menstruating women (Study No. 2) suggested that both follicular and luteal phase length were reasonably well correlated *within* subjects (Fig. 4.14) but of the two phases, luteal phase length appeared more consistent. In fact analyses of variance applied to the results of this study and to similar results from the study of 17 normally menstruating British women (Study No. 5) showed that the variation *between* subjects was, like the equivalent endocrine data, much more significant than the variation *within* subjects (Table 4.7).

Table 4.7 Analyses of variance (and the significance) of the lengths of the follicular and luteal phases of the cycle *between* pairs of cycles in 17 normally menstruating British women or *between* five cycles per subject in 14 normally menstruating Swedish women (Study Nos. 5 and 2 respectively)

	F-value	Significance
British Women		
Follicular phase	4.26	$P < 0.002$
Luteal phase	18.66	$P < 0.0001$
Swedish Women		
Follicular phase	7.64	$P < 0.001$
Luteal phase	7.98	$P < 0.001$
Cycle length	2.67	ns

ns = not significant.

Correlations between hormones and phase lengths

It is of interest to note that for the subjects illustrated in Fig. 4.14, the individuals with a short follicular phase tended to be those with a longer luteal phase and conversely long follicular phases were associated with shorter luteal phases. This association was highly significant as indicated by the strong negative correlation ($r = -0.76$, $P < 0.001$) between follicular and luteal phase lengths (Diczfalusy & Landgren, 1981).

In the study of 65 normally menstruating women (Study No. 1) some other correlations between hormone levels and cycle length were noted. For instance LH concentrations (mean value LH−7 to LH−3; mean LH throughout the cycle; LH surge maximum) correlated positively with cycle length ($r = 0.45$, $P < 0.001$; $r = 0.35$ $P < 0.01$; $r = 0.35$ $P < 0.01$ respectively). Similarly oestradiol concentrations (mean value M+1 to M+6; mean follicular phase concentration; mean oestradiol throughout the cycle) correlated negatively with cycle length ($r = 0.44$ $P < 0.001$; $r = 0.41$ $P < 0.001$; $r = 0.35$ $P < 0.01$ respectively). It seemed that LH and oestradiol levels influenced the duration of the follicular phase (and hence cycle length) but that FSH and progesterone were not correlated with the length of the cycle or with any particular phase (see Diczfalusy & Landgren, 1981) and it is tempting to speculate that the combination low oestradiol and high LH leads to relatively long cycles, whilst high oestradiol and low LH is associated with shorter cycles. However, similar correlations in the group of 14 normally menstruating women failed to show any significant trends.

Prolactin concentrations during the normal cycle

No review of the normal menstrual cycle would be complete without mentioning prolactin although it wouId take a complete chapter to do justice to this particular subject. there is a vast amount of literature on the effects of hyperprolactinaemia in anovulatory women with or without galactorrhoea and with or without pituitary microadenomas. This review is however concerned only with the normal cycle as this occurs in regularly menstruating women. The role of prolactin in the regulation of ovarian function in normally menstruating women is poorly understood; certainly information obtained in hyperprolactinaemic-anovulatory women cannot be applied to the regularly cycling women.

Since the introduction of prolactin radioimmunoassay the pattern of prolactin concentration throughout the menstrual cycle has been extensively studied (Friesen et al, 1972; L'Hermite et al, 1972; Vekemans et al, 1972; Ehara et al, 1973; Tamura & Igarashi, 1973; Epstein et al, 1975; McNeilly & Chard, 1975; Schmidt-Gollwitzer & Saxena, 1975; Franchimont et al, 1976; Lenton et al, 1979). The problems associated with the gonadotrophin assays mentioned earlier, also apply to prolactin radioimmuno-assays which make it difficult to compare numerically results obtained by different investigators. Essentially these problems are (i) use of various standard preparations (ii) small numbers of subjects and (iii) invalid methods of mathematical analysis (cf. example quoted earlier in this chapter). Mean prolactin concentrations change little throughout the cycle except for a diffuse elevation at mid-cycle (Vekemans et al, 1972; Tamura & Igarashi, 1973; Lenton et al, 1979). Small but significant differences between mean follicular and luteal prolactin concentration have been observed Vekemans et al, 1972; Franchimont, 1976). Unfortunately daily prolactin concentrations have been determined in only 53 of the 62 women (Study No. 5) and in ten of the 17 women (Study No. 5) described in this chapter. The radioimmunoassay used has been described previously (Lenton et al, 1979) and utilised the First International Reference Preparation for prolactin (75/504) supplied by the World Health Organization through the National Institute for Biological Standards and Control, London. Geometric means, 68 per cent and 95 per cent confidence limits of plasma prolactin determined daily throughout the cycle for the 53 women are shown in Fig. 4.15. Very little alteration in mean prolactin concentrations was observed; the lowest mean concentration of 250 mu/l occurred on

LH−11 and the highest mean concentration of 475 mu/l on LH−0. Minimum and maximum values for the 68 per cent and 95 per cent confidence limits ranged from 125 to 850 mu/l and 50 to 1450 mu/l respectively. These ranges are relatively larger than equivalent concentration ranges of the other reproductive hormones (see Fig. 4.3) and this coupled with the lack of any specific change in prolactin profile throughout the cycle serves to emphasise the indirect role of prolactin in the reproductive cycle.

There are two practical reasons why the concentration ranges of prolactin are greater than for the other hormones. Firstly prolactin concentrations are much more variable from day to day. There are frequent apparently random fluctuations as well as a diurnal or sleep associated prolactin secretion (Ehara et al, 1973; Schmidt-Gollwitzer & Saxena, 1975) and both these changes are of greater magnitude than changes related to the stage of the menstrual cycle. The second reason for the large 'normal' concentration range is the variability between individuals. Some subjects have relatively low concentrations throughout the cycle whilst others have concentrations that would be considered by some investigators to be abnormally high. Since these high concentrations occur in apparently normal women and in spontaneous conception cycles (Lenton et al, 1982c) it is probably true to say that absolute levels of prolactin are not critical in the normally menstruating woman.

Prolactin concentrations between subjects

An alternative method from that shown in Fig. 4.15, for assessing the normal range of prolactin concentration is to look at the range of mean prolactin concentrations per cycle. This gives a measure of the variation between individuals rather than a measure of the variation with the stage of the cycle. Taking the mean prolactin from LH−12 to LH+12 (i.e. a mean of 25 individual prolactin determinations) for each of the 53 women gave an overall range of 130 mu/l to 1002 mu/l. Thus the difference in mean

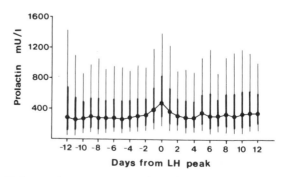

Fig. 4.15 Geometric mean concentrations of circulating plasma concentrations of prolactin in 53 of the 62 British women (Study No. 3, see text). Sixty-eight per cent confidence limits are indicated by the heavy bars and 95 per cent confidence limits by the light bars. The prolactin standard was 75/504 (unpublished data)

prolactin/cycle between the lowest and the highest individual in the series was approximately 8-fold. Clearly prolactin is more variable than the other four hormones. Geometric mean prolactin concentration/subject was 340 mu/1 with 68 per cent and 95 per cent confidence limits of 216–530 mu/1 and 138–832 mu/1 respectively. The subject with the greatest mean prolactin concentration/cycle (of 1002 mu/1), was a woman with regular cycles and normal progesterone secretion. She conceived spontaneously shortly after these samples were collected.

Prolactin concentrations within subjects

There is little published information on the consistency of prolactin concentrations between successive cycles in one individual (Lenton et al, 1983a). The only available data are from the study of 17 regularly menstrauating women (Study No. 5) reported here. Prolactin concentrations were available for ten of these 17 women and applying one way analysis of variance for the three phases of the cycle (i.e. from LH−12 to LH−4; LH−4 to LH+4; LH+4 to LH+12) it was possible to again show that there was significantly more $P < 0.001$) variation *between* subjects than *within* subjects. Mean prolactin concentrations/cycle are characteristic of the individual although single isolated prolactin estimations would not be anything like as representative.

Prolactin and the other reproductive hormones

Again there are no published data on possible associations between prolactin and the other reproductive hormones. Using the technique described earlier of selecting cycles with high or low concentrations of one hormone and then comparing the profiles of the other hormones using a data base of 186 cycles (Study No. 7) it is possible to show that in a population study of this kind there is no association between prolactin and either LH, oestradiol and progesterone (Fig. 4.16). In particular it should be noted that the group of subjects with high prolactin concentrations did not have a greater incidence of cycles with short or defective luteal phases (Corenblum et al, 1976; Coutts et al, 1978). Both groups showed evidence of a mid-cycle increase in prolactin concentration. These data should be interpreted with some caution because although no clear associations between prolactin and the other hormones were demonstrated between these two populations, it does not necessarily follow that pharmacological manipulation of prolactin concentrations will not affect ovarian function. In fact reduction of circulating prolactin concentrations in regularly cycling women has been shown to alter both the length of the follicular phase (Smith et al, 1983) and luteal function (Cooke & Lenton 1980; Cooke et al, 1981). Thus the possible endocrinological significance of changing

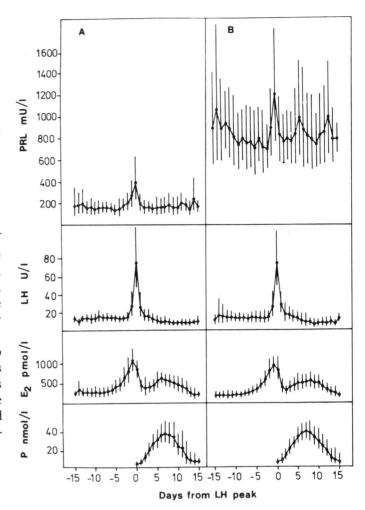

Fig. 4.16 Geometric mean levels (with 68 per cent confidence limits) of prolactin LH, oestradiol progesterone in two groups of normally menstruating women (Study No. 7, see text). The groups were selected from a data bank of 186 fully documented spontaneous cycles on the basis of specific features such as (A) a 'low' mean prolactin concentration over the interval LH−12 to LH + 12 (n = 22) and (B) a 'high' mean prolactin (unpublished data)

prolactin levels during the menstrual cycle remains to be elucidated.

Follicle scanning as an extra dimension

Until this point the word 'ovulation' has hardly been used. Subjects have been described as having 'normal' cycles where normal implies regular menstruation although this does not guarantee normal ovulation. In the past a cycle was considered to be 'ovulatory' provided there was a mid-cycle LH surge followed by certain minimum levels of progesterone secretion (Abraham et al, 1972; Black et al, 1972; Israel et al, 1972). These threshold progesterone concentrations were considered to be in the range 3–5 ng/ml (9.6–16 nmol/1). In fact what these earlier authors were doing was attempting to distinguish those cycles with minimum amounts of progesterone secretion and an orderly sequence of cyclical endocrine changes from those more bizarre cycles with grossly disturbed hypothalamic-pituitary-ovarian relationships. Since it was obvious that these latter cycles were also anovulatory (and the subjects were not infrequently also amenorrhoeic), cycles with some progesterone secretion, obtained from women who were menstruating were naturally termed ovulatory.

Although a suggestion was made by Arrata & Iffy in 1971 that certain women may not ovulate despite apparently normal endocrine profiles (the ovum being trapped inside the follicle), this idea did not receive widespread recognition until he work of Koninckx et al, (1978) and Marik & Hulka (1978). When more exacting conditions for describing 'ovulation' were imposed such as visualisation of the stigma on the surface of the follicle/corpus luteum, it became apparent that significant numbers of women were not ovulating despite cyclical steroid profiles that would have appeared compatible with the earlier criteria of ovulation. In fact although the absence of an ovulation stigma shortly after the LH peak would appear to be strong evidence that ovulation has *not* occurred, the converse, the presence of a stigma indicates only that the follicule has ruptured but does not prove that the ovum has been relased. It has yet to be shown that follicular rupture is *always* synonymous with ovulation (extrusion of the oocyte). As has been stated before probably the only irrefutable evidence of spontaneous follicular rupture and ovulation is conception.

Recently a number of groups have been attempting to use ultrasound to define follicular rupture (Queenan et al, 1980; Renaud et al, 1980; Smith et al, 1980; Kerin et al, 1981; Wetzels & Hoogland, 1982) This unfortunately is not as simple as it sounds. The ultrasonic appearances of a large pre-ovulatory follicle — a well defined cystic structure — are easy to demonstrate but the changes associated with rupture/ovulation are more variable. There are, as far as we are aware, no published data attempting to correlate ultrasonic appearances with proven rupture such as could be obtained by careful scanning of patients before and after follicular aspiration for *in vitro* fertilisation. Until such data

are available we have to rely on our previously described standard for the normal cycle and for normal ovulation, and describe the ultrasound appearances of follicles in *spontaneous* conception cycles. This procedure simultaneously fulfils a secondary objective, namely that of establishing the normal size of the pre-ovulatory follicle in spontaneously fertile cycles.

As with studies to establish endocrine profiles in *spontaneous* conception cycles the greatest problem is obtaining sufficient numbers of cycles. Despite actively trying to recruit potentially fertile cycles we have so far only obtained four. In each case maximum follicular diameter was observed on LH-0 and ranged from 17.5 through 18.75, 18.75 to 19.0 mm respectively. This was followed by a marked decrease in follicle size on LH+1 or, in one case on LH+2. In this latter patient the ultrasonic appearance although not the size of the follicle, altered on LH+1, the follicle showing 'spongy' echoes (Wetzels & Hoogland, 1982).

A typical follicular growth profile obtained daily in a subject with normal mid-luteal progesterone concentrations is shown in Fig. 4.17. Blood samples obtained simultaneously allowed the pattern of follicular growth and rupture to be synchronised with the endocrine changes. On LH-2, the mean longitudinal diameter of a follicle in the left ovary were 17.25 mm, by LH-1, this had increased to 19 mm and LH concentrations were beginning to rise ($\times 2.5$ follicular levels). The pre-ovulatory follicle was still clearly visible on LH-0 (LH concentrations were now $\times 7$ follicular levels), its size had not increased much further (diameter 19.5 mm) but its appearance had changed slightly — the borders of the follicle are not as clearly demarcated as on LH-2. By LH+1 the follicle had altered dramatically, the size had reduced, the outline had become irregular although a clear fluid centre was still visible. The approximate size of the follicle remnant was 13.5 mm with a central cystic core of 9.3 mm. We assume that a dramatic decrease in the size of a large pre-ovulatory follicle is a result of folliclar rupture and consequent loss of follicular fluid. By LH+2, the structure had 'filled in', it was no

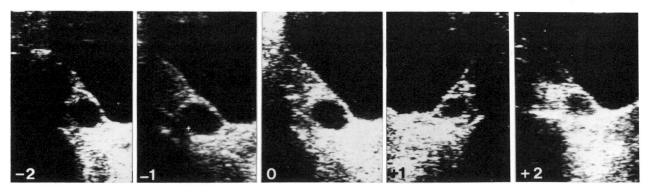

Fig. 4.17 Daily ultrasonographic records of the final stages of growth of the dominant follicle (LH − 2; LH − 1; LH − 0), its probable rupture (LH + 1) and finally formation of a corpus luteum (LH + 2). The days relative to the LH peak (LH − 0) are as indicated (unpublished data)

longer cystic and although its size could be determined as approximately 13.5 mm it was quite obviously a corpus luteum. Indeed plasma progesterone by this time was already 18 nmol/l.

Although it is relatively simple (particularly with some of the more advanced ultrasound scanners now available) to quantitate the growth of the pre-ovulatory follicle, it is more difficult to describe qualitative changes and to show whether these synchronise with endocrine signals. One method of decumenting both the changes in size and appearance of the follicle with changes in endocrine parameters is shown in Table 4.8. This subject also appeared to

Table 4.8 Synchronisation of the endocrine parameters (LH, oestradiol and progesterone concentrations) with the day of the cycle and the diameter and appearance of the dominant follicle as determined by ultrasound in an apparently normal cycle. The dominant follicle was on this occasion in the right ovary

Cycle day	LH (u/l)	E_2 (pmol/l)	P (nmol/l)	FD (mm)	Follicle appearance
9	9.0	96	1.6	11.3	
10	9.3	271	0.8	12.3	
11	9.6	299	1.6	13.3	Cystic
12	9.1	578	0.8	15.5	Cystic
13	22.0	1028	6.0	18.0	Clearly cystic
14	81.0	677	7.6	17.5	Cystic but edges not clear
15	14.5	179	12.0	*	No cystic structure
16	8.8	131	20.7	8.8	Irregular shape
18	6.3	215	43.0	6.3	Irregular
20	5.9	271	63.7	9.3	Irregular

* No measurable structure in the ovary.

have a normal cycle, with folliclar rupture on LH+1 followed by the formation of a corpus luteum whose size could be determined only approximately. The reason for attempting to identify and define follicular rupture and then to attribute a size to the corpus luteum in potentially normal cycles is to provide a standard against which to compare potentially abnormal cycles particularly those where the follicle luteinises but does not rupture. Thus although the quantitative measurement of a corpus luteum can only at best be inexact, nonetheless it should be possible to distinguish between a structure of 10 mm diameter and one of 20 mm. This information taken in conjunction with the previous daily growth pattern of the follicle when synchronised with *daily* blood samples may be sufficient to identify potentially abnormal (infertile) cycles.

In order to define a 'normal' group containing sufficient numbers of observations to have some validity, we matched features of a conception cycle — i.e. a follicle with a minimum maximum diameter ≥17.5 mm, rupture on LH+1 or LH+2 and mid-luteal progesterones within the fertile range — with a group of non-pregnant cycles. In the absence of any definitive evidence to the contrary a log-normal distribution of follicular diameters was assumed

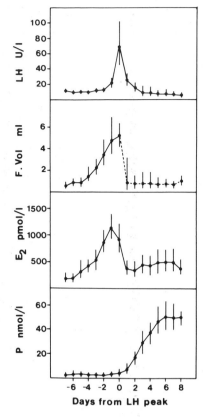

Fig. 4.18 Geometric means (with 68 per cent confidence limits) for the parameters LH, oestradiol, progesterone and follicular volume in a group of 16 non-conception cycles which 'matched' four spontaneous conception cycles with respect to maximum follicular diameter (>17.5 mm); clear evidence of follicular rupture (on LH + 1 or LH + 2) and normal mid-luteal progesterone concentrations (PI > 40 nmol/l) (Study No. 8, see text). At the present time this group of 20 cycles is the best representation we have of cycles which are both putatively 'normal' endocrinologically and 'normal' with respect to follicle growth and ovulation (unpublished data)

(Gaddum, 1945) and geometric means and 68 per cent confidence limits calculated (Fig. 4.18). Geometric mean LH, oestradiol and progesterone concentrations match those features in a group of conception cycles (Fig. 4.4) so it is assumed that this group of cycles were at least endocrinologically normal. Mean maximumum follicular diameter (on LH−0) was 19.5 mm corresponding to a volume of 3.86 ml. Ninety-five per cent confidence limits were 17.0–22.4 mm or 2.55–5.84 ml respectively. However the possibility remains that these cycles, even though they 'matched' the small number of spontaneous conception cycles with respect to three parameters (follicle size, timing of rupture, progesterone index), might not have been really 'normal' or might not have adequately represented the 'normal' range because they were too highly selected. For example, the results of an unstimulated cycle in a 39-year-old woman who has experienced at least six spontaneous abortions over a period of 4 years are shown in Table 4.9.

It would appear that despite normal progesterone levels (mid-luteal levels not shown, but PI = 39.2 nmol/1), this

Table 4.9 Synchronisation of the endocrine parameters (LH, oestradiol and progesterone concentrations) with the day of the cycle and the diameter and appearance of the dominant follicle as determined by ultrasound. The dominant follicle was in the left ovary, the right being inactive. This subject had experienced six abortions during the previous 4 years

Cycle day	LH (u/l)	E$_2$ (pmol/l)	P (nmol/l)	FD (mm)	Follicle appearance
13	9.2	408	0.8	13.3	
14	8.4	683	0.8	16.3	
15	10.0	647	0.8	17.0	Clearly cystic
16	12.0	812	0.8	19.0	Cystic
17	15.5	1431	2.1	15.3	Filled in
18	78.0	1046	4.0	9.0	Small cystic areas only
19	13.5	541	14.3	*	Irregular shape
20	8.4	303	15.9	*	Irregular shape
21	4.2	339	30.3		No scan

* No measurable structure in the ovary.

Table 4.11 Distribution of normal (i.e. with potentially fertile mid-luteal progesterone concentrations) non-conception cycles with respect to their maximum follicular diameter and time of apparent follicular rupture (ovulation)

| Follicle diameter (mm) | Apparent rupture relative to the LH peak | | | |
	Early Before or on LH − 0	Normal LH + 1 or LH + 2	Delayed* On or after LH + 3	Total
Normal (≥17.5)	3	20†	0	23
Small (16.0 to 17.4)	2	3	0	5
Very small (< 16.0)	1	3	0	4
Total	6	26	0	32

* Delayed also includes follicles which did not apparently rupture at all (Luteinised unruptured follicle) or in which it was difficult to determine whether rupture occurred.

† This group alone matches the features observed in four spontaneous conception cycles.

follicle ruptured prematurely. No other active follicles in either ovary greater than 10 mm diameter were seen despite daily scans over 11 consecutive days. The cause of the recurrent abortions was initially thought to be due to a uterine abnormality (subseptate uterus) but in three instances the abortion was of an anembryonic pregnancy, and in another instance, although a fetus was present, it was grossly abnormal. The question then arises — is this 'premature' ovulation? Is it merely a normal variant? Does it perhaps signify an abnormal infertile cycle in an otherwise normal individual or might this type of profile actually be compatible with conception even if not a normal pregnancy?

Although we have described some information on the cycle to cycle variability of endocrine parameters within an individual, as far as we are aware there are no comparable data on the consistency of follicular growth and rupture from cycle to cycle. Table 4.10 gives the results of one-way analysis of variance between pairs of cycles in a small series of subjects where observations on follicle growth were obtained simultaneously with endocrine information (Study No. 9). Consistency in follicular volume or diameter was not as marked as the equivalent endocrine features, as these parameters just failed to reach statistical significance. Further corroborative data are required to show whether

Table 4.10 Analyses of variance (and the significances) of LH and oestradiol concentrations and follicular diameter and volume *between* cycles (*within* individuals) compared with *between* individuals in 12 normally menstruating British women (Study No. 9 see text). The mean of the two greatest LH, follicular diameters or follicular volumes and the three greatest oestradiol concentrations were used to minimise technical and operator variability

	F-Value	Significance
LH — maximum	6.33	$P < 0.01$
E$_2$ — maximum	5.89	$P < 0.01$
Follicular diameter	2.47	ns
Follicular volume	2.38	ns

this could be a reflection of intrinsic variability or of the technical limitations of ultrasonography.

Finally in order to emphasise that premature follicle rupture was not the only unexpected finding when women with *normal* mid-luteal progesterone concentrations were submitted to serial follicular scans, Table 4.11 shows the numbers of subjects who 'matched' the conception cycles in two out of the three parameters only and who were not included in the calculations for Fig. 4.18. Are these cycles also 'normal'? Are they ovulatory? Are they fertile? It is hoped that over the next few years as experience with ultrasonic visualisation of the follicle increases the answers to these questions will be forthcoming.

CONCLUDING REMARKS

This chapter is not a review of the normal cycle in the conventional sense of comparing and contrasting all available endocrine data. Pertinent reasons are that data from many investigators are of limited comparability (due to variance in methodology and mathematical analysis) and, given the marked variability between individuals, are generally based on insufficient numbers of subjects. But the most important reason for not describing endocrine profiles such as those shown in Fig. 4.3 in great detail, is that the information is not particularly informative and can be misleading; mean hormone profiles from a group of subjects based on samples taken every 24 h give at best an over-simplified version of the normal menstrual cycle and at worst disguise individual variability in, for example, cycle phase length.

The normal cycle. What is a *normal* cycle? Here again there are a number of philosophical difficulties associated with subject selection. The choice of subjects must depend on what aspect of reproduction is being investigated. For example if the question is 'to define a *normal-fertile* cycle' then only subjects who conceive *during* the study can be used; if the question is 'to define a *normal-ovulatory* cycle' then the physical process of follicular rupture and ovulation must be demonstrated. This is actually much more difficult than it sounds. One way would be to again use conception cycles, alternatively ovulation stigma could be visualised directly by appropriately timed laparoscopies. Introducing an operative procedure will inevitably restrict numbers and visualisation of the stigma may still be insufficient evidence for *normal-ovulation* as it now seems likely that ovulation (as detected by ultrasound, Tables 4.9 and 4.11) may not always be normally synchronised with endocrine events; the mere presence of an ovulation stigma cannot provide information about when follicular rupture occurred. The data described in Fig. 4.3 do not show normal-fertile cycles, nor do they show normal-ovulatory cycles, they merely illustrate the range of endocrine values to be found in a population of women who are neither very old nor very young and who have regular cycles. Not surprisingly comparison of these profiles with those of conception cycles (Fig 4.4) which are after all cycles of both normal-ovulation and normal-fertility, reveals some differences. We suggest that 'the normal cycle' does not exist; cycles should be described as normal with respect to ovulation, or to fertility, or to luteal phase length, or to prolactin concentrations, etc and as we have shown, there are many versions of the normal cycle, not only within a non-conception group and also within conception cycles themselves. There are marked qualitative and quantitative differences in endocrine function *between* women but not *within* a woman, where cycles will generally be very reproducible with respect to endocrine features (Table 4.3) although less so when follicular growth dynamics are considered (Table 4.10).

Progesterone index. There are dangers in extrapolating from data obtained in population studies to the results obtained in an individual, but clinically there is considerable pressure to do just this. Unfortunately all hormone secretion is episodic and blood levels may vary quite considerably from minute to minute (Fig. 4.5). This means that assessing reproductive status using single endocrine measurements will be very imprecise — particularly at an individual level, slightly less so in population studies (Hull et al, 1982) Integrated endocrine functions over sections of the cycle (e.g. the Progesterone Index, PI + 5 to + 8) offer an improved method of assessment. The index described here based on mean progesterone concentrations over the interval LH + 5 to LH + 8 is more difficult to use clinically than some of the other published methods (Abraham et al, 1974; Coutts et al, 1982) but is more precise and more relevant physiologically. For ease of comparison, it would be an advantage if one particular method of integration was adopted by all investigators.

The fertile cycle. There are no marked differences (up to LH + 8, around the time of implantation) between control

(Fig. 4.3) and conception cycles (Fig. 4.4) except in progesterone secretion. It is possible that real differences in gonadotrophin secretion may exist but these are not detectable with current radioimmunoassays. It seems unlikely that there are any real differences in oestradiol and so the only point requiring explanation is the progesterone differences. The first impression is that progesterone secretion in conception cycles is actually greater than in control cycles but careful study of Table 4.2 shows that in fact conception cycle PI (+ 5 to + 8) values are not better than *all* control cycle PI (+ 5 to + 8) values but in fact merely occupy the top half of the PI (+ 5 to + 8) range observed in women who were not attempting to conceive. In other words conception cycles form a self-selected sub-group of cycles within the general population. This impression is strengthened by the observation that the distribution of conception cycle PI (+ 5 to + 8) values is log-normal, unlike control cycle PI (+ 5 to + 8) values where the distribution is normal.

Why should there be such a wide range of PI (+ 5 to + 8) values in a group of control women and does the difference between these cycles and conception cycles indicate that progesterone may be associated with fertility? It is well known that women (Cooke et al, 1981) do not all have the same fertility potential, some will be highly fertile whilst others will have much reduced fertility. However, even though a woman is of low fecundity, she may still conceive a number of times during her reproductive life. Nonetheless cycle for cycle she would have conceived less readily than a highly fecund woman. Accepting that there are individual differences in fertility, then is it possible that there is some endocrine or ovarian reason for this? Quantitative differences in progesterone secretion (monitored using a progesterone index) form an attractive hypothesis because (i) conception cycles occur only above a minimum PI (+ 5 to + 8) concentration and (ii) regularly-cycling women complaining of infertility show a greater than expected incidence of low PI + 5 to + 8 concentrations.

Differences in progesterone secretion could not affect the fertility of individual women unless these differences were present in every cycle. When the consistency of PI (+ 5 to + 8) values were assessed in two small studies (Tables 4.4 and 4.5), it was found that progesterone secretion was extraordinarily consistent from cycle to cycle. Two points should be noted: consistency was least in the women who overall showed the worst luteal function, and that no matter what their characteristic PI (+ 5 to + 8) value, some women would occasionally have an atypical cycle. These facts give support to the hypothesis because they show that quantitatively, luteal function is characteristic of the women; some women will always have good function while others will always have poor function. Despite this, none of the normal volunteers in these studies failed to have at least one cycle where conception would theoretically have been possible.

Progesterone and fertility. Efficient reproduction is more likely to occur in 'good' cycles which are those where follicular growth, timing of ovulation and luteinisation are optimal. Progesterone secretion, as a measure of luteinisation, is only the last of a sequence of events and so it is improbable that decreased progesterone alone is the cause of an infertile cycle. In fact the converse may also be true, some cycles may be infertile even though progesterone secretion is within the conception cycle range (Tables 4.9 and 4.11). Thus fertility or potential fertility is probably directly related to the incidence of 'good' cycles and it is only because progesterone secretion (the final common pathway) is quantitatively affected in 'poor' cycles that progesterone secretion per se seems to be associated with fertility.

Unfortunately blood samples taken at 24 h intervals can only show what is happening in the peripheral circulation at one moment in time. Using a progesterone index we may be able to discriminate between 'good' cycles and 'bad' cycles but we cannot tell why a cycle should be suboptimal. Longitudinal studies across the cycle do not give any information about how the dominant follicle interacts with the hypothalamic-pituitary axis to initiate an LH surge, nor how well this event synchronises with follicular rupture and ovulation. In short, we are only just beginning to understand the complexities of the control and regulation of human reproductive function, and to be able to distinguish *normal* from *abnormal*. Hopefully over the next decade, carefully designed studies paying meticulous attention to methodological and analytical techniques, will markedly change this situation.

REFERENCES

Abraham G E, Swerdloff R S, Tulchinsky D, Hopper K, Odell W D 1971 Radioimmunoassay of plasma 17-hydroxyprogesterone and estradiol-17β during the menstrual cycle. Journal of Clinical Endocrinology and Metabolism 33: 42–46

Abraham G E, Odell W D, Swerdloff R J, Hopper K 1972 Simultaneous radioimmunoassay of FSH, LH, progesterone, 17-hydroxyprogesterone and estradiol-17β during the menstrual cycle. Journal of Clinical Endocrinology and Metabolism 34: 312–318

Abraham G E, Maroulis G B, Marshall J R 1974 Evaluation of ovulation and corpus luteum function using measurements of plasma progesterone. Obstetrics and Gynecology 44: 522–525

Aedo A-R, Landgren B-M, Cekan Z, Diczfalusy E 1976 Studies on the pattern of circulating steroids in the normal menstrual cycle. 2. Levels of 20-dihydroprogesterone, 17-hydroxyprogesterone and 17-hydroxypregnenolone and the assessment of their value for ovulation prediction. Acta Endocrinologica 82: 600–616

Aedo A-R, Nunez M, Landgren B-M, Cekan S Z, Diczfalusy E 1977 Studies on the pattern of circulating steroids in the normal menstrual cycle: 3 Circadian variation in the periovulatory period. Acta Endocrinologica 84: 320–332

Arrata W S M, Iffy L 1971 Normal and delayed ovulation in the human. Obstetric and Gynaecological Survey 26: 675–689

Aso T, Guerrero G, Cekan Z, Diczfalusy E 1975 A rapid 5 hour radioimmunoassay of progesterone and oestradiol in human plasma. Clinical Endocrinology 4: 173–182

Black W P, Martin B T and Whyte W G 1972 Plasma progesterone concentrations as an index of ovulation and corpus luteum function in normal and gonadotrophin-stimulated menstrual cycles. Journal of Obstetrics and Gynaecology of the British Commonwealth 79: 363–372

Briggs M H, Briggs M 1972 Steroid hormone concentrations in blood plasma from residents of Zambia, belonging to different ethical groups. Acta Endocrinologica 70: 619–624

Brosens I A, Koninckx P R, Corveleyn P A 1978 A study of plasma progesterone, oestradiol 17β, prolactin and LH levels and of luteal phase appearance of ovaries in patients with endometriosis and infertility. British Journal of Obstetrics and Gynaecology 85: 246–250

Cargille C M, Ross G T, Yoshimi T 1969 Daily variations in plasma follicle stimulating hormone, luteinizing hormone and progesterone in the normal menstrual cycle. Journal of Clinical Endocrinology and Metabolism 29: 12–19

Cekan S 1976 Reliability of Steroid Radioimmunoassays. Doctoral thesis, Uppsala University

Chiazze L, Brayer F T, Macisco J J, Parker M P, Duffy B J 1968 The length and variability of the human menstrual cycle. Journal of the American Medical Association 203: 377–380

Cooke I D, Lenton E A 1980 The use of bromocriptine in ovulatory infertility. Scottish Medical Journal, 25: 583–588

Cooke I D, Lenton E A, Sulaiman R, Sobowale O 1981 Ovulatory infertility and the role of bromocriptine. In: Insler V, Bettendorf G. (eds) Advances in Diagnosis and Treatment of Infertility, pp 85–95. Elsevier N Holland Amsterdam

Cooke I D, Sulaiman R, Lenton E A, Parsons R J 1981 Fertility and infertility statistics: their importance and application In: Hull M (ed) Clinics in Obstetrics and Gynaecology, Vol 8, pp 531–548. W B Saunders Ltd, London

Corenblum B, Pairaudeau N, Schewchuk A B 1976 Prolactin hypersecretion and short luteal phase defects. Obstetrics and Gynecology 47: 486–488

Coutts J R T Fleming R, Carswell W, Black W P, England P, Craig A, McNaughton M C 1978 The defective luteal phase. In: Jacobs H S (ed) Advances in Gynaecological Endocrinology pp 65–91. Proceedings of the Sixth Study Group of the Royal College of Obstetricians and Gynaecologists, London

Coutts J R T, Adam A H, Fleming R 1982 The deficient luteal phase may represent an anovulatory cycle. Clinical Endocrinology 17: 389–394

Diczfalusy E, Landgren B-M 1977 Hormonal changes in the menstrual cycle. WHO Symposium on Advances in Fertility Regulation, pp 21–71. Scriptor, Copenhagen

Diczfalusy E, Landgren B-M 1981 How normal is the normal cycle? In: Crosignani P G, Rubin B L (eds) Endocrinology of human infertility New Aspects. Proceedings of the Serono Clinical Colloquia on Reproduction, Number 2, pp 1–25. Academic Press, London

Dodson K S, Coutts J R T, Macnaughton M N C 1975 Plasma sex steroid and gonadotrophin patterns in human menstrual cycles. British Journal of Obstetrics and Gynaecology 82: 602–614

Dyrenfurth I, Jewelewicz R, Warren M, Ferin M, Vande Wiele R L 1974 Temporal relationships of hormonal variables in the menstrual cycle. In: Ferin M, Halberg F, Richart R M, Van de Wiele R L (eds) Biorhythms and Human Reproduction, pp 171–202. John Wiley, New York

Edqvist L-E, Johannsson E D B 1972 Radioimmunoassay of oestrone and oestradiol in human and bovine peripheral plasma. Acta Endocrinologica (Kbh) 71: 716–730

Ehara Y, Siler T, Van der Berg G, Sinha Y N, Yen S S C 1973 Circulating prolactin levels during the menstrual cycle: episodic release and diurnal variation. American Journal of Obstetrics and Gynecology 117: 962–970

Epstein M T, McNeilly A S, Murray M A F, Hockaday T D R 1975 Plasma testosterone and prolactin in the menstrual cycle. Clinical Endocrinology 4: 531–535

Fisher R A, Yates F 1963 Statistical Tables for Biological, Agricultural and Medical Research, 6th end. Longman, London

Franchimont P, Burger H 1975 Human Growth Hormone and Gonadotrophins in health and Disease. pp 327–335. North-Holland Publishing Company, Amsterdam

Friesen H, Hwang P, Guyda H, Tolis G, Tyson J, Myers R 1972 A radioimmunoassay for human prolactin; physiological, pathological and pharmacological factors which affect the secretion of prolactin. In: Boyns A R, Griffiths K (eds) Prolactin and Carcinogenesis, pp 64–80. Alpha Omega Publishing, Cardiff

Frölich M, Brand E D, Van Hall E V 1976 Serum levels of unconjugated aetiolocholanolone, androstenedione, testosterone, dehydroepiandrosterone, aldosterone, progesterone and oestrogen during the normal menstrual cycle. Acta Endocrinologica 81: 548–562

Gaddum J H 1945 Lognormal distributions. Nature 156: 463–466

Guerrero R, Aso T, Brenner P F, Cekan Z, Landgren B-M, Hagenfeldt K, Diczfalusy E 1976 Studies on the pattern of circulating steroids in the normal menstrual cycle. 1. Simultaneous assays of progesterone, pregnenolone, dehydroepiandrosterone, testosterone, dihydrotestosterone, androstenedione, oestradiol and oestrone. Acta Endocrinologica 81: 133–149

Hackeloer B J, Fleming R, Robinson H P, Adam H P, Coutts J R T 1979 Correlation of ultrasonic and endocrinologic assessment of human follicular development. American Journal of Obstetrics and Gynecology 135: 122–128

Holmdahl T H, Johansson E D B 1972 Peripheral plasma levels of 17-hydroxyprogesterone, progesterone and oestradiol during normal menstrual cycles in women. Acta Endocrinologica 71: 743–754

Hodgen G D 1982 The dominant ovarian follicle. Fertility and Sterility 38: 281–300

Hull M G R, Savage P E, Bromham D R, Ismail A A A, Morris A F 1982 The value of single serum progesterone measurement in the mid-luteal phase as a criterion of a potentially fertile cycle "ovulation") derived from treated and untreated conception cycles. Fertility and Sterility 37: 355–360

Instructions to Authors 1974 The validation of assays and the statistical treatment of results. Journal of Endocrinology 63: 1–4

Israel R, Mishell D R, Stone S C, Thorneycroft I H, Moyer D L 1972 Single luteal phase serum progesterone assay as an indicator of ovulation. American Journal of Obstetrics and Gynecology 112: 1043–1046

Johannsson E D B, Wide L, Gemzell C 1971 Luteinizing hormone (LH) and progesterone in plasma and LH and oestrogens in urine during 42 normal menstrual cycles. Acta Endocrinologica 68: 502–512

Jones G S, Aksel S, Wentz A C 1974 Serum progesterone values in the luteal phase defects. Obstetrics and Gynecology 44: 26–34

Kerin J F, Edmonds D K, Warnes G M, Cox L W, Seamark R F, Matthews C D, Young,, G B, Baird D T 1981 Morphological and functional relations of Graafian follicle growth to ovulation in women using ultrasonic, laparoscopic and biochemical measurements. British Journal of Obstetrics and Gynaecology 88: 81–90

Kletzy D A, Nakamura R M, Thorneycroft I H, Mishell D R 1975 Lognormal distribution of gonadotrophins and ovarian steroid values in the normal menstrual cycle. American Journal of Obstetrics and Gynecology 121: 668–694

Koninckx P R, Heyns W, Corveleyn P A, Brosens I A 1978 Delayed onset of luteinisation as a cause of infertility. Fertility and Sterility 29: 266–269

Landgren B-M, Campo S, Cekan S Z, Diczfalusy E 1977 Studies on the pattern of circulating steroids in the normal menstrual cycle. 5. Changes around the onset of menstruation. Acta Endocrinologica 86: 608–620

Landgren B-M, Unden A-L, Diczfalusy E 1980 Hormonal profiles in the cycles in 68 normally menstruating women. Acta Endocrinologica 94: 89–98

Landgren B-M, Aedo A-R, Diczfalusy E 1982 Hormonal changes associated with ovulation and luteal function. In: Flamigni C, Givens J R (eds) The gonadotrophins. Basic Science and Clinical Aspects in Females. Proceedings of the Serono Symposia, Vol. 42, pp 187–201. Academic Press, London

Lehmann F, Just-Nastansky I, Czygan P J, Bettendorf G 1976 Effects of 17-ethinyl-19-nortestosterone (ENT) on corpus luteum function. European Journal of Obstetrics and Gynaecology and Reproductive Biology 6: 219–224

Lenton E A, Cooke I D 1981 Investigation and assessment of the infertile woman by comparison with the endocrine parameters of a fertile cycle. In: Spira A, Jouannet P (eds) Facteurs de la fertilité humaine. Les colloques de l'Inserm, 103, pp 383–408

Lenton E A, Adams M, Cooke, I D 1978 Plasma steroid and gonadotrophin profiles in ovulatory but infertile women. Clinical Endocrinology 8: 241–255

Lenton E A, Brook L M, Sobowale O, Cooke I D 1979 Prolactin concentrations in normal menstrual cycles and conception cycles. Clinical Endocrinology 10: 383–391

Lenton E A, Neal L M, Sulaiman R 1982a Plasma concentrations of human chorionic gonadotrophin from the time of implantation until the second week of pregnancy. Fertility and Sterility 37: 773–778

Lenton E A, Sulaiman R, Sobowale O, Cooke I D 1982b The human menstrual cycle: plasma concentrations of prolactin, LH, FSH, oestradiol and progesterone in conceiving and non-conceiving women. Journal of Reproduction and Fertility 65: 131–139

Lenton E A, Cripps K A, Sulaiman R, Sobowale O, Ryle M, Cooke I D 1982c Plasma prolactin concentrations during conception and the first ten weeks of human pregnancy. Acta Endocrinologica 100: 295–300

Lenton E A, Lawrence G F, Coleman R A, Cooke I D 1984 Individual variation in gonadotrophin and steroid concentrations and in lengths of follicular and luteal phases in women with regular menstrual cycles. Clinical Reproduction and Fertility 2: 143–150

Lenton E A, Landgren B-M, Sexton L, Harper R 1983b Normal variation in the length of the follicular phase of the menstrual cycle. Effect of chronological age. British Journal of Obstetrics and Gynaecology In press

Lenton E A, Landgren B-M, Sexton L 1983c Normal variation in the length of the luteal phase of the menstrual cycle: identification of the short luteal phase. British Journal of Obstetrics and Gynaecology In Press

Leyendecker G, Hinckers K, Nocke W, Plotz E J 1975 Hypophysäre Gonadotropine und ovarielle Steroide im Serum während des normalen menstruellen Cyclus und bei Corpus-luteum-Insuffizienz Arch Gynäk 218: 47–52

L'Hermite M, Delvoye P, Nokin J, Vekemans N, Robyn C 1972 Human prolactin secretion, as studied by radioimmunoassay in some aspects of its regulation. In: Boyns A R, Griffiths K (eds) Prolactin and Carcinogenesis, pp 81–97. Alpha Omega Alpha Publishing, Cardiff

McIntosh J E A, Matthews C S, Crocker J M, Broom J J, Cox L W 1980 Predicting the luteinising hormone surge: Relationship between the duration of the follicular and luteal phases and the length of the human menstrual cycle. Fertility and Sterility 34: 125–130

McNeilly A S, Chard T 1974 Circulating levels of prolactin during the menstrual cycle. Clinical Endocrinology 3: 105–112

Marik J, Hulka J 1978 Luteinised unruptured follicle syndrome: a subtle cause for infertility. Fertility and Sterility 29: 270–274

Martin Ritzen E, Fröysa B, Gustafsson B, Westerholm G, Diczfalusy E 1982 Improved in vitro bioassay of follitropin. Hormone Research 16: 42–48

Midgley A R Jr, Jaffe R B 1968 Regulation of human gonadotropins: IV Correlation of serum concentrations of follicle stimulating and luteinizing hormones during the menstrual cycle. Journal of Clinical Endocrinology 28: 1699–1703

Milewich L, Gomez-Sanchez C, Crowley G, Porter J C, Madden J D, MacDonald P C 1977 Progesterone and 5 -pregnane-3, 20-dione in peripheral blood of normal young women. Daily measurements throughout the menstrual cycle. Journal of Clinical Endocrinology and Metabolism 45: 617–622

Mishell D R, Nakamura R M, Crosignani P G, Stone S, Kharma K, Nagata Y, Thorneycroft I 1971 Serum gonadotropin and steroid patterns during the normal menstrual cycle. American Journal of Obstetrics and Gynecology 111: 60–65

Moghissi K S, Syner F N, Evans T N 1972 A composite picture of the menstrual cycle. American Journal of Obstetrics and Gynecology 114: 405–418

Mortimer D, Lenton E A 1983 Distribution of sperm counts in suspected infertile men. Journal of Reproduction and Fertility 68: 91–96

Neil D, Johansson E D B, Catta J K, Knobil E 1967 Relationship between the plasma levels of luteizing hormone and progesterone during the normal menstrual cycle. Journal of Clinical Endocrinology 27: 1167–1173

Parker D C, Rossman L G, Vanderllan E F 1973 Sleep related nyctohemeral and episodic variation in human plasma prolactin concentrations. Journal of Clinical Endocrinology and Metabolism 36: 1119–1124

Pizarro M A 1975 Plasma profile and the role of progesterone during the course of the menstrual cycle. In: Vokaer R, De Bock G, (eds) Reproductive Endocrinology, pp 113–121. Pergamon Press, Oxford

Queenan J T, O'Brien G D, Bains L M, Simpson S, Collins W P, Campbell S 1980 Ultrasound scanning of ovaries to detect ovulation in women. Fertility and Sterility 34: 99–105

Rajalakshmi M, Robertson D M, Choi S K, Diczfalusy E 1979 Biologically active luteinizing hormone (LH) in plasma. Acta Endocrinology 90: 585–598

Renaud R L, Macler J, Dervain I, Ehret M-C, Aron C, Plas-Roser S, Spira A, Pollack H 1980 Echographic study of follicular maturation and ovulation during the normal menstrual cycle. Fertility and Sterility 33: 272–276

Robertson D M, Diczfalusy E 1977 Biological and immunological characterization of human luteinzing hormone II. A comparison of the immunological and biological activities of pituitary extracts after electrofocussing using different standard preparations. Molecular and Cellular Endocrinology 9: 57–67

Roger M, Veinante A, Soldat M C, Tardy J, Tribondeau E, Scholler R 1975 Étude simultanée des gonadotrophines, des oestrogénes, de las progestérone et de la 17-hydrosyprogesterone plasmatique au cours du cycle ovulatoire. Nouve Presse Méd 4: 2173–2178

Romani P, Robertson D M, Diczfalusy E 1977 Biogically active luteinizing hormone (LH) in plasma. II Comparison with biologically active LH lelvels throughout the human menstrual cycle. Acta Endocrinology 84: 697–712

Ross G T, Cargille C M, Lipsett M B, Rayford P L, Marshall J R, Strott, C A, Robard D 1970 Pituitary and gonadal hormones in women during spontaneous and induced ovulatory cycles. Recent Progress in Hormone Research 26: 1–62

Runnebaum B, Rieben W, Bierwirth-v. Münstermann A-M, Zander J 1972 Circadian variations in plasma progesterone in the luteal phase of the menstrual cycle and during pregnancy. Acta Endocrinologica 69: 731–738

Salmon J A, Chew P C T, Ratnam S S 1976 Plasma hormone concentrations during the menstrual cycle of normal Chinese women. Acta Obstetrica et Gynecologica Scandinavia 55: 239–243

Saxena B B, Demura H, Gandy H M, Peterson R E 1968 Radioimmunoassay of human follicle stimulating and luteinsing hormones in plasma. Journal of Clincial Endocrinology and Metabolism 28: 519–534

Saxena B N, Dusitsin N, Poshyachinda V, Smith I 1974 Luteinizing hormone, oestradiol and progesterone levels in the serum of menstruating Thai women. Journal of Obstetrics and Gynaecology of the British Commonwealth 81: 113–119

Schulz K-D, Geiger W, del Pozo E, Künzig H J 1978 Pattern of sexual steroids, prolactin, and gonadotropic hormones during prolactin inhibition in normally cycling women. American Journal of Obstetrics and Gynecology 132: 561–566

Schmidt-Gollwitzer M, Saxena B B 1975 Radioimmunoassay of human prolactin (PRL) Acta Endocrinologica 80: 262–274

Shaaban M M, Klopper A 1973 Plasma oestradiol and progesterone concentration in the normal menstrual cycle. Journal of Obstetrics and Gynaecology of the British Commonwealth 80: 776–782

Sherman B M, Korenman S G 1974 Measurement of plasma LH, FSH, estradiol and progesterone in disorders of the human menstrual cycle: the short luteal phase. Journal of Clinical Endocrinology and Metabolism 38: 89–93

Sherman B M, Korenman S G (1975) Hormonal characteristics of the human menstrual cycle throughout reproductive life. Journal of Clinical Investigation 55: 699–706

Shumin X, Johannisson E, Landgren B-M, Diczfalusy E 1983

Pituitary, ovarian and endometrial effects of progesterone released prematurely during the proliferative phase. Contraception In press

Smith D H, Picker R H, Sinosich M, Saunders D M 1980 Assessment of ovulation by ultrasound and estradiol levels during spontaneous and induced cycles. Fertility and Sterility 33: 387–390

Smith S K S, Sobowale O, Lenton E A, Cooke I D 1983 Effect of bromocriptine on menstrual cycle length. British Journal of Obstetrics and Gynecology In press

Spona J 1973 Serumspiegel des Luteinisierenden hormons (LH) in der Zyklusmitte. Endokrinologie 62: 41–47

Storring P L, Zaidi A A, Mistry Y G, Froysa B, Stenning B E, Diczfalusy E 1981 A comparison of preparations of highly purified human pituitary follicle stimulating hormone (FSH): differences in the FSH potencies as determined by in-vivo bioassay, in-vitro bioassay and immunoassay. Journal of Endocrinology 91: 353–362

Storring P L, Zaidi A A, Mistry Y G, Lindberg M, Stenning B E, Diczfalusy E 1982 A comparison of preparations of highly purified human pituitary luteinizing hormone: differences in the luteinizing hormone potencies as determined by in vivo bioassays, in vitro bioassay and immunoassay. Acta Endocrinologica 101: 339–347

Strott C A, Lipsett M B 1968 Measurement of 17-hydroxyprogesterone in human plasma. Journal of Clinical Endocrinology and Metabolism 28: 1426–1430

Strott, C A, Cargille C M, Ross G T, Lipsett M B 1970 The short luteal phase. Journal of Clinical Endocrinology and Metabolism 30: 246–251

Tamura S, Igarashi M 1973 Serum prolactin levels during ovulatory menstrual cycle and menstrual disorders in women. Endocrinology Jap 20: 483–488

Taymor M L Aono T, Pheteplace C, Page G 1968 Follicle-stimulating hormones and luteizing hormone in serum during the menstrual cycle determined by radioimmunoassay. Acta Endocrinological 59: 298–306

Thorneycroft I H, Mishell D R Jr, Stone S C, Kharma K M, Nakamura R M 1971 The relation of serum 17-hydroxygesterone and estradiol 17β levels during the human menstrual cycle. American Journal of Obstetrics and Gynecology 111: 947–951

Treloar A E, Boynton R E, Benn B G, Brown R W 1967 Variation of the human menstrual cycle throughout reproductive life. International Journal of Fertility 12: 77–126

Van Damme M-P, Robertson D M, Diczfalusy E 1974 An improved in vitro bioassay method for measuring luteinizing hormone (LH) activity using mouse leydig cell preparations. Acta Endocrinology 77: 655–671

Vekemans M, Delvoye P, L'Hermite M, Robyn O 1977 Serum prolactin levels during the menstrual cycle. Journal of Clinical Endocrinology and Metabolism 44: 959–1003

Vollman R F 1977 In: The Menstrual Cycle: Major Problems in Obstetrics and Gynaecology, Vol 7. W B Saunders, Philadelphia

West C D, Mahajan D K, Chauvré V J, Nabros C J, Tyler F H 1973 Simultaneous measurement of multiple plasma steroids by radioimmunoassay demonstrating episodic secretion. Journal of Clinical Endocrinology and Metabolism 36: 1230–1236

Wetzels L G G, Hoogland H J 1982 Relation between ultrasonographic evidence of ovulation and hormonal parameters: luteinizing hormone surge and initial proogesterone rise. Fertility and Sterility 37: 336–341

Wide L 1976 Human pituitary gonadotrophins In: Loraine J A, Bell E T (eds), Hormone Assays and their Clinical Applications, 4th edn, pp 87–140. Churchill Livingstone, Edinburgh

Wide L, Nillius J, Gemzell C, Roos P 1973 Radioimmunsorbent assay of follicle-stimulating hormone and luteinizing hormone in serum and urine from men and women. Acta Endocrinologica Suppl 174: 1–58

World Health Organization (WHO) Task force on methods for the determination of the fertile period. Special programme of Research Training in Human Reproduction 1980. Temporal relationships between ovulation and defined changes in concentration of plasma estradiol-17β, luteinising hormone, follicle-stimulating hormone and progesterone. American Journal of Obstetrics and Gynecology 138: 383–390

Wu C-H, Prazak L, Flickinger G L, Mikhail G 1974 Plasma 20-

hydroxypregn-4-3-one in the normal menstrual cycle. Journal of Clinical Endocrinology and Metabolism 39: 536–539

Yen S S C, Vandenberg G, Tsai C C, Parker D C 1974 Ultradian fluctuations of gonadotropins In: M Ferin, F Halberg, R M Richart, R L Van de Wiele (eds) Biorythms and Human Reproduction pp 203–218. John Wiley, New York

Yen S S C, Vela P, Rankin J, Littell A S 1970 Hormonal relationships during the menstrual cycle. Journal of the American Medical Association 211: 1513–1517

Younglai E V, Smith S L, Cleghorn J M, Steiner D L 1975 Variations in ovarian steroid levels during the luteal phase of the menstrual cycle. Clinical Biochemistry 8: 234–239

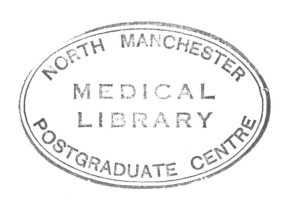

Endocrine response in the female genital tract

INTRODUCTION: STRATIFICATION OF ENDOCRINE RESPONSE

Endocrine events are brought about when a hormone acts on a tissue that is sensitive to it. Sensitivity of a tissue to a hormone generally means that the tissue has hormone-specific receptors — in the plasma membrane, in the cytoplasm, or perhaps in the nucleus — the chemical and physical properties of which are altered by the hormone binding. Conformational changes in the receptors have effects on the immediate intracellular environment of the receptors, so that the cell's intermediary metabolism is redirected to effect a transient or permanent change in the cell's function. Cellular endocrine response may then become integrated into a tissue or organ response, with consequent alterations in body economy and physiology.

Hormonal actions can be simple or complicated, depending not so much on the hormone as on the response a cell chooses to have to that hormone. So whereas the number of hormones available to act on the genital tract is limited, the contrary is true of the qualitative and quantitative range of responses that can be elicited. Of the main responsive tissues in the genital tract, this is especially the case with the *epithelium*, regional specialisation of which in the Fallopian tube, endometrium, cervix, vagina and vulva (including local glandular epithelial derivatives) causes enormous differences in structure and function; even within a single organ or tissue different responses occur to the same hormone (in the endometrium, for example, quite different things happen in deep and superficial epithelial cells when oestrogen reasserts its effect in the early proliferative phase).

Other responsive tissues in the genital tract include the *smooth muscle* of the muscularis, which constitutes the bulk of the wall of the hollow genital tract and which is more limited than the epithelium in its expression of endocrine action, and the *connective tissue stroma*, the response of which has not received much attention outside the endometrium and, more recently, the cervix.

Disentanglement of the intricate tiers of endocrine influences and responses in the human genital tract is far from complete. It has depended on painstaking experiments on individual tissues in humans and other mammals, with additional clues coming from generalisations, analogies and homologies within and between species. After an examination of the intracellular mechanisms by which a hormonal stimulus is translated into action, this chapter aims to introduce the integration of endocrine response that takes place within the individual organs and tissues of the female genital tract.

Peptide hormones, biogenic amines, and prostaglandins

Membrane receptors

The water-soluble hormones that act on the genital tract include the peptide hormones such as oxytocin, the catecholamines adrenalin and noradrenalin, and the (locally-produced) prostaglandins, together with their pharmacologically administered analogues. They are all able, as their mechanism of action, to bind to specific receptors that are located on the periphery of the cell. These cell-membrane receptors are composed of membrane proteins that extend through the lipid bilayer (Singer & Nicolson, 1972) of the membrane. The external portion of the receptor protein is glycosylated (and therefore constitutes part of the cell-surface carbohydrate layer, the glycocalyx); the internal part of the protein is able to make physicochemical contact with enzymes in the cell cytoplasm, either directly or indirectly, via other membrane proteins. Binding of a hormone to those carbohydrate and amino acid groups that form the receptor on the cell-surface produces a conformational change in the membrane protein that the interior of the cell perceives as a signal for a change in enzymatic activity — and, in some cases, an eventual change in transcriptional activity at the cell nucleus.

Binding of the hormone to the cell-membrane receptor is specific and tight. Although it is possible, experimentally, to exchange labelled exogenous hormones for bound hormones (indicating that the hormone-receptor reaction is not strictly irreversible but is an equilibrium reaction between association and dissociation), the vast bulk of bound hormone stays bound. The cell internalises the receptor and its hormone, which then ultimately finds its way into the cell's lysozome system for destruction. New plasma membrane with empty receptors takes the place of the internalised portions for the cell to regain sensitivity to new hormone. Although this process causes the hormone to enter the cell, it is important to recognise that this is merely a way of getting rid of it and replenishing receptors. Information transfer (i.e. hormone action) takes place at the cell membrane and is a virtually instantaneous consequence of hormone binding. Internalisation of the receptor probably terminates the information transfer (Kaplan, 1981).

Adenylate cyclase and protein kinase

Most peptide hormones, many biogenic amines, and some prostaglandins activate their target cells by stimulating adenylate cyclase to convert ATP to cyclic AMP (cAMP). The adenylate cyclase system is the best understood among several membrane systems that exist for translating hormone binding into cellular biochemical activity and there are very few, if any, cellular functions that are not directly or indirectly under the influence of an adenylate cyclase system (Birnbaumer, 1977).

According to a model proposed by Rodbell (1980), the adenylate cyclase enzyme complex has at least three components (Fig. 5.1): a receptor or R component; a nucleotide-regulatory or coupling component (N), which may be either stimulatory (N_s or inhibitory (N_i); and a catalytic component (C), which actually effects the conversion of [magnesium-ion-containing] ATP to cAMP. Association of R and N to form an RN complex increases the affinity of R for its specific hormone. When not linked to C, RN units associate to form oligomers and resist binding GTP. Hormone binding to R allows N to bind GTP, the RN units dissociate, and the individual GTP-RN units react with C to form the holoenzyme depicted in Fig. 5.1. Opposing regulation of C by independent types of RN complexes may occur, for example with alpha-adrenergic receptors inhibiting and beta-adrenergic receptors stimulating cAMP production in myometrium (cAMP in this tissue inhibits contractility).

Protein phosphorylation and dephosphorylation is now recognised to be a major general mechanism by which intracellular events in mammalian tissues are controlled by hormonal and neural stimuli (Cohen, 1982). The enzymes that phosphorylate and dephosphorylate proteins are known, respectively, as kinases and phosphorylases, the *protein kinases* transferring a phosphate group from ATP to the particular protein. Multiple phosphorylation of some enzymes is possible, causing gradual or sudden changes in substrate specificity. Some enzymes are more active in

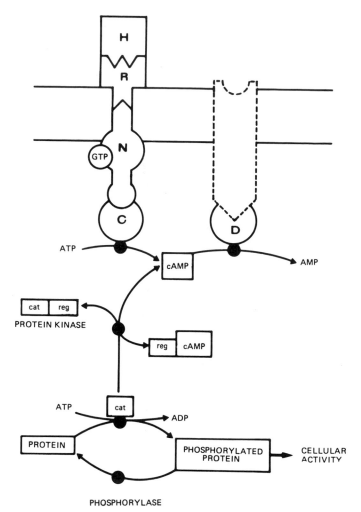

Fig. 5.1 Adenylate cyclase holoenzyme complex in the plasma membrane after Rodbell (1980). Binding of the water-soluble hormone (H) to the membrane receptor (R) allows its coupling component (N) to bind GTP and to react with the catalytic component (C) of the complex to increase or decrease cyclic AMP formation. Cyclic AMP removes the regulatory subunit (reg) from protein kinase, enabling its catalytic subunit (cat) to phosphorylate enzymes and other proteins; phosphorylated enzymes may have more or less activity than their unphosphorylated parent forms, and cellular biochemical activity is thereby modified. Dissociation of cyclic AMP from the regulatory subunit of protein kinase allows it to recombine with the catalytic subunit, terminating protein kinase activity. Free cyclic AMP concentration and hence protein kinase activity is governed by the rate of formation by adenylate cyclase versus the rate of degradation by phosphodiesterase (D), which is subject to similar extracellular controls

phosphorylated form; some in dephosphorylated form. The C-component of adenylate cyclase itself is, in some systems at least, subject to phosphorylation in order to acquire activity.

Cyclic AMP owes its intracellular action to the stimulation of a single group of closely related protein kinases, which can be membrane-bound or soluble. Cyclic AMP-dependent protein kinase (cAMP-PrK) is composed of a regulatory and a catalytic subunit. Binding of cAMP, which is soluble, to the regulatory subunit causes it to dissociate from the catalytic subunit, which is then free to phosphorylate a further series of protein kinases. Dissociation of cAMP from the catalytic subunit allows the subunit to recombine with the regulatory subunit and kinase activity stops. The amount of free cAMP about depends on its production rate from adenylate cyclase and on its intracellular clearance rate through hydrolysis by the enzyme *phosphodiesterase* — an enzyme itself subject to complex intracellular and extracellular (hormonal) control. The activity of adenylate cyclase is not just regulated by hormone-receptor binding or exogenous stimulation: tachyphylaxis can occur in adenylate cyclase systems so that a cell, presumably by producing some feedback substance that acts on the C component, can reduce its cAMP production even though receptor numbers and substrate are maintained.

Cyclic AMP has a substantial phylogenetic history, being first encountered in bacteria, in which adenylate cyclase is a soluble, cytoplasmic enzyme; in all animals, invertebrate and vertebrate, adenylate cyclase is present only in the cell membrane — a position ideally suited for reacting to signals from water-soluble hormones. Depending on the protein kinases the cell makes available to cAMP-PrK, a variety of metabolic pathways can be activated, deactivated or modified. Included among the possibilities are regulation of transcriptional activity in the cell nucleus. Some of these effects will be seen only after prolonged stimulation. The shortest time required for endocrine effects to become clinically apparent through the adenylate cyclase-cyclic AMP system is probably in the range of seconds to minutes. For quicker results, different means are necessary.

Calcium and calmodulin

Entry of Ca^{2+} into a cell or release of Ca^{2+} from sarcoplasmic reticulum under a neural stimulus is a well-known trigger for physiological activity. Most of the intracellular actions of Ca^{2+} are mediated by the calcium-binding protein calmodulin, acting as a second-messenger similar to cAMP.

Calmodulin is a monomer of MW 17 000 and contains four calcium-binding sites, the affinity of which for calcium varies considerably and the fractional occupancy of which may dictate the precise systems regulated (Means & Dedman, 1980). Calmodulin is a molecule of very ancient lineage: its highly conserved structure and function through the plant and animal kingdoms implies fundamental roles in cellular function.

Calmodulin accounts for several known protein kinases that are not stimulated by the cAMP system, including *smooth muscle myosin light chain kinase*, which is essential both for assembly of myosin into filaments and for actin-activated actomyosin ATPase and smooth muscle contraction; inactivation of this enzyme by cAMP-PrK may be how adrenalin, acting through beta-receptors, relaxes smooth muscle of the uterus (Cohen et al, 1980). Calmodulin also effects Ca^{2+}-dependent *secretory processes*, a role that may prove to be important in genital tract epithelium.

The calmodulin system intertwines with the adenylate cyclase system both synergistically and antagonistically. Calmodulin can regulate cAMP levels by affecting phosphodiesterase activity, and cAMP-PrK often phosphorylates calmodulin-dependent enzymes (Cohen et al, 1980).

The stimulus for Ca^{2+} is often neural and can occur in milliseconds. The duration of the Ca^{2+}-mediated signal is limited, especially in smooth muscle, as Ca^{2+} is pumped out of the cell or taken up again by the endoplasmic reticulum; the enzyme for this, Ca^{2+}/Mg^{2+}-dependent ATPase, is itself stimulated by activated calmodulin.

Other protein kinase activators

A number of physiological stimuli elevate neither cAMP nor intracellular Ca^{2+}, but nevertheless appear to work through protein kinases. Acetylcholine, acting through muscarinic receptors in smooth muscle, apparently induces rapid hydrolysis of membrane phosphytidylinositol to yield inositol cyclic phosphate and *diacylglycerol*; protein kinase-C, which is ubiquitous in mammalian cells, requires diacylglycerol for activity (Cohen, 1982).

Cyclic GMP has long been known to be present in cells and attempts have been made to elucidate second-messenger systems comparable to those involving cAMP — but without success. Cyclic GMP-dependent protein kinase is known, but there is no physiological process that has an absolute requirement for guanylate cyclase in cell-free systems (Murad et al, 1979). It used to be thought that muscarinic effects of acetylcholine on smooth muscle were mediated through cGMP (Lee et al, 1972), but more recent evidence indicates that smooth muscle contraction can be induced with choline esters in the absence of increases in cGMP; instead, increases in cGMP have been found in smooth muscle *after* contractility has increased, a phenomenon that has led Murad and colleagues to propose that cGMP is formed as a result of altered redox potential in a cell, and that it may feed back negatively to influence one or more redox reactions and steer the cell's redox potential back to normal — therefore implying a role for cGMP in prevention of oxidative damage to proteins and lipids (Murad et al, 1979).

Membrane phospholipid methylation

So far we have encountered several chemical means by which the conformation, and hence the activity, of enzymes can be modified. These means have included phosphorylation and dephosphorylation, addition of nucleotide (as in the binding of GTP to the regulatory component of adenylate cyclase), and binding of a cation (Ca^{2+}-activated calmodulin). Another potent and prominent means of altering chemical properties is *enzymatic methylation*.

Methylation of membrane phospholipids, causing their translocation from the cytoplasmic side to the outer surface of cell membranes and reducing viscosity within the lipid bilayer, has been shown to play an important enhancing role in the transduction of receptor-mediated signals (Hirata & Axelrod, 1980). As a chemical process it is not necessarily incompatible with the model of receptor-adenylate cyclase coupling described earlier. Reduced viscosity within the membrane allows the receptors to have greater lateral mobility, both improving the efficiency with which cAMP is generated and increasing Ca^{2+}-permeability of the membrane. Methylation of phospholipids may allow receptors previously masked to become available for binding.

Phospholipid methylation is also closely coupled to activation of phospholipase A_2, which releases arachidonic acid from membrane phospholipids. Arachidonic acid is the precursor of the prostaglandins and thromboxanes. In this way prostaglandin generation can accompany membrane receptor activation. The prostaglandins, in turn, may have their own membrane receptors, activation of which can either enhance or limit the original hormonal stimulus.

The stage is therefore set for infinite fine-tuning of cellular endocrine response.

Acetylcholine and neurogenic stimuli

Cholinergic actions

Acetylcholine is the main neurotransmitter of the autonomic nervous system, being present in preganglionic fibres of the sympathetic and parasympathetic nervous systems, the postganglionic fibres of the parasympathetic system, and parts of the postganglionic sympathetic system. Acetylcholine receptors have been very well characterised and in classical neurophysiology are divisible into those receptors that respond also to nicotine (nicotinic receptors) or to muscarine (muscarinic receptors).

Nicotinic receptors are not directly relevant to the genital tract, but provide a useful contrast to the endocrine receptors we have encountered so far — although, strictly speaking, there is no clear division between the chemistry of neural stimulation and that of humoral or endocrine stimulation. Nicotinic cholinergic receptors are found in autonomic ganglia and skeletal muscle motor endplates. In contrast to peptide hormone binding to cell-membrane receptors, which favours association over dissociation to the point that the hormone is likely to get carried into the cell as the membrane is internalised for replacement, acetylcholine binding to the receptor is very reversible: the duration of stimulation is fleeting (a few milliseconds) and is ended by enzymatic degradation of acetylcholine by cholinesterase in the synaptic space. Intra-

cellular response accords this brief exposure by being explosively quick: cell-membrane proteins undergo conformational changes that open channels in the membrane to small ions, so depolarising what in excitable cells was a previously polarised cell-membrane (a membrane carrying a transmembrane potential); excitable cells are then able to propagate a wave of depolarisation that can be regarded as a second-messenger translating surface-receptor activation into intracellular biochemical activity.

Examination of slower *muscarinic receptors* brings us closer to humoral stimulation. These cholinergic receptors are found on visceral smooth muscle cells throughout the genital tract, and stimulation causes changes in calmodulin and cyclic nucleotide concentrations intracellularly, putting neural stimulation into direct competition with endocrine stimulation in influencing intracellular second-messenger systems.

Catecholaminergic actions

In fluorimetric studies of catecholamine content of the human ovary, tube and uterus, *noradrenalin* is the main catecholamine detected (Owman et al, 1967); adrenalin, if present at all, constitutes less than 5 per cent of total catecholamines, and dopamine is undetectable. Noradrenalin is present in granules in sympathetic nerve endings, rather than in chromaffin cells, which are rare in the genital tract. The noradrenalin can be released both through nerve stimulation and by the action of other hormones, including acetylcholine.

Unlike the nicotinic acetylcholine receptor, which has been substantially conserved through vertebrate phyla at least, whole families of receptors exist for the catecholamines noradrenalin and adrenalin. There are two broad categories of adrenergic receptors: *alpha receptors*, which react to both adrenalin and noradrenalin, but only weakly or not at all to isoprenalin; and *beta receptors*, which react to isoprenalin at least as well as, and often more than, they do to adrenalin and noradrenalin. Alpha receptors in the genital tract are generally stimulatory, beta-receptors inhibitory. The pregnant myometrium is especially sensitive to the contracting effects of ergometrine, which acts mainly through adrenergic alpha-receptors.

The β-receptors in the genital tract are subcategorised as β_2-receptors because they are stimulated more by adrenalin than by noradrenalin, β_1-receptors in cardiac muscle being equally sensitive to adrenalin and noradrenalin (Lefkowitz, 1976), thus conferring on the genital tract musculature, especially the myometrium during menstruation or pregnancy, clinically-exploitable sensitivity to the smooth muscle-relaxing properties of β_2-agonists such as ritodrine, salbutamol and terbutaline. Although these pharmacological properties are very useful clinically, the physiological function of the receptors is less clear, since noradrenalin, the chief catecholamine of the genital tract, is among the weakest of catecholamines in stimulating β_2-receptors.

Although few comparative studies that relate to the genital tract are available, visceral adrenergic innervation generally, and β-receptor responsiveness in particular, are rather late evolutionary developments among the vertebrates (Coupland, 1979). Even among mammals the relative distribution of α- and β-receptors in the genital tract varies, with, for example, α-receptors predominating in the Fallopian tube musculature of the rabbit (which therefore contracts in response to adrenalin) and β-receptors predominating in the human tube (which relaxes in response to adrenalin).

The intracellular mode of action of the catecholamines is intimately involved with adenylate cyclase. Cyclic AMP was discovered in studies of catecholamine action in the liver, and relaxation of the myometrium through stimulation of beta adrenergic receptors remains one of the best characterised adenylate cyclase systems. The effect is rapid and, in at least some systems, coupling between receptor-occupancy and adenylate cyclase activation is through methylation of membrane phospholipids (Hirata & Axelrod, 1980).

Much less is known about the second messenger for α-adrenergic stimulation. In situations where cAMP production is significant, α-adrenergic stimulation decreases cAMP production; but, since phylogenetically it is older than the β-adrenergic system, it would be surprising if α-adrenergic stimulation did not have its own potent means of effecting intracellular biochemical events. Recent studies in cardiac muscle and vascular smooth muscle have now shown that adrenergic stimulation of contractility is the result of progressive recruitment of receptor-operated slow Ca^{2+} channels, which permit diffusion of Ca^{2+} down its concentration gradient into the cell, raising the free cytoplasmic Ca^{2+} concentration (Braunwald, 1982).

Genital tract innervation

The visceral part of the genital tract is supplied with parasympathetic and sympathetic nerves.

Parasympathetic preganglionic fibres originate in spinal segments S2 to S4 and traverse the pelvic splanchnic branches (nervi erigentes) of the corresponding spinal nerves to terminate in ganglia close to the organs innervated: the isthmus of the tube, the uterus and cervix, and the vagina and clitoris. The outer part of the tube (the ampulla) and the ovary receive parasympathetic supply from terminal branches of the vagus nerve. Parasympathetic fibres are cholinergic and appear to have functions that are phylogenetically well established, being particularly active during sexual arousal; parasympathetic activity is associated with vasodilatation, clitoral engorgement and lower genital tract secretion. The role of acetylcholine in the upper genital tract, where acetylcholinesterase-containing fibres are sparse (Sjöberg, 1967), is difficult to determine, both because of overlaying of more sophisticated and obvious control mechanisms and because exogenous acetylcholine applied to these tissues *in vitro* may act through releasing noradrenalin from sympathetic nerve endings. As in the lower genital tract, cholinergic nerves in the uterus and tubes are restricted to blood vessels; they may play especially important roles in the genital tract's response to sexual stimulation (see below).

Sympathetic preganglionic fibres from spinal segments T12 to L2 or L3 traverse the lumbar splanchnic branches of the sympathetic trunk and synapse with postganglionic neurons in the inferior mesenteric plexus (Barr, 1974); these supply the pelvic viscera with 'long' adrenergic neurons. Preganglionic fibres also run in the hypogastric nerves, to synapse in ganglia near the cervicovaginal junction with 'short' adrenergic neurons (Sjöberg, 1967). The tubes, uterus and vagina thus receive innervation through both short and long noradrenergic neurons. Many of these fibres are vasomotor, and experiments in rabbits with 6-hydroxydopamine, which selectively destroys adrenergic nerve endings, have not shown that their loss causes any substantial disturbance in fertility (Pauerstein et al, 1974; Johns et al, 1974). Noradrenalin distribution in the genital tract stops short of the epithelium, although the epithelium does contain the principal degrading enzyme of the catecholamines, monoamine oxidase (Kubo et al, 1970).

Peptidergic actions

A number of recent studies have demonstrated peptidergic neurons containing *vasoactive intestinal polypeptide* (VIP) in the human genital tract, particularly the isthmus of the Fallopian tube, the cervix and the vagina (Walles et al, 1980; Helm et al, 1981; Ottesen, 1983). Distribution within these organs is to blood vessels, smooth muscle and epithelium. *In vitro* studies have shown that smooth muscle from both the tubal isthmus and the cervix responds to VIP with a concentration-dependent reduction in contractile activity, whereas the myometrium, which does not receive VIP innervation, is unresponsive (Helm et al, 1981).

Many peptides, including somatostatin, substance P, gastrin/cholecystokinin, enkephalin and neurotensin, have been identified in neurons of the gut — often with amine neurotransmitters identifiable in the same nerve endings (Hökfelt et al, 1980). VIP has been found in association with acetylcholine — an association that may be a general feature of secretomotor neurones. The importance of these peptides in peripheral nerves is quite unknown. No systematic search for peptides other than VIP has been made in the genital tract and no comment can yet be made on the contribution of peptidergic innervation of the genital tract to its function.

Steroid hormone responsiveness

The most stable humoral stimulation that cells enjoy comes not from the water-soluble hormones and the membrane receptors we have considered so far, but from fat-soluble hormones that act on receptors inside the cell cytoplasm: the steroid hormones. Compared with the peptides, prostaglandins and biogenic amines, the steroids — or rather their actions — are phylogenetically rather new, finding definitive and specialised expression in regulating reproductive function only in the vertebrates, although the molecules we recognise as sex-steroids do occur in invertebrates and even plants (Barrington, 1975; Sandor & Mehdi, 1979).

The structure of the steroid hormones among the vertebrates is very inflexible, with a high degree of specificity of action dependent on relatively minor structural differences (Bentley, 1976); such secondary experimentation and adaptation that has occurred through evolution has presumably been restricted to the development of sophisticated and highly specific receptor systems. It is noteworthy that progesterone, which is a precursor for both androgen and oestrogen synthesis, has been one of the newest recruits among hormones that act specifically on the genital tract: it is essential for the gestation of developing young within the genital tract of mammals, but it has no consistent comparable role among viviparous fish, amphibians or reptiles (Amoroso et al, 1979).

Despite these relatively late adaptations of the genital tract to steroid hormone control, the ovarian steroids have come to exert an overwhelming impact on all segments of the tract and affect every aspect of growth, differentiation and function; and steroids also affect both quantitative and qualitative responses to other hormones. The onset of response to steroids (usually hours or days) is much slower than responses to the water-soluble hormones; but the stability of this response is virtually unprecedented, often being measured in days or weeks. The variety of different responses that take place in different parts of the tract is infinite — the result of subtle differences in receptors and gene transcription that are only just beginning to be understood.

Oestrogen and progesterone cytosol and nuclear receptors

Oestrogens exert a pronounced proliferative effect on the Fallopian tubes, uterus, cervix and vagina. Progesterone either supplements or antagonises many actions of oestrogens. With the exception, possibly, of progesterone's anti-androgen action, tissue effects of progesterone require previous or concomitant exposure to oestrogen (Brotherton, 1976).

Entry of steroids into cells from the extracellular space occurs by diffusion at a rate directly proportional to free (i.e. dissociated from plasma carrier proteins) steroid

concentration (for review, see Clark & Peck, 1977). Retention of the steroid in the cell then depends on two types of binding: (a) high affinity, high specificity, low capacity, saturable binding — known as *steroid receptors*; and (b) low affinity, high capacity, non-saturable binding — known as *non-specific binding*. Non-specific intracellular steroid binding may be quite important in maintaining a pool of immediately available steroid close to the receptors. The

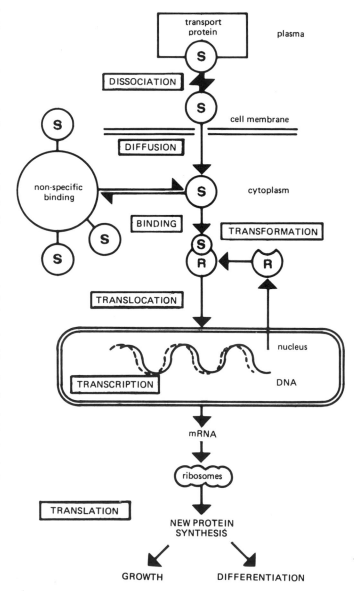

Fig. 5.2 Steroid hormone action depends on *dissociation* of the lipid-soluble steroid (S) from its plasma transport protein and *diffusion* into the cell cytoplasm, where retention of the steroid is encouraged by nonspecific *binding*, as well as specific binding to cytoplasmic steroid receptors (R). The *transformed* steroid-receptor complex *translocates* to the nucleus, where binding to specific chromatin acceptor sites enables DNA-dependent mRNA synthesis, or *transcription*, to take place; mRNA diffuses to the cytoplasm where it instructs the ribosomes to *translate* steroid action into protein synthesis for growth and differentiation

cellular action of the sex steroids is through binding to these specific, high affinity receptors, which, when bound and activated, cause transcriptional induction of the synthesis of regulating and differentiating proteins (Milgrom et al, 1973; Chan & O'Malley, 1976).

The first of a number of discrete steps needed for steroid action (Fig. 5.2) after *binding* with cytoplasmic receptors is induction of a conformational change in the receptor (Bailly et al, 1978). This receptor *transformation*, in the case of the oestrogen receptor (E-R) but not the progesterone receptor (P-R) (Chan & O'Malley, 1976; Kasid & Laumas, 1981), produces an increase in sedimentation rate and confers on the steroid-receptor (RS) complex the ability to bind to the nucleus (Notides & Nielson, 1974). *Translocation* of the steroid-receptor complex to the nucleus occurs within minutes and is not rate-limiting. In the nucleus the RS complex binds to high affinity chromatin acceptor sites (Yamamoto & Alberts, 1975), after which *transcription* (DNA-dependent messenger-RNA synthesis) begins within 10 minutes (Chan & O'Malley, 1976). *Translation* of this action into protein synthesis is discernible in 30 to 40 minutes (Chan & O'Malley, 1976) and eventually produces growth and/or differentiation of the target tissue.

Cells of the immature rat uterus each contain about 15 000 to 20 000 cytoplasmic oestrogen receptors (R_c) (Clark et al, 1977b). After a single high-dose injection of radioactive oestradiol, cytosol E-R content decreases quickly, but then slowly rises to a level higher than its initial concentration (Jensen et al, 1969). The quick fall in cytosol receptor reflects translocation of RE complexes from the cytoplasm (R_cE) to the nucleus (R_nE), where the receptor is then inactivated; the subsequent rise takes place because oestradiol induces further synthesis of its own receptor (Milgrom et al, 1973). In this way oestrogens increase tissue oestrogen-sensitivity. Progesterone, on the other hand, partly owes its oestrogen-antagonist action to its ability to prevent replenishment of E-R (Hsueh et al, 1976; Koligian & Stormshak, 1977; Okulicz et al, 1981).

Activation of cytoplasmic E-R prior to translocation depends not only on binding with oestrogen; a rather more substantial change in the receptor takes place, as is reflected by the change that occurs in its sedimentation coefficient from 4s to 5s, and is due to its complexing with a *receptor activator*, which appears to be a basic, 3s cytoplasmic protein (Thampan & Clark, 1981). It is this activating protein that is able to bind E-R to the nucleus. By stabilising the receptor-activator complex, the steroid molecule thus shifts the distribution equilibrium of the receptor from the cytoplasm to the nucleus, which acts as a sink for the receptor complex. A corollary of this equilibrium model of receptor translocation is that a small fraction of receptor-activator complexes at any one time will, by chance, have formed without a stabilising steroid molecule and so be found in the nucleus. That this does indeed occur, and that free receptors can be detected in the

nucleus, is now quite clear (e.g. Jungblut et al, 1978; Sheridan et al, 1979).

Clark and colleagues have also described a nuclear oestrogen receptor that is different from the translocated cytoplasmic receptor in that it has a lower affinity for oestrogen, but a much higher capacity, in those tissues in which it occurs. It is not known whether this Type II receptor binds the native steroid or the R_nE complex. The Type II receptor is only found in tissues that *grow* in response to oestrogen, so it is present in uterine tissues, but absent in the pituitary and hypothalamus, which do contain classical or Type I E-R (Clark & Markeverich, 1981). The Type II sites appear to be associated with the nuclear matrix and may play a role in DNA replication. Both progesterone and corticosteroids inhibit uterine growth: they appear to do so by selectively interfering with these Type II sites (Markeverich et al, 1981).

DNA synthesis does not necessarily accompany oestrogen exposure, even in tissues that are capable of responding to oestrogen this way; rather, a sustained presence of oestrogen in the nucleus is needed (Stormshak et al, 1977). Continuous exposure of the uterine cell to oestrogen, on the other hand, is not accompanied by infinite self-perpetuating responsiveness: a dose-dependent state of refractoriness eventually develops in the tissue, apparently due to accumulation of polypeptide chalones.

Oestradiol binds strongly to target tissues and is the most potent oestrogen: it dominates tissue oestrogen influence in the reproductive years. Oestradiol is subject to metabolism to oestrone in the cytoplasm of endometrial epithelium through the action of oestradiol 17β-dehydrogenase, an enzyme induced by progesterone and synthetic progestogens — so providing a second mechanism for progesterone's anti-oestrogen effects (Gurpide et al, 1977; King et al, 1980). *Oestrone* has specific roles in the central nervous system, but its peripheral oestrogenic action, which becomes predominant after the menopause, results from conversion to oestradiol in the target tissue (Gurpide & Welsh, 1969; Gurpide et al, 1977); labelled oestrone appears not to translocate to the nucleus and may therefore itself be devoid of transcriptional oestrogenic activity (Tseng & Gurpide, 1973).

Oestriol is the weakest oestrogen. Demonstration that after a bolus injection it interferes with subsequent oestradiol action has led to proposals that endogenous oestriol may be important in protecting against oestrogen-dependent neoplasia. This concept is misleading. Oestriol has been shown to bind normally to oestrogen receptors, to translocate to the nucleus, and to initiate transcription; but its retention by the nucleus is of short duration: premature destruction of the receptor occurs and oestrogen action terminates early (Clark et al, 1977a). Oestriol given as a bolus does not bind to the nuclear Type II sites that are associated with true uterine growth (Clark & Markaverich, 1981). An oestriol bolus therefore depletes cytoplasmic E-R without producing a full realisation of oestrogen action and compromises a subsequent response to oestradiol. But in steady state conditions that allow replenishment of cytoplasmic E-R, for example with a subcutaneous oestriol implant, oestriol is a potent oestrogen without antagonistic properties (Clark et al, 1977a); Type II sites become occupied, and true uterine growth occurs (Clark & Markaverich, 1981).

Progesterone receptors (P-R) are induced by oestrogen (Milgrom et al, 1973), which explains sensitisation of tissues to progesterone by oestrogens. After a single injection of oestradiol, the half-life of P-R in the guinea-pig uterus in the absence of progesterone is about 5 days; but when progesterone is injected on the day after the oestradiol injection, a very marked fall in cytosol P-R follows immediately, and is sustained (Hsueh et al, 1976). This deleterious effect of progesterone on its own receptors is the result of enhanced receptor inactivation after translocation to the nucleus, without progesterone itself supplying any stimulus for receptor replenishment. Progesterone also selectively reduces the concentration of the occupied form of the nuclear oestrogen receptor (Okulicz et al, 1981), preventing the means by which oestradiol normally replenishes its own receptor. The clinical correlate of these phenomena is the often transitory nature of endometrial differentiation induced by progestogens: a secretory change may be followed by endometrial necrosis in both normal and neoplastic endometrium (Bonte, 1972).

Data from different animal and human tissues, and from autoradiographic studies within tissues, indicate that the principles of hormone-receptor physiology outlined above have general relevance (Reel, 1976; Hsueh et al, 1976; Gurpide et al, 1977) and that similar mechanisms probably regulate receptor concentration in most or all of the various cell types of the uterus, the cervix, and the vagina. The physicochemical properties of endometrial and myometrial progesterone receptors in a number of different mammalian species appear to be identical, although the endometrial stromal or decidual progesterone receptor may be different (Leavitt et al, 1977); the endometrial stroma is also unique among genital tract tissues in that progesterone may cause a wave of mitosis in the luteal phase.

Receptor assays, or measurements of sensitivity of a tissue such as the endometrium to oestrogens and progesterone, are fraught with difficulties (in contrast, say, to assaying the hormones themselves in plasma). The usual practice is to estimate free cytoplasmic receptor content. The uptake of tritiated steroid by the cytosol fraction of tissue homogenates is measured at low temperatures (e.g. 4°C), under circumstances that allow one to subtract nonspecific binding from total steroid binding to give an asymptotic curve that indicates saturable binding (Evans et al, 1974; Pollow et al, 1975; Clark & Peck, 1977). By ignoring steroid-receptor complexes (including the complexes still in the cytoplasm and those translocated to the nucleus), such assays estimate only what could be called the *latent receptor capacity*: measuring in reality not what the steroid is doing at any instant, but rather what it is not yet doing. Moreover, assays even of the empty receptors become difficult to do if nonspecific binding is a high proportion of total binding (see Clark & Peck, 1977).

Total receptor population assays, measuring both free and bound receptors in both the cytosol and nuclear fractions of tissue homogenates, are possible with exchange assays performed at higher temperatures (30°–37°C), which allow displacement of endogenous bound steroid by the labelled steroid (Bayard et al, 1978). New problems arise, however, because the higher temperatures needed for steroid-receptor dissociation also allow receptor degradation; careful control studies must be done for each tissue and for each steroid receptor to determine optimal conditions (Clark & Peck, 1977). But, no matter how well receptor assays are performed, none of these measurements will indicate the receptor turnover rate — and so, by inference, receptor activity — in situations where hormone levels are changing, because not only is time required for receptors to be replenished after a hormone surge but the resynthesis rate also varies under different conditions. Sequential experiments that determine nuclear retention time of receptors and measurements of specific messenger-RNAs are designed to give truer estimates of quantitative hormone action.

Assays of cytosol oestrogen and progesterone receptors in the endometrium through the menstrual cycle (Fig. 5.3) provide a practical illustration of these problems. Cytosol available E-R peaks early in the follicular phase, then falls in concentration first as the plasma oestradiol rise translocates receptors to the nucleus and second as progesterone rises to stop replenishment. It should be remembered, though, that this represents the behaviour of receptor *concentration* and not the total receptor *content* of the proliferating tissue. Cytosol P-R rises in the follicular phase under the influence of plasma oestradiol, and then falls quickly in the luteal phase as plasma progesterone both utilises the receptors and prevents replenishment. These receptor profiles clearly do not coincide with biological activity as reflected histologically, endometrial proliferation becoming more intense as plasma oestradiol rises up to the time of ovulation. A better correlation is provided by measurement of nuclear (translocated) receptor concentrations: nuclear E-R concentration peaks in the late follicular phase, and nuclear P-R concentration peaks in the early luteal phase (Bayard et al, 1978).

Genital tract androgen receptors

Androgen receptors are found throughout the femal genital tract, but their significance outside the vulva (see p. 154) is quite unknown.

Possible non-cytosol-receptor steroid actions

Cyclic AMP may be involved in some oestrogen actions. Oestrogen administration to ovariectomised rats causes an early increase in adenylate cyclase activity (Rosenfeld & O'Malley, 1971) that is prevented by the β-adrenergic receptor blocker, propranolol. The significance of these observations is not yet clear. The earliest detectable response in the uterus to oestrogen administration is an increase in wet weight due to fluid accumulation; this response is so quick that it might be considered a candidate for a membrane site of oestrogen action, but this seems not to be the case (Tchernitchin et al, 1977) and there is evidence for it being mediated by Type I receptors in the nucleus (Clark & Markeverich, 1981). The significance of cAMP modulation by oestrogen, if this can be shown to be a direct effect, is unknown. Meanwhile, evidence from the use of fluorescein-labelled steroids indicates that specific binding sites for oestrogen may be present on target cell membranes (Nenci et al, 1981). Progesterone (and some of its water-soluble metabolites) has also been suggested to have a cell membrane effect and, because of its rapid action, a membrane action of progesterone has been hypothesised to be involved with the general depressive action this hormone has an excitable cells of the central nervous system and smooth muscle; the few empirical data available to support this hypothesis are discussed below.

THE FALLOPIAN TUBES

Cyclical changes in steroid exposure

Cyclical changes in steroid receptors

The Fallopian tube, like the endometrium and myometrium (see below), is able to concentrate oestradiol and progesterone to many times circulating plasma levels, indicating that high affinity tissue binding proteins or receptors are present (Batra et al, 1980; Devoto et al, 1980).

Sedimentation and binding characteristics of human Fallopian tube oestradiol and progesterone receptors are similar to those of steroid receptors in the endometrium (Verhage et al, 1980; Pollow et al, 1981). Binding in the cytoplasm followed by translocation of the receptor-steroid complex to the nucleus, as described for steroid receptors in the previous section, has been reported (Pollow et al, 1981). In a non-human primate it has been shown that cytoplasmic E-R concentration is increased by oestradiol and decreased by progesterone (Brenner et al, 1974). Furthermore, progesterone action in the early luteal phase promotes, as it does in the uterus, the activity of oestradiol dehydrogenase, which metabolises oestradiol to its inactive metabolite oestrone (Wu et al, 1977). Cyclical changes in Fallopian tube structure and function can therefore be considered to be mediated by ovarian steroids acting through specific receptors that are chemically comparable to those of other parts of the genital tract.

The *ampulla* is the lateral part of the tube; it has a thin muscular wall and a wide lumen with complicated mucosal folds; the ratio of epithelium to smooth muscle is high. The *isthmus* is situated between the ampulla and the uterus; it has a thick muscular wall and a very narrow lumen with only a few mucosal folds; its ratio of epithelium to smooth muscle is low. Cytosol E-R and P-R concentrations are greater in the ampulla than in the isthmus (Robertson & Landgren, 1975; Flickinger et al, 1977; Pollow et al, 1981). At first sight, therefore, it may be that receptor content in the tube is a reflection of the proportion of the tissue composed of epithelium. There are indications (Fuentealba et al, 1976) that the endosalpinx has a higher concentration of steroid binding sites than the myosalpinx (a situation similar to that in the uterus, where endometrium has a higher steroid receptor content than the myometrium). However, a number of studies have shown that the *fimbrial end* of the tube, which has the highest epithelium: smooth muscle ratio of all, has the lowest concentration of steroid receptors at all stages of the cycle (Flickinger et al, 1977; Pollow et al, 1981).

Because steroid receptor concentrations are usually expressed numerically as 'binding sites per unit weight of tissue protein', and because the muscular isthmus contains so much protein and so little epithelium, it can be concluded from these receptor concentration data that (a) tubal steroid receptors are predominantly located in the epithelium, and (b) the concentration of receptors in the epithelium becomes greater with increasing distance from the ovary. This second conclusion may have important functional implications.

Figure 5.3 shows the relationship of total (free plus bound) cytoplasmic E-R and P-R to nuclear (translocated) E-R and P-R during the menstrual cycle (Pollow et al, 1981). Oestrogen receptors are high early in the follicular phase and most are in the cytoplasm, untranslocated; the ratio between tissue and plasma oestradiol levels is greatest at this stage, being around 12:1 for the isthmus and 8:1 in the ampula (Batra et al, 1980). With the pre-ovulatory rise in plasma oestradiol, late in the follicular phase, the proportion of E-R that has translocated to the nucleus rises considerably; progesterone receptors are in high concentration in the cytoplasm and the peri-ovulatory period, as ovarian progesterone production starts to rise, is the time of highest tissue:plasma ratios for progesterone — about 26:1 for the isthmus and 18:1 for the ampulla (Batra et al, 1980). After ovulation, with the luteal phase rise of plasma progesterone, E-R and P-R fall, and there is a predominance of nuclear receptors over cytoplasmic receptors (Pollow et al, 1981). A curious observation, one for which there is no obvious explanation and one that needs confirming, is the relative abundance of translocated progesterone receptors in the early part of the follicular phase.

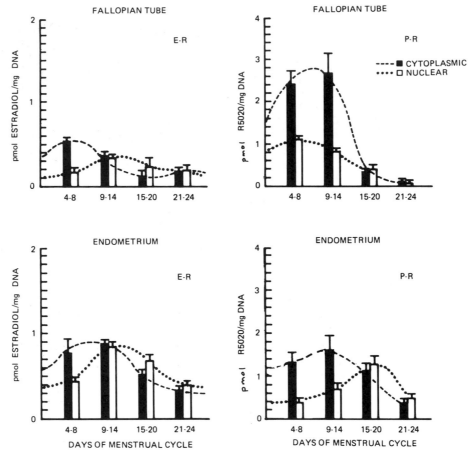

Fig. 5.3 Relationship between Fallopian tube and endometrial total, cytosol and nuclear oestradiol receptor (E-R) and progesterone receptor (P-R) concentrations through the menstrual cycle. Receptor concentrations peak earlier in the Fallopian tube than in the endometrium. (Redrawn from Pollow et al, 1981)

The origin of the tube's steroid milieu

The data of Pollow and colleagues (Fig. 5.3) show that the distribution of cytoplasmic versus nuclear receptors is slightly — perhaps significantly — different in the Fallopian tube and the uterus. It is as if steroid events in the menstrual cycle happen sooner in the tube than in the uterus. Although it is possible that this reflects inherent differences in steroid-responsiveness in the two organs, it is also possible that it is the steroid milieu that is different: that it is not merely circulating plasma levels of oestradiol and progesterone to which the tube, in particular, is exposed. There are now a number of lines of evidence to show that this is indeed the case.

An early observation to indicate that ovarian steroids may have routes of access to the tube that are more direct than the peripheral circulation was the discovery of asymmetry in oestrogen receptor concentration between the fimbrial ends on each side after ovulation, E-R levels on the side of the corpus luteum being much lower (Flickinger et al, 1977); this asymmetry was barely apparent (and the difference not statistically significant) in the more medial parts of the tube. Further, the discrepancy between

fimbrial and ampullary E-R levels is much greater in women with ovulatory cycles than it is in women on oral contraceptives, who have a systemic rather than a local source of oestrogen and progestogen (Flickinger et al, 1977).

Studies on monkey tubal fluid have shown that ovarian steroid hormones are found there in total concentrations that are about the same as plasma levels before ovulation, but are present in tubal fluid in greater concentrations than in plasma after ovulation. Significantly, however, the concentration of steroid binding proteins is very much lower in tubal fluid than in plasma at all stages of the cycle, so *free* or diffusible steroids — including androstenedione, testosterone, oestrone, oestradiol and progesterone — are *all* present in several-fold higher concentrations in tubal fluid, both before and after ovulation (Wu et al, 1977).

Peritoneal fluid in women also contains high levels of ovarian steroids (Koninckx et al, 1980a,b; Donnez et al, 1982; Jansen, 1983). Progesterone concentrations are higher than in plasma throughout the cycle, and show a very substantial and sudden increase with rupture of the ovulating follicle (Fig. 5.4). Oestradiol levels are also some-

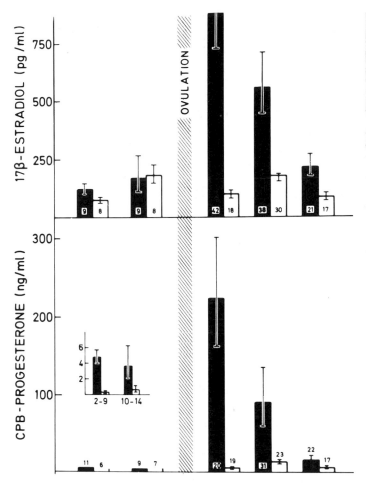

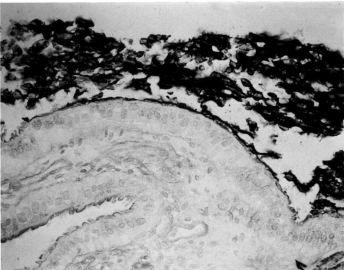

Fig. 5.5 Cumulus tissue in the monkey Fallopian tube lumen after ovulation (Jansen, previously unpublished). *In vitro* studies indicate that cumulus cells secrete oestradiol, progesterone and prostaglandins, all of which may have a marked and direct effect on the tube's endocrine milieu. High iron diamine (pH 1), alcian blue (pH 2.5), nuclear fast red

Fig. 5.4 Oestradiol and progesterone concentrations in peritoneal fluid (solid bars) and plasma (open bars) through the menstrual cycle. Oestradiol concentrations in peritoneal fluid increase dramatically with follicular rupture; progesterone concentrations do too, but levels in peritoneal fluid are also higher than plasma levels during the follicular phase. (From Koninckx et al (1980), with the permission of the author and the Journal of Clinical Endocrinology and Metabolism)

through the ovulatory stigma (Koninckx et al, 1980a,b). But it is also possible that the extruded granulosa cells, which can enter both Fallopian tubes (Fig. 5.5), themselves continue to produce oestradiol and progesterone (McNatty et al, 1980; Shutt & Lopata, 1981) and so create for the Fallopian tube, and the events that take place in its lumen, a steroid environment of very considerable dimensions.

Cyclical changes in tubal morphology and function

Cyclical epithelial changes

There are two main types of differentiated cells in the tubal epithelium, non-ciliated *secretory cells* and *ciliated cells* (Fig. 5.6 & 5.7). Ciliated cells predominate in the fimbriae whereas secretory cells predominate in the isthmus. Both types of cell undergo changes in structure and function with cyclical changes in oestradiol and progesterone. Mature, differentiated cells are seen only at midcycle (Verhage et al, 1979), under the influence of oestradiol. Mitosis is rare in the adult Fallopian tube at any stage of the menstrual cycle, so there is little or no cyclical change in cell number. Distinction between the two types of cells is not absolute and occasional differentiating cells display both cilia and secretory granules (Jansen & Bajpai, 1982). Under the prolonged influence of progestogens, cells dedifferentiate, so that those that have lost their cilia cannot be distinguished from those that have lost their secretory granules; progestogens therefore increase the proportion of non-ciliated cells in relation to cells that are still ciliated.

The thickness and general morphology of the endosal-

what greater in peritoneal fluid before ovulation, though the difference narrows just before ovulation (Donnez et al, 1982); after follicle rupture again a sudden rise in peritoneal fluid steroid concentration occurs, with oestradiol levels far exceeding those in plasma (Fig. 5.4). These differences are all the more significant when the lower sex hormone binding globulin levels of peritoneal fluid are taken into account.

In summary, the ovaries create around them a steroid milieu that is quite different to the steroid environment provided by circulating blood plasma. Before ovulation it is presumed that follicular-peritoneal fluid steroid exchange is at least as important to adjacent structures as exchange between the follicle and its circulation. With follicular rupture at ovulation an explosive increase in oestradiol and progesterone takes place in the local peritoneal and tubal environment. This increase has been interpreted as coming from the still open follicle — production from the developing corpus luteum directly entering the peritoneal cavity

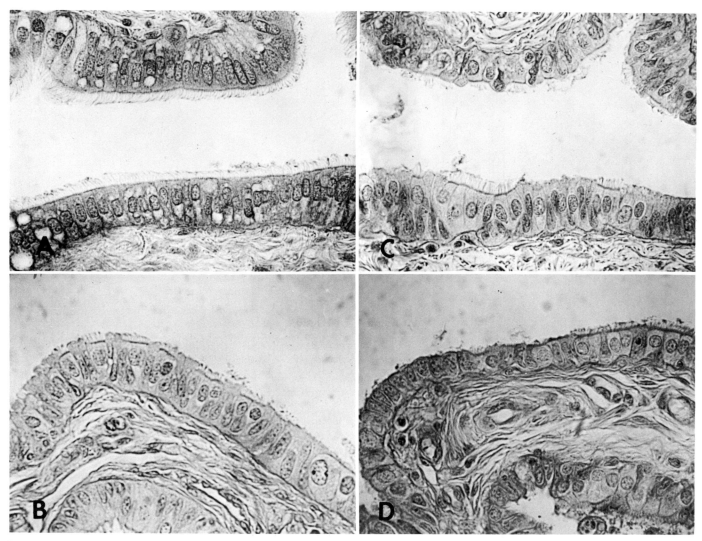

Fig. 5.6 Ampullary tubal epithelium through the normal menstrual cycle, showing cyclical changes in epithelial height, secretory cell activity and cilial prominence. [A] proliferative phase, [B] preovulatory, with distended secretory cells, [C] postovulatory, with discharged secretory cells, [D] late luteal phase. Periodic acid-Schiff, haematoxylin

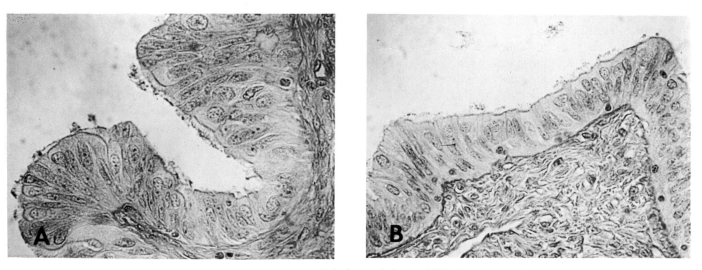

Fig. 5.7 Isthmic tubal epithelium showing [A] distended secretory cells before ovulation, and [B] cilial prominence after ovulation. Periodic acid-Schiff, haematoxylin

pinx varies during the cycle, but the variations are much less conspicuous than the changes the endometrium undergoes (see below). The changes are qualitatively similar in different parts of the tube, although there are quantitative differences.

Light microscopy (LM) shows that the ampullary epithelium reaches maximum height (30–35 μm) at midcycle (Fig. 5.6), at which time ciliated cells and the secretory cells are of equal height, with secretory cell apices forming domes between tufts of cilia; the epithelium in the isthmus is taller, though less uniform (Fig. 5.7). For a short time after ovulation the cilia become more prominent as the secretory cells discharge their apical secretions. The epithelium then loses height as ciliated cells become broader and lower. With menstruation — and especially during pregnancy — the epithelial cells are uniformly low (10–15 μm) (Snyder, 1923; Novak & Everett, 1928; Woodruff & Pauerstein, 1969).

The greater resolution of transmission electron microscopy (TEM) and scanning electron microscopy (SEM) has generally confirmed and extended LM observations. The secretory cells show the most conspicuous cyclical changes, especially in the isthmus (Fig. 5.8). Early in the cycle the apices of the secretory cells have prominent microvilli and the cilia of ciliated cells appear discrete and healthy (Fig. 5.8A). With the high oestrogen stimulation of midcycle, apocrine secretion appears to be taking place and secretory material obscures the cilia (Fig. 5.8B). At this time, serous granules are evident in the apical cytoplasm of the secretory cells on TEM (Bjorkman & Fredricsson, 1962; Clyman, 1966). Histochemical and TEM studies in primates have indicated, however, that endoplasmic reticulum vacuoles and not serous granules contain the secre-

tion that dominates the tubal isthmic lumen at midcycle — a secretion that is composed of glycogen and acid mucus glycoproteins (Jansen & Bajpai, 1983).

This luminal secretion persists through the time of ovulation and, although it is particularly pronounced in the isthmus (Fig. 5.8C; Jansen, 1978, 1980a), it can also be recognised in the ampulla (Ferenczy & Richart, 1974; Ludwig & Metzger, 1976; Orlandini & Pacini, 1978). As ovarian progesterone production becomes established, secretory activity stops, granules are no longer seen and ribosomes leave the endoplasmic reticulum to lie free in the cytoplasm (Bjorkman & Fredricsson, 1962); SEM shows cilia again to be conspicuous (Fig. 5.8D) as the secretion disappears.

With loss of hormonal support from the endosalpinx at the end of the luteal phase, numerous lysozomes are found in the cytoplasm (Hashimoto et al, 1964; Clyman 1966). Cilia give the SEM appearance of having lost vigour (Patek et al, 1972) and microvilli become sparse on the nonciliated cell surfaces (Fig. 5.8E).

Exogenous *oestrogens* stimulate differentiation of secretory cells in the fimbriae and ampulla, with appearance of numerous vesicles containing material that is less electrondense than the contents of the serous granules (Fredricsson & Björkman, 1973). These vesicles have also been demonstrated, though to a lesser extent, during midcycle of spontaneous cycles (Hashimoto et al, 1962). In rhesus monkeys they constitute a major, if fleeting, midcycle secretory phenomenon (Jansen & Bajpai, 1983).

Progestogens counteract these effects of oestrogens. When progestogens are administered long-term, irrespective of concomitant oestrogen administration, atrophy and deciliation of the endosalpinx can be produced (Fig. 5.8F).

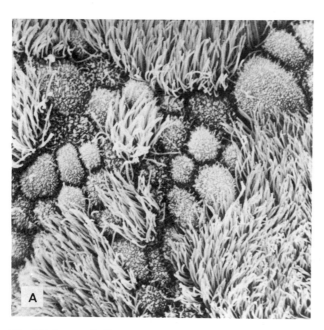
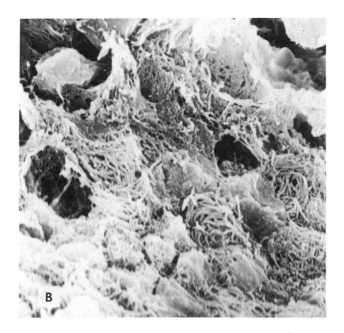

Fig. 5.8 (see overleaf)

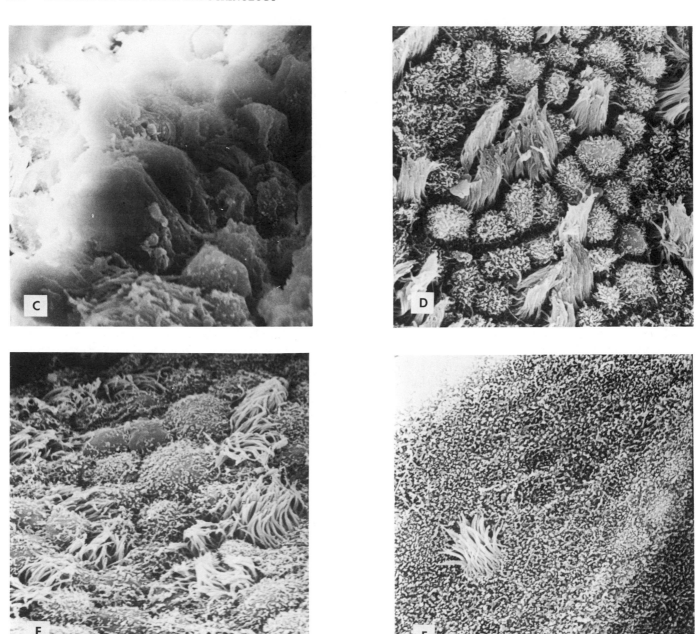

Fig. 5.8 Human Fallopian tube isthmic secretion as visualized by scanning electron microscopy. From Jansen (1980a), with permission of The American Journal of Obstetrics and Gynecology. [A] Late menstrual phase. Early oestrogen effect after recovery from progestogenic influence. Secretory cells with surface microvilli lie among ciliated cells. [B] Late follicular phase. Extracellular secretion produced under the influence of oestradiol blankets the cell surfaces, so that cilia are indistinct. [C] Postovulation. Abundant extracellular secretion fills the isthmic lumen at a time that the ovum is still confined to the ampulla. [D] Four days after ovulation. Secretions have disappeared and cilia regain prominence under the influence of progesterone at about the time of ovum transport through the isthmus to the uterus. [E] Late luteal phase. Progesterone withdrawal causes a loss of hormonal support from the endosalpinx at the same time that menstruation starts in the uterus. [F] Prolonged progestogen therapy leads to atrophy and deciliation

Myosalpingeal structure and function

Visceral smooth muscle cells are arranged in sheets. In the Fallopian tube these sheets generally constitute (a) an *inner circular layer* and (b) an *outer longitudinal layer*, which merges with the spirally orientated fibres of the myometrium at the uterotubal junction (UTJ); the isthmus near the UTJ also has (c) an *inner longitudinal layer* (Daniel et al,

1975b; Wilhelmsson et al, 1979). As mentioned above, the muscular coat of the ampulla is very thin, whereas the muscular coat of the more medial isthmus is relatively thick; orientation of muscle bundles in the thinner parts of the ampulla shows a loss of distinct layering (Daniel et al, 1975b). The junction between ampulla and isthmus is the ampullary-isthmic junction (AIJ), a region that is not as sharply defined histologically as palpation of the tube at laparotomy would suggest.

Much of the interpretation of myosalpingeal function has been based on assumptions that tubal smooth muscle has electrical properties similar to other visceral smooth muscle. The mechanism of excitation-coupling of the myosalpinx, for instance, is presumed to be similar to that of the myometrium, described below. Intracellular recordings of tubal smooth muscle electrical activity have only recently been performed. Human tubal smooth muscle cells have been studied with intracellular electrodes only in tissue culture; a resting potential of -35 mV was recorded, which is less than expected on the basis of smooth muscle properties elsewhere; in some cells action potentials were recorded, in others there were slow ('pacemaker') waves of amplitude 5–20 mV (Sinback & Shain, 1979).

Travel of electrical activity along the tube has been demonstrated in a number of species, including the human (Daniel et al, 1975a; Talo & Pulkkinen, 1982), giving the opportunity for pacemaker activity and integrated, propagated contractions. The extent to which smooth muscle cells form a functional syncytium depends on the frequency with which points of very close contact occur. These points of contact allow propagation of action potentials, whether endogenous or induced by acetylcholine from nerve endings, to spread from cell to cell by ephaptic conduction. The myosalpinx, unlike the myometrium, does not have gap junctions, but it does have *simple contacts*, points of

very close opposition, which, though less efficient than gap junctions, do allow electrical transmission. Conduction velocity in the tube is correspondingly slow, with velocities of 1–3 mm/s reported in human tubes (Talo & Pulkkinen, 1982).

Before considering autonomic and short-acting endocrine influences on tubal musculature in detail, we should examine the patterns of spontaneous or myogenic contractility in the tube under different steroid-hormone environments.

Telemetric studies in rhesus monkeys *in vivo* using external force transducers have produced results probably applicable to humans (Fromm et al, 1976). During menses and the early follicular phase, contractions were sporadic and of variable amplitude. As the follicular phase progressed, bursts of activity were noted. Plasma oestrogens were assayed daily, and those monkeys with the highest plasma oestrogen levels (but whose plasma progesterone levels were low) showed much more regular contractions of larger amplitude; exogenous oestrogen administration also increased contraction frequency. When plasma progesterone was high, contractions were much less regular and of small amplitude. This steroid-dependent contractile activity is superimposed on changes in oestradiol-dependent circular muscle tone in the tubal isthmus — at least in rabbits, but probably also in humans (Fig. 5.9).

Noradrenergic innervation is prominent in the circular smooth muscle of the isthmus (Paton et al, 1978). Ultrastructural studies in human tubes confirm the presence of

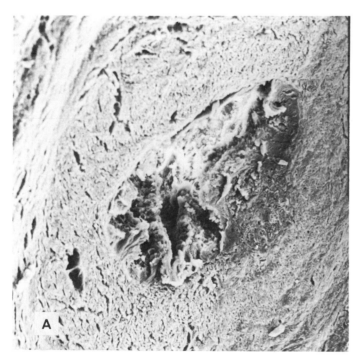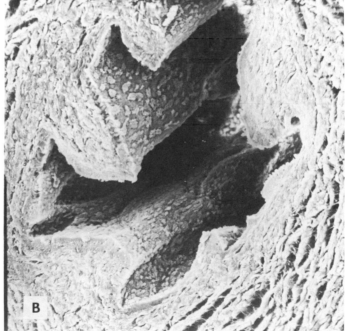

Fig. 5.9 Fallopian tube isthmic contraction [A] before ovulation under the unopposed influence of oestradiol, and relaxation [B] under the opposing influence of progesterone after ovulation. Low power scanning electron micrographs (from Jansen, 1980a, with permission of The American Journal of Obstetrics and Gynecology)

nerve bundles among the circular muscle of the isthmus; few close contacts between nerves and muscle cells are present and noradrenalin-containing varicosities are located down the length of the terminal axons (Hodgson & Eddy, 1975), so noradrenalin released from nerve endings has a diffuse effect. Innervation of the ampulla is much less substantial; ultrastructurally, nerves are associated only with blood vessels. Chemical determinations of noradrenalin concentrations also give higher values for the isthmus than for the ampulla in human tube (Owman et al, 1976).

Beta-receptors generally predominate in human isthmic circular muscle; noradrenalin causes relaxation at all stages of the menstrual cycle except around the time of ovulation, under the influence of high plasma oestradiol levels, when it causes contraction (Owman et al, 1976; Moawad et al, 1977). A rise in plasma progesterone above 2 ng/ml reverses the response to noradrenalin (Moawad et al, 1977) and marked isthmic relaxation is apparent *in vitro* several days after ovulation (Owman et al, 1976). Longitudinal smooth muscle from the isthmus, on the other hand, usually contracts in response to noradrenalin and so presumably is mostly under α-adrenergic influence (Owman et al, 1976); contraction in response to noradrenalin after ovulation aids dilatation of the isthmic lumen.

Reactivity of the human isthmus to noradrenalin therefore fits in well with the increase in isthmic tone that occurs with the midcycle oestradiol peak (leading up to ovulation) and for a short time afterwards (while the egg is retained in the ampulla). Progesterone production then establishes the dominance of β-receptors: relaxation in response to noradrenalin then coincides with isthmic dilatation and ovum transport down the isthmus to the uterus.

A number of *in vivo* observations, however, cast serious doubt on noradrenergic nerves having any monopoly on regulation of normal tube function or on mediation of steroid action, at least in experimental animals such as the rabbit. Fertility in rabbits is not jeopardised significantly (a) by depletion of noradrenalin from nerve endings with reserpine (Hodgson et al, 1975); (b) by adrenergic blockade with guanethidine or with phenoxybenzamine and propranol together (Hodgson et al, 1975); (c) by surgical denervation (Pauerstein et al, 1974); or (d) by pharmacological denervation with 6-hydroxydopamine (Pauerstein et al, 1974; Johns et al, 1974). If noradrenalin-content is increased with the monoamine oxidase inhibitor iproniazid, the rate of ovum transport is marginally increased; and if noradrenalin-content is decreased with reserpine, ovum transport is retarded slightly; but these effects are much less than those achievable by manipulating oestradiol and progesterone concentrations (Bodkhe & Harper, 1972). At most, therefore, noradrenergic control of tubal function can be seen as a modulating activity consistent with optimal function.

Cyclic nucleotides have been implicated in smooth muscle physiology since the discovery that cAMP relaxes intestinal smooth muscle. Dibutyryl cAMP, a cAMP analogue, induces relaxation of the musculature of isthmus and ampulla (Maia et al, 1976). The effect is not blocked by β-adrenergic blockade with propranolol, indicating a site of action distal to the β-adrenergic receptor. Theophylline, which inhibits phosphodiesterase and increases intracellular cAMP, enhances the relaxing effects of β-adrenergic stimulants.

Prostaglandins appear to have centrally-important effects on tubal contractility. In vivo studies in rabbits have shown that exogenous $PGF_{2\alpha}$ stimulates tubal contractility and accelerates egg transport; PGE_2, on the other hand, inhibits tubal contractility. Similar studies in humans have given similar results (Coutinho & Maia, 1971), although increased contractility in response to $PGF_{2\alpha}$ is not necessarily accompanied by accelerated ovum transport (Croxatto et al, 1978a).

Further characterisation of human tubal response to prostaglandins *in vitro* has indicated that their site of action is proximal to adenylyl cyclase and probably at the cell membrane: $PGF_{2\alpha}$ has its contractile effects decreased by β-adrenergic stimulants and by phosphodiesterase inhibitors. PGE_2's inhibition of isthmic circular muscle contractility is accompanied by an increase in cAMP (Maia et al, 1976). However, the intracellular mechanism by which $PGF_{2\alpha}$ mediates an increase in contractility is not known; it is additive to α-adrenergic stimulation with phenylephrine, maximal stimulation by either alone being augmentable by addition of the other (Tonpe & Lindblom, 1979).

Whether prostaglandins are necessary for spontaneous myogenic activity *in vivo* and whether steroid effects on myogenic contractility are mediated through changes in prostaglandin production or metabolism remain unanswered questions. At present the data are compatible (a) with steroids affecting smooth muscle directly, (b) with changes in adrenergic activity and response, and (c) with changes in prostaglandin synthesis, metabolism and response.

Ciliary activity

If the cumulus mass, stained supravitally with methylene blue, is placed on the fimbriae of the rabbit tube, movement of the cumulus is slow and steady for the first few minutes over the fimbriae and for the initial few millimetres into the ampullary lumen. After this, movement changes to a complex pattern of quick forward and backward jumps associated visually with segmental contractions of the tubal wall. Nevertheless net forward progress takes place until the AIJ is reached, at which point forward and backward movements continue, but net forward progress stops for some time. In primates, including humans, these segmental contractions are much less evident: ampullary transport of the egg is slower and steadier than in the rabbit (Blandau et al, 1979).

The importance of cilia in ovum-pickup from the ovary and in these transport phenomena can be demonstrated by observing their persistence or failure (a) with complete inhibition of muscular activity, and (b) with selective interference with ciliary activity. Complete inhibition of tubal contractions can be accomplished with the β-adrenergic agonist isoprenalin. In rabbits *in vivo*, infusion of isoprenalin has no impact on total transit time of the ampulla, although rapid to-and-fro movements of the cumulus are abolished (Halbert et al, 1976); by implication, cilia provide the sole propellant force for the cumulus under these conditions.

Ciliary activity in the rabbit *ampulla* can be manipulated by resecting a 1 cm segment of ampulla, twisting it 180° on its mesosalpingeal pedicle, and reinserting it by microsurgical anastomosis (Eddy et al, 1978). Segmental reversal of a piece of proximal, middle or distal ampulla in this way effectively prevents pregnancy, although fertility is maintained in control animals treated by microsurgical segmental reinsertion without reversal. Segmental reversal of rabbit *isthmic* segments, on the other hand, does not disturb fertility in comparison with controls, so isthmic cilia are not thought to be very important in the isthmic phase of ovum transport.

The rabbit fimbrial end and ampulla have a higher proportion of ciliated cells than the same parts of the human tube do, and this may account for the much quicker ampullary transit time of the rabbit ovum (6 minutes) (Halbert et al, 1976) compared with the human ovum (about 30 minutes) (Blandau et al, 1979).

A number of studies have sought a change in *cilial beat frequency* in the tubal mucosa before and after ovulation. In human tubes an 18 per cent increase in beat frequency in the luteal phase compared with the follicular phase has been described (Critoph & Dennis, 1978); the increase in beat frequency after ovulation occurred in the ampulla and the isthmus, and brought their cilial beat frequency up from about 6/s to the 7/s frequency that characterised fimbrial cilia both before and after ovulation. Prostaglandins E_2 and $F_{2\alpha}$ both stimulate cilial beat frequency in mucus-free rabbit fimbrial mucosa in organ culture (Verdugo et al, 1980). Preliminary evidence suggests that the mechanism for this increase is through the release of intracellular Ca^{2+} (Verdugo et al, 1976a). Provision of progesterone in a high-oestradiol environment, which happens just after ovulation, increases histochemically demonstrable ATP in human isthmic endosalpinx (Kugler et al, 1976).

Ciliogenesis in the Fallopian tube is an oestrogen-dependent process; it is antagonised by progesterone. Recent detailed TEM studies have confirmed that ciliogenesis takes place during the follicular phase (Verhage et al, 1979; Cornier et al, 1980). Mature ciliated cells are seen only at mid-cycle; deciliation and atrophy accompany the postovulatory rise of plasma progesterone, and careful quantitative studies indicate that 10–12 per cent of cells then lose their cilia; these cells regenerate their cilia in the next follicular phase (Verhage et al, 1979). During human pregnancy deciliation is variable by the time of delivery, but commonly progresses further in the puerperium (Andrews, 1951; Jansen, 1980a).

Verhage and colleagues noted that plasma oestradiol levels were higher during periods of atrophy and deciliation than they were during periods of hypertrophy and reciliation (Verhage et al, ,1980); they concluded that ciliogenesis is a process that is sensitive to low amounts of oestradiol and that serum oestradiol levels are probably sufficient at all stages of the human menstrual cycle to maintain ciliated cells, but that progesterone, when present, is able to block this oestrogen effect and also requires a recovery phase to follow its withdrawal. There are indications that even minipill doses of progestogens (norethisterone 350 μg or levonorgestrel 30 μg per day) are enough to antagonise oestradiol's maintenance of ciliated cells (Oberti et al, 1974) and cause partial deciliation of the endoslapinx.

Steroid influence on ciliary activity may be summarised, therefore, as being oestrogen-dependent in the sense that oestradiol causes differentiation of ciliated cells, including ciliogenesis. A change from an oestrogen to a progesterone-dominated environment may increase the ciliated cells' ability to provide cilial dynein with ATP from apically located mitochondria, which are increased in concentration immediately after ovulation. Stimulation of increased cilial beat frequency might then be triggered by local release of prostaglandins in the tubal mucosa or by prostaglandins synthesized by cumulus cells in the tubal lumen, acting through the release of Ca^{2+} ions from intracellular storage sites or entry from the extracellular space. More prolonged exposure to the antagonistic effects of prosgesterone, after the time of ovum transit, eventually causes cilial regression.

Tubal impedance to ovum transport

After sperm ascent distally and fertilisation of the newly ovulated egg in the ampulla, the egg has its proximal transport delayed in the ampulla at or near the ampullary-isthmic junction (AIJ) for at least 48 hours before the isthmus is passed and the ovum reaches the uterus (Croxatto et al, 1978b). The physiological explanation for this ovum transport delay at the AIJ is controversial.

Myosalpingeal activity is undoubtedly responsible for the almost instantaneous to-and-fro movements the egg displays in the tubal lumen (Talo, 1980). It is also possible that these contractions may be subject to slight directional bias, perhaps imposed by ciliary activity, so that net movement of tubal contents can be effected in one direction or the other (Portnow et al, 1977; Verdugo et al, 1976b). The evidence indicates that this bias may be quantitatively and qualitatively different at different stages of the human menstrual cycle. But notwithstanding these subtle changes in myosalpingeal contractility, muscular activity imparts a high degree of randomness on the immediate position of the ovum (Chatkoff, 1975), in spite of which there is surprisingly little variability in overall transport rates to the uterus between different ova in the same Fallopian tube, between ova in the right and left tube of the same animal, between ova in different animals in similar endocrine states, and even, in a broad sense, between ova of quite distantly related mammalian species. Despite more or less inexorable beating of cilia towards the uterus, temporary delay of ovum transport at the ampullary-isthmic junction (AIJ) seems to be an almost universal feature among mammals. This constancy suggests imposition of a well-defined system of control of ovum transport for which neither the mechanism of statistical bias among segmenting contractions nor the mechanism of minor changes in ciliary beat frequency qualify as serious candidates.

The endosalpingeal lining of the tube is normally in close apposition to itself (Blandau et al, 1979); there is little waste space in the lumen. The ovum, when present in the tubal lumen, causes distortion of the endosalpingeal folds in the ampulla and an increase in the lumen's internal dimensions in the isthmus (Pauerstein, 1974). It is apparent, therefore, that the tube might impede ovum transport by the rigidity of its walls or the viscosity of its luminal secretions. Both tubal wall compliance and tubal luminal contents are normally dependent on hormonal control.

Scanning electron micrographs of the rabbit and the human isthmus give the distinct impression that there is an increase in luminal diameter after ovulation in comparison with the pre-ovulatory phase (Fig. 5.9). This implies that there is relaxation of circular smooth muscle, contraction of longitudinal smooth muscle, a reduction in mural bulk through decreased interstitial fluid (Hodgson, 1978), or all three.

Relaxation of isthmic circular muscle with the onset of progesterone dominance is accompanied by a shift from α-adrenergic to β-adrenergic sensitivity to noradrenalin and by a shift away from dominance of the contractile effects of $PGF_{2\alpha}$ to the relaxing effects of PGE_2; longitudinal isthmic muscle, on the other hand, is stimulated by PGE_2 and therefore actively augments the increase in isthmic diameter.

Moreover, as acid mucus glycoproteins accumulate and persist in the isthmic lumen under the influence of oestradiol around the time of ovulation, their presumably highly expanded and negatively charged state *in vivo* could be expected to impede entry into the isthmus of either the acid proteoglycan-rich cumulus mass or the acid glycoproteinaceous zona pellucida of the ovum. (The chemical structure

Table 5.1 Properties of complex carbohydrates important in reproduction

	Serum glycoproteins	Mucus glycoproteins	Proteoglycans

Occurrence	circulating glycoproteins
	  FSH, LH, hCG
	  immunoglobulins
	  transport proteins (eg SHBG)
	cell membrane integral proteins
	  receptor proteins
	  Ca^{2+}-dependent ATPase
		urogenital mucosal surfaces
		  cervical mucus
		  ?tubal secretions
		?zona pellucida
		cell membrane peripheral proteins
		  tubal, endometrial, &
		  trophoblast glycocalyx
			connective tissue stroma
			  cumulus mass around oocyte
			
			hyaluronic acid, * chondroitin
			  sulphate, dermatan sulphate,
			  heparin, heparan sulphate etc.

Carbohydrates
  Proportion
  Configuration
	less than 25%
	branched oligosaccharide
	  (<10 sugars)
		50%; often 80%
		branched oligosaccharide
		  (<10 sugars)
			95%
			glycosaminoglycan
			  long linear repeating disaccharide
			  units of sugar + hexuronic
			  acid (exc. keratan
			  (<50 units)

Sugar composition	fucose, galactose, sialic acid,
	  N-acetyglucosamine,
	  N-acetylgalactosamine,
	  mannose, & arabinose
		fucose, galactose, sialic acid,
		  N-acetylglucosamine, &
		  N-acetylgalactosamine
		ester sulphate groups
		rich in serine & threonine
		  (contain -OH groups)
			hexuronic acids: glucuronic or
			  iduronic acid
			sugars: glucosamine or galactosamine
			ester sulphate groups add to acidity
			  (except hyaluronic acid)

Polypeptide Amino acids	typical first-class protein composition	cysteine present	

CHO-polypeptide linkage	N-glycosidic
	  (N-ac.glucosamine-asparagine)
		O-glycosidic
		  (N-ac.galactosamine-serine
		  -theonine)
			xylose linkage

* a glycosaminoglycan without protein.

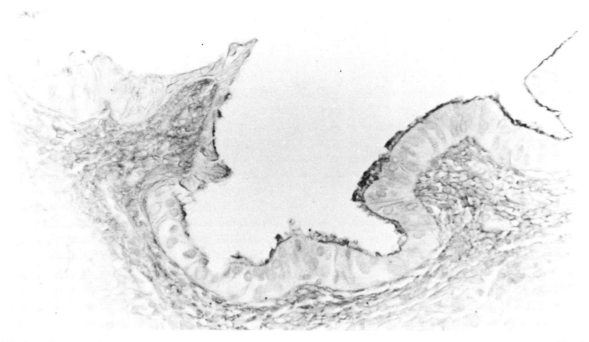

Fig. 5.10 Fallopian tube glycocalyx present over normal epithelium but deficient over abnormal epithelium in fallopian tube damaged by chronic salpingitis; if transport of an early embryo through the tube is delayed by damage to smooth muscle and cilia, absence of glycocalyx could facilitate ectopic implantation. Alcian blue (pH 3.5), nuclear fast red, red filter

of these egg-coats in comparison with that of the genital tract secretions is given in Table 5.1.)

Endocrine resistance in the Fallopian tube

Chronic salpingitis

Damage of the Fallopian tubes caused by infection and luminal occlusion, with a consequent increase in hydrostatic pressure adding to mucosal damage produced by the infection, is a common cause of infertility. Technically successful reparative surgery (in the sense that tubal patency is restored) is accompanied by a high incidence of tubal pregnancy, spontaneous abortion and persisting infertility (Jansen, 1980b, 1981, 1982). Endorgan resistance to oestradiol may be part of the pathophysiology of these persistently abnormal tubes, manifesting morphologically as a disturbance of myosalpingeal architecture, ciliation and secretory function (Fig. 5.10), and endocrinologically as a decrease in cytosol E-R (O. Petrucco, personal communication).

ENDOMETRIUM

The endometrium is the most dramatically responsive of the genital tract tissues to cyclical changes in ovarian steroid production. Periodic menstruation in humans and other primates is direct evidence of cyclical ovarian activity. In contrast to the Fallopian tube and myometrium, however, little is known of the endometrium's response to water-soluble hormones and the role of their intracellular second messengers as effectors of physiological change.

Cyclical changes in endometrial steroid receptors

The endometrium concentrates oestradiol and progesterone from the plasma against a concentration gradient (Porias et al, 1978) by binding these hormones both to specific low-capacity receptors and to nonspecific sites of high capacity. The ovary's *follicular phase*, dominated by production of oestradiol, manifests in the endometrium as the *proliferative phase*, during which glands and stroma grow and the endometrium becomes thicker. Progesterone of the ovary's *luteal phase* stops epithelial and stromal proliferation in the endometrium and causes morphological appearances in endometrial glands that give this phase of the menstrual cycle in the endometrium the name *secretory phase*. The biochemistry of endometrial steroid metabolism and response, together with a description of the practical problems associated with the measurement of oestrogen receptors (E-R) and progesterone receptors (P-R), is treated in detail in the Introduction to this chapter.

Endometrial cytosol available E-R peaks early in the proliferative phase; E-R then falls in concentration first as the plasma and tissue oestradiol-rise translocates receptors to the nucleus, and second as progesterone becomes available to stop E-R replenishment (Fig. 5.3). It should be remembered that this represents the behaviour of receptor *concentration*, and not necessarily the total cytosol receptor *content*, of the proliferating tissue, the volume of which increases steadily during this phase. Cytosol P-R rises in the proliferative phase under the influence of plasma oestradiol, and then falls quickly in the secretory phase as plasma progesterone both utilises the receptors and prevents replenishment. These receptor profiles do not coincide with biological activity as reflected histologically: endometrial proliferation becomes more intense as plasma oestradiol rises up to the time of ovulation (see below). Measurement of nuclear (translocated) receptor concentrations provide a better correlation: nuclear E-R peaks in the late follicular phase and nuclear P-R peaks early in the luteal phase (Bayard et al, 1978).

Cyclical changes in endometrial morphology [by Elisabeth Johannisson]

Introduction: problems with dating the endometrial biopsy

Present knowledge of the cyclical morphological changes of the endometrium rests mainly on the classic human and rhesus monkey studies that appeared between 1913 and 1951 (Schröder, 1913; Bartelmez, 1933; Sturgis & Meigs, 1936; Markee, 1940; Noyes et al, 1950; Bartelmez et al, 1951), at which time modern assays of steroids and gonadotrophins in urine and plasma had not been developed and endometrial changes could be related only to basal body temperature and the onset of menstruation (Noyes et al, 1950; Noyes & Haman, 1953). With the advent of chemical and radioimmunological assays a plethora of data accumulated in which the by-then-established histological dating provided by the endometrial biopsy was used as the point of reference for 'dating' corresponding plasma steroid levels.

Paradoxically, therefore, studies in which the hormone profile of the normal menstrual cycle has been used as the point of reference for endometrial morphology have not been prominent (Moghissi et al, 1973; Tredway et al, 1973; Lundy et al, 1974; Koninckx et al, 1977; Genz et al, 1980). The morphological criteria of a 'normal' menstrual cycle are still based on the ideal cycle of 28 days (Noyes et al, 1950), in which ovulation occurs on day 14 and divides the cycle into proliferative and secretory phases of equal length; specific morphological day-to-day changes, particularly during the secretory phase, could allow dating of the endometrium in relation to the cycle day selected for the biopsy. This concept is still very much in use. If the histological dating corresponds to the cycle day selected, the endometrium is considered to represent a normal endocrine response, irrespective of the hormone profile in the plasma during that cycle; if the histological dating does not correspond, the endometrium is considered to be 'out-of-phase' (Cline, 1979; Sulewski et al, 1980; Wentz, 1980a).

Correlation between endometrial morphology and circulating steroid levels has been questioned (Cooke et al, 1972; Rosenfeld & Garcia, 1976; Shepard & Senturia, 1977; Trevoux et al, 1979) and, indeed, the range of allowable morphology has been emphasised, if not exactly delineated, by Noyes himself (Noyes, 1973).

Recent studies have shown that, in normally menstruating women of previous fertility who exhibit a cycle length of 25 to 36 days, the follicular phase varies between 9 and 23 days and the luteal phase between 8 and 17 days (Landgren et al, 1980). Among the 68 women in this study, only 32 (47 per cent) had an endocrinologically-determined luteal phase length that corresponded to the ideal secretory phase of 14 to 15 days. A certain cycle day selected for an endometrial biopsy may therefore vary considerably from the standard 28-day cycle and still the cycle may fulfill the hormonal criteria of a normal one (Johannisson et al, 1982). Indeed, when the cycle days selected for the biopsy were related to the midcycle LH-surge in another 68 cycles, biopsies taken on cycle days 15 and 16, intended to be immediately after ovulation, turned out to have been timed anywhere between LH −7 days and LH +6 days; those obtained on cycle days 21 and 22 corresponded to anything from LH +1 to LH +12; and variability was equally marked on cycle days 25 and 26. A given cycle day *per se* is therefore an unreliable guide for selection of the appropriate time for assessment of secretory activity of the endometrium.

Accordingly, uncritical comparison between histological dating and the cycle day selected for the biopsy risks false interpretation of the endocrinological response of the endometrium. Especially marked differences can exist between the levels of the plasma steroids and endometrial biopsy findings in women near the menopause (see Endometrial Resistance, p. 140)

Proliferative phase

In 91 per cent of women studied (Landgren et al, 1980; and see Ch. 4) the hormone profile of the follicular phase is characterised by an average oestradiol level between 150 and 370 pmol/l (40–100 pg/ml) during the first 6 days of the cycle, and by a pre-ovulatory peak value higher than 690 pmol/l (190 pg/ml). The mean levels of progesterone during the first 6 days of the follicular phase do not exceed 4.4 nmol/l (1.4 ng/ml). Taking into account the complexity of steroid receptor mechanisms, it is improbable that a simple correlation should exist between circulating plasma steroids, concentration of cytosol steroid receptors, and morphological events in the endometrium. Comparisons between plasma oestradiol and endometrial oestradiol receptors (E-R) have certainly given variable results. Some authors have found a positive correlation between endometrial E-R and circulating plasma oestradiol levels during the entire proliferative phase (Levy et al, 1980; Baulieu et

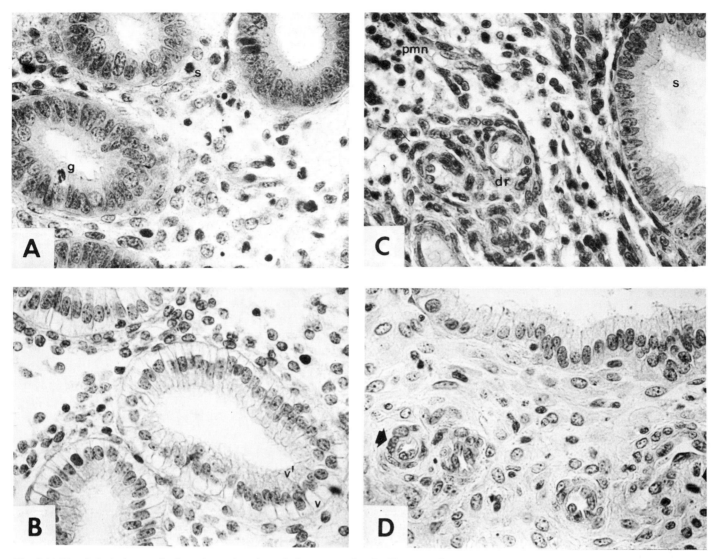

Fig. 5.11 Morphological events in the endometrium through the menstrual cycle. Haematoxylin and eosin. [A] Proliferative phase. Glandular (g) and stromal (s) mitoses under the influence of estradiol. [B] Early secretory phase. Subnuclear vacuolation (v) and supranuclear vacuolation (v') in glandular epithelium, with cessation of mitosis, are evidence of progesterone action; early stromal oedema (oe). [C] Mid-late secretory phase. Ragged apical borders of glandular epithelium and intraluminal secretion (s); early predecidual reaction (dr) around spiral arteries is evidence of prolonged progesterone action; loss of stromal oedema; early polymorphonuclear infiltration (pmn) signals progesterone decline. [D] Late secretory phase. Pronounced predecidualisation of stroma extends between spiral artery (arrow) and gland

al, 1980); others have claimed that such a correlation exists only for the first seven days (Genz et al, 1980).

Data on progesterone receptors are more consistent. Progesterone receptors (P-R) increase during the proliferative phase and correlate positively with plasma oestradiol levels (Kreitmann et al, 1979; Spona et al, 1979; Genz et al, 1980; Levy et al, 1980).

The stimulatory influence of oestradiol on endometrial growth through mitosis is well known (Fig. 5.11A). Early autoradiographic studies of human endometrium following *in vitro* incorporation of tritiated-thymidine indicated that nucleic acid synthesis was highest during the first 7 days of the cycle (Fettig, 1965), whereas more recent investigations have shown that greatest labelling occurs on cycle days 8 to 10 and is associated with a maximum number of mitoses in both stromal and glandular cellular elements of the uterine mucosa at that time (Ferenczy et al, 1979); these studies have not related results to plasma oestradiol levels.

Our studies (Figs. 5.12–5.14; Johannisson et al, 1982b), in which the number of glandular and stromal mitoses were estimated in 68 biopsies from 14 women during five menstrual cycles monitored by daily steroid and gonadotrophin assays, showed that the number of mitoses per 1000 glandular *epithelial cells* was fairly uniform from day LH−11 onwards through the follicular phase; in the *stromal cells* a peak mitosis rate occurred 2 to 3 days before the LH surge. No significant correlation was found between the rate of glandular or stromal mitoses and the mean levels of oestradiol in the peripheral plasma of the 72 hour period prior to the biopsy.

Lack of correlation between number of mitoses and circulating oestradiol levels may be misleading, however, since light-microscopic (LM) examination only allows observation of metaphase, anaphase or telophase of a cell's division; these three stages together represent only about one-tenth of the duration of the cell cycle. Cell nuclei synthesising DNA — considered to be an oestradiol-dependent process (see Introduction) — cannot be detected by conventional LM methods. Microspectrophotometric analysis of isolated endometrial cells has certainly revealed an increasing number of cell nuclei synthesising DNA during the proliferative phase (Vokaer, 1951; Hughes et al. 1963; Johannisson & Hagenfeldt, 1971) and other cytochemical studies have shown a gradual increase in nuclear RNA per endometrial cell during the same period (Johannisson, 1980), but these methods are not available for routine use.

Accepting the premise that the endometrium should display some degree of histologically apparent differentiation before it can react structurally to progesterone, it is reasonable, by quantification, to try to identify criteria for dating the proliferative phase in relation to the midcycle surge of LH (Johannisson et al, 1982b). But, in view of the considerations above, any morphometric index of oestrogen effect would need to reflect endometrial growth in a more accurate way than the number of mitoses does.

In a proliferative endometrium, *glandular size and volume* reflect growth (Vokaer, 1951; Delforge & Ferin, 1970). Indeed, when the diameter of the glands is compared with circulating oestradiol levels during the entire proliferative phase, a significant correlation is found ($P < 0.01$). Large gland openings can be seen on SEM (Fig. 15A). *Pseudostratification* of the glandular epithelium is significantly increased at days LH −5 and −4, and *glandular mitoses* are significantly *decreased* at days LH −1 and LH 0, when compared with LH −3 and −2.

These data suggest that the proliferative phase could be

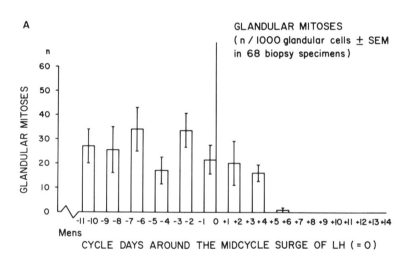

A

GLANDULAR MITOSES
(n / 1000 glandular cells ± SEM
in 68 biopsy specimens)

CYCLE DAYS AROUND THE MIDCYCLE SURGE OF LH (= 0)

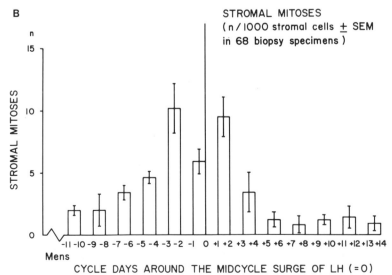

B

STROMAL MITOSES
(n / 1000 stromal cells ± SEM
in 68 biopsy specimens)

CYCLE DAYS AROUND THE MIDCYCLE SURGE OF LH (= 0)

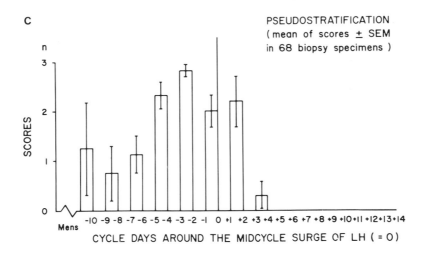

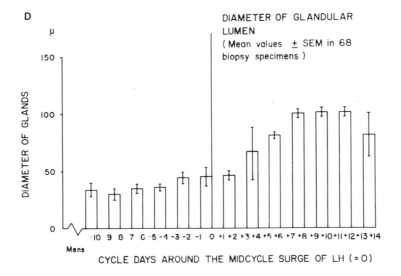

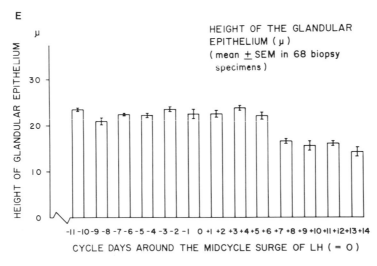

Fig. 5.12 Morphometric indices from 68 endometrial biopsies with a known relation to the LH peak (see text for details). [A] Glandular mitoses per 1000 glandular cells in 30 microscopic fields in each of three biopsy specimens obtained from three different sites in the uterus. [B] Stromal mitoses. [C] Pseudostratification evaluated semiquantitatively by the following scoring system: 0 = none; 1 = slight; 2 = moderate; 3 = marked. Evaluation in groups of 48-hour periods. [D] Diameter of glands in microns, measured in 70–100 glands in each biopsy. [E] Glandular epithelial height in microns; quantitation as for [D]

dated with acceptable accuracy from days LH −5 and −4 to the day of the LH surge, whereas biopsies obtained before LH −5 reveal morphological variations, particularly gland size, that will, during this phase of the cycle, be as variable as the levels of oestradiol they depend on.

Secretory phase

The midcycle LH surge is the central reference point of the menstrual cycle because it initiates progesterone production and ovulation. We prospectively studied endometrial morphology in relation to the day of the midcycle LH peak and to circulating levels of oestradiol and progesterone (Figs. 5.12–5.14; Johannisson et al, 1982b). Plasma progesterone levels reaching a maximum of 32–92 nmol/l (10–30 ng/ml) and exceeding 16 nmol/l (5 ng/ml) for a minimum of 5 days were used as criteria to define endocrinologically normal ovulation and adequate luteal function (Landgren et al, 1980; and see Ch. 4).

The appearance of basal, subnuclear vacuoles in the glandular epithelium (Fig 5.11B) is commonly regarded as the first sign of *progesterone* effect in the endometrium. These vacuoles apparently contain glycogen and glycoproteins (McKay et al, 1956). Analysis of glycogen metabolism is difficult, because both synthesis and degradation of glycogen occur during the (progesterone-dominated) post-

ovulatory phase (Hackl et al, 1971); most of the enzymes involved in glycogen metabolism appear in the cytoplasm or are attached to the glycogen molecules and so cannot easily be observed (Nilsson et al, 1974). The vacuoles on TEM seem to be filled by a homogenous substance containing only a few scattered glycogen granules (Fig. 5.16.).

Histochemically and electronmicroscopically, however, glycogen appears at the basal part of the cytoplasm of glandular cells as early as the sixth to the tenth day of the cycle (Hughes et al, 1963; Schmiedt-Matthieson, 1963; Themann & Schunke, 1963) and accumulates as the preovulatory phase progresses (Gompel, 1962; Wynn & Harris, 1967). In this respect it is noteworthy that basal vacuolation has also been reported in the presence of an excess of *oestrogens* in endometrial cystic glandular hyperplasia, in ovariectomised women, in post-menopausal women treated with a combination of oestrogen and testosterone propionate (Ferin, 1971), and in ovariectomised rhesus monkeys treated with oestrogens (Jansen, unpublished data).

Subsequent further accumulation of glycogen in the subnuclear vacuoles after ovulation undoubtedly takes place and may be the result of a synergistic effect of oestrogen and progesterone (Hughes et al, 1963; Milwidsky et al, 1980; Shapiro et al, 1980; Mimori et al, 1981). In our own study (Johannisson et al, 1982b), regular basal vacuolation was seen in the glandular epithelium as early as 24 h after the LH surge, but could also still be absent 48 h after the mid-cycle LH peak, despite a hormonally normal luteal phase subsequently. During the first 4 days after the LH surge the number of basal vacuoles is negatively correlated with plasma oestradiol levels ($P < 0.02$) and positively correlated with plasma progesterone levels ($P < 0.02$) — consistent with a view that maximum development of the basal vacuoles depends on the oestradiol:progesterone ratio.

With the LM appearance of basal vacuolation, mitotic activity of the glandular epithelium stops. The speed with which it does so is inversely related to the amount of oestradiol still circulating, as a significant positive correlation ($P < 0.05$) is found between the number of mitoses per 1000 glandular cells and plasma oestradiol values during the period LH + 1 to LH + 4. No pseudostratification is seen after LH + 3. Stromal mitoses are also significantly decreased by LH + 3 to + 4; a negative correlation was found between stromal mitoses and circulating plasma progesterone levels ($P < 0.01$) during the remainder of the secretory phase.

These observations are consistent with the principle that progesterone interferes with growth of the endometrium (Nordqvist, 1970; Gerulath & Borth, 1977). Accordingly, one would expect a decrease in nucleoprotein content under the influence of progesterone. Quantitative measurements of RNA and DNA-content carried out by cytochemical, histochemical and biochemical methods in normal

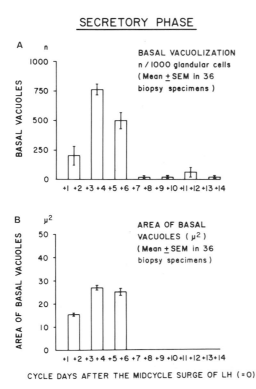

Fig. 5.13 Morphometric indices from 68 endometrial biopsies with a known relation to the LH peak (continued; see text for details). [A] Frequency of basally vacuolated cells; quantitation as for Fig. 5.12A. [B] Area of basal vacuoles measured in 30 to 40 glandular cells with basal vacuolation; quantitation as for Fig. 5.12A

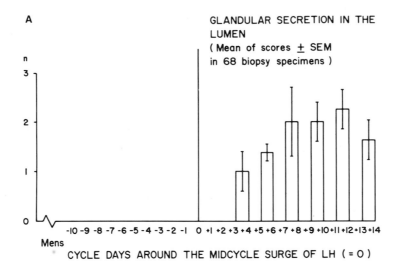

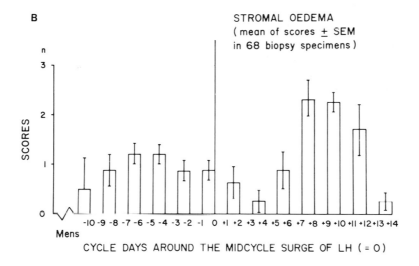

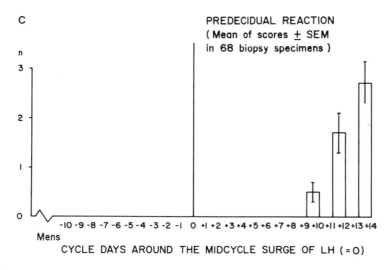

Fig. 5.14 Morphometric indices from 68 endometrial biopsies with a known relation to the LH peak (continued; see text for details). [A] Glandular secretion in glandular lumens; semiquantitative scoring system as for Fig. 5.12C. [B] Stromal oedema assessed as for Fig. 5.12C. [C] Predecidual reaction assessed as for Fig. 5.12C

endometrium have shown that nuclear RNA remains at high levels from LH 0 to LH + 5 (Hughes et al, 1963; Johannisson, 1980), coinciding with the time glycogen is deposited in the cytoplasm of the glandular cells (Johannisson & Hagenfeldt, 1971).

A number of studies have shown a lack of precise correlation between endometrial development and plasma progesterone levels during the luteal phase (Cooke et al, 1972; Rosenfeld & Garcia, 1976; Shepard & Senturia, 1977; Rosenfeld et al, 1980). Doubtless this lack of correlation is partly explained by the fact that a single plasma measurement of a steroid whose concentrations are known first to rise and then to fall is of little value as an indicator of its overall production, and hence of normal corpus luteum function. But it may also be true that endometrial response to progesterone is an individually determined phenomenon that depends as much on endometrial P-R concentration as it does on circulating plasma levels. Since oestradiol stimulates synthesis of progesterone receptors (Kreitmann et al, 1979; Levy et al, 1980; Genz et al, 1980), the morphology of the secretory phase may depend not just on plasma progesterone levels of the ovarian luteal phase but also on oestradiol levels of the follicular phase. It is clear that no simple relationship exists between plasma levels of oestradiol and progesterone, the tissue concentrations of these steroids, and cytosol concentrations of E-R and P-R.

Whereas the histological changes that take place in the human endometrium during the first 6 days after ovulation can be dated with a reasonably high degree of accuracy (83%) by the method of Noyes et al (1950), the error in dating a biopsy this way increases with the distance from the day of the LH surge (Johannisson et al, 1982b). This is consistent with the observation that the length of the luteal phase in normally menstruating women varies between 9 and 17 days (Landgren et al, 1980).

At day LH + 6 the apical cell-surfaces of the epithelium lining the uterine cavity are bulging, probably due to the accumulation of secretory products (Fig. 5.15B). Then, as the glandular diameter increases in size, secretory products are seen in the glandular lumina of the functionalis layer — the phenomenon that gives the secretory phase its name.

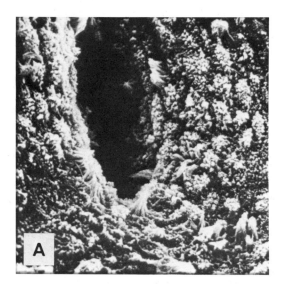

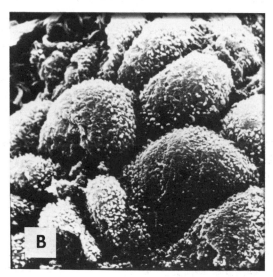

Fig. 5.15 [A] Endometrial gland opening on SEM. Note the abundance of ciliated cells surrounding the opening. [B] Secretory phase endometrium, day LH +6. Apical cell surfaces on SEM are bulging into the cavity, apparently due to accumulation of secretion

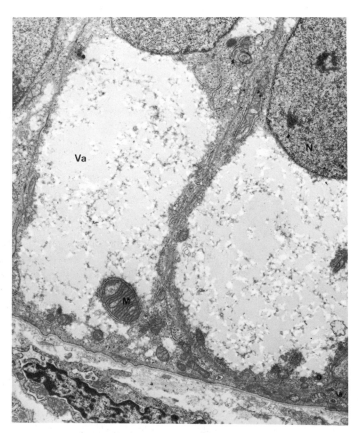

Fig. 5.16 Endometrial gland epithelium, TEM, day LH + 4, showing basal vacuoles containing glycogen

During the late secretory phase one of the criteria for dating the endometrium is the development of the stromal predecidual reaction, which is not likely to occur before day LH + 9. The predecidual change in the stroma seems to be correlated with the occurrence of *progestogen-dependent endometrial protein* (PEP) (Joshi et al, 1980). Prolactin has also been reported to be synthesised by the endometrium during the normal menstrual cycle, and the appearance and degree of this synthesis correspond to decidualisation (Masler & Riddick, 1979).

Menstrual phase

Premenstrually, total concentrations of E-R and P-R are lowest (Levy et al, 1980) and DNA-synthesising activity is negligible (Johannisson & Hagenfeldt, 1971; Ferenczy et al, 1979). Endometrial thickness is decreased, glandular diameter is diminished, and regressive changes take place with an infiltration of neutrophil leucocytes 48 to 24 hours before the onset of menstruation (Fig. 5.11C; Daly et al, 1982). The signs of regression have been thought to indicate irreversible cell injury of the functionalis layer, but it is probable that only a minority of the cells actually undergo necrosis; most remain viable and are remodelled to participate in the next cycle (Flowers & Wilborn, 1978).

Regional variations in endometrial steroid response

Circumferentially, biopsies from the lateral uterine mucosa are histologically indistinguishable from those of the anterior wall at any stage of the cycle (Johannisson, 1982 unpublished data); proliferation kinetic studies, however, indicate that the uterine angles and the uterine isthmus (the lower uterine segment, just above the endocervix) show lower rates of cell division (Ferenczy et al, 1979). Pathologists are well aware that the lower uterine segment does not display the complete manifestations of oestradiol and progesterone effect that the fundal endometrium shows (Novak & Woodruff, 1979). The endocrinological correlate of this phenomenon is that there is a steep, decreasing and continuous gradient in E-R and P-R concentrations within the endometrium from the fundus downwards at all stages of the menstrual cycle (Tsibris et al, 1981); the steadiness and continuity of this decline is in apparent contrast with the general uniformity of secretory change above the lower uterine segment.

Cyclical changes in endometrial function

Endometrial fluid production

The 'secretory' phase is in one way a misnomer. The *volume* of endometrial transudation and secretion increases during the proliferative phase and is maximal at midcycle (Aitken, 1979): quantitatively it is oestradiol, not proges-terone, that produces the bulk of endometrial fluid. Indeed, the first discernible action of oestradiol on the uterus of immature or ovariectomised rats is an increase in uterine blood flow and an increase in capillary permeability (Clark & Markerivich, 1981). Transendometrial potential is increased (Levin & Edwards, 1968), perhaps due to oestradiol stimulation of Na^+/K^+-dependent ATPase; histochemically, maximal alkaline phosphatase activity is found at the apical borders of epithelial cells at this time (Boutselis, 1973; Wilborn & Flowers, 1979).

The reduction of fluid in the endometrial cavity that starts after ovulation and continues through the time of entry of the early embryo into the uterus (Clemetson et al, 1973) is thought to be important in effecting the first stage of implantation — apposition of the blastocyst to the endometrial surface. Water resorption is apparently brought about the sodium resorption, with the conse-quence that potassium concentration of the endometrial fluid at the time of implantation is about 38 mEq/l (Clemetson et al, 1973) — much higher than serum levels.

Endometrial glandular secretion

The endometrial secretion that gives its name to the second half of the menstrual cycle, despite the considerations of fluid production above, is clearly a progesterone-dependent series of phenomena. Much of the preparation for it takes place, however, during the proliferative phase under the influence of oestradiol.

Glycogen synthesis, demonstrated by diastase-labile histo-chemical reactivity with periodic acid-Schiff reagent (PAS), is first evident in the early proliferative phase and increases up to and through the time of ovulation; it is, initially at least, an oestradiol action. Progesterone seems to affect the distribution of the glycogen. Subnuclear accumulation takes place first (and causes the subnuclear vacuolation that is the first endometrial sign of progesterone effect; Fig. 5.11B); then there is passage to the supranuclear portion of the cytoplasm; and finally the glycogen is extruded from the cell into the lumen in the mid-secretory phase.

Acid mucus glycoproteins, PAS-positive but diastase-resistant, are not produced and secreted before day LH + 3. Although glycogen in the endometrium can be seen as having a potential embryotrophic role, no function is ascribable yet to the glycoproteins, which are secreted in substantial amounts and are most abundant at the time of implantation. At least one species of progesterone-dependent glycoprotein can be identified electrophoretically in secretory phase uterine washings (Sylvan et al, 1981). Both glycogen and mucus glycoproteins are particularly abundant in the endometrium during pregnancy (McKay et al, 1956; Wilborn & Flowers, 1979).

Free ribosomes reach a maximum in the late proliferative phase, then decline as glycogen accumulates (Cavasos &

Lucas, 1973). The *rough endoplasmic reticulum* reaches a maximum early in the secretory phase, after which there is progressive dilatation of cisternae. The *Golgi apparatus*, situated above the nucleus and responsible for packaging the products of the endoplasmic reticulum before secretion, is most developed in the mid-secretory phase, the time of maximal secretion.

Lipids vary in inverse proportion to the abundance of specific secretion, being present early only to disappear until the end of the cycle, after secretion has stopped and menstruation is due (Cavasos & Lucas, 1973). Lipids presumably represent a metabolic alternative to glycogen and glycoprotein synthesis.

Stromal decidual reaction to progesterone

After a wave of mitosis among the stromal cells in the midluteal phase (Fig. 5.12B), thought but not proven to be due to the midcycle rise of oestradiol (Ferenczy et al, 1979), the stromal cells undergo differentiation to decidual cells (Fig. 5.11D). Whereas the stromal fibroblasts before the decidual reaction are widely separated, are spindle-shaped, and contain rough endoplasmic reticulum for collagen synthesis, the post-mitotic decidual cells are plump and tend to exclude intervening ground substance by forming junctional complexes, including tight junctions and gap junctions, with each other; the abundant cytoplasm contains lysozomes, smooth endoplasmic reticulum engaged in glycogen synthesis, and glycogen granules (Finn & Porter, 1975; Wynn, 1977).

The epithelioid stromal decidual reaction reaches full development only with pregnancy or with prolonged administration of exogenous progestogens (Eichner et al, 1951), but the qualitatively identical, if quantitatively incomplete, 'predecidua' of the normal menstrual cycle is a morphological landmark of the last few days of the secretory phase. The predecidual reaction is not seen before day LH+9 (Fig. 5.14C); it first appears around endometrial spiral arterioles (Fig. 5.11C) and then forms, as well, under the superficial epithelium; it occupies a major part of the endometrial stroma by the time leucocyte invasion takes place to signal progesterone withdrawal and impending menstruation. If conception and implantation are successful, and progesterone production from the corpus luteum does not decrease, development of the decidua continues (Fig. 5.11D).

The role the decidua plays in the menstrual cycle or in pregnancy has not been worked out. Trophoblast nutrition and resistance to trophoblast invasion are functions that have been suggested for many years, but remain phenomenological hypotheses rather than tested theories. Several possible endocrine functions are attracting attention.

The discovery that amniotic fluid contains large amounts of *prolactin*, chemically and immunologically indistinguishable from pituitary prolactin but unlike circulating prolactin in pregnancy not suppressed by bromocriptine, led to identification of prolactin in the decidua of the pregnant uterus (Bigazzi et al, 1979). It is now clear that existence of adjacent trophoblast is not needed for prolactin synthesis by decidual cells: prolactin is present in the stroma after treatment with progestogens (Meuris et al, 1980) and in the predecidua of the normal menstrual cycle (Maslar & Riddick, 1979). Decidual prolactin production increases very quickly if pregnancy takes place, irrespective of whether the pregnancy is uterine or tubal (Maslar et al, 1980).

No physiological role for decidual prolactin has been established. A possible effect in concert with hCG on luteal function has been observed (Fried & Rakoff, 1952), but no comparable recent studies have been done. An *in vitro* study suggesting a stimulatory effect on myometrial contractility (Bigazzi & Nardi, 1981) is teleologically difficult because decidual prolactin, if conception has occurred, is increasing just at the time that myometrial quiescence is needed, although the same authors have also identified *relaxin* in the decidua of pregnancy and ascribe to it an important inhibitory action on myometrial contractility. This finding has not been confirmed by others, and perhaps the most plausible role for decidual prolactin is in regulation of fluid transport across the fetal membranes (Healy et al, 1983).

Lysozomes, prostaglandin synthesis and endometrial bleeding

Acid phosphatase is one of more than 50 hydrolases contained in lysozomes; most of these hydrolases are active at acidic pH (Wilson, 1980). Histochemically, acid phosphatase activity during the proliferative phase is present only in the apical part of the epithelial cells, whereas in the mid to late secretory phase activity is detectable throughout the cell cytoplasm and, prior to menstruation, in the stromal cells (Wilborn & Flowers, 1979; Flowers & Wilborn, 1979). For most of the cycle, staining is particulate, presumably localised to *lysozomes* and to the Golgi apparatus, which is most prominent in the mid-secretory phase (Cavasos & Lucas, 1973); but just before menstruation diffuse cytoplasmic activity is present — an observation that has been interpreted as indicating increased lysozomal permeability during this time (Bitensky & Cohen, 1965). Morphologically, giant lysozomes of the autophagocytic type, which digest material from inside their own cell and which contain acid phosphatase (Henzl et al, 1972), are most abundant at the extreme ends of the menstrual cycle and during menstruation (Cavasos & Lucas, 1973).

These observations give rise to the attractive hypothesis that release of lysozomal enzymes from endometrial cells follows a fall in plasma progesterone and is responsible for the tissue dissolution that accompanies menstruation. Lysozomal phospholipases could then be invoked to account for increased prostaglandin synthesis and, ultimately, menstruation itself (Wilson, 1980). Prostaglandin $F_{2\alpha}$ synthesis in the endometrium increases substantially premenstrually (Hagenfeldt, 1980) and endometrial bleeding can be produced by exogenous $PGF_{2\alpha}$ infusions without there necessarily being a fall in plasma progesterone (Lehmann et al, 1972); conversely, the clinical symptom of premenstrual spotting, which may occur with an intra-uterine device and also occurs in endometriosis (Wentz, 1980b), may have abnormal $PGF_{2\alpha}$ exposure of the endometrium as its pathogenic mechanism. For these and no doubt other reasons, the plasma progesterone level at which bleeding actually starts in the normal menstrual cycle is very variable (Landgren et al, 1977).

Differences in endocrine response within the endometrium

Epithelium of the endometrial surface, epithelium of the glands, and stromal cells all seem to differ slightly in their response to oestradiol and progesterone. Surface epithelial cells accumulate glycogen during the proliferative phase several days earlier than glandular epithelial cells, but during the remainder of the luteal phase morphological changes lag behind those in the glandular cells in timing and in degree (Wynn, 1977). Stromal cells differ qualitatively from epithelial cells in displaying a wave of mitosis in the mid-to-late secretory phase (see below). Studies in mice show that oestradiol alone produces many mitoses in luminal and glandular epithelia, but not among stromal cells, in this species; after pretreatment with progesterone, oestradiol produces many mitoses among stromal cells, but few among the epithelial cells (Martin & Finn, 1968).

Although the clinical relevance of this differential sensitivity has not been explored directly, observations on anomalies produced in the embryonic reproductive tract by non-steroidal oestrogen analogues, including clomiphene and diethylstilboestrol (DES), may be very pertinent. Clomiphene administration to pregnant rats causes a bizarre range of hyperplastic epithelial abnormalities in the developing reproductive tract of the pups (McCormack & Clark, 1979); these abnormalities manifest after birth as disorganisation of the uterus and fallopian tubes, reminiscent of the effects produced in humans by fetal DES exposure (Kaufmann et al; 1977). Clomiphene, which has an oestrogenic action in these rats, has in common with DES a prolonged nuclear retention time after binding with E-R. Because oestradiol administered to pregnant animals has none of these detrimental developmental effects, it is plausible that it is the differential response of different components of the endometrium and other reproductive tract tissues to oestrogens that is exploited by those oestrogens with abnormally long durations of action to produce abnormal differential growth, and hence abnormal anatomical development.

Endometrial response to abnormal ovarian function and exogenous steroids

Oestrogens alone

Oestrogen unopposed by progesterone causes proliferation and hyperplasia of the endometrium up to and including atypical adenomatous hyperplasia (Gusberg, 1967). By so setting the stage for further progression to neoplasia, it is highly likely that oestrogen is a necessary, though probably insufficient, cause of endometrial adenocarcinoma. Endometrial hyperplasia and adenocarcinoma are therefore most likely to occur (a) after the menopause, when ovulation and cyclical progesterone production has finished; (b) following prolonged anovulation during the reproductive years due to conditions such as the polycystic ovary syndrome; and (c) with oestrogen therapy unaccompanied by sufficient progestogen administration. Hyperplasia and carcinoma can rarely occur despite exposure to what would normally be considered sufficient progesterone or progestogen.

Most *endogenous and exogenous oestrogens* are active in the endometrium through oestradiol (Whitehead et al 1981). Oestradiol's orally effective C-17 ethinyl derivative, ethinyloestradiol, is itself active and binds directly to E-R. Mestranol requires metabolism in the liver to ethinyloestradiol for activity and is therefore less active in the endometrium than the same amount of ethinyloestradiol (Delforge & Ferin, 1970). Esterified oestradiol preparations (which are metabolised to oestrone during gastro-intestinal absorption), and conjugated oestrones such as oestrone sulphate, owe their activity to the equilibrium oestrone has with oestradiol in target tissues.

Postmenopausal oestrogen therapy (see also Ch. 7) is the commonest clinical use of exogenous oestrogens alone. The extent to which an oestrogen stimulates the endometrium depends less on the type of oestrogen than it does on the dose. For example, conjugated oestrogen 1.25 mg per day taken cyclically (3 weeks out of 4) has been shown to produce endometrial hyperplasia — ranging in degree from cystic glandular to atypical hyperplasia — in 26 per cent of patients in whom aspiration curettage has been possible (Campbell & Whithead, 1977). The considerable incidence of endometrial hyperplasia and the occurrence of endometrial carcinoma on 1.25 mg per day has been substantiated in several prospective studies (Sturdee et al, 1978; Buchman et al, 1978). Reducing the dose to 0.625 mg per day has on occasion allowed reversion of hyperplastic endometrium to proliferative endometrium (Campbell & Whitehead, 1977); but the observation that bleeding is common with this dose administered cyclically (Campbell & Whitehead, 1977; Sturdee et al, 1978) indicates that endometrial growth does take place, and cystic glandular hyperplasia has been reported with this dose (Sturdee et al, 1978).

The relative risk for endometrial cancer in patients who received oestrogen after the menopause in three large retrospective studies (Smith et al, 1975; Ziel & Finkle, 1975; Mack et al, 1976) was between 4 and 8 to 1. According to Doll, risks of the size demonstrated in these studies are likely to be real (Doll et al, 1977). Patients with endometrial cancer and a history of oestrogen use tend to have less advanced disease compared with non-users (Studd, 1976), but the association in the retrospective studies persisted when analyses were confined to patients with invasive cancer (Ziel & Finkle, 1976; Mack et al, 1976). Deaths from the consequences of oestrogen-deprivation after the menopause, particularly osteoporosis, greatly out-number those from endometrial carcinoma (Greenblatt, 1977), so oestrogen replacement therapy, quite apart from its more immediate symptomatic benefits, has a firmly established place; but it must be administered safely.

If there is no withdrawal bleeding on a low-dose cyclical oestrogen regimen, such as ethinyloestradiol 10–20 μg or conjugated oestrogen 0.3–0.625 mg per day, endometrial samples are either too scanty for histological assessment or show a normal proliferative pattern (Sturdee et al, 1978). Endometrial hyperplasia is no less likely with cyclical oestrogen regimens overall than with continuous ones, but if no withdrawal bleeding takes place with low dose cyclical administration it is reasonable to conclude that the regimen is a safe one for that patient, although in practice periodic endometrial aspiration curettage would be an advisable additional safeguard.

Cyclical provision of a progestogen may logically be expected to prevent endometrial proliferation and hyperplasia when a clinically indicated dose of cyclical oestrogen is such that scheduled or unscheduled uterine bleeding takes place. Empirical data are available to show that adequate progestogen administration with oestrogen therapy actually reduces the risk of endometrial carcinoma below that expected if neither oestrogens or progestogens are given (Hammond et al, 1980). Important evidence is now also available that the duration of progestogen therapy is of paramount importance if endometrial proliferation is to be blocked, and that the presence of regular withdrawal bleeding is no guarantee that hyperplasia or even carcinoma is not present (Buchman et al, 1978; Sturdee et al, 1978).

Progestogen treatment for the last 5 days of oestrogen therapy is not enough to guarantee prevention of hyperplasia and carcinoma in postmenopausal women (Buchman et al, 1978; Sturdee et al, 1978). Past reports of endometrial hyperplasia and carcinoma in young women on sequential oral contraceptive regimens that included progestogens for 5 to 7 days (Lyon, 1975; Silverberg & Makowski, 1975; Jansen & Elliott, 1977) both substantiate the data on post-menopausal women and indicate that 7 days' progestogen is also likely to be insufficient. On the other hand, only two cases of endometrial hyperplasia have been reported in postmenopausal women who received progestogens for 10 days (Paterson et al, 1980) and no cases

have been reported with treatment lasting more than 10 days (Nachtigall et al, 1976; Sturdee et al, 1978; Paterson et al, 1980). Therefore a cyclical regimen that produces withdrawal bleeding should incorporate at least a 10-day course of progestogen. The minimum dose required is probably much less than has been usual with shorter courses in the past: maximal suppression of endometrial oestrogen action is seen with norethisterone 1 mg or D/L-norgestrel 150 μg per day (Whitehead et al, 1981). Again, periodic endometrial biopsy would constitute an additional safeguard with long-term treatment.

Amenorrhoea or oligomenorrhoea is common in the *polycystic ovary syndrome* (PCOS; see Ch. 20), but some patients have dysfunctional uterine bleeding (Goldzieher & Green, 1962). Patients are usually well oestrogenised and are at risk of developing endometrial hyperplasia and carcinoma (Shearman & Cox, 1965; Wood & Boronov, 1975; McDonald et al, 1977; Eddy, 1978) — prevention of which demands regular endometrial secretory change, either with exogenous progestogens or by establishing regular ovulation. Exogenous progestogens can be administered alone for at least 10 days per month or, if ovarian suppression for hyperandrogenism is indicated, as a low dose oestrogen–progestogen combination oral contraceptive. Alternatively, in patients attempting pregnancy, ovulation can be induced with clomiphene or exogenous low-LH gonadotrophin. The presence of endometrial hyperplasia is not a contra-indication to ovulation induction: even endometria diagnosed as highly differentiated carcinoma have sometimes reverted to normal with establishment of cyclical endogenous progesterone production (Kistner, 1970; Fechner & Kaufmann, 1974).

Cytoplasmic E-R concentrations in *endometrial hyperplasia* are variable (Evans et al, 1974; Elliott et al, 1980), but generally comparable to levels found in proliferative endometrium (Evans et al, 1974; Muechler et al, 1975; Elliott et al, 1980). In 9 cases studied in our laboratory, cytoplasmic P-R was present in concentrations equal to or greater than those of late proliferative endometrium (Elliott et al, 1980) — an observation that agrees with the well known response of hyperplastic endometrium to treatment with progestogens (Kistner, 1970).

E-R levels in *endometrial adenocarcinoma* are particularly variable (Evans et al, 1974; Pollow et al, 1977; Gurpide et al, 1977; Martin & Hähnel, 1978). The value of E-R and especially P-R determinations in breast cancer as an index of the likelihood of response to endocrine ablation therapy (Lippman & Allegra, 1978) has stimulated work on associating endometrial adenocarcinoma receptor levels with likelihood of response to progestogens. There is a general tendency for tumours of higher differentiation to contain higher concentrations of P-R (Pollow et al, 1977), but highly differentiated tumours without demonstrable P-R have been reported (Haukkamaa et al, 1971; MacLaughlin & Richardson, 1976). Work is proceeding to correlate clinical progestogen-responsiveness to P-R content: in one series seven of eight P-R positive tumours responded to progestogens, whereas only one of 16 P-R negative tumours responded (Ehrlich et al, 1981). Another intriguing possibility that has attracted interest on the basis of receptor theory is the induction of tumour progestogen-responsiveness with a short course of oestrogen; fragmentary clinical data exist to support this concept (Sherman, 1966; Smith et al, 1966; Collins, 1972).

Regular provision and withdrawal of progesterone or a progestogen would normally be supposed to protect the endometrium from the hyperplastic and neoplastic consequences of oestrogen, provided that the duration of administration is more than 10 days. However, endometrial carcinomas have very occasionally been described in women with *normal menstrual cycles* (Jones & Brewer, 1941; Jansen & Shearman, 1981) and in women on *combined oral contraceptives* (Silverberg & Maksowski, 1975; Cohen & Deppe, 1977; Muechler et al, 1975). These are anomalies that demand explanation. The old observation that during the luteal phase of the menstrual cycle areas of proliferative endometrium may persist as islands of endometrium apparently resistant to the normal secretory change that occurs elsewhere (Novak & Martzloff, 1924) may be a clue to the paradox. One may speculate that such areas of endometrium fail to respond because of a localised deficiency in P-R. The relative incidence of carcinoma in such women would then depend on the amount of circulating oestrogen and, where the P-R deficiency was relative rather than absolute, on the brevity of progesterone or progestogen exposure.

On this basis, highly-differentiated carcinomas in such patients might be expected to have high E-R, which has been reported (Muechler et al, 1975), but low or absent P-R; they would also be expected not to respond to high-dosage progestogen treatment. We have seen two moderately-differentiated adenocarcinomas in regularly ovulating women: cytosol E-R and P-R were both very low, which implies that oncogenesis in these cases was accompanied by the acquisition of autonomy from both oestradiol and progesterone.

Progestogens alone

Progestogens alone, administered continuously, are used for endometriosis (Ch. 22), for contraception (Chs 33, 34, 35) and, in high dosages, for amelioration of endometrial adenocarcinoma (Kistner et al, 1965; Bonte, 1972). Cyclical progestogen therapy is used for controlling oestrogen-induced dysfunctional uterine bleeding (Ch. 31) and for prophylaxis against endometrial hyperplasia in anovulatory, high-oestrogen situations.

Progestogen in adequate dosage, given alone but in an environment of prior oestrogen exposure, initially arrests endometrial proliferation and induces a secretory change similar to that of the secretory phase of the normal menstrual cycle. If treatment is prolonged, menses are delayed, the secretory effects in the epithelium are lost, and the glands atrophy; with long-term low-dose progestogen therapy accompanied by amenorrhoea, the endometrium tends to be scant and the glands are dilated (Ludwig, 1982; Johannisson et al, 1982a). Compared with the epithelium, the stroma takes much longer to lose its responsiveness (Dallenbach-Hellweg, 1980) and decidualisation of the stroma is a consistent effect of long-term progestogen therapy (Ludwig, 1982). When the stroma does atrophy, necrosis and bleeding may occur — a phenomenon that places troublesome clinical limitations on progestogen-only therapy and was responsible, during the development of oral contraceptives, for the addition of oestrogens to pill formulations.

Both major groups of synthetic, orally effective progestogens — the 19-nortestosterone derivatives norethisterone and norgestrel, and the 21-carbon progestrogens such as medroxyprogesterone acetate — exert their progestogenic effects by direct binding to P-R (Shapiro et al, 1978), often with nuclear retention times that are significantly longer than when progesterone binds and translocates P-R (Kasid & Laumas, 1981). The 19-nortestosterones also appear to bind to androgen receptors (DHT-R). The endocrinological correlate of the endometrial atrophy that eventually takes place with progestogens is thought to be progestogen-induced loss of progesterone receptor (P-R).

Oestrogens and progestogens in combination

With the oestrogen-progestogen combinations used for oral contraception, the proliferative phase is shortened, presumably as oestrogen action through E-R allows synthesis of P-R, which, because progestogen has been administered simultaneously with the oestrogen, then allows expression of progestogen action within days. Glands and stroma fail to develop completely; mitoses are rare; there is premature appearance of persistently deficient secretory change in the glands, which remain uncoiled; and stromal oedema occurs early and persists until a distinct predecidual or decidual reaction takes place around the 15th to 20th day (Fechner, 1971; Dallenbach-Hellweg, 1980).

Prolonged contraceptive use results in further changes. The abortive secretory changes gradually subside and disappear; the glands themselves decrease in number; and the endometrium generally becomes thin and atrophic, with a reduction in or even failure of periodic withdrawal bleeding. Patchy necrosis sometimes occurs, as with progestogen only therapy, and may manifest as inter-menstrual bleeding. Occasionally a hyperplastic and hypersecretory response can occur to combination preparations, similar to the Arias-Stella reaction of pregnancy, which is a focal endometrial epithelial reaction characterised by irregular nuclear enlargement and hyperchromasia, proliferation, and cytoplasmic vacuolation suggestive of secretion (Oertel, 1978).

Endometrial resistance to hormone action

Luteal phase defects

Insufficient corpus luteum progesterone production as a cause of otherwise unexplained infertility or recurrent abortion has been controversial for more than 30 years. Two conclusions are certain: (1) if the ovarian luteal phase ends and the endometrium starts to bleed before implantation of the blastocyst takes place (normally about 7 days after ovulation and fertilisation), then fertility is not possible; and (2) if the corpus luteum, or the ovary containing it, is surgically excised before the 36th day after ovulation, before the placenta takes over from the corpus luteum responsibility for maintenance of pregnancy, abortion will follow (Csapo et al, 1973). All other definitions of luteal phase adequacy or inadequacy, whether based on luteal phase length, plasma progesterone levels or endometrial histology, are arbitrary.

The concept of luteal phase deficiency is tempered by at least three observations: (1) that fertility in many animals is hindered more by endometrial *over*development than *under*development (McLaren & Michie, 1956; Noyes, 1959); (2) that extreme degrees of luteal dysfunction are usually the product of grossly defective follicular development and ovulation, introducing doubt as to whether progesterone deficiency is cause or consequence of the reproductive problem in a particular instance; and (3) that if progesterone deficiency is aetiologically important in reproductive dysfunction then the endometrium would not be alone among the tissues to be compromised, but tubal and myometrial dysfunction could be important too (Jones, 1968).

The concept that endometrial expression of progesterone action, or lack of it, can jeopardise fertility finds its strongest empirical support in identification of populations of women with otherwise unexplained infertility who have either peak or integrated luteal phase progesterones that are more than two standard deviations lower than those of women with infertility of obvious cause, such as azoospermia or tubal occlusion (Radwanska & Swyer, 1974; Dodson et al, 1975a; Lenton et al, 1978). Some of these studies, unfortunately most without controls, have indicated that therapy aimed at increasing progesterone levels in these women causes an increase in the number of successful pregnancies that occur among them. Limited success has been claimed, on the one hand, for regimens that involve stimulation of follicular development with clomiphene and/or gonadotrophins (Radwanska & Swyer, 1974; Cooke et al, 1977; Quagliarello & Weiss, 1979) and, on the other, for regimens that assume normal ovulation and add exogenous progesterone during the luteal phase (Mosz-

kowski et al, 1962; Soules et al, 1977; Rosenberg et al, 1980) — indicating that luteal phase deficiency is more than one clinical entity. The corollary to this conclusion is that the endometrium is not necessarily responsible for mediating the reproductive disturbance that can accompany real or imagined progesterone deficiency, especially when the luteal phase is short.

Nevertheless premenstrual endometrial sampling is particularly useful in screening patients for progesterone insufficiency. Because of the progressive nature of the changes progesterone causes in endometrial morphology (see above), demonstration of obvious predecidua in the stroma prior to menses implies not just that integrated progesterone levels in the plasma have been reasonable, but that progesterone has found the reproductive tissues to be sufficiently responsive to allow manifestation of its biological actions. But it should be emphasised: (1) that comparisons must be made with the time of subsequent menses and not the previous menstrual period; (2) that criteria for normality have not been rigorously defined; (3) that biopsies should be taken from high in the endometrial cavity, since less developed secretory changes are usual in the lower uterine segment; (4) that an apparently abnormal biopsy should be repeated before attaching substantial significance to the abnormality (Jones, 1976); and (5) that there are no studies that prove that treatment of diagnosed defects in women with normal luteal phase lengths makes a difference to reproductive performance.

Primary endometrial resistance to progesterone action rather than deficiency of progesterone production and exposure has been described (Keller et al, 1979), but is probably rare. A 23-year-old woman with infertility demonstrated repeated failure of her endometrial stroma to undergo a predecidual reaction late in the luteal phase, despite normal serum progesterone levels and despite exogenous progesterone administration; cytosol P-R levels were measured and found to be low, although the cytosols were from late in the luteal phase rather than immediately before ovulation, when discrimination would have been more reliable. Her husband had an embryonal cell carcinoma of the testis, so there is doubt about the endometrium's sole responsibility for her infertility. Although endometrial resistance to progesterone occurs in the uterus of aged rodents and correlates with an increased incidence of pregnancy failure (Hsueh et al, 1979), the relevance of this phenomenon to declining human fertility with age (Jansen, 1984) is not known.

Secondary endometrial resistance due to the anti-oestrogen *clomiphene* can be inferred from a number of observations. Clomiphene's anti-oestrogenic effects may last well into the follicular phase, as indicated by a reduction in cervical mucus production (McBain & Pepperell, 1980) and by reduced mitotic activity in late proliferative endometrium (Lamb et al, 1972). Oestradiol-induced synthesis of E-R and P-R, and hence ability to respond to oestradiol and progesterone, can therefore be compromised (Kokko et al, 1981). Clomiphene cycles are characterized by higher than normal plasma progesterone levels (Dodson et al, 1975b; Hammond et al, 1980), but by a high prevalence of retarded progesterone response on endometrial biopsy (Jones et al, 1970). Uterine bleeding can even fail altogether despite ovulation (and in the absence of conception) when prolonged, incrementally-increasing regimens of clomiphene are used (O'Herlihy et al, 1981).

Endometrial atrophy

Loss of responsive endometrium and amenorrhoea can occur from excessive curettage and consequent regional or (rarely) total obliteration of the uterine cavity from *intra-uterine adhesions* between the anterior and posterior walls. The recently pregnant uterus, especially if infected, is particularly susceptible; curettage for secondary post-partum haemorrhage or missed abortion is therefore a common cause. Vigorous attempts at curettage in hypo-oestrogenic states, such as investigation of primary amenor-rhoea, is occasionally aetiological. Loss of endometrium is usually only partial, so therapy aimed at increasing reproductive performance involves surgical lysis of adhesions accompanied by stimulation of the residual endometrium's growth with oestrogen (Jansen, 1982, and see Ch. 25).

Polishuk has described a related condition in which traumatic amenorrhoea after curettage is unaccompanied by adhesions, but is associated with profound *endometrial fibrosis* (Yaffe et al, 1978). These cases may be resistant to treatment. Chronic endometritis, for example tuberculous or schistosomiatic endometritis, may also occasionally be accompanied by endometrial sclerosis that is extensive enough to be associated with amenorrhoea. These lesions are rare, however, and even in the presence of stromal calcification an apparently normal response to progesterone has been reported (Untawale et al, 1982).

MYOMETRIUM

The myometrium is the most specialised region of the genital tract's muscle coat. Its hormonal responses and pharmacology are of singular clinical importance in the menstrual cycle and in pregnancy.

Control of myometrial activity

Anatomy and physiology of myometrial smooth muscle

Visceral smooth muscle cells generally are arranged in bundles and sheets. In the myometrium these constitute an interlacing network of substantial intricacy: attempts to distinguish layers of different orientation or composition have not produced a uniform view (Finn & Porter, 1975).

Within the bundles are fusiform smooth muscle cells, running along the axis of the bundle.

The extent to which smooth muscle cells form a functional syncytium depends on the frequency with which points of very close contact, called *gap junctions* or *nexuses*, occur. Gap junctions are specialised regions that bridge adjacent cells, allowing ionic cytoplasmic continuity and propagation of action potentials between cells. Action potentials, whether endogenous or induced by acetylcho-line from nerve endings, can spread from cell to cell by ephaptic conduction in the absence of gap junctions — e.g. the points of simple close contact between cells that occur in the myosalpinx allow propagation — but without the facility gap junctions allow.

Actin and myosin filaments of smooth muscle are dispersed quite differently to those of striated muscle. The actin filaments are attached to dense bodies to form a network; some of the dense bodies are attached to the cell membrane. Myosin filaments, dispersed among the actin filaments, are outnumbered by them. Chemical interaction between the actin and myosin filaments is brought about through stimulation of myosin ATPase by Ca^{2+}-activated calmodulin. The free Ca^{2+} ions can be of external or internal origin, the internal compartment being endo-plasmic reticulum (or sarcoplasmic reticulum, to the extent this is present). Contraction is both slow to develop and slow to dissipate because of the time needed for Ca^{2+} to be extruded from the cytoplasm, but the fibre arrangement is so efficient that smooth muscle achieves about the same maximum strength of contraction per unit cross-sectional area as striated muscle. Moreover the long duration of smooth muscle contraction means that much less energy expenditure is necessary to maintain the same tension as striated muscle (Guyton, 1981). Because the arrangement of actin and myosin filaments in smooth muscle is so loose, smooth muscle fibres can shorten with contraction much more than striated fibres do. In the uterus this helps the extreme change of uterine dimensions that follow expulsion of products of conception to take place.

Entry of Ca^{2+} into smooth muscle cells or release from the endoplasmic reticulum is associated both with contraction and with depolarisation and the generation of action potentials. Although calcium release and excitation-contraction coupling follows depolarisation, there is no fixed relationship between action potentials and contractions. Smooth muscle contraction neither depends on action potentials nor is it an all-or-none phenomenon. Calcium release and either the occurrence of a contraction or a change in tone (depending on the time frame) can, in the myometrium, be elicited by: (a) *neurotransmitters* (e.g. acetylcholine, or noradrenalin acting on α-receptors); (b) *other hormones* (including prostaglandins, polypeptides such as oxytocin, and steroids — at least indirectly but, as discussed below, perhaps directly); (c) *spontaneously* (waxing and waning of Ca^{2+}-dependent membrane ATPase due to pacemaker activity or in response to *stretch*); and (d) *experimentally* by electrical nerve, field or muscle stimulation.

The greater the depolarisation of a smooth muscle cell the more chance there is, generally, of an action potential being produced. The action potential may have the form of a *spike* (duration 10–50 msec) or a *spike-and-wave* (lasting, in the myometrium, anywhere from 200 ms to 30 s). Action potentials may occur in clusters or bursts, at the apices of *slow* or '*pacemaker*' *waves* of periodic background depolarisation, to produce rhythmic contractions (Talo, 1976). In other tissues a number (say 30 or 40) of smooth muscle cells must depolarise simultaneously for self-propagating action potentials and propagated waves of contraction to follow, and the same presumably applies to the uterus. The speed of propagation of electrical activity in the non-pregnant uterus is slow — in the range 1 to 10 cm/s. Impulses in the myometrium can travel independently of each other and the velocity of travel longitudinally within a bundle is much faster than lateral spread, particularly between bundles (Kao, 1977).

The occurrence in the uterus of myometrium with fast intrinsic activity that might act as pacemaker for other parts of the myometrium has not been shown to be restricted to any particular anatomical region. Contractions accompany bursts of spikes in the human myometrium and the intensity of the contraction locally depends partly on the frequency of spikes in each burst. The extent of propagation of the contraction, and hence the intensity of the contraction of the uterus as a whole, may depend on the extent gap junctions have formed — which, together with the other basic myometrial properties described in this section, is very much a phenomenon regulated by hormones, and is discussed below.

The intracellular second-messengers of these hormonal influences have been considered in the Introduction to this chapter. *Calcium*, through calmodulin and myosin light chain kinase, is the chief determinant of contraction; *cyclic AMP*, through cAMP-protein kinase, inhibits myosin light chain kinase and causes relaxation; and *cyclic GMP* may be produced as part of reestablishment of the cell's redox potential after contraction.

Non-steroid endocrine responsiveness of myometrium

Prostaglandins may be produced in the uterus or may be exogenous, delivered to the uterus either pharmacologically or as part of the semen with insemination. Prostaglandin production in the uterus takes place mainly in the endometrium, including, during pregnancy, the decidua of the endometrial stroma; the prostaglandins then diffuse into the myometrium (Fuchs et al, 1982). As introduced in the first section of this chapter, prostaglandin production from cell membranes, through membrane phospholipid methylation, can be self-generating: once substantial myometrial activity is underway it is likely that further prostaglandin release takes place from cell membranes in the myometrium itself.

Prostaglandin receptors are present in myometrium but not in endometrium (Wakeling & Wyngarden, 1974). The mechanism of action of prostaglandins is almost certainly through increasing the availability of free Ca^{2+} in the smooth muscle cytoplasm; although the molecular details of their action has not been worked out precisely, inhibition of Ca^{2+}-binding to the ATP-dependent enzyme that extrudes Ca^{2+} from the cytoplasm and enhanced release of Ca^{2+} from the sarcoplasmic reticulum may be involved (Carsten, 1973). Exogenous Ca^{2+} potentiates the effects of prostaglandins clinically (Weinstein et al, 1976) and *diazoxide*, which is thought to act by preventing Ca^{2+}-release from the sarcoplasmic reticulum, is one of the few drugs (*magnesium sulphate* is another) that acts sufficiently distally to inhibit prostaglandin and Ca^{2+}-induced myometrial contractility (Wilson et al, 1974; Elliott, 1983).

Prostaglandin $F_{2\alpha}$ is a powerful stimulant of myometrial contraction and is the critical endogenous physiological effector for myometrial contractions with initiation of menstruation and during labour, at which times it is present in high concentrations in the myometrium (Vijayakumar & Walters, 1981).

Prostaglandin E_2 instilled into the uterine cavity, at doses similar to those found in secretory endometrium generally or those found in semen, also has a stimulatory action on the myometrium. This is true for all stages of the cycle except midcycle, when in normal, fertile women it is inhibitory (Martin & Bygdeman, 1975; Toppozada et al, 1977); in a subgroup of women with unexplained infertility, PGE_2 instillation at midcycle had a paradoxical stimulatory effect on the myometrium (Toppozada et al, 1977). PGE_2's concentration in the myometrium is maximal at midcycle (Vijayakumar & Walters, 1981).

Oxytocin in physiological doses initiates action potentials in quiescent cells whose excitability was previously borderline and it increases the frequency of action potentials, as well as the frequency of pacemaker activity (slow wave depolarisations that lead to bursts of action potentials), in active myometrium (Marshall, 1974). Its mechanism of action is presumably through opening ionic channels in the smooth muscle cell membrane, though decreased Ca^{2+}-binding has been described (Carsten, 1979); overall, however, its physiological effects are qualitatively different from those of $PGF_{2\alpha}$ (Seitchik et al, 1977). At pharmacological doses oxytocin induces a sustained depolarisation of the cell membrane, which is accompanied by tetanic contraction (Marshall, 1974). Plasma membrane oxytocin receptors are found in the myometrium and in the decidual stroma of the pregnant uterus; as well as stimulating myometrium directly, oxytocin in the endometrium of term pregnancy acts on decidual membrane receptors to release arachidonic acid and allow prostaglandins to be produced (Fuchs et al, 1982), which then further stimulate myometrial contractility. The actions of oxytocin are considered fully in Chapter 10.

Alpha-adrenergic receptors in smooth muscle mediate contraction through the opening of slow Ca^{2+}-channels in the cell membrane, permitting Ca^{2+} to diffuse down its concentration gradient into the cell to increase excitability (Braunwald, 1982). Although this mechanism has been worked out chiefly for vascular smooth muscle and cardiac muscle, drugs such as *nifedipine* that specifically block these Ca^{2+} channels have a marked tocolytic effect on human myometrium *in vitro* and *in vivo* (Ulmsten et al, 1978). *Ergometrine* owes its stimulatory action on the myometrium to binding with α-receptors. *Beta$_2$-adrenergic receptors* in the myometrium inhibit contractility, through production of cAMP. Beta-adrenergic agonists, including *salbutamol*, *terbutaline*, *ritodrine* and *isoxuprel*, have great clinical usefulness in inhibiting unwanted uterine contractions.

Despite these clinically useful ways of exploiting myometrial adrenergic receptors, their physiological significance is quite unknown. *Adrenergic innervation* of the myometrium additional to vasomotor innervation is quite conspicuous, though less dense than in the tubal isthmus or the cervix (Owman et al, 1967; Zuspan et al, 1981); the neurotransmitter these adrenergic nerves contain is noradrenalin. The overall importance of adrenergic innervation is thought at best to be slight, however, because functional denervation with the nerve poison tetrodotoxin in experimental animals has no effect on the course of labour. *Cholinergic nerves* are sparse and mainly related to blood vessels (Coupland, 1960).

Steroid hormone responsiveness of myometrium

Oestrogen and progesterone profoundly modify the myometrium's response to the water-soluble hormones. The myometrium contains specific oestradiol and progesterone receptors that are very similar physically to those of endometrium; concentrations are comparable to those in endometrium and, qualitatively, vary through the menstrual cycle with the same pattern (Soules & McCarty, 1982). Myometrium, like the Fallopian tube and the endometrium, is therefore able to concentrate oestradiol and progesterone from plasma (Runnebaum et al, 1978).

The muscle layer of the genital tract is unique among smooth muscle tissues of the body in requiring oestrogen for acquisition of spontaneous activity and rhythmicity. *Oestrogen* treatment of immature or oophorectomised rabbits causes an increase in resting membrane potential from about -30 mV to about -50 mV and, with it, a loss of quiescence; one injection of oestradiol in oophorectomised rabbits, for example, results in the appearance of myometrial action potentials within 24 hours (Kao, 1977). Trains of action potentials of high amplitude and low

frequency and initiation of regular, rhythmic contractions of the myometrium follow (Heap et al, 1973). Accompanying this electrophysiological response to oestrogens is an increase in uterine blood flow and an increase in dry weight of the uterus, as hyperplasia and hypertrophy of smooth muscle cells take place. Although actin and myosin are present in oestrogen-deprived myometrial cells, their concentrations as well as their total amounts double with administration of oestrogen. Glycogen is deposited.

The action of *progesterone* is greatly influenced by the extent to which the myometrium has been primed with oestrogen. Its effect on oestrogen-deprived myometrium is negligible, whereas the propagated electrical activity of a stimulated strip of myometrium from an oestradiol-treated rabbit can be changed, with progesterone treatment, to a pattern where only the immediate segment stimulated contracts (Heap et al, 1973). *In vivo* studies show that progesterone can completely block myometrial activity induced by ovariectomy in pregnant rabbits. Observations such as these led Csapo to propose that a '*progesterone block*' during pregnancy allowed uterine quiescence up to the time of labour.

The mechanism by which progesterone has this inhibitory effect on myometrial contractility is still not clear. Csapo originally thought that progesterone block was due to depolarisation; empirical studies published by him in 1959 caused this to be revised (Goto & Csapo, 1959). Immature rabbit myometrium, stabilised with oestrogen at a resting potential of -45 mV (as determined by intracellular electrodes) showed an increase to -60 mV with two injections of progesterone. Kao was unable to confirm this and believes that any apparent increase is explainable by an improvement in the success of impalement of cells with recording electrodes under the influence of progesterone, so artificially increasing the mean of recorded values (Kao, 1977). Whether or not progesterone increases myometrial resting membrane potential remains unsettled.

Intra-uterine pressure monitoring in oestrogen-treated ovariectomized ewes, before, during and after progesterone treatment, has shown that progesterone reduces the frequency and amplitude of myometrial activity; moreover progesterone can abolish uterine reactivity to both oxytocin and $PGF_{2\alpha}$ (Lye & Porter, 1978). These observations imply that the cellular action of progesterone on the myometrium is very close, molecularly, to the contractile mechanism or to the coupling of excitation and contraction. In this regard it is interesting that 5β-pregnanolone, a water-soluble progesterone metabolite with a pronounced hypnotic effect, also has an inhibitory effect on the myometrium (Gyermek, 1968). It would therefore seem possible that progesterone metabolites, as well as progesterone itself (Figdor et al, 1957), might be responsible for progesterone's inhibitory effect on excitable tissue (Heap et al, 1973). A recent study has shown that progesterone has a direct effect in promoting Ca^{2+}-binding by *microsomal* fractions of myometrial homogenates prepared from pregnant and from non-pregnant uteri (Carsten, 1979) — an observation that, because the nuclear and cytosol fractions are largely excluded, implies a mechanism of steroid action other than through cytoplasmic and nuclear receptors.

A remarkable morphological phenomenon, one that has profound electrophysiological significance for integrated uterine contractions, accompanies the withdrawal of progesterone and the introduction of $PGF_{2\alpha}$ to the myometrium of the rat — a combination of events that accompanies labour. Electron microscopy shows a precipitate and highly significant increase in the number, size and area of *gap junctions*, which, by establishing direct cytoplasmic electrical contact between myometrial smooth muscle cells, may transform the myometrium into a functional syncytium, with generation of low-resistance pathways of current flow and promotion of coordinated contractions that involve the entire uterus (Garfield et al, 1982). Similar studies in humans have shown that gap junctions form with the establishment of labour (Garfield & Hayashi, 1981) and are also present during the menstrual cycle in women with dysmenorrhoea (Garfield & Hayashi, 1980).

Cyclical changes in myometrial activity

The resting pressure in the uterine cavity is about 10–15 mmHg. Conflicting studies on changes in myometrial contractility have been reviewed by Finn & Porter (1975), who conclude that the data of Csapo, which follow, are the most thorough and reliable available.

Menstruation is attended by low frequency (25–35 per hour), high amplitude (70–75 mm) contractions, which by day 6 have given rise to more frequent (80/h), lower amplitude (15 mm) contractions (Csapo, 1970, cited by Finn & Porter, 1975). Midcycle, under the influence of oestradiol, is characterised by low amplitude (10 mm or less), high frequency (over 200/h) contractions. The frequency of contractions falls very quickly (by day 26 about 80/h) as progesterone rises after the time of ovulation, but the amplitude stays low (15 mm). During this time the myometrium is especially resistant to the effects of exogenous oxytocin. Contraction frequency keeps falling until, with the marked increase in $PGF_{2\alpha}$ production in the endometrium that precedes menstruation, the amplitude of contractions rises dramatically.

Cause and effect relationships between circulating oestradiol and progesterone levels and these changes in myometrial activity are not in doubt in principle, but the pathways and intermediaries by which these steroids, especially progesterone, ultimately exert their actions are still controversial.

Excessively painful uterine contractions with menstruation, *dysmenorrhoea*, can be effectively treated with a number of drugs, including prostaglandin synthesis inhibitors such as mefenamic acid and naproxen, β_2-adrenergic agonists such as salbutamol, and Ca^{2+}-channel blockers such as nifedipine (Ch. 31). All have been shown to decrease the amplitude of uterine contractions substantially. $PGF_{2\alpha}$ production is increased in women with dysmenorrhoea, but the reason for this increase is not clear. Plasma levels of vasopressin are said to be four times higher at the time of menstruation in women with dysmenorrhoea, even after effective treatment with naproxen to rule out pain as the cause of the vasopressin elevation, and vasopressin has a significant oxytocic action on the myometrium (Strömberg et al, 1981).

Myometrial activity in pregnancy and labour

The uterus enlarges in pregnancy and its chemical composition changes due to two major influences: (a) the chemical action of hormones; and (b) the physical stimulus to the myometrium of an enlarging conceptus (Heap et al, 1973). Myometrial growth in pregnancy is almost entirely brought about by hypertrophy rather than hyperplasia. It is clear that oestrogens and progesterone alone are insufficient to account for this hypertrophy (which accompanies an increase in uterine weight during pregnancy from about 10–15 g to 800–1000 g; Heap et al, 1973), and that other factors must operate; but it is not known to what extent the stimulus for hypertrophy is physical (Csapo et al, 1965) or to what extent somatotropic hormones from the placenta might play a part.

A detailed review of the physiology of the myometrium during pregnancy and labour is beyond this chapter's scope. Intra-uterine pressure recordings are easier to perform during pregnancy than during the menstrual cycle, owing to the greater volume available in the uterine cavity, and the empirical data are not controversial (Finn & Porter, 1975). By 7 weeks' gestation the frequency of contractions is high (132/h) and the amplitude low (less than 10 mmHg). At 14 weeks the pattern is the same, but after this there is a gradual increase in amplitude and frequency — slow at first, and then, towards term, very quickly. Labour is characterised by regular, highly coordinated, high amplitude (50–100 mm) contractions with a frequency of 3–10 per 10 minutes (Caldeyro-Barcia & Poseiro, 1965; Csapo, 1969; Finn & Porter, 1975).

The hormone-induced accommodation the uterus shows to its contents as pregnancy progresses is all the more remarkable when one considers that stretch is a powerful stimulus to smooth muscle contraction. The mechanism by which myometrial activity is blocked is controversial in humans, although in species such as the rabbit progesterone clearly has both the ability and the likely predominant role (Heap et al, 1973; Finn & Porter, 1975; Kao, 1977). The situation in humans is complicated by the fact that, unlike the rabbit, plasma progesterone concentrations do not fall in any indisputable manner prior to the onset of labour, and nor do even massive amounts of exogenous progesterone inhibit labour once it has begun. The molecular mechanisms by which progesterone might exert any gestation-promoting effect are certainly still not clear. But it is also reasonable to state that the importance of its withdrawal in the onset of labour cannot finally be settled until it is known precisely what happens to its receptor-binding and to its metabolism in the term uterus. Meanwhile it is true that there is no single exception to the rule that complete withdrawal of progesterone at any stage of human pregnancy promptly terminates the pregnancy — and for this reason alone it would seem that the etymological foundations of the name 'progesterone' are firm.

THE CERVIX

Morphology and biochemistry of the endocervix

Introduction: mucus glycoprotein biochemistry

Cyclical changes in cervical mucus are among the best known quantitative and qualitative alterations in genital tract responsiveness that occur during the menstrual cycle. These changes, consisting of an increase in volume, decrease in viscosity, increase in spinnbarkeit (stretchiness), and acquisition of a property known as ferning when the mucus is dried on a slide, all take place with follicular development leading up to the time of ovulation and correlate with development of sperm-penetrability of the mucus. Their cause is clearly endocrine: the same mucus characteristics can be induced with exogenous oestrogens. Progesterone and synthetic progestogens, on the other hand, reverse these oestrogen-dependent effects.

The chemical basis for these steroid hormone actions on cervical mucus is still not properly understood. An examination of some possibilities, however, gives important insights into cervical mucus physiology as well as suggestions for endocrine response in other parts of the genital tract. Some knowledge of the chemistry of cervical mucus — and of complex carbohydrates in general — is essential.

Table 5.1 lists the important properties of the major groups of carbohydrate-protein conjugates. These groups comprise the *serum glycoproteins* (constituting most circulating proteins other than albumin), the *mucus glycoproteins* (the glycoproteins of mucosal surfaces, including cervical mucus), and the *proteoglycans* (present in connective tissue and the cumulus matrix, and formerly termed mucopolysaccharides).

The general structure of mucus glycoproteins (MGPs) is thought to be similar in the gastrointestinal tract, respiratory tract and genital tract (see Table 5.2). The backbone of the MGP molecule is a linear polypeptide chain rich in the amino acids serine and threonine, both of which contain hydroxyl groups, to which oligosaccharides are linked through the amino-sugar N-acetylgalactosamine

(Carlson, 1977; Reid & Clamp, 1978; Clamp et al, 1978). The sugars that make up the oligosaccharide side chains often include sialic acid; in some cases, ester sulphates, which are even more acidic than sialic acid, may also be found. These acidic groups are dissociated and highly anionic at neutral pH, causing the oligosaccharides to be mutually repellent and to organise about themselves a huge domain of water and cations. The 'naked' parts of the polypeptide chain, which do not bear carbohydrate substitutuions, may be connected to each other through cysteine residues and disulphide bonds, causing the subunits (typically of MW $c.500\,000$) to form aggregates (at least in the case of pig gastric mucin, which is the MGP best characterised chemically — Allen, 1978) of MW $c.2 \times 10^6$. It is these aggregates that then interact with each other through hydrogen bonds to give solutions of MGPs their mucus-like properties of viscosity, stretchiness and reparability — properties that can chemically be destroyed with disulphide bond-splitting agents such as mercaptoethanol or by digesting the naked parts of the polypeptide chains with peptidases (Allen, 1978).

Synthesis of mucus glycoproteins in endocervical cells and elsewhere begins with production of the polypeptide chain in the rough endoplasmic reticulum (Phelps, 1978). The polypeptide is transported through a series of smooth-membrane components into the Golgi apparatus, where sugars (previously linked to phosphorylated nucleotides in the cytoplasm) are transfered to serine and threonine residues on the polypeptide chain with great precision, through glycosyltransferases, sialyltransferase and sulphotransferase. Packaging into secretory granules (or 'secretory droplets', since these acidic and expanded molecules are not packed nearly so tightly as the neutral proteins and glycoproteins of electron-dense, serous granules are) is accompanied by further modification of sugars in the oligosaccharide side-chains; in the rabbit endocervical mucus cell, granules become more acidic and more

Table 5.2 Mucus glycoprotein structure

Primary	amino acids rich in serine and threonine (contain –OH groups); cysteine present (–SH groups to allow disulphide bonds); 5 sugars (see Table 5.1), including sialic acid and ester sulphates
Secondary	linear polypeptide forms extended chain in glycosylated part, alpha-helix in non-glycosylated part branched oligosaccharide side chains linked to polypeptide chain
Tertiary	molecular unit resembles a 'bottle brush', with mutually-repellant acidic oligosaccharide 'bristles' on part of the chain, and a carbohydrate-free portion represented by the 'handle'
Quaternary	subunit aggregation occurs at two levels: (i) disulphide bonds link through 'handles' to form tetramers (ii) hydrogen bonds form between carbohydrate 'bristles' to cause viscosity and gelation

electron-lucent as they reach the apical part of the cell (Chilton et al, 1980).

Secretion occurs through exocytosis (a calmodulin-mediated function), preceded often by coalescence of droplets in the cytoplasm, giving, overall, a combined merocrine and apocrine pattern of secretion ultrastructurally, and accounting for the presence of membrane and cellular fragments amidst the mucus produced (Philipp & Overbeck, 1969; Shingleton & Lawrence, 1976). Further molecular modification may well take place after secretion as the need for at least some degree of close packaging is shed, abundant evidence having long existed for the presence of ectoglycosyltransferases on cell-surfaces. Unknown mechanisms then compose the secreted acid MGPs into extracellular mucus.

The mucus glycoproteins constitute the high viscosity component of cervical mucus. Although mucus is a gel, it can be solubilised by physical or chemical means in the laboratory; moreover, even as a gel, mucus contains a soluble or low viscosity component, the proportion of which increases under the influence of oestrogen (see below). Dissolved in this low viscosity solution are the various components of plasma, though in altered concentration: salts, sugars, amino acids and soluble proteins, including albumin, enzymes and immunoglobulins — all of which have the potential for chemical interaction with the mucus glycoproteins of the gel, so changing the gel's properties.

Histochemistry and ultrastructure of the endocervix

The transition between endometrial cells of the uterine isthmus and the glandular cells of the endocervix is abrupt (Sorvari & Laakso, 1970): the cells quite suddenly display strong cytoplasmic staining for acid MGPs, with affinity for periodic acid-Schiff (PAS) reagent, which stains most carbohydrates, whether acidic or neutral, and for cationic dyes such as Alcian blue and iron diamine (for review see Jansen & Bajpai, 1982), which selectively stain acidic substances. As in endometrium, both non-ciliated, secretory and (rather fewer) ciliated cells are present in the endocervix; the ciliated cells move the secreted mucus towards the vagina; they do not change in ultrastructural appearance through the menstrual cycle (Philipp & Overbeck, 1969).

Oestrogen is clearly needed for synthesis of acid MGPs in the endocervix, as shown by the substantial reduction in stainable MGP that takes place after the menopause and by stimulation of incorporation of ^{14}C-N-acetylglucosamine into MGPs in oestrogen-treated ovariectomised rabbits (Chilton et al, 1980). However, few morphological changes in the endocervix are observable light microscopically through the menstrual cycle, other than some increase in epithelial cell height around midcycle (Nillson & Westman, 1961) and some restriction in the amount of stainable intra-cellular acid MGP during menstruation (Kellett et al, 1969).

Transmission electronmicroscopy (TEM) of endocervical mucus-producing cells shows that secretory activity continues throughout the menstrual cycle, implying a low threshold of sensitivity of mucus-production to oestrogen, but there does seem to be a discernible increase in secretory activity between day 11 and day 15 of the cycle (Philipp & Overbeck, 1969). Mucus content of endocervical cells decreases quite markedly in the puerperium (Philipp, 1972). TEM studies have also indicated a number of interesting features among secretion droplets themselves, including heterogeneity of density of their contents (Nilsson & Westman, 1961) and the appearance of filaments in some apical droplets but not others (Philipp & Overbeck, 1969; Philipp, 1972), implying that more than one type of mucus may be produced.

Cyclical changes in cervical structure and function

Both the substantive nature of cervical mucus and the central importance of its structure to normal reproductive function make it clear that studies of genital tract morphology should not stop at mucosal surfaces. The marked cyclical changes that occur in cervical mucus are in dramatic contrast to the inconspicuousness of changes in the more solid tissues of the endocervix.

Cervical mucus structure: physical and ultrastructural studies

It has long been known that most biological fluids — and particularly cervical mucus — deviate from ideal or Newtonian behaviour when *viscosity*, or resistance to flow, is measured (Clift, 1979). A Newtonian fluid with dissolved spherical particles will exhibit the same viscosity irrespective of the shear rate, or deforming velocity gradient, at which the viscosity is determined. Cervical mucus, on the other hand, shows less viscosity with a sudden shear than it does when a slow rate of shear is maintained over a period of time. It also shows *elasticity*, the ability to recoil from a small deformation and resume initial dimensions. With a more substantial deformation, mucus shows spinability (*spinnbarkeit*), or the capacity to be drawn out into long threads before losing continuity. Furthermore mucus can recover its properties, though in a new shape, to respond to a second occasion of deformation in precisely the same way as to the first: it shows *reparability*. With the exception of viscosity (which for native cervical mucus is *least* at midcycle), these parameters are maximal under the influence of oestrogen at midcycle, when it is unopposed by progesterone (Clift, 1979).

All these rheological properties of mucus follow directly from its molecular structure. From the standpoint of molecular biophysics, Odeblad has interpreted these observations to be the result of entanglement of long, high MW molecules through hydrogen bonds (Odeblad, 1968), which would be expected to show the great ease of rupture and the fairly long recovery time (of the order of seconds) observed. Similar conclusions have been reached more recently by others (Wolf et al, 1977a–c).

Perhaps the best known property of midcycle mucus is *ferning* — the crystallisation of sodium chloride on expanded MGPs that occurs when cervical mucus is allowed to dry on a microscope slide. The phenomenon is almost entirely a product of sodium chloride concentration and available space in which to form crystals, with the MGP molecules imposing direction on the sodium chloride crystals as they grow, in the watery mucus produced by oestrogen unopposed by progesterone, to produce the arborisation pattern that is typical of midcycle (Saga et al, 1977).

Information on the degree and type of hydration of large molecules can be obtained rather more precisely with nuclear magnetic resonance (NMR) techniques, which Odeblad has used to devise a physical model for cervical mucus that has helped greatly in understanding its composition, its properties and the changes it undergoes during the cycle (Odeblad, 1968). NMR permits a study of proton mobility and bonding in water, and results indicate large hydration volumes, particularly in midcycle mucus, with hydration again predominantly through hydrogen bonding; in the luteal phase there is evidence of qualitatively different interactions, with fewer but more strongly bound water molecules. NMR also shows a great difference between flow viscosity (see above) and molecular viscosity of the aqueous phase, an observation that not only has led Odeblad to conclude that mucus has the structure of a gel, but has allowed him to make rather precise predictions of its internal structural dimensions.

Odeblad has concluded (Odeblad, 1968, 1976) that midcycle mucus — also referred to as *type E*, or oestrogenic, mucus — is composed of micelles with a diameter of about 0.5 μm and each containing 100–1000 molecular chains; the distance between micelles is of the order of 1–10 μm; micelles are arranged parallel with each other within long rods of mucus, up to several millimetres in length, with each rod originating, perhaps, from a separate cervical gland or cleft. At some points the micelles may have branches connecting them to neighbouring micelles (Fig 5.17). Midcycle mucus is, according to Odeblad, composed almost (but not quite) entirely of type E mucus. Type E mucus is 97–98.5 per cent water and allows sperm migration between at least some of its micelles.

During prolonged or intense exogenous oestrogen stimulation, an even more watery mucus, referred to by Odeblad as type H mucus, forms; it is exceptionally fluid, has a very high water content and low water binding capacity; sperm migration through it is irregular.

Luteal phase mucus — *Type G*, or gestagenic (progestogenic) mucus (Fig. 5.17) — on the other hand, has little

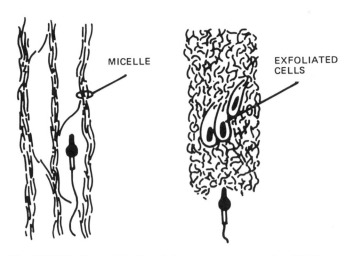

Fig. 5.17 Micellar model of cervical mucus structure, after Odeblad (1968). Ovulatory mucus (left) allows sperm migration through intermicellar spaces. Early follicular or luteal mucus (right) has a tight non-micellar structure that excludes sperm penetration

or no micellar arrangement; the chains form a rather tight meshwork, with a mesh size of only about 0.3 μm; and there is no parallel or directional arrangement of the chains. Type G mucus, which is only 87–95 per cent water and is much more viscous, constitutes about 90 per cent of cervical mucus during the luteal phase.

Not only would luteal mucus arranged this way impede sperm migration through it, but Odeblad has also proposed that advantageous oscillations could occur in midcycle micellar mucus that would allow resonance between sperm flagellation and the molecular lattice of the mucus to produce a 'surfing mechanism' of rapid sperm transport. No similar confirmatory studies from other laboratories exist, unfortunately, but nor do any negative studies; so the idea, if unproven, remains attractive. Empirical studies show that sperm injected into the vagina can reach the tubes in 5 minutes (Fordney Settlage et al, 1973; Tredway et al, 1975).

TEM examination of unfixed cervical mucus has tended to confirm Odeblad's predictions. Singer & Reid (1970a) collected cervical mucus with minimum distortion directly onto copper specimen grids at colposcopy, stained the mucus with ammonium molybdate, and with TEM showed midcycle mucus to consist of positively-stained parallel fibres of 5–15 micron diameter, separated by distances of 5–20 microns, and each apparently composed of smaller fibres; in luteal phase mucus the parallel pattern was replaced by a denser meshwork. Similar conclusions were reached by Elstein et al (1971).

When glutaraldehyde-fixed endocervical mucosa is prepared for SEM by critical-point drying, its surface mucus assumes a granular-filamentous appearance (Ludwig & Metzger, 1976). A similar appearance is obtained with glutaraldehyde-fixed aspirated mucus dried either the same way (Zanefeld et al, 1975) or by cold lyophilisation ('freeze drying') (Chretien et al, 1973). These studies also support

Odeblad's predictions, in that early follicular phase mucus, luteal phase mucus, pregnancy mucus, and postmenopausal mucus all appear to be composed of dense networks of filaments, whereas midcycle mucus shows more open areas where the filaments are much less entangled (Chretien et al, 1975; Zanefeld et al, 1975); but the range of appearances published suggests that considerable distortion and artefact is produced by these methods.

A somewhat different picture of cyclical changes in cervical mucus has come from SEM techniques that have been gentler than those used in the studies described above. Daunter et al (1976) (Fig 5.18) fixed aspirated mucus briefly in weak glutaraldehyde solution and freeze-dried it slowly, to demonstrate a degree of structure in cervical mucus that is without precedent: an interconnecting system of thin membranous walls giving a honeycomb structure with no free filaments. Channel size in the honeycomb was around 30–35 nm at midcycle, but only 2–6 nm in the early follicular phase and the luteal phase (Elstein & Daunter, 1976).

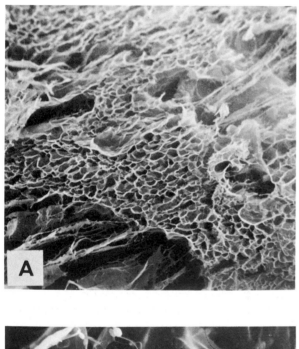
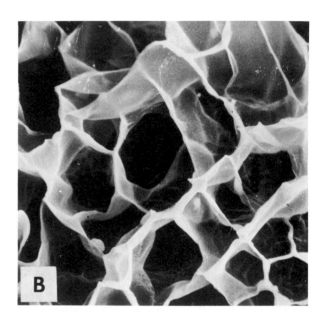
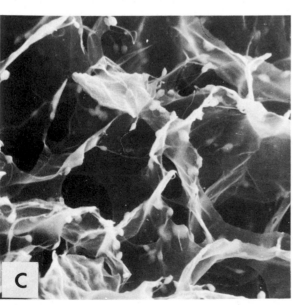
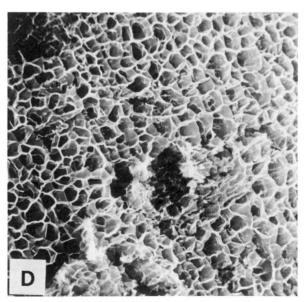

Fig. 5.18 Honeycomb structure of cervical mucus visualised by SEM after gentle fixation and preparation. [A] Early proliferative phase; channel diameter 2–6 μm. [B] Mid-proliferative phase; channel diameter 14–25 μm. [C] Late proliferative phase showing sperm migration; channel diameter 30–35 μm. [D] Luteal phase; channel diameter 4–6 μm. Original magnification × 900. (From Daunter, with the permission of Dr Daunter and the British Journal of Obstetrics and Gynaecology)

Chemical basis of cyclical changes in cervical mucus

Despite accumulating knowledge both of the chemical nature of cervical mucus and of the physical changes it undergoes through the menstrual cycle, the link between the two — the chemical basis of mucus changes or, following Odeblad, the difference between type E and type G mucus — is still not clear. Changes in the molecular structure of the MGPs themselves (either among the polypeptides or the oligosaccharide sugars), changes in the soluble proteins associated with the MGPs, changes in electrolytes and pH, and direct interactions between steroid hormones and the mucus have all been suggested to be the primary determinant of conformational changes in the MGPs.

Wolf and colleagues have indicated that there may be both quantitative and qualitative changes in the MGPs during the cycle (Wolf et al, 1977a–c, 1978, 1979). Cervical mucus samples from different patients were dialysed and freeze-dried, so removing from the mucus all but the nondialysable solids (soluble proteins plus MGPs), before being reconstituted with a fixed amount of electrolyte solution of standard ionic strength and pH. Comparing wet mucus weight with dry weight confirmed that the bulk of the increase in mucus volume that occurs at midcycle is due to an increase in water content of the mucus, with, after an initial rise in the early follicular phase, little or no change in dry weight during the cycle (Wolf et al, 1977b). But they were also able to show that, after correction for dilution, mucus at midcycle shows an *increase* in viscoelasticity, which they interpreted as being due to a qualitatively different MGP, an increase in MGP:soluble protein ratio (Wolf et al, 1977b), or both (Wolf et al, 1977c).

A qualitative change in MGP could arise from a change in the *amino acid* sequence of the polypeptide backbone of the molecule or from a change in sugar composition of the oligosaccharide side chains. An early study indicated an increase in serine and threonine among the amino acids of cervical mucus in the luteal phase and in pregnancy, accompanied by an increase in *sialic acid* at these times (Iacobelli et al, 1971). On the other hand, *in vitro* studies on salivary MGP show that sialic acid contributes greatly to the viscosity of a standard preparation of MGP (Gottschalk, 1960), which (from Wolf's studies described above) is what might be expected to occur in midcycle mucus. Sialic acid content at midcycle has been thought to increase in bonnet monkey cervical mucus, despite a remarkably constant amino acid composition (Hatcher et al, 1977), and in human cervical mucus (Daunter, 1978); Daunter also showed that removal of sialic acid residues with neuraminidase caused the SEM appearance of midcycle mucus to change to that of early follicular or luteal mucus. Meyer, however, removed 80 per cent of sialic acid from bovine cervical mucus without producing any change in its viscosity (Meyer, 1976). Gibbons (1978) has also discounted structural changes in MGPs as being necessary for altered physical properties.

In a particularly careful recent study in which gas-liquid chromatography was used for sugar analysis, and sugar contributions from non-MGP proteins were excluded (van Kooij et al, 1980), no cyclical variations were detected in sugar or sialic acid content. There was also no change in electrophoretic behaviour of the MGPs after solubilisation with the disulphide bond-splitting agent dithiothreitol, which could be interpreted as indicating no change in the degree of acidification (sulphation) of sugar residues of the MGPs through the cycle.

The *soluble proteins* in mucus all decrease in concentration at midcycle (Schumacher et al, 1977), an event that is likely to be at least partly the result of the increased hydration of the mucus that occurs then. Because these proteins include immunoglobulins as well as some of the protease inhibitors, this decrease may be important in allowing sperm to penetrate the mucus. But the presence or absence of small proteins may also directly affect the physical properties of the mucus (Tam & Verdugo, 1981). The viscosity of purified mucus can be increased *in vitro* by addition of albumin (List et al, 1978), so a relative increase in MGP secretion by the cervix compared with, say, a constant amount of albumin transudation could be enough to explain cyclical changes in mucus properties (van Kooij et al, 1980). Irrespective of whether this phenomenon is important or not in determining changes in cervical mucus in the normal cycle, it could be a mechanism by which mucus viscosity is increased in pathological conditions such as cervicitis.

The *electrolyte* environment in which the MGPs exist may influence their conformation. The degree of expansion of acid MGPs and hence their physical properties depend on the mutual repulsion of acidic groups. In an electrolyte solution, partial neutralisation of these acidic, anionic groups will occur as cationic 'counterions' are attracted to them electrostatically: the MGP molecule will be more contracted in a solution of salt than in distilled water (Allen, 1978). Divalent cations are more effective than monovalent ions in acting as counterions and contracting the MGPs. A qualitative change in cationic composition of cervical mucus effected by endocervical cells could therefore cause substantial changes in its physical characteristics. Sodium chloride content of cervical mucus is maximal at midcycle, either as a proportion of whole mucus or as a proportion of dry weight (Kopito et al, 1973a). Studies at midcycle on divalent cations such as Ca^{2+} and Zn^{2+} have, however, produced inconsistent results (perhaps because of irregular contributions from ejaculated semen). There is no firm indication that electrolyte changes of sufficient magnitude to substantially alter MGP properties could occur physiologically to be the major factor behind the cyclical changes in the mucus that take place (Meyer, 1967).

Although *pH variations* in cervical mucus could also be expected to influence the degree of expansion of the MGPs and the hydration of the mucus (Tam & Verdugo, 1981), there is evidence that such variations in pH that occur in cervical mucus are chiefly the result of variable contamination of the mucus with acidic vaginal secretions: pH is lower and percentage of nondialyzable solids higher in the first of several sequential samples taken during any particular day (Wolf et al, 1978).

Oestrogen appears to have no direct effect on cervical mucus *in vitro* compared with water, but several studies have suggested that addition of *progesterone* or progestogens to aspirated cervical mucus can induce thickening and an increase in viscosity independent of any action on the endocervix itself (Martin et al, 1978; Cheng & Boettcher, 1981). The physiological significance of these observations is quite unknown.

Cervical response to oral contraception

Oral contraceptives that contain a progestogen have an important antifertility effect on the cervix. Cyclical variations are eliminated and the mucus does not acquire the hydrated midcycle state that is required for sperm penetration (Bowman, 1968; Diczfalusy, 1968).

These clinical observations have been supported by TEM (Singer & Reid, 1970b), SEM (Chretien et al, 1980), biochemical (Kosasky et al, 1973) and rheological studies (Wolf et al, 1979). Wolf and colleagues were not able to show any qualitative differences between purified MGPs obtained from women on combined oestrogen–progestogen oral contraceptives compared with MGPs recovered from ovulatory women. Even low-dose progestogen-only 'minipill' formulations containing 350 μg norethisterone or 30 μg laevonorgestrel consistently (although perhaps only for slightly less than 24 h after tablet ingestion) alter cervical mucus to make it impenetrable to sperm, despite, in most cases, continuation of ovulation and normal cyclical oestrogen production (e.g. Moghissi & Marks, 1971); this effect on cervical mucus constitutes their main contraceptive action.

Histologically, Kellett found an increase in stainable acid MGP in endocervical cells of women on high-dose oestrogen sequential oral contraceptives (Kellett et al, 1969); the histochemical effect of more modern combined preparations is not known.

Cervical stromal response to relaxin

During the late luteal phase and during pregnancy the cervix comes under the influence of a non-steroidal hormone, relaxin. Relaxin is a polypeptide produced by the corpus luteum in small amounts during the menstrual cycle and in much larger amounts during the third trimester of pregnancy (Bryant-Greenwood, 1982). Relaxin may be

produced by the decidua, and Bryant-Greenwood has proposed that the dispersed origin of this molecule, which is chemically related to insulin and the insulin-like growth factors, may imply a widespread role in remodelling connective tissue. The high levels of relaxin found in pregnancy, which are thought to result in relaxation of the pelvic ligaments in preparation for parturition, give it the status of a true hormone. In the cervix it is thought to soften the fibromuscular tissue to allow cervical dilatation (Bryant-Greenwood, 1982).

Investigations of cervical function

Cervical score

The changes the cervix undergoes in response to oestrogen stimulation in the menstrual cycle can be assessed clinically in a semi-quantitative scoring system — the *cervical score* (Insler et al, 1972) — that is very useful in practice (Table 5.3).

Table 5.3 Cervical score (after Insler et al, 1972). Each parameter receives a score from 0 to 3; the maximum score is 12; with abundant oestrogen most women have a score equal to or greater than 8 (McBain & Pepperell, 1980)

Parameter	Score 0	1	2	3
Amount of mucus	none	scant	dribble	cascade
Spinnbarkeit	none	slight	moderate	pronounced
Ferning	amorphous	linear	partial	complete
Cervical os	closed		partly open	gaping

The cervical score has been used to predict the time of ovulation in the treatment of infertility, particularly with artificial insemination, when it serves as a bioassay of ovarian follicular oestrogen production; however, although there is a direct and predictable relationship between plasma oestradiol and cervical score for an individual, the correlation between the two is very poor in a population of women (McBain & Pepperell, 1980; Zegers et al, 1981). A low cervical score can result from a low amount of oestrogen, from antagonism of oestrogen-effect with progesterone or a progestogen, or from resistance of the cervix to the effects of oestrogen (see below).

Modifications have been suggested to this method of cervical scoring to take into account mucus cellularity, the number of leucocytes being high in the early follicular and luteal phases, and low at midcycle (Moghissi, 1979; Rezai et al, 1979).

Postcoital test (PCT)

Microscopic examination of cervical mucus aspirated from the endocervical canal by a tuberculin or insulin syringe (or similar device) for sperm is a very basic investigation, but there are a number of essential requirements, often forgotten or ignored, for the test to be interpreted correctly.

From the discussion in this chapter so far it should be clear that sperm are to a greater or lesser extent unable to penetrate mucus that is not under a strong oestrogenic influence: only midcycle mucus, from about day −2 to day +1 in relation to the LH peak and with a cervical score of 8 or more, may allow normal sperm penetration (Zegers et al, 1981). Timing in relation to ovulation is therefore critical and the test should, in doubtful cases, be repeated daily through midcycle until the patient has clearly entered the luteal phase. It has also been shown that the act of aspirating cervical mucus can easily contaminate the mucus with vaginal contents, introducing into the mucus dead sperm, debris and vaginal acidity, so spuriously lowering the pH (Wolf et al, 1978; Versteegh & Shade, 1979); removing the outermost part of the cervical mucus column with a swab is an important prerequisite to a reasonably accurate test.

If these precautions are taken, and if mucus is sampled from close to the internal os (Davajan & Kunitake, 1969), there is good correlation between the number of inseminated sperm and sperm density in the mucus for about 24 h — and particularly over the first 150 minutes — from the time of insemination (Tredway et al, 1975). The median number of motile sperm under these optimal conditions is 15 per microscopic high-power field (HPF), with a lower 95 per cent confidence limit of 5 or 6 per HPF (Tredway, 1976). There is also a definite relationship between sperm survival in the mucus for 48 h or more and the chance of conception (Hanson et al, 1982).

There may be substantial discrepancies between the results of the PCT expressed in motile and non-motile sperm per HPF and the numbers of sperm present in peritoneal fluid aspirated from the pouch of Douglas at laparoscopy. The latter test has rather restricted application, but produces results that correlate much better with subsequent fertility than does a negative cervical mucus PCT (Asch, 1978; Templeton & Mortimer, 1980).

In practice a wide range of observed sperm densities, including values lower than 5 sperm per HPF, is compatible with previous (Kovacs et al, 1978) or subsequent (Jette & Glass, 1972; Giner et al, 1974) fertility. The PCT is most useful when it is clearly normal — particularly when sperm density stays high for many hours after intercourse. On the other hand, a negative or poor PCT in the presence of a good cervical score indicates a need for further assessment of semen quality and coital technique, and a search for antisperm antibodies in both partners; a poor PCT with a low cervical score indicates a need for further assessment of ovulatory function or for correct timing of the test, and for assessment of cervical mucus responsiveness to normal preovulatory oestrogen exposure (see below).

In vitro sperm-cervical mucus interaction testing

In vitro tests of cervical mucus that involve observation of sperm penetration are clinically indicated when negative or poor PCTs are hard to interpret or when one wants information on sperm-cervical mucus interaction associated with an artificial insemination programme.

The simplest of these tests is the *slide test*, carried out by placing a droplet of mucus and a droplet of semen on a microscope slide and then bringing them into contact along an interface under the weight of a cover-slip (Moghissi et al, 1964). Finger-like projections, or phalanges, of seminal fluid develop at the interface within minutes and push into the mucus. Spermatozoa penetrate the apex of the phalangeal canal and enter the mucus; after initial resistance has been overcome by the leading sperm others follow more quickly (Moghissi, 1979). The junctional area is examined microscopically and the number of sperm in the first (F_1) and second (F_2) fields away from the interface are counted at intervals of 5, 10 and 30 minutes. Some degree of quantitative assessment is possible in this way, but reproducibility of the test is variable.

The *capillary penetrability test* as developed by Kremer is both more accurate and more reproducible (Kroeks & Kremer, 1980). The mucus needs to be sufficiently fluid to be drawn into fine, 6 cm-long capillary tubes. Air bubbles in the mucus must be avoided. One end of the horizontal tube is then placed in a drop or reservoir of semen, the system is kept at 37°C, and penetration by spermatozoa is assessed microscopically in terms of distance travelled in 30 or 60 minutes, sperm density, and duration of forwardly-progressive movement. Normal results include more than 4 cm penetration in 30 minutes and motility persistent for 24 h. The interested reader is referred elsewhere (Kroeks & Kremer, 1980) for further technical details and for information and refinements possible with capillary testing.

When the result of a capillary penetrability test is unsatisfactory, either the mucus or the semen may be at fault. By simultaneously testing donor semen and donor mucus in a three- or four-way cross with the semen and mucus of the couple being investigated, useful further information can be obtained; a decision can usually be made on whether it is the mucus or the semen (or both) that is abnormal — at least on the day of testing. Practical experience with the test shows that poor results are much more often the result of real or artifactual mucus problems (Matthews et al, 1980) than sperm problems, which, such as the presence of semen sperm antibodies (Morgan et al, 1977), need to be severe for a negative test (Matthews et al, 1980; Kroeks & Kremer, 1980).

Antisperm antibodies

Local iso-immunity to sperm can occur in the genital tract

in either the presence or absence of readily detectable serum sperm antibodies (Moghissi et al, 1980; Jones, 1980; Leading Article, 1981). Antisperm antibodies generally fall into one of two categories: *immobilising antibodies*, which, if present in sufficiently high titre, are a potent cause of infertility in women and can be screened for with a postcoital test; and *agglutinating antibodies*, which usually do not cause either infertility or an abnormal PCT in women (Friberg, 1981a), but which, if present in semen, may markedly reduce the number and survival of sperm that invade cervical mucus (Friberg, 1981b).

As with most soluble proteins in cervical mucus, the concentration of antisperm antibodies in cervical mucus is least at midcycle, but this is when mucus is most abundant and most easily collected; in practice this means that the time of mucus collection for detection of sperm antibodies is not critical. Separation of the antibodies from the structural components of the mucus to allow immunological studies can be achieved with bromelin (a proteolytic enzyme) or, preferably, simply by centrifugation and collection of supernatant (Jones, 1980).

Cervical resistance to hormone action

Resistance of the cervix to normal circulating levels of steroids, particularly oestrogen, can cause manifestations of oestrogen deficiency in the cervix, with poor development of cervical mucus, a persistently low cervical score, poor or absent sperm penetration, and infertility.

Anatomical defects

Occasional patients are seen who have had a substantial part of the endocervix removed or damaged by cone biopsy or extensive diathermy of the cervix. Other patients may have cervical stenosis or adhesions in the endocervical canal. In both groups of patients cervical mucus needs to be either completely absent or grossly deficient in quantity to cause infertility. Cases of endocervical stenosis or adhesions may respond to dilatation followed by exogenous oestrogen administration (ethinyloestradiol 100 μg per day). Colposcopy may be useful to assess the endocervical mucosa in the remaining cases. A reduced amount of mucosa may allow response to a pharmacological dose of oestrogen (Check, 1980; and see below), whereas a complete absence of mucosa, often with direct access into the uterus, would indicate a need for treatment with intra-uterine artificial insemination, which is not often successful.

Tests and treatment for cervical oestrogen resistance

In most cases where cervical resistance to oestrogen is suspected as the cause of infertility, the true problem lies with poor ovarian follicular development and suboptimal oestrogen production. There are several pathological conditions of the cervix, however, in which cervical mucus production is either faulty or resistant to normal midcycle circulating levels of oestradiol. Distinguishing between the two is possible by administering exogenous oestrogens, preferably from the time of menstruation, in order to rule out the concomitant presence of progesterone, which if present will prevent normal oestrogen action on the cervix.

Insler (1977) has defined conditions he calls 'relative and absolute dysmucorrhoea', characterised by the response of the cervix to two doses of ethinyloestradiol: *relative resistance* means (a) a failure of the cervical score to exceed 8 and (b) a persistence of poor sperm penetration despite administration of ethinyloestradiol 75 μg per day for 8 days; *absolute resistance* is present when the same lack of response also occurs with 150 μg per day for 7 days. Patients with *apparent cervical resistance* respond to the lower of these two dosage regimens and are presumed to have an ovulatory problem.

The treatment of apparent cervical resistance, then, is by inducing better follicular maturation, usually with clomiphene or exogenous gonadotrophins. Gonadotrophins have the advantage of stimulating oestradiol secretion from more than one follicle, whether or not more than one follicle goes on to ovulate, and plasma oestradiol levels in treated cycles that allow a good chance of pregnancy are higher than they are in spontaneous cycles; the extra oestradiol is usually reflected by excellent pre-ovulatory mucus. Clomiphene is an anti-oestrogen and its effects may persist in the genital tract several days after the drug, given at the beginning of the cycle, is stopped; this may manifest as a reduction in the cervical score despite a considerable increase in pre-ovulatory oestrogen production (McBain & Pepperell, 1980). Nevertheless clomiphene has a place in well selected cases.

Attempting to supplement pre-ovulatory follicular oestrogen production with oral oestrogens does not make sense when the cause of the problem is poor follicular development, but does have some logic when relative cervical resistance is diagnosed. Unfortunately even low doses of exogenous oestrogens, such as ethinyloestradiol 10–20 μg, conjugated oestrogens 0.3–0.625 mg, oestriol 0.25 mg, or stilboestrol 0.1–0.2 mg per day, given through the late follicular phase, will prevent ovulation in a proportion of cases, and either a lack of success (McBain & Pepperell, 1980) or only sporadic success (e.g. Scott et al, 1977; Rezai et al, 1979) has been reported with such regimens; the dose of oestrogens used is clearly much less than the 75–150 μg per day needed to diagnose cervical resistance. One study with stilboestrol has given rather better results: although there was no control group, all the pregnancies that occurred (11/63) did so within the first four treatment cycles (Moran et al, 1974).

The treatment of true cervical resistance is therefore likely to require substantial doses of oestrogens — doses that inhibit ovulation unless given in association with exogenous gonadotrophins (Check, 1980). As mentioned above, it is worth studying the effect gonadotrophins have alone before the exogenous oestrogens are added in treating these patients.

VAGINA

Cyclical changes in vaginal morphology and physiology

Steroid effects on vaginal morphology

The vagina is unique in its response to sex steroids. *Oestradiol* is the active endogenous oestrogen in the vagina (Morse et al, 1979), as it is elsewhere in the genital tract. Oestradiol stimulates growth, maturation and desquamation of the stratified squamous epithelium (Fig. 5.19) that constitutes the vaginal mucosal surface, whereas *progesterone* inhibits maturation at the upper mid-zone level of the epithelium (Ferenczy & Guralnick, 1979).

Oestradiol-dependent mitosis takes place mainly in the parabasal cells and to a lesser extent in the basal cells

(Averette et al, 1970). The transit time from basal and parabasal layers to the superficial layers is 4 days. Although oestradiol increases the total number of cells, the transit time through the epithelium is unchanged. Glycogen synthesis begins when the cells are in the parabasal layer and continues in the intermediate layer. The glycogen content of the epithelium is constant during the menstrual cycle, reflecting either independence from oestradiol action or the combined effect of stimulation plus increased cell turnover (Gregoire et al, 1971). The most superficial cells under oestrogen dominance have pyknotic nuclei and contain keratin: they are cornified. *Progestogens*, including progesterone, prevent this final maturation and cornification of the epithelium. Epithelium under progesterone dominance cannot easily be distinguished from epithelium stimulated by only low levels of oestradiol.

Exfoliative cytology

For a thorough exposition on vaginal cytology the reader is referred elsewhere (Frost, 1979) and the following is meant only to be a brief summary. Cells exfoliated from

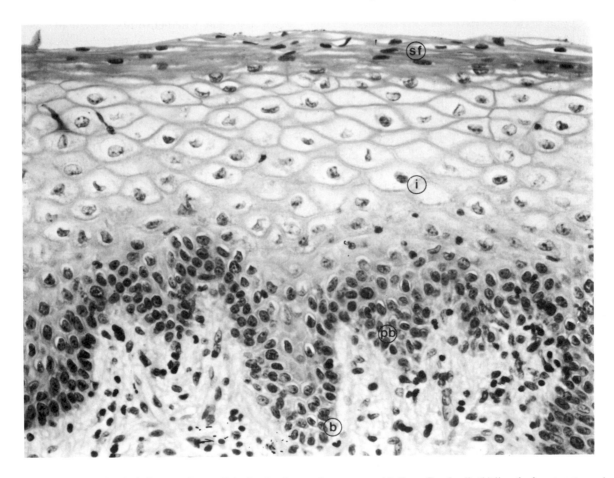

Fig. 5.19 Vaginal mucosa under the influence of oestradiol, showing layers of squamous epithelium. Basal cells (b) line the basement membrane separating epithelium from underlying connective tissue; adjacent cuboidal parabasal cells (pb) are desquamated under conditions of estradiol lack; flattened intermediate cells (i) with vacuolated nuclei are desquamated with moderate estradiol effect or under the influence or progesterone; superficial cells (sf) with pyknotic nuclei are desquamated under conditions of substantial and unopposed oestradiol exposure.

the vaginal epithelium are flattened and squamous in shape, with central nuclei. The size and density of the nucleus, the relative abundance of cytoplasm and, less reliably, the staining properties of the cells indicate from which layer of the stratified squamous epithelium they are derived; by inference, the relative proportions of each cell-type indicate the level of maturity that has been reached by the epithelium as it exfoliates its uppermost cells.

Parabasal cells dominate smears from prepubertal girls and from most postmenopausal, oestrogen-deficient women; they are recognised by their still rather spherical shape, which manifests as cytoplasmic thickness in comparison with the flattened nature of the more superficial cells; the nucleus is round or oval. *Intermediate cells* have very thin cytoplasm from nucleus to cell margin; the nucleus remains vesicular, with a discernible chromatin pattern. Intermediate cells dominate smears when oestradiol influence is only moderate or when its effects are opposed by progesterone. *Superficial cells* have equally thin cytoplasm, but the nucleus is pyknotic; the cytoplasm changes to become acidophilic, but this tinctorial reaction is less reliable than the nature of the nucleus in identifying these cells. Superficial cells dominate the vaginal smear under the unopposed influence of oestradiol; under extreme oestradiol influence, cells become anuclear.

Several systems are in use for quantitating steroid influence on vaginal cytology from the vaginal pool or from the lateral vaginal wall. The *karyopyknotic index* is the percentage of squamous cells with nuclear pyknosis; its value is limited by not taking into account the presence or absence of parabasal cells. The *maturation index* is more informative, being a differential count of the three possible types of exfoliated cells: parabasal/intermediate/superficial.

Cyclical changes in vaginal secretion

The vagina is kept moist by transudation of fluid through the vaginal epithelium and by cervical secretion (Moghissi, 1979). The cervical component of vaginal moisture is increased by oestradiol, as described earlier, but in women who have had a hysterectomy and bilateral ovariectomy it is clear that vaginal transudation is also increased by oestrogens (Perl et al, 1959). The mechanism of oestrogen-induced vaginal transudation at midcycle is thought simply to be increased mucosal blood flow.

Sexual arousal and orgasm

Four levels of sexual arousal have been described (Masters & Johnson, 1966). The first physiological evidence of the human female's response to any form of sexual stimulation occurs during the *excitement phase* and is the production of vaginal lubrication, which is a transudate increased by marked vasocongestion in the vaginal mucosa. Transudation decreases slightly in the second or *plateau phase*, during which vasocongestion becomes localised and extreme in the lower third of the vagina. The explosive physiological entity of orgasm is centred on this area during the *orgasmic phase*, during which regular contractions of the vagina's muscle coat occur at 0.8 second intervals. Muscle contractions stop and vasocongestion subsides during the *resolution phase*.

The cervix participates in sexual arousal only by gaping during the resolution phase. The myometrium shows activity that is to some extent coordinated, but less so than during menstruation or early labour; regular fundal contractions start 2 to 4 seconds after subjective awareness of the onset of the orgasmic experience; the contractions may be painful, especially in multiparas (Masters & Johnson, 1966).

The neurohumoral mechanisms behind the events of sexual excitement are not precisely understood, but parasympathetic innervation is probably important. Recent studies imply an important role for vasoactive intestinal polypeptide (VIP) peptidergic neurons: VIP-containing nerve fibres are more abundant in the vagina and clitoris than in any other part of the reproductive tract; VIP-infusion produces vasodilation and an increase in vaginal blood flow; and VIP concentrations in peripheral venous blood increase during sexual arousal (Ottesen, 1983). The reactions described, including lubrication and smooth muscle contraction, can take place after bilateral ovariectomy, so are independent of oestradiol, and increased vaginal transudation with sexual arousal can also take place in a surgically-produced artificial vagina.

VULVA

Cutaneous androgen action

Although the main steroid influence on the adult internal genitalia comes from oestrogen and progesterone, the adult vulva and surrounding pubic skin depend considerably on androgens for maintenance. (Androgen receptors are found in the endometrium, but their role is unknown–Rose et al, 1978.)

The main circulating androgen, in women as well as in men, is testosterone; the weaker circulating androgens androstenedione and dehydroepiandrosterone (DHA) appear to owe their action to conversion to testosterone in the skin. The ability of DHA and the $\Delta5$ steroid $\Delta5$-androstenediol to act as androgens depends on tissue expression of the 3β-ol dehydrogenase/$\Delta5,4$-isomerase enzyme — unlike androstenedione, which in addition to being a testosterone precursor in target tissues also contributes to circulating testosterone (Thomas & Oake, 1974; Givens, 1978; Mauvis-Jarvis, 1977). However, the most potent androgen, and the androgen for which most peripheral tissue receptors (Chan & O'Malley, 1976) are specific, is testosterone's reduced metabolite: *dihydrotestosterone*

(DHT) (Wilson & Walker, 1969). The distribution of testosterone 5α-reductase, which converts testosterone to DHT, shows great regional variation, being concentrated in the derivatives of the urogenital ridge (the clitoris and the labia majora) (Wilson & Walker, 1969) and also in regions bearing ambosexual hair (the lower pubic triangle and the axillae, which are sensitive to low levels of androgens) (Parker, 1981).

Just as the internal genitalia govern oestradiol action by the rate of metabolism of oestradiol to oestrone, so the external genitalia govern androgen exposure by adjusting the balance between testosterone and androstenedione, by governing the rate of DHT formation from testosterone, and by influencing the metabolism of testosterone and DHT to the 5α-androstanediols (Liang et al, 1977). Oestradiol and progesterone both have anti-androgenic actions peripherally, the effects of which may be lost after the menopause: oestradiol competes with testosterone for 17β-oxidoreductase; progesterone, and C-21 progestogens such as medroxyprogesterone acetate, compete with testosterone for 5α-reductase (Parker, 1981).

DHT is by no means the obligatory androgen. Not only is there a clear distinction between different regions of skin in response to androgens as a group, but the further one looks down the delta of intracellular cutaneous androgen metabolic transformations the greater are the qualitative and quantitative differences likely to be observed in steroid metabolism, which can vary enormously in different cutaneous appendages only microscopic distances apart (Liang et al, 1977; Givens, 1978). It has been suggested that metabolites such as 5α-androstane-3α, 17β-diol may act as potent androgens on their own specific receptors in certain systems (Evans & Pierrepoint, 1975). Finally the skin also contains conjugating enzymes, so metabolites do not need further processing by the liver for inactivation before being being excreted.

Chalones and vulval dystrophy

In addition to their action on skin appendages such as hair follicles and sebaceous sweat glands, androgens affect epidermal cell turnover. Observation on the local effect of steroids on axillary skin (Papa & Kligman, 1965) indicate a hyperplastic action for testosterone and an atrophic action for corticosteroids (and little action at all for oestrogens). It is now thought that this expression of steroid action is mediated through changes in the production of *dermal growth factors* and tissue specific *chalones* (Friedrich, 1976), which are high MW polypeptides that inhibit mitosis in the cell line they arise from and so control cell numbers in that tissue (Rytömaa, 1976; Marks, 1976). Friedrich has proposed that effects on such mechanisms explain the therapeutic effect of testosterone and corticosteroids on, respectively, *lichen sclerosis et atrophicus* and *hypertrophic vulval dystrophy*.

Post-menopausal women with lichen sclerosis do not differ in plasma oestrogens or androgens from normal post-menopausal women (Baird, 1979) and so this condition can be seen as being a manifestation of *end-organ resistance* in the vulva.

The further exploration of locally-acting polypeptides, which are similar in structure to insulin and included among which is relaxin (mentioned earlier as being an important hormone in softening connective tissues during pregnancy), constitute a new dimension for the future in the exploration of endocrine responses in the genital tract. The receptor system (or systems) for this class of polypeptides is still quite uncharacterised (Cohen, 1982).

REFERENCES

Aitken R J 1979 Tubal and uterine secretions; the possibilities for contraceptive attack. Journal of Reproduction and Fertility 55: 247–254

Allen A 1978 Structure of gastrointestinal mucus glycoproteins and the viscous and gel-forming properties of mucus. British Medical Bulletin 34: 28–33

Amoroso E C, Heap R B, Renfree M B 1979 Hormones and the evolution of viviparity In: Barrington E J W (ed) Hormones and Evolution, pp 925–989. Academic Press, New York

Andrews M C 1951 Epithelial changes in the puerperal fallopian tube. American Journal of Obstetrics and Gynecology 62: 28–37

Asch R H 1978 Sperm recovery in peritoneal aspirate after negative Sims-Huhner test. International Journal of Fertility 23: 57–60

Averette H E, Weinstein G D, Frost P 1970 Autoradiographic analysis of cell proliferation kinetics in human genital tissues. I. Normal cervix and vagina. American Journal of Obstetrics and Gynecology 108: 8–17

Bailly A, Savourer J-F, Sallas N, Milgrom E 1978 Factors modifying the equilibrium between activated and non-activated forms of steroid-receptor complexes. European Journal of Biochemistry 88: 623–632

Baird P 1979 Ph.D. Thesis. University of Sydney, Australia

Barr M L 1974 The Human Nervous System. An Anatomical Viewpoint, pp 343–344. Harper and Row, Hagerstown

Barrington E J W 1975 An Introduction to General and Comparative Endocrinology, 2nd edn, pp 106–128. Clarendon Press, Oxford

Bartelmez G W 1933 Histological studies on the menstruating mucous membrane of the human uterus. Contributions to Embryology, Carnegie Institution of Washington 24: 143–187

Bartelmez G W, Corner G W, Hartman C G 1951 Cyclic changes in the endometrium of the Rhesus monkey (Macaca mulatta). Contributions to Embryology, Carnegie Institution of Washington 34: 99–146

Batra S, Helm G, Owman C, Sjöberg N-O, Walles B 1980 Female sex steroid concentrations in the ampullary and isthmic regions of the human fallopian tube and their relationship to plasma concentrations during the menstrual cycle. American Journal of Obstetrics and Gynecology 136: 986–991

Baulieu E E, Mortel R, Robel P 1980 Oestrogen and progesterone receptors in human endometrium: regulatory and pathophysiological aspects. In: Diczfalusy E, Fraser I S, Webb F T G (eds) WHO Symposium on Steroid Contraception and Mechanism of Endometrial Bleeding, pp 266–290. Pitman, Bath

Bayard F, Damilano S, Robel P, Baulieu E-E 1978 Cytoplasmic and nuclear estradiol and progesterone receptors in human endometrium. Journal of Clinical Endocrinology and Metabolism 46: 635–648

Bentley P J 1976 Comparative Vertebrate Endocrinology. Cambridge University Press, Cambridge

Bigazzi M, Nardi E 1981 Prolactin and relaxin: antagonism on the sponataneous motility of the·uterus. Journal of Clinical Endocrinology and Metabolism 53: 665–667

Bigazzi M, Pollicino G, Nardi E 1979 Is human decidua a specialized endocrine organ? Journal of Clinical Endocrinology and Metabolism 49: 847–850

Birnbaumer L 1977 The actions of hormones nucleotides on membrane-bound adenylyl cyclases: an overview. In: O'Malley B W, Birnbaumer L (eds) Receptors and Hormone Action, Volume I, pp 485–547. Academic Press, New York

Bitensky L, Cohen S 1965 The variation of endometrial acid phosphatase activity with the menstrual cycle. Journal of Obstetrics and Gynaecology of the British Commonwealth 72: 769–774

Bjorkman N, Fredricsson B 1962 Ultrastructural features of the human oviduct epithelium. International Journal of Fertility 7: 259–266

Blandau R J, Bourdage R, Halbert S 1979 Tubal transport. In: Beller F K, Schumacher G F B (eds) The Biology of the Fluids of the Female Genital Tract, pp 319–333. Elsevier/North Holland, New York

Bodkhe R R Harper M J K 1972 Changes in the amount of adrenergic neurotransmitter in the genital tract of untreated rabbits, and rabbits given reserpine or iproniazid during the time of egg transport. Biology of Reproduction 6: 288–299

Bonte J 1972 Medroxyprogesterone in the management of primary and recurrent or metastatic uterine adenocarcinoma. Acta Obstetrica et Gynecologica Scandinavica 19: 21–24

Boutselis J G 1973 Histochemistry of the normal endometrium. In: Norris H J, Hertig A T, Abell M R (eds) The Uterus, pp 175–184 Williams and Wilkins, Baltimore

Bowman J A Jr 1968 The effect of norethindrone-mestranol on cervical mucus. American Journal of Obstetrics and Gynecology 102: 1039–1040

Braunwald E 1982 Mechanism of action of calcium-channel-blocking agents. New England Journal of Medicine 307: 1618–1627

Brenner R M, Resko J A, West N B 1974 Cyclic changes in oviductal morphology and residual cytoplasmic estradiol binding capacity induced by sequential estradiol-progesterone treatment of spayed rhesus monkeys. Endocrinology 95: 1094–1104

Brotherton J 1976 Sex Hormone Pharmacology, pp 127–129. Academic Press, New York

Bryant-Greenwood G D 1982 Relaxin as a new hormone. Endocrine Reviews 3: 62–90

Buchman M I, Kramer E, Feldman G B 1978 Aspiration curettage for asymptomatic patients receiving estrogen. Obstetrics and Gynecology 51: 339–341

Caldeyro-Barcia R, Poseiro J J 1965 The powers and the mechanism of labor. In: Greenhill J P (ed) Obstetrics. 13th edn, pp 278–304. WB Saunders, Philadelphia

Campbell S, Whitehead M 1977 Oestrogen therapy and the menopausal syndrome. Clinics in Obstetrics and Gynaecology 4: 31–47

Carlson D M 1977 Chemistry and biosynthesis of mucin glycoproteins. Advances in Experimental Medicine and Biology 89: 251–273

Carsten M 1973 Prostaglandins and cellular calcium transport in the pregnant human uterus. American Journal of Obstetrics and Gynecology 117: 824–832

Carsten M E 1979 Calcium accumulation by human uterine microsomal preparations: effects of progesterone and oxytocin. American Journal of Obstetrics and Gynecology 133: 598–601

Cavasos F, Lucas F V 1973 Ultrastructure of the endometrium. In: Norris H J, Hertig A T, Abell M R (eds) The Uterus, pp 136–174. Williams and Wilkins, Baltimore

Chan L, O'Malley B W 1976 Mechanism of action of the sex steroid hormones. New England Journal of Medicine 294: 1322–1328, 1372–1381, 1430–1437

Chatkoff M L 1975 A biophysicist's view of ovum transport Gynecologic Investigation 6: 105–122

Check J H 1980 Treatment of cervical factor with combined high-dose estrogen and human menopausal gonadotropins. Fertility and Sterility 33: 562–563

Cheng C Y, Boettcher B 1981 Effects of steroids on the in vitro forward migration of human spermatozoa. Contraception 24: 183–188

Chilton B S, Nicosia S V, Laufer M R 1980 Effect of estradiol-17β on endocervical cytodifferentiation and glycoprotein biosynthesis in the ovariectomized rabbit. Biology of Reproduction 23: 677–686

Chretien F C, Gernigon C, David G, Psychoyos A 1973 The ultrastructure of human cervical mucus under scanning electron microscopy. Fertility and Sterility 24: 746–757

Chretien F C, Cohen J, Borg V, Psychoyos A 1975 Human cervical mucus during the menstrual cycle and pregnancy in normal and pathological conditions. Journal of Reproductive Medicine 14: 192–196

Chretien F C, Sureau C, Neau C 1980 Experimental study of cervical blockage induced by continuous low-dose oral progestogens. Contraception 22: 445–456

Clamp J R, Allen A, Gibbons R A, Roberts G P 1978 Chemical aspects of mucus. British Medical Bulletin 34: 25–41

Clark J H Peck E J Jr 1977 Steroid hormone receptors: basic principles measurement. In: O'Malley B W, Birnbaumer L (eds) Receptors and Hormone Action. Volume I. pp 383–410. Academic Press, New York

Clark J H, Markeverich B M 1981 Relationships between Type I and Type II estradiol binding sites and estrogen induced responses. Journal of Steroid Biochemistry 15: 49–54

Clark J H, Paszko Z, Peck E J Jr 1977a Nuclear binding and retention of the receptor estrogen complex: relation to the agonistic and antagonistic properties of estriol. Endocrinology 100: 91–96

Clark J H, Peck E J Jr, Hardin J W, Eriksson H 1977b The biology and pharmacology of estrogen receptor binding: relationship to uterine growth. In: O'Malley B W, Birnbaumer L (eds) Receptors and Hormone Action. Volume II, pp 1–31. Academic Press, New York

Clemetson C A B, Kim J K, de Jesus T P S, Mallikarjuneswara V R, Wilds J H 1973 Human uterine fluid potassium and the menstrual cycle. Journal of Obstetrics and Gynaecology of the British Commonwealth 80: 553–561

Clift A F 1979 Early studies on the rheology of cervical mucus. American Journal of Obstetrics and Gynecology 134: 829–832

Cline D L 1979 Unsuspected subclinical pregnancies in patients with luteal phase defects. American Journal of Obstetrics and Gynecology 134: 438–444

Clyman M J 1966 Electronmicroscopy of the human fallopian tube. Fertility and Sterility 17: 281–301

Cohen P 1982 The role of protein phosphorylation in neural and hormonal control of cellular activity. Nature 296: 613–620

Cohen C J, Deppe G 1977 Endometrial carcinoma and oral contraceptive agents. Obstetrics and Gynecology 49: 390–392

Cohen L F, di Sant'Agnese P A, Friedlander J 1980 Cystic fibrosis and pregnancy. A national survey. Lancet ii: 842–844

Collins J 1972 Combined hormone therapy for recurrent adenocarcinoma of the endometrium. American Journal of Obstetrics and Gynecology 113: 842–843

Cooke I D, Morgan C A, Parry T E 1972 Correlation of endometrial biopsy and plasma progesterone levels in infertile women. Journal of Obstetrics and Gynaecology of the British Commonwealth 79: 647–650

Cooke I D, Lenton E A, Adams M, Pearce M A, Fahmy D, Evans C R 1977 Some aspects of pituitary-ovarian relationships in women with ovulatory infertility. Journal of Reproduction and Fertility 51: 203–213

Cornier E, Chatelet F, Grenier J, Valade S, Salat-Baroux J, Roland J 1980 Epithelium cilie de la trompe de Fallope chez la femme. Etude ultrastructurale. Journal de Gynecologie, Obstetrique et Biologie de la Reproduction (Paris) 9: 505–511

Coupland R E 1960 The distribution of cholinesterase-positive nerve fibres in the human uterus [Abstract]. Journal of Anatomy 94: 289

Coupland R E 1979 Catecholamines In: Barrington E J W (ed) Hormones and Evolution, pp 309–341. Academic Press, New York

Coutinho E M, Maia H S 1971 The contractile response of the human uterus, Fallopian tubes and ovary to prostaglandins in vivo. Fertility and Sterility 22: 539–544

Critoph F N, Dennis K J 1978 Ciliary activity in the human oviduct. British Journal of Obstetrics and Gynaecology 84: 216–218

Croxatto H B, Ortiz M-E, Guiloff E, Ibarra A, Salvatierra A-M, Croxatto H-D, Spilman C H 1978a Effect of 15(S)-15-methyl prostaglandin F$_{2\alpha}$ on human oviductal motility and ovum transport. Fertility and Sterility 30: 408–414

Croxatto H B, Ortiz M E, Diaz S, Hess R, Balmaceda J, Croxatto H-D 1978b Studies on the duration of egg transport by the human oviduct. II. Ovum location at various intervals following luteinizing hormone peak. American Journal of Obstetrics and Gynecology 132: 629–634

Csapo A, Erdos T, de Mattos C R, Gramms E, Moscowitz C 1965 Stretch-induced uterine growth, protein synthesis and function. Nature 207: 1378–1379

Csapo A I, Pulkkinen M O, West W G 1973 Effects of luteectomy and progesterone replacement therapy in early pregnant patients. American Journal of Obstetrics and Gynecology 115: 759–765

Dallenbach-Hellweg G 1980 The influence of contraceptive steroids on the histological appearance of the endometrium. In: Diczfalusy E, Fraser I S, Webb F T G (eds) Endometrial Bleeding and Steroid Contraception, pp 153–173. Pitman, Bath

Daly D C, Tohen N, Doney T J, Maslar I A, Riddick D H 1982 The significance of lymphocytic-leukocytic infiltrates in interpreting late luteal phase endometrial biopsies. Fertility and Sterility 37: 786–791

Daniel E E, Lucien P, Posey V A, Paton D M 1975a A functional analysis of the myogenic control systems of the human Fallopian tube. American Journal of Obstetrics and Gynecology 121: 1046–1053

Daniel E E, Posey V A, Paton D M 1975b A structural analysis of the myogenic control systems of the human Fallopian tube. American Journal of Obstetrics and Gynecology 121: 1054–1066

Daunter B 1978 Sialic acid levels and scanning electronmicroscopy of cervical mucus. Contraception 17: 27–34

Daunter B, Chantler E N, Elstein M 1976 The scanning electronmicroscopy of human cervical mucus in the non-pregnant and pregnant states. British Journal of Obstetrics and Gynaecology 83: 783–743

Davajan V, Kunitake G M 1969 Fractional in-vivo and in-vitro examination of postcoital cervical mucus. Fertility and Sterility 20: 197–

Delforge J P, Ferin J 1970 A histometric study of two estrogens: ethinyl-estradiol and its 3-methyl-ether derivative (mestranol); their comparative effect upon the growth of the human endometrium. Contraception 1: 57–72

Devoto L, Soto E, Magofke A M, Sierralta W 1980 Unconjugated steroids in the fallopian tube and peripheral blood during the normal menstrual cycle. Fertility and Sterility 33: 613–617

Diczfalusy E 1968 Mode of action of contraceptive drugs. American Journal of Obstetrics and Gynecology 100: 136–163

Dodson K S, Macnaughton M C, Coutts J R T 1975a Infertility in women with apparently ovulatory cycles. I. Comparison of their plasma sex steroid and gonadotrophin profiles with those in the normal cycle. British Journal of Obstetrics and Gynaecology 82: 615–624

Dodson K S, Macnaughton M C, Coutts J R T 1975b Infertility in women with apparently ovulatory cycles. II. The effects of clomiphene treatment on the profiles of gonadotrophin and sex steroid hormones in peripheral plasma. British Journal of Obstetrics and Gynaecology 82: 625–633

Doll R, Kinlen L J, Skegg D C G, Smith P G, Vessey M P 1977 Hormone replacement therapy and endometrial carcinoma. Lancet i: 745

Donnez J, Langerock S, Thomas K 1982 Peritoneal fluid volume and 17β-estradiol and progesterone concentrations in ovulatory, anovulatory, and postmenopausal women. Obstetrics and Gynecology 59: 687–692

Eddy C A, Flores J J, Archer D R, Pauerstein C J 1978 The role of cilia in fertility: an evaluation by selective microsurgical modification of the rabbit oviduct. American Journal of Obstetrics and Gynecology 132: 814–821

Eddy W A 1978 Endometrial carcinoma in Stein-Leventhal syndrome treated with hydroxyprogesterone caproate. American Journal of Obstetrics and Gynecology 131: 581–582

Ehrlich C E, Young P C M, Cleary R E 1981 Cytoplasmic progesterone and estradiol receptors in normal, hyperplastic, and carcinomatous endometria: therapeutic implications. American Journal of Obstetrics and Gynecology 141: 539–546

Eichner E, Goler G G, Reed J, Gordon M B 1951 The experimental production and prolonged maintenance of decidua in the nonpregnant woman. American Journal of Obstetrics and Gynecology 61: 253–264

Elliott J P 1983 Magnesium sulfate as a tocolytic agent. American Journal of Obstetrics and Gynaecology 147: 277–284

Elliott P M, Krozowski Z, Jansen R P S 1980 Cytosol oestradiol and progesterone receptors in endometrial hyperplasia and adenocarcinoma. Australian and New Zealand Journal of Obstetrics and Gynaecology 20: 199–204

Elstein M, Daunter B 1976 The structure of cervical mucus. In: Jordan J A, Singer A (eds) The Cervix, pp 137–147. W B Saunders, London

Elstein M, Mitchell R F, Syrett J T 1971 Ultrastructure of cervical mucus. Journal of Obstetrics and Gynaecology of the British Commonwealth 78: 180–183

Evans L H, Martin J D, Hähnel R 1974 Estrogen receptor concentration in normal and pathological human uterine tissues. Journal of Clinical Endocrinology and Metabolism 38: 23–32

Evans C R, Pierrepoint C G 1975 Demonstration of a specific cytosol receptor in the normal and hyperplastic canine prostate for 5 α-androstane-3-α, 17β-diol. Journal of Endocrinology 64: 539–

Fechner R E 1971 The surgical pathology of the reproductive system and breast during oral contraceptive therapy. Pathology Annual 6: 299–319

Fechner R E, Kaufmann H K 1974 Endometrial adenocarcinoma in Stein-Leventhal syndrome. Cancer 34: 444–452

Ferenczy A, Bertrand G, Gelfand M M 1979 Proliferation kinetics of human endometrium during the normal menstrual cycle. American Journal of Obstetrics and Gynecology 133: 859–867

Ferenczy A, Richart R M 1974 Female Reproductive System: Dynamics of Scan and Transmission Electron Microscopy, pp 213–254. Wiley, New York

Ferenczy A, Guralnick M S 1979 Morphology of the human vagina. In: Beller F K, Schumacher G F B (eds) The Biology of the Fluids of the Female Genital Tract, pp 3–12. Elsevier/North-Holland, New York

Ferin J 1971 The effects of progesterone on the human uterovaginal tract. International Encyclopedia of Pharmacology and Therapeutics, Volume 1, Ch 22

Fettig O 1965 Autoradiographische Untersuchungen der DNS-RNS-und Protein Synthese im menschlichen Endometrium in Abhangigkeit von der Ovulation. Archiv für Gynäkologie 202: 246–251

Finn C A, Porter D G 1975 The Uterus, pp 204–229. Elek Science, London

Flickinger G L, Elsner C, Illingworth D V, Muechler E K, Mikhail G 1977 Estrogen and progesterone receptors in the female genital tract of humans and monkeys. Annals of the New York Academy of Sciences 286: 180–189

Flowers C E, Wilborn W H 1978 New observations on the physiology of menstruation. Obstetrics and Gynecology 51: 16–24

Flowers C E, Wilborn W H 1979 Histoenzymology of the human endometrium during menstruation (II). In: Beller F K, Schumacher G F B (eds) The Biology of the Fluids of the Female Genital Tract, pp 203–223. Elsevier/North-Holland, New York

Fordney Settlage D S, Motoshima M, Tredway D R 1973 Sperm transport from the external cervical os to the fallopian tubes in women: a time and quantitation study. Fertility and Sterility 24: 655–661

Fredriksson B, Björkman N 1962 Studies on the ultrastructure of the human oviduct epithelium in different functional states. Zeitschrift für Zellforschung 58: 387–402

Fredriksson B, Björkman N 1973 Morphologic alterations in the human oviduct epithelium induced by contraceptive steroids. Fertility and Sterility 24: 19–30

Friberg J 1981a Postcoital testing in relation to circulating sperm-agglutinating antibodies in women. American Journal of Obstetrics and Gynecology 139: 587–591

Friberg J 1981b Postcoital tests and sperm-agglutinating antibodies in men. American Journal of Obstetrics and Gynecology 141: 76–80

Fried, P H, Rakoff A E 1952 The effects of chorionic gonadotropin and prolactin on the maintenance of corpus luteum function. Journal of Clinical Endocrinology and Metabolism 12: 321–337

Friedrich E G 1976 Lichen sclerosus. Journal of Reproductive Medicine 17: 147–154

Fromm E, Garcia C-R, Jeutter D C 1976 Physiologic assessment of oviductal motility — extraluminal telemetric subject evaluation. In: Harper M J K, Pauerstein C J, Adams C E, Coutinho E M, Croxatto H B, Paton D M (eds) Ovum Transportation and Fertility Regulation, pp 107–125. Scriptor, Copenhagen

Frost J K 1979 Gynecologic and obstetric clinical cytopathology. In: Novak E R, Woodruff J D (eds) Novak's Gynecologic and Obstetric Pathology with Clinical and Endocrine Relations, pp 689–781. W B Saunders, Philadelphia

Fuchs A-R, Fuchs F, Husslein P, Soloff M S, Fernström M J 1982 Oxytocin receptors and human parturition: a dual role for oxytocin in the initiation of labor. Science 215: 1396–1398

Fuentealba B E, Escudero G, Swaneck G E 1976 Progesterone binding protein in cytosol fraction from human oviduct. In: Harper M J K, Pauerstein C J, Adams C E, Coutinho E M, Croxatto H B, Paton D M (eds) Ovum Transport and Fertility Regulation, pp 527–538. Scriptor, Copenhagen

Garfield R E, Hayashi R H 1980 Presence of gap junctions in the myometrium of women during various stages of menstruation. American Journal of Obstetrics and Gynecology 138: 569–574

Garfield R E, Hayashi R H 1981 Appearance of gap junctions in the myometrium of women in labor. American Journal of Obstetrics and Gynecology 140: 254–260

Garfield R E, Puri C P, Csapo A I 1982 Endocrine, structural, and functional changes in the uterus during premature labor. American Journal of Obstetrics and Gynecology 142: 21–27

Genz T, Eiletz J, Kreuzer G, Pollow K, Schmidt-Gollwitzer M 1980 Untersuchungen zur endokrinen Regulation des Endometriums wahrend des mensuellen Zyklus. Geburtshilfe und Fraunheilkunde 40: 990–999

Gerulath A H, Borth R 1977 Effect of progesterone and estradiol-17β on nucleic acid synthesis in vitro in carcinoma of the endometrium. American Journal of Obstetrics and Gynecology 128: 772–776

Gibbons R A 1978 Mucus of the mammalian genital tract. British Medical Bulletin 34: 34–38

Giner J, Merino G, Luna J, Aznar R 1974 Evaluation of the Sims-Huhner postcoital test in fertile couples. Fertility and Sterility 25: 145–148

Givens J R 1978 Normal and abnormal androgen metabolism. Clinical Obstetrics and Gynecology 21: 115–123

Goldzieher J W, Green J A 1962 The polycystic ovary. I. Clinical and histologic features. Journal of Clinical Endocrinology and Metabolism 22: 325–338

Gompel C 1962 The ultrastructure of the human endometrial cell studied by electronmicroscopy. American Journal of Obstetrics and Gynecology 84: 1000–1009

Goto M, Csapo A 1959 The effect of the ovarian steroids on the membrane potential of uterine muscle. Journal of General Physiology 43: 455–467

Gottschalk A 1960 Correlation between composition, structure, shape and function of a salivary mucoprotein. Nature 186: 949–951

Gould K G, Ansari A H 1983 Chemical alteration of cervical mucus by electrolytes. American Journal of Obstetrics and Gynecology 145: 92–99

Greenblatt R B 1977 Estrogens and endometrial cancer — gross exaggeration or fact? Geriatrics 32: 60–72

Gregoire A T, Kandil O, Ledger W J 1971 The glycogen content of human vaginal epithelial tissue. Fertility and Sterility 22: 64–68

Gurpide E, Tseng L, Gusberg S B 1977 Estrogen Metabolism in normal and neoplastic endometrium. American Journal of Obstetrics and Gynecology 129: 809–816

Gurpide E, Welch M 1969 Dynamics of uptake of estrogens and androgens by human endometrium. Journal of Biological Chemistry 244: 5159–5169

Gusberg S B 1967 Hormone-dependence of endometrial cancer. Obstetrics and Gynecology 30: 287–293

Guyton A C 1981 Textbook of Medical Physiology, 6th edn, pp 138–148. W B Saunders, Philadelphia

Hackl H 1971 Zur hormonellen Steuerung der Glykogensynthese im humanen Endometrium. Archiv für Gynäkologie 211: 617–626

Hagenfeldt K 1980 Prostaglandins and related compounds and their metabolism in normal and steroid-exposed endometrium. In: Diczfalusy E, Fraser I S, Webb F T G (eds) Endometrial Bleeding and Steroidal Contraception, pp 222–245 Pitman, Bath

Halbert S A, Tam, P Y, Blandau R J 1976 Egg transport in the rabbit oviduct: the roles of cilia and muscle. Science 191: 1052–1053

Hammond M G, Radwanska E, Talbert L M 1980 Effect of clomiphene citrate on corticosteroid-binding globulin and serum progesterone levels during ovulation induction. Fertility and Sterility 33: 383–386

Hanson F W, Overstreet J W, Katz D F 1982 A study of the relationship of motile sperm numbers in cervical mucus 48 hours after artificial insemination with subsequent fertility. American Journal of Obstetrics and Gynecology 143: 85–90

Hashimoto M, Shimoyama T, Kosaka M, Komori A, Hirasawa T, Yokoyama Y, Akashi K 1962 Electron microscopic studies on the epithelial cells of the human fallopian tube (Report I). Journal of the Japanese Obstetrical and Gynecological Society 9: 200–209

Hashimoto M, Shimoyama T, Kosaka M, Komori A, Hirasawa T, Yokoyama Y, Kawase N, Akashi K 1964 Electron microscopic studies on the epithelial cells of the human fallopian tube (Report II). Journal of the Japanese Obstetrical and Gynecological Society 11: 92–100

Hatcher V B, Schwarzmann G O H, Jeanloz R W, McArthur J W 1977 Changes in the sialic acid concentration in the major cervical glycoprotein from the bonnet monkey (Macaca radiata) during a hormonally induced cycle. Fertility and Sterility 28: 682–688

Haukkamaa M, Karjalainen O, Luukkainen T 1971 In vitro binding of progesterone by the human endometrium during the menstrual cycle and by hyperplastic, atrophic, and carcinomatous endometrium. American Journal of Obstetrics and Gynecology 111: 205–210

Healy D L, Herington A C, O'Herlihy C 1983 Chronic idiopathic polyhydramnios: evidence for a defect in the chorion laeve receptor for lactogenic hormones. Journal of Clinical Endocrinology and Metabolism 56: 520–523

Heap R B, Perry J S, Challis J R G 1973 Hormonal maintenance of pregnancy. In: Astwood E, Grey R (eds) Handbook of Physiology. Section 7, Volume II, Part 2, pp 217–260. Baltimore: American Physiological Society

Helm G, Otteson B, Fahrenkrug J, Larsen J-J, Owman C, Sjöberg N-O, Stolberg B, Sundler F, Walles B 1981 Vasoactive intestinal polypeptide (VIP) in the human female reproductive tract: distribution and motor effects. Biology of Reproduction 25: 227–234

Henzl M R, Smith R E, Boost G, Tyler E T 1972 Lysosomal concept of menstrual bleeding in humans. Journal of Clinical Endocrinology and Metabolism 34: 860–875

Hirata F, Axelrod J 1980 Phospholipid methylation and biological signal transmission. Science 209: 1082–1090

Hodgson B J 1978 Post-ovulatory changes in the water content and inulin space of the rabbit oviduct. Journal of Reproduction and Fertility 53: 349–351

Hodgson B J, Eddy C A 1975 The autonomic nervous system and its relationship to tubal ovum transport — a reappraisal. Gynecologic Investigation 6: 162–185

Hodgson B J, Fremming B D, Daly S 1975 Effects of adrenergic drugs administered during ovum transport and chemical sympathectomy of the oviduct on fertility in rabbits. Biology of Reproduction 13: 142–146

Hökfelt T, Johansson O, Ljungdahl A, Lundberg J M, Schultzberg M 1980 Peptidergic neurones. Nature 284: 515–521

Hsueh A J W, Peck E J Jr Clark J H 1976 Control of uterine estrogen receptor levels by progesterone. Endocrinology 98: 438–444

Hsueh A J W, Erickson G F, Lu K H 1979 Changes in uterine estrogen receptor and morphology in aging female rats. Biology of Reproduction 21: 793–800

Hughes E C, Jacobs R D, Rubulis A, Husney R M 1963 Carbohydrate pathways of the endometrium: effects on ovular growth. American Journal of Obstetrics and Gynecology 85: 594–609

Iacobelli S, Garcea N, Angeloni C 1971 Biochemistry of cervical mucus: a comparative analysis of the secretion from preovulatory, postovulatory, and pregnancy periods. Fertility and Sterility 22: 727–734

Insler V 1977 The evaluation and treatment of cervical mucus diseases leading to infertility. Advances in Experimental Medicine and Biology 89: 477–488

Insler V, Melmed H, Eichenbrenner I, Serr D M, Lunenfeld B 1972 The cervical score. A simple semiquantitative method for monitoring of the menstrual cycle. International Journal of Gynaecology and Obstetrics 10: 223–228

Jansen R P S 1978 Fallopian tube isthmic mucus and ovum transport. Science 201: 349–351

Jansen R P S 1980a Cyclic changes in the human fallopian tube isthmus and their functional importance. American Journal of Obstetrics and Gynecology 136: 292–308

Jansen R P S 1980b Abortion incidence following fallopian tube repair. Obstetrics and Gynecology 56: 499–502

Jansen R P S 1981 Fallopian tube secretions: implications for tubal microsurgery. Australian and New Zealand Journal of Obstetrics and Gynaecology 21: 140–142

Jansen R P S 1982 Spontaneous abortion incidence in the treatment of infertility. American Journal of Obstetrics and Gynecology 143: 451–473

Jansen R P S 1983 Peritoneal and plasma estradiol and progesterone levels in mild and moderate endometriosis: a serach for luteinized unruptured follicles [Abstract]. Fertility and Sterility 39: 394

Jansen R P S 1984 Fertility in older women. International Planned Parenthood Federation Medical Bulletin, 18(2): 4–6

Jansen R P S, Bajpai V K 1983 Periovulatory glycoprotein secretion in the macaque fallopian tube. American Journal of Obstetrics and Gynecology 147: 598–608

Jansen R P S, Bajpai V K 1982 Oviduct acid mucus glycoproteins in the estrous rabbit: ultrastructure and histochemistry. Biology of Reproduction 26: 155–168

Jansen R P S, Elliott P M 1977 Oral contraceptives and endometrial carcinoma: case for progesterone-receptor defect. Lancet i: 602–603

Jansen R P S, Shearman R P 1981 Oncological endocrinology. In: Coppleson M (ed) Gynecologic Oncology, pp 96–120. Churchill Livingstone, Edinburgh

Jensen E V, Suzuki T, Numata M, Smith S, de Sombre E R 1969 Estrogen-binding substances of target tissues. Steroids 13: 417–427

Jette N T, Glass R H 1972 Prognostic value of the postcoital test. Fertility and Sterility 23: 29–32

Johannisson E 1980 The influence of contraceptive steroids on the histochemistry and cytochemistry of the normal endometrium. In: Diczfalusy E, Fraser I S, Webb T T G (eds) WHO Symposium on Steroid Contraception and Mechanism of Endometrial Bleeding, pp 174–190 Pitman Press, Bath

Johannisson E, Hagenfeldt K 1971 Isolation and cytochemical properties of human endometrial cells. In: Diczfalusy E (ed) Karolinska Symposia on Research Methods in Reproductive Endocrinology, 3rd Symposium : In Vitro Methods in Reproductive Cell Biology, pp 81–108 Acta Endocrinologica, Copenhazen

Johannisson E, Landgren B-M, Diczfalusy E 1982a Endometrial morhology and peripheral steroid levels in women with and without intermenstrual bleeding during contraception with 300 ug norethisterone (NET) minipill. Contraception 25: 13–30

Johannisson E, Parker R A, Landgren B-M, Diczfalusy E 1982b Morphometric analysis of the human endometrium in relation to peripheral hormone levels. Fertility and Sterility 38: 564–571

Johns A, Chlumecky J, Paton D M 1974 Role of adrenergic nerves in ovulation and ovum transport [Letter]. Lancet ii: 1079

Jones G 1968 Luteal phase defects. In: Behrman S J, Kistner R W (eds) Progress in Infertility, pp 299–325. Little Brown, Boston

Jones G E S, Maffezzoli R D, Strott C A, Ross G T, Kaplan G 1970 Pathophysiology of reproductive failure after clomiphene-induced ovulation. American Journal of Obstetrics and Gynecology 108: 847–865

Jones G S 1976 The luteal phase defect. Fertility and Sterility 27: 351–356

Jones H W, Brewer J I 1941 Studies of ovaries and endometrium of patients with fundal adenocarcinoma. American Journal of Obstetrics and Gynecology 42: 207

Jones W R 1980 Immunologic infertility — fact or fiction? Fertility and Sterility 33: 577–586

Joshi S G, Henriques E S, Smith R A, Szarowski D H 1980 Progestogen-dependent endometrial protein in women: tissue concentration in relation to developmental stage and to serum hormone levels. American Journal of Obstetrics and Gynecology 138: 1131–1136

Jungblut P W, Kallweit E, Sierralta W, Truitt A J, Wagner R K 1978 The occurrence of steroid-free, "activated" estrogen receptor in target cell nuclei. Hoppe-Seyler's Zeitschrift für Physiologische Chemistrie 359: 1259–1268

Kao C Y 1977 Electrophysiological properties of uterine smooth muscle. In: Wynn R M (ed) Biology of the Uterus, pp 423–496. Plenum, New York

Kaplan J 1981 Polypeptide-binding membrane receptors: analysis and classification. Science 212: 14–20

Kasid A, Laumas K R 1981 Nuclear progestin receptors in human uterus. Endocrinology 109: 553–560

Kaufmann R H, Binder G L, Gray P M Jr Adam E 1977 Upper genital tract changes associated with exposure in utero to diethylstilbestrol. American Journal of Obstetrics and Gynecology 128: 51–59

Keller D W, Wiest W G, Askin F B, Johnson L W, Strickler R C 1979 Pseudocorpus luteum insufficiency: a local defect of progesterone action on endometrial stroma. Journal of Clinical Endocrinology and Metabolism 48: 127–132

Kellett W W III Hester L L Jr Spicer S S, Williamson H O 1969 Effects of a sequential oral contraceptive on endocervical carbohydrate histochemistry. Obstetrics and Gynecology 34: 536–544

King R J B, Dyer G, Collins W P, Whitehead M I 1980 Intracellular estradiol, estrone and estrogen receptor levels in endometria from postmenopausal women receiving estrogens and progestins. Journal of Steroid Biochemistry 13: 377–382

Kistner R W 1970 The effects of progestational agents on hyperplasia and carcinoma in situ of the endometrium. International Journal of Gynaecology and Obstetrics 8: 561–572

Kistner R W, Griffiths C T, Craig J M 1965 Use of progestational agents in the management of endometrial cancer. Cancer 18: 1563–1579

Kokko E, Jänne O, Kauppila A, Vihko R 1981 Cyclic clomiphene citrate treatment lowers cytosol estrogen and progestin receptor concentrations in the endometrium of postmenopausal women on estrogen replacement therapy. Journal of Clinical Endocrinology and Metabolism 52: 345–349

Koligian K B, Stormshak F 1977 Progesterone inhibition of estrogen receptor replenishment in ovine endometrium. Biology of Reproduction 17: 412–416

Koninckz P R, Goddeeris P G, Lauweryns J M, de Hertogh R C, Brosens I A 1977 Accuracy of endometrial biopsy dating in relation to the midcycle luteinizing hormone peak. Fertility and Sterility 28: 443–445

Koninckx P R, Heyns W, Verhoeven G, van Baelen H, Lissens W D, de Moor P, Brosens I A 1980a Biochemical characterization of peritoneal fluid in women during the menstrual cycle. Journal of Clinical Endocrinology and Metabolism 51: 1239–1244

Koninckx P R, de Moor P, Brosens I 1980b Diagnosis of the luteinized unruptured follicle syndrome by steroid hormone assays on peritoneal fluid. British Journal of Obstetrics and Gynaecology 87: 929–934

Kopito L E, Kosasky H J, Sturgis S H, Lieberman B L, Swachman H 1973a Water and electrolytes in human cervical mucus. Fertility and Sterility 24: 499–506

Kopito L E, Kosasky H J, Swachman H 1973b Water and electrolytes in cervical mucus from patients with cystic fibrosis. Fertility and Sterility 24: 512–516

Kosasky H J, Kopito L E, Sturgis S H, Shwachman H 1973 Changes in water and electrolytes in human cervical mucus during treatment with chlormadinone acetate. Fertility and Sterility 24: 507–511

Kovacs G T, Newman G B, Henson G L 1978 The postcoital test: what is normal? British Medical Journal i: 818

Kreitmann B, Bugat R, Bayard F 1979 Estrogen and progestin regulation of the progesterone receptor concentration in human endometrium. Journal of Clinical Endocrinology and Metabolism 49: 926–929

Kroeks M V A M, Kremer J 1980 The role of crevical factors in infertility. In: Pepperell R J, Hudson B, Wood C (eds) The Infertile Couple, pp 113–125. Churchill Livingstone, Edinburgh

Kubo K, Kawano J, Ishii S 1970 Some observations on the autonomic innervation of the human oviduct. International Journal of Fertility 15: 30–35

Kugler P, Wrobel K-H, Wallner H J, Heinzmann U 1976 Hitochemische und histologische Untersuchungen am menslicher Eileiter unter verschiedenen hormonellen Einflüssen. I. ATPase-Nachweis mit besonderer Berücksichtigung reaktiver Zilienzellen. Archiv für Gynäkologie 221: 345–366

Lamb E J, Colliflower W W, Williams J W 1972 Endometrial histology and conception rates after clomiphene citrate. Obstetrics and Gynecology 39: 389–396

Landgren B M, Unden A L, Diczfalusy E 1980 Hormonal profile of the cycle in 68 normally menstruating women. Acta Endocrinologica 94: 89–98

Landgren B-M, Johannisson E, Masironi B, Diczfalusy E 1977 Studies on the pattern of circulating steroids in the normal menstrual cycle. Changes around the onset of menstruation. Acta Endocrinologica 86: 608–620

Leading Article 1981 Antisperm antibodies and fertility. Lancet i: 136–138

Leavitt W W, Chen T J, Do Y S, Carlton B D, Allen T C 1977 Biology of progesterone receptors. In: O'Malley B W, Birnbaumer L, (eds) Receptors and hormone action. Volume II, pp 157–188. Academic Press, New York

Lee T-P, Kuo J F, Greengard P 1972 Role of muscarinic cholinergic receptors in regulation of guanosine 3':5'-cyclic monophosphate content in mammalian brain, heart muscle, and intestinal smooth muscle. Proceedings of the National Academy of Sciences (USA) 69: 3287–3291

Lefkowitz R J 1976 β-adrenergic receptors: recognition and regulation. New England Journal of Medicine 295: 323–328

Lehmann F, Peters F, Breckwoldt M, Bettendorf G 1972 Plasma progesterone levels during infusion of prostaglandin F$_{2\alpha}$ in the human. Prostaglandins 1: 269–277

Lenton E A, Adams M, Cooke I D 1978 Plasma steroid and gonadotrophin profiles in ovulatory but infertile women. Clinical Endocrinology 8: 241–255

Levin R J, Edwards F 1968 The transuterine endometrial potential difference, its variation during the oestrous cycle and its relation to uterine secretion. Life Sciences 7: 1019–1036

Levy C, Robel P, Gautray J P, De Brux J, Verma U, Descomps B et al 1980 Estradiol and progesterone receptors in human endometrium. American Journal of Obstetrics and Gynecology 136: 646–651

Liang T, Tymoczko J L, Chan K M B, Hung S C, Liao S 1977 Androgen action: receptors and rapid responses. In: Martini L and Motta M (eds) Androgens and Antiandrogens, pp 77–89. Raven Press, New York

Lippman M E, Allegra J C 1978 Receptors in breast cancer. New England Journal of Medicine 299: 930–933

List S J, Findlay B P, Forstner G G, Forstner J F 1978 Enhancement of the viscosity of mucin by serum albumin. Biochemical Journal 175: 565–571

Ludwig H 1982 The morphologic response of the human endometrium to longterm treatment with progestational agents. American Journal of Obstetrics and Gynecology 142: 796–808

Ludwig, H, Metzger H 1976 The human female reproductive tract. A Scanning Electron Microscopic Atlas, pp 28–29, 79–10. Springer verlag, Berlin:

Lundy L E, Lee S G, Levy W, Woodruff J D, Wu C H, Abdalla M 1974 The ovulatory cycle: a histologic, thermal, steroid and gonadotropin correlation. Obstetrics and Gynecology 44: 14–25

Lye S J, Porter D G 1978 Demonstration that progesterone 'blocks' uterine activity in the ewe in vivo by a direct action on the myometrium. Journal of Reproduction and Fertility 52: 87–94

Lyon F A 1975 The development of adenocarcinoma of the endometrium in young women receiving long term sequential oral contraception. American Journal of Obstetrics and Gynecology 123: 299–301

MacLoughlin D T, Richardson G S 1976 Progesterone binding by

normal and abnormal human endometrium. Journal of Clinical Endocrinology and Metabolism 42: 667–678

Mack T M, Pike M C, Henderson B E, Pfeffer R I, Gerkins V R, Arthur M, Brown S C 1976 Estrogen and endometrial cancer in a retirement community. New England Journal of Medicine 294: 1262–1267

Maia H Jr Barbosa I, Coutinho E M 1976 Relationship between cyclic A M P levels and oviductal contractility. In: Harper M J K, Pauerstein C J, Adams C E, Coutinho E M, Croxatto H B, Paton D M (eds) Ovum Transportation and Fertility Regulation, pp 168–181. Scriptor, Copenhagen

Markee J E 1940 Menstruation in intraocular endometrial transplants in the Rhesus monkey. Contributions to Embryology, Carnegie Institute of Washington 28: 219–308

Markeverich B M, Upchurch S, Clark J H 1981 Progesterone and dexamethasone antagonism of uterine growth: a role for a second nuclear binding site for estradiol in estrogen action. Journal of Steroid Biochemistry 14: 125–132

Marks F 1976 Epidermal growth control mechanisms, hyperplasia, and tumor promotion in skin. Cancer Research 36: 2636–2643

Marshall J M 1974 Effects of neurohypophyseal hormones on the myometrium. In: Greys R, Astwood E (eds) Handbook of Physiology. Section 7, Volume IV, Part 1, pp 469–492. American Physiological Society, Baltimore

Martin G P, Marriott C, Kellaway I W 1978 The interaction of steroidal hormones with mucus glycoproteins. Journal of Pharmacy and Pharmacology 30 Suppl: 10P

Martin J D, Hähnel R 1978 Oestrogen receptor studies in carcinoma of the endometrium, carcinoma of the uterine cervix and other gynaecological malignancies. Australian and New Zealand Journal of Obstetrics and Gynaecology 18: 55–59

Martin J N Jr, Bygdeman M 1975 The effect of locally administered PGE$_2$ on the contractility of the nonpregnant human uterus in vivo. Prostaglandins 10: 253–265

Martin L, Finn C A 1968 Hormonal regulation of cell division in epithelial and connective tissues of the mouse uterus. Journal of Endocrinology 41: 363–371

Maslar I A, Riddick D H 1979 Prolactin production by human endometrium during the normal menstrual cycle. American Journal of Obstetrics and Gynecology 135: 751–754

Maslar I A, Kaplan B M, Luciano A A, Riddick D H 1980 Prolactin production by the endometrium of early human pregnancy. Journal of Clinical Endocrinology and Metabolism 51: 78–83

Masters W H, Johnson V E 1966 Human Sexual Response, pp 68–100. Little Brown, Boston

Matthews C D, Makin A E, Cox L W 1980 Experience with in vitro sperm penetration testing in infertile and fertile couples. Fertility and Sterility 33: 187–192

Mauvais-Jarvis P 1977 Androgen metabolism in human skin: mechanisms of control. In: Martini L, Motta M (eds) Androgens and Antiandrogens, pp 229–245. Raven Press, New York

McBain J C, Pepperell R J 1980 Unexplained infertility. In: Pepperell R J, Hudson B, Wood C (eds) The Infertile Couple, pp 164–181. Churchill Livingstone, Edinburgh

McCormack S, Clark J H 1979 Clomid administration to pregnant rats causes abnormalities of the reproductive tract in offspring and mothers. Science 204: 629–631

McDonald T W, Malkasian G S, Gaffey T A 1977 Endometrial cancer associated with feminizing ovarian tumor and polycystic ovarian disease. Obstetrics and Gynecology 49: 654–658

McKay D G, Hertig A T, Bardawil W A, Velardo J T 1956 Histochemical observations on the endometrium. I. Normal endometrium. Obstetrics and Gynecology 8: 22–39

McLaren A, Michie D 1956 Studies on the transfer of fertilized mouse eggs to uterine foster-mothers. I. Factors affecting the implantation and survival of native and transferred eggs. Journal of Experimental Biology 33: 394–416

McNatty K P, Smith D M, Makris A, Osathanondh R, Ryan K J 1980 Steroidogenesis by the human oocyte-cumulus cell complex in vitro. Steroids 35: 643–651

Means A R Dedman J R 1980 Calmodulin — an intracellular calcium receptor. Nature 285: 73–77

Meuris S, Soumenkoff G, Malengreau A, Robyn C 1980

Immunoenzymatic localization of prolactin-like immunoreactivity in decidual cells of the endometrium from pregnant and nonpregnant women. Journal of Histochemistry and Cytochemistry 12: 1347–1350

Meyer F A 1976 Mucus structure: relation to biological transport function. Biorheology 13: 49–58

Milgrom E, Thi M L, Baulieu E E 1973 Control mechanisms of steroid hormone receptors in the reproductive tract. Transactions, 6th Karolinska symposium on research methods in reproductive endocrinology "Protein synthesis in reproductive tissue", Geneva, pp 380–403

Milwidsky A, Palti Z, Gutman A 1980 Glycogen metabolism of the human endometrium. Journal of Clinical Endocrinology and Metabolism 51: 765–770

Mimori H, Fukuma K, Matsuo I, Nakahara K, Maeyama M 1981 Effects of progestogen on glycogen metabolism in the endometrium of infertile patients during the menstrual cycle. Fertility and Sterility 35: 289–295

Moawad A H, Kim M H, Zuspan F P, Chagrasulis R, Pishotta F T, Zuspan K J 1977 Effects of progesterone on the adrenergic mechanisms of the genital tract. Annals of the New York Academy of Sciences 286: 287–303

Moghissi K S 1979 The cervix in infertility. Clinical Obstetrics and Gynecology 22: 27–42

Moghissi K S, Marks C 1971 Effects of microdose norgestrel on endogenous gonadotropic and steroid hormones, cervical mucus properties, vaginal cytology, and endometrium. Fertility and Sterility 22: 424–434

Moghissi K S, Darich D, Lebine J, Neuhaus O W 1964 Mechanism of sperm migration. Fertility and Sterility 15: 15–

Moghissi K, Syner F N, McBride L C 1973 Contraceptive mechanism of microdose norethindrone. Obstetrics and Gynecology 41: 585–594

Moghissi K S, Sacco A G, Borin K 1980 Immunologic infertility. I. Cervical mucus antibodies and postcoital test. American Journal of Obstetrics and Gynecology 136: 941–950

Moran J, Davajan V, Nakamura 1974 Comparison of the fractional post-coital test with the Sims-Huhner post-coital test. International Journal of Fertility 19: 93–96

Morgan H, Stedronska J, Hendry W F, Chamberlain G V P, Dewhurst C J 1977 Sperm/cervical-mucus crossed hostility testing and antisperm antibodies in the husband. Lancet ii: 1228–1230

Morse A R, Hutton J D, Jacobs H S, Murray M A F, James V H T 1979 Relation between the karyopyknotic index and plasma oestrogen concentrations after the menopause. British Journal of Obstetrics and Gynaecology 86: 981–983

Moszkowski E, Woodruff J D, Jones G E S 1962 The inadequate luteal phase. American Journal of Obstetrics and Gynecology 83: 363–372

Mueehler E K, Flickinger G L, Mangan C E, Mikhail G 1975 Estradiol binding by human endometrial tissue. Gynecologic Oncology 3: 244–250

Murad F, Arnold W P, Mittal C K, Braughler J M 1979 Properties and regulation of guanylate cyclase and some proposed functions for cyclic G M P. Advances in Cyclic Nucleotide Research 11: 175–204

Nachtigall L E, Nachtigall R H, Nachtigall R D, Beckman E M 1976 Estrogens and endometrial carcinoma [Letter]. New England Journal of Medicine 204: 848

Nenci I, Fabris G, Marzola A, Marchetti E 1981 The plasma membrane as an additional level of steroid-cell interaction. Journal of Steroid Biochemistry 15: 231–234

Nilsson O, Westman A 1961 The ultrastructure of the epithelial cells of the endocervix during the menstrual cycle. Acta Obstetrica et Gynecologica Scandinavica 40: 223–233

Nilsson O, Hagenfeldt K, Johannisson E 1974 Ultrastructural signs of an interference in the carbohydrate metabolism of human endometrium produced by the intrauterine Copper-T device. Acta Obstetrica et Gynecologica Scandinavica 53: 139–149

Nordqvist S 1970 The synthesis of DNA and RNA in normal human endometrium in short-term incubation in vitro and its response to estradiol and progesterone. Journal of Endocrinology 48: 17–38

Notides A C, Nielsen S 1975 A molecular acid kinetic analysis of estrogen receptor transformation. Journal of Steroid Biochemistry 6: 483–486

Novak E, Everett H S 1928 Cyclical and other variations in the tubal epithelium. American Journal of Obstetrics and Gynecology 16: 499–530

Novak E, Martzloff K H 1924 Hyperplasia of the endometrium — a clinical and pathological study American Journal of Obstetrics and Gynecology 8: 385–

Novak E R, Woodruff J D 1979 Novak's Gynecologic and Obstetric Pathology with Clinical and Endocrine Relations, pp 689–781. W B Saunders, Philadelphia

Noyes R W 1959 The underdeveloped secretory endometrium. American Journal of Obstetrics and Gynecology 77: 929–945

Noyes R W 1973 Normal phases of the endometrium. In: Norris H J, Hertig A T, Abell M R (eds) The Uterus, pp 110–135. Williams and Wilkins, Baltimore

Noyes R W, Haman J O 1953 Accuracy of endometrial dating: correlation of endometrial dating with basal body temperature and menses. Fertility and Sterility 4: 504–509

Noyes R W, Hertig A T, Rock J 1950 Dating the endometrial biopsy. Fertility and Sterility 1:3–25

O'Herlihy C, Pepperell R J, Brown J B, Smith M A, Sandri L, McBain J C 1981 Incremental clomiphene therapy: a new method for treating persistent anovulation. Obstetrics and Gynecology 58: 535–542

Oberti C, Dabancens A, Garcia-Huidobro M, Rodriguez-Bravo R, Zanartu J 1974 Low-dosage oral progestogens to control fertility. II. Morphologic modifications in the gonad and oviduct. Obstetrics and Gynecology 43: 285–294

Odeblad E 1968 The functional structure of human cervical mucus. Acta Obstetrica et Gynecologica Scandinavica 47 Suppl 1: 59–79

Odeblad E 1976 The biophysical aspects of cervical mucus. In: Jordan J A, Singer A (eds) The cervix pp 155–163. W B Saunders, London

Oertel Y C 1978 The Arias-Stella reaction revisited. Archives of Pathology and Laboratory Medicine 102: 651–654

Okulicz W C, Evans R W, Leavitt W W 1981 Progesterone regulation of the occupied form of nuclear estrogen receptor. Science 213: 1503–1505

Orlandini G E, Pacini P 1978 L'épithelium de la trompe uterine humaine au microscope a balayage. Bulletin de l'Association des Anatomistes (Nancy) 62: 115–120

Ottesen B 1983 Vasoactive intestinal polypeptide as a neurotransmitter in the female genital tract. American Journal of Obstetrics and Gynaecology 147: 208–224

Owman Ch, Falck B, Johansson E D B, Rosengren E, Sjöberg N O, Sporrong B, Svensson K-G, Walles B 1976 Autonomic nerves and related amine receptors mediating motor activity in the oviduct of monkey and man. Histochemical, chemical and pharmacological study. In: Harper M J K, Pauerstein C J, Adams C E, Coutinho E M, Croxatto H B, Paton D M (eds) Ovum Transportation and Fertility Regulation, pp 256–275. Scriptor, Copenhagen

Owman Ch, Rosengren E, Sjöberg N-O 1967 Adrenergic innervation of the human female reproductive organs: a histochemical and chemical investigation. Obstetrics and Gynecology 30: 763–773

Papa C M, Kligman A M 1965 The effect of topical steroids on the aged human skin. Biology of Skin 6: 177–19

Parker F 1981 Skin and hormones. In: Williams R H (ed) Textbook of Endocrinology pp 1080–1098. W B Saunders, Philadelphia

Patek E, Nilsson L, Johannisson E 1972 Scanning electron microscopic study of the human fallopian tube. Report I. The proliferative and secretory stages. Fertility and Sterility 23: 459–465

Paterson M E L, Wade-Evans T, Sturdee D W, Thom M H, Studd J W W 1980 Endometrial disease after treatment with oestrogens and progestogens in the climacteric. British Medical Journal ii: 822–824

Paton D M, Widdicombe J H, Rheaume D E, Johns A 1978 The role of the adrenergic innervation of the oviduct in the regulation of mammalian ovumtransport. Pharmacological Reviews 29: 67–102

Pauerstein C J 1974 The Fallopian Tube: a Reappraisal, pp 29–68. Lea & Febiger, Philadelphia

Pauerstein C J, Hodgson B J, Fremming B D, Martin J E 1974 Effects of sympathetic denervation of the rabbit oviduct on normal ovum transport and on transport modified by estrogen and progesterone. Gynecologic Investigation 5: 121–132

Perl J I, Milles G, Shimozato Y 1959 Vaginal fluid subsequent to panhysterectomy. American Journal of Obstetrics and Gynecology 78: 285–289

Phelps C F 1978 Biosynthesis of mucus glycoprotein. British Medical Bulletin 34: 43–48

Philipp E 1972 Uber den granulofilamentären Umbau von Sekretgranula im schleimbildenden Epithel der Endocervix der Frau. Zeitschrift für Zellforschung 134: 555–563

Philipp E, Overbeck L 1969 Die Ultrastrukture des Zervixepithels. Zeitschrift für Geburtshilfe und Gynaekologie 171: 159–171

Pollow K, Lubbert H, Boquoi E, Kreuzer G, Pollow B 1975 Characterization and comparison of receptors for 17β-estradiol and progesterone in human proliferative endometrium and endometrial carcinoma. Endocrinology 96: 319–328

Pollow K, Schmidt-Gollwitzer M, Nevinny-Stickel J 1977 Progesterone receptors in normal human endometrium and endometrial carcinoma. In: McGuire W L, Raynava J-P, Baulieu E-E (eds) Progesterone Receptors in Normal and Neoplastic Tissues, pp 313–338. Raven Press, New York

Pollow K, Inthraphuvasak J, Manz B, Grill H-J, Pollow B 1981 A comparison of cytoplasmic and nuclear estradiol and progesterone receptors in human fallopian tube and endometrial tissue. Fertility and Sterility 36: 615–622

Porias H, Sojo I, Carranco A, Gonzalez-Martinez R, Cortes-Gallegos V 1978 A simultaneous assay to quantitate plasma and endometrial hormone concentrations. Fertility and Sterility 30: 66–69

Portnow J, Hodgson B J, Talo A 1977 Simulation of oviductal ovum transport. Canadian Journal of Physiology and Pharmacology 55: 972–997

Quagliarello J, Weiss G 1979 Clomiphene citrate in the management of infertility associated with shortened luteal phases. Fertility and Sterility 31: 373–377

Radwanska E, Swyer G I M 1974 Plasma progesterone estimation in infertile women and in women under treatment with clomiphene and chorionic gonadotrophin. Journal of Obstetrics and Gynaecology of the British Commonwealth 81: 107–112

Reel J R 1976 The mode of action of progestagens on endometrial carcinoma. In: Menon K M J, Reel J R (eds) Steroid Hormone Action and Cancer, pp 85–94. Plenum, New York

Reid L, Clamp J R 1978 The biochemical and histochemical nomenclature of mucus. British Medical Bulletin 34: 5–8

Rezai P, Dmowski W P, Auletta F, Scommegna A 1979 Effect of oral estriol on cervical secretions and on ovulatory response in infertile women. Fertility and Sterility 31: 627–633

Robertson D M, Landgren B-M 1975 Oestradiol receptor levels in the human fallopian tube during the menstrual cycle and after the menopause. Journal of Steroid Biochemistry 6: 511–513

Rodbell M 1980 The role of hormone receptors and GTP-regulatory proteins in membrane transduction. Nature 284: 17–22

Rose L I, Reddy V V, Biondi R 1978 Reduction of testosterone to 5α-dihydrotestosterone by human and rat uterine tissues. Journal of Clinical Endocrinology and Metabolism 46: 766–769

Rosenberg S M, Luciano A A, Riddick D H 1980 The luteal phase defect: the relative frequency of, and encouraging response to, treatment with vaginal progesterone. Fertility and Sterility 34: 17–20

Rosenfeld M G, O'Malley B W 1970 Steroid hormones: effects on adenyl cyclase activity and adenosine 3′,5′-monophosphate in target tissues. Science 168: 253–255

Rosenfeld D L, Garcia L R 1976 A comparison of endometrial histology with simultaneous plasma progesterone determinations in infertile women. Fertility and Sterility 27: 1256–1266

Rosenfeld D L, Chudow S, Bronson R A 1980 Diagnosis of luteal phase inadequacy. Obstetrics and Gynecology 56: 193–196

Runnebaum B, Klinga K, von Holst T, Junkerman H 1978 Steroids in human myometrium and peripheral blood during the menstrual cycle. American Journal of Obstetrics and Gynecology 131: 628–631

Rytömaa T 1976 The chalone concept. International Review of Experimental Pathology 16: 153–206

Saga M, Okigaki T, Davajan V, Nakamura R M 1977 Mechanism of crystallization of purified human cervical mucus. American Journal of Obstetrics and Gynecology 129: 154–158

Sandor T, Mehdi A Z 1979 Steroids and evolution. In: Barrington E J W (ed) Hormones and Evolution, pp 1–72. Academic Press, New York

Schmiedt-Matthieson H 1963 Histochemie, p 149 Goerg Thieme, Stuttgart

Schröder R 1913 Der normale menstruelle Zyklus der Uterusschleimhaut. Hirschwald, Berlin

Schumacher G F B, Kim M H, Hosseinan A H, Dupon C 1977 Immunoglobulins, proteinase inhibitors, albumin and lysozyme in human cervical mucus. American Journal of Obstetrics and Gynecology 129: 629–636

Scott J Z, Nakamura R M, Mutch J, Davajan V 1977 The cervical factor in infertility: diagnosis and treatment. Fertility and Sterility 28: 1289–1294

Seitchik J, Chatkoff M L, Hayashi R H 1977 Intrauterine pressure waveform characteristics of spontaneous and oxytocin-or prostaglandin $F_{2\alpha}$-induced active labor. American Journal of Obstetrics and Gynecology 127: 223–227

Shapiro S S, Dyer R D, Colas A E 1978 Synthetic progestins: In vitro potency on human endometrium and specific binding to cytosol receptor. American Journal of Obstetrics and Gynecology 132: 549–554

Shapiro S S, Dyer R D, Colas A E 1980 Progesterone-induced glycogen accumulation in human endometrium during organ culture. American Journal of Obstetrics and Gynecology 136: 419–425

Shearman R P, Cox R I 1965 Clinical and chemical correlations in the Stein-Leventhal syndrome. American Journal of Obstetrics and Gynecology 92: 747–754

Shepard M K, Senturia Y D 1977 Comparison of serum progesterone and endometrial biopsy for confirmation of ovulation and evaluation of luteal formation. Fertility and Sterility 28: 541–548

Sheridan P J, Buchanan J M, Anselmo V C, Martin P M 1979 Equilibrium: the intracellular distribution of steroid receptors. Nature 282: 579–582

Sherman A I 1966 Progesterone caproate in the treatment of endometrial cancer. Obstetrics and Gynecology 28: 309–314

Shingleton H M, Lawrence W D 1976 Transmission electron microscopy of the physiological epithelium. In: Jordan J A, Singer A (eds) The Cervix, pp 6–43. W B Saunders, London

Shutt D A, Lopata A 1981 The secretion of hormones during the culture of human preimplantation embryos with corona cells. Fertility and Sterility 35: 413–416

Silverberg S G, Malowski E L 1975 Endometrial carcinoma in young women taking oral contraceptive agents. Obstetrics and Gynecology 46: 503–506

Sinback C N, Shain W 1979 Electrophysiological properties of human oviduct smooth muscle cells in dissociated cell culture. Journal of Cell Physiology 98: 377–390

Singer A, Reid B 1970a The ultrastructure of cervical mucus. Journal of Reproduction and Fertility 21: 377–378

Singer A, Reid B L 1970b Effect of oral-contraceptive steroids on the ultrastructure of human cervical mucus — a preliminary communication. Journal of Reproduction and Fertility 23: 249–255

Singer S J, Nicolson G L 1972 The fluid mosaic model of the structure of cell membranes. Science 175: 720–731

Sjöberg N-O 1967 The adrenergic transmitter of the female reproductive tract: distribution and functional changes. Acta Physiologica Scandinavica Suppl 305: 1–32

Smith J P, Rutledge F, Soffar S W 1966 Progestins in the treatment of patients with endometrial adenocarcinoma. American Journal of Obstetrics and Gynecology 94: 977

Smith D C, Prentice R, Thompson D J, Herrman W L 1975 Association of exogenous estrogen and endometrial carcinoma. New England Journal of Medicine 293: 1164–1167

Snyder F F 1923 Changes in the fallopian tube during the ovulation cycle and early pregnancy. Johns Hopkins Hospital Bulletin 34: 121–125

Sorvari T E Laakso L 1970 Histochemical investigation of epithelial mucosubstances in the uterine isthmus. Obstetrics and Gynecology 36: 76–81

Soules M R, McCarty K S Jr 1982 Leiomyomas: steroid receptor content. Variation within normal menstrual cycles. American Journal of Obstetrics and Gynecology 143: 6–11

Soules M R, Wiebe R H, Aksel S, Hammond C B 1977 The diagnosis and therapy of luteal phase deficiency. Fertility and Sterility 28: 1033–1037

Spona J, Ulm R, Bieglmayer C, Huysslein P 1979 Hormone serum levels and hormone receptor contents of endometria in women with normal menstrual cycles and patients bearing endometrial carcinoma. Gynecologic Investigation 10: 17–80

Stormshak F, Harris J N, Gorski J 1977 Nuclear estrogen receptor and DNA synthesis. In: O'Malley B W, Birnbaumer L (eds) Receptors and Hormone Action, Volume II, pp 63–81. Academic Press, New York

Strömberg P, Forsling M L, Akerlund M 1981 Effects of prostaglandin inhibition on vasopressin levels in women with primary dysmenorrhea. Obstetrics and Gynecology 58: 206–208

Studd J 1976 Oestrogens as a cause of endometrial carcinoma [Letter]. British Medical Journal i: 1144–1145

Sturdee D W, Wade-Evans T, Paterson M E L, Thom M, Studd J W W 1978 Relations between bleeding pattern, endometrial histology, and oestrogen treatment in menopausal women. British Medical Journal i: 1575–1577

Sturgis S H, Meigs J V 1936 Endometrial cycle and mechanism of normal menstruation. American Journal of Surgery 33: 369–379

Sulewski J M, Ward S P, McGaffic W 1980 Endometrial biopsy during a cycle of conception. Fertility and Sterility 34: 548–551

Sylvan P E, Maclaughlin D T, Richardson G S, Scully R E, Nikrui N 1981 Human uterine luminal fluid proteins associated with secretory phase endometrium: progesterone-induced products? Biology of Reproduction 24: 423–429

Talo A 1976 Electrophysiology of the oviduct. In: Harper M J K, Pauerstein C J, Adams C E, Coutinho E M, Croxatto H B, Paton D M (eds) Ovum Transportation and Fertility Regulation, pp 161–167. Scriptor, Copenhagen

Talo A 1980 Myoelectrical activity and transport of unfertilized ova in the oviduct of the mouse in vitro. Journal of Reproduction and Fertility 60: 53–58

Talo A, Pulkkinen M O 1982 Electrical activity in the human oviduct during the menstrual cycle. American Journal of Obstetrics and Gynecology 142: 135–147

Tam P Y, Verdugo P 1981 Control of mucus hydration as a Donnan equilibrium process. Nature 292: 340–342

Tchernitchin A, Tchernitchin X, Rodriguez A, Mena M A, Unda C, Mairesse N, Galand P 1977 Effect of propranolol on various parameters of estrogen stimulation in the rat uterus. Experientia 33: 1536–1537

Templeton A A, Mortimer D 1980 Laparoscopic sperm recovery in infertile women. British Journal of Obstetrics and Gynaecology 87: 1128–1131

Thampan T N R V, Clark J H 1981 An oestrogen receptor activator protein in rat uterine cytosol. Nature 290: 152–154

Themann H, Schunke W 1963 Die Feinstruktur der Drüsenepithelien des menschlichen Endometrium: elektronenoptische Morphologie. In: Schmiedt-Matthiesen H (ed) Das Normale Menschliche Endometrium, p 111. Georg Thieme, Stuttgart

Thomas J P, Oake R J 1974 Androgen metabolism in the skin of hirsute women. Journal of Clinical Endocrinology and Metabolism 38: 19–22

Tonpe N, Lindblom B 1979 The influence of prostaglandin synthetase inhibition on the spontaneous contractile activity and induced responses of the human oviduct. Acta Physiologica Scandinavica 107: 181–183

Toppozada M, Khowessah M, Shaala S, Osman M, Rahman H A 1977 Aberrant uterine response to prostaglandin E_2 as a possible etiologic factor in functional infertility. Fertility and Sterility 28: 434–439

Tredway D R 1976 The interpretation and significance of the fractional postcoital test. American Journal of Obstetrics and Gynecology 124: 352–355

Tredway D R, Mishell D R Jr Moyer D 1973 Correlation of endometrial dating with luteinizing hormone peak. American Journal of Obstetrics and Gynecology 117: 1030–1033

Tredway D R, Fordney Settlage D S, Nakamura R M, Motoshima M, Umezaki C U, Mishell D R Jr 1975 Significance of timing for the postcoital evaluation of cervical mucus. American Journal of Obstetrics and Gynecology 121: 387–393

Trevoux R, De Brux J, Grenier J, Roger M, Bailleul S, Scholler R 1979 Etude histo-hormonale de 399 perimenopauses et menopauses confirmees. Journal de Gynecologie, Obstetrique et de Biologie de la Reproduction 8: 13–22

Tseng L, Gurpide E 1973 Effect of estrone and progestone on the nuclear uptake of estradiol by slices of human endometrium. Endocrinology 93: 245–248

Tsivris J C M, Fort F L, Cazenave C R, Cantor B, Bardawil W A, Notelovitz M, Spellacy W N 1981 The uneven distribution of estrogen and progesterone receptors in human endometrium. Journal of Steroid Biochemistry 14: 997–1003

Ulmsten U, Andersson K-E Forman A 1978 Relaxing effects of nifedipine on the nonpregnant human uterus in vitro and in vivo. Obstetrics and Gynecology 52: 436–441

Untawale V G, Gabriel J B Jr Chauhan P M 1982 Calcific endometritis. American Journal of Obstetrics and Gynecology 144: 481–483

Verdugo P, Lee W F, Rumery R E, Tam P Y 1976a Control of oviductal ciliary activity. Effect of prostaglandins (sic) E_2 [Abstract] Biophysical Journal 16: 120a

Verdugo P, Blandau R J, Tam P Y, Hablert S A 1976b Stochastic elements in the development of deterministic models of egg transport. In: Harper M J K, Pauerstein C J, Adams C E, Coutinho E M, Croxatto H B, Paton D M (eds) Ovum Transportation and Fertility Regulation, pp 126–137. Scriptor, Copenhagen

Verdugo P, Rumery R E, Tam P Y 1980 Hormonal control of oviductal ciliary activity: effect of prostaglandins. Fertility and Sterility 33: 193–196

Verhage H G, Bareither M L, Jaffe R C, Akbar M 1979 Cyclic changes in ciliation, secretion and cell height of the oviductal epithelium in women. American Journal of Anatomy 156: 505–521

Verhage H G, Akbar M, Jaffe R C 1980 Cyclic changes in cytosol progesterone receptor of human fallopian tube. Journal of Clinical Endocrinology and Metabolism 51: 776–780

Versteegh L R, Shade A R 1979 The fractional postcoital test: a reappraisal. Fertility and Sterility 31: 40–44

Vijayakumar R, Walters W A W 1981 Myometrial prostaglandins during the human menstrual cycle. American Journal of Obstetrics and Gynecology 141: 313–318

Vokaer R 1951 Observations sur l'histologie, l'histophotometrie de l'endometre humain. Gynecologie et Obstetrique 50: 372–385

Vu Hai M T, Milgrom E 1978a Characterization and assay of the progesterone receptor in rat uterine cytosol. Journal of Endocrinology 76: 21–31

Vu Hai M T, Milgrom E 1978b Characterization and assay of the progesterone receptor in rat uterine nuclei. Journal of Endocrinology 76: 33–41

Vu Hai M T, Logeat F, Warembourg M, Milgrom E 1977 Hormonal control of progesterone receptors. Annals of the New York Academy of Sciences 286: 199–209

Wakeling A E, Wyngarden L J 1974 Prostaglandin receptors in the human, monkey and hamster uterus. Endocrinology 95: 55–64

Walles B, Hakanson R, Helm G, Owman Ch, Sjöberg N-O, Sundler F 1980 Relaxation of human female genital sphincters by the neuropeptide vasoactive intestinal polypeptide. American Journal of Obstetrics and Gynecology 138: 337–338

Weinstein L, Droegemueller W, Greer B 1976 The synergistic effect of calcium and prostaglandin $F_{2\alpha}$ in second trimester abortion. Obstetrics and Gynecology 48: 469–471

Wentz A C 1980a Endometrial biopsy in the evaluation of infertility. Fertility and Sterility 33: 121–124

Wentz A C 1980b Premenstrual spotting: its association with endometriosis but not luteal phase inadequacy. Fertility and Sterility 33: 605–607

Whitehead M I, Lane G, Dyer G, Townsend P T, Collins W P, King R J B 1981 Oestradiol: the predominant intranuclear oestrogen in the endometrium of oestrogen-treated postmenopausal women. British Journal of Obstetrics and Gynaecology 88: 914–918

Wilborn W H, Flowers C E 1979 Histoenzymology of human endometrium during the proliferative and secretory phases (I). In: Beller F K, Schumacher G F B (eds) The Biology of the Fluids of the Female Genital Tract, pp 73–87. Elsvier/North-Holland, New York

Wilhelmsson L, Lindblom B, Wiqvist N 1979 The human uterotubal junction: contractile patterns of different smooth muscle layers and the influence of prostaglandin E_2, prostaglandin $F_{2\alpha}$, and prostaglandin I_2 in vitro. Fertility and Sterility 32: 303–307

Wilson E W 1980 Lysosome function in normal endometrium and endometrium exposed to contraceptive steroids. In: Diczfalusy E, Fraser I S, Webb F T G (eds) Endometrial Bleeding and Steroidal Contraception, pp 201–221 Pitman, Bath

Wilson J D, Walker J D 1969 The conversion of testosterone to 5α-androstan-17β-ol-3-one (dihydrotestosterone) by skin slices of man. Journal of Clinical Investigation 48: 371–379

Wilson K H, Lauerson N H, Raghavan K S, Fuchs F, Niemann W H 1974 Effects of diazoxide and beta adrenergic drugs on spontaneous and induced uterine activity in the pregnant baboon. American Journal of Obstetrics and Gynecology 118: 499–509

Wolf D P, Blasco L, Khan M A, Litt M 1977a Human cervical mucus. I. Rheological characteristics. Fertility and Sterility 28: 41–46

Wolf D P, Blasco L, Khan M A, Litt M 1977b Human cervical mucus. II. Changes in viscoelasticity during the ovulatory menstrual cycle. Fertility and Sterility 28: 47–52

Wolf D P, Blasco L, Khan M A, Litt M 1978 Human cervical mucus. IV. Viscoelasticity and sperm penetrability during the ovulatory menstrual cycle. Fertility and Sterility 30: 163–169

Wolf D P, Blasco L, Khan M A, Litt M 1979 Human cervical mucus. V. Oral contraceptives and mucus rheologic properties. Fertility and Sterility 32: 166–169

Wolf D P, Sokoloski J, Khan M A, Litt M 1977c Human cervical mucus. III. Isolation and characterization of rheologically active mucin. Fertility and Sterility 28: 53–58

Wood G P, Boronov R C 1976 Endometrial adenocarcinoma and the polycystic ovary syndrome. American Journal of Obstetrics and Gynecology 124: 140–142

Woodruff J D, Pauerstein C J 1969 The Fallopian Tube, pp 46–66. Williams and Wilkins, Baltimore

Wu C H, Mastroianni L Jr, Mikhail G 1977 Steroid hormones in monkey oviductal fluid. Fertility and Sterility 28: 1250–1256

Wynn R M 1977 Histology and ultrastructure of the human endometrium. In: Wynn R (ed) Biology of the Uterus, pp 341–376. Plenum Press, New York

Wynn R M, Harris J A 1967 Ultrastructural cyclic changes in the human endometrium. I. Normal preovulatory phase. Fertility and Sterility 18: 632–648

Yaffe H, Ron M, Polishuk W Z 1978 Amenorrhea, hypomenorrhea, and uterine fibrosis. American Journal of Obstetrics and Gynecology 130: 599–601

Yamamoto K R, Alberts B 1975 The interaction of estradiol-receptor protein with the genome: an argument for the existence of undetected specific sites. Cell 4: 301–310

Zanefeld L J D, Tauber P F, Port C, Propping D, Schumacher G F B 1975 Structural aspects of human cervical mucus. American Journal of Obstetrics and Gynecology 122: 650–654

Zegers F, Lenton E A, Sulaiman R, Cooke I D 1981 The cervical factor in patients with ovulatory infertility. British Journal of Obstetrics and Gynaecology 88: 537–542

Ziel H K, Finkle W D 1975 Increased risk of endometrial carcinoma among users of conjugated estrogens. New England Journal of Medicine 293: 1167–1170

Ziel H K, Finkle W D 1976 Estrogens and endometrial cancer [Letter]. New England Journal of Medicine 294: 848

Zuspan F P, O'Shaughnessy R W, Vinsel J, Zuspan M 1981 Adrenergic innervation of uterune vasculature in human term pregnancy. American Journal of Obstetrics and Gynecology 139: 678–680

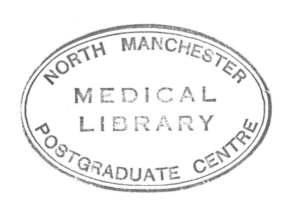

Endocrinology of ovulation prediction

INTRODUCTION

Ovulation is the central event in reproduction and all other phenomena, such as the fertile phase, the duration of sperm survival, age of the corpus luteum and onset of menstruation should strictly be timed from this event. In the majority of animal species, sexual behaviour is rigidly linked to ovulation by the phenomenon of oestrus. This is a very characteristic behaviour pattern in which the female allows copulation with the male for a limited period of time before ovulation. The time interval between the onset of oestrus and ovulation is approximately constant for each animal species. Therefore, the moment of ovulation can be calculated with an accuracy of a few hours when the onset of oestrus is known. For example, in the sheep, onset of oestrus is determined as the time when the ewe first allows the ram to mount and complete service. Ovulation occurs approximately 24 hours after this event. Oestrus is initiated by the rise in oestrogen production which precedes ovulation and is rapidly suppressed by the rise in progesterone production which follows ovulation.

During evolution, the human female has largely lost the phenomenon of oestrus, probably in return for a stable monogamous relationship. However, vistigial remnants of the state still persist in that female initiated sexual activity is more common just after cessation of menstruation, before ovulation and before menstruation, times when progesterone production is low; the pre-ovulatory sexual activity is suppressed by oral contraceptives containing progesterone (Adams et al, 1978). Because the human female has lost the phenomenon of oestrus, it has been necessary to develop alternative methods for determining the times of fertility and ovulation during the menstrual cycle. The advances in this area during the past 50 years have been as spectacular as those which have occurred in other branches of medicine and of human endeavour.

By analogy with the dog, it was first thought that fertility and ovulation occurred immediately following menstruation. Ogino (1930) on the basis of timed inspection of the ovaries at laparotomy and pregnancy following timed acts of intercourse, and Knaus (1933) using the latter criterion, showed that ovulation occurs at mid-cycle with a constant time relationship to the onset of the next menstruation. Knaus concluded that this time interval was always 14 days whereas Ogino considered more correctly that it was 11 to 15 days (Table 6.1) Although these calculations give only the approximate time of ovulation and depend on the date of the next menstrual period, which cannot be predicted with certainty, they are applied in all other methods of pinpointing ovulation as the determinant of when to commence observations. The information was immediately applied to natural family planning as a means of determining the days required for abstinence. This procedure became known as the Ogino-Knaus Rhythm or Calendar Method, and although its effectiveness may seem poor by modern standards, it was one of the few methods available at the time and it has been widely used because of its simplicity.

As soon as ovulation could be dated to within a few days by the Ogino-Knaus calculations, it became clear that several phenomena which had been noted for many years were closely related to ovulation. Thus the biphasic temperature pattern of the ovulatory cycle had been known since the mid-nineteenth century, but the relationship of the temperature shift to ovulation was not appreciated until 1928. Detection of this temperature shift became the main marker of ovulation for the next 40 years. The test was simple and could be performed by the patient herself. However, recent work has shown that timing of ovulation by the temperature shift may be in error by up to 4 days. Nevertheless, papers are still being published in which ovulation is timed by the temperature record. The temperature method was first applied to natural family planning by Wilhelm Hillebrand in 1935 (Historical Note 1971) and is still being widely used for this purpose. The main disadvantage is that the temperature shift occurs after ovulation and therefore provides retrospective information only.

The characteristic changes which occur in the production and quality of the cervical mucus during the ovulatory cycle of all mammals has probably been known

Table 6.1 Time intervals between cycle markers and ovulation seen by direct inspection at laparotomy or laparoscopy or serial ultrasound examinations

Visualisation method — marker — no. of observations — reference | Incidence of ovulation at each interval

Numbers of women ovulated/total women observed

Laparotomy, next menstruation, (N = 78), Ogino (1930)

	>17	16	15	14	13	12	≤11	Days
Days before next menstruation	0/21	2/2	2/4	3/5	2/2	6/7	37/37	

Laparotomy and histology, plasma LH peak, (N = 103), WHO (1980)

	≤8	16	24	32	40	≥48	Hours
Hours after LH peak	0/22	3/6	2/2	8/8	5/7	58/58	

median 16.5 hrs (9.5–23.0 hrs)*

Laparotomy and histology, plasma LH rise, (N = 98), WHO (1980)

	≤16	24	32	40	48	56	≥64	Hours
Hours after LH rise	0/18	0/3	1/5	5/5	5/5	10/11	51/51	

median 32.0 hrs (24–38 hrs)*

Laparoscopy, plasma LH rise, (N = 26), Garcia et al (1981)

	26	27	28	29	30	31	>36	Hours
Hours after LH rise	0/1	0/2	2/10	3/4	3/7	1/2	4/4	

Laparoscopy, plasma LH rise, (N = 30), Testart et al (1981)

	30–32	33–35	36–38	Hours
Hours after LH rise	0/3	0/17	2/10	

Serial ultrasound, urine LH rise (Higonavis), (N = 9), de Crespigny et al (1981)

	<27	28	32	33	34	35	
Hours after LH rise when ovulation occurred	2	1	1	2	2	1	Hours / Ovulations

* 95% confidence limits.

since pre-history. Smith (1855) reported that a woman is most fertile when the cervical mucus is most fluid and shortly afterwards Sims (1868) described the postcoital test for sperm penetration. However, the symptom was largely ignored until interest was renewed following the work of Ogino and Knaus. Shettles (1949) gave a complete description of the mucus symptom and predicted all of its modern applications. The symptom is widely used in fertility studies because of its simplicity and its predictive value; it is also extensively used in natural family planning. Thus by 1949 all of the symptomatic markers of ovulation including mid-cycle pain (mittelschmerz) and vaginal cytology were fully appreciated and were being applied clinically. However, the exact relationships between these markers and the moment of ovulation had still to be determined.

The next advances occurred during the 1950's with the development of quantitative methods for measuring ovarian and pituitary hormone production. These early assay methods utilised urine which contained the hormone metabolites in a relatively concentrated form. The broad pattern of urinary oestrogen excretion had already been determined by bioassay (Smith et al, 1938) and of pregnanediol excretion by chemical measurement. The mid-

cycle peak of luteinising hormone (LH) had also been well documented by biossay. The new chemical methods for measuring urinary oestrogen and pregnanediol excretion provided details of ovarian oestrogen and progesterone production which had not been obtained before. It was shown that serial measurements provided an accurate picture of cyclic ovarian activity and the assays were applied to the documentation of normal and abnormal ovarian function, to the study of ovarian stimulation and suppression and to many probelms relating to fertility and infertility. The correlations between the oestrogen, progesterone and LH patterns were established together with the correlations between these and the symptomatic markers. Rapid assays were developed suitable for the monitoring of ovarian activity as it happens and these proved to be of considerable value in further studies aimed at establishing control over ovarian function (Brown, 1955; Brown et al, 1958; Brown & Matthew, 1962; Townsend et al, 1966; Burger et al, 1968; Billings et al, 1972; Brown & Beischer, 1972).

The mid-cycle oestrogen peak and early pregnanediol rise were the first mid-cycle hormone markers of ovulation to be applied to any extent. However their precise relationship to the moment of ovulation was still unknown. At first it was thought that the precipitate fall in oestrogen values after the mid-cycle peak was caused by the cataclysm of ovulation. However, this possibility was soon shown to be unlikely since inseminations performed up to 2 days after the oestrogen peak still resulted in pregnancy (Brown & Matthew, 1962). Data obtained from timed laparotomy were inconclusive. Animal models were investigated. Raeside (1963) showed that the sow has a pre-ovulatory peak of urinary oestrone similar to that of the human. He attempted to correlate this peak with the moment of ovulation by inserting a plastic window and pulling the ovary into view from time to time (Raeside, personal communication). However, near ovulation, the follicular structures were so fragile that it was impossible to state whether the rupture had been spontaneous or had been initiated by the procedure, a problem which had been encountered earlier during inspection of human ovaries at laparotomy. In another study, oestradiol and progesterone were measured in ovarian-vein blood collected from ewes at various times of the oestrous cycle (Moore et al, 1969) A well defined elevation of oestrogen production was identified 24–36 hours before ovulation. By analogy, it was therefore argued that ovulation occurred in the human during the period 24–48 hours after the oestrogen peak. This agreed with the insemination data; it also agreed with the emerging evidence that ovulation occurred during the 24-hour period after the LH peak or after the day on which urinary pregnanediol excretion first began to rise to exceed twice the mean value for the preceding follicular phase (Billings et al, 1972). A more precise statement on the relationship of these markers to ovulation has been made recently (WHO Report, 1980).

The methods for measuring urinary oestrogen and pregnanediol excretion were applied extensively in only a few laboratories. For the majority, the Ogino-Knaus calculations and the shift in basal body temperature remained the standard methods for timing ovulation. The next major advance came with the development of radioimmunoassays (RIA). These were applied to the measurement in blood of the two pituitary hormones, LH and FSH (follicle stimulating hormone), and the two major ovarian hormones, oestradiol and progesterone. The first comprehensive study of these hormones throughout the ovulatory cycle using RIA was reported by Ross et al (1970). The procedure of RIA proved to be universally acceptable. The identification of the mid-cycle surge of LH in serum of plasma rapidly became the accepted mid-cycle hormonal marker for timing ovulation and the reference point for relating all the other mid-cycle events. The hormonal patterns throughout the menstrual cycle as determined by RIA have already been considered in detail in Chapter 4.

Two other advances in timing ovulation were required before the hormonal markers could be precisely related to the moment of rupture. Jacobaeus (1910) described an instrument termed a laparoscope which was inserted through the abdominal wall into the peritoneal cavity thus allowing the various structures to be visualised. The technique was not generally accepted until it was popularised by Steptoe (1967). This procedure allowed inspection of the ovaries with much less trauma to the patient than was involved in laparotomy. The actual observation of follicle rupture using culdotomy was first reported by Doyle (1951). With the widespread use of laparoscopy, observation of this event has become much more common. Steptoe (1974) stated that 'there can be no better indication of the moment of ovulation than watching the rupture of the follicle, nor anything more dramatic'. He observed that the follicle did not burst explosively from the apex of the stigma, but that the follicular fluid flowed gently from the base as described in other species. He also considered the possibility that rupture might have been stimulated artificially by the formation of the pneumoperitoneum during laparoscopy, or by the manipulation of the ovaries; however he never observed rupture in any patient examined before the follicles were mature. Edwards & Steptoe (1975) observed that ovulation usually occurs within 24 hours of the peak LH value and emphasised the difficulty of timing the peak even with frequent sampling.

Ultrasound scanning has also been applied to the monitoring of follicular growth and rupture. The procedure is completely non-invasive and can be repeated serially in the same subject. Many workers have measured growth rate patterns of the ovarian follicles and have shown a close correlation between follicular diameter and serum oestradiol values (Hackeloer et al, 1979). O'Herlihy et al (1980a) reported that the follicular diameter just before ovulation can range from 17 to 24 mm (mean 20 mm) and therefore follicular size is not a reliable predictor of ovulation. They considered that ovulation had occurred when a previously well circumscribed follicle, seen on ultrasound, disappeared leaving a much less distinct area containing low-level echoes. Such evidence of ovulation was usually observed during the same day as the LH peak or during the next 24 hours.

O'Herlihy, in this department, recorded the above events on video tape. He performed ultrasound scans for several days before ovulation to document the progressive enlargement of the dominant follicle. The patient was being scanned when the follicle ruptured. The rapid reduction in follicular size was clearly recorded together with moving pockets of escaping follicular fluid. Ovulation in the human had been filmed before using culdotomy but this required anaesthesia and exposure for 4–5 hours (Doyle 1951, 1954). The present study using a completely non-invasive procedure and a conscious subject had been the dream of many workers for more than 50 years. Yet those who had not lived through those 50 years were surprisingly unexcited by this final achievement. It should be added that with all the technology involved, the placement of the ultrasound probe just before ovulation still involved a large element of chance and depended considerably on the subject's own intuition of impending ovulation, her understanding of her mucus symptoms and her ability to cope with a full bladder. It is apparent that collapse of the follicle occurs over an interval of approximately 15 minutes. Therefore the moment of ovulation when the ovum is extruded occurs sometimes during this interval, but the exact timing is unknown.

In considering the future of natural family planning, it is clear that ultrasound examination could be very helpful in determining the fertile period of the cycle. Abstinence would be practiced while a follicle was visible and for a prescribed period after rupture. The high cost of ultrasound equipment could be drastically reduced by mass production and it is possible that it could be used in the home in conjunction with a television screen.

APPLICATIONS OF OVULATION PREDICTION

The latitude allowable in ovulation prediction depends on the application. The following applications are listed in increasing order of refinement required.

Natural family planning

This is potentially the largest application of ovulation prediction. The aim is to identify the period of possible fertility during the cycle, and to abstain from intercourse during this time if pregnancy is to be avoided. Time is allowed for the fertilising life of the sperm in the female genital tract and for the fertilisable life of the ovum after ovulation. In most couples the maximum fertilising life of the sperm is 3–4 days but it may reach 7 days in very fertile couples. The fertilisable life of the ovum is considered to be approximately 12 hours (Fig. 6.1). Thus, for the majority of couples, the unsafe period spans approximately 5 days but the present errors involved in identifying this

period with certainty require a 9-day period of abstinence for safety. Thus the ability to time ovulation with certainty together with a 5-day predictive period would be of great value in making natural family planning more reliable and acceptable. In this application timing ovulation to within 24–48 hours is adequate.

Timed insemination for conception

There is no doubt that in some sub-fertile couples, the period of fertility is restricted to 24–48 hours or less before ovulation and that concentration of intercourse within this fertile period greatly increases the chances of conception. The period of fertility is even more restricted when insemination is performed artificially into the uterus using frozen sperm. Here the reservoir effect of the cervix is bypassed and timing of insemination is critical. Much of the recent interest in hormonal markers of ovulation has been for the better timing of artifiical insemination and the improved pregnancy rates achieved provide evidence for the accuracy of the procedures. A prediction of the time of ovulation to within a 24-hour period is adequate for this application.

Provision of a mid-cycle marker of ovulation

Accurate information on the time of ovulation is basic to many studies of human reproduction. Up till recently, most phenomena observed during the menstrual cycle were dated to ovulation through the basal body temperature shift or even the Ogino-Knaus calculations. The primitive timing methods were forgotten and the phenomena were then used circuitously to time ovulation. This applied particularly to dating ovulation by histological examination of the endometrium (Noyes et al, 1950). A reliable mid-cycle marker of ovulation is essential for studies of corpus luteum function: a short luteal phase of less than 10–11 days is a bar to conception, a prolonged natural luteal phase of 17 days or more indicates pregnancy and reliable dating of the endometrium is necessary for diagnosing luteal phase insufficiency. Timing of ovulation to within 24 hours is adequate for this application.

Collection of pre-ovulatory oocytes for *in vitro* fertilisation and embryo transfer (IVF)

This is the most demanding application of ovulation prediction. Indeed, the success of an IVF programme depends largely on the accuracy with which ovulation can be predicted so that the ova are collected reproducibly within 0–2 hours before the follicle would have ruptured naturally. This requirement has stimulated the recent advances in precise ovulation prediction. However, in spite of these advances correct timing of ovum pick-up still involves a considerable element of chance.

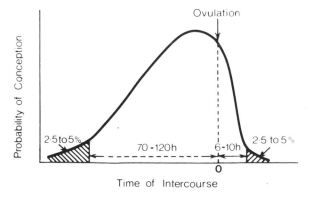

Fig. 6.1 Graph of the probability of conception versus the time of intercourse relative to ovulation in the human (from Austin, 1975)

ASSAY RELIABILITY

Assay reliability has been the subject of much study and debate for more than 50 years. It is unfortunate that the subject still requires consideration here.

The detailed patterns of blood hormone concentrations during the menstrual cycle were obtained using precise RIAs employing lengthy equilibration times. These took 3–4 days for completion and were clearly unsuitable for the daily monitoring of hormone concentrations. Therefore, there has been a marked swing to rapid 1–3 hour assays, particularly for the key hormone, LH. These rapid assays employ short incubation times and less than ideal equilibration conditions. Comparison with the original optimised assay showed excellent agreement of results with high correlation coefficients. However, considerable sensitivity and precision were sacrificed in the process. Often a rapid RIA which had been developed for plasma or serum was applied to the measurement of LH in urine without further checking that the optimum conditions applied; consequently the urinary results were poor or meaningless. In fact, no completely satisfactory RIA has yet been developed for urine, probably because no one has yet studied the optimum equilibration and separation conditions required. In the earlier studies, it was customary to analyse all samples from an experiment in the one assay run to avoid interassay variation. This practice was not possible with daily monitoring so that interassay variation was further added to the imprecision of a suboptimal method. The problems were further enhanced by the almost universal adoption of commercial RIA kits designed for use by unskilled workers. The result has been a marked deterioration of assay performance. For example, at the present time it is impossible to state whether imprecision in the prediction of ovulation to within a 0–3 hour period is due to imprecision in the identification of the LH surge caused by poor assays or whether it is due to a real biological variation. There is no substitute for continual vigilance in ensuring impecable assay performance and the routine inclusion of adequate controls.

The well recognised criteria of assay reliability are specificity, accuracy, precision, sensitivity and convenience. All methods of hormone analysis have an assay blank contributed by the biological sample and the solvents used. The assay blank affects the specificity and sensitivity of the method, and these determine its applicability. It is a general truism that provided allowance is made for procedural losses, the method which gives the lowest result is likely to be the most specific. This test is readily applied when measuring the marked fluctuations in hormone levels during the menstrual cycle, because the method which gives the greatest difference between the lowest and highest values is likely to be the most specific. Thus the mean rise in plasma progesterone values from the follicular phase to the mid luteal phase is 50-fold (see later). The corresponding increase in urinary pregnanediol is 15-fold and in saliva progesterone 6-fold. Thus, of these three methods, assay of progesterone in plasma provides the most specific measure of progesterone production during the cycle. The lower increment provided by the urinary pregnanediol assays is due to the production of small amounts of pregnanediol precursors other than progesterone and not to errors in the assay. The poor performance of the salivary assay is best explained by a high level of non-specific interference. This is the iceberg effect described by Chard (personal communication) in which the true progesterone values are apparent only during the luteal phase when they rise significantly above a general high level of non-specific interference. Many believe that the salivary values reflect the levels of the free and therefore active hormone in blood. However, this may not be true because recent work indicates that the protein bound fraction may be the active hormone (Siiteri et al, 1982). In the case of oestrogen assay, the mean rise in serum oestradiol from early follicular phase levels to the preovulatory peak is 4.5-fold whereas the increment for total urinary oestrogens is 7-fold. These figures show that the serum values suffer from an iceberg effect in which the true early follicular phase values are obscured by the noise level of the assay. This iceberg effect is small and invalidates only the early follicular phase measurements.

THE HORMONAL MARKERS OF OVULATION

The principal hormone markers of ovulation are the mid-cycle surge of pituitary LH, the pre-ovulatory peak of ovarian oestradiol and the ovulatory rise of ovarian progesterone. These will be considered in detail. As described in Chapter 4, other hormones show cyclic changes during the menstrual cycle. These include pituitary production of FSH and perhaps prolactin, and ovarian production of 17-hydroxyprogesterone. The first significant rise in 17-hydroxyprogesterone occurs 32 to 48 hours before the LH peak and this could be useful predictor of the moment of ovulation (Landgren et al, 1982). The patterns of LH, FSH, oestrogen and progesterone production during the ovulatory cycle and their temporal relationships are summarised in Fig. 6.2. It should be emphasised that the figure shows mean values and that the actual ranges of values found between different individuals and even in the same individual between different cycles are considerable. The patterns for the steroid hormones shown are characteristic of the fertile ovulatory cycle. However, cycles have been reported in which normal oestrogen and progesterone patterns were found in the absence of a well defined LH surge (Landgren et al, 1982). This agrees with the view that the trigger for ovulation occurs at a relatively low blood concentration of LH.

The cyclic changes in oestrogen and progesterone

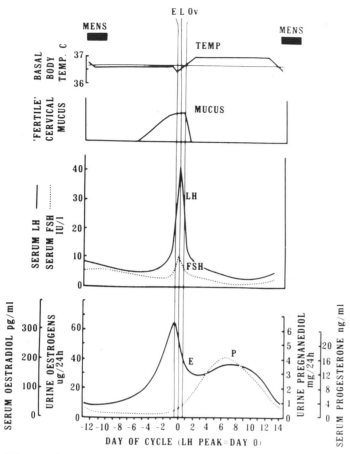

Fig. 6.2 Mean values for serum LH, FSH, oestradiol and progesterone and urinary oestrogens and pregnanediol throughout the menstrual cycle. Basal body temperatures, and times of mucus production and menstruation are shown. The vertical lines represent the times of the pre-ovulatory oestrogen peak (E), the LH peak (L) and ovulation (Ov)

production are reflected by many somatic changes, some of which can be observed by the woman herself. These include changes in the production and consistency of the cervical mucus, the appearance of the cervical os, a shift in basal body temperature, changes in the endometrium, changes in the cells lining the vagina, changes in the nipples and breasts, mid-cycle bleeding and mid-cycle pelvic pain (mittelschmerz). Since these symptoms are secondary to the underlying hormonal changes and are used as markers of ovulation and of the fertile period, the more important of them are also considered in this chapter.

The mid-cycle LH surge

The mid-cycle surge of LH and its role in the initiation of the final stages of ovulation have been known for many years. A biological test for identifying this surge was described by Farris (1946). Urine was injected into an immature female rat and the ovaries were inspected several hours later for a hyperaemic reaction which indicated that ovulation was imminent. The LH surge was readily detected in urine by a variety of bioassay systems which

measured LH specifically or as mixtures of FSH and LH (total gonadotrophin). However these bioassays were laborious and time consuming and it was not until LH could be measured in blood by RIA that it became the most important hormonal marker of ovulation.

LH is measurable in blood and urine throughout the menstrual cycle, the general levels being significantly lower during the luteal phase than during the follicular phase (Fig. 6.2). The values rise markedly at mid-cycle, the mean increase above the general base-line levels being approximately 8-fold (5 iu/l to 40 iu/l). The values are usually elevated for 3 days in the human and the interval between the first detectable rise (doubling of base-line values) and the peak value is approximately 16 hours. The fall after the peak is equally abrupt. The values therefore increase 4-fold in a 16-hour period. This rise is usually clearly visible even with 3-hourly sampling when an increase of at least 5 iu/l per sample is expected, a value which is well within the discrimination of most assay methods. Thus the mid-cycle peak of LH is the most dramatic of the mid-cycle hormonal markers and is the one which is most commonly used. Similar or greater quantitative changes occur in the urinary oestrogen and plasma progesterone values but these take place over longer intervals of time and appear as less marked phenomena than the LH surge. In other animal species, the LH peak is even more evanescent. For example, in the sheep, the peak occurs over a 1–2 hour interval and 20 minute sampling is required for its positive identification. The LH peak in the human is almost always detectable by daily sampling. However, for the most accurate timing of ovulation, serial monitoring every 3–4 hours is required. It is now recognised that the signal which triggers ovulation occurs during the early part of the surge and that the peak itself is inconsequential. Difficulties are involved in identifying the exact moment of the peak value. For the most precise timing of ovulation, as in IVF programmes, it is usual to count from the beginning of the surge when the first increase above base-line is recorded using 3-hourly sampling. However, for other purposes it is usually sufficient to time the peak value on the basis of daily sampling.

Midgley & Jaffe (1971) and Yen et al (1972) showed that the serum concentrations of LH fluctuate in a pulsatile fashion throughout the menstrual cycle. Blood samples were collected either at hourly intervals or every 10–15 minutes over selected periods of the cycle. The periodicity of the fluctuations was every 1–2 hours during the early follicular phase, the mid-cycle surge, and the early luteal phase. A pulse was defined as a rise of at least 5 iu/l which was well within the discrimination of the assay method. Fluctuations in which the concentrations changed by a factor of 2 were common, and over the mid-cycle surge the changes in absolute concentrations were large. For example, in one subject cited, the successive spikes and troughs over a 6-hour period were 63, 46, 70, 45, 78, 50,

80 (peak value), 58, 67, 42 and 62 iu/1 and in another over a 30-hour period, they were 26, 19, 30, 21, 40, 30, 46, 37, 56, 40, 67, 41, 77, 47, 95 (peak value), 82 iu/1. Yen et al (1972) showed that the shape of the spikes was consistent with a pulsatile release of LH, the rise to the spike being rapid and the decline being relatively slow with a calculated half-time of 30–45 minutes, consistent with the known serum half-life of LH. These fluctuations interfere considerably in the timing of the initial LH rise and peak and contribute greatly to the error in pin-pointing ovulation by these criteria. Several methods for integrating the values have been proposed. They include continuous blood collection from an indwelling catheter and pooling the sample collected over a 4-hour period (Urban et al, 1979), collection of three equally spaced blood samples taken at 6–18 minute intervals and pooling the specimens (Goldzieher et al, 1976) and collection of timed urine samples over 3-hour periods (Kulin et al, 1975).

Numerous rapid RIAs for LH in venous blood, fingerprick blood and urine which provide results in 1 day (Younger et al, 1978), 3½ hours (Djahanbakhch et al, 1980), 3 hours (Kerin et al, 1980), 2 hours (Hay et al, 1981) and 1½ hours (Kilpatrick et al 1981) have been developed. The increased speed was obtained by using higher concentrations of antibody and antigen and higher incubation temperatures to reduce equilibration times, and faster procedures for separating antibody complexes. The rapid assays were not as sensitive as the original assays but they were considered adequate for detecting the mid-cycle surge of LH. Several 2-hour urine tests based on the haemagglutination end-point are available commercially, the most widely used being the Hi-Gonavis Assay marketed by Mochida Pharmaceutical Co. Ltd, Tokyo, Japan.

Measurement of LH in urine has several potential advantages over blood measurement in ovulation prediction. Firstly, serial collections of urine are less invasive and more readily tolerated than frequent venipunctures and avoid the stress of multiple blood collection which may inhibit or delay the ovulatory events in some women. Secondly, urine collections overcome the problem of fluctuating LH values in blood. However, the quality of results obtained from urine compared with serum or plasma differs widely among different laboratories. Thus, Djahanbakhch et al (1980) found that the Hi-Gonavis kit gave erroneous information on the beginning of the LH surge in four out of ten patients when compared with their rapid assay for serum LH. On the other hand, Varma et al (1982) found an excellent correlation between the results provided by the Hi-Gonavis test on urine and those provided by RIA on serum.

Kerin et al (1980) found that the urine LH levels measured by their 3-hour assay paralleled almost exactly the serum values during the rise to the peak. They expressed their values in terms of iu/1 instead of the customary iu/h, which is puzzling since urine volumes per hour can fluc-

tuate considerably during the approach to ovulation. Hay et al (1981) expressed their urinary LH values in terms of iu/h and found no correlation between the concentrations of LH in serum and urine in 11 of 30 cycles studied. All these workers performed the assays directly on unprocessed urine. Urban et al (1979) concentrated the gonadotrophin from urine by precipitation with acetone and failed to find a correlation between the LH values found in serial specimens of urine collected during the day and corresponding serum specimens but found a correlation in the specimens collected overnight. No one has provided a satisfactory explanation for these conflicting findings. The problems may be due to errors in the assay methods used. For example, some workers claim that direct RIA of LH in urine is satisfactory (Bagshawe et al, 1966) whereas others consider that valid assays are only obtained following kaolin adsorption or acetone precipitation (Baghdassarian et al, 1970). It is clear that further work is required for optimising an RIA system for application to urine. The renal clearance of LH may be dependent not only on time but may vary at different times of the day or the metabolites might be recognised differently by different antisera. The delay between pituitary release of LH and its appearance in the urine has not yet been measured although it is likely to be short because of the rapid serum half-life of LH. Nevertheless, the urinary Hi-Gonavis test has proved to be reliable for identifying the beginning of the LH surge in our IVF programme although a more quantitative measure would be desirable. Details of our use of this test are given later.

Relationship between the beginning of the LH surge, the LH peak and the moment of ovulation.

The time intervals between the beginning of the LH surge, the LH peak and the moment of ovulation have been determined by several groups of workers. In most cases the ovaries have been inspected at laparotomy or laparoscopy performed at timed intervals after the LH surge and peak and the presence of a mature follicle, a recently ruptured follicle or a corpus luteum noted. Serial ultrasound was used by one group of workers to time ovulation. The results are summarised in Table 6.1. The WHO group comprised ten participating centres and studied 127 women. The ovaries were inspected at laparotomy and the structures observed were excised for confirmation by histological examination. Blood was collected three times a day and the first significant rise in circulating LH was defined as the first value which was 1.5 times the mean of the preceding base-line values and which was followed by a continuous rise to the peak. The peak was defined as the highest value reached that was preceded and followed by lower values and was at least three times the preceding mean base-line value for LH. The statistical technique of probit analysis was used to analyse the results. Whether ovulation had or had not occurred was assessed by the surgeon at operation, by colour photographs taken at the time and by independent histological assessment of the structure excised at operation. Testart et al (1981) collected blood four times a day and went to considerable lengths to allow for the pulsatile LH values when defining the 'serum LH surge-initiating rise (LHSIR)'. They considered that these pulses could cause changes of up to 250% in the LH values determined 5 hours apart. They found that this variation was reduced to 80% by averaging the results for the four preceding assays. They defined the LHSIR as any value which exceeded 180% of the mean value for the four preceding assays. The actual time when this occurred was calculated by interpolation. Garcia et al (1981) collected blood every 4 hours and defined the beginning of the LH surge as being the first specimen which exceeded 60 iu/l of LH by their assay procedure. De Crespigny et al (1981) collected urine at 3-hourly intervals and recorded the beginning of the urinary LH surge as being the first specimen to give a rising value in the Hi-Gonavis test. Follicular growth was monitored by ultrasound. Ovulation was diagnosed when a previously clearly defined follicle suddenly became smaller and disappeared with collections of fluid appearing around the ovary and in the cul-de-sac. The corpus haemorrhagicum then formed quickly, as early as 1 hour after ovulation in some cases, and was seen as a structure with smooth edges containing a fine granular echo pattern. Over the subsequent few days, the corpus luteum became gradually more difficult to identify because of increasing internal echo density. They found that ovulation could occur at any stage between a follicular diameter of 17–25 mm but no other better marker could be found of impending ovulation.

The results are summarised in Table 6.1; they are very important because they form the basis for all the predictions of ovulation calculated from the mid-cycle hormonal and symptomatic markers. The time intervals between the beginning of the LH surge and the LH peak are shown in relation to laparoscopy and the operative findings at each time interval are shown, whether no follicles had ruptured, a proportion of the follicles had ruptured or all follicles had ruptured. The WHO group (Table 6.1) calculated that ovulation occurred at a mean interval of 32 hours after the first significant rise of LH or 16.5 hours after the LH peak with 95 per cent confidence limits of 24–38 hours and 9.5–23 hours respectively. These confidence limits are probably unduly wide because three ovulations occurred at 40 and 56 hours, well outside the distribution of the others. Garcia et al (1981) considered that a 28-hour interval from the first significant rise in LH was the 'ideal time' for ovum pick-up for IVF because only a few recent ovulations had occurred by then. Testart et al (1981) found that ovulations were just being encountered by 36 hours after the beginning of the LH rise whereas the WHO group (1980) found that ovulations were just being ecountered by

32 hours after the beginning of the rise. On the other hand, de Crespigny et al (1981), using ultrasound, were just beginning to encounter ovulations by 27 hours after the beginning of the LH rise and all subjects had ovulated by 35 hours. Thus all groups agreed that ovulation commenced in the period 27–36 hours after the beginning of the LH surge and the majority of subjects had ovulated by 40 hours after the rise. The 9-hour range found for the onset of ovulation is disappointing in view of the aim of predicting ovulation to within 0–3 hours. The different findings are almost certainly due to the use of different criteria for defining the beginning of the surge and the methodological problems involved. The relative contributions of true biological differences and methodological errors to these ranges are still unknown. The mean interval from the LH peak to ovulation was 16.5 hours in the WHO study and 10 ± 5 hours in the study reported by Garcia et al (1981). Testart et al (1981) remarked that the process of ovulation must set in very early during the LH surge when the plasma LH values are still comparatively low. This probably occurs when a serum spike reaches 10–20 iu/l (Fig. 6.2). This is equivalent to a pulse of 400–800 iu of LH being produced by the pituitary. For comparison, the dose of hCG commonly used for initiating ovulation is 5000 iu.

Timing ovulation following administration of hCG

In IVF programmes, the difficulties involved in timing ovulation by the LH surge in spontaneous cycles have stimulated interest in the alternative approach of inducing the ovulatory mechanism by administering hCG. This is usually performed following ovarian hyperstimulation with clomiphene citrate and /or human menopausal gonadotrophin (hMG). The procedure has several advantages. Firstly multiple follicles are produced and several ova are available for fertilisation even when some follicles are inaccessible. Secondly the administration of hCG can be timed so that ovum pick-up is performed at a convenient time. Thirdly, pregnancy rates are increased by transferring more than one embryo to the mother.

Many protocols for inducing hyperstimulation with clomiphene and/or hMG have been proposed. All seem to be equally successful in achieving pregnancies in IVF programmes. The main problems encountered involve the maturity of the follicles when the hCG is given and the time interval between the injection and ovulation. These two factors are closely related. Follicular growth is usually monitored by daily urinary oestrogen or serum oestradiol assays and by ultrasound.

The time interval between the injection of hCG and ovulation has been studied by Edwards & Steptoe (1975) using laparoscopy performed between 32 and 42 hours after the injection of hCG. They found that ovulation seldom occurred before 36 hours. They observed the actual process of rupture in two patients at 37 and 38.5 hours and a third had just ovulated at this time. At 40–42 hours two of the three patients examined had ovulated and the third showed no large follicles or corpus luteum. Several women had ovulated prematurely: evidence that a spontaneous LH surge had occurred was obtained in each case. Thus the study was not completely conclusive but subsequent experience has shown that 36 hours is the optimum time for ovum pick-up following the injection of hCG. A similar time interval applies when ovulation is induced with hCG in unstimulated cycles.

These procedures are not without their problems. The multiple follicles produced during a hyperstimulation programme usually develop at different rates and are at different stages of maturity when the hCG is given. They are referred to as first order, second order, third order, etc. follicles which yield mature ova 36 hours later and the sensitivities to hCG differ and that the timing of the hCG dose is optimal for only some of the follicles. These are the follicles which yeild mature ova 36 hours later and the other follicles yield ova which are either still immature or are post mature. Compensation for these errors is achieved by pre-incubating the ovum before insemination to simulate the conditions which would have existed if it had remained in the follicle for the correct period of time. In this procedure, the less mature ova require the longer incubation times. However, no method has yet been devised for determining the maturity of each ovum so that it is incubated for the optimum period of time. Edwards & Steptoe (1975) considered the possibility that the procedure of laparoscopy, particularly the pneumoperitoneum, might cause premature rupture of fragile follicles when ovulation is imminent. This could also apply to the pressure exerted by the full bladder necessary for visualising the follicles by ultrasound. Although this effect in producing premature ovulation is probably small, it could explain the frequency with which ovulation is actually observed during these techniques which would seem to be greater than would be expected by pure chance.

A protocol for timing ovum pick-up in an IVF programme

The principles of ovulation timing are illustrated in practice by the following protocol used in the IVF programme at the Royal Women's Hospital, Melbourne. This protocol is continually being updated. The aim is to devise the optimum conditions for follicular development for each individual woman.

Clomiphene citrate 50–150 mg per day is given starting on day 3 or 5 of the cycle. The clomiphene is continued until day 9 or longer and in some cases hMG (150–300 iu) is given on cycle days 7, 8 and 9 or longer, depending on the response. Ultrasound examination is performed on day 9 and repeated at intervals as required. Follicular response is monitored by daily rapid RIA of serum oestradiol

performed on blood collected at 0800 hours. Stimulation with climiphene citrate is discontinued when the largest follicle on ultrasound is $\geqslant 14$ mm (usually day 9). When hMG is used to supplement clomiphene citrate, it is discontinued when the leading follicle is $\geqslant 18$ mm (usually day 11). The patient is then admitted to hospital and blood is collected twice daily at 0800 hours and 1800 hours and urine is collected 3 hourly. LH is measured in the blood specimens by a rapid RIA, the results of the evening specimen for the previous day and the morning specimen of that day being available at 1330 hours. Selection of the urines to be assayed for the LH surge depends on the results obtained from the blood specimens. For example, if the LH values for both blood specimens are at basal levels ($\leqslant 20$ iu/1) only the urine collections subsequent to the last blood collection (0800 hours) are assayed for LH by the Hi-Gonavis test. This test has been modified slightly so that 50 assays are obtained from one kit of ten. These assays are performed to detect a spontaneous LH surge which may occur before administering the hCG. Usually a spontaneous LH surge does not occur and hCG (5000 iu) is given as a single injection when the leading follicle exceeds 20 mm diameter or the serum oestradiol value reaches 500 pg/ml per follicle greater than or equal to 15 mm in diameter or 60 hours after the last injection of hMG. Ovum pick-up is performed 36 hours later. However, if the Hi-Gonavis test shows that a spontaneous LH surge has commenced as indicated by a continuing rise above the usual urinary base-line excretion of 3 iu/hour, hCG is not given and ovum pick-up is performed 24–27 hours after this rise, counting from the mid-point of the urine collection.

The results obtained from this protocol (Table 6.2) reflect the efficiencies of the various monitoring procedures and the accuracy of ovulation prediction. Of a total of 250 cycles, 46 (18 per cent) required management on the basis of the spontaneous LH surge which occurred, and the remainder were managed by hCG control of ovulation. Although successful recovery of ova was higher in the hCG

Table 6.2 IVF results for 1982.
250 Laparoscopies — 32 pregnancies

	All cycles N = 250	hCG controlled cycles N = 204	Spontaneous LH surge N = 46
Number of patients from whom ova were collected	224 (90%)	192 (94%)	34 (74%)
Fertilised	64%	64%	64%
Cleaved	80%	75%	95%
Embryo transfer	174 (70%)	146 (72%)	28 (61%)
Pregnancies	32	27	5
Pregnancies/ laparoscopy	13%	13%	11%
Pregnancies/ embryo transfer	18%	18%	18%

controlled group the pregnancy rates were identical. Ovulation of one or more follicles had occurred spontaneously before ovum pick-up in 29 of the 205 cycles (14 per cent) controlled by hCG and in five of the 46 cycles (11 per cent) controlled by a spontaneous LH surge. One pregnancy resulted from an ovum obtained from one of the latter five cycles. During 1980, 122 laparoscopies were performed in unstimulated cycles 28 hours after the onset of the LH surge as determined by the Hi-Gonavis test: ovulation had already occurred in 18 cycles (15 per cent).

The data provided by the 1982 study allowed the results obtained by the Hi-Gonavis assay on urine to be compared with those obtained by the rapid LH assay on serum. The validity of these results could then be checked by the findings at ovum pick-up and the subsequent pregnancy rates. The Hi-Gonavis test and the rapid LH assay gave consistent results in all but eight of the 250 cycles. These eight cycles were all managed according to the finding of a spontaneous LH surge identified by the Hi-Gonavis assay. In these eight anomolous cycles the serum LH values were already elevated above 20 iu/1 when the blood collections were commenced, yet the beginning of the LH surge was identifiable by the Hi-Gonavis assay. On checking the serum LH values against the laboratory optimised assay, the high values were confirmed in four, the remainder being explained by the loss in precision and sensitivity of the rapid assay. The high values in the remainder were attributable to the clomiphene therapy used; they showed an additional rise in line with the Hi-Gonavis values and returned to normal base-line values after discontinuing the clomiphene. Thus the basic time intervals between observed events and ovulation are largely correct and the Hi-Gonavis assay is giving valid results. Nevertheless, there is room for considerable improvement.

The preovulatory oestrogen peak and the pre- and post-ovulatory progesterone rise

The preovulatory oestrogen peak was first accurately documented by measuring urinary oestrogen excretion throughout the menstrual cycle (Brown, 1955). Daily urinary oestrogen and pregnanediol values throughout 61 ovulatory menstrual cycles are shown in Fig. 6.3, together with the 10th, 50th and 90th percentiles.

The patterns of daily plasma or serum oestradiol and oestrone concentrations together with those of FSH, LH and progesterone have been documented throughout the ovulatory menstrual cycle by many workers (Abraham et al, 1972; Korenman & Sherman, 1973; Saxena et al, 1974; Dhont et al, 1974; Guerrero et al, 1976; Wu, 1978; and others).

When comparing the urine values with the plasma values it is necessary to consider the underlying processes involved. The ovaries secrete both oestradiol, the most potent oestrogen, and oestrone cyclically throughout the

menstrual cycle. Oestrone is also produced constantly by the extraglandular aromatisation of adrenal androgens. Consequently, the ratio of oestradiol to oestrone in blood varies during the cycle being approximately one during the early follicular phase, more than two at the mid-cycle peak, one at the nadir and approximately 1.5 during the luteal phase (Guerrero et al, 1976). Thus the measurement of oestradiol provides the best assessment of the pre-ovulatory peak in plasma or serum. The oestradiol and oestrone are metabolised by identical pathways so that the urine oestrogen values reflect the sum of the two. The principal urinary oestrogens commonly measured are the glucuronides of oestradiol, oestrone and oestriol. The excretion of oestradiol and oestrone glucuronides is prompt but the excretion of the oestriol glucuronides is delayed by approximately 12 hours by a complex enterohepatic circulation involving biliary excretion and re-absorption (the oestriol 'lag' phenomenon; Brown, 1955). Thus, when monitoring ovarian events by the assay of urinary oestrogens, the changes in urinary oestradiol or oestrone provide the closest relationship in time to the changes occurring in ovarian oestrogen production. Although the analysis of serum oestradiol should theoretically provide the best definition of the pre-ovulatory oestrogen peak, in practice, analyses on urine show the greater changes because of the absence of the iceberg effect encountered with blood. Blood assays have an advantage that they provide immediate values for the moment of collection whereas urine assays provide the median value for the period of collection, which for valid results should not be less than 3 hours. On the other hand, blood oestradiol values fluctuate in a pulsatile fashion and the errors caused by this phenomenon are obviated by performing assays on urine (Korenman & Sherman, 1973). These differences between blood and urine assays are stressed because rapid chemiluminescence-immunoassays for urinary oestrone glucuronide and pregnanediol glucuronide have been reported (Lindner et al, 1981) and a very simple 5 minute enzyme-immunoassay suitable for home use has been developed for pregnanediol glucuronide in our laboratory. Thus monitoring ovarian function by simple and rapid urine assays could well replace blood assays in the near future.

The blood and urine assays give almost identical patterns of oestrogen values during the menstrual cycle. The values are low during the first week of a 28-day cycle (Figs 6.2 & 6.3), they begin to rise about 6 days before the LH peak (day −6) and increase logarithmically at a daily incremental rate of 1.3–1.4 until the peak is reached usually on LH day −1. In individual cycles monitored by urinary assays, an early follicular phase base-line is usually recognisable and commencing follicular activity is seen as a rise above this base-line, the rise continuing to the pre-ovulatory peak. Identification of the beginning of the oestrogen rise has important practical applications because it coincides with the increase in cervical mucus production,

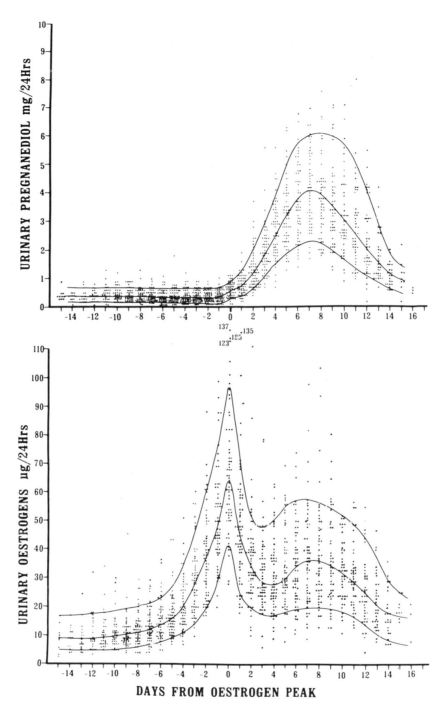

Fig. 6.3 Daily urinary oestrogen and pregnanediol values in 61 ovulatory menstrual cycles from 26 parous and 14 nulliparous women aged 20–24 years. All values are plotted and the 10th, 50th and 90th percentile lines are shown. The mid-cycle oestrogen peak was defined for every cycle and days are numbered from this day (= day 0) (from Brown et al, 1981)

it occurs 11–4 days (means 6 days) before ovulation and it is the most likely hormone marker available for detecting the beginning of the fertile period (Fig. 6.4). Some deviations from this general pattern are observed. The rise is sometimes interrupted by falling values for several days and then the rise commences again. In 13 per cent of cycles, two oestrogen peak values are seen separated by an intervening lower values. In this case, the actual pre-

ovulatory peak is determined by alignment with the accompanying pregnanediol values and the LH peak. The mean rise from the early follicular phase base-line to the pre-ovulatory peak is 7-fold by urine analyses (Fig. 6.3) and 4.5-fold by blood analyses (Guerrero et al, 1976).

After the peak value is reached, the oestrogen values fall rapidly. This prompt fall is an intrinsic feature of the ovulatory response to LH. When the LH surge fails to

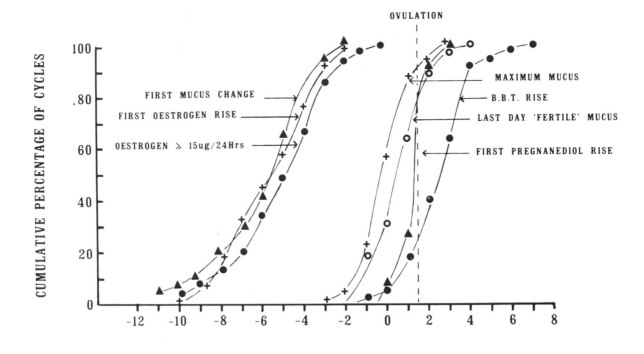

Fig. 6.4 Cumulative percentage of cycles in which the events had occurred by a particular day. Days are numbered from the day of the pre-ovulatory oestrogen peak = day 0. The vertical dotted line indicates the best estimate of the moment of ovulation which has a degree of uncertainty of approximately ± 12 hours. The last day of fertile mucus represents the 'peak' symptom (from Brown et al, 1981)

initiate ovulation the rise is accelerated and very high oestrogen peaks may be seen in anovulatory cycles (Brown, 1978). The values reach a nadir usually of less than 50 per cent of the peak value approximately 3 days after the peak, and then rise again during the luteal phase and fall before onset of menstruation.

The time intervals between the LH peak in plasma and the oestrogen peak in plasma or urine reported in the literature are summarised in Table 6.3. The oestrogen peak in plasma occurred between LH days 0 to −3, with the majority occurring on day −1. The peak in urine occurred approximately 12 hours later as would be expected because oestriol was included in the assay. The WHO Report (1980) showed that the mean interval between the plasma oestrogen peak and ovulation was 24 hours (95 per cent confidence range 17–32 hours) and between the plasma oestrogen peak and the LH peak was 7.5 hours, a shorter time than that indicated by the values shown in Table 6.3.

Progesterone production during the ovulatory cycle shows a characteristic pattern. The values are low during the follicular phase and reach a nadir 3 days before the LH peak (Fig. 6.2). They then begin to rise: this rise is small at first but is usually clearly apparent by day 0; it accelerates during the post ovulatory period and the values reach a maximum on days 6–8 after the LH peak. At this time the corpus luteum reaches its peak of functional activity (Corner, 1956). Thereafter degeneration commences, progesterone output gradually falls, and menstruation occurs on approximately day 14. The beginning of the

progesterone rise provides an important marker of imminent ovulation (Yussman & Taymor, 1970) and the high luteal phase values provide the best biochemical evidence that ovulation has occurred. Guerrero et al (1976) described the peri-ovulatory changes in plasma progesterone values as follows. During days −7 to −2 the mean plasma progesterone concentrations remained close to 0.3 ng/ml. The mean values then increased reaching 0.33 ng/ml on day −2, 0.49 ng/ml on day −1, 1.17 ng/ml on day 0 and 1.80 ng/ml on day +1 relative to the LH peak. All of these daily differences were highly significant from one day to the next. The mean plasma progesterone concentration reached 17 ng/ml on day +7, a total rise of 50-fold. This

Table 6.3 Relationship between the day of the preovulatory oestrogen peak and the day of the LH peak

Reference and Fluid Assayed	Numbers of cycles/day on which the oestrogen peak occurred (day 0 plasma LH peak)			
	Day −3	−2	−1	0
Korenman & Sherman (1973) (N32) Plasma	2 (6%)	7 (22%)	13 (41%)	10 (31%)
Guerrero et al (1976) (N17) Plasma	–	2 (12%)	9 (53%)	6 (35%)
Burger et al (1968) (N11) Urine		1 (9%)	5 (45.5%)	5 (45.5%)
Brown et al (1981) (N20) Urine		2 (10%)	7 (35%)	11 (55%)

is by far the greatest change seen in the concentrations of any hormone during the human ovulatory cycle. The pre-ovulatory rise in plasma progesterone is being used along with the LH surge in several IVF and artificial insemination programmes to time ovulation (Djahanbakhch et al, 1981; Fleming & Coutts, 1982). Urinary pregnanediol values measured by specific methods also show definite pre-ovulatory increases (Fig. 6.3). Billings et al (1972) used the day on which the urinary pregnanediol values had more than doubled the mean follicular phase levels as one of their criteria of the day of ovulation. Documentation of this early rise in progesterone production is particularly useful in identifying the day of ovulation when ambiguity exists in the other markers, for example when double peaks occur in the LH or oestrogen values. The progesterone values before ovulation seem to be critical for fertility. We have encountered several women who failed to conceive during cycles in which the pregnanediol values were raised above 1 mg per 24 hours at this time but conceived immediately when the levels were half this value. The finding of a plasma progesterone concentration of 5 ng/ml or more on days 5 to 8 after the LH peak (Guerrero et al, 1976) or of a urinary pregnanediol value of 2 mg per 24 hours or more (Pepperell et al, 1975) provides important confirmation that ovulation did in fact occur after identification of the mid-cycle events.

The ovary rather than the pituitary is the organ most intimately involved in ovulation. Thus it might have been expected that production of the ovarian hormones, oestradiol and progesterone would have been more closely related in time with the process of rupture. However, this has not proven to be the case and the LH surge is the better criterion. Attempts to define the precise time of the pre-ovulatory oestrogen peak in urine by sampling more frequently than every 24 hours, for example every 3 hours, makes the rise from sample to sample so small that it is completely obscured. This is because the oestrogen rise occurs over a much longer period of time (6 days) than the LH rise (1 day) and the latter is clearly visible on frequent sampling. Furthermore, it is probable that the follicular productions of oestradiol and progesterone are secondary to the main ovulatory events and the oestradiol levels may be inconsequential once they have triggered the LH surge; they have fallen markedly by the time rupture occurs.

Progesterone occurs in saliva at approximately one hundredth the concentration found in plasma. Measurement of this by RIA has been proposed as a test for ovulation (Walker et al, 1979). The concentrations during the follicular phase fluctuate from values which are too low for accurate measurement (< 20 pg/ml) to values not exceeding 30 pg/ml; they reach a maximum during the luteal phase of 70–170 pg/ml and fall before the onset of menstruation. This represents a mean rise of approximately 6-fold between the follicular and the luteal phase compared with 50-fold for plasma, which indicates a large iceberg effect. The ease of collecting serial specimens of saliva makes this procedure very attractive. Several large programmes of ovulation detection by salivary analysis are planned. It will be interesting to see whether the loss of discrimination between the follicular and luteal phase levels leads to serious errors in interpretation, or whether the information obtained is any better than would be provided by measuring basal body temperature.

THE SYMPTOMATIC MARKERS OF OVULATION

Basal body temperature (BBT)

The BBT shows a biphasic pattern during the ovulatory cycle, the luteal phase levels being approximately 0.3°C higher than the follicular phase levels due to the thermogenic effect of the raised progesterone production. Considerable variations in this pattern are found. Some patterns show a dip which has been ascribed to the action of oestrogen before the main rise occurs (Fig. 6.2): others show a definite rise which is easily interpreted, others show a slow and indefinite rise, and in others the rise occurs in a step-wise fashion. These variations in patterns may not be important when the sole objective is to determine whether ovulation has occurred, but they are important when the temperature shift is used to time ovulation, such as is required in natural family planning programmes. Many rules have been formulated to deal with the problem. Thus Billings et al (1972) drew a line just above the general levels of the follicular phase (the 'marginal' line) and considered that the temperature rise had commenced when the first persistent value above this line was encountered. Other workers define the thermal change as the first of three consecutive daily readings which are 0.2°C higher than the previous 6 daily temperatures (Moghissi, 1980).

Women are instructed to record their temperature with the same thermometer every morning upon awakening and before getting out of bed. A period of 6 to 8 hours uninterrupted rest is recommended. The majority record oral temperature but this route is most susceptible to external factors and the variable results reported are partly due to these errors. Vaginal or rectal readings provide more exact information on deep body temperature but are not without their complications. During vaginal recordings care is required to ensure that the thermometer is inserted in the vagina (loose) and not in the urethra (tight) because thermometers have been lost in the bladder; furthermore, at maximum mucus production the thermometer readily slips out of the vagina before the temperature reaches equilibrium and falsely low values are recorded. Depth of insertion is also important. Most women dislike taking temperatures rectally (Abrams & Royston, 1981). Recently electronic devices for recording BBT have been developed. An instrument marketed under the name 'Bioself 101' is available at the beginning of 1983 from Bioself, Geneva.

This instrument records the cycle day and measures and records the BBT taken either orally, vaginally or rectally, stores the temperature readings for 62 consecutive days and the lengths of the last six menstrual cycles, and from an analysis of the results indicates whether the woman is in a phase of low fertility, high fertility, or infertility (late safe-days indicated by the 3-day rule). The instrument ensures that the temperature is measured for a standard period of time and should eliminate all patient errors from the BBT recording and from its use in natural family planning. Furthermore, the information stored in its memory can be printed out for inspection using a printer. This instrument would appear to be the ultimate in BBT recording.

In its earliest applications for timing ovulation, the accuracy of the BBT record was much over-rated. Its first comparison with the hormonal markers indicated some gross discrepancies (Brown et al, 1958). Of eight cycles which were ovulatory by the hormonal criteria, one showed a completely monophasic BBT record, in one the temperature rise was so gradual that identification of the day of the shift was impossible and in two the shift occurred 4 days after the other markers indicated that ovulation had occurred. In an earlier study of eight cycles, the agreement between the temperature shift and the hormone marker was excellent (Brown, 1955). However, it was not until methods for the measurement of LH by RIA became widely established that the errors in the BBT became fully recognised. An unjustified over-reaction has occurred particularly from those who firmly believed that the rise in temperature coincided with ovulation or that ovulation always occurs within 27–72 hours of the thermal shift. Three types of error have been identified. Firstly, some women who ovulate do not show a biphasic temperature record. Lenton et al (1977) encountered this error in 20 per cent of ovulatory cycles, Bauman (1981) found it in 35 per cent of ovulatory cycles and Moghissi (1976) found it in 20 per cent of ovulatory cycles. Thus the finding of a monophasic temperature record is not proof that the cycle was anovulatory. Secondly, the time relationship between the temperature shift and ovulation was found to be much more variable than was first thought. This invalidated all the conclusions based on timing ovulation by the temperature shift, such as lengths of the luteal phase, and optimum times for insemination. These errors were well recognised by those who used the BBT method for natural family planning because of the accidental pregnancies which resulted. Lenton et al (1977) found that the BBT shift indicated the day of ovulation correctly to within 2 days in only 43 per cent of charts from normal subjects and in only 25 per cent of charts from infertility patients. Lotan & Diamant (1979) found that the BBT shift agreed with the day of ovulation as judged by the LH peak in only 26 per cent of cycles, and that the span was greater than 1 day before or 1 day after in 53 per cent of cycles. Bauman (1981) found that the BBT shift occurred within ±1 day of the LH peak in 38 per cent of cycles and ±2 days or more of the LH peak in another 27 per cent of cycles. Billings et al (1972) studied 19 ovulatory cycles and found that the temperature shift occurred on the same day as the LH peak (= day 0) in one cycle, on day +1 in four cycles, on day +2 in ten cycles, on day +3 in three cycles and on day +4 in one cycle; all these temperature records were biphasic. Similar results are summarised in Fig. 6.4 which shows that the temperature shift is the least accurate of all the mid-cycle markers in identifying the day of ovulation. These results were obtained from normal women practicing natural family planning. The third error involves differences in the interpretation of a BBT record by different observers or even the same observer at different times. Thus Lenton et al (1977) found such inconsistencies in interpretation in approximately 40 per cent of cycles and that this effect occurred most commonly in infertility patients. This error illustrates the difficulties involved in interpreting BBT charts in many cases. While some of these problems will be minimised by the use of electronic recording and interpretation, the great variation in the day of the temperature shift in relation to the day of ovulation is likely to remain.

The BBT record identifies only the late safe days for natural family planning. These commence when the BBT has been elevated for 3 consecutive days (the '3-day rule'). It is generally agreed that the fertilisable life of the ovum after ovulation is at the most 24 hours. The 3-day rule was formulated from extensive experience; the requirement is due to the intrinsic error of the BBT method in pinpointing ovulation. Marshall (1968) studied 321 couples who confined coitus to the late safe days through 4749 cycles. The failure rate was 6.6 pregnancies per 100 women-years.

Dating of ovulation by histological examination of the endometrium

The histological appearance of the endometrium obtained by curettage during the luteal phase is widely used as a test that ovulation has occurred and that the endometrium is responding normally to the action of progesterone. Frequently it is used to diagnose the presence of the inadequate luteal phase. This is defined as an endometrium which lags 2 days or more behind normal development in two or more cycles (Jones & Madrigal-Castro, 1970). The dating of the endometrium is based on eight major criteria described by Noyes et al (1950). These criteria were dated on the assumption that ovulation occurred 14 days before the onset of the next menstruation. Later, Noyes & Haman (1953) showed that the criteria were equally accurate when the shift in BBT was taken as the time of ovulation. This dating has recently been checked against the LH peak.

Tredway et al (1973) studied 11 normally ovulating women and found that the date determined by endometrial biopsy agreed with that determined by the LH peak with an accuracy of ±2 days in ten out of 11 cycles. In five of the 11 subjects, the histological pattern lagged 2 days behind the true date indicating an impossibly high incidence of the luteal phase defect. Similar results were reported by Koninckx et al (1977). These recent findings support Novak's (1954) original criticism of the dating procedure, in that it was based on 'very tenuous' and 'insecure' timing of ovulation, that large variations in the histological picture occurred in different endometria obtained on the same day of the luteal phase and that noting the time of the succeeding period was much more precise for dating the endometrium than reliance on stereotyping of histological changes.

Dating of ovulation by biopsy of the corpus luteum

Corner (1956) established the criteria for dating the ages of corpora lutea by histological examination based on 213 carefully selected biopsy specimens. Ovulation was timed by the menstrual history and endometrial dating. More importantly, the histological appearance of a structure excised 1 hour after an ovulation witnessed by Doyle (1954) provided the description for +1 hours, and the macroscopic appearances of the recently ruptured follicles and early corpora lutea described by the surgeons and pathologists could be related to timed events in the Rhesus monkey and other animals. Thus the dating of the corpus luteum for the first 2 days of its development could be stated to within hours.

Yussman & Taymor (1970) related the serum levels of FSH, LH, and progesterone to the time of ovulation as determined by biopsy of the corpus luteum. Blood was collected at 8-hour intervals over a 5-day period before scheduled laparotomy which was performed in the early post-ovulatory phase in eight subjects. A fresh corpus luteum less than 48 hours old was recovered from five subjects and these were utilised for the report. It was concluded that these early corpora lutea could be dated with an undoubted accuracy of ±12 hours or a total range of 24 hours. In all five subjects the time of ovulation determined by biopsy occurred 24–36 hours after the first rise in LH, 12–24 hours after the LH peak and 16–24 hours after the first rise in progesterone. In relation to the peak of LH (= 0 hours), the rise in progesterone was seen at −8 hours in three subjects, and at 0 hours in two subjects. This was the first accurate documentation of the early rise of plasma progesterone and of the temporal relationships between the values for LH and progesterone and ovulation. The results agreed perfectly with those described earlier in this chapter.

Changes in the cervix and in cervical mucus production

During the ovulatory menstrual cycle, characteristic changes occur in the production and quality of the cervical mucus and in the appearance of the cervix and of the cervical os. These changes are under the control of the ovarian hormones; mucus production begins with the first secretion of oestradiol by the growing follicle, it reaches a maximum at the time of the pre-ovulatory oestrogen peak and then regresses rapidly under the influence of progesterone produced by the developing corpus luteum. This regression occurs even in the presence of raised oestrogen secretion and is a more sensitive measure of the rising progesterone production than the shift in BBT. The day before this rapid change occurs coincides with the day of ovulation in the majority of cycles (Fig. 6.4).

The changes in the mucus and cervical os can be followed readily by daily inspection by a physician and by collection of the mucus for laboratory examination. Alternatively the mucus symptoms can be observed by the woman herself simply by noting sensations of wetness or dryness in the vulval area. Most modern methods of natural family planning utilise the mucus symptoms either alone (the Ovulation Method, Billings) or in conjunction with the BBT record and the Ogino-Knaus calculations (the Sympto-thermal Method). Self palpation of the cervical os provides additional information and is advocated by some centres.

Cervical mucus has been studied extensively by Odeblad (1978) who has described two main types named E type (oestrogenic) and G type (oestrogen negative or progestogenic). Odeblad has identified many subgroups of the E type. The G type mucus occurs early in the cycle when the oestrogen values are low and during the luteal phase when the progesterone values are high: it is viscous, has a low water content, is secreted in small amount, is opaque and is impenetrable by sperm. The cervical os is closed when G type mucus is being produced and this is readily felt on digital palpation; the consistency of the cervix at this time is hard like the tip of the nose.

As oestrogen production increases, the amount of E type mucus increases. At its maximum production this mucus is seen pouring from an open os; the size of the opening is apparent by digital palpation and the cervix feels soft like the lips and is high in the vagina and difficult to reach. This fertile E type mucus has a high water content, is acellular and brilliantly clear, has a low viscosity and is highly lubricative, appearing like raw egg white. This mucus has the capacity of being stretched into threads ('spinnbarkeit') and when allowed to dry on a microscope slide it forms channels and produces a characteristic fern-like pattern ('ferning'). At this time the mucus reaches its highest pH, its highest glucose content and its highest salt content. These characteristics occur in all mammals and it is likely that the saltiness of the mucus along with the characteristic odours indicate to the male that oestrus is approaching. This mucus is highly receptive to sperm and several methods are available for testing this capacity, for example the post-coital test and the slide sperm penetration test. The mucus is made up of glycoprotein fibrils which form a micellar structure orientated along the direction of the cervical canal: this directs sperm migration along channels towards the uterine cavity and into crypts in the endocervix where reservoirs of sperm are formed. These properties reach a maximum just before ovulation and shortly afterwards the cervical os closes and the production of E type mucus ceases abruptly and is replaced by G type mucus for the remainder of the cycle.

Insler et al (1972) described a method for scoring the cervical mucus; scores of 1, 2 or 3 are given to the appearance of the cervical os, the amount of mucus, its spinnbarkeit and its ferning ability. A score of 9 or more indicates the time of peak fertility during the cycle. This scoring system is used widely in determining the optimum time for insemination.

An important advance in natural family planning was made by Drs John and Evelyn Billings when they showed that these changes in cervical mucus at the os were readily detected by the women themselves by noting sensations in the vulval area (Billings, 1964). These sensations are described briefly as follows. In the majority of women, unless the cycle is short, the cessation of menstrual bleeding is followed by a series of 'dry days' during which nothing is coming from the vagina and there is a positive sensation of dryness outside the vagina. In other women there is minimal continuing discharge. When this phase is prolonged as in long cycles, these symptoms persist day after day indicating lack of underlying cyclic ovarian activity and therefore infertility. As oestrogen production commences the mucus symptoms change; this change has different characteristics for different women and tuition is required for recognising them; the change indicates the commencement of the fertile period. The sensation becomes one of dampness. The mucus symptoms increase and reach the characteristics already described. These characteristics are obvious to the woman herself without the need for exploring the vagina or cervix. The last day of this fertile mucus is noted; it is termed the 'peak' day; it is the day of maximum fertility and coincides with or is immediately followed by ovulation. After ovulation, the mucus becomes minimal, thick and tacky once more (France, 1981, 1982). The fertile period is considered to commence with the first change from infertile to fertile type mucus; it ends and the late safe days commence on the evening of the fourth day after the 'peak' symptom in line with the 3-day rule for the BBT. Intercourse obscures the mucus symptoms for a period of 24 hours. It has been shown that the mucus symptoms as recorded by the woman herself correlate almost exactly with observations of mucus production made by a physician by vaginal and cervical examination (Hilgers & Prebil, 1979). Rules have been formulated in which these mucus symptoms are utilised for natural family planning (Billings & Westmore 1980; Billings 1981). Teaching women to recognise the mucus symptoms is best carried out by specially trained women instructors who are themselves observing their own symptoms for natural family planning.

The World Health Organization has recently completed a multicentre, cross-cultural trial of the Ovulation Method Billings. Centres in Auckland, Bangalore, Dublin, Manila and San Miguel have participated. In the teaching phase of the trial it was shown that 94 per cent of women were soon able to recognise and record their mucus symptoms. In the application phase, 725 subjects participated for a total of 7500 cycles. The average number of days of abstinence required by the method was 17. The effectiveness varied with the centre. High rates of method failure were found in the two most socially developed centres, Auckland and Dublin. The Pearl rates for method failure ranged from 9.4 per 100 women years in Auckland to 1.1 in Manila and 0 in Bangalore and San Miguel. As might be expected the greatest number of pregnancies were due to

Table 6.4 The beginning of 'fertile' mucus and the 'peak' mucus symptom related to the day of ovulation determined by hormone analyses

| | | Number of cycles in which the symptom occurred on a prescribed day dated to ovulation = day 0 | | | | | | | | | | | | |
| | | Beginning of fertile mucus | | | | | | 'Peak' day | | | | | | |
Day of Symptom		$\geq$ -11	-10 -9	-8 -7	-6 -5	-4	-3	Mean	-3	-2	-1	0	+1	+2	Mean
Reference and number of cycles studied															
Billings et al (1972)	N = 22	0	5	6	3	4	4	-6.2	2	4	9	5	1	1	-0.9
Cortesi et al (1981)	N = 31:32		1	8	19	2	1	-6.0		1	4	21	6		0.0
Hilgers et al (1978)	N = 63							-5.9	1	4	9	24	13	12	-0.3
Brown et al (1981)	N = 19									1	7	10	–	1	-0.6
	N = 43	4	7	11	17	3	1	-7.0	3	6	12	13	6	3	-0.5
Total	96:179	4	13	25	39	9	6	-6.3	6	16	41	73	26	17	-0.3

conscious departure from the rules of the method for avoiding pregnancy (Report, 1982).

The time-relationships between the self-observed mucus symptoms and the hormone markers of fertility from four studies are summarised in Table 6.4. All used the Billings' classifications and the results obtained in the four studies were almost identical. The 'peak' symptom occurred within ±1 day of the estimated day of ovulation in 78 per cent of cycles and ±2 days in 96 per cent of cycles.

The mean interval between the day of the peak symptom and ovulation was −0.35 days. The beginning of the fertile mucus symptom gave at least 5 days warning of ovulation in 83 per cent of cycles (mean 6.2 days). These figures were obtained by women who had been taught to recognise their symptoms and the results show a high degree of correlation between the symptoms and the hormonal findings.

The mucus symptoms were correlated with urinary oestrogen and pregnanediol values during short and prolonged follicular phases, during anovulatory cycles and during the spectrum of ovarian activity which occurs post-partum, during breast feeding and after weaning and during the climacteric. Fertile type mucus was observed whenever the urinary oestrogen values exceeded 10 μg per 24 hours, the dividing line between base-line extraglandular production of oestrogen and superimposed ovarian production of oestradiol. Patches of fertile type mucus were observed whenever the oestrogen values exceeded this base-line. Thus, mucus production is a very sensitive indicator of even trace production of ovarian oestradiol and provides an immediate warning of commencing ovarian activity. However, the mucus symptoms do not reach the full characteristics of the pre-ovulatory phase unless a rise equivalent to a pre-ovulatory oestrogen peak eventuates. Furthermore the characteristic phenomenon of the 'peak symptom' does not take place unless ovulation and its accompanying rise in progesterone occurs. A woman who was observing increasing frequency of fertile type mucus production during prolonged breast feeding had no difficulty in recognizing the 'peak' symptom which showed that the first ovulation following childbirth was occurring (Brown et al, 1981). This study also demonstrated that the mucus symptoms observed post-partum and during lactation could give many false positive indications that ovulation might be imminent but they gave no false negatives. Thus the mucus symptoms provide predictions of possible ovulation which are useful for natural family planning during the post-partum period, lactation and the climacteric when all other methods based on retrospective ovulation detection such as the BBT record are not applicable.

Other symptomatic markers of ovulation

Midcycle pain

Some women experience lower abdominal pain (mittelschmerz) at the approximate time of ovulation. The pain may be sharp or it may be a dull dragging ache; it is not proof of ovulation and may be recorded in anovulatory cycles. The symptom when it occurs has been widely used for timing ovulation and was applied in the early studies of Ogino (1930).

O'Herlihy et al (1980b) investigated 96 ovulating women and found that 34 (35 per cent) recorded mid-cycle lower abdominal pain. This pain, which usually lasted for 6 to 12 hours, was correlated with the LH peak in serum and with the time of ovulation determined by ultrasound. In 27 women, the discomfort was localised to one or other iliac fossa which in all but two cases corresponded to the side of the developing follicle. In 26 women (77 per cent), the pain was felt on the day of the serum LH peak and in 31 (91 per cent) the pain occurred 24–48 hours before ovulation assessed by ultrasound. In all but one woman, the intact follicle could still be seen by ultrasound after the pain had disappeared. Therefore mittelschmerz is a symptom experienced by approximately one-third of women and it occurs during the 24-hour period before ovulation. O'Herlihy et al (1980b) considered that the pain was due to the action of LH which increases the contractility of ovarian peri-follicular smooth muscle probably through the action of prostaglandin.

Vaginal blood flow

A close correlation between vaginal blood flow and plasma oestradiol levels has been found during the oestrous cycle in sheep and cows. The blood flow is estimated by measuring the rate of removal of heat from the vaginal wall by a cooled probe inserted in the vagina. Vaginal probes similar to those used in sheep were applied to a study of six normally ovulating women to determine whether changes in blood flow also occur in the human before ovulation. Plasma levels of oestradiol, progesterone, LH, and FSH, vaginal temperature and blood pressure were measured. No definite pattern of blood flow was detected which correlated significantly with any of the other parameters measured. This was an unexpected negative finding and the possible reasons were discussed (Abrams et al, 1978).

Changes in body electric potential

Evidence that body electric potentials change near the time of ovulation is conflicting. An instrument called the Ovutron has been marketed by Ovutron Corporation, Las Vegas, Nevada, U.S.A. to measure these changes. This is a digital voltmeter which measures the voltage difference between the index fingers of the two hands. The manufacturers claim that a swinging voltage showing both positive and negative readings of up to ±10 mV ('voltage mix') during five measurements performed over 10 minutes indicate approaching ovulation. This device was tested against the serum LH, oestradiol and progesterone measurements and the BBT record in ten normally ovulating women (Roy & Mishell, 1981). A voltage mix was observed in eight of the ten women during days 0–4 before the LH peak and in two women during days 2–4 after the peak. The voltage mix was unimpressive in most cases and the device would appear to have little merit.

ADDENDUM

The present chapter is a very incomplete account of the history of ovulation detection and timing by hormone assays or hormone effects. In researching the early work, the reader is impressed by the amount of information which was then available but which has not become general knowledge until recently. Thus Sims in 1868 was well aware that maximum fertility occurred at mid-cycle when the cervical mucus was easily penetrated by spermatozoa. However, the occurrence of ovulation at mid-cycle was not generally appreciated until Ogino completed his classical studies in 1930 and another 30–40 years passed before the mucus symptoms became widely used clinically for identifying the optimum time for insemination and for natural family planning. Furthermore, an impressive number of women have wittingly or unwittingly allowed themselves to be operated upon or have contributed daily or hourly specimens so that this information could be accumulated.

Hormone assays have only recently been widely applied clinically to the prospective monitoring of ovarian activity and to the timing of ovulation. Their use has greatly improved the understanding and treatment of infertility, the timing of insemination, the collection of pre-ovulatory oocytes for IVF and the development of methods of natural family planning. However, their cost is causing concern because of the spiralling health bill. Furthermore, the increasing demand for RIAs is causing a discharge of radiochemicals which is reaching the allowable limits in some areas. Thus a great need is developing for cheaper non-radioactive methods for hormone monitoring. The World Health Organization has been supporting such developments but this has been discontinued because of lack of funds. As a preliminary in this area we have developed a simple and very cheap enzyme immunoassay for pregnanediol glucuronide in urine aimed at home use by the women themselves. After 2 years' trial, during which the method has performed excellently in the laboratory, the conclusion has been reached that women without scientific training have great difficulty in making correct objective measurements on themselves. They are strongly biased towards interpreting the results by what they think they should be rather than what they clearly see. Thus this cheap and easy method is not practicable without further simplification. Nevertheless such simple and cheap methods for measuring hormones or their metabolites in urine are likely to be developed and widely applied providing that the results obtained are as accurate and precise as the best RIAs available at the present time.

REFERENCES

Abraham G E, Odell W D, Swerdloff R S, Hopper K 1972 Simultaneous radioimmunoassay of plasma FSH, LH, progesterone, 17-hydroxyprogesterone, and estradiol-17β during the menstrual cycle. Journal of Clinical Endocrinology and Metabolism 34: 312–318

Abrams R M, Royston J P 1981 Some properties of rectum and vagina as sites for basal body temperature measurement. Fertility and Sterility 35: 313–316

Abrams R M, Kalra P S, Wilcox C J 1978 Vaginal blood flow during the menstrual cycle. American Journal of Obstetrics and Gynecology 132: 396–399

Adams D B, Gold A R, Burt A D 1978 Rise in female-initiated sexual activity at ovulation and its suppression by oral contraceptives. The New England Journal of Medicine 299: 1145–1150

Austin C R 1975 Sperm fertility, viability and persistence in the female tract. Journal of Reproduction and Fertility Supplement 22: 75–89

Baghdassarian A, Gyda H, Johanson A, Migeon C J, Blizzard R M 1970 Urinary excretion of radioimmunoassayable luteinizing hormone (LH) in normal male children and adults, according to age and stage of sexual development. Journal of Clinical Endocrinology and Metabolism 311: 428–435

Bagshawe K D, Wild C E, Orr A H 1966 Radioimmunoassay of human chorionic gonadotropin and luteinizing hormone. Lancet i: 1118–1121

Bauman J E 1981 Basal body temperature: unreliable method of ovulation detection. Fertility and Sterility 36: 729–733

Billings E, Westmore A 1980 The Billings Method. Anne O'Donovan, Richmond, Victoria, Australia

Billings E L, Billings J J, Brown J B, Burger H G 1972 Symptoms and hormonal changes accompanying ovulation. Lancet i: 232–234

Billings J J 1964 The Ovulation Method. Advocate Press, Melbourne, Australia

Billings J J 1981 Cervical mucus, the biological marker of fertility and infertility. International Journal of Infertility 26: 182–195

Brown J B 1955 Urinary excretion of oestrogens during the menstrual cycle. Lancet i: 320–323

Brown J B 1978 Pituitary control of ovarian function — concepts derived from gonadotrophin therapy. Australian and New Zealand Journal of Obstetrics and Gynaecology 18: 47–54

Brown J B, Beischer N A 1972 Current status of estrogen assay in obstetrics and gynecology. Part 1: Estrogen assays in gynecology and early pregnancy. Obstetrical and Gynecological Survey 27: 205–235

Brown J B, Matthew G D 1962 The application of urinary estrogen measurements to problems in gynecology. Recent Progress in Hormone Research 18: 337–385

Brown J B, Klopper A I, Loraine J A 1958 The urinary excretion of oestrogens, pregnanediol and gonadotrophins during the menstrual cycle. Journal of Endocrinology 17: 411–424

Brown J B, Harrisson P, Smith M A, Burger H G 1981 Correlations between the mucus symptoms and the hormonal markers of fertility throughout reproductive life. Published by the Ovulation Method Research and Reference Centre, 127 Alexandra Parade, North Fitzroy, Melbourne, Victoria 3068, Australia

Burger H G, Catt K J, Brown J B 1968 Relationship between plasma luteinizing hormone and urinary estrogen excretion during the menstrual cycle. Journal of Clinical Endocrinology and Metabolism 28: 1508–1512

Corner G W Jr 1956 The histological dating of the human corpus luteum of menstruation. American Journal of Anatomy 98: 377–401

Cortesi S, Rigoni G, Zen F, Sposetti R 1981 Correlation of plasma gonadotrophins and ovarian steroids pattern with symptomatic changes in cervical mucus during the menstrual cycle in normal cycling women. Contraception 23: 629–641

de Crespigny L Ch, O'Herlihy C, Robinson H P 1981 Ultrasonic observation of the mechanism of ovulation. American Journal of Obstetrics and Gynecology 139: 636–639

Dhont M, VandeKerckhove D, Vermeulen A, Vandeweghe M 1974 Daily concentrations of plasma LH, FSH, estradiol, estrone and progesterone throughout the menstrual cycle. European Journal of Obstetrics, Gynecology and Reproductive Biology Supplement S153–S159

Djahanbakhch O, Templeton A A, Hobson B M, McNeilly A S 1980 Prediction of ovulation by measurement of luteinizing hormone. Lancet i: 1199–1200

Djahanbakhch O, Swanton I A, Corrie J E T, McNeilly A S 1981 Prediction of ovulation by progesterone. Lancet ii: 1164–1165

Doyle J B 1951 Exploratory culdotomy for observation of tubo-ovarian physiology at ovulation time. Fertility and Sterility 2: 475–486

Doyle J B 1954 Ovulation and the effects of selective uterotubal denervation — direct observations by culdotomy. Fertility and Sterility 5: 105–130

Edwards R G, Steptoe P C 1975 Induction of follicular growth, ovulation and luteinization in the human ovary. Journal of Reproduction and Fertility Supplement 22: 121–168

Farris E J 1946 A test for determining the time of ovulation and conception in women. American Journal of Obstetrics and Gynecology 52: 14–27

Fleming R, Coutts J R T 1982 Prediction of ovulation in women using a rapid progesterone radioimmunoassay. Clinical Endocrinology 16: 171–176

France J T 1981 Overview of the biological aspects of the fertile period. International Journal of Fertility 26: 143–152

France J T 1982 The detection of ovulation for fertility and infertility. In: Bonnar J (ed). Recent Advances in Obstetrics and Gynaecology, pp 215–239. Churchill Livingstone, Edinburgh

Garcia J E, Seegar Jones G, Wright G L 1981 Prediction of the time of ovulation. Fertility and Sterility 36: 308–315

Goldzieher J W, Dozier T S, Smith K D, Steinberger E 1976 Improving the diagnostic reliability of rapidly fluctuating plasma hormone levels by optimized multiple-sampling techniques. Journal of Clinical Endocrinology and Metabolism 43: 824–830

Guerrero R, Aso T, Brenner P F, Cekan Z, Landgren B-M, Hagenfeldt K, Diczfalusy E 1976 Studies on the pattern of circulating steroids in the normal menstrual cycle. 1. Simultaneous assays of progesterone, pregnenolone, dehydroepiandrosterone, testosterone, dihydrotestosterone, androstenedione, oestradiol and oestrone. Acta Endocrinologica 81: 133–149

Hackelöer B J, Fleming R, Robinson H P, Adam A H, Coutts J R T 1979 Correlation of ultrasonic and endocrinologic assessment of human follicular development. American Journal of Obstetrics and Gynecology 135: 122–128

Hay D L, Tasker P A, Johnston W I H, Horacek I 1981 Two-hour assay for lutropin during ovulation. Clinical Chemistry 27: 727–730

Hilgers T W, Prebil A M 1979 The Ovulation Method — vulvar observations as an index of fertility/infertility. Obstetrics and Gynecology 53: 12–22

Hilgers T W, Abraham G E, Cavanagh D 1978 I. The peak symptom and estimated time of ovulation. Obstetrics and Gynecology 52: 575–581

Historical Note 1971 Dr Med H C Wilhelm Hillebrand. Journal of Biosocial Science 3: 331–337

Insler V, Melmed H, Eichenbrenner I, Serr D M, Lunenfeld B 1972 The cervical score: a simple semiquantitative method for monitoring of the menstrual cycle. International Journal of Gynaecology and Obstetrics 10: 223–228

Jacobaeus H C 1910 Ueber die Möglichkeit die Zystoskopie bei

Untersuchung seröser Höhlungen anzumenden. Muenchener Medizinische Wochenschrift 57: 2090–2092

Jones G S, Madrigal-Castro V 1970 Hormonal findings in association with abnormal corpus luteum function in the human: the luteal phase defect. Fertility and Sterility 21: 1–13

Kerin J F, Warnes G M, Crocker J, Broom T G, Ralph M M, Matthews C D, Seamark R F, Cox L W 1980 3-hour urinary radioimmunoassay for luteinizing hormone to detect onset of preovulatory LH surge. Lancet ii: 430–431

Kilpatrick M J, Collins P O, Marinho A O, Collins W P 1981 Capillary blood luteinizing hormone levels to predict ovulation. Lancet ii: 1165

Knaus H 1933 Die periodische Frucht-und Unfruchtbarkeit des Weibes. Zentralblatte für Gynäkologie 57: 1393–1408

Koninckx P R, Goddeeris P G, Lauweryns J M DeHertogh R C, Brosens I A 1977 Accuracy of endometrial dating in relation to the midcycle luteinizing hormone peak. Fertility and Sterility 28: 443–445

Korenman S G, Sherman B M 1973 Further studies of gonadotropin and estradiol secretion during the preovulatory phase of the human menstrual cycle. Journal of Clinical Endocrinology and Metabolism 36: 1205–1209

Kulin H E, Bell P M, Santen R J, Ferber A J 1975 Integration of pulsatile gonadotropin secretion by timed urinary measurement: an accurate and sensitive 3-hour test. Journal of Clinical Endocrinology and Metabolism 40: 783–789

Lenton E, Weston G A, Cooke I D 1977 Problems in using basal body temperature recordings in an infertility clinic. British Medical Journal 1: 803–805

Landgren B-M, Aedo A-R, Diczfalusy E 1982 Hormonal changes associated with ovulation and luteal function. In: Flamigni C, Givens J R (eds) The Gonadotropins: Basic Science and Clinical Aspects in Females, Serono Symposia Vol. 42, pp 187–201. Academic Press London

Lindner H R, Kohen F, Eshar Z, Kim J B, Barnard G, Collins W P 1981 Novel assay procedure for assessing ovarian function in women. Journal of Steroid Biochemistry 15: 131–136

Lotan Y, Diamant Y Z 1979 The value of simple tests in the detection of human ovulation. International Journal of Gynaecology and Obstetrics 16: 309–313

Marshall J 1968 A field trial of the basal-body-temperature method of regulating births. Lancet i: 8–10

Midgley A R, Jaffe R B 1971 Regulation of human gonadotropins: X. Episodic fluctuation of L H during the menstrual cycle. Journal of Clinical Endocrinology and Metabolism 33: 962–969

Moghissi K S 1976 Accuracy of basal body temperature for ovulation detection. Fertility and Sterility 27: 1415–1421

Moghissi K S 1980 Prediction and detection of ovulation. Fertility and Sterility 34: 89–98

Moore N W, Barrett S, Brown J B, Schindler I, Smith M A, Smyth B 1969 Oestrogen and progesterone content of ovarian vein blood of the ewe during the oestrous cycle. Journal of Endocrinology 44: 56–62

Novak E 1954 Editor's note. Obstetrical and Gynecological Survey 9: 727

Noyes R W, Haman J O 1953 Accuracy of endometrial dating: correlation of endometrial dating with basal body temperature and menses. Fertility and Sterility 4: 504–517

Noyes R W, Hertig A I, Rock J 1950 Dating of the endometrial biopsy. Fertility and Sterility 1: 3–25

Odeblad E 1978 Cervical factors. In (ed) Keller P J. Contributions to Gynecology and Obstetrics, pp 132–142. Karger, Basel

Ogino K 1930 Ovulationstermin und Konzeptionstermin. Zentralblatt für Gynäkologie 54: 464–479

O'Herlihy C, de Crespigny L J Ch, Robinson H P 1980a Monitoring ovarian follicular development with real-time ultrasound. British Journal of Obstetrics and Gynaecology 87: 613–618

O'Herlihy C, Robinson H P, de Crespigny L J Ch 1980b Mittelschmerz is a preovulatory symptom. British Medical Journal 280: 986

Pepperell R J, Brown J B, Evans J H, Rennie G C, Burger H G 1975 The investigation of ovarian function by measurement of urinary oestrogen and pregnanediol excretion. Journal of Obstetrics and Gynaecology of the British Commonwealth 82: 321–332

Raeside J I 1963 Urinary oestrogen excretion in the pig at oestrus and during the oestrous cycle. Journal of Reproduction and Fertility 6: 421–426

Report 1982. Trials of the ovulation method of natural family planning. Research in Reproduction, Published by The International Planned Parenthood Federation 14: 1

Ross G T, Cargille C M, Lipsett M B, Rayford P L, Marshall J R, Strott C A, Rodbard D 1970 Pituitary and gonadal hormones in women during spontaneous and induced ovulatory cycles. Recent Progress in Hormone Research 26: 1–62

Roy S, Mishell 1981 Correlation of Ovutron readings and basal body temperature (BBT) with serum sex-hormone and luteinizing hormone levels. Contraception 24: 635–646

Saxena B N, Dusitsin N, Poshyachinda V 1974 Luteinizing hormone, oestradiol, and progesterone levels in serum of menstruating Thai women. Journal of Obstetrics and Gynaecology of the British Commonwealth 81: 113–119

Shettles L B 1949 Cervical mucus: cyclic variations and their clinical significance. Obstetrical and Gynecological Survey 4: 614–621

Siiteri P K, Murai J T, Hammond G L, Nisker J A, Raymoure W J, Kuhn R W 1982 The serum transport of steroid hormones. Recent Progress in Hormone Research 38: 457–510

Sims J M 1868 Illustrations of the value of the microscope in the treatment of the sterile condition. British Medical Journal ii: 465–466, 492–494

Smith G V S, Smith O W, Pincus G 1938 Total urinary estrogen, estrone and estriol during a menstrual cycle and pregnancy. American Journal of Physiology 121: 98–106

Smith W T 1855 The Pathology and Treatment of Leucorrhoea. Churchill, London

Steptoe P C 1967 Laparoscopy in Gynaecology. Churchill Livingstone, Edinburgh

Steptoe P 1974 Clinical and physiological studies on human conception. In: Phillips J M, Keith L (eds) Gynecological Laparoscopy, pp 27–41. Grune & Stratton, New York

Testart J, Frydman R, Feinstein M C, Thebault A, Rodger M, Scholler R 1981 Interpretation of plasma luteinizing hormone assay for the collection of mature oocytes from women: definition of a luteinizing hormone surge-initiating rise. Fertility and Sterility 36: 50–54

Townsend S L, Brown J B, Johnstone J W, Adey F D, Evans J H, Taft H P 1966 Induction of ovulation. Journal of Obstetrics and Gynaecology of the British Commonwealth 73: 529–543

Tredway D R, Mishell D R, Moyer D L 1973 Correlation of endometrial dating with luteinizing hormone peak. Amercian Journal of Obstetrics and Gynecology 117: 1030–1033

Urban M D, Lee P A, Kowarski A, Plotnick L, Migeon C J 1979 Comparison of estimates of gonadotropin levels by isolated blood samples, integrated blood concentrations, and timed urinary fractions. Journal of Clinical Endocrinology and Metabolism 48: 732–735

Varma T R, Patel R H, Everard D 1982 Determination with Hi-Gonavis of luteinizing hormone levels in urine compared with those in plasma. British Journal of Obstetrics and Gynaecology 89: 87–90

Walker R F, Read G F, Riad-Fahmy D 1979 Radioimmunoassay of progesterone in saliva: application to the assessment of ovarian function. Clinical Chemistry 25: 2030–2033

World Health Organization Report 1980 Temporal relationships between ovulation and defined changes in the concentration of plasma estradiol17β, luteinizing hormone, follicle-stimulating hormone and progesterone 1. Probit analysis. American Journal of Obstetrics and Gynecology 138: 383–390

Wu C H 1978 Monitoring of ovulation induction. Fertility and Sterility 30: 617–630

Yen S S C, Tsai C C, Naftolin F, Vandenberg G, Ajabor L 1972 Pulsatile patterns of gonadotropin release in subjects with and without ovarian function. Journal of Clinical Endocrinology and Metabolism 34: 671–675

Younger J B, Boots L R, Coleman C 1978 The use of a one-day luteinizing hormone assay for timing of artificial insemination in infertility patients. Fertility and Sterility 30: 648–653

Yussman M A, Taymor M L 1970 Serum levels of follicle stimulating hormone and luteinizing hormone and of plasma progesterone related to ovulation by corpus luteum biopsy. Journal of Clinical Endocrinology and Metabolism 30: 396–399

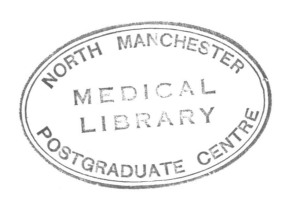

Endocrine aspects of the menopause

Many of the physiological changes which occur at the end of a woman's reproductive life affect multiple organ systems and have a common basis — the depletion of gonadotrophin responsive primordial ovarian follicles and consequent diminution of oestrogen production. This dramatic endocrine change, unique among mammals, has received a significant amount of attention. Recent studies have expanded dramatically our understanding of this important interval in a woman's life. This chapter will review our current understanding of the relevant endocrine physiology.

The term *climacteric* refers to the interval of time during which diminished reproductive potential manifests clinically and marks the transition from the reproductive stage of life. This period, also referred to as the *perimenopause*, usually spans several years and may or may not be accompanied by symptoms including menstrual abnormalities, vasomotor symptoms and genital atrophy. The vague term *'menopausal syndrome'* encompasses these findings plus additional features which are probably coincident with the climacteric rather than a consequence of it. These problems include emotional lability, insomnia, depression, and psychosocial changes. The term *menopause* should be reserved specifically for the occurrence of the last menstrual period which usually occurs several years into the climacteric. The diagnosis of menopause is usually established with certainty after 1 year has elapsed. The *postmenopause* is characterised by further endocrine changes and is significant clinically; osteoporosis may develop during this interval and pre-existing symptoms may become more severe.

EPIDEMIOLOGY

The median age of menopause varies in different parts of the world (Table 7.1) and there is much confusion regarding the effects of various factors. Age at menopause is related to familial patterns and possibly race. Higher socio-economic status, living at lower altitudes, high parity and pathological conditions including diabetes, uterine fibroids, endometrial and breast adenocarcinoma and carcinoma of the cervix have been related to delayed age of menopause. Carcinomas of the vulva and ovaries and cigarette smoking have been associated with earlier loss of menstrual function. Current estimates of the mean age of menopause range from 50.1 to 50.78 years (Frommer, 1964; Frere, 1971; McKinlay et al, 1972) and the actual mean age has probably not changed appreciably over the past several hundred years. About 8 per cent of women will have cessation of menses before the age of 40.

Few topics in medicine have incited as much early interest yet have been so delayed in having the essential physiological principles elucidated. The relationship of diminished fertility to age has been appreciated since biblical times. In Genesis, Abraham expressed surprise when told that he and his wife would be parents (Frommer, 1964) . . . 'shall a child be born unto him that is an hundred years old? And shall Sara that is ninety years old bear?' Percival Pott was probably the first to realise a critical function of the ovaries when he described the case of a 23-year-old servant woman who presented with bilateral inguinal ovaries producing pain with motion. He reported in 'Chirurgical Observations' in 1775 that after removal of both ovaries: 'She has enjoyed good health ever since, but is become thinner and apparently muscular — her breasts which were large are gone; nor has she ever menstruated since the operation, which is now some years' (Pott, 1775).

Brown-Sequard (1890) was an early proponent of hormone replacement therapy for postmenopausal women in the late 1800's. He gave testimony from personal experience with guinea-pig and dog testicular extracts and claimed that they enhanced intellectual function, improved defecation, and produced greater strength of micturition, not to mention the effects on virility. He applied similar ovarian extracts to 'ovariectomised and hysterical' women and allegedly found a spectacular response. His prominence as 'president of the Societe de Biologie' in France did much to popularise endocrine treatment for meno-

Table 7.1 Estimates of the age of menopause from selected studies (Gray, 1976)

Country and year of study	Race	Mean or median age at menopause in years	Study design	Source
Scotland 1970	Caucasian	50.1 median	Cross sectional	Thompson et al (1973)
England 1965	Caucasian	50.78 median 47.49 mean	Cross sectional	McKinley et al (1972)
England 1951–61	Caucasian	49.82 median	Cross sectional	Frommer (1964)
U.S.A. 1934–7	Caucasian	49.8 median 49.5 mean	Cohort	Treloar (1974)
U.S.A. 1966	Caucasian Negro Both races	50.02 median 49.31 median 49.8 median	Cross sectional	MacMahon & Worcester (1966)
Germany 1972	Caucasian	49.06 mean	Retrospective	Hofmann & Soergel (1972)
Finland 1961	Caucasian	49.8 mean	Retrospective	Hauser et al (1961)
Switzerland 1961	Caucasian	49.8 mean	Retrospective	Hauser et al (1961)
Israel 1963	Caucasian	49.5 mean	Retrospective	Hauser et al (1963)
Netherlands 1969	Caucasian	51.4 median	Cross sectional	Jaszmann et al (1969)
New Zealand 1967	Caucasian	50.7 median	Cross sectional	Burch & Gunz (1967)
South Africa 1971	Caucasian Negro	50.4 median 49.7 median	Cross sectional	Frere (1971)
South Africa 1960	Negro	48.1 median 47.7 mean	Retrospective	Abramson et al (1960)
South Africa 1960	Caucasian	48.7 mean	Retrospective	Benjamin (1960)
Punjah 1966	Asian	44.0 median	Cohort & cross sectional	Wyon et al (1966)
New Guinea 1973	Melanesian	47.3 median (non-malnourished) 43.6 median (malnourished)	Cross sectional	Scragg (1973)

pausal symptoms long before the specific effects of sex steroids had been adequately characterised.

Butenandt (1929) succeeded in isolating and purifying the first oestrogen, oesterone, in 1929 and his work was later acknowledged when he received the Nobel prize in chemistry. This work lay the foundations for more effective oestrogen compounds. Oestrogens were conclusively proven to be effective clinically in treating vasomotor symptoms and atrophic vaginitis in the menopause in 1935 (Mazer & Israel, 1935; Davis, 1935). The development and accessibility of the orally active oestrogens diethylstilboestrol and ethinyl oestradiol in 1938 made oestrogen replacement therapy available to large numbers of women. Albright et al (1941) noted the benefit of oestrogen replacement therapy in 'postmenopausal osteoporosis' and this became an additional indication.

The popularity of oestrogen replacement therapy flourished and perhaps reached its apex in the early 1960's when the menopause itself was described as a 'preventable disease state' in Robert A. Wilson's book, *Feminine Forever* (1966). In this text he advocated oestrogen therapy to maintain youthfulness among other reasons. The interest of the public was reflected in the sharp increase in the sales of oestrogen compounds, in particular of conjugated oestrogens. This was tempered abruptly in 1975 with the publication of two papers and an editorial in the New England Journal of Medicine reporting an increased risk of endometrial adenocarcinoma in oestrogen users (Smith, et al, 1975; Ziel & Finkle, 1975; Weiss, 1975). An attempt has been made over the past few years to place the risk-benefit ratio of oestrogen therapy in its proper perspective and to devise methods to reduce the apparent risks of endometrial neoplasia. During the same interval considerable effort has demonstrated the potential benefits of oestrogen therapy in the treatment of postmenopausal osteoporosis, a common disease with considerable morbidity and mortality.

PHYSIOLOGY OF THE MENOPAUSE

The menopause is the consequence of an amount of oestradiol inadequate to induce endometrial proliferation and subsequent withdrawal bleeding. This, in turn, results from the relative absence of primordial ovarian follicles capable of responding to gonadotrophins with follicular maturation, oestradiol production, ovulation and progesterone production.

While variable, the earliest manifestation of the approaching menopause is usually shortening of the menstrual cycle. This is accomplished by a progressive reduction of the mean follicular phase to 8 to 10 days and preservation of the length of the luteal phase. This is probably a consequence of a greater amount of FSH being produced earlier in the cycle which is in turn necessary to ensure that an adequate number of follicles are recruited for the cohort. It may reflect an early subtle disruption of the negative feedback effect of oestradiol and inhibin on FSH production. The increased FSH secretion appears to result in accelerated follicular maturation and earlier ovulation. The length of the luteal phase is usually not affected during this initial period of the perimenopause. Later in this process, however, an increased frequency of cycles with luteal dysfunction does occur. When the remaining, progressively fewer follicles become less responsive to gonadotrophin stimulation, less oestradiol is produced and a longer follicular phase may be required to achieve the critical oestradiol level that is essential to exert a positive feedback induction of the LH surge. Still later this critical stimulus is not produced at all and anovulatory cycles result. Oligomenorrhoea is common, as is dysfunctional uterine bleeding. Finally, when there are no longer any responsive follicles left to produce oestradiol and endometrial development, the true menopause is reached.

Primary manifestations

Ovaries

The ovary begins development in embryonic life during the seventh week, and the migration of the germ cells by amoeboid movement from the posterior portion of the yolk sac along the dorsal mesentery of the hindgut to the gonadal ridge is usually completed by the beginning of the sixth week of life. The primordial germ cells then undergo differentiation into oogonia and subsequently begin multiple mitotic divisions. The maximum number of germ cells, approximately six million, is reached by 5 months through mitosis. Some of the oogonia differentiate into primary oocytes which enter prophase of the first meiotic division. This begins between day 60 and 65. They remain at the diplotene stage until some time in the distant future when meiosis resumes after puberty and immediately prior to ovulation. However, most oocytes undergo atresia, and this process begins in the sixth month of life, such that a birth only 1 000 000 to 2 000 000 remain. During embryogenesis the oogonia are invested with epithelial cells from the coelomic epithelium and primordial follicles are formed beginning at the tenth week. This process is critical to the survival of the oocytes as all oogonia not transformed into primordial follicles are resorbed through atresia by the time of birth.

Atresia is an inexorable process that occurs, irrespective of ovulation, throughout a woman's life until menopause. This process results in the number of primordial follicles being reduced to an average of 380 000 by puberty and to

8000 by the time a woman reaches her early forties. Although residual follicles may be present after the time of the last menses, these follicles are thought to be abnormal in their inability to respond to gonadotrophins or their ability to resist atresia.

The depletion of follicles at menopause results in the transformation of the gross appearance of the ovary from its typical appearance in reproductive life to a shrunken, pitted organ after the menopause. The cortex becomes atrophic but the amount of medullary stroma and interstitium increase. There may be a few remaining follicles present but these are almost invariably atretic.

The major oestrogen of reproductive age women secreted by the ovaries is 17β-oestradiol and the mean serum levels fall from 120 to 18 ng/l after the menopause (Judd, 1976) (Table 7.2). A subtle reduction in the amount

Table 7.2 Oestrogen metabolism before and after spontaneous menopause

	Mean circulating level (ng/l)	Daily production rate	MCR (l/24 h)
Premenopause			
Oestradiol	35–500	40–675 µg/24 h	1350
Oestrone	30–200	65–450 µg/24 h	2210
Oestriol	7–12		
Postmenopause			
Oestradiol	13–18	12 mcg/24 h	910
Oestrone	30–60	45–55 mcg/24 h	1600
Oestriol	6		

of circulating oestradiol and an intermittent, modest elevation of FSH are the earliest endocrine changes in the perimenopause. During reproductive life 95 per cent of oestradiol is produced directly by the ovaries and the remainder by peripheral aromatisation of oestrone and testosterone. The menopause is associated with the loss of the ability to synthesise oestradiol from pregnenolone via the $\triangle^5$β-hydroxysteroid or the $\triangle^4$ 3 ketosteroid pathways. The ovary continues to produce significant quantities of androgens, specifically androstenedione and testosterone, but the ability to convert these products to oestradiol via the aromatase system in the granulosa cells is lost. The majority of the remaining oestradiol is produced by peripheral conversion of oestrone to oestradiol (Judd et al, 1982). Evidence for this comes from studies which report the suppression of oestradiol levels after administration of dexamethasone or adrenalectomy (Veldhuis et al, 1978). The metabolism of oestradiol is modulated after the menopause by a 30 per cent reduction in the metabolic clearance rate (Longcope, 1971). Oestradiol is bound to sex hormone binding globulin (SHBG) and albumin but is probably not biologically available when bound to SHBG (Pardridge & Meitus, 1979).

Oestrone is the principle oestrogen produced after the menopause and the mean serum level is 35 ng/l (Longcope et al, 1969). An inactive conjugated metabolite, oestrone sulfate, is actually the most abundant postmenopausal oestrogen, having a mean serum concentration of 178 ng/l. Oestrone is primarily derived from the peripheral conversion of androstenedione. The mean conversion rate is 2.8 per cent (Chang & Judd, 1981) and this process correlates directly to weight. There have been conflicting data concerning the relationship of age to oestrone synthesis (Hemsell et al, 1974; Judd et al, 1980). This aromatisation process has been demonstrated in adipose tissue, liver, kidney, brain, and adrenals (Longcope et al, 1978). A small amount of oestrone is produced by the post menopausal ovary (Chang & Judd, 1981) Oestrone is not bound to SHBG. Oestrone is transported into cell nuclei where it initiates RNA and protein synthesis but it is not as effective an oestrogen receptor activator as is oestradiol (Barnea & Gorski, 1970).

Progesterone synthesis becomes impaired during the perimenopause and this is manifested by the increased incidence of luteal dysfunction preceeding the menopause. This may be a consequence of perturbations in gonadotrophin secretion prior to the formation of the corpus luteum or impaired steroidogenesis subsequent to abnormalities in the remaining follicles. After the menopause progesterone levels remain in the follicular phase range.

The climacteric is also characterised by dramatic changes in androgen production. The abundant postmenopausal ovarian stroma and remaining nests of theca cells continue to produce testosterone and some androstenedione in response to the greatly increased circulating levels of LH. Androstenedione, the predominant ovarian androgen in premenopausal women, decines from a circulating mean of 1500 ng/l during reproductive life to a mean of 800–900 ng/l after the menopause (Judd et al, 1974). Androstenedione is produced in roughly equal quantities by the ovaries and adrenals in the premenopausal state but the postmenopausal ovarian contribution is approximately 20 per cent (Chang & Judd, 1981). It is produced in a circadian pattern suggesting an adrenal influence. The amount of testosterone produced by the ovaries is increased after menopause but the total amount of testosterone is actually decreased since the amount of the primary source, peripheral conversion of androstenedione, is reduced (Chang & Judd, 1981) (Table 7.3). Menopause does not

affect the metabolic clearance rates of testosterone or androstenedione and both are bound to SHBG, testosterone with much greater affinity. Dehydroepiandrosterone (DHEA) and dehydroepiandrosterone sulfate (DHEA-S) are two adrenal androgens which are normally diminished in the menopause but are increased by an increase of SHBG with exogenous oestrogen administration (Abraham & Maroulis, 1975).

Pituitary and hypothalamus

The pathognomonic laboratory sign heralding the onset of ovarian failure or the menopause is a sustained elevation of FSH. Recent studies have reported individuals with isolated elevations of gonadotrophins who subsequently recovered normal menstrual function and have even conceived (Rebar, 1982). However, these individuals are rare and this phenomenon seems unique to women with premature ovarian failure.

The FSH elevation usually precedes a rise in LH. Since FSH is more sensitive to the negative feedback effect of oestrogen, an additional ovarian factor such as inhibin has been postulated to explain why FSH is not suppressed in an oestrogenic milieu that is capable of exerting a negative feedback effect on LH release. Such an ovarian compound has not yet been fully characterised. The increased serum FSH level is a result of increased release of FSH. There is no change in the metabolic clearance rate of FSH or LH at the menopause (Kohler et al, 1968).

As the climacteric progresses, there are wide oscillations in FSH and, less notably, in LH as well which reach maximum levels 2 to 3 years after the menopause. The FSH/LH ratio becomes greater than one, a phenomenon that does not normally occur in reproductive life. FSH is a more sensitive index of ovarian function at this time since an LH elevation may be associated with ovulation or polycystic ovarian syndrome. Later in the climacteric there may be a gradual decline of LH and FSH. In one large study of gonadotrophins in post-menopausal women mean plasma LH and FSH basal levels were 93.8 ± 5.4 and 132.4 ± 5.6 miu/ml, respectively (Scaglin et al, 1976). LH and FSH are released in a pulsatile fashion at 10 to 20 min intervals in menopausal women, a frequency more rapid than that present in normally cycling women (Odell, 1976). The apparent difference in circulating levels of the two hormones is a reflection of their different half-lives: 21 min for LH and 3.9 h for FSH. The increased frequency of pulsatile release in the menopause probably represents the removal of the negative feedback of oestrogen at the level of the hypothalamus. Although current methodology — specifically lack of a suitable assay — precludes accurate assessment of changes in gonadotrophin releasing hormone (GnRH) metabolism, it is known that the pituitary is much more responsive to exogenously administered GnRH after the menopause (Fig. 7.1) The increased release of LH and

Table 7.3 Androgen metabolism before and after spontaneous menopause

	Mean circulating level (ng/l)	Daily production rate	MCR (l/24 h)
Premenopause			
Testosterone	325	250 mcg/24 h	600
Androstenedione	1500	3 mg/24 h	1800
Postmenopause			
Testosterone	250	150 mcg/24 h	600
Androstenedione	800–900	1.6 mg/24 h	1800

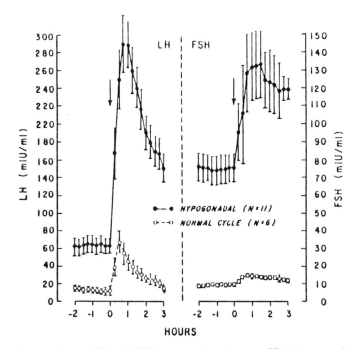

Fig. 7.1 Serum LH and FSH concentration (mean ± SE) 2 h pre- and 3 h post-LRF (150 μg, i.v.) for hypogonadal women is compared with normal women in the early follicular phase of the cycle. The differences were significant (P < 0.001) at all points for both LH and FSH (Siler & Yen, 1973)

FSH may result from heightened pituitary sensitivity of GnRH and an actual increase in frequency or amplitude of GnRH release. Prolactin, another pituitary hormone, is produced in reduced quantities after the menopause possibly in response to the decreased oestrogen level (Vekemans & Robyn, 1975)

Other primary manifestations of the menopause

Coincident with the endocrine changes of the climacteric are other multiple physiological changes in various organ systems. Many of these changes have historically been causally related to the menopause, but it now appears most are only temporally linked. Most of these alterations more correctly represent senescent processes that continue independently of the hormonal environment. The physiology of ageing is a fascinating area that only recently has attracted legitimate scientific interest. Two general sets of theories have been proposed to address the process of senescence. The classical thesis maintains that senectitude is the summation of a lifetime of environmental insults and random errors in cell replication. The other hypothesis suggests that ageing represents a genetically predetermined orderly event that has critical evolutionary significance — the survival of the species. There is now a body of data that supports the thesis that all species have a maximum life expectancy and any individual has the potential to realise this posibility if life is not interrupted by a genetic disease, intercurrent fatal disease or accidental death (Calkins,

1981). In 1961 Hayflick reported the results of a classic experiment in which he cultured human embryonic fibroblasts (Hayflick & Moorehead, 1961). He found that such cells were capable of replicating only about 50 times before the cells died. This process was related to the age of the donor and when older cells were cultured, they were capable of fewer cell divisions. Adult cells divided an average of 20 times before additional doubling ceased. All division stops either when additional DNA is no longer synthesised (G1 block) or the process of mitosis is arrested (G2 block). Blocked cells may either reverse the process and resume proliferation or succumb. Gelfant & Smith (1972) maintain that this non-cycling state, which is unique to ageing cells, is reversible.

Alternatively or concurrently, cell death may result from primary errors in DNA synthesis which become more common in the older cell or as a result of the accumulation of toxic macromolecules which undergo collagen linking. Burnet (1970) has proposed that mutated immunocytes and a compromised or 'exhausted' thymus dependent immune system gives rise to cancer and autoimmune disorders in the aged. He maintains that since each physiological system has 'an inbuilt biologic clock,' the organ that dissipates its genetic quota first is most vulnerable to the effects of ageing.

Virtually all organ systems are affected by the process of ageing. The nervous system undergoes several different changes including the progressive loss of neurons, most notably in the cerebral cortex; the impairment of nerve transmission; delaying of reflexes; and diminished sensitivity of the senses. Investigators have also noted deterioration of fine motor skills, difficulty with coordination resulting in more frequent accidents and diminished ability to learn new psychomotor skills and assimilate new information.

A specific neurological change associated with ageing is the progressive failure of the dopaminergic system. Clinically this may be associated with the onset of Parkinson's disease or it may be a sub-clinical phenomenon except for a hypothetical acceleration of the ageing process. Old rats treated with L-dopa experience resumption of vaginal cycling (Linnoila & Cooper, 1976). This study and other similar ones have been cited as evidence for the existence of a central 'biological clock' in the suprachiasmatic nucleus of the hypothalamus controlling various codons and genes at different ages of life which could potentially activate self destruction mechanisms or deactivate homeostatic controls at the end of an individual's life (Romero, 1978). By extension of this thesis, the menopause may be a neuroendocrine mediated event with follicle depletion being a consequence of changes in gonadotrophin output. However, there are little conclusive data to support this thesis.

Other organ systems undergo less dramatic senescent changes. A feature common to most tissues is the progressive loss of cells. This phenomenon has been observed in skin, cardiac myofibrils, and lung. There is also a decrease in tissue elasticity which can be of clinical concern when respiration is jeopardised by the increased compliance. In the kidney, there is a progressive decrease in renal plasma flow probably as a result of decreasing cardiac output and a direct reduction of blood flow in the renal vascular system (Calkins, 1981). The amount of creatinine produced daily decreases secondary to a decrease in the body muscle mass but serum creatinine values usually remain the same since creatinine clearance is reduced. This latter observation has clinical significance in that elderly individuals may be predisposed to overdoses of medication since their ability to excrete drugs is impaired.

In contrast to the changes in the ovary and gonadotrophin compartment of the adenohypophysis, the remainder of the endocrine system is relatively unaffected by the ageing process. The ability of the pituitary to respond to stress with the release of ACTH remains the same, as does the release of TSH in women (Calkins, 1981). There is some impairment of pancreatic ability to respond to a glucose load with the release of an appropriate amount of insulin. This may result in an apparent abnormality in the glucose tolerance that may be distinguished from true adult onset diabetes mellitus by a special nomogram that adjusts for age.

Summary of primary manifestations

The most clinically visible physiological changes in the ageing female are a consequence of senescent changes in the ovary, chiefly characterised by an absence of developing follicles. This in turn causes dramatic changes in steroid production, the principle features include: (1) the abrupt decline of oestradiol production in the ovary and the role of primary oestrogen synthesis being assumed by the peripheral conversion of androstenedione to oestrone with much less total biological potency and (2) alterations in androgen production resulting in a reduction in total androstenedione and testosterone synthesis but increased ovarian production of testosterone with greater potential androgenic activity subsequent to the decline in oestrogen and SHBG. The end product of this synthesis is the availability of more free biologically active androgen. These effects results in the loss of a negative feedback effect and gonadotrophins and probably LH-RH rise in response to this lack of suppression. This sequence of events progresses concomitantly with the development of senescent changes in other organs. The physiology of ageing is poorly understood but current data suggest that individual cells and whole organisms have a genetically programmed life span that may be determined by a limited number of cell replications. The overall control of the ageing process may be mediated by the neuroendocrine system. Much more work

in this area needs to be done before a clear picture can emerge.

Secondary manifestations of the climacteric
(symptoms of oestrogen deficiency)

Features of the climacteric which are most apt to come to clinical attention are those that are related to the relatively abrupt decrease in oestrogen production. Indeed the efficacy of oestrogen replacement therapy has been so great in ameliorating some of the symptoms of menopause that it has been viewed as a veritable panacea for all symptoms of the climacteric. Oestrogen deficiency directly affects target tissues, those organs that are known to possess oestrogen receptors. Oestrogen receptors have been identified in a variety of tissues including ovary, endometrium, vaginal epithelium, hypothalamus and skin. Other tissues without oestrogen receptors may be secondarily affected by oestrogen deficiency if oestrogen modulates another effector. For example, although oestrogen receptors have not been identified in bone, oestrogen may play a role in calcium metabolism. Presently there are only three symptom complexes which have been clinically proven to be improved by oestrogen replacement therapy: vasomotor symptoms, urogenital atrophy and osteoporosis.

Vasomotor symptoms

Vasomotor symptoms — principally the hot flash or hot flush — have been the oldest indication for oestrogen replacement therapy and are generally the most bothersome component of the menopausal syndrome, afflicting 75 to 85 per cent of women experiencing a natural menopause (Bates, 1981). The onset of the hot flash may begin several years prior to the actual menopause and it uniquely improves with time as the climacteric progresses. Subjectively, it is described as the sudden onset of warmth and vasodilatation, visible as a red flush which is most apparent over the face and chest. They occur more frequently in warmer ambient temperatures. Hot flashes are frequently accompanied by other vasomotor symptoms including: nausea, dizziness, headaches, palpitations, diaphoresis and night sweats. Following the hot flash many individuals experience chills associated with a vasoconstriction component. Perhaps their most troublesome associated symptom is the high incidence of sleep disturbances. In nine postmenopausal women studied in a sleep laboratory, 47 objectively documented hot flashes were recorded and 45 of these were associated with awakening episodes (Erlik et al, 1981).

The investigation of the pathophysiology of the hot flash has been hindered until recently by the absence of a suitable method to quantitate objectively its frequency, duration and intensity. The development of a skin sensor that is capable of detecting a temperature elevation associated with subjectively perceived hot flashes by Molnar (1979) and Meldrum et al (1979) has provided a valuable research tool. A temperature rise greater than 1°C on the dorsum of the finger is consistently associated with the subjective experience of a hot flash. Studies using this monitor have correlated hot flashes with hormonal changes and have noted an association between hot flashes and an increase in circulating LH (Tataryn et al, 1979). Increases in DHEA, androstenedione and cortisol have been noted 10 to 20 min after a hot flash is objectively perceived (Meldrum et al, 1981). The significance of these latter findings is unknown and the adrenal production of steroids may be the consequence of the stress of the hot flash or a common pathway in the neurotransmitter initiation of the hot flash and ACTH release. The association of the hot flash with increased LH secretion is more directly related, however. LH itself does not seem to be the effector of hot flashes since patients with pituitary insufficiency and previous hypophysectomy may experience hot flashes in the absence of detectable LH release (Meldrum et al, 1981; Mulley et al, 1977). These data, coupled with observations regarding the oestrogen suppression of hypothalamic factors suggest that the hot flash is associated with the release of GnRH or other modulators of LH release. The proximity of the GnRH neurons to the temperature regulating centres in the preoptic portion of the hypothalamus make the existence of a common defect more possible. GnRH secretion is modulated, in part, by α-adrenergic stimulation — an observation which supports the concept that hot flashes are caused by alterations in the autonomic nervous system. Evidence for a role for the autonomic system in triggering the hot flash includes the observations that hot flashes spread along the pattern of distribution of the cervical sympathetic pathways and the administration of clonidine — an α-adrenergic agonist which decreases central sympathetic outflow — reduces the frequency and intensity of hot flashes (Clayden et al, 1974). Current data suggests that hot flashes are centrally mediated, they are probably controlled by hypothalmic releasing factors which may include GnRH and central catecholamine concentrations may in turn modulate their release.

Genito-urinary changes

The most obvious feature of the menopause — amenorrhoea — results from the lack of oestrogen stimulation of the endometrium. Prior to the cessation of menses there may be intervals of oligomenorrhoea interspersed with bleeding episodes that are usually anovulatory. At times these irregular menses are characterised by menorrhagia and metrorrhagia which may mimic endometrial adenocarcinoma, a disease which becomes increasingly more prevalent after the menopause. This concern frequently dictates more intensive histological surveillance with endometrial biopsy and dilatation and curettage. Following the meno-pause, the endometrium may persist in one of the following patterns: weakly proliferative, senile atrophic, cystic hyperplasia, adenomatous hyperplasia, frankly neoplastic or most uncommonly, secretory. The overall hormonal milieu is the specific determinant of the histological pattern. A recent study (Strathy et al, 1982) reports that a significant fraction of uterine oestrogen receptors becomes biologically inactive (incapable of nuclear binding) during the menopause. This may result from the change in circulating oestrogen concentrations or it may be mediated by a yet unidentified process. The myometrium shrinks during this interval and the total uterine weight decreases from the premenopausal mean of 120 g to the postmenopausal average of 25–50 g. The endocervical glands contract and there is a marked reduction in cervical mucus production.

The vagina undergoes progressive thinning and foreshortening and loss of the rugose pattern. The premenopausal oestrogenised vagina is characterised by a thick epithelium with four distinct layers: basal, parabasal, intermediate and superficial. Oestrogen stimulation results in epithelial growth and a preponderance of cells from the superficial layers on vaginal smear. With the decline in oestrogen production, the parabasal and intermediate cells predominate. This effect may be followed clinically by a variety of cytological indices which compare the relative percentages of the three most superficial cell layers. These include: the maturation index, the ratio of parabasal, intermediate and superficial cells; the Karyopyknotic index, the ratio of superficial to intermediate cells; the eosinophilic index, the relative proportion of mature eosinophilic to mature cyanophilic cells; and the folded cell index, the ratio of mature folded to mature flat cells (Utian, 1980). They are all of limited value in assessing the adequacy or necessity of oestrogen replacement treatment.

Symptomatically, the atrophic changes result in dyspareunia and an increased susceptibility to vaginal trauma and infection. The aetiology of post menopausal vaginitis may include any of the organisms implicated in premenopausal vaginitis in addition to sterile atrophic vaginitis. The latter condition may be prevented or retarded by regular intercourse.

Features of pelvic relaxation including cystocoele with stress urinary incontinence, rectocoele with constipation, and descensus may become more prominent after the menopause. Considerable controversy exists over the role of oestrogen in treating these conditions. The pelvic floor is composed of striated muscle that is not derived from the Müllerian system. Oestrogen receptors have not been demonstrated in these tissues and theoretically oestrogen should not be of value. Although some authors continue to recommend the use of oestrogen (Greenhill, 1972), objective controlled studies have not demonstrated their advantage (Stark et al, 1978). The urethra does appear to undergo changes with oestrogen deprivation and urethral caruncular and urethral shortening may become prominent. The 'urethral syndrome' (recurrent abacterial urethritis) with consequent dysuria, frequency, urgency, nocturia and post-voiding dribbling is improved with oestrogen therapy. Stress incontinence and rectocoele are not improved by oestrogen therapy and birth trauma, multiparity and obesity are probably more significant factors than diminished oestrogen production in their aetiology. The vulva undergoes classic changes after the menopause which are not affected by oestrogen replacement therapy, although it is endowed with oestrogen receptors. Senescent changes including progressive hair loss, thinning of the overlying skin, resorption of the labia minora and thinning of the subcutaneous layers occur. Vulvar dystrophies and pruritus develop more commonly and some varieties (hypertrophic vulvar dysplasia) are improved with oestrogen but there are no data to suggest that hypooestrogenism may be a causative factor.

Skeletal

Postmenopausal osteoporosis is the most significant of the oestrogen deficiency symptoms and the scope of the problem is vast. Although the actual incidence of osteoporosis is difficult to estimate, its sequellae are not. The three principal complications of osteoporosis are vertebral compression fractures, distal forearm fractures and hip fractures. Approximately 25 per cent of Caucasian women over 60 years of age will have a spinal compression fracture. After age 90, three out of 100 women sustain a fracture of the femoral head each year in the United Kingdom (Gallannaugh et al, 1976). One-fifth of these individuals die in hospital and the average stay is over 1 month. Total estimates of the various costs of hip fractures in Europe and North America exceed two billion dollars annually (Anonymous, 1978).

Fuller Albright coined the term postmenopausal osteoporosis (Albright et al, 1940) to describe the process of progressive loss of bone mass which progresses more rapidly after the cessation of ovarian function. The association of oestrogen lack and osteoporosis (as manifested by loss of height) was strengthened in 1957 when Henneman & Wallach (1957) reported positive therapeutic and prophylactic effects of oestrogen treatment on the course of osteoporosis in menopausal women. Although a wealth of clinical data suggests a link between oestrogen and the stabilisation of bone structure, a detailed understanding of bone and oestrogen physiology has been slow in forthcoming.

Bone density gradually increases until age 35 to 40 then gradually declines in both sexes (Garn, 1970). The declivity in bone mass in women is greater than in men and averages 1–1.5 per cent per year such that by age 80 a Caucasian woman will have lost 30–50 per cent of her original bone mass (Krane & Holick, 1980). This process is more rapid and more severe in individuals who are Caucasian, seden-

tary, underweight and smokers. Osteoporosis affects the axial skeleton with its preponderance of trabecular bone before cortical bone, the major component of long bones, but ultimately affects the entire skeleton. A recent study described bone loss in the vertebral column as beginning in young adulthood and remaining linear while loss of mineral density in the appendicular skeleton began at age 50 and was accelerated between ages 51 to 65 (Riggs et al, 1980). This may explain the increase in hip fractures observed after the menopause. It also highlights the limitations of following the course of osteoporosis with serial studies performed on accessible bone such as a metacarpal and extrapolating changes seen radiographically to another bone such as a vertebra with possibly different rates of demineralisation.

Primary osteoporosis is a heterogeneous group of disorders with multiple cuases (Table 7.4). These various factors reflect the variety of potential sites of effect of bone metabolism. Bone simultaneously undergoes opposite dynamic effects — bone formation governed by the osteoblasts and bone resorption controlled by the osteoclasts. Bone formation is thought to be normal in individuals with osteoporosis but bone resorption is enhanced and this leads to disordered bone remodelling with demineralised bone. Bone resorption is predominantly modulated by parathormone (PTH) which is released in response to hypocalcaemia. PTH serves to raise serum calcium levels by

Table 7.4 Causes of osteoporosis

Physiological
  Immobilisation or weightlessness

Pharmacological
  Corticosteroids
  Cytotoxic agents
  Heparin
  Anticonvulsants
  Isoniazid
  Tetracycline

Endocrinological
  Hypoestrogenism or hypoandrogenism
  Hyperthroidism
  Primary hyperparathyroidism
  Cushing's syndrome
  Growth hormone deficiency
  Acromegaly

Nutritional
  Vitamin D deficiency
  Calcium deficiency
  Intestinal malabsorption syndromes
  Upper gastrointestinal surgery
  Vitamin C deficiency
  Alcoholism

Hereditary
  Osteogensis imperfecta

Miscellaneous
  Rheumatoid arthritis
  Chronic renal failure
  Diabetes mellitus
  Malignancy
  Idiopathic

causing the release of calcium from bone or resorption, reducing renal excretion and promoting tubular reabsorption of calcium and catalysing the conversion of 25-hydroxyvitamin D to its active metabolite, 1α, 25-hydroxyvitamin D, by 1α-hydroxylation. The last effect is critical for the intestinal absorption of calcium. The calcium elevating effects of PTH are antagonised by the thyroid hormone calcitonin. It is obvious that there are numerous points of vulnerability in the bone remodelling process that may lead to hypocalcaemia and osteoporosis including: decreased dietary intake of calcium, impaired intestinal absorption of calcium, vitamin D deficiency states, other vitamin deficiencies such as vitamin C which is necessary for normal osteoblastic activity, and use of drugs which increase calcium excretion including corticosteroids, isoniazid, and tetracycline.

The putative role of oestrogen in arresting or preventing osteoporosis has not been clearly elucidated. Several epidemiological studies have demonstrated a strong relationship between menopause or bilateral oophorectomy (Garn, 1970; Nordin, 1971; Aitken et al, 1973) and bone loss. Oestrogen does not stimulate osteoblastic formation of new bone. This has been documented only in the case of formation of medullary egg bone in the bird. Oestrogen receptors have not been demonstrated in bone.

Oestrogen deficiency is associated with the increased urinary excretion of calcium (Hammond & Maxson, 1981) and hydroxyproline (Nordin et al, 1975), an amino acid found almost exclusively in collagen. Both of these features have been ascribed to increased bone resorption and the processes are reversed with oestrogen replacement therapy. This does not seem to be a consequence of absolute oestrogen levels or an alteration in the binding of sex steroids (Davidson et al, 1980).

Studies of PTH levels after the menopause have usually demonstrated a decrease in the immunoreactive fraction of PTH (Riggs et al, 1976). This finding has lead to the premise that PTH decreases secondarily in response to hypercalcaemia caused by a yet to be identified factor (Riggs et al, 1976). Alternatively, preliminary results from a recently developed cytochemical bioassay suggest that the bioactive fraction of PTH may actually be elevated after the menopause and is even higher in individuals with severe osteoporosis (Posillico et al, 1981, unpublished data).

Gallagher et al (1980) have suggested that oestrogen's major effect in the treatment of osteoporosis is to increase calcium absorption by increasing serum 1,25 dihydroxyvitamin D. This suggests that oestrogen might counter the effects of osteoporosis by increasing renal tubular absorption of calcium and increasing gastrointestinal absorption of calcium by increasing the amount of active vitamin D retained and inhibiting bone resorption. Other theories have suggested that oestrogen may act by antagonising GH (Klotz, 1980) and osteoporotic women may have impeded secretion of GH (Rico et al, 1979).

Much of the difficulty in investigating the physiology of osteoporosis stems from the relative unavailability of reliable, inexpensive, non-invasive tests to follow the course of the disease. Also, the effects of both disease and therapy may require years to become obvious. There are a number of techniques that are currently available to diganose and follow osteoporosis (Utian, 1980). Conventional radiography of the spine and long bones is of little value in assessing bone density because of numerous technical limitations.

The Barnett-Nordin index may be derived by calculating the cortical area of bone and dividing this by the total area of a long bone. This calculation may be performed on data obtained from conventional radiographs and is more accurate than an uncorrected X-ray but still has an unacceptably high reproducibility error. Bone biopsy and histological analysis is a very accurate, highly reproducible technique but it is invasive and costly. The Singh index consists of grading the trabecular bone pattern in the proximal femur. There is considerable potential error in the interpretation since the bone pattern is correlated to bone density and the two do not always change consistently. X-ray densitometry using an aluminum equivalent standard offers an accurate reproducible estimate of bone density but this technique is best suited to evaluating small accessible bones such as the metacarpals and they may not be reflective of osteoporotic changes occurring at more vulnerable sites, i.e. the hip or vertebra. Photon absorptiometry is a simple non-invasive method that relies on the measuring of the γ-radiation that is blocked by bone which varies with density. A radioisotope such as ^{125}I or ^{241}Am and a scintillation detector are used. Assessment of mineral content is theoretically accurate to within 2 per cent of the actual value (Cameron et al, 1968) but when used serially there may be considerably greater error stemming from difficulties encountered in relocating the original site (Utian, 1980). Total body neutron activation analysis may be used to quantitate accurately the total calcium content of the entire skeleton but has little utility in following changes in specific bones. Perhaps the most promising technique currently available is computed tomography (CT) of both cancellous and trabecular bone (Cann et al, 1980). This method is available in most centres, is very accurate and permits assessment of a variety of different bones.

Long-term clinical studies with reliable techniques to evaluate risk factors of disease and efficacy of different therapies are still forthcoming. It is hoped that this information will permit appropriate selection for treatment of the many millions of women afflicted with osteoporosis.

Other systems

The assessment of the effects of reduced circulating oestrogen concentrations upon the skin is often complicated by other simultaneous senescent changes which are independent of hormonal effects. Oestrogen receptors have been identified in skin and they may be involved in the regulation of collagen metabolism. Other changes with age that are probably not oestrogen-mediated include: progressive thinning of the epidermis with loss of epidermal ridges and dermal papillae, less scalp and body hair and a decrease in sebaceous gland production.

The breast undergoes significant changes in size after the menopause. The glandular system of the glandular tissues becomes more atrophic and the nipples become smaller, sometimes losing their erectile properties. Cooper's ligament becomes less elastic causing the breast to lie more flatly against the chest wall.

Manifestations possibly related to oestrogen deficiency

Oestrogen was inferred to be a protective factor in the genesis of various atherosclerotic cardiovascular diseases and was recommended for prophylaxis after the menopause on the basis of several epidemiological observations. Women rarely suffer myocardial infarctions prior to the menopause (Kannel et al, 1976). Following the menopause a woman's risk of cardiovascular disease rapidly approximates that of a man's. Further, some studies demonstrated that women who underwent an early surgical menopause (before age 40) were found to have a greater incidence of coronary artery disease than their age-matched controls (Parrish et al, 1967). This finding has not been substantiated by other studies and most reports addressing this question have been criticised for deficiencies in design (Roberts & Giraldo, 1979). The association of oestrogen deficiency and cardiovascular disease was also challenged by reports showing a linear increase in the incidence of coronary heart disease in women between the ages of 30 and 90 with no apparent change at the menopause (Furman, 1973). Although serum cholesterol levels — an established risk factor for heart disease — rise throughout life, the relationship to endogenous oestrogen production is obscure. The apparent decrease in the male:female ratio for cardiovascular risk after the menopause may be a consequence of the relative amelioration of a male risk factor such as a reduction in the oestrogen:testosterone ratio production or loss of another female factor such as progesterone production. Obviously, this area needs much more study before clinically proven conclusions may be available.

A variety of psychological problems including depression anxiety, emotional lability, neuroses and psychoses have been attributed to the menopause as well. Few of these conclusions have survived objective scrutiny in terms of their having a hormonal aetiology. However, there is an increased incidence in the number of hospital admissions for depression in postmenopausal women (Spicer et al, 1973). This period of a woman's life coincides with several major life transitions including loss of reproductive potential, waning youth and beauty, the departure of one's children from the home, changes in a spouse's career and frequently the death, major illnesses or physical dependencies of her own parents and in-laws. This combination of stresses increases the likelihood of all psychiatric illnesses and declining oestrogen production is probably the least significant factor. However, the association between hot flashes and waking episodes or insomnia is well established and this may aggravate an already difficult situation (Erlik et al, 1981). Oestrogen is also reported to exert a 'mental tonic' effect which is associated with a greater sense of wellbeing (Utian, 1972). This may result from the modifying of brain metabolism of serotonin and dopamine.

OESTROGEN (AND PROGESTIN) REPLACEMENT THERAPY

Pharmocology of oestrogens

Oestrogens may be defined as compounds capable of increasing the uterine weight or vaginal cornification. They can be steroid derivatives of cyclopentanoperhydrophenanthrene, as are the three naturally occurring human oestrogens: oestrone, oestradiol and oestriol. Alternatively, compounds with oestrogenic activity may be chemically unrelated to steroids but capable of exerting similar biological effects. Such compounds include diethylstilboestrol (DES), a stilbene derivative, and methallenestrill, a naphthylene derivative. Naturally occurring oestrogens are not active when absorbed through the gastrointestinal tract and all orally active agents are either synthetically modified natural oestrogens, usually by attaching an ethinyl group at the 17 position or are chemically unrelated to the natural oestrogens (Fig. 7.2).

Oestrogens circulate in free, protein-bound or conjugated forms. The free fraction is the biologically active one and easily passes through cell membranes and remains in equilibrium with the protein-bound portion. The latter is bound to SHBG and to a lesser extent albumin and is confined to the vascular compartment. Recent evidence suggests that SHBG minimally influences clearance of oestrogen and albumin-bound oestradiol may cross capillary endothelium (Loriaux et al, 1974; Pardridge & Meitus, 1979). These findings suggest that the bound fraction may have more biological activity than was previously surmised. Oestrogens are metabolised in the liver by conjugation with sulphate or glucuronate before being excreted into urine or bile. Conjugated oestrogens are water soluble, biologically inactive and may be orally absorbed. Sulphated oestrogens are well suited for replacement therapy as they are readily absorbed and made biologically active in the liver by the enzymatic clevage of the sulphate group by sulphatases.

Oestrogens exert their metabolic effects at the cellular

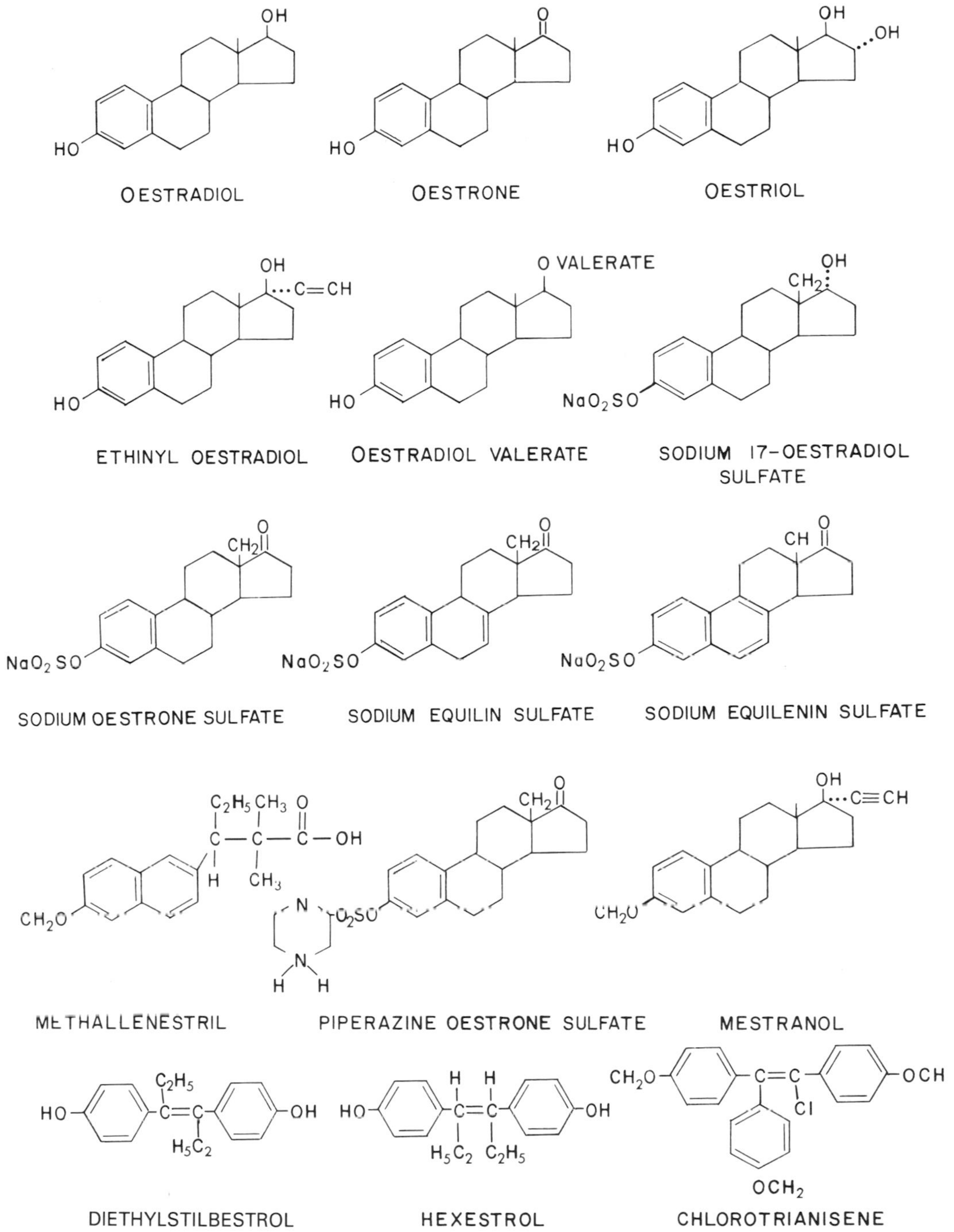

Fig. 7.2 Oestrogen structures

level via a large (sedimentation rate 8 S), high-affinity protein receptor in the cytosol. After binding to the receptor the complex is transported to the nucleus where it attaches to the nucleus. Messenger RNA is then produced and this secondarily results in increased protein synthesis which can be observed several hours following exposure to oestrogen. Oestrogen induces its own receptor formation. There appears to be a gradient which favours oestradiol's entry into the cell nucleus regardless of the peripheral oestrone:oestradiol ratio. Whitehead et al

(1981b) recently reported that oestradiol remains the predominant intranuclear oestrogen even when peripheral oestrone levels far exceed plasma oestradiol concentrations, i.e. after the menopause. These data possibly exonerate oestrone as an endometrial carcinogen, as had been previously proposed (Ziel & Finkle, 1976). Oestrogenic potency is probably dependent on the length of time the oestrogen molecule occupies the oestrogen receptor. This governs the amount of protein synthesised and hence the intensity of the biological effect. Oestriol demonstrates the shortest interval of nuclear occupation (1–4 h), oestradiol and diethylstilboesterol remain in the nucleus for 6–24 h and triphenylethylene compounds such as tamoxifen and nafoxidine are present for 24–48 h (Clark et al, 1978). The latter compounds act as oestrogen agonists initially but when administered repeatedly they accomplish down-regulation of the oestrogen receptors and function as oestrogen antagonists. *In vitro* assessment of oestrogenic activity varies greatly with the target organ observed, the type of oestrogen administered, the dose of oestrogen and the route of administration, the metabolic clearance rate and the relative number of oestrogen receptors present. One oestrogen may manifest different effects at different doses. All responses are subjectively interpreted and there may be considerable variation among observers. All of these factors make grading the potencies of various oestrogens very difficult.

Systemic effects of oestrogen therapy

Hypothalamic-pituitary

Perhaps oestrogen replacement therapy's most dramatic effect during the menopause is to reduce the frequency of hot flashes. Although clinicians have long concluded that oestrogen is efficacious in reducing the frequency of hot flashes, objective documentation has been made available only recently. Using the skin temperature sensor, Judd's group has objectively demonstrated less frequent hot flashes after oestrogen treatment (Tataryn et al, 1981). Oestrogen therapy presumably suppresses the release of GnRH from the hypothalamus, and this may be mediated by a direct effect of oestrogen or catechol oestrogens or other neurotransmitters. However, peripheral GnRH levels have not been adequately quantitated and GnRH levels in the peripheral circulation may not be reflective of fluctuations in the hypothalamic portal system. Consequently the true mechanism of action remains unknown. Oestrogen replacement does suppress FSH and LH but it is dosage- and drug-dependent and symptomatic relief does not correlate consistently with gonadotrophin suppression. Thus, gonadotrophin determination has not been a clinically useful guide for adjusting the dosage of oestrogen.

Genito-urinary effects

Oestrogen's primary genito-urinary effect is to re-establish the continuity of the epithelial surface of the endometrium after menstruation. This process is accomplished rapidly and is essentially complete by the fourth postmenstrual day. With continuous oestrogen stimulation there is additional proliferation of the endometrium and this is apparent microscopically as increased mitotic activity. The endometrium becomes thicker and the glands develop in a straight tubular pattern which becomes more tortuous as ovulation approaches. Oestrogen increases RNA synthesis and alters water transport to permit greater availability of materials necessary for RNA synthesis, including energy stores, and the enzymes, alkaline phosphatase and serum aldolase (Kistner, 1973). These events are grossly manifested by hyperaemia and weight gain. If oestrogen exposure continues and is not interrupted by ovulation or progestin exposure the proliferative response becomes more intense and endometrial hyperplasia may ensue. Kistner demonstrated the development of endometrial hyperplasia in 43 per cent of a small population of young, previously ovulatory women who were treated with an average dose of 48 mg of tri-p-anisyl-chloroethylene (TACE), a synthetic oestrogen, for 45 to 100 days (Kistner et al, 1956). The role of oestrogen in inducing more severe degrees of hyperplasia and neoplasia is less clear. There is an association between continuous oestrogen administration and progressive changes from proliferative endometrium to cystic hyperplasia and to adenomatous hyperplasia.

Oestrogen does not improve symptoms of pelvic relaxation except perhaps cases of mild stress urinary incontinence. Individuals suffering from 'atrophic cystitis' with frequency and dysuria may also be improved (Smith, 1977). Oestrogen administered either topically or systemically improves atrophic vaginitis and reduces the attendant pruritus and discharge. This may be observed objectively by noting a change in the karyopyknotic index to favour a more superficial, oestrogen mediated pattern (Hammond & Maxson, 1981). This is accompanied by a thickening in the vaginal mucosa and a decrease in the pH of vaginal secretions. Four to 12 weeks of treatment may be required to note an effect.

Osteoporosis

Oestrogen is effective in retarding the development of osteoporosis after the menopause. Several studies have demonstrated stabilisation of bone structure with a variety of methods for evaluating density including photon absorption densitometry, radiogrammetry and metacarpal densitometry when various oestrogens were administered after the menopause (Meema & Meema, 1976; Aitken et al, 1976). Bone mineral loss may actually be prevented when treatment is begun within two months of cessation of ovarian function (Aitken et al, 1973). Perhaps more persuasively, the incidence of fractures of the radius and hip are markedly reduced during the menopause by oestrogen replacement therapy (Hammond et al, 1979b; Weiss et al, 1980; Paganini-Hill et al, 1981).

The role of oestrogen in the treatment of established osteoporosis is less clear, however. Most investigators have failed to demonstrate an increase in bone density after oestrogen is given to individuals with symptomatic disease (Gallagher et al, 1972). There does appear to be a decrease in calcium excretion and restoration of a positive calcium balance for the first few months. This effect is short-lived, though, and is actually a manifestation of the different sensitivities to oestrogen of the bone resorption and remodelling mechanisms (Heaney, 1976). In other words, oestrogen induces bone remodelling initially and bone resorption ensues several months after initiation of oestrogen therapy to restore the normal equilibrium of bone homeostasis and bone density does not change further. Several investigators have described an increase in bone density after oestrogen therapy in younger women following oophorectomy (Lindsay et al, 1976) and in menopausal patients being treated with conjugated oestrogens (Nachtigall et al, 1979).

When treatment is delayed for 6 years or more from the time of menopause, oestrogen is probably ineffective in preventing subsequent demineralisation (Aitken et al, 1973). Oestrogen must be given for a protracted period of time (cyclically or continuously) to maintain this effect. The necessary dose of oestrogen to maintain bone stabilisation is considerably less than that required to treat other symptoms of the menopause. Mestranol 20 μg and conjugated oestrogens 0.6 mg, both daily, are known to be effective doses (Gordon & Genant, 1978) and studies are currently in progress to assess the adequacy of lower doses.

Cardiovascular

Exogenously administered oestrogen may affect cardiovascular risk factors in a variety of ways depending on the type of oestrogen given, dosage and route of administration. A period of early enthusiasm for a purported protective role of oestrogen from cardiovascular disease (Wilson, 1966) was followed by an interval during which oestrogen was implicated as a risk factor for cardiovascular disease, specifically in regard to the increased risk of thrombophlebitis and cerebrovascular accidents among oral contraceptive users. Cardiovascular disease is known to have numerous risk factors including ageing, obesity, hypertension, cigarette smoking, diet, diabetes and family history. Studies assessing the relative significance of a single risk are inherently limited by other complicating factors.

Serum lipids, specifically cholesterol and triglycerides, have been consistently correlated with risk of myocardial infarction. The high density lipoprotein (HDL) fraction of cholesterol is inversely related to ischaemic heart disease, being highest in populations with low risk such as Nordic skiers and long-distance runners (Hulley et al, 1977). The low density lipoprotein (LDL) portion correlates directly with risk for atherosclerotic heart disease and is frequently noted to be elevated in individuals with a previous history of myocardial infarction. Total serum cholesterol, which rises throughout life, is also directly related to risk for cardiovascular disease. Individuals with serum cholesterol values greater than 250 mg/100 ml have significantly

greater risk of heart disease at all ages. These factors have been used to gauge indirectly the cardiovascular effects of oestrogen since they are easily measured and can be obtained serially through the course of oestrogen treatment. Clinical correlation is, however, limited.

Oestrogen is thought to affect cholesterol and the lipoprotein fractions through its rate of synthesis and the rate of degradation and excretion (Boyd, 1963). 'Natural' oestrogens such as conjugated equine oestrogens decrease the LDL fraction and raise the HDL portion (Coronary Drug Project Research Group, 1970). Oral contraceptives containing ethinyl oestradiol produce the opposite pattern (Philips, 1978) and normal women given parenteral oestradiol do not demonstrate any change. Synthetic oestrogens increase serum triglyceride levels in males being treated for prostate cancer whereas this effect was not noted with natural oestrogens (Wallentin & Varenhorst, 1978).

Epidemiological studies addressing the relationship of oestrogen use and myocardial infarction have yielded contradictory results. Various investigators have reported clinical benefit with oestrogen therapy (Hammond et al, 1979; Ross et al, 1981), deterioration (Gordon et al, 1978) and no effect on the development of coronary artery disease (Oliver & Boyd, 1961). Most studies have shown no change or a slight clinical advantage with treatment. Young women with ovarian failure or following oophorectomy may derive greater cardiovascular benefit from oestrogen replacement therapy since their risk of acquiring cardiovascular disease is much greater (Parrish et al, 1967). Otherwise, there is no justification currently for using oestrogen therapy for prophylaxis of coronary artery disease. Conversely, oestrogen replacement therapy as currently practiced with low dose 'natural' oestrogens does not appear to confer significant risk of accelerating cardiovascular disease.

Putative effects of oestrogen

In addition to the previously mentioned mental tonic effect oestrogen has been said to produce numerous other beneficial effects which are documented less adequately. These include the arrest of the ageing process, relief from depression and enhancement of libido. Although oestrogen was once enthusiastically administered for these indications current data no longer support oestrogen use for these reasons.

Pharmacology of progestins

Progesterone — the most potent natural progestin — was first isolated from the corpora lutea of rabbits and was found to have a critical role in the maintenance of pregnancy. Progesterone has multiple systemic effects including stimulation of the development of the alveoli and lobules in the breast, induction of secretory changes in the endometrium and alteration of cervical mucus. Progesterone suppresses the release of hypothalamic factors and it, or a metabolite, has a thermogenic effect capable of producing the characteristic 0.5°C basal body temperature elevation noted after ovulation. It is a potent agent for relaxation of smooth muscle. Progesterone competes with aldosterone in the renal tubule and decreases sodium reabsorption. It produces a reduction in plasma amino acids which results in increased urinary nitrogen excretion (Meyers et al, 1972).

Progesterone is synthesised from corticoids, oestrogens and androgens. In addition to being produced in the ovary, the testis, adrenal and placenta are capable of progesterone

synthesis. Pregnanediol is the principle metabolite and urinary values may be determined to infer a reasonably accurate index of serum production rates. Although progesterone is rapidly absorbed from any site it is almost completely metabolised to pregnanediol and conjugated to glucuronic acid after its first passage through the liver. This renders oral administration ineffective.

To circumvent difficulties with oral administration numerous molecular alterations have been carried out to yield orally active progestins. Most of these compounds are 17α-hydroxyprogesterone or 17α-acetoxyprogesterone derivatives such as 17α-hydroxyprogesterone acetate,

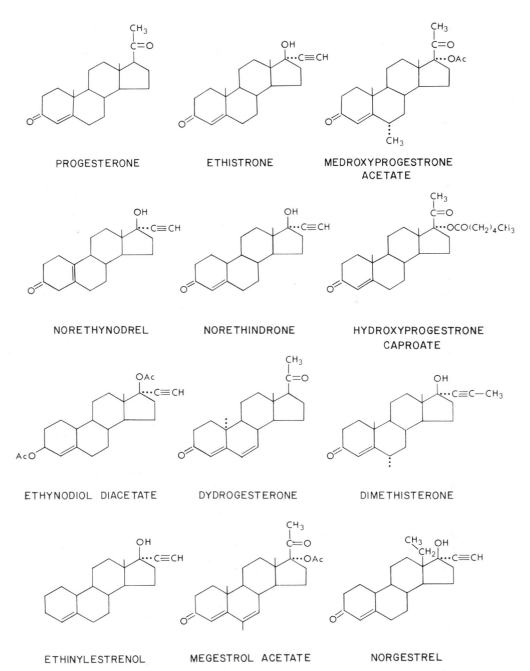

Fig. 7.3 Progestin structures

medroxyprogesterone acetate (6α-methyl-17α-acetoxyprogesterone) and megestrol acetate (6α-methyl-Δ⁶-17α-acetoxyprogesterone), or 19-nortestosterone derivatives including norethynodrel (17α-ethinyl-Δ⁵(10)-19-nortestosterone), norethindrone also known as nor-ethisterone (17α-ethinyl-19-nortestosterone), norethindrone acetate, dimethisterone (6α-methyl-17α[1-propynyl]testosterone) and ethynodiol diacetate (Fig. 7.3). The former group has properties more similar to natural progesterone. The 19-nortestosterone derivatives demonstrate progestational activity but also have varying androgenic effects and are primarily used in oral contraceptives.

Systemic effects of progestins

Although progestins are clearly inferior to oestrogen for the treatment of most symptoms of the menopause, they do effectively suppress some symptomotology. They are capable of alleviating vasomotor symptoms (Schiff et al, 1980; Morrison et al, 1980) and, in preliminary studies, have been demonstrated to prevent bone loss in osteoporotic individuals (Lindsay et al, 1978).

Although progestin therapy is inadequate treatment of genito-urinary atrophic changes of hypo-oestrogenism it produces a host of effects in Müllerian derived structures. Progestins presently have their greatest values in being used in associated with oestrogens to reduce the risk of endometrial adenocarcinoma. Progesterone produces a relatively unvarying sequence of changes in endometrium that, from a teleologic perspective, prepare the endometrium for the implantation of a blastocyst. This chain of events, first described by Noyes et al (1950), begins 2 days after ovulation with the appearance of basal vacuoles around the glands. This is followed by migration of the vacuoles through the glands and culminates in the extrusion of their material by day 21. The next series of changes occurs in the stroma and consists of increasing oedema and predecidualisation which initially appears around the spiral arterioles on day 23, below the capsule by day 25 and coalesces through the whole endometrium by day 27. The final changes are the appearance of stromal mitoses and a leucocytic infiltrate which precede menses by 2 days and 1 day, respectively.

Progestins induce the above secretory changes in endometrium after a short duration of exposure but produce atrophic changes with longer exposure (Kokko et al, 1982). Progestins, 17-aceto-oxyprogesterone and 19-nortestosterone derivatives, produce similar effects in endometrium but the former compounds are apparently less potent. The specific response of the endometrium to progestin varies with the prior stage of development (degree of oestrogenisation), duration of exposure, individual specificity, specific areas of the endometrium and different agents (Hammond & Ory, 1982). A reduction in stromal proliferation after oestrogen exposure is one of the earliest effects

of progestins. Subsequently the cytoplasmic volume increases and a generalised pseudodecidual reaction appears. This finding may be confused with the histological pattern of early pregnancy but the presence of atrophic glands serves to distinguish it. Later the venules dilate and become prominent while the arterioles recede. Some compounds produce unusual effects such as norethindrone which arrests endometrial development.

There progestational effects are associated with several ultrastructural changes as well. Progestins block the production of oestradiol receptors (Tseng & Gurpide, 1975a). Oestradiol dehydrogenase, the enzyme that converts oestradiol to the weaker oestrogen oestrone, is induced by progestins (Tseng & Gurpide, 1975b). Progestins also increase the rate of sulphurylation of oestrogen in the endometrium (Pack et al, 1979). All of these effects tend to limit the endometrium's exposure to oestrogen.

Progestational agents have been known to be effective in reversing endometrial hyperplasia (Kistner, 1959) and even carcinoma (Nilsen & Kolstad, 1971) for over 20 years. It has been established more recently that progestins reduce the risk of endometrial adenocarcinoma incurred with oestrogen therapy (Hammond et al, 1979; Gambrell et al, 1980). Moreover, recent studies have demonstrated that the maximal progestational effect on postmenopausal endometrium occurs after 6 days of continuous treatment with norethindrone or d/l-norgestrel (Whitehead et al, 1981a). This finding may explain why women taking sequential contraceptives with 6 days of exposure to a weak progestin had an increased risk of endometrial carcinoma (Weiss & Sayvetz, 1980) while individuals taking standard combination oral contraceptives have been found to have a decreased chance of developing the same malignancy (Hulka et al, 1982b).

Progestins have numerous systemic effects which are unrelated to their effects on the reproductive system. Most of the metabolic studies have been performed with medroxyprogesterone acetate (MPA) and 19-nortestosterone derivatives given in conjunction with oestrogens, i.e. oral contraceptives. These latter data are not suitable for assessing the effects of pure progestin or sequential oestrogen-progestogen therapy. MPA produces a slight increase in fasting glucose and enhances the insulin response to a glucose load (Spellacy et al, 1972). Most studies have not reported any change in serum triglyceride or cholesterol levels (Fraser & Weisberg, 1981) but one study did report a modest (15 per cent below controls) reduction in the HDL cholesterol fraction when 50 mg of MPA were administered weekly (Briggs & Briggs, 1979). Norgestrel and norethindrone acetate, 19-nortestosterone derivatives, are reported to produce greater reductions in HDL fractions (Hammond & Maxson, 1982). Medroxyprogesterone acetate administered at high doses is also capable of adrenal suppression and this effect is probably accomplished by the quenching of ACTH. Adrenal insufficiency resulting from MPA has not been described and this is probably due to its own weak intrinsic glucocorticoid activity (Fraser & Weisberg, 1981).

ADVERSE EFFECTS OF HORMONE REPLACEMENT THERAPY

Endometrial adenocarcinoma

The primary risk of oestrogen replacement therapy remains adenocarcinoma of the endometrium. The association of oestrogen and uterine cancer may have first been made by Schoeder (1922) when he reported an individual developing endometrial adenocarcinoma in conjunction with a granulosa cell (oestrogen secreting) tumour of the ovary. Gusberg reported 23 patients with endometrial adenocarcinoma in 1961 and stated that oestrogen played a role in the development of their disease (Mahboubi et al, 1982). As oestrogen use became more prevalent there were increasing numbers of case reports and small uncontrolled series which were flawed but suggested a link between oestrogen use and uterine adenocarcinoma. The publication of two large case control series in 1975 (Smith et al, 1975; Ziel & Finkle, 1975) and several subsequent reports (Antunes et al, 1979; Weiss et al, 1979) seemed to establish oestrogen use as a definite risk factor in the evolution of endometrial adenocarcinoma (Table 7.5).

To date research in this area has principally been directed towards two lines of investigation: epidemiological investigations and histological or biochemical *in vitro* studies. Most of the currently published epidemiological studies have been criticised for multiple methodological deficiencies. Most of these have examined intervals of time during which relevant medical practices have significantly changed including: the more frequent performance of hysterectomies, the increase and subsequent decrease in the prevalence of oestrogen use, and the availability of new procedures to obtain and examine endometrium. These factors, in addition to changes in prescription patterns — such as choice of oestrogen compounds, varying dosages, duration of exposure and the sequential use of progestins — have greatly complicated the interpretation of data and undoubtedly partially explain the reported variation in relative risk. Nevertheless, most reports have described a 4 to 8 fold increase in the incidence of endometrial adenocarcinoma in long-term oestrogen users. The general risk of endometrial carcinoma is reported to be 1/1000 per year (Weiss, 1975). Some researchers have described much larger risks and others have found no increased risk with oestrogen use (Dunn & Bradbury, 1967; Horwitz & Feinstein, 1978). Differences in the choice of controls and assessment of other known risk factors such as obesity and dietary fat intake probably account for some of these differences.

Additional support for oestrogen being a contributing factor in the development of endometrial carcinoma is derived indirectly from the established association of uterine adenocarcinoma with other chronic hyperoestrogenic states such as polycystic ovarian disease and other anovulatory states, oestrogen secreting ovarian tumours and hepatocellular disease resulting in impaired oestrogen metabolism (MacDonald & Siiteri, 1974). Also, Jick et al (1979) have described a recent reduction in the incidence of endometrial adenocarcinoma which has paralleled the decreased use of oestrogen for replacement therapy; they have inferred that this circumstantially incriminates oestrogen therapy.

Histological reports reviewing the association between oestrogen and endometrial carcinoma have generally consisted of: (1) review of endometrial biopsies obtained prior to the diagnosis of endometrial adenocarcinoma; (2) prospective studies conducted on patients with endometrial hyperplasia; or (3) studies of hyperplastic tissue contiguous with foci of cancerous areas. These studies have been deficient because of difficulties in follow-up, lack of availability of appropriate biopsies and the understandable reluctance of physicians not to intercede and therefore permit the study of the natural course of the disease. Most of these investigations have found a consistent relationship between continuous oestrogen exposure and progression of disease through the various endometrial hyperplasias to hyperplasia with atypia and adenocarcinoma. There does not appear to be any reduction in risk of developing endometrial hyperplasia with cyclic (3 weeks out of 4) therapy rather than continuous therapy (Schiff et al, 1982). The probability of an individual developing an adenocarcinoma subsequent to an endometrial biopsy interpreted as 'hyperplastic' has been reported to range from 1.57 to 25 per cent depending on the characteristics of the population (Gore, 1973). *In vitro* studies using endometrial adenocarcinoma cell cultures have not been technically feasible to date.

Currently, it appears from a variety of studies that oestrogen use is a risk factor for the development of adenocarcinoma of the endometrium. This risk appears to be directly related to the dose and duration of exposure. Other factors, such as following oestrogen therapy with progestin therapy, may curtail the risk or even reduce the risk below that of the general population (Gambrell et al, 1980; Morrison et al, 1980). Some authors have expressed the concern that adding a progestin to oestrogen replacement therapy may confer the same risk of cardiovascular disease incurred by oral contraceptive users on a more vulnerable population — menopausal patients (MacDonald, 1981). Much further work is necessary before a clear estimate of risk in optimal circumstances — i.e. minimum dose of oestrogen for minimum interval of time and accompanied by progestin therapy — will be forthcoming.

Table 7.5 Epidemiological studies examining the association between oestrogen replacement therapy and endometrial adenocarcinoma (modified from Davies et al, 1981)

Reference	Period covered	Population	No. of cases	No. of controls	Type of controls	Matching factors	Oestrogen exposure	Relative risk	95% confidence limits
Jensen Ostergaard (1954)	1939–1952	Denmark (Fredericksburg): Hospitalised Patients	105	52	Diseases not biasing results	none	Any oestrogen	1.9	
Wynder et (1959)	1959	U.S. (N.Y.) Hosp. patients	112	200	No breast or gynecological disease	None	Any oestrogen	0.6	
Dunn & Bradbury (1967)	1963–1965	U.S. (Iowa) Hosp. patients	56	83	Postmenopausal bleeding with atrophic endometrium	None	Any oestrogen		
Smith et al (1975)	1960–1972	U.S. (Wash.) Clinic & hosp. patients	317	317	Other gynecological malignancies	Age of, diag., year of diag.	Any oestrogen use ≥ 6 mos.	7.5	4.4–14.4
Ziel & Finkie (1975)	1970–1974	U.S. (Calif.) members of a health plan	94	188	No hysterectomy	Age, length of membership	Conjugated equine	7.6	4.3–13.4
Mack et al (1976)	1971–1975	U.S. (Calif.) Residents of retirement community	63	252	No hysterectomy	Age, marital status	Any oestrogen / Conjugated equine	8.0 / 5.6	3.5–18.1 / 2.6–11.1
McDonald et al (1976)	1945–1974	U.S. (Minn.) Residents of a single community	145	580	No hysterectomy	Age, duration of medical care	Any oestrogen / Conjugated equine	0.9 / 2.0	0.6–1.4 / 1.1–3.3
Gray et al (1977)	1947–1976	U.S. (Ken.) patients from private practice	205	205	Hysterectomy to benign disease	Age, partly weight	Any oestrogen use ≥ 3 months Conjugated oestrogen use ≥ 3 months	3.1	1.5–6.8
Antunes et al (1975)	1973–1978	U.S. Maryland Hosp. patients	509	435	No hysterec., gynecocal disorder	Race, age at diag., adm. date	Any pure oestrogen preparation	2.0	1.4–2.8
				450	No hysterec., nongynecological disorder			6.0	3.7–9.7
Horwitz & Feinstein (1978)	1974–1975	U.S. (Conn.) postmenopausal hosp. patients	119	119	Other gynecological cancer	Age, race	Conjugated oestrogen dose — 0.30.3 mg–6 months	12.0	4.0–47.7
			149	149	D & C or hysterectomy in study			2.3	1.3–4.6
Weiss et al (1979)	1975–1976	U.S. (Wash.) Residents of a single county	322	289	No hysterec.	Age range	Any oestrogen	6.0	
Hulka et al (1980)	1970–1976	U.S. (North Carolina) Residents of a state	256	22 321	Gynecological patients community controls	Race, age year of admission	Any oestrogen	6.0	0.7–1.8 1.4–1.5
									0.3–2.5 0.4–5.1

Breast carcinoma

Breast carcinoma, the most common malignancy of women, is influenced by sex steroids (Chapter 36). Currently there is no clear association between oestrogen replacement therapy and the likelihood of developing breast cancer. There have been many more risk factors elucidated for carcinoma of the breast than for endometrial carcinoma, data which have complicated the evaluation of a single risk factor such as exogenous oestrogen therapy.

If a risk exists it is a small one (Hammond et al, 1979a). Ross et al (1980), prospectively and retrospectively, examined the incidence of breast carcinoma in a retirement community and found a risk ratio of 2.5 in women with intact ovaries who had received a total dose of oestrogen of 1500 mg. Hulka et al (1982a) recently reported that oestrogen therapy was not associated with increased risk of breast malignancy in women having previously undergone surgical menopause and it was associated with a relative risk of breast cancer of 1.7 or 1.8 in women undergoing natural menopause with both groups receiving all types of oestrogen. This risk was only 1.2–1.3 (depending on which control group was compared) when women receiving injectable oestrogens were excluded. This latter figure is not statistically significant. Gambrell & Vasquez (1982) described an actual reduction in risk of breast malignancy, particularly when oestrogen was combined with progestin therapy, in a prospective study involving over 5000 women.

Thromboembolism

Thromboembolism and pulmonary embolism are not increased in menopausal women receiving low or modest dosage oestrogen replacement (Boston Collaborative Drug Surveillance Program, 1974; Studd et al, 1978). Although these complications are associated with oral contraceptive use and one would expect individuals in this age group to be more susceptible to thromboembolic disorders, this has not been the case. Differences in dosage and use of 'natural' rather than 17-ethinyl derived oestrogens may ameliorate the risk. There may be other unknown physiological changes at the menopause which account for these observed differences.

Natural and synthetic oestrogens produce a variety of changes in blood clotting factors most of which are of unknown significance. Plasma antithrombin III levels, a good index of risk for thrombophlebitis, are unchanged in patients receiving conjugated oestrogens (Notelovitz & Greig, 1976) while they are decreased (favouring development of thrombophlebitis) in patients on oral contraceptives (Howie et al, 1970).

Hypertension

The association between oral contraceptive therapy and mild and reversible hypertension is well established (Fisch & Frank, 1977) but a comprehensive understanding of the mechanism of this pathophysiology is still awaited. Synthetic oestrogens, and to a lesser extent natural oestrogens, enhance renin activity, renin substrate and aldosterone secretion (Crane et al, 1971). Oral contraceptive users have a 2 to 2.5 times increased risk over non-users of developing hypertension (Royal College of General Prac-

titioners, 1974). The epidemiological data addressing hypertension in menopausal oestrogen users are less clear. Two studies conducted by Pfeffer demonstrated small but statistically significant increases in non-diabetic women (Pfeffer & Van den Noort, 1976; Pfeffer, 1978). A third, more recent study using a variety of analytic methods in an attempt to exclude complicating variables did not find an increased risk of developing hypertension in women over 67 who used oestrogen for short intervals in low doses (average 0.6 mg of conjugated oestrogens) (Pfeffer et al, 1979). Von Eiff (1975) demonstrated a decrease (mean 6 mmHg) in diastolic blood pressure and heart rate (eight beats per minute) in individuals receiving oestradiol valerate following bilateral oophorectomy. The physiological significance and implications of increased risk of vascular disease consequent to such changes in blood pressure in the elderly is unknown.

Glucose tolerance

Most investigators have described slight deterioration in glucose tolerance in individuals treated with conjugated oestrogens (Yen & Vela, 1968; Notelovitz, 1974), ethinyl oestradiol (Yen & Vela, 1968) and mestranol (Gow & MacGillivray, 1971). This effect appears to be more prominent in patients treated with synthetic oestrogens than patients receiving conjugated oestrogens and patients taking oestradiol valerate may not have any change in their glucose tolerance curves (Larsson-Cohn & Wallentin, 1977). Addition of a progestin may have a synergistic effect producing glucose intolerance (Thom et al, 1977). Oestrogen therapy has not been reported to induce glucose intolerance in a previously normal individual. Goldzieher et al (1978) have proposed that the distinction between mild glucose intolerance and frank diabetes may be the absence of long-term diabetic sequellae in the former group. Thus oestrogen therapy may be a concern in patients with established diabetes, but it need not be avoided to prevent producing diabetes in non-diabetics.

Cholelithiasis

Individuals receiving oestrogen replacement therapy are at an increased risk of developing gallstones as are pregnant patients, women taking oral contraceptives and menstruating women in general. The Boston Collaborative Drug Surveillance report (1974) found a 2.5 times greater risk in oestrogen users than in controls. Women age 45–49 had an annual incidence of 87 per 100 000 of cholelithiasis in controls and 218 per 100 000 in oestrogen users. The alteration in high density lipoprotein cholesterol secondary to oestrogen has been implicated as a probable factor in the genesis of cholelithiasis. Progestational agents alone have also been associated with increased risk of gallstones.

Side effects

Uterine bleeding is the most troublesome associated feature of oestrogen replacement therapy. Although bleeding is usually infrequent and minimal most women object to therapy which produces uterine bleeding after the menopause. Oestrogen-progesterone withdrawal bleeding which occurs at the end of a treatment cycle typically consists of light flow which is self-limited and is usually benign. This can usually be distinguished from pathological bleeding which occurs at variable times during the cycle and may be protracted and heavy. The occurrence of abnormal bleeding frequently necessitates sampling of the endometrium to eliminate the possibility of an endometrial malignancy or precancerous condition. The best means of accomplishing this remains fractional dilatation and curettage. Irregular bleeding is a dose-related phenomenon. Individuals taking 1.25 mg of conjugated oestrogens have a 2–12 per cent incidence of uterine bleeding while patients receiving 0.625 mg/day have a 1–4 per cent incidence (Lauritzen, 1976).

Approximately 6 to 10 per cent of women taking ethinyl oestradiol experience nausea and vomiting but this is uncommon with patients using conjugated oestrogens (Lebech, 1976). Mastodynia occurs in 12 per cent of women treated with ethinyl oestradiol (Hammond & Maxson, 1981) but may be more common in women treated with continuous oestrogen regimens. Additional reported side-effects include weight gain, oedema, and heartburn (Lauritzen, 1976).

TREATMENT OF THE MENOPAUSE

There is a considerable variety of oestrogen preparations available worldwide. Conjugated oestrogens are the most commonly prescribed oestrogen compound in the United States and they constitute over 80 per cent of presciptions for replacement oestrogens (Schiff & Ryan, 1980). This formulation consists of sodium oestrone sulphate (48–51 per cent), sodium equilin sulphate (22–26 per cent), sodium 17α-dihydroequilin (15–16 per cent), and smaller quantities of sodium sulphates of 17α-dihydroequilin and of 17α-oestradiol (Howard & Keaty, 1971; Adams et al, 1979). These preparations are derived from pregnant mare's urine and are formulated in 0.3 mg, 0.625 mg, 1.25 mg, and 2.5 mg tablets. Conjugated oestrogens are also formulated as vaginal creams which may achieve serum levels approximating those of the orally administered drug (Riggs et al, 1978). The standard dose in the United States is currently 0.625 mg orally and this amount is capable of suppressing FSH levels in menopausal women by 40 per cent and LH levels in the same population by 25 per cent (Schiff & Ryan, 1980).

Esterified oestrogens are similar to conjugated oestrogens but they contain 75 to 85 per cent sodium oestrone sulphate and less than 15 per cent sodium equilin sulphate (Utian, 1980). They also contain proportionately less 17α-oestradiol, 17α-dihydroequilin, and 17α-dihydroequilinon. They are available in the same dosages as conjugated oestrogens and have no established advantage or disadvantage in comparison to them. Piperazine oestrone sulphate is a crystalline oestrone solution available in the same formulations as conjugated and esterified oestrogens. The relative serum oestrone:oestradiol ratio remains consistant with conjugated oestrogens, 1.25 mg, piperazine oestrone sulphate, 1.8 mg, and oestradiol valerate, 2.0 mg, (Hammond & Maxson, 1982). The relative potencies have been inferred from these data.

Additional 'natural' oestrogen compounds include oestradiol valerate, a fatty acid ester of oestradiol, which is popular in Europe and Australia, oestriol hemisuccinate, and micronised oestradiol which is readily absorbed but extensively metabolised in the liver to oestrone prior to its appearance in the peripheral circulation. All of these compounds are manufactured in 1 and 2 mg tablets. Oestriol has also been used to treat climacteric symptoms although its efficacy is not as well established (Schiff & Ryan, 1980). It was previously thought to be associated with a reduced risk of developing breast carcinoma, since multiparous women are known to have a reduced incidence of breast cancer. This concept is probably not valid (Vorherr & Messer, 1978; Schiff & Ryan, 1980). Oestriol is available in 1 and 2 mg tablets.

Synthetic oestrogens, including diethylstilboestrol (DES) benzestrol, chlorotrianisene (TACE), dienoestrol, hexoestrol, methallenstril, quinestrol, and promesthestrol dipropionate are available in a variety of formulations. The only advantage of their use is the low cost. They are associated with a variety of physiological changes, many poorly characterised, that confers an unacceptably high risk with their use. Ethinyl oestradiol, most commonly used in combination oral contraceptives, is available in 10 μg, 20 μg and 50 μg tablets but has the same disadvantage as the other synthetic oestrogens. Combination oral contraceptives should not be used for oestrogen replacement therapy because their dose is usually excessive and menopausal patients are at high risk for their associated vascular complications.

Considerable controversy has continued over the choice of the route of administration. Orally administered preparations may be stopped rapidly, the dose can be more easily regulated, and they may be given cyclically. Parenterally administered oestrogens and long-acting, slow release oestrogen pellet systems may be effective in treating climacteric symptoms with lower and less variable serum oestrogen levels. They may also be advantageous in avoiding the extensive hepatic metabolism and the associated deleterious changes in lipids and hepatic proteins following oral administration. Investigations are currently in progress to assess the feasibility of these systems for oestrogen replacement and contraception.

Contraindications to oestrogen replacement therapy include: (1) patients with known or suspected oestrogen-dependent neoplasia, specifically breast and endometrial carcinoma; (2) undiagnosed abnormal genital bleeding; (3) history of significant thrombophlebitis or thromboembolic disorders; and (4) active hepatic disease. Relative contraindications to therapy are: (1) strong family history of breast carcinoma; (2) uterine leiomyomata; (3) history of liver disease; (4) severe varicose veins; (5) diabetes mellitus; (6) significant hypertension; and (7) porphyria.

There are fewer choices for a suitable progestational agent than for oestrogens. Medroxyprogesterone acetate has been used most commonly for the purpose of inducing endometrial regression in the United States. It is formulated in 2.5 mg and 10 mg tablets. Megestrol acetate in 20 and 40 mg tablets and norethindrone and norethindrone acetate in 5 mg tablets have been used, as well. The latter two compounds are 19-nortestosterone derivatives and they are generally associated with more undesirable effects. The contraindications to progestational therapy are essentially the same as for oestrogen therapy excluding endometrial carcinoma. However, most of the data addressing the risk of progestins have been derived from studies examining the risk in patients taking combination oral contraceptives in which it has not been possible to separate effects of progestins from those of oestrogens. Thus, a meaningful set of contraindications to progestin therapy after the menopause is not yet available.

Recommendations

The decision to initiate hormonal therapy for symptoms of the climacteric must be made after a careful assessment of risks versus potential benefits. It seems reasonable to provide oestrogen therapy for those individuals who do not have contraindications to oestrogen and are genuinely discomfited by vasomotor symptoms or genital atrophy. Treatment should be started at the lowest effective dose of oestrogen and continued for the shortest period of time possible. In practice, 0.6 mg or 1.25 mg of conjugated oestrogens or an equivalent dose of another non-synthetic oestrogen may be given for 21 to 25 days of the month. If this dose is not effective in relieving vasomotor symptoms it may be increased. Most individuals will tolerate having their dose reduced after a few months of high dose therapy without recurrence of symptomotology. It is usually possible gradually to decrease therapy so that it may be stopped altogether after 3 years with minimal persistence of symptoms. Obviously, some individuals will require more protracted therapy. Medroxyprogesterone acetate 10 mg should be added for the last 7–10 days of oestrogen treatment to induce endometrial regression.

Individuals who are unable to take oestrogen may obtain relief from vasomotor symptoms with progestin-only therapy (20 mg medroxyprogesterone acetate daily), other progestins, androgens, or clonidine. Traditional measures such as barbituates, sedatives and minor tranquilisers are frequently used as adjunctive treatment but do not have well-established efficacy for treatment of vasomotor symptoms. Currently, there is no satisfactory alternative to oestrogen for treatment of genito-urinary atrophy.

The issue of intermittent sampling of the endometrium has not been settled. Until a comprehensive assessment of risk of endometrial adenocarcinoma with lower doses of oestrogen and added progestins is available, it seems wise to consider endometrial biopsy at intervals. Currently, there are little data available relating to the topic of optimal frequency to sample endometrium. Any individual with abnormal vaginal bleeding on oestrogen therapy should be promptly evaluated with dilatation and curettage.

Treatment of osteoporosis is a more complex topic. Oestrogen has been demonstrated to be effective prophylaxis for the development of postmenopausal osteoporosis. However, it is neither desirable nor necessary to treat all individuals at risk, i.e. all postmenopausal women. Presently, there are no parameters known to be sensitive predictors of risk of osteoporosis. It seems desirable to treat patients with established disease to arrest progression and individuals with a high probability of developing disease. This group includes sedentary, thin, lightly pigmented women. The greatest beneficiaries of this treatment, however, are patients who undergo surgical menopause prior to the time of expected menopause. They would otherwise be hypooestrogenic for the longest interval and would hence have more opportunity to develop osteoporosis. Oestrogen therapy for osteoporosis must be continued indefinitely to remain effective, but these individuals require less oestrogen to stabilise bone density. The dose of 0.6 mg daily for conjugated oestrogens or 20 μg of mestranol are known to be effective for this purpose and studies are in progress to evaluate the efficacy of lower doses. The role of adjunctive treatments such as calcium supplementation, fluoride, calcitonin, exercise and vitamin D is not clear, but they may be helpful in the therapy of osteoporosis, as well. They should be prescribed when oestrogen is contraindicated.

SUMMARY

The primary endocrine feature of the climacteric is the loss of ovarian function and the resultant diminution in oestradiol production. The direct and indirect effects of hypooestrogenism which have only recently attracted intensive scientific scrutiny involve multiple organ systems and may be accompanied by profound psychological and sociological changes, as well. These physiological changes which are obligatory for the transition from reproductive life to a life

2

beyond reproduction have critical evolutionary significance. However they may be associated with sequellae that impair the quality of life or are life threatening themselves. Oestrogen replacement therapy has been shown to be effective in alleviating some of this symptomotology including vasomotor symptoms and genital atrophy and is effective in preventing postmenopausal osteoporosis. However, this treatment carries with it certain risks, endometrial adenocarcinoma being the most significant

one. Current data suggest that this risk can be significantly reduced by using 'natural oestrogens,' at lowest dose, in a cyclic regimen, with 7 to 10 days of progestational therapy. Following these guidelines it appears that the potential benefits significantly outweigh the hazards. Hopefully, the resolution of many of the unanswered questions described in this chapter will permit therapy to be further optimised in the future.

REFERENCES

Abraham G E, Maroulis G B 1975 Effect of exogenous estrogen on serum pregnenolone, cortisol and androgens in postemenopausal women. Obstetrics and Gynecology 45: 271–274

Abramson J H, Gampel B, Slome C, Scotch N 1960 Age at menopause of urban Zulu women. Science 132: 356–357

Adams W P, Hasegawa J, Johnson R N, Haring R 1979 Conjugated estrogens bioinequivalence: comparison of our products in postmenopausal women. Journal of Pharmacologic Science 68: 986

Aitken J M, Hart D M, Lindsay R 1973a Oestrogen replacement therapy for prevention of osteoporosis after oophorectomy. British Medical Journal 3: 515–518

Aitken J M, Hart D M, Anderson J B, Lindsay R, Smith D A, Speirs C F 1973b Osteoporosis after oophoreetomy for non-malignant disease in premenopausal women. British Medical Journal 2: 325–328

Aitken J M, Hart D M, Lindsay R 1976 Long term oestrogens for the prevention of post-menopausal osteoporosis. Postgraduate Medical Journal 52: 18–25

Albright F, Bloomberg F, Smith D H 1940 Postmenopausal osteoporosis. Transactions of the Association of American Physicians 55: 298–305

Albright F, Smith D H, Richardson A M 1941 Postmenopausal osteoporosis: its clinical features. Journal of the American Medical Association 116: 2465–2474

Anonymous 1978 Treatment of osteoporosis. British Medical Journal 1: 1303

Antunes C M G, Stolley P D, Rosenshein N B, Davies J L, Tonascia J A, Brown C, et al 1979 Endometrial cancer and estrogen use: report of a large case control study. New England Journal of Medicine 300: 9–13

Barnea A, Gorski J 1970 Estrogen-induced protein: time course of synthesis. Biochemistry 9: 1899–1904

Bates G W 1981 On the nature of the hot flash. Clinical Obstetrics and Gynecology 24: 231–241

Benjamin F 1960 The age of menarche and of the menopause in white South African women and certain factors influencing these times. South African Medical Journal 34: 316–320

Boston Collaborative Drug Surveillance Program, Boston University Medical center 1974 Surgically confirmed gallbladder disease, venous thromboembolism and breast tumors in relation to postmenopausal estrogen therapy. New England Journal of Medicine 290: 15–19

Boyd G S 1963 Hormones and cholesterol metabolism. Biochemical Society Symposium 24: 79–98

Briggs M H, Briggs M 1979 Plasma lipoprotein changes during oral contraception. Current Medical Research and Opinion 6: 249–254

Brown-Sequard C E 1890 Remarques su les effets produits sur la femme par des injections sous-cutanees d'un liquide retire d'ovaires d'animaux. Archives de Physiologie Normale et Pathologique 2: 456–457

Burch P R J, Gunz F W 1967 The distribution of menopausal age in New Zealand. An exploratory study. New Zealand Medical Journal 66: 6–10

Burnet F M 1970 An immunological approach to aging. Lancet ii: 358–360

Butenandt A 1929 Untersuchungen uber das weibliche sexual hormon.

darstellung und eigen schaften des kristallisierten progynons. Deutsche Medizinische Wochenschrift 55: 2171–2174

Calkins E 1981 Aging of cells and people. Clinical Obstetrics and Gynecology 24: 165–179

Cameron J R, Mazess R B, Sorenson J A 1968 Precision and accuracy of bone mineral determination by direct photon absorptiometry. Investigative Radiology 3: 141–150

Cann C E, Genant H K, Ettinger B, Gordan G S 1980 Spinal mineral loss in oophorectomized women, determination by quantitative computed tomography. Journal of the American Medical Association 244: 2056–2059

Chang R J, Judd H L 1981 The ovary after menopause. Clinical Obstetrics and Gynecology 24: 181–191

Clark J H, Hardin J W, McCormack S A 1978 Estrogen receptor binding and growth of the reproductive tract. Pediatrics 62: 1121–1127

Clayden J R, Bell J W, Pollard D 1974 Menopausal flushing: double blind trial of a nonhormonal medication. British Medical Journal 1: 409–412

Coronary Drug Project Research Group 1970 The coronary drug project: initial findings leading to modifications of its research protocol. Journal of the American Medical Association 214: 1303–1313

Crane M G, Harris J J, Windsor W 1971 Hypertension, oral contraceptive agents and conjugated estrogens. Annals of Internal Medicine 74: 13–21

Davidson B J, Riggs B L, Coulam C B, Toft D O 1980 Concentration of cytosolic estrogen receptors in patients with postmenopausal osteoporosis. American Journal of Obstetrics and Gynecology 136: 130–134

Davies J L, Rosenshein N B, Antunes C M, Stolley P D 1981 A review of the risk factors for endometrial carcinoma. Obstetrical and Gynecological Survey 36: 107–116

Davis M E 1935 Treatment of senile vaginitis with ovarian follicular hormone. Surgical Gynecology and Obstetrics 61: 680–686

Dunn L J, Bradbury J T 1967 Endocrine factors in endometrial carcinoma. American Journal of Obstetrics and Gynecology 97: 465–471

Erlik Y, Tataryn I V, Meldrum D R, Lomax P, Bajorek J G, Judd H L 1981 Association of waking episodes with menopausal hot flushes. Journal of the American Medical Association 245: 1741–1744

Fisch I R, Frank J 1977 Oral contraceptives and blood pressure. Journal of the American Medical Association 237: 2499–2503

Fraser I S, Weisberg E 1981 A comprehensive review of injectable contraception with special emphasis on depot medroxyprogesterone acetate. The Medical Journal of Australia 1 suppl: 3–19

Frere G 1971 Mean age at menopause and menarche in South Africa. South African Journal of Medical Science 36: 21–24

Frommer D J 1964 Changing age of menopause. British Medical Journal 2: 349–351

Furman R H 1973 Coronary heart disease and the menopause. In: Ryan K J, Gibson D C (eds) Menopause and Aging: Summary Report and Selected Papers from a Research Conference on Menopause and Aging, DHEW Publication Number (NIH 73–319), pp 39–55. U S Government Printing Office, Washington D C

Gallagher J C, Young M M, Nordin B E C 1972 Effects of artifical menopause on plasma and urine calcium and phosphate. Clinical Endocrinology 1: 57–64

Gallaher J C, Riggs B L, DeLuca H F 1980 Effect of estrogen on calcium absorption and serum vitamin D metabolites in postmenopausal osteoporosis. Journal of Clinical Endocrinology and Metabolism 51: 1359–1364

Gallannaugh S C, Martin A, Millard P U 1976 Regional study of femoral neck fractures. British Medical Journal 2: 1496–1497

Gambrell R D, Vasquez J M Estrogen therapy and breast cancer — is the verdict in? Contemporary Obstetrics and Gynecology 19: 38–45

Gambrell R D, Massey F M, Castaneda T A, Ugenas A J, Ricca C A, Wright J M 1980 Use of progestogen challenge test to reduce the risk of endometrial cancer. Obstetrics and Gynecology 55: 732–738

Garn S M 1970 The earlier Gain and Later Loss of Cortical Bone in Nutritional Perspective. Charles C. Thomas, Springfield, Illinois

Gelfant S, Smith J G 1972 Aging noncycling cells: an explanation. Science 178: 357–361

Goldzieher J W, Chenault CgG, de la Pena A, Dozier T S, Knauer D C 1978 Comparative studies of the ethinyl estrogen used on oral contraceptives. VI Effects with or without progestational agents on carbohydrate metabolism in humans, baboons and beagles. Fertility and Sterility 30: 146–153

Gordan G S, Genant H K 1978 Postmenopausal osteoporosis is a preventable disease. Contemporary Obstetrics and Gynecology 11: 47–59

Gordon T, Kannel W B, Hjortland M C, McNamara P M 1978 Menopause and coronary heart disease: the Framingham study. Annals of Internal Medicine 89: 157–161

Gore H 1973 Hyperplasia of the endometrium. In: Norris A J, Hertig A T, Abell M R (eds) The Uterus, pp 255–275. Williams and Wilkins, Baltimore

Gow S, MacGillivray I 1971 Metabolic hormonal and vascular changes after oestrogen therapy in oophorectomized women. British Medical Journal 2: 73–77

Gray R H 1976 The menopause/epidemiological and demographic considerations. In: Beard R J (ed) The Menopause pp 25–40. University Part Press, Baltimore

Gray L A, Christopherson W M, Hoover R N 1977 Estrogens and endometrial carcinoma. Obstetrics and Gynecology 49: 385–389

Greenhill J P 1972 The non-surgical management of vaginal relaxation. Clinical Obstetrics and Bynecology 15: 1083–1097

Hammond C B, Maxson W S 1981 Current status of estrogen therapy for the menopause. Fertility and Sterility 37: 5–20

Hammond C B, Ory S J 1982 Endocrine problems in the menopause. Clinical Obstetrics and Gynecology 25: 19–38

Hammond C B, Jelovsek F R, Lee K L 1979a Effects of long-term estrogen replacement therapy: II Neoplasia. American Journal of Obstetrics and Gynecology 133: 537–547

Hammond C B, Jelovsek F R, Lee K L, Creasman W T, Parker R T 1979b Effects of long-term estrogen replacement therapy. I. Metabolic effects. American Journal of Obstetrics and Gyneclogy 133: 525–536

Hauser G A, Oribi J A, Valaer M, Erb H, Muller T, Remen U, et al 1961 Der einfluss des menarchealters auf das menopausealter. Gynaecologia 152: 279–286

Hauser G A, Remen U, Valaer M, Erb H, Muller T, Oribi J 1963 Menarche and menopause in Israel. Gynaecologia 155: 39–47

Hayflick L, Moorhead P S 1961 The serial cultivation of human diploid cell strains. Experimental Cell Research 25: 585–621

Heaney R P 1976 Estrogens and postmenopausal osteoporosis. Clinical Obstetrics and Gynecology 19: 791–803

Hemsell D L, Grodin J M, Brenner D F, Siiteri P K, MacDonald P C 1974 Plasma precursors of estrogens: II Correlations of the extent of conversion of plasma androstenedione to estrone with age. Journal of Clinical Endocrinology and Metabolism 38: 476–479

Henneman P H, Wallach S 1957 A review of the prolonged use of estrogens and androgens in postmenopausal and senile osteoporosis. Archives of Internal Medicine 100: 715–723

Hofmann D, Soergel T 1972 Studies on the age of menarche and the age of menopause. Geburtshilfe Trauenheilkd 32: 969

Horwitz R I, Feinstein A R 1978 Alternative analytic methods for case-control studies of estrogens and endometrial cancer. New England Journal of Medicine 199: 1089–1094

Howard R P, Keaty E C 1971 Evaluation of equilin 3 monosulfate and other estrogens. Archives of Internal Medicine 128: 229–234

Howie P W, Prentice C R M, Mallinson A C, Horne C H W, McNichol C P, 1970 Effect of combined oestrogen-progestogen oral contraceptives, oestrogen and progestgen on anti-plasmin and anti-thrombin activity. Lancet ii: 1329–1332

Hulka B S, Chambless L E, Deubner D C, Wilkinson W E 1982a Breast cancer and estrogen replacement therapy. American Journal of Obstetrics and Gynecology 143: 638–644

Hulka B S, Chambless L E, Kaufman D G, Fowler W C, Greenberg B G 1982b Protection against endometrial carcinoma by combination-product oral contraceptives. Journal of the American Medical Association 247: 475–477

Hulley S B, Cohen R, Widdowson G 1977 Plasma high-density lipoprotein cholesterol level. Influence of risk factor intervention. Journal of the American Medical Association 238: 2269–2271

Jaszmann L, Van Lith N D, Zaat J C A 1969 The age at menopause in the Netherlands. International Journal of Fertility 14: 106–117

Jelovsek F R, Hammond C B, Woodard B H, Draffin R, Lee K L, Creasman W T, et al 1980 Risk of exogenous estrogen and endometrial cancer. American Journal of Obstetrics and Gynecology 137: 85–91

Jenson E I, Ostergaard E 1954 Clinical studies concerning the relationship of estrogens to the development of cancer of the corpus uteri. American Journal of Obstetrics and Gynecology 67: 1094–1102

Jick H, Watkins R N, Hunter J R, Dinan B J, Madsen S, Rothman K, et al 1979 Replacement estrogens and endometrial cancer. New England Journal of Medicine 300: 218–222

Judd H L 1976 Hormonal dynamics associated with the menopause. Clinical Obstetrics and Gynecology 19: 775–788

Judd H L, Lucas W E, Yen S S C 1974 Effects of oophorectomy on circulating testosterone and androstenedione levels in patients with endometrial cancer. American Journal of Obstetrics and Gynecology 118: 793–798

Judd H L, Davidson B J, Frumar A J, Shamonki I M, Lagasse L D, Ballon S C 1980 Serum androgens and estrognes in postmenopausal women with and without endometrial cancer. American Journal of Obstetrics and Gynecology 136: 859–871

Judd H L, Shamonki I M, Frumar A M, Lagasse L D 1982 Origin of serum estradiol in postmenopausal women. Obstetrics and Gynecology 59: 680–686

Kannel W B, Hjortland M C, McNamara P M, Gordon T 1976 Menopause and coronary heart disease: the Framingham study. Annals of Internal Medicine 85: 447n–452

Kistner R W 1959 Histological effects of progestins on hyperplasia and carcinoma-in-situ of the endometrium. Cancer 12: 1106–1122

Kistner R W 1973 Endometrial alterations associated with estrogen and estrogen-progestin cambinations. In: Norris A J, Hertig A T, Abell M R (ed) The Uterus, pp 227–253. Williams and Wilkins, Baltimore

Kistner R W, Duncan C J, Mansell H 1956 Suppression of ovulation by tri-p-anisyl-chloroethylene (TACE). Obstetrics and Gynecology 8: 399n407

Klotz H P 1980 The corrections by estrogens of calcium disorders induced by estrogne deficient states. In: Pasetto N, Paoletti R, Ambrus J L (eds) The Menopause and Postmenopause. Proceedings of an International Symposium held in Rome, June 1979 pp 157–161. MTP Press, Lancaster

Kohler P O, Ross G T, Odell W D 1968 Metabolic clearance and production rates of human luteinizing hormone in pre- and postmenopausal women. Journal of Clinical Investigation 47: 38–47

Kokko E, Janne O, Kauppila A, Vihko R 1982 Effects of tamoxifen, medroxyprogesterone acetate, and their combination on human endometrial estrogen and progestin receptor concentrations. 17α-hydroxy-steroid dehydrogenase activity, and serum hormone concentrations. American Journal of Obstetrics and Gynecology 143: 382–388

Krane S M, Holick M F 1980 Metabolic bone disease. In: Isselbacher K J, Adams R D, Braunwald E, Peterdorf R G, Wilson J D (eds)

Harrison's Principles of Internal Medicine, 9th edn, pp 1849–1860. McGraw-Hill, New York

Larsson-Cohn U, Wallentin L 1977 Metabolic and hormonal effects of postmenopausal oestrogen replacement treatment. I Glucose, insulin and human growth hormone levels during oral glucose tolerance tests. Acta Endocrinologica (Copenhagen) 86: 583–596

Lauritzen C H 1976 The female climacteric syndrome: significance, problems, treatment. Acta Obstetricia et Gynecologica Scandinavica (Stockholm) (Supplement) 51: 47

Lebech P E 1976 Effects and side-effects of estrogen therapy. In: van Keep P A, Greenblatt R B, Albeaux-Fernet M (eds) Consensus on Menopause Research, pp 44–47. University Park Press, Baltimore

Lindsay R, Hart D M, Aitken J M, MacDonald E B, Anderson J B, Clarke A C 1976 Longterm prevention of postmenopausal osteoporosis by oestrogen. Lancet i: 1038–1041

Lindsay R, Hart D M, Purdie D, Ferguson M M, Clark A S, Kraszewski A 1978 Comparative effects of estrogen and progestogen on bone loss in post-menopausal women. Clinical Science and Molecular Medicine 54: 193–195

Linnoila M, Cooper R L 1976 Reinstatement of vaginal cycles in aged female rats. Journal of Pharmacology and Experimental Therapeutics 199: 477–482

Longcope C 1971 Metabolic clearance and blood production rates of estrogens in postmenopausal women. American Journal of Obstetrics and Gynecology 111: 778–781

Longcope C, Kato T, Horton R 1969 Conversion of blood androgens to estrogens in normal adult men and women. Journal of Clinical Investigation 48: 2191–2201

Longscope C, Pratt J H, Schneider S H, Fineberg S E 1978 Aromatization of androgen by muscle and adipose tissue in vivo. Journal of Clinical Endocrinology and Metabolism 46: 146–152

Loriaux D L, Kono S, Lipsett M B 1974 Plasma estradiol binding and renal clearance: the effect of testosterone binding globulin (TeBG) (abstract 92) Endocrine Society Abstracts of the 56th Annual Meeting, Atlanta, p. A–101

MacDonald P C 1981 Estrogen plus progestin in postmenopausal women. New England Journal of Medicine 305: 1644–1645

MacDonald P C, Siiteri P K 1974 The relationship between the extraglandular production of estrone and the occurrence of endometrial neoplasia. Gynecologic Oncology 2: 259–263

Mack T, Pike M, Henderson B, Pfeffer R, Gerkins V, Arthur M, et al 1976 Estrogens and endometrial cancer in a retirement community. New England Journal of Medicine 294: 1262–1267

MacMahon B, Worcester J 1966 Age at Menopause: United States 1960–62. U.S. Vital and Health Statistics, Series II, No 19

Mahboubi E, Eyler N, Wynder E L 1982 Epidemiology of cancer of the endometrium. Clinical Obstetrics and Gynecology 25: 5–17

Mazer C, Israel S L 1935 Symptoms and treatment of the menopause. Medical Clinics of North America 19: 205–211

Meema S, Meema H E 1976 Menopausal bone loss and estrogen replacement. Israeli Journal of Medical Science 12: 598–606

Meldrum D R, Shamonki I M, Frumar A J, Tataryn I V, Chang R J, Judd H L 1979 Elevations in skin temperature of the finger as an objective index of postmenopausal hot flashes: standardization of the technique. American Journal of Obstetrics and Gynecology 135: 713–717

Meldrum D R, Tataryn I V, Frumar A M, Erlik Y, Lu K H, Judd H L 1980 Gonadotropins, estrogens and steroids during the menopausal hot flash. Journal of Clinical Endocrinology and Metabolism 50: 685–689

Meldrum D R, Erlik Y, Lu J K, Judd H L 1981 Objectively recorded hot flashes in patients with pituitary insufficiency. Journal of Clinical Endocrinology and Metabolism 52: 684–687

Meyer W J, Henneman D H, Keiser H R, Bartler F C 1976 17@-estradiol: separation of estrogen effect on collagen from other clinical and biochemical effects in man. Research Communications in Chemical Pathology and Pharmacology 13: 685–695

Meyers F H, Jawetz E, Goldfien A 1972 The gonadal hormones and inhibitors. In: Review of Medical Pharmacology, 3rd edn, Ch 38, pp 362–388. Lange Medical Publications, Los Altos

McDonald T W, Annegers J R, O'Fallon W M, Dockerty M G, Malkasian G D, Kurland L T 1977 Exogenous estrogen and endometrial cancer: case-control and incidence study. American Journal of Obstetrics and Gynecology 127: 572–580

McKinlay S, Jefferys M, Thompson B 1972 An investigation of the age of menopause. Journal of Biosocial Science 4: 161–173

Molnar G W 1979 Investigation of hot flashes by ambulatory monitoring. American Journal of Physiology 237: R306–310

Morrison J C, Martin D C, Blair R A, Anderson G D, Kincheloe B W, Bates G W, et al 1980 The use of medroxyprogesterone acetate for relief of climacteric symptoms. American Journal of Obstetrics and Gynecology 138: 99–104

Mulley G, Mitchell J R A, Tattersall R B 1977 Hot flashes after hypophysectomy. British Medical Journal 2: 1062

Nachtigall L E, Nachtigall R H, Nachtigall R D, Beckman E M 1979 Estrogen replacement therapy I: A 10-year prospective study in the relationship to osteoporosis. Obstetrics and Gynecology 53: 277–281

Nilsen P A, Kolstad P 1971 Hormonal treatment of pre-invasive and invasive carcinoma of the corpus uteri. In: Brush M G et al (eds) Symposium on Endometrial Cancer, p. 115. Heinemann, London

Nordin B E C 1971 Clinical significance and pathogenesis of osteoporosis. British Medical Journal 1: 571–576

Nordin B E C, Gallagher S C, Aaron J F, Horsman A 1975 Postmenopausal osteoporosis and osteopenia. Frontiers of Hormonal Research 3: 131

Notelovitz M 1974 Metabolic effect of conjugated oestrogen on glucose tolerance. South African Medical Journal 48: 2599–2603

Notelovitz M, Greig H B W 1976 Natural estrogen and anti-thrombin: III Activity in postmenopausal women. Journal of Reproductive Medicine 16: 87–90

Noyes R W, Hertig A T, Rock J 1950 Dating the endometrial biopsy. Fertility and Sterility 1: 3–25

Odell W D 1976 Releasing factors in the menopause. In: Greenblatt R B, Albeaux-Fernet M (eds) Consensus on Menopause Research, pp 9–10. University Park Press, Baltimore

Oliver M G, Boyd G S 1961 Influence of reduction of serum-lipids on prognosis of coronary heart disease. A five year study using oestrogen. Lancet ii: 499

Pack B A, Tovar R, Booth E, Brooks S C 1979 The cyclic relationship of estrogen sulfurylation to the nuclear receptor level in human endometrial curettings. Journal of Clinical Endocrinology and Metabolism 48: 420–424

Paganini-Hill A, Ross R K, Gerkins V R, Henderson B E, Arthur M, Maak T M 1981 Menopausal estrogen therapy and hip fractures. Annals of Internal Medicine 95: 28–31

Pardridge W M, Mcitus L J 1979 Transport of steroid hormones through the rat blood brain barrier: primary role of albumin bound hormone. Journal of Clinical Investigation 64: 145–154

Parrish H M, Carr C A, Hall D G, King T M 1967 Time interval from castration in premenopausal women to development of excessive coronary atherosclerosis. American Journal of Obstetrics and Gynecology 99: 155–162

Pfeffer R I 1978 Estrogen use, hypertension and stroke in post-menopausal women. Journal of Chronic Diseases 31: 389–398

Pfeffer R I, Van den Noort S 1976 Estrogen use and stroke risk in postmenopausal women. American Journal of Epidemiology 103: 445–456

Pfeffer R I, Kurosaki T T, Charlton S K 1979 Estrogen use and blood pressure in later life. American Journal of Epidemiology 110: 469–478

Philips G B 1978 Sex hormones, risk factors and cardiovascular disease. American Journal of Medicine 65: 7–11

Pott P 1775 Chirurgical Observations. London

Rebar R W, Erickson G F, Yen S S C 1982 Idiopathic premature ovarian failure: clinical and endocrine characteristics. Fertility and Sterility 37: 35–41

Rico H, del Rio A, Vila T, Patino R, Carrera F, Espinos D 1979 The role of growth hormone in the pathogenesis of postmenopausal osteoporosis. Archives of Internal Medicine 139: 1263–1265

Riggs B L, Jowsey J, Kelly P J, Arnaud C D 1976 Role of hormonal factors in the pathogenesis of postmenopausal osteoporosis. Clinical Obstetrics and Gynecology 19: 615–619

Riggs L A, Hermann H, Yen S S C 1978 Absorption of estrogens from vaginal creams. New England Journal of Medicine 298: 195–197

Riggs B L, Wahner H W, Dunn W L, Mazess R B, Offord K P, Melton L J 1980 Differential changes in bone mineral density of the appendicular and axial skeleton with aging. Journal of Clinical Investigation 67: 328–335

Roberts W C, Giraldo A A 1979 Bilateral oophorectomy in menstruating women and accelearated coronary atherosclerosis: an unproved connection. American Journal of Medicine 67: 363–365

Romero J A 1978 Biologic rhythms and sympathetic neural control of pineal metabolism. Advanced Experimental Medical Biology 108: 235

Ross R K, Paganini-Hill A, Gerkins V R, Mack T M, Pfeffer R, Arthur M, et al 1980 A case control study of menopausal estrogen therapy and breast cancer. Journal of the American Medical Association 243: 1635–1639

Ross R K, Paganini-Hill A, Mack T M, Arthur M, Henderson B E 1981 Menopausal oestrogen therapy and protection from death from ischemic heart disease. Lancet i: 858–860

Royal College of General Practitioners 1974 Oral contraceptives in health: an interim report from the oral contraception study of the Royal College of General Practitioners. Pitman Medical Publishers, London

Scaglia H, Medina M, Pinto-Ferreira A L, Vazques G, Gual C, Perez-Palacios G 1976 Pituitary LH and FSH secretion and responsiveness in women of old age. Acta Endocrinologica (Kbh) 81: 673–684

Schiff I, Ryan K J 1980 Benefits of estrogen replacement. Obstetrical and Gynecological Survey (supplement) 35: 400–411

Schiff I, Tulchinsky D, Cramer D, Ryan K J 1980 Oral medroxyprogesterone in the treatment of postmenopausal symptoms. Journal of the American Medical Association 244: 1443–1445

Schiff I, Sela H K, Cramer D, Tulchinsky D, Ryan K J 1982 Endometrial hyperplasia in women on cyclic or continuous estrogen regimens. Fertility and Sterility 37: 79–82

Schroeder R 1922 Granulosazelltumor des ovars mit glandularcystischer hyperplasia des endometrium und beginnendem karzinom auf diesern. Zentrab Gynaekol 46: 195

Scragg R F R 1973 Menopause and reproductive span in rural Niugini. Presented at the Annual Symposium of the Papua New Guinea Medical Society, Port Moresbry, p 126

Siler T M, Yen S S C 1973 Augmented response to synthetic LRF in the hypogonadal state. Journal of Clinical Endocrinology and Metaboli sm 37: 491–494

Smith D C, Prentice R, Thompson D J, Herrmann W 1975 Association of exogenous estrogens and endometrial carcinoma. New England Journal of Medicine 293: 1164–1167

Spellacy W N, MacLeod A G W, Buhi W C, Birk S A 1972 The effects of medroxyprogesterone acetate on carbohydrate metabolism: measurements of glucose, insulin and growth hormone after twelve months of use. Fertility and Sterility 23: 239–244

Spicer C C, Hare S A, Slater E 1973 Neurotic and psychotic forms of depressive illness. British Journal of Psychiatry 123: 535–541

Stark M, Adoni A, Milwidsky A, Gilon G, Palti A 1978 Can estrogens be useful for treatment of vaginal relaxation in elderly women? American Journal of Obstetrics and Gynecology 131: 585–586

Strathy J H, Coulam C B, Spelburg T C 1982 Comparison of estrogen receptors in human premenopausal and postmenopausal uteri: indication of biologically inactive receptor in postmenopausal uteri. American Journal of Obstetrics and Gynecology 142: 372–382

Studd J, Dubiel M, Kakkar V V, Thom M, White P J 1978 The effect of hormone replacement therapy on glucose tolerance, clotting factors, fibrinolysis, and platelet behaviour in postmenopausal women. In: Cooke I D (ed) The Role of Estrogen/Progestogen in the Management of The Menopause, pp 41–59. Proceedings of a Symposium held at the University of Sheffield on March 16, 1978. University Park Press, Baltimore

Tataryn I V, Meldrum D R, Lu K H, Frumar A M, Judd H L 1979 LH, FSH and skin temperature during the menopausal hot flash. Journal of Clinical Endocrinology and Metabolism 49: 152–154

Tataryn I V, Lomax P, Meldrum D R, Bajorek J G, Chesarek W, Judd H L 1981 Objective techniques for the assessment of postmenopausal hot flashes. Obstetrics and Gynecology 57: 340–344

Thom M, Chakravarti S, Oram D H, Studd J W W 1977 Effect of hormone replacement therapy on glucose tolerance in postmenopausal women. British Journal of Obstetrics and Gynaecology 84: 776–783

Thompson B, Hart S A, Durno D 1973 Menopausal age and symtomatology in a general practice. Journal of Biosocial Science 5: 71–82

Treloar A E 1974 Menarche, menopause and intervening fecundability. Human Biology 46: 89–107

Tseng L, Gurpide E 1975a Effect of progestins on estradiol receptor levels in human endometrium. Journal of Clinical Endocrinology and Metabolism 41: 402–404

Tseng L, Gurpide E 1975b Induction of human estradiol dehydrogenase by progestins. Endocrinology 97: 825–833

Utian W H 1972 The mental tonic effect of oestrogens administered to oophorectomized females. South African Medical Journal 46: 1079–1082

Utian W H 1980 Menopause in Modern Perspective. Appleton-Century Crofts, New York

Vehemans M, Robyn C 1975 Influence of age on serum prolactin in women and men. British Medical Journal 4: 738–739

Veldhuis J D, Santen R J, Santner S 1978 Unique Pharmacologic Estrogen Deprivation by Aminoglutethimide, p 201. Proceedings of the 60th Annual Meeting of the Endocrine Society, Miami

Von Eiff A W 1975 Blood pressure and estrogens. Frontiers of Hormone Research 3: 177

Vorherr H, Messer R H 1978 Breast cancer: potentially predisposing and protecting factors. American Journal of Obstetrics and Gynecology 130: 335–358

Wallentin L, Varenhorst E 1978 Changes of plasma lipid metabolism in males during estrogen treatment for prostatic carcinoma. Journal of Clinical Endocrinology and Metabolism 47: 596–599

Weiss N S 1975 Risks and benefits of estrogen use. New England Journal of Medicine 293: 1200–1202

Weiss N S, Sayvetz T A 1980 Incidence of endometrial cancer in relation to the use of oral contraceptives. New England Journal of Medicine 302: 551–554

Weiss N S, Szekeley D, English D, Schweid A 1979 Endometrial cancer in relation to patterns of menopausal estrogen use. Journal of the American Medical Association 242: 261–264

Weiss N S, Ure C L, Ballard J H, Williams A R, Daling J R 1980 Decreased risk of fractures of the hip and lower forearm with postmenopausal use of estrogen. New England Journal of Medicine 303: 1195–1198

Whitehead M I, Townsend P T, Pryse-Davies J, Ryder T A, King R J B 1981a Effects of estrogens and progestins on the biochemistry and morphology of the post-menopausal endometrium. New England Journal of Medicine 305: 1599–1606

Whitehead M I, Lane G, Dyer G, Townsend P T, Collins W P, King R J B 1981b Oestradiol: the predominant intranuclear oestrogen in the endometrium of oestrogen-treated postmenopausal women. British Journal of Obstetrics and Gynecology 88: 914–918

Wilson R A 1966 Feminine Forever. Mayflower–Dell, New York

Wyan J B, Finner S L, Gordon J E 1966 Differential age at menopause in the rural Punjab, India. Population Index 32: 328

Wynder E, escher G, Mantel N 1966 An epidemiological investigation of cancer of th endometrium. Cancer 19: 489–520

Yen S S C, Vela P 1968 Effects of contraceptive steroids on carbohydrate metabolism. Journal of Clinical Endocrinology and Metabolism 28: 1564–1570

Ziel H K, Finkle W D 1975 Increased risk of endometrial carcinoma among users of conjugated estrogens. New England Journal of Medicine 293: 1167–1170

Ziel H K, Finkle W D 1976 Association of estrone with the development of endometrial carcinoma. American Journal of Obstetrics and Gynecology 124: 735–740

8

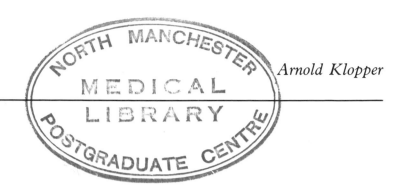

Arnold Klopper

Steroids in pregnancy

INTRODUCTION

When the planning of this chapter began it was intended to have a description of the steroids of the fetus and placenta. It was difficult enough to stick to steroids when often half the story lay with proteins. To keep only to the fetus and placenta was too unnatural a limitation. It would leave out the role of the ovary and ignore the signals which shuttle to and fro between the uterus and conceptus before and during implantation. It was decided to embark upon the larger concept of the steroids of pregnancy; thus getting free of the shackles of anatomy, only to find that now the title was too embracing. To do it justice would use disproportionate space. Of necessity this chapter will not embark on all that might be subsumed under its title. It can do no more than pick out a few likely growth areas. That is always a dangerous activity. Time will overtake us and in any case any selection of topics is only a matter of taste and experience. I shall consider only what seems to me changing and growing at the present moment and hope that the matter may still be of some interest in the near future.

Historical note

The story does not spring into being suddenly. In a way it is as old as science itself. How old is that? As good a point to start as any other, is the early thirties of this century. This was the era of the biochemists; of men like Butenandt and Marrian who crystallised the steroids from the urine of pregnant women and bit by bit worked out their molecular construction. In terms of pregnancy steroids; perhaps the best example of work published at that time was Marrian's description in 1930 of oestriol; a gem of scientific writing that never got the acclaim it merits (Marrian; 1930).

The next stage took steroids from the biochemical laboratory into the ward. It was the time when methods for urinary steroid measurements were being developed.

To do so, methods for measuring microgram amounts of steroid had to be devised — a great challenge at a time when biochemists had never dealt with quantities so small as to be nearly invisible to the naked eye and a decade before radioimmunoassay enlarged our horizon. The challenge was met by developing colour reactions for steroids — Kober for oestrogens, Zimmerman for 17 oxosteroids and a yellow sulphuric acid colour for pregnanediol. None of these colour reactions was specific and they had to be preceded by a great deal of laborious purification; mainly by chromatographic adsorption on alumina columns. The pregnancy field was dominated by the urinary method of Brown (1955) for the measurement of urinary oestrogens.

Progesterone is not excreted in measurable quantities and could not be determined in urine but the development of a method for measuring its main metabolite, pregnanediol, told substantially the same story as appeared many years later when progesterone was measured in blood (Klopper et al, 1955). Indeed blood measurements were for long a kind of El Dorado in the steroid field. When, finally, radioimmunoassay ushered in the era of plasma hormone assay it turned into a chimera. In terms of clinical application, blood assays told no more than did the urinary measurements. This is not the place to rehearse the arguments of plasma versus urinary assays; it has been done at some length elsewhere (Klopper 1976).

Woven in with the search for clinical usefulness, with all attention directed toward the use of steroid assays in obstetric decision making, was a thread of scientific curiosity. What do steroids do in pregnancy? Why does the placenta pour such a torrent of progesterone and oestrogen into the mother? We have long known the answer in general terms — myometrial contractility, uterine and breast growth, fluid changes, etc. The discovery of receptor proteins in target cells helped to spell the answer more clearly. Before we can manipulate steroids in pregnancy to our advantage we need to know much more clearly what they do, how and where. That way lies tomorrow.

EARLY PREGNANCY

Fertilisation

There are two views about fertilisation in the human. One is that it is accidental, but a statistical probability. When a woman is having intercourse two or three times a week there is bound to come an occasion when fresh sperm are released in the vagina at just the right moment to reach a recently ovulated ovum at the right stage of development at the right position in the tube. Given that happy accident it is likely that sufficient numbers of sperm will swim in the right direction and certainly enough to enable one to penetrate the zona pellucida. The other view is purposive: that she is more likely to have intercourse at the right time, that the sperm receive signals leading them to the ovum. When an event, however complex, depends on one sperm among many millions carrying through the right sequence of actions, it is statistically probable that the accident will happen. But the tightly coordinated series of events which carry the fertilised ovum through the next stage depends on a single entity — the tiny cluster of cells that is the proliferating ovum. It can only do what it does by being programmed; by giving and receiving signals. If we are willing to accept that the transport and nidation of the fertilised egg is programmed, it seems probable that fertilisation is also programmed. The central thesis is that the whole process of gestation from fertilisation to parturition is a sequence of coordinated events. There is a constant exchange of information between embryo and mother. We are just beginning to decipher some of the signals which flicker back and forth between the mother and her conceptus. Some of those signals are undoubtedly steroid in nature.

Transport of the fertilised ovum

There are three stages in the progress of the egg down the tube. It is rapidly transported through the ampulla by a combination of muscular contractions and ciliary action. It is then retained for 1–2 days at the junction of the ampulla and the isthmus as though some functional block exists at this site. It is here that fertilisation takes place. It is then fairly rapidly transported through the isthmus although it may be held at the utero-tubal junction for a short while as fluid accumulates until a contraction pushes a gush into the uterine cavity.

The fertilised egg has to reach the uterus at the right stage of development. Its 3 day stay in the oviduct is under the control of ovarian steroids, but the experimental findings which point to this are disconnected observations, often species- and dose-dependent, and cannot yet be put together to form an integrated description of the events. The critical locking of the egg at the ampullary-isthmic junction is probably under oestrogen control (Greenwald, 1961). The effect of progesterone on egg transport is exerted by its restraining effect on tubal contractions but in animal experiments the rate of egg transport is much affected by the dose of progesterone and the stage of the cycle (Harper, 1965).

It is likely that the fertilised ovum in some manner signals its presence to the mother and thus conditions her endocrine responses. Thus Sobowale et al (1978) found that the progesterone levels in the early luteal phase were higher in cycles in which conception occurred than in those when it did not. Very likely this is a response of the mother to the presence of a fertilised ovum. The signals being emitted from the ovum are more difficult to read, the more so as they have to be discriminated from the 'noise' of maternal signals and particularly as the embryonic signals may be of the same steroid nature as the maternal ovarian ones. Certainly rabbit blastocycsts contain both progesterone and oestradiol, increasing in amount as the blastocyst grows (Borland et al, 1977). It is a fine point, quite unresolved, whether such steroid accumulations represent uptake by the blastocyst of maternal steroid, or de novo synthesis of steroid by the conceptus. We are well past the point of believing that the elaboration of progesterone or oestradiol is the prerogative of acknowledged endocrine tissues such as the granulosa cells of the ovary. The capacity of the blastocyst to synthesise progesterone and oestradiol from labelled precursors has been demonstrated (Dickmann et al, 1976).

Decidualisation

The probability that an exchange of signals takes place between ovum and host before implantation becomes greater when one examines the process of decidualisation. Admittedly we are a great deal more advanced at reading these signals in the rat than in the woman, but it is reasonable to suppose that such a fundamental mechanism will be similar in all mammals. The story as set forth for the rat by Shelesnyak et al (1967) runs roughly as follows: a surge of oestrogen precedes implantation, and is essential for it. This is less easy to demonstrate in the human although it is agreed that a secondary peak of oestrogen occurs in the luteal phase. The decidual reaction is fully dependent on progesterone; luteëctomy prevents it. The breakdown of the decidual reaction induced by ovariectomy is prevented by the administration of progesterone. The rest of the story is somewhat more speculative but it hangs together. Decidualisation is induced by the local release of histamine where it comes into contact with the fertilised ovum. Why should this be? As a kind of immune reaction, the endometrium having previously been sensitised by contact with paternal antigens in the seminal fluid which are also expressed on the surface of the blastocyst. Be that as it may, one thing is sure — decidualisation is essential for implantation and decidualisation is induced by progesterone. The whole sequence of events involves only ovum, ovary and uterus. Once ovulation has been induced in a hypophysectomised woman decidualisation and implantation will proceed normally without further administration of pituitary hormones.

Implantation

The processes of decidualisation and of implantation are so interwoven that a description of the endocrine control of one is largely a description of the sequence of endocrine events in the other. If, however, one takes implantation rather than decidualisation as the marker event the focus shifts somewhat and a repeat description of the previous section with implantation in mind may make the endocrinology more clear. The ovum reaches the uterine cavity 3–4 days after fertilisation, and in the human, starts to penetrate the endometrium 3 days later. This is a very precisely timed process, both as far as the egg is concerned and also the endometrium. The egg has to be in the blastocyst stage and the endometrium has to be receptive. If the endometrium is not receptive, the human blastocyst will rapidly degenerate. In other species the blastocyst has the capacity to arrest its development; indeed in the roe deer this is the normal process. The fact that we can, at will, induce or abolish uterine receptivity in experimental animals has given some insight into the endocrine control of implantation. The receptive state is induced by at least 48 hours exposure to progesterone. After that oestrogen will induce implantation. The chronology of the events is not entirely conditioned by the endometrial state. In the last few hours before implantation the blastocyst makes contact with the underlying endometrium and probably signals its presence in some way, for oedema and areas of localised increased capilliary permeability of the endometrium develop in the vicinity of the blastocyst (Psychoyos, 1969). The sequence of 48 hours progesterone followed by oestrogen comes from the ovary and it is very likely that it is somehow aware of the blastocyst. Although it is only recently that we can describe the events in molecular terms, endocrinologists have long entertained the concept that the fertilised ovum signals its presence in the uterus. Eighty years ago Halban asked: 'How does the corpus luteum know that this is a pregnancy?' (Halban, 1904).

The oestrogen surge is as essential to implantation as the preceding progesterone. In an ovariectomised animal, implantation is delayed until oestrogen is given even if the animal is given frequent large doses of progesterone. The oestrogen affects both endometrium and blastocyst; causing oedema and areas of localised increased capilliary permeability in the former and lysis of zona pellucida in the latter — the somewhat fancifully named 'hatching' of the egg. After implantation the continued action of progesterone causes a second period of unreceptivity in the endometrium where it will not receive further implantation. This second period of unreceptivity can again be overcome by oestrogen. Suitable endocrine manipulation of experimental animals can produce the interesting situation of a second asynchronous implantation. This is a laboratory curiosity. In the human there is no evidence of a second period of receptivity.

We can now go a stage further in our understanding of the endocrinology of implantation. The initial progesterone causes the formation of a macromolecular oestrogen binder — an increase in oestrogen receptors (Toft & Gorski, 1966). When the newly available receptors are saturated with oestrogen a stage of endometrial unreceptivity supervenes. The bound oestrogens promote the synthesis of new protein in the endometrium (Miller & Emmens, 1969) which leads to implantation.

This complex interplay of precisely timed signals between the ovary, the endometrium and the blastocyst is susceptible to disarray. The story depends on laboratory work in experimental animals where we can examine and manipulate these tissues directly. In the human we can only read a few faint echoes in the peripheral blood of the mother and we have no idea how much reproductive failure may be due to disarray in these signals. Although there is no doubt that the effect of oral contraceptives is mainly due to suppression of ovulation, the fearful crash of false signals in the genital tract must play some part. Perhaps we shall soon learn how to block the endogenous signals without offering such an extensive endocrine insult as oral contraceptives.

THE CORPUS LUTEUM IN PREGNANCY
Formation of corpus luteum of pregnancy

In early pregnancy there is no detectable difference between the corpus luteum of pregnancy and the corpus luteum of the luteal phase which preceded it, although they presumably subserve somewhat different functions. The lifespan of the corpus luteum of the menstrual cycle is simply extended. There are two ways in which this could happen: a luteotrophic stimulus may prolong the life of the menstrual corpus luteum or a luteolytic process may be abrogated. There are several candidates for the role of luteotrophic stimulus. The pituitary hormones LH and prolactin both show luteotrophic properties. In some mammals, e.g. the cow (LH) and the rat (prolactin) such a luteotrophic role is very likely. This of course raises Halban's question one gland higher in the endocrine hierarchy — how does the pituitary know that the cow or the rat is pregnant? In the human, where the signal of pregnancy is directed at the ovary, it comes from the conceptus itself in the form of chorionic gonadotrophin. The pituitary has been removed in early pregnancy without terminating the pregnancy (Kaplan, 1961). More convincingly, pregnancy can be maintained without further endocrine treatment in hypophysectomised women who have had ovulation induced by menopausal gonadotrophin and chorionic gonadotrophin.

The alternative, i.e. stopping a luteolytic process, applies in some mammals but probably not in the human. In many animals, such as the guinea-pig, the life of the corpus luteum is ended by a signal from the uterus. If the animal becomes pregnant or a hysterectomy is done soon after ovulation, that signal does not come and the corpus luteum continues secreting oestrogen and progesterone long after it should have stopped. Almost certainly this uterine signal is a prostaglandin, probably $PGF_{2\alpha}$. On the other hand, if a hysterectomy is done on a woman in the luteal phase the corpus luteum involutes at the expected time, just before menstruation would have occurred. In species where a luteolytic mechanism is operative the prostaglandin exerts a vasoconstrictive effect, reducing ovarian blood flow below the level necessary for the maintenance of the corpus luteum. These findings led to the somewhat optimistic use of prostaglandin as a luteolytic agent for the termination of early pregnancy. It did not work, possibly because the injection of a bolus of prostaglandin into a peripheral vein is not the equivalent of constant secretion of prostaglandin into the uterine vein.

There is, however, no doubt about the luteotrophic effect of chorionic gonadotrophin. Stock et al (1971) showed that chorionic gonadotrophin, alone or together with placental lactogen, would extend the life of the corpus luteum if given 2 or 3 days before the period is due — just about when involution of the corpus luteum normally starts and when the first traces of chorionic gonadotrophin can be detected if the woman is pregnant. The blastocyst is hardly more than 32 cells at this stage — A speck of tissue, yet able to generate a signal so strong that, diluted and at a distance, it can still alter the course of steroidogenesis. It may be that chorionic gonadotrophin is not the whole story of the signals produced by the early conceptus. Certainly it releases other proteins into the maternal circulation, notably Schwangerschaftsprotein 1 (SP_1) and possibly pregnancy-associated plasma protein A (PAPP-A). Also the levels of hCG fall sharply after 12 weeks gestation but there is no concomitant change in the histology of the corpus luteum, and the other placental proteins such as SP_1 and PAPP-A continue to rise.

The lifespan of the corpus luteum of pregnancy

It is difficult to know what to make of the secretory activity of the corpus luteum after the first 5 or 6 weeks of pregnancy. Although some cystic, possibly degenerative changes, can be found in the human corpus luteum by midpregnancy there is good evidence that it continues to secrete progesterone right up to term (Mikhail & Allen, 1967). The anatomical arrangements and degree of persistence of the corpus luteum is very much a matter of the species. Thus esoteric animals such as the black rhinocerus or some African bats have proved to be a happy hunting ground for zoologists to find all manner of unusual arrangements (Amoroso & Perry, 1977). In some animals the corpus luteum disappears early in pregnancy, in others it persists throughout. In the pregnant mare the corpus luteum persists only for about as long as the normal cyclic one. New corpora lutea are formed throughout the pregnancy by luteinisation of unruptured follicles. The formation of additional luteal tissue to provide additional steroid secretion in pregnancy is a common mechanism in other species.

The corpus luteum of pregnancy produces at least one polypeptide — relaxin — and a number of steroids, in particular progesterone and other progestins, 17α-hydroxyprogesterone and various oestrogens. There are not many

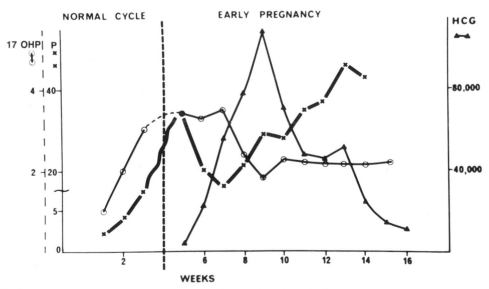

Fig. 8.1 Plasma chorionic gonadotrophin (▲–▲), plasma progesterone (x–x) and 17α-hydroxyprogesterone in early pregnancy

observations on ovarian progesterone production in pregnancy. Much of the early pregnancy data is derived from studies of women in whom ovulation has been induced. This is not a good model as the ovary may be overstimulated. In any case it soon becomes impossible to distinguish between ovarian and placental secretion. A generally accepted version of the changes is shown in Fig. 8.1. This of course shows a mixture of ovarian and placental products. The hCG is placental in origin, the 17α-hydroxyprogesterone is ovarian and progesterone is a mixture of the two. If, as is generally assumed, the 17α-hydroxyprogesterone levels can be taken as an index of ovarian steroidogenesis, it suggests that ovarian activity slows at 6 weeks but persists at a steady reduced level for the rest of the pregnancy.

The data on oestrogen production during early pregnancy are even more sparse. For the most part early pregnancy studies make no distinction between ovarian and placental oestrogen. The corpus luteum does produce oestradiol-17β and it is a reasonable guess that the ovarian production follows the line suggested by 17α-hydroxyprogesterone.

THE CHANGEOVER FROM CORPUS LUTEUM TO PLACENTA

It has long been known that in some mammals the ovary, and by implication the corpus luteum, is essential for the maintenance of pregnancy throughout gestation. This is not the case in the human; here the ovary is necessary only in early pregnancy. Soon the placenta takes over the function of producing oestrogen and progesterone and the ovary is no longer necessary. It is generally assumed that some pregnancy failures can be ascribed to a fault in the timing of this takeover, ovarian function declining before placental steroid production can substitute for it. This reasoning may be fallacious. It has already been pointed out that there is no good reason to suppose that ovarian steroid secretion stops naturally at a given point in pregnancy. If a decline in ovarian hormone secretion is ever implicated in abortion it is more likely to be a primary inadequacy rather than the premature occurrence of a normal programmed event.

Our understanding of the timing of placental takeover derives largely from two pieces of work, the first done more than 20 years ago. In 1961 Diczfalusy & Borell encountered the rare situation of a woman with only one ovary having to have it removed in early pregnancy. This occurred on the 78th day after her last menstrual period. They were therefore presented with an example of what would happen to hormone levels if the ovarian input was suddenly completely removed. The answer was nothing much. The urinary output of oestrone, oestradiol, oestriol and pregnanediol was essentially unchanged. From this they inferred that by 11 weeks of pregnancy the ovary was no longer making a significant contribution to the total production of oestrogen and progesterone. The experiments of Csapo & Pulkinen (1978) were more deliberately designed to determine at what point in pregnancy the placenta could substitute for the ovary and which hormone deficiency could cause abortion. They performed luteëctomies on women admitted for therapeutic abortion some days before the scheduled operation. They found that the critical time was between 6 and 7 weeks from the last menstrual period. If the luteëctomy was done before this time the woman aborted; if done after, the pregnancy persisted until it was surgically terminated. It would appear therefore that the indispensable lifespan of the corpus luteum in pregnancy was only 4–5 weeks. They then tested the effect of treatment with oestrogen or progesterone when the corpus luteum was removed before the critical period. If oestrogen was given, the plasma oestradiol stayed up but the progesterone fell and abortion occurred. If progesterone was given, the oestrogens fell but progesterone stayed up and abortion did not occur. They inferred that it was progesterone secretion from the ovary before the 7th week which was essential to the maintenance of pregnancy.

The clinical implications of these findings are obvious. One clear conclusion is that the only category of patient in whom a primary ovarian failure can be compensated by progesterone treatment is that rare group which comes under surveillance before 7 weeks gestation. Almost all trials of progestational compounds in the treatment of abortion have involved patients who did not come under treatment before 8–10 weeks pregnancy. If there is an element of primary progesterone deficiency in women who abort after 7 weeks, it is a deficiency of placental production and one for which it may be very difficult to compensate. Placental progesterone is probably directed at the endometrium and the myometrium and is continuously produced. Administering progesterone discontinuously by mouth or by injection will result in very little active hormone reaching the target site. Progesterone has a plasma half-life of the order of 5–8 minutes. If, on the other hand, it is intended to make good an ovarian deficiency before 7 weeks it would be more logical to stimulate the failing corpus luteum with hCG and hope that it will maintain progesterone levels by continuous secretion.

STEROID PRODUCTION BY THE FETOPLACENTAL UNIT

The steroid nucleus

Clinicians are apt to show a stout resistance to the charms of the benzene ring, much beloved of the biochemist. A brief exposure to 6 hydroxy-chickenwire is however essential for understanding how the fetoplacental unit produces the hormones of pregnancy. The first prerequisite is a map

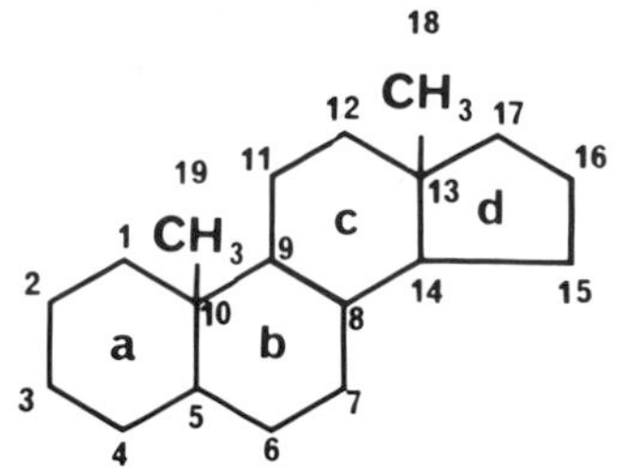

Fig. 8.2 The steroid skeleton

reference to the parts of the skeleton which, when fleshed, makes up progesterone or the oestrogens. The complete map, numbered and lettered, is shown in Fig. 8.2. It is built up of four carbon rings fused together. Three of them, rings A, B, and C are six-membered. The fourth, ring D, has only five carbon atoms. Carbon is tetravalent and the spare valencies, not taken up by their attachment to neighbouring carbon atoms, are satisfied by hydrogen. Each meeting point of the lines in Fig. 8.2 represents a carbon atom with one, two or three attached hydrogen atoms. Each carbon atom is numbered, the logical sequence of which is evident only to the initiated. This numbering system does, however, give an essential grid reference by which particular parts of the steroid nucleus can be designated. Thus if you wish to refer to some substituent attached to the third carbon atom from the

peak of ring A you refer to it as on C_3. The ring structures contain altogether 17 carbon atoms, numbered as shown in Fig. 8.2. In addition there are methyl groups (carbons with three attached hydrogens) on C_{10} and C_{13}. If you imagine the steroid nucleus laid flat on this paper the angular methyl groups would project upward toward your eye. Any substituent attached to the nucleus projecting in the same direction is said to be α-orientated; one on the opposite side of the molecule is β-orientated. In this way the grid reference is three dimensional. Oestriol, for instance, has a hydroxyl attached to C_{16} and pregnanediol, the main metabolite of progesterone, has one on C_3. In steroid nomenclature they are described as 16αOH and 3βOH respectively.

The steroid molecule is modified to form progesterone. Its characteristic features are twofold: the first is in ring A where there is a double bond between C_4 and C_5 (designated $\Delta 4$), and an oxo group on C_3. The $\Delta 4$-3-oxo is a linked structure present in other steroids, e.g. testosterone and is metabolised as a unit. As a rule the double bond is saturated and the oxo group simultaneously reduced to hydroxyl as when progesterone is inactivated to pregnanediol. The $\Delta 4$-3-oxo configuration is an essential feature of progesterone; without it the molecule is biologically inactive. The second feature of the progesterone molecule is a side chain of two carbon atoms attached to C_{17}. By the

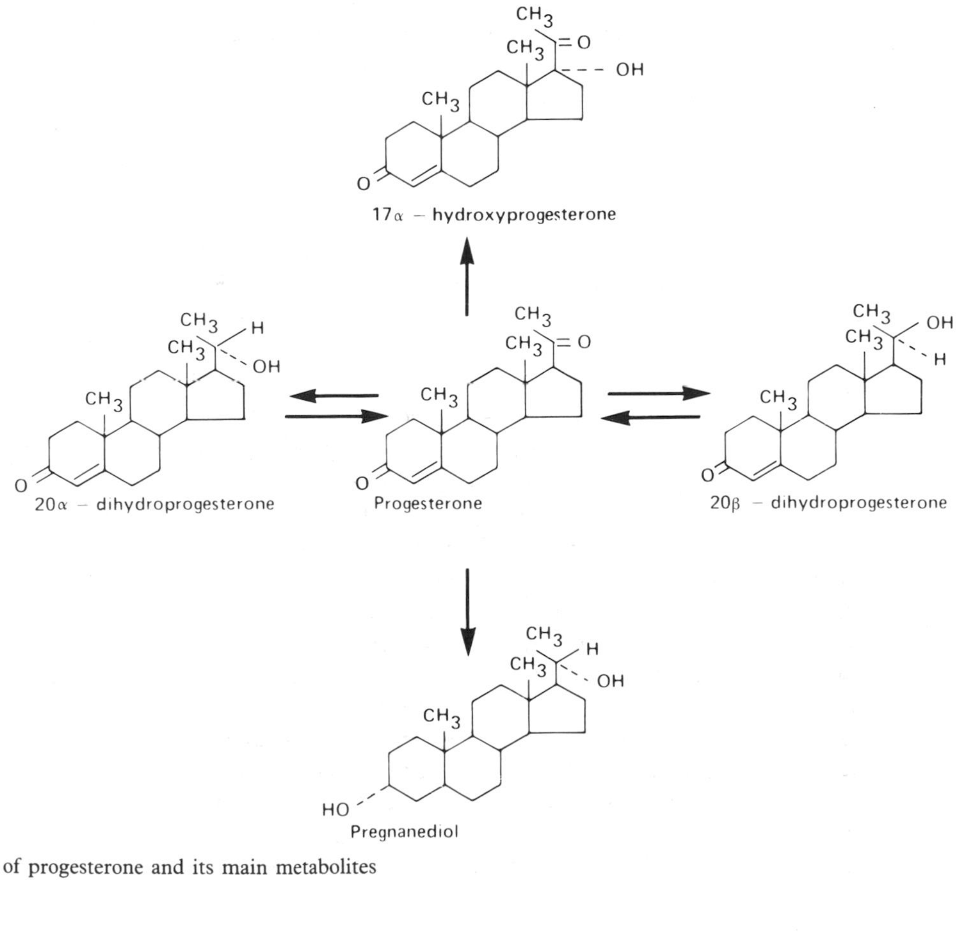

Fig. 8.3 The structure of progesterone and its main metabolites

obscure logic of our map reference these become C_{20} and C_{21}. Progesterone and all chemically related compounds (the pregnane series) have 21 carbon atoms; two more than the basic nucleus (the androstane series). The structure of progesterone and its main metabolites are shown in Fig. 8.3. Progesterone has an oxo group attached to C_{20}. This is less essential to the biological activity of the molecule than the $\Delta 4$-3-oxo grouping and when it is reduced to a hydroxyl grouping the resulting compounds still have some progestational activity. The formation of oestrogens involves a reduction in the number of carbon atoms in the basic C_{19} androstane nucleus. The angular methyl at C_{19} is removed, so all oestrogens are 18 carbon compounds. A further essential feature is that ring A becomes aromatic, having double bonds between alternate carbon atoms. In addition there is a hydroxyl group on C_3. This structure — an unsaturated six carbon ring with a hydroxyl group is a feature common to a large group of natural compounds, the phenols. Oestrogens are the only phenolic steroids. This gives them some special chemical characteristics which biochemists have used to advantage. Phenols ionise and act as though they were weak acids. They are therefore much more water soluble than the neutral steroids and will be separated from all other steroids by partition between an organic solvent and aqueous NaOH. Oestrogens also have substituents elsewhere on the steroid nucleus, notably on C_{17}. The structure of the three 'classical' oestrogens, oestrone, oestradiol and oestriol is shown in Fig. 8.4. Oestrone has an oxo group on C_{17}. Such groups are designed -one in steroid nomenclature, hence the -one in oestrone. Oestradiol has the obligatory hydroxyl on C_3 and a second one at C_{17}. Hydroxyl groups are indicated by the suffix -ol and oestradiol having two hydroxyls is therefore a -diol. The hydroxyl on C_{17} can be either α or β in orientation. Some mammals produce the α compound but the human product is overwhelmingly oestradiol-17β. The remaining oestrogen in Fig. 8.4 has a third hydroxyl, an α-orientated substituent on C_{16}, hence the designation oes*triol*. There is an unsolved mystery about this steroid, the main oestrogen of pregnancy. In non-pregnant women it is formed by C_{16} hydroxylation of oestradiol, but the fetal liver and to a lesser extent the fetal adrenal has the capacity to 16 hydroxylate steroids other than oestrogens. The fetoplacental unit therefore makes

oestriol directly by a route not involving oestradiol and does so in very large amounts compared to the production of other steroids. The mystery lies in why it should do so. So far nobody has been able to find a biological function for oestriol which is peculiar to it and not equally well performed by other oestrogens.

Each step in steroid synthesis and metabolism is carried out by enzymes. Steroid producing glands such as the adrenal, the testis, the ovary and the placenta possess an array of enzymes which, starting from simple two-carbon fragments, can synthesise complex steroids. Particular enzyme systems attach, remove or transform particular substituents at particular sites in the molecule. The main end products of the gland depends on the relative amounts of various enzyme systems in the tissue. Thus the placenta has high concentrations of aromatase, the enzyme system which removes the angular methyl (CH_3) at C_{19} and inserts alternate double bonds in ring A. Another important enzyme system in the placenta is 3β hydroxysteroid dehydrogenase, the system which produces the $\Delta 4$-3-oxo grouping or progesterone. Other organs, notably the liver and the kidney also have enzymes which metabolise steroids. These are different in kind for they attach other radicals to the hydroxyl substituents of steroids. Commonly these groups are either glucuronic acid or sulphuric acid, forming glucuronides and sulphates by a process known as conjugation. The fetal liver is rich in sulphuryl transferase and most of the steroids in the fetal circulation are transformed into sulphates. Such conjugates are biologically inactive and conjugation is an essential step in the catabolism and excretion of steroids.

Steroid synthesis by the fetoplacental unit

If a steroid producing tissue such an adrenal slice or a placental homogenate is incubated with acetate — a two carbon fragment — small amounts of radioactive steroids are produced. The main steroid so produced is an all too familiar compound not often considered in endocrine terms. It is cholesterol. Although there is no doubt about the ability of the placenta to synthesise cholesterol from acetate (van Leusden & Villee, 1965), *in vivo* the placenta utilises preformed cholesterol for the synthesis of progesterone and oestrogens. Cholesterol exists in a variety of

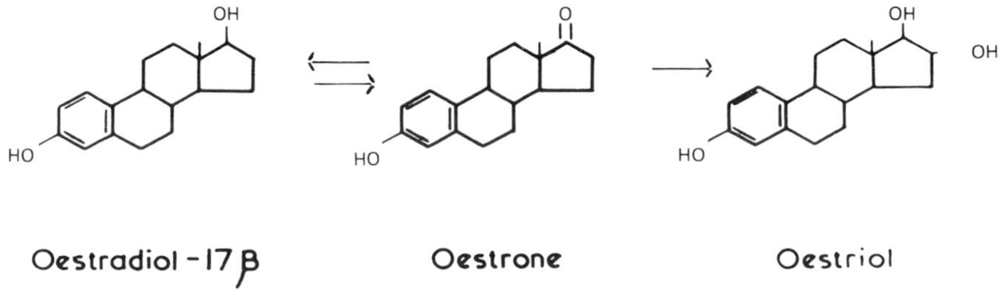

| Oestradiol -17 β | Oestrone | Oestriol |

Fig. 8.4 The structure of the three 'classical' oestrogens

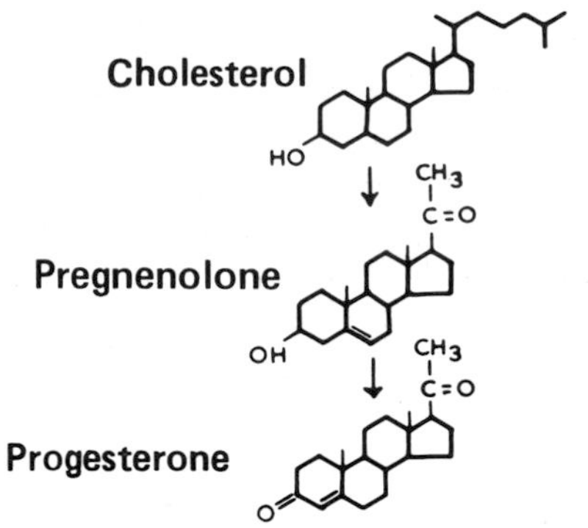

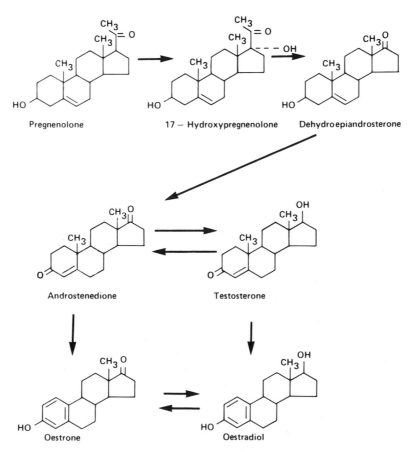

Fig. 8.5 The biosynthesis of progesterone from cholestrol

combinations in the mother but recent work suggests that only the cholesterol of the low density lipoprotein fraction is utilised by the placenta (Winkel et al, 1980).

Cholesterol is a steroid which has a long side chain with eight carbon atoms attached at C_{17}. The first step in the synthesis of progesterone which has 21 carbon atoms is to remove six carbon atoms from cholesterol, a C_{27} steroid. This is shown schematically in Fig. 8.5. Removing six carbons from the side chain of cholesterol is a complex process involving several intermediate steps. The critical enzyme in this process is a desmolase present in the fetal

adrenal. Although the placenta is able also to split cholesterol this step in the main is carried out in the fetus and the placenta utilises the C_{21} steroid, pregnenolone, so formed as a substrate for the generation of progesterone.

Figure 8.5 shows also the characteristic features of pregnenolone. It is worth dwelling on them for a moment, for pregnenolone is not only the precursor of progesterone, it is the raw material from which all steroid hormones, from cortisol to testosterone, is made. Pregnenolone is the last common point in all steroid pathways. From here they branch off along lines determined by the pattern of enzymes in the hormone-producing tissue. Pregnenolone is a C_{21} steroid with an oxo group (at C_{20}) as the -one part of the name indicates. It also has a hydroxyl (-ol-) at C_3, and a double bond at C_5. This $\Delta 5$-$3\beta OH$ configuration is a feature common to a number of steroids and their metabolism depends on an enzyme system, 3β-hydroxysteroid dehydrogenase, which has a central role in the synthesis of steroid hormones. It is the rate-limiting step which determines the production of progesterone from pregnenolone by transforming the $\Delta 5$-$3\beta OH$ of the latter into the $\Delta 4$-3-oxo of the former.

There are two pathways leading to the formation of oestrogens. One branches off from pregnenolone, the other goes via progesterone. The former pathway is the major

Fig. 8.6 The biosynthesis of oestrogens from pregnenolone via androgens

one in the fetoplacental unit and as it carries many clinical implications it is necessary to look at it in more detail.

Pregnenolone has 21 carbon atoms and oestrogens have 18. The transformation of pregnenolone into an oestrogen therefore involves the loss of three carbon atoms, and the acquisition of the characteristic features of oestrogens shown in Fig. 8.4 — an aromatic ring A and a substituent on C_{17}. The reduction in carbons proceeds in two stages: first the removal of the two carbon side chain, C_{21} and C_{20}, of pregnenolone and then the elimination of the angular methyl at C_{19} (for once the numbers follow an arithmetical order). Removing the side chain of pregnenolone produces 19 carbon steroids many of which are androgens. In terms of steroid synthesis at least, the male precedes the female and the main difference between the two is one carbon atom.

An essential step, prior to cleavage of the side chain is 17α-hydroxylation, as shown in Fig. 8.6. The 17–20 desmolase can then act to convert 17α-hydroxypregnenolone into dehydroepiandrosterone, the corresponding C_{19} androgen which retains the Δ5-3βol configuration of pregnenolone. The enzymes (17α-hydroxylase and 17–20 desmolase) which convert pregnenolone into dehydroepiandrosterone are present in the fetal adrenal and it is here that dehydroepiandrosterone (DHA) is generated. As can be inferred from Fig. 8.6 this C_{19} androgen is central in oestrogen biosynthesis and we shall have to explore its clinical implications later.

The next step in oestrogen biosynthesis involves again the important enzyme system 3α-hydroxysteroid dehydrogenase for the Δ5-3αol of dehydroepiandrosterone has to be changed into Δ4-3-oxo giving a potent C_{19} androgen, testosterone. The placenta has a high concentration of 3β-hydroxysteroid dehydrogenase and the conversion of pregnenolone into progesterone or of dehydroepiandrosterone into androstenedione takes place in the trophoblast. As shown in Fig. 8.6, androstenedione retains the C_{17} oxo group of the parent androgen, dehydroepiandrosterone. Transhydrogenase systems which convert a C_{17} oxo into a hydroxyl group and *vice versa*, are widely distributed. Androstenedione is therefore rapidly converted into the corresponding C_{17} hydroxy androgen, testosterone. The testosterone so formed is also converted back into androstenedione, so these two androgens differing only by one hydrogen atom form a dynamic equilibrium mixture. As we shall see, exactly the same situation arises with the oestrogens.

A complex linked system of enzymes carry out the last step of the conversion of androgens into oestrogens, removing the C_{19} angular methyl and inserting the double bonds and C_3 hydroxyl in ring A. This step also is largely carried out in the placenta and the main enzyme, aromatase is very oxygen sensitive. The lowered oestrogen production associated with placental insufficiency may be due to reduced aromatase activity engendered by oxygen lack.

When testosterone serves as substrate for oestrogen synthesis the product is oestradiol-17β. When androstenedione is the precursor, the product is oestrone. Oestradiol and oestrone, like testosterone and androstenedione, differ by one hydrogen atom and are readily interconvertible. Like the androgens they exist as an equilibrium mixture.

So far little has been said about the main pregnancy oestrogen, oestriol. Figure 8.4 shows that it differs from oestradiol in having a third hydroxyl, attached to C_{16}. One might suppose therefore that it is derived by hydroxylation of oestradiol and indeed in non-pregnant women this is probably the case. The fetal liver and adrenal, however, possess enzymes capable of 16α-hydroxylating neutral steroids such as pregnenolone and dehydroepiandrosterone. These 16 hydroxylated precursors are fed into the oestrogen biosynthetic pathway. They retain the 16 hydroxyl group throughout and emerge as oestriol or as 16α hydroxyl oestrone, an oestrogen which is rapidly reduced to oestriol.

When Diczfalusy (1962) enunciated the thesis of the fetoplacental unit he had the distribution of oestrogen synthesising enzymes in mind. Both placenta and fetus are incomplete biosynthetic units; incapable of carrying out the full synthesis outlined here. But what one lacks the other possesses and by shuttling substrates to and fro between them they are able to complete the pathway. The fetal adrenal can 17-hydroxylate and has the desmolase for removing the side chain of 17α-hydroxypregnenolone. It can therefore convert pregnenolone to dehydroepiandrosterone. Given a supply of dehydroepiandrosterone from the fetus, the placenta has the 3β hydroxysteroid dehydrogenase and aromatase to convert dehydroepiandrosterone to oestrogen. On the other hand 16-hydroxylation is a purely fetal activity. It is because of this special fetal role in its biosynthesis that oestriol has won a reputation as an index of fetal wellbeing.

There is another pair of enzymes of which fetus and placenta hold one each. The fetal liver is rich in sulphuryl transferase, an enzyme which attaches sulphate radicles to suitable hydroxyl substituents. There is a high concentration of oestrogen, mainly oestriols, in the fetus, but it is held as a pool of inactive oestriol-3-sulphate. It has been argued that the high sulphurylation capacity of the fetus is a means for protecting it against biologically active steroids. This seems reasonable in the case of pregnenolone and of dehydroepiandrosterone which are metabolised as the sulphate. Large amounts of dehydroepiandrosterone sulphate can therefore be processed for the synthesis of oestrogens without exposing the fetus to a biologically active steroid. The sulphurylation of oestriol which is an endpoint, is less easy to understand. Why make large amounts of the steroid in the first place if all you do with it is inactivate it?

The placenta has the opposing enzyme systems — sulphatases which cleave both neutral and oestrogen sulphates. In the case of oestrogen cleaving sulphates this is the means by which oestrogens are transferred from fetus to mother. Sulphates are very slowly transmitted, free steroids pass the placenta rapidly. The neutral sulphatases serve another important function. Dehydroepiandrosterone sulphate requires to be hydrolysed before it can be converted to oestrogen. Placental sulphatase therefore determines the availability of an essential substrate for oestrogen synthesis and may so constitute a rate limiting step. In the rare interesting case of sulphatase deficiency this enzyme is lacking in the placenta. Oestrogen synthesis is much retarded and oestriol levels are low without there being any special fetal jeopardy.

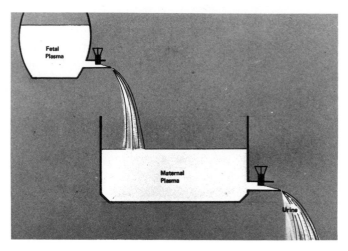

Fig. 8.7 An idealised concept of the factors which determine plasma steroid concentration

THE DISTRIBUTION OF STEROIDS IN PREGNANCY

The maternal compartment

Clinicians are familiar with the notion of measuring urinary steroid excretion. When radioimmunoassay swept in a tide of plasma assays, it was assumed, without much reflection, that these were a sort of sophisticated urinary assay. They are nothing of the kind. For one thing urinary assays are the end of the line; there is nowhere for a steroid to go and nothing more can happen to it once it is in the urine. The plasma is a kaleidoscope with steroids moving hither and thither, changing from moment to moment. To pick a single molecular species and freeze it in a number is to put your finger on a blob of mercury. Urinary excretion is a summary of the events of 24 hours, plasma assays are a moment in time — that moment when the needle was put into the vein. Most of all plasma assays are a shifting balance between input and outflow with the volume of the intravascular compartment as a third independent variable. It behoves us to look a little more closely at the dynamic situation represented by the figure for plasma oestriol or progesterone concentration.

The assumption, not always clearly realised, behind plasma assays is that the maternal plasma steroid concentration bears a direct relationship to the rate of production of the steroid by the fetoplacental unit. In its simplist state the concept is illustrated in Fig. 8.7. This supposes that say, oestriol, is produced in the fetoplacental unit, runs into the maternal plasma, and is excreted in the urine. The concentration in the plasma is therefore a direct reflection of the rate of synthesis in the fetoplacental unit. But a moments reflection serves to show there is not a single stream of oestriol flowing into the mother. There is oestriol in the fetal circulation being transmitted to the mother. There is oestriol, newly synthesised in the placenta being secreted into the retroplacental blood. Most of the oestriol coming from the placenta is unconjugated but small amounts of oestriol conjugates cross at rates very different from the free steroid. The rate of synthesis itself may be

controlled by the supply of substrate, say 16 OH dehydroepiandrosterone sulphate or by 3β-hydroxysteroid dehydrogenase converting it to 16 OH androstenedione or by aromatase converting it to oestriol or by sulphatase determining the rate at which oestriol sulphate is transmitted across the placenta. At the very least we have to assume a multiple inflow, the individual components of which represent very different processes and which have very different rates of inflow.

The second oversimplification is that of a single compartment into which the oestriol flows. Oestriol passes from the maternal intravascular space into the interstitial space, into the body fat and into the intracellular space. There is a constant ebb and flow from these spaces into and out of the plasma compartment. Most important of all more than half the oestriol produced by the fetoplacental unit finds its way into the bile (Adlercreutz, 1974). Here it is completely sequestered from the plasma until it finds its way back by readsorption from the gut. The oestriol you measure in the mother may not have come directly from the fetus but may largely represent readsorption from the gut and only more distantly fetal synthesis. Bacterial enzymes in the gut are essential for readsorption of oestriol. If the gut is sterilised as when a pregnant woman is treated with ampicillin for a urinary infection, the readsorption does not take place and plasma oestriol concentration falls, although the fetoplacental production is not impaired.

The importance of the multicompartment model for oestriol distribution in the mother is well illustrated by the post partum decline in plasma oestriol. As can be seen in Fig. 8.8 the mother's plasma oestriol falls by half, 8 minutes after delivery of the placenta. If it were simply the plasma compartment emptying itself after all inflow had been stopped by delivery of the placenta, the plasma oestriol concentration would be down to a trace well within the hour. But 4 or 5 days later it is still running at 20 per cent of its initial value as shown in Fig. 8.9. This is because

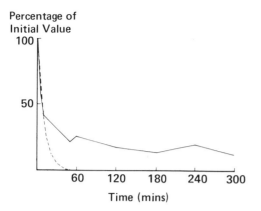

Fig. 8.8 Post-partum decline in oestriol expressed as a percentage of the value at delivery. Solid line represents mean value in 12 subjects. Dotted line represents the theoretical rate of decline based on a half-life of 8 minutes

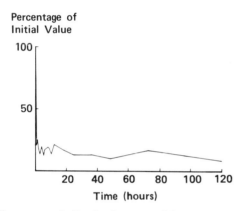

Fig. 8.9 Post-partum decline in plasma oestriol expressed as a percentage of the value at delivery. Mean of 12 subjects

inflow from adjacent communicating compartments takes over and prevents the plasma compartment concentration declining at its initial rate.

The outflow situation, the neglected part of the balance, is hardly less complicated. Outflow of steroid takes place not only into the urine but via the gut and into the other communicating compartments. Steroid is also removed by metabolism within the plasma compartment. Thus very little progesterone is excreted, most of it is removed by metabolism into pregnanediol. These routes of outflow are independent and one or other may exert a dominant influence on the plasma concentration without any change of inflow from the fetoplacental unit. The real situation concerning plasma assays is more accurately represented by Fig. 8.10 than by Fig. 8.7.

The fetal compartment

There are high concentrations of oestrogens and progesterone in the fetal as well as in the maternal circulation. If a labelled steroid is injected into either, radioactivity soon appears in the other compartment. But the two are not in equilibrium. A high concentration of progesterone or oestrogen in one does not imply the same in the other. It is an open question as to which is the primary compartment. Does the placenta secrete first into the fetal blood and later transmit the steroid from fetal to maternal blood? Or does it secrete in both directions simultaneously? If the latter is the case, what determines the proportion of any steroid which goes into the mother compared to the amount passing to the fetus? There are interesting physiological implications in the question. If the placenta is actively secreting hormones to the fetus it is likely that they

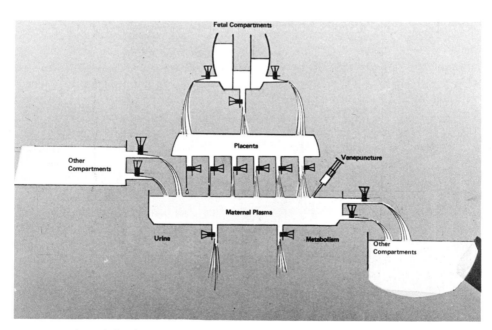

Fig. 8.10 Plasma hormone assay — the real situation

have a function in the fetus. Perhaps we have for too long been looking at the mother and ignoring her fetus. Perhaps the real target of the placental steroid is in the fetus. The fetus certainly consumes progesterone. The concentration of progesterone in the fetal vein is well above that in the artery (Maynard et al, 1981).

THE VARIABILITY OF PREGNANCY STEROIDS

Variability with gestation

Once the fetoplacental synthesis of steroids is established their plasma concentration and urinary excretion increases steadily with advancing gestation. By the end of pregnancy the urinary output of oestriol is 1000 to 10 000 times greater than before the woman became pregnant. For most steroids in man the pregnancy curve is S-shaped. If the mean placental weight curve is plotted during pregnancy, the same type of S-shaped curve is obtained. It is thus deduced that the plasma concentration or urinary excretion (they are fairly closely related) is determined by the functional mass of the trophoblast. There is indeed a statistically significant correlation between steroid levels and placental weight. This applies equally to such purely placental products as progesterone and fetoplacental hormones such as oestradiol. This implies that in normal circumstances the supply of substrates such as dehydroepiandrosterone is adequate and the rate of oestrogen synthesis is determined by placental factors such as 3β-hydroxysteroid dehydrogenase and aromatase. When placental growth and function decline in late pregnancy the steroid output flattens out and may decline if the pregnancy goes past term.

There is one exception to the late pregnancy plateau of steroids. This is oestriol. Twenty years ago Klopper & Billewicz (1963) observed that at about 34 weeks gestation there was an increase in the rate of oestriol excretion and the curve became steeper instead of flattening off. They surmised that in late pregnancy some new factor, probably fetal in origin, became operative in oestriol production. This phenomenon has often been commented on since and indeed it has been suggested that the late pregnancy surge in plasma oestriol could be a measure of the stage of gestation and a useful index of fetal wellbeing (Buster et al, 1976).

Variability from subject to subject

Even when the variation due to gestation is allowed for by comparing patients all at the same stage of gestation, there is a great deal of difference between one normal woman and the next. This is brought out in Table 8.1 which shows that, regardless of whether you are measuring urinary excretion of a metabolite or the plasma concentration of a free or conjugated steroid the co-efficient of variation is around 30 per cent. Put in another way, a value 60 per cent

Table 8.1 Subject-to-subject variation in plasma and urinary steroids at 38 weeks gestation (From Klopper et al, 1974)

Assay	Co-efficient of variation (%)
24 h urinary oestriol excretion	28
Total plasma oestriol	34
Unconjugated plasma oestriol	32
Unconjugated plasma oestradiol	37
Plasma progesterone	31
Urinary pregnanediol	38

above or below the mean value could still be in the normal range. Such a large normal spread carries the implication that there will be a large overlap between normal and abnormal. It is unlikely that you can even diagnose fetal growth retardation with any security on the basis of a low plasma oestriol simply because so many women carrying a fetus of normal weight for gestation will also have a plasma oestriol well below the mean normal value.

This somewhat gloomy prognosis is somewhat lightened by an odd feature of the normal distribution of plasma steroid concentration or of urinary excretion. This is that some wild high values occur in every survey. They pull the mean value up unduly and leave more values below than above the mean. In other words the distribution is not a normal bell-shaped Gaussian distribution but is skewed. Such a distribution is not adequately described in terms of a normal mean and standard deviation but requires the values to be plotted as logarithms, square roots or squares. Perhaps more understandably from the point of view of those who are not mathematically minded the point can also be met by describing the normal range in terms of median and centiles. Any of these devices have the effect of raising the lower normal limit, thus increasing the discrimination between the highest abnormals and the lowest normals. Of course it also has the effect of increasing the upper normal limit, but there is no prize for clinical application of hormone assay to be gained at that end. Those who have wondered why some women have wild high values have always come away with a dusty answer.

There is another consequence of the large normal range. It should make it easy to identify what maternal or fetal characteristics are associated with high or low steroid values. Apart from the obvious factors of placental and fetal size (they are probably the same thing and hold true convincingly only for oestriol), no other factor such as parity or age appears to influence steroid production. This is most disappointing, for it means we have no lead to any factor which might determine placental activity. To all intents and purposes the placenta is running free with no feedback control. It lends weight to Professor Chard's despairing thesis that placental proteins and steroids have no function; the placenta is simply coded to produce them and pours them out without control other than uterine blood flow and placental mass (Gordon & Chard, 1979).

Variability from time to time

In view of the many factors bearing on the plasma concentration of steroids it is to be expected that there will be a good deal of short term variation. When one considers that to the physiological variation must be added an element of variability due to the experimental error of the method (the interassay precision of most radioimmunoassay is 6–10 per cent) the variability of plasma steroids is not great. The day-to-day coefficient of variation for plasma unconjugated oestriol in late pregnancy is 16.5 per cent (Masson et al, 1977). Other plasma oestrogens such as oestradiol have similar variabilities but progesterone with a coefficient of variation at 21 per cent is somewhat more variable (Klopper et al, 1974). Surprisingly the urinary excretion of oestriol (28 per cent) is distinctly more variable than the plasma concentration.

Steroid levels are sufficiently variable to give rise to some difficulty when using them as a measure of fetal wellbeing. Because of the large subject-to-subject variation stress is usually laid on serial estimations where each patient acts as her own control and the absolute value is less significant than the change with time. It then becomes a matter of concern to define how large a drop in, say oestriol, concentration is significant. A more or less empirical judgement suggests that a drop more than 30 per cent below the previous value suggests that there is a real change in oestriol production.

CLINICAL APPLICATIONS OF STEROID HORMONE ASSAY

There is a mood of disenchantment about the usefulness of steroid assays in the assessment of fetal wellbeing. There has never been any great enthusiasm for progesterone assays and the disappointment is mainly with oestriol assays. This subject had been reviewed at some length (Chard & Klopper, 1982) and the findings will not be repeated. Suffice to point out that the expectations were in some respects unreasonable. The assays have been applied without regard to the cause of the fetal hazard, or to the nature of the variability of steroid concentration. It is inherently unlikely that conditions as diverse as maternal diabetes, pre-eclamptic toxaemia, Rh incompatibility and fetal growth retardation will all affect oestriol production equally. Yet the criteria for oestriol change in each of these is the same.

Two specialised tests have met with some acclaim and deserve closer consideration. The first is the dehydroepiandrosterone sulphate loading test. When this steroid (DHAS) is injected into the circulation of a pregnant woman it is rapidly removed by the placenta which converts it in part to oestradiol. The rate at which the injected DHAS is removed from the circulation is decreased in pre-eclamptic toxaemia and this decline in the clearance of DHAS has been used as a test of placental function (Gant et al, 1971). Subsequently other workers used not the disappearance of DHAS but the appearance of the product oestradiol as a test of placental function. This test has become standard practice in some maternity units (Lauritzen et al, 1975) but its reception in Britain has not been so favourable (Korda et al, 1975; Klopper et al, 1976). The response varies so much from one normal woman to another that it is not a discriminating test of placental function. It is however a powerful tool for investigating the physiology of oestrogens in pregnancy and it is a pity that it has fallen into disuse before this aspect was explored.

The second test has met with no better success. Oestetrol is a highly hydroxylated oestrogen formed in the fetal liver from oestradiol (Gurpide et al, 1966). Because of its purely fetal origin it was supposed that it would reflect the fetal state very accurately and indeed in the beginning clinicians regarded oestetrol assays very favourably (Tulchinsky, 1975). Subsequent authors did not view the test with so much enthusiasm and it has failed to gain a place in the clinical armentarium (Notation & Tagatz, 1977).

THE PHYSIOLOGICAL ACTIONS OF OESTROGENS AND PROGESTERONE

Twenty-two years ago Diczfalusy & Lauritzen (1961) wrote a book about oestrogens. It gave a detailed account of the effects of oestrogens on 32 tissues and listed 2207 references. One might suppose that by now the role of oestrogens in pregnancy would be clearly understood. Not so; we are not even sure how necessary they are. Every pregnancy needs progesterone, lots of progesterone, but women with placental sulphatase deficiency produce very little oestrogen. Yet fetal growth and differentiation proceeds apace, and pregnancy is to all intents and purposes normal except for a tendency for the failure of onset of labour. If the steroids of pregnancy are fulfilling some vital functions one would expect the steroid level to have some bearing on the matter. Yet oestrogen concentrations cover an enormous range from one woman to another with no detectable differences to go with the differences in oestrogen levels. Most of all there is no evidence of any feedback control from a site of action. There is nothing which tells the fetoplacental unit when it is producing too much or too little oestrogen. If you raise someone's insulin by 20 per cent their plasma glucose plummets; if you quadruple the output of oestradiol from the placenta by injecting 50 mg of dehydroepiandrosterone nothing happens.

Of course in very general terms we know the message that the oestrogen molecule carries. In pregnancy, as in the non-pregnant, it says to target cells: 'make new protein, grow, proliferate'. So the breasts and the uterus grow to keep pace with the needs of pregnancy. But some 27 variations on the theme of C_{18} phenolic steroids have been recognised in the urine of pregnant women. Do some do one thing and some another? There is precious little evidence to show much physiological difference between one oestrogen and another and none to suggest that any one oestrogen is unique. Tantalising glimpses of special functions for particular oestrogens appear from time to time. Oestriol appears to home in on the cervix (Puck et al, 1957) and may play a large part in the changes in composition and architecture of this tissue which are a feature of pregnancy. On the other hand catechol oestrogens, i.e. oestrogens haveing C_2 substituents such as 2-hydroxyoestrone, 2-methoxyoestrone and 2-hydroxyoestradiol, have none of the uterotropic activity of oestrone, oestradiol, oestriol and oestetrol (Martucci & Fishman, 1977), and one is at a loss to assign any activity in pregnancy to them although pregnant women poduce them in quantity.

The role of the steroid hormones in parturition

Women with a sulphatase-deficient placenta produce very little oestrogen but the growth of the breasts, the uterus and other presumed oestrogen-dependent pregnancy changes are normal. The only fault lies in parturition — the onset of labour is delayed and its progress halting and uncertain. It might be presumed therefore that steroid hormones, or at least oestrogens play a part in parturition. If so, their role might be elucidated by a close examination of the changes which take place at the onset and during labour. This is an area where controversy has raged for a long time. There is little profit in rehearsing the arguments between those who believe that consistent changes can be found in plasma oestrogens, progesterone and cortisol when a woman goes into labour and those who have failed to demonstrate such changes. There is little doubt about the changes in some other mammals such as rabbits and sheep; the problem is with the human female. It is, of course, always more difficult to prove a positive but the weight of negative evidence is now formidable. That does not, however, preclude the possibility of local uterine changes which cannot be read in the peripheral circulation.

Oestrogens and progesterone act at receptor sites in responsive tissues. The increase of these hormones during pregnancy is massive and it is likely these receptors are fully saturated and not responsive to fluctuations of the steroids well above the critical level. But parturition may depend on steroid actions of a somewhat different kind.

There is sound evidence that the switch which turns on labour is in the fetoplacental unit, not in the mother (Anderson & Turnbull, 1973). Very likely the mechanism consists of an activation of the fetal pituitary-adrenal axis in late pregnancy with a surge cortisol and dehydroepiandrosterone sulphate synthesis in the fetal adrenal. Cortisol stimulates aromatase activity in the placenta and the increased oestrogen synthesis is further enhanced by the increased substrate. All these changes are taken up in a recent hypothesis about the onset of labour by Fuchs (1982). He points out that the changes in oestradiol, progesterone and cortisol, although not manifest in the maternal peripheral circulation bring about changes in the decidua, myometrium and membranes. The rise in oestrogens stimulate the formation of binding sites for oxytocin in the myometrium and alter lysosomal membrane stability resulting in the release of lipases in the endometrium with consequent liberation of arachidonic acid from the lipids. Arachidonic acid is the substrate for prostaglandin synthesis and the result is an increased local production and release of these compounds. The same type of oestrogen action also leads to the release of proteolytic enzymes which break down the collagen fibrils in the cervix and change the composition of its glycosaminoglycans, thus causing ripening of the cervix and possibly making the membranes more liable to rupture. The increased dehydroepiandrosterone sulphate also has the effect of decreasing conversion of pregnenolone to progesterone thus altering the electro-chemical properties of the myometrium by altering the resting potential of the progesterone-dominated myometrium.

ENVOY

The role of steroids in pregnancy has for some years been in the shadows. Estimations of steroid hormones have not been as helpful in the management of pregnancy as had been hoped, and the elucidation of the receptor mechanism did not bring a great leap forward in our understanding of the part they play in pregnancy. Now there is movement again. At both ends of pregnancy — implantation and parturition — the roles of steroids are being elucidated. They turn out to be complex, highly integrated processes like immunosuppression and enzyme activity involving the co-ordination of many factors in a localised context. This growing understanding greatly increases the possibilities of control over conception and delivery.

REFERENCES

Adlercreutz H 1974 Hepatic metabolism of oestrogens in health and disease. New England Journal of Medicine 290: 1081–1084

Amoroso E C, Perry J S 1977 Ovarian activity during pregnancy. In: Zuckerman S, Weir B (eds) The Ovary, p. 316. Academic Press, New York

Anderson A B M, Turnbull A C 1973 Comparative aspects of factors involved in the onset of labour in ovine and human pregnancy. In: Klopper A, Garner J (eds) Endocrine Factors in Labour, pp 141–162. Cambridge University Press, Cambridge

Borland R M, Erickson G F, Ducibella T 1977 Accumulation of

steroids in rabbit preimplantation blastocysts. Journal of Reproduction and Fertility 49: 219–224

Brown J B 1955 A chemical method for the determination of oestriol, oestrone and oestradiol in human urine. Biochemical Journal 60: 185–189

Buster J E, Sakakini J, Killam A P, Scragg W 1976 Serum unconjugated estriol levels in the third trimester and their relationship to gestational age. American Journal of Obstetrics and Gynecology 125: 672–680

Chard T, Klopper A 1982 Placental Function Tests. Springer Verlag, Heidelberg

Csapo A, Pulkinen M 1978 Indispensability of the human corpus luteum in the maintenance of early pregnancy. Obstetrical and Gynecological Survey 33: 69–81

Dickmann Z, Dey S K, Gupta J S 1976 A new concept: control of early pregnancy by steroid hormones originating in the preimplantation embryo. Vitamins and Hormones 34: 215–42

Diczfalusy E 1962 Endocrinology of the fetus. Acta Obstetrica Gynecologica Scandinavica 41: Suppl. 1: 45

Diczfalusy E, Borell U 1961 Influence of oophorectomy on steroid excretion in early pregnancy. Journal of Clininal Endocrinology and Metabolism 21: 1119–1121

Diczfalusy E, Lauritzen Ch 1961 Oestrogene beim Menschen. Springer Verlag, Heidelberg

Fuchs F 1982 The onset of labour. In: Fuchs F, Klopper A (eds) The Endocrinology of Pregnancy, 3rd edn. Harper and Row, New York

Gant N F, Hutchinson H T, Siiteri P K, MacDonald P 1971 Study of the metabolic clearance rate of dehydroepiandrosterone sulfate in pregnancy. American Journal of Obstetrics and Gynecology 111: 555–562

Gordon Y B, Chard T 1979 The specific proteins of the human placenta: some new hypotheses. In: Klopper A, Chard T (eds) Placental Proteins, p. 1. Springer Verlag, Heidelberg

Greenwald G S 1961 A study of the transport of ova through the rabbit oviduct. Fertility and Sterility 12: 80–95

Gurpide E, Schwers J, Welch M T, Vande Wiele R L, Lieberman S 1966 Fetal and maternal metabolism of estradiol during pregnancy. Journal of Clinical Endocrinology and Metabolism 26: 1355–1365

Halban J 1904 Discussion of L Fraenkel's report. Quoted by Psychoyos A 1973 Endocrine control of egg implantation. In: Greep R O (ed) Handbook of Physiology, 11, Part 2, p 194. American Physiological Society, Washington

Harper M J 1965 Transport of eggs in cumulus through the ampulla of the rabbit oviduct in relation to day of pregnancy. Endocrinology 77: 114–123

Kaplan N M 1961 Successful pregnancy following hypophysectomy during the twelfth week of gestation. Journal of Clinical Endocrinology and Metabolism 21: 1139–1141

Klopper A 1976 The choice between assays on blood or on urine. In: Loraine J A, Bell T (eds) Hormone Assays and their Clinical Application. 4th edn, Ch 2, pp 73–86. Churchill Livingstone, Edinburgh

Klopper A, Billewicz Z 1963 Urinary excretion of oestriol and pregnanediol during pregnancy. Journal of Obstetrics and Gynaecology of the British Commonwealth 70: 1024–1035

Klopper A, Michie E, Brown J B 1955 A method for the measurement of pregnanediol in urine. Journal of Endocrinology 12: 209–217

Klopper A, Wilson G, Masson G 1974 The variability of plasma hormone levels in late pregnancy. In: Scholler R (ed) Exploration Hormonale de la Grossesse, p 77. Edition Sepe, Paris

Klopper A, Varela-Torres R, Jandial V 1976 Placental metabolism of

dehydroepiandrosterone sulphate in normal pregnancy. British Journal of Obstetrics and Gynaecology 83: 478–483

Korda A R, Challis J J, Anderson A B, Turnbull A C 1975 The DHAS conversion test. British Journal of Obstetrics and Gynaecology 82: 656–661

Lauritzen Ch, Strecker J, Lehmann W D 1975 Dynamic tests of placental function: some findings on the conversion of DHAS and oestrogens. In: Klopper A (ed) Plasma Hormone Assays in Evaluation of Fetal Wellbeing, pp 113–135. Churchill Livingstone, Edinburgh

Marrian G F 1930 The chemistry of oestrin. Biochemical Journal 24: 1021–1023

Martucci C, Fishman J 1977 Direction of oestradiol metabolisms as a control of its hormonal action — uterotrophic activity of oestradiol metabolites. Endocrinology 101: 1709–1715

Maynard P V: Stein P E, Symonds E M 1981 Umbilical cord plasma at term in relation to mode of delivery. British Journal of Obstetrics and Gynaecology 87: 864–868

Masson G M, Klopper A I, Wilson G R 1977 Plasma oestrogens and pregnancy-associated plasma proteins. A study of their variability in late pregnancy. Obstetrics and Gynaecology 50: 435–438

Mikhail G S, Allen W M 1967 Ovarian function in human pregnancy American Journal of Obstetrics and Gynecology 99: 308–311

Miller B G, Emmens C V 1969 The effect of oestradiol and progesterone on the incorporation of tritiated uridine into the genital tract of the mouse. Journal of Endocrinology 43: 427–436

Notation A D, Tagatz E M 1977 Unconjugated estriol and 15α-hydroxy estriol in complicated pregnancies. American Journal of Obstetrics and Gynecology 128: 747–753

Psychoyos A 1969 Hormonal factors governing decidualisation. Excerpta Medica Foundation. International Congress Series 184: 935–938

Puck A, Korte W, Hubner K A 1957 Die Wirkung des Oestriol auf Corpus uteri, Cervix uteri und Vagina der Frau. Deutche Medizinische Wochenschrift 82: 1–15

Shelesnyak M C, Marcus G J Kraicer P F, Lobel B L 1967 Experimental study of decidualisation. International Journal of Fertility 12: 391–397

Sobowale O, Lenton E, Francis B, Cooke I D 1978 Comparison of plasma steroid and gonadotrophin profiles in spontaneous cycles in which conception did or did not occur. British Journal of Obstetrics and Gynaecology 85: 460–468

Stock R J, Josimovich J B, Kosor B, Klopper A, Wilson G R 1971 The effect of chorionic gonadotrophin and of chorionic somatomammotrophin on steroidogenesis in the corpus luteum. Journal of Obstetrics and Gynaecology of the British Commonwealth 78: 549–560

Toft D, Gorski J 1966 A receptor molecule for estrogens; isolation from the rat uterus and preliminary characterisation. Proceedings of the National Academy of Science of the USA 55: 1574–1581

Tulchinsky D, Frigoletto F D, Ryan K J, Fishman J 1975 Plasma estetrol as an index of fetal wellbeing. Journal of Clinical Endocrinology 40: 560

Van Leusden H, Villee C A 1965 De novo synthesis of sterols and steroids from acetate by preparation of human term placenta. Steroids 6: 31–37

Winkel C A, MacDonald P C, Simpson E R 1980 The role of maternal circulating low density lipoprotein in regulating placental cholesterol metabolism. In: Klopper A, Genazzani A, Crosignani P G (eds) The Human Placenta: Proteins and Hormones, pp 401–406. Academic Press, London

Placental proteins

INTRODUCTION

The human placenta contains a wide range of proteins and small peptides. Some of these appear to be actually produced by this organ, while others — for example, some of the plasma binding globulins — appear simply as a consequence of the fact that the placenta contains a large volume of maternal blood and will thus reflect the general increased synthesis of these molecules in other organs during pregnancy. Reviews on placental proteins have dealt extensively with this subject (Chard & Klopper, 1982; Grudzinskas et al, 1982). This chapter addresses aspects of pregnancy-associated proteins relevant to clinical practice.

Chemistry

Placental proteins present a variety of chemical structures, at least as disparate as that of the whole range of adult plasma proteins. One generalisation is possible: each protein can exist in a number of different forms. In some cases, for example hCG and its subunits, the different forms and their inter-relationships have been clearly defined. In others, e.g. placental protein 5 (PP5), the relationships are less clearly defined, but the study of different types had led to a better understanding of the biological significance of the compound.

Synthesis

There is general consensus that the principal site of synthesis of the placental proteins in late pregnancy is the syncytiotrophoblast. In early pregnancy the cytotrophoblast may also contribute. However, the ability to synthesise these molecules is not limited exclusively to the trophoblast and other cells must carry the code albeit in a repressed state. De-repression may occur with tumours. Furthermore, high concentrations of placental proteins are found in seminal plasma (Ranta et al, 1981; Lee et al, 1983; Bischof

et al, 1983); the origin appears to be in the ampullary part of the vas deferens and the seminal vesicle (Wahlstrom et al, 1982).

Investigation of the exact site of protein synthesis within the trophoblast has revealed a differentiation between 'thick' and 'thin' areas (Burgos & Rodriguez, 1966). The thick areas are rich in endoplasmic reticulum and microvilli, and may therefore be specialised for protein synthesis; the thin areas ('vasculosyncytial membranes') overlie fetal capillaries and may be specialised for transport of nutrients and waste products. This dissociation of function could be of considerable practical significance since it is possible to envisage a condition which interferred with the all-important 'transfer' areas but left the 'synthetic' zones intact.

Placental proteins are secreted almost exclusively into the maternal circulation. With the possible exception of hCG, their presence in other compartments seems to have little or no functional significance unlike the complex distribution and excretion of the fetoplacental steroids, a simple generalisation is possible for the metabolism of placental proteins: they are cleared principally in the kidneys and liver, and a small proportion is excreted in the urine. An aspect of metabolism which is relevant to clinical measurement is the half-life: in principle, the shorter the half-life of a molecule the more rapidly will its levels reflect a decrease in placental function.

But this theoretical advantage is not found in clinical practice: the efficiency of estimation of human placental lactogen (hPL) and pregnancy specific beta-1 glycoprotein (SP1) is comparable in the detection of fetal intra-uterine growth retardation, while the half-lives are vastly different (hPL 15 minutes, SP1 40 hours). The reason is that most situations where placental function tests are of value are long-standing rather than acute.

Since there is no evidence of any feedback control or pulsatile release of most proteins from the placenta, it is likely that the major control mechanism is uterine blood-flow (Chard, 1981; Houghton et al, 1982).

HUMAN CHORIONIC GONADOTROPHIN (hCG)

Chemistry and synthesis

Human chorionic gonadotrophin is a glycoprotein (molecular weight 38 400) which consists of two dissimilar non-covalently linked subunits designated alpha(α) and beta(β). Whereas the α subunit (92 amino acids) is nearly identical to that of the other human glycoprotein hormones (TSH, LH and FSH), the β subunit (145 amino acids) only shares structural and antigenic characteristics with the β subunit of LH. The major difference is the presence in hCG of an additional 30 amino acid sequence at the N-terminus. The source of hCG is the trophoblast, and it can be detected in the maternal circulation as early as the time of implantation, i.e. several days before the missed period. The maternal blood levels rise logarithmically to reach a peak between 56 and 68 days of gestation, maximum concentrations in the fetal blood and amniotic fluid being seen at 11–14 weeks. Maternal levels decline by some 90 per cent to a nadir at 16–18 weeks; relatively constant levels are maintained throughout the remainder of pregnancy. The chorionic tissue concentrations of hCG parallel those in maternal serum, the synthesis of α and β subunits being independent, i.e. there are quite separate messenger RNAs. The two subunits combine in the cell prior to release as intact hCG and for this reason only small quantities of the free subunits are secreted into the circulation. Whereas β subunit levels parallel those of intact hCG, the concentrations of the α subunit increase as pregnancy advances (Reuter et al, 1980). hCG is metabolised by the liver and kidneys, only a fraction of the total being excreted in urine. The half-life of hCG in the circulation, as estimated from serial samples following removal of the placenta, shows an initial rapid phase (T $\frac{1}{2}$ 5–10 hours) followed by a phase of slower decline (T $\frac{1}{2}$ 30–50 hours). Although there is some evidence that cyclic adenosine monophosphate or luteinising hormone-releasing factor will stimulate hCG production in placental explants, it has proved difficult to identify control mechanisms *in vivo*. A number of functions have been proposed for hCG (Table 9.1; for review see Gaspard, 1980), but it must be emphasised that it is important to distinguish between a 'function' (i.e. the physiological role of hCG) and an 'effect' (i.e. the action of hCG in experimental conditions)

Table 9.1 Suggested biological functions of hCG

Maintenance of corpus luteum and steroid production of the corpus luteum
Stimulation of progesterone synthesis
Trophic action on fetal adrenal
Stimulation of fetal gonads, especially testosterone production by the testis
Immunosuppression

Measurement

hCG has been widely used as the standard pregnancy test since the time of its discovery in 1927. Immunochemical techniques have rendered biological assays obsolete and the commonest current techniques utilise particle agglutination in tubes or on slides. These methods are largely qualitative, providing a 'yes' or 'no' answer to the presence of an early pregnancy. Quantitative results, yielding a number for comparison with a normal range, require more elaborate techniques such as radioimmunoassay (RIA), radioreceptor assays or more recently fluoroimmunoassay. Since assays for intact hCG are very liable to interference by pituitary LH, assays directed to the β subunit alone are considerably more specific and are the method of choice (for review see Bagshawe et al, 1979).

Clinical application of hCG measurement

The largest application of hCG measurement is as a qualitative test for the presence of pregnancy; quantitative measurements for monitoring patients with trophoblastic disease is another major use. The introduction of highly sensitive and specific assays (RIA) represents a significant advance in the earliest possible diagnosis of pregnancy and related disorders such as ectopic gestation. However, such tests also present problems of interpretation. Thus, Miller et al (1980) have estimated that only 60 per cent of pregnancies diagnosed biochemically at the time of the first missed period will proceed beyond 20 weeks. This observation adds support to the hypothesis that some 80 per cent of all pregnancies are lost within a few weeks of conception (Roberts & Lowe, 1975). The availability of specific evidence for conception soon after implantation provides a valuable diagnostic test in certain categories of patients (e.g. those undergoing therapy for subfertility). However, in routine use the highly sensitive assays may detect a substantial group of pregnancies with an abnormal outcome: this is undesirable on pragmatic grounds, and the use of rapid and less sensitive agglutination systems remains more appropriate for the population as a whole.

A recent and most interesting application of hCG measurement is its use to determine the stage of gestation in early pregnancy. A single level of hCG (or hPL or SP1) at 30–60 days provides an estimate of gestational age equivalent or superior to that which can be achieved by ultrasonic measurement of crown-rump length (Lagrew et al, 1983; Whittaker et al, 1983; Westergaard et al, 1983d). In addition, an hCG level can be used to predict the day of spontaneous delivery with an accuracy equivalent to that of an unambiguous menstrual history.

In patients with vaginal bleeding in early pregnancy the measurement of hCG may be of prognostic significance. Normal levels of hCG are associated with satisfactory outcome in 90 per cent of patients, while the majority of patients with low levels will miscarry. Serial estimations can be of particular value in this situation; if levels do not increase or actually fall over a period of 1 week, during which time they would normally be expected to increase three-fold or more, then pregnancy is likely to be abnormal. Levels of hCG in excess of 25 U/l are found in 90 per cent of patients with ectopic pregnancy. In 100 consecutive patients with lower abdominal pain or vaginal bleeding 25 per cent gave a positive result (i.e. >25 U/l hCG), the diagnosis being ectopic or uterine pregnancy in 22 patients (Seppala et al, 1980). Since a positive result was obtained by routine urine testing in only 6.5 per cent of these patients, the rapid RIA for hCG may be of great value in the differential diagnosis of lower abdominal pain in women of reproductive age. By contrast, the general conclusion is that hCG assays in late pregnancy are not especially helpful in clinical management complications (Obiekwe & Chard, 1982a).

Chorionic gonadotrophin is the most sensitive biochemical index in the management of patients with trophoblastic disease. After the evacuation of a molar pregnancy, quantitative estimation of hCG is routinely used to ascertain the prognosis and the need or otherwise for additional therapy.

HUMAN PLACENTAL LACTOGEN (hPL)

Chemistry and synthesis

The presence of a placental protein with chemical and biological similarities to growth hormone and prolactin was first shown by Josimovich & McLaren (1962). The term human placental lactogen (hPL) is the most commonly used for this protein although several other designations have been suggested including human chorionic somatomammotrophin, choriomammotropin and pregnancy-associated plasma protein C. Placental lactogen has a molecular weight of 21 000 with a single chain of 191 amino-acids. A number of biological activities has been demonstrated including stimulation of lactogenesis, growth promotion, an effect on carbohydrate and lipid metabolism, stimulation of the corpus luteum, erythropoiesis, inhibition of fibrinolysis and immunosuppression. However, the observation of a normal outcome in pregnancies in which hPL cannot be detected, either in the circulation or trophoblastic tissue, emphasises the importance of distinguishing between activity and function. Indeed, it has been suggested that hPL and other placental proteins may have no extra-placental function but instead are waste products of intrinsic metabolic activities of the placenta (Gordon & Chard, 1979).

As with all placental products, the evidence for the existence of control mechanisms similar to other endocrine systems is sparse and ambiguous. It has been proposed that the rate of synthesis of proteins and steroids by the trophoblast is a function of trophoblast mass and uteroplacental blood flow; this would explain why products which depend on fetal precursors, such as oestriol, often show changes which parallel hPL in pathological pregnancies (Chard, 1982).

In common with other placental proteins and hormones, hPL is a product of the syncytiotrophoblast. The half-life of hPL in the maternal circulation is 10–20 min, and the rate of synthesis in late pregnancy is 1–2 g/24 h. This is greater than that of any other hormone in any site in the non-pregnant state, an interesting observation in view of the dispute as to whether it has any function. There is general agreement that maternal levels of hPL show no circadian rhythm, but instead show random fluctuations (Houghton et al, 1982). For this reason serial samples yield greater diagnostic accuracy than single samples (Obiewke et al, 1984). The levels of hPL in the fetal circulation are 100-fold less than those in the mother; levels in amniotic fluid are 10-fold less.

Clinical applications of measurement

Human placental lactogen can be detected by RIA in maternal blood from 6 weeks gestation, and the levels rise to reach a plateau after the 35th week (Fig. 9.1). The increase follows a sigmoid curve which closely reflects the growth of the placenta. Circulating hPL does not alter in relation to the time of onset of labour. In common with other placental products the variation of levels around the mean during normal pregnancy shows a positively skewed distribution (Fig. 9.1). Consequently, the best estimate of the true mean and standard deviation is obtained after logarithmic transformation of the data. Alternatively, the range can be expressed as a median and centiles which make no assumption about the distribution and which are relatively simple to interpret for clinical purposes (Chard & Klopper, 1982).

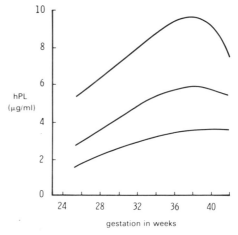

Fig. 9.1 Normal range (80 per cent confidence limits) for hPL in late pregnancy

Placental lactogen is merely one of a number of biochemical products of the fetoplacental unit, any of which might serve as an index of fetal wellbeing. Two factors may explain its present acceptance and use. Firstly, the method of measurement is technically simple and therefore readily available. Secondly, the literature on its clinical applications is comprehensive (for a detailed review see Chard, 1982, 1983), so that interpretation is straightforward. In the clinical situation, the routine use of hPL or oestriol estimations probably provides as much information as it is possible to obtain from this type of test: in essence, the identification of fetal growth retardation (Lilford et al, 1983) and the prediction of acute fetal problems during labour (Obiekwe & Chard, 1982b).

Given the fairly widespread acceptance of this type of test, the following questions may also be posed: (1) are tests of placental function worthwhile? (2) what is the value of an hPL result compared to other parameters recorded as part of antenatal care? and (3) can the information lead to a reduction in morbidity and mortality? The first two questions have been answered in recent publications (Gordon et al, 1978; Grudzinskas et al, 1981). Using a 'relative risk factor', low hPL levels found as part of a routine screening programme of an entire obstetric population were as efficient a predictor of poor fetal outcome as the occurrence of severe hypertensive disorders, low maternal weight and heavy smoking by the mother. All were better than many other 'risk' factors considered to be of great value in antenatal diagnosis. Several years ago, Spellacy et al (1975) investigated a large group of subjects regarded as 'at risk' and divided these into two randomised groups, one in which clinicians were aware of the results, and the other in which they were not. In the first group the perinatal death rate was 3.5 per cent, in the second 15 per cent, a clear indication of the clinical relevance of hPL estimations. Since a considerable proportion of perinatal morbidity and mortality cannot be identified by current clinical procedures, a sound argument can be presented for the routine application of hPL measurement or a similar test in all pregnancies.

PLACENTAL ENZYMES

The variety of enzymes contained in the human placenta represent the range of structural and metabolic enzymes found in all mammalian cells. However, this general category of enzymes does not distinguish the trophoblast from other organs as these enzymes are not secreted by the placenta and their levels do not change in the peripheral circulation. By contrast, the serum levels of hydrolytic enzymes may increase substantially during pregnancy: some of these are synthesised and secreted by the placenta and may therefore be regarded as specific for pregnancy. The most notable are heat stable alkaline phosphatase (HSAP; also known as placental alkaline phosphatase, PLAP), and cystine aminopeptidase (CAP; also referred to as oxytocinase). Both HSAP and CAP are candidates for placental function tests as they are specific products of the placenta. However, studies of their clinical value have been limited in scope and estimations of these enzymes is not widely used in this context (for review see Chard & Klopper, 1982).

Chemistry and metabolism

HSAP occurs as a number of genetically determined variants, all of which are resistant to heating to 50–70 °C. The molecular weight is 116 000 and a similar isoenzyme is found in the blood and tissues of some patients with carcinoma. By contrast, CAP is a single molecular species (molecular weight 290 000). The general function of these substances is concerned with active transport across cell membranes but no function in the peripheral circulation has been proposed.

Clinical applications of enzyme measurement

Clinical enzyme measurements are fraught with methodological problems (e.g. the necessity for exact conditions of ionic strength, pH, and temperature; the presence of non-specific inhibitors in serum). This rather than any inherent biological factor is probably why clinical experience with placental enzymes has been generally unfavourable (Chard & Klopper, 1982). Nevertheless, there may be renewed interest in enzyme activity in the placenta as the evidence for the biological function of some of the 'new' placental proteins (see below) indicates their involvement in intra- rather than extra-placental metabolic events.

NEW PLACENTAL PROTEINS

A number of pregnancy-specific proteins of placental origin have recently been identified in and extracted from the maternal circulation (Table 9.2). In addition, several soluble placental tissue proteins have been described (Bohn et al, 1982). A considerable literature has been generated on schwangerschafts protein 1 (also known as pregnancy-specific beta-1 glycoprotein), pregnancy-associated plasma protein A, and placental protein 5, and only these molecules will be considered here (for review see Grudzinskas et al, 1982).

Table 9.2 New placental proteins (For extensive reviews see Grudzinskas et al, 1982)

Pregnancy-specific beta-1 glycoprotein (SP1) also known as
pregnancy-associated plasma protein C (PAPP-C) and PSbG
Pregnancy-associated plasma protein A (PAPP-A)
Pregnancy-associated plasma protein B (PAPP-B)
Placental protein 5 (PP5)

Schwangerschafts protein 1

Schwangerschafts protein 1 (SP1 or SP1-beta) was the first of a group of apparently functionless molecules extracted from placental tissue or late pregnancy blood. It is now clear that SP1 or proteins with anti-SP1 antigenic determinants exist in at least three molecular forms. Although authentic SP1 (SP1-beta) has a beta-1 electro-phoretic mobility and a molecular weight of 90 000, at least two forms of higher molecular mass and alpha electrophoretic mobility have been described (Teisner & Bach, 1982). The larger molecular weight forms have a striking effect on the quantitation of authentic SP1 by gel precipitation immuno-assays, whereas estimations obtained by competitive assays, such as RIA or EIA, do not seem to be significantly affected.

SP1 can be detected in the maternal circulation from an early stage of pregnancy (Grudzinskas et al, 1977); positive levels have been claimed as early as 6–14 days after ovulation (Ahmed & Klopper, 1983) the levels rising exponentially to reach concentrations of 10–20 mg/l at the end of the first trimester (Fig. 9.2). Thereafter a progressive

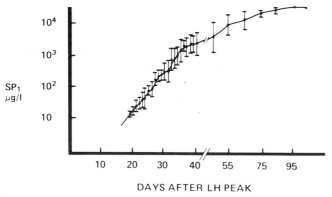

Fig. 9.2 Circulating SPl during the first trimester (n = 10) (Lenton et al, 1981)

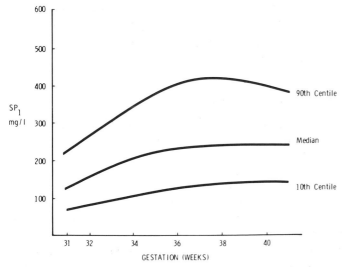

Fig. 9.3 Median, 10th and 90th centiles of maternal SP1 levels after the 30th week of pregnancy (Gordon et al, 1977)

increase to a plateau at 34–36 weeks is observed with a median level variously estimated at between 95 and 250 mg/l (Fig. 9.3). The time to time variation is 10 per cent or less, and there is no change in concentration during labour.

SP1 is produced by the syncytiotrophoblast and secreted largely into the maternal circulation; levels are 1000 and 100-fold less in the fetal circulation and amniotic fluid respectively. After birth, SP1 disappears from the circulation with a half-life of 20–40 hours. There has been much speculation on the biological function of this protein, including a role in the regulation of carbohydrate metabolism, iron transport, binding of steroid hormones and feto-maternal immunological interactions. However, the evidence for any of these is inconclusive and the role of SP1 is still to be defined.

Although SP1 is unlikely to supplant hCG for detection of early pregnancy there are two situations in which its measurement may prove to be a valuable ancillary test. First, hCG levels may sometimes be ambiguous (because of cross-reaction with LH) and second, if hCG has been administered for therapeutic reasons (e.g. for ovulation induction), SP1 assays may provide the only indisputable biochemical evidence of early pregnancy. SP1 measurements may be of diagnostic value in complications of early pregnancy, such as threatened abortion (Jouppila et al, 1980); depressed levels of SP1 are associated with early pregnancy failure, but whether this information is of prognostic value in cases in which ultrasound results are also available is uncertain. The use of SP1 assays in patients with trophoblastic tumours is also under evaluation; it may provide a valuable additional parameter to measurement of hCG (Lee et al, 1981; Tsakok et al, 1983). In complications of late pregnancy, there is general agreement that depressed levels of SP1 are associated with an increased risk of intra-uterine growth retardation. In common with hPL, low SP1 values presumably indicate diminished placental function and are only indirectly related to fetal growth. The predictive value of depressed SP1 levels during the third trimester is comparable to that of hPL (for review see Grudzinskas & Sinosich, 1982). Nevertheless, the high circulating levels of SP1 during the third trimester offer the advantages of low cost, simplicity and ease of measurement, permitting the use of simple immunodiffusion assays; by contrast, hPL assays are usually RIAs.

Pregnancy-associated plasma protein-A (PAPP-A)

This large glycoprotein (molecular weight 800 000, alpha-2 electro-phoretic mobility) is antigenically distinct from, but physicochemically similar to, alpha-2 macroglobulin (Lin et al, 1974; Bischof, 1979). There are two characteristics which distinguish it from other placental proteins. First, it is confined to the surface of the syncytiotrophoblast; second, the circulating levels in the mother continue

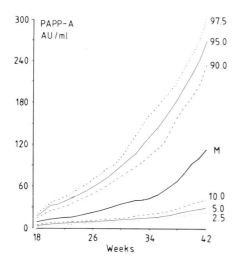

Fig. 9.4 A normal range (80–95 per cent confidence limits) for serum PAPP-A (Westergaard & Teisner, 1982)

to rise until parturition (Fig. 9.4). In common with alpha-2 macroglobulin, PAPP-A is a potent protease inhibitor (Sinosich et al, 1982) and has inhibitory effects on both the complement and coagulation systems. In addition, PAPP-A has a high affinity for heparin (Westergaard et al, 1983a), a property which has been successfully exploited in its purification and also implies that serum is the appropriate fluid for clinical measurements. Though the precise function of PAPP-A is unknown, it is of great interest to note that a pregnancy with an apparent total deficiency of PAPP-A led to the delivery of a child with Cornelia de Lange syndrome (Westergaard et al, 1983b).

Circulating PAPP-A can be detected by RIA 3–4 weeks after conception. In later pregnancy, less sensitive procedures are adequate. An early claim that elevated PAPP-A levels may be predictive of hypertension has not been substantiated. Furthermore, PAPP-A levels are of no value in the prediction of growth retardation, antepartum haemorrhage, or premature labour (Westergaard & Teisner, 1982). However, studies on early pregnancy complications hold great promise (Masson et al, 1983). Low levels of PAPP-A are associated with spontaneous abortion in patients with painless bleeding during the first half of pregnancy *even* when fetal heart action is evident by ultrasound (Westergaard et al, 1983c) (Fig. 9.5). This distinction cannot be made by other tests; if these data are confirmed, then PAPP-A measurements will provide a valuable clinical tool in those patients previously beyond the reach of any diagnostic measure.

Placental protein 5 (PP5)

Placental protein 5 (molecular weight 36 600, beta-1 electrophoretic mobility) can be detected in maternal blood during the first trimester and rises progressively to reach a plateau during late pregnancy (30–40 g/l). Like PAPP-A, it has a high affinity for heparin and it has been suggested

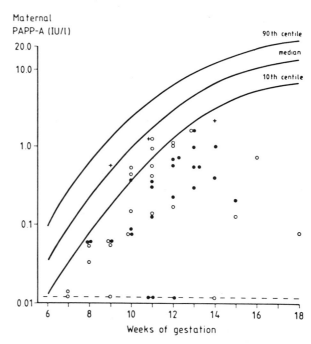

Fig. 9.5 The 80 per cent confidence limits of circulating PAPP-A in 40 normal pregnancies. PAPP-A levels in patients with (o) and without (•) ultrasonic evidence of fetal life and one twin pregnancy with live fetuses (+) who subsequently miscarried

that the molecule is a placental analogue of antithrombin III (Salem et al, 1981a; Rice & Chard, 1983). Clinical studies have provided further circumstantial evidence for a complex relationship with the coagulation and fibrinolytic system, including the observation of an elevation of PP5 levels in women prior to abruption of the placenta (Fig. 9.6) (Salem et al, 1982), and also in association with pre-eclampsia (Nisbet et al, 1981; Salem et al, 1982; Salem & Chard, 1982). Though general evaluation of PP5 as a clinical marker of placental function has been disappointing, some preliminary observations suggest that elevated levels in mid-trimester may be predictive of premature labour (Salem et al, 1981b). Further studies are awaited with interest, once technical difficulties encountered in purification of adequate amounts of PP5 for assay have been solved.

Early pregnancy factor

Early pregnancy factor (EPF) is detected by an *in vitro* rosette inhibition test, which measures the capacity of antilymphocyte serum (ALS) to inhibit rosette formation between T-lymphocytes and heterologous erythrocytes (Fig. 9.7). Rosette inhibition is enhanced by pregnancy serum or the use of lymphocytes incubated in pregnancy serum and the material responsible for this phenomenon is called early pregnancy factor (Morton et al, 1977). The physicochemical characteristics of EPF are unknown and, indeed, it is not certain whether it is a single factor or a complex of factors. If the existence of EPF can be firmly

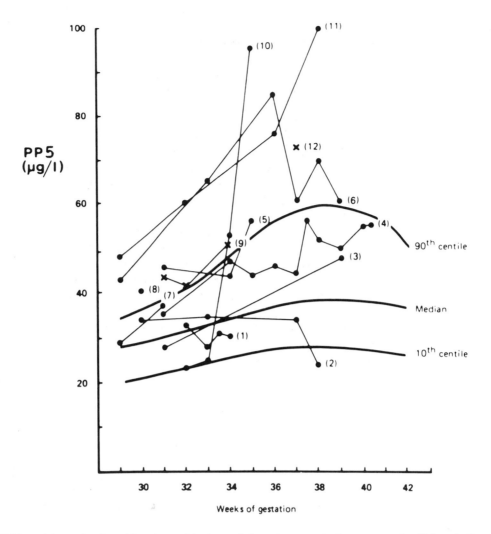

Fig. 9.6 Circulating PP5 in serial samples from 12 patients with placental abruption: ● = singleton; x = twins (Salem & Chard, 1982)

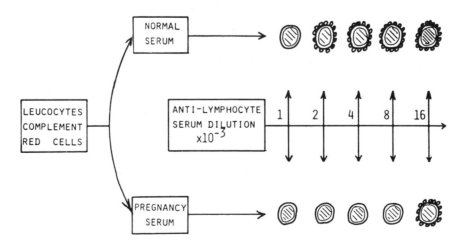

Fig. 9.7 Test for early pregnancy factor (Smart et al, 1981)

proven, then the claims that it appears in maternal serum within 24 hours of conception offer great potential as a diagnostic marker for fertilisation. However, at the present time the specificity of EPF is in some doubt and further appraisal must await the presentation of additional data.

RELAXIN

Relaxin is a polypeptide hormone produced by the ovaries during pregnancy in a number of mammalian species including the human (for review, see Anderson, 1982). It has a molecular weight of 6 300 and is structurally similar to insulin, nerve growth factor and insulin-like growth factor; all four molecules presumably arise from the same primitive precursor. The site of synthesis is probably the corpus luteum (O'Byrne et al, 1978), although significant quantities have also been found in seminal plasma (Loumaye et al, 1980) and both pregnancy (Bigazzi et al, 1980) and non-pregnant endometrium (Quagliarello et al, 1980). It is

Table 9.3 Proposed roles of relaxin during pregnancy

Relaxation of pelvic ligaments
Remodelling of uterine stroma
Suppression of myometrial contractility
Ripening of the cervix
Mammary growth

secreted into the circulation in pulses and is rapidly cleared with a half-life of less than 1 min. Relaxin influences collagen metabolism in most target tissues. It is thought to be responsible for the relaxation of the interpublic ligament in pregnancy and, in humans, for the cervical ripening which precedes labour at term. Other possible biological roles during pregnancy are listed in Table 9.3 and an involvement in ovulation has been proposed. The control mechanisms are unknown, but in humans it is considered that hCG may be a trophic stimulus. Circulating relaxin in humans can be measured using a RIA based on porcine relaxin, but it is likely that full exploration of the role in normal pregnancy must await a fully homologous assay.

REFERENCES

Ahmed A G, Klopper, A 1983 Diagnosis of early pregnancy by assay of placental proteins. British Journal of Obstetrics and Gynaecology 90: 604–611

Anderson L 1982 Relaxin. Plenum Press, New York

Bagshawe K D, Searle F, Wass M 1979 Human chorionic gonadotrophin. In: Gray C H, James V H T (eds) Hormones in Blood, pp 364–411. Academic Press, London

Bigazzi M, Nardi E, Bruni P, Petrucci F 1980 Relaxin in human decidua. Journal of Clinical Endocrinology and Metabolism 51: 939–941

Bischof P 1979 Purification and characterisation of pregnancy associated plasma protein A (PAPP-A). Archives of Gynaecology 227: 315–321

Bischof P, Martin-du-Pan R, Lauber K, Girard J P, Hermann W L, Sizonenko P C 1983 Human seminal plasma contains a protein that shares physicochemical, immunochemical and immunosuppressive properties with pregnancy-associated plasma protein-A. Journal of Clinical Endocrinology and Metabolism 56: 359–362

Bohn H, Kraus W, Winkler W 1982 Pregnancy specific beta 1 glycoprotein (SPl) and other soluble placental tissue proteins (PPs). In: Grudzinskas J G, Teisner B, Seppala M (eds) Pregnancy Proteins: Chemistry, Biology and Clinical Application, pp 195–204. Academic Press, Sydney

Burgos M H, Rodriguez E M 1966 Specialized zones in the trophoblast of the human term placenta. American Journal of Obstetrics and Gynecology 96: 342–348

Chard T 1981 Synthesis of placental lactogen by human placentae. In: Fotherby K, Pal, S B (eds) Hormones in Normal and Abnormal Human Tissues, pp 409–428. Walter de Gruyter, Berlin

Chard T 1982 Placental Lactogen: Biology and Clinical Applications. In Grudzinskas J G, Teisner B, Seppala M (eds) Pregnancy Proteins: Chemistry, Biology and Clinical Application, pp 101–118. Academic Press, Sydney

Chard T 1983 Human placental lactogen. Current Topics in Experimental Endocrinology 4: 167–191

Chard T, Klopper A 1982 Placental Function Tests. Springer Verlag, Heidelberg

Gaspard W 1980 Les Hormone Proteiques Placentaires. Masson, Paris

Gordon Y B, Grudzinskas J G, Lewis J D, Jeffrey D, Letchworth A T 1977 Circulating levels of pregnancy specific beta-1 glycoprotein and human placental lactogen in the third trimester of pregnancy their relationship to parity birth weight and placental weight. British Journal of Obstetrics and Gynaecology 84: 642–647

Gordon Y B, Chard T 1979 The specific proteins of the human placenta; some new hypotheses. In: Klopper A, Chard T (eds) Placental Proteins, 1–22. Springer-Verlag, Heidelberg

Gordon Y B, Lewis J D, Pendlebury D J, Leighton M, Gold J 1978 Is the measurement of placental function and maternal weight worthwhile? Lancet i: 1001–1003

Grudzinskas J G, Sinosich M J 1982 Pregnancy specific beta 1 glycoprotein in normal and abnormal late pregnancy. In: Grudzinskas J G, Teisner B, Seppala M (eds) Pregnancy Proteins: Chemistry, Biology and Clinical Application, pp 251–262. Academic Press, Sydney

Grudzinskas J G, Lenton E A, Gordon Y B, Kelso I M, Jeffrey D, Sobowale O, Chard T 1977 Circulating levels of pregnancy-specific beta-1 glycoprotein in early pregnancy. British Journal of Obstetrics and Gynaecology 84: 740–742

Grudzinskas J G, Gordon Y B, Wadsworth J, Menabawey M, Chard T 1981 Is placental function testing worthwhile? An update on placental lactogen. Australian and New Zealand Journal of Obstetrics and Gynaecology 21: 103–106

Grudzinskas J G, Teisner B, Seppala M 1982 Pregnancy Proteins: Biology, Chemistry and Clinical Application. Academic Press, Sydney

Houghton D J, Newnham J P, Lo K, Rice A, Chard T 1982 Circadian variation of four placental proteins. British Journal of Obstetrics and Gynaecology 89: 831–835

Josimovich J B, McLaren J A 1962 Presence in the human placenta and term serum of a highly lactogenic substance immunologically related to pituitary growth hormone. Endocrinology 71: 209–220

Jouppila P, Seppala M, Chard T 1980 Pregnancy specific beta-1 glycoprotein in complications of early pregnancy. Lancet i: 662–688

Lagrew D C, Wilson E A, Jawad M J 1983 Determination of gestational age by serum concentrations of human chorionic gonadotrophin. Obstetrics and Gynecology 62: 37–40

Lee J N, Salem H T, Al-Ani ATM, Huang S C, Ouyand P C, Chard T 1981 Circulating concentrations of specific placental proteins (hCG, SPl and PP5) in untreated gestational trophoblastic tumours. American Journal of Obstetrics and Gynecology 139: 702–704

Lee J N, Lian J D, Lee J H, Chard T 1983 Placental proteins (human chorionic gonadotrophin, human placental lactogen, pregnancy specific beta 1 glycoprotein, and placental protein 5) in seminal plasma of normal men and patients with infertility. Fertility and Sterility 39: 704–706

Lenton E A, Grudzinskas J G, Gordon Y B, Chard T, Cooke I D 1981 Pregnancy specific beta-1 glycoprotein and chorionic gonadotrophin in early human pregnancy. Acta Obstetricia et Gynaecologica Scandinavica 60: 489–492

Lilford R J, Obiekwe B C, Chard T 1983 Maternal blood levels of human placental lactogen in the prediction of fetal growth retardation: choosing a cutoff point between normal and abnormal. British Journal of Obstetrics and Gynaecology 90: 511–515

Lin T M, Halbert S P, Keifer D, Spellacy W N, Gall S 1974 Characterisation of four pregnancy associated plasma proteins. American Journal of Obstetrics and Gynecology 118: 223–226

Loumaye E, Cooman S, Thomas K 1980 Immunoreactive relaxin-like substance in human seminal plasma. Journal of Clinical Endocrinology and Metabolism 50: 1142–1143

Masson G M, Anthony F, Wilson M S 1983 Value of schwangerschafts-protein (SP1) and pregnancy-associated plasma protein-A (PAPP-A) in the clinical management of threatened abortion. British Journal of Obstetrics and Gynaecology 90: 146–149

Miller J F, Williamson E, Glue J, Gordon Y B, Grudzinskas J G, Sykes A 1980 Fetal loss after implantation. Lancet i: 554–556

Morton H, Rolfe B, Clunie C J A, Anderson M J, Morrison J 1977 An early pregnancy factor detected in human serum by the rosette inhibition test. Lancet i: 394–397

Nisbet A D, Bremner R D, Jandial V, Sutherland H W, Horne C H W, Bohn H 1981 Placental protein 5 (PP5) in complicated pregnancies. British Journal of Obstetrics and Gynaecology 88: 492–499

Obiekwe B C, Pendlebury D J, Gordon Y B, Grudzinskas J G, Chard T, Bohn H 1979 The radioimmunoassay of placental protein 5 and circulating levels in maternal blood in the third trimester of normal pregnancy. Clinica Chimica Acta 95: 509–516

Obiekwe B C, Chard T 1982a Human chorionic gonadotrophin levels in maternal blood in late pregnancy: relation to birthweight, sex and condition of the infant at birth. British Journal of Obstetrics and Gynaecology 89: 543–546

Obiekwe B C, Chard T 1982b What do placental function tests predict? Observations on placental lactogen levels in growth retardation and fetal distress. European Journal of Obstetrics, Gynaecology and Reproductive Biology 14: 69–73

Obiekwe B C, Sturdee D W, Cockrill B L, Chard T 1984 The value of serial estimations in fetoplacental function testing: placental lactogen levels in the diagnosis of intra-uterine growth retardation. Journal of Obstetrics and Gynaecology 4, 157–160

O'Byrne E M, Flitcraft J F, Sawyer W K, Hochman J, Weiss G, Steinetz B G, 1978 Relaxin bioactivity and immunoactivity in human corpora lutea. Endocrinology 102: 1641–1644

Quagliarello J, Goldsmith L, Steinetz B G, Lustig D S, Weiss G 1980 Induction of relaxin secretion in non-pregnant women by human chorionic gonadotropin. Journal of Clinical Endocrinology and Metabolism 51: 74–77

Ranta T, Siiteri J E, Koistinen R, Salem H T, Bohn H, Koskimies A I, Seppala M 1981 Human seminal plasma contains a protein that shares physicochemical and immunochemical properties with placental protein 5 from the human placenta. Journal of Clinical Endocrinology and Metabolism 53: 1087–1089

Reuter A M, Gaspard U J, Deville J L, Vrindts-Gevaert Y, Franchimont P 1980 Serum concentrations of human chorionic gonadotrophin and its alpha and beta subunits. I. During normal singleton and twin pregnancies. Clinical Endocrinology 13: 305–318

Rice A, Chard T 1983 A method for the purification of placental protein 5 (PP5) from placental extracts. Clinica Chimca Acta 131: 289–294

Roberts C J, Lowe C R 1975 Where have all the conceptions gone? Lancet i: 498–499

Salem H T, Seppala M, Chard T 1981a The effect of thrombin on serum placental protein 5 (PP5): is thrombin the naturally occurring antithrombin III of the human placenta? Placenta 2: 205–210

Salem H T, Lee J N, Vaara L, Aula P, Al-Ani A T M, Chard T 1981b Measurement of placental protein 5, placental lactogen and pregnancy specific beta 1 glycoprotein in mid-trimester as a predictor of outcome of pregnancy. British Journal of Obstetrics and Gynaecology 88:371–374

Salem H T, Chard T 1982 Placental protein 5 (PP5): biological and clinical studies. In: Klopper A (ed) Immunology of Human Placental Proteins, pp 103–114. Praeger, London

Salem H T, Westergaard J G, Hindersson P, Lee J N, Grudzinskas J G, Chard T 1982 Maternal serum levels of placental protein 5 in complications of late pregnancy. Obstetrics and Gynaecology 59: 467–471

Seppala M, Tontti K, Ranta T, Stenman U-H, Chard T 1980 Use of a rapid hCG-beta-subunit radioimmunoassay in acute gynaecological emergencies. Lancet i: 165–166

Sinosich M J, Davey M W, Ghosh P, Grudzinskas J G 1982 Specific inhibition of human granulocyte elastase by human pregnancy associated plasma protein A. Biochemistry International 5: 777–786

Smart Y C, Roberts T K, Clancy R L, Cripps A W 1981 Early pregnancy factor: its role in mammalian reproduction-research review. Fertility and Sterility 35: 397–402

Spellacy W N, Buhi W C, Birk S A 1975 The effectiveness of human placental lactogen as an adjunct in decreasing perinatal deaths. American Journal of Obstetrics and Gynaecology 121: 835–844

Teisner B, Bach A 1982 Pregnancy specific beta-1 glycoprotein (SP1): molecular forms. In: Grudzinskas J G, Teisner B, Seppala M (eds) Pregnancy Proteins: Chemistry Biology and Clinical Application, pp 205–214. Academic Press, Sydney

Tsakok F H M, Koh S, Chua S E, Ratnam S S, Teisner B, Jones G R D, Sinosich M, Grudzinskas J G 1983 Prognostic significance of the new placental proteins in trophoblastic disease. British Journal of Obstetrics and Gynaecology 90: 473–486

Wahlstrom T, Bohn H, Seppala M 1982 Immunohistochemical demonstration of placental protein 5 (PP5)-like material in the seminal vesicle and the ampullar part of the vas deferens. Life Sciences 31: 2723–2725

Westergaard J G, Teisner B 1982 Pregnancy associated plasma protein A in normal and abnormal late pregnancy. In: Grudzinskas J G, Teisner B, Seppala M (eds) Pregnancy Proteins: Chemistry Biology and Clinical Application, pp 345–354 Academic Press, Sydney

Westergaard J G, Hau J, Teisner B, Grudzinskas J G 1983a Specific and reversible interaction between pregnancy-associated plasma protein A and heparin. Placenta 4: 13–18

Westergaard J G, Chemnitz J, Teisner B, Poulsen H K, Ipsen L, Beck B, Grudzinskas J G 1983b Pregnancy-associated plasma protein A: a possible marker in the classification and prenatal diagnosis of Cornelia de Lange syndrome. Prenatal Diagnosis 3, 225–232

Westergaard J G, Sinosich M J, Bugge M, Madsen L T, Teisner B, Grudzinskas J G 1983c Pregnancy associated plasma protein A (PAPP-A) in the prediction of early pregnancy failure. American Journal of Obstetrics and Gynecology 145, 67–69

Westergaard J G, Teisner B, Grudzinskas J G, Chard T 1983d Accurate assessment of early gestational age by measuring serum hCG or SP1. Lancet ii: 567–568

Whittaker P G, Aspillaga M O, Lind T 1983 Accurate assessment of early gestational age in normal and diabetic women using serum human placental lactogen. Lancet ii: 304–306

Oxytocin

INTRODUCTION

The posterior pituitary gland is the storage site from which the two neurohypophysial hormones — oxytocin and vasopressin — are released. As early as 1828, the human hypophysis cerebri was known to be made up of two lobes: one derived from an ectodermal dorsal invagination of the oral epithelium which becomes the anterior lobe or adenohypophysis and the other derived from a ventral process from the floor of the diencephalon constituting the posterior lobe or neurohypophysis. In contrast to the anterior lobe which is connected with the cerebrum through vascular channels, the posterior lobe is the end point of axons from specialised nerve cells in various areas of the hypothalamus. The oxytocic activity of pituitary extracts was first shown by Dale (1906), but Oliver & Schafer (1895) had earlier found posterior pituitary extracts to have vasopressor activity. Subsequently, posterior pituitary extracts were found to have galactokinetic (Ott & Scott, 1910) and antidiuretic properties (Konschegg & Schuster, 1915) which were shown to be due to two separate hormones, oxytocin and vasopressin, respectively (Dudley, 1919). Du Vigneaud et al (1954) carried out the structural analysis and synthesis of oxytocin and in 1956, the presence of the binding proteins, neuro-physins, was demonstrated (Acher et al, 1956).

Bargmann & Scharrer (1951) showed that the neurohypophysial hormones are synthesised in the hypothalamus and transported to the pituitary for storage and release. This provided one of the first examples of neurosecretion and the concept of endocrine roles of neural tissues.

STRUCTURE AND CHEMISTRY

Figure 10.1 shows the structures of oxytocin, vasotocin, and vasopressin for comparison. Both oxytocin and vasopressin consist of nine amino acid residues, of which two are half cystines forming a disulphide bridge between the positions 1 and 6. In the animal kingdom, there are six

posterior pituitary hormones with oxytocic properties — oxytocin, mesotocin, isotocin, glumitocin, valitocin and aspargtocin. In all these hormones, substitutions have occurred only in positions 3, 4, and 8, thus suggesting that the amino acid residues in positions 1, 2, 5, 6, 7, and 9 are essential for oxytocic function and could be the original

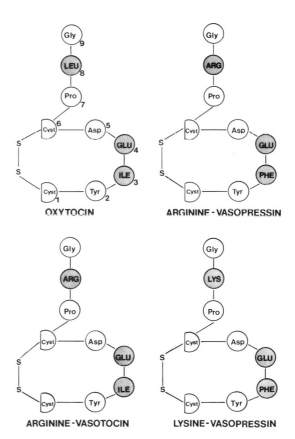

Fig. 10.1 Structure of oxytocin, arginine-vasopressin, lysine-vasopressin and arginine-vasotocin. Changes in amino acid have occurred only in positions 3, 4 and 8. Oxytocin and arginine-vasopressin are found in human beings, vasotocin in the human foetus and fish, and lysine-vasopressin in the pig, hippopotamus and the peccary. (From Dawood, M Y 1982 Neurohypophysial Hormones. In: Fuchs F, Klopper A (eds), Endocrinology of Pregnancy, 3rd edn, JB Lippincott & Co, Philadelphia)

ancestral molecule that has evolved to become oxytocin in mammals. Vasotocin, which has potent oxytocic and vasopressor properties, is present in fish and in human fetal posterior pituitary and pineal glands. It is probable that vasotocin subserves both oxytocic and vasopressor activities in lower aquatic species but evolved into two separate molecules, oxytocin and vasopressin, to separate out these two functions in higher species where they are not required simultaneously (Sawyer, 1964). The molecular weight of oxytocin is 1007.

Neurophysins are polypeptides with a molecular weight of about 10 000. In the human, there are two forms of circulating neurophysins, the oestrogen-stimulated neurophysin (ESN) or neurophysin I which binds to oxytocin, and nicotine-stimulated neurophysin (NSN) or neurophysin II, binding vasopressin (Robinson, 1975).

SYNTHESIS, STORAGE, AND SECRETION

Oxytocin is synthesised in the perikarya of the neurons present mainly in the paraventricular nucleus of the hypo-

thalamus but in the rat, recent evidence indicates that oxytocin is also produced in the supra-optic nucleus (George, 1978). Although oxytocin and vasopressin are produced in both the supraoptic and paraventricular nuclei, the individual neurons are specialised to produce either oxytocin or vasopressin only. Thus, oxytocinergic and vasopressinergic neurons are found in the paraventricular and supraoptic nuclei, with oxytocinergic cells clustered more rostrally and vasopressin-containing cells located more caudally (Swaab et al, 1975). Each hormone is produced in a set of neuronal cells specialised to synthesise only that hormone together with its own binding protein, the neurophysin, to which it is specifically bound. In the cow, rat and human, neurophysin I is located exclusively in the neurons that contain oxytocin and neurophysin II exclusively in neurons that contain vasopressin (Dierickx & Vandesande, 1979; Dierickx et al, 1976; Vandesande et al, 1975a,b). Oxytocin is synthesised as a larger molecule, a form of prohormone, which is then cleaved into oxytocin (Fig. 10.2). Oxytocin is then bound to neurophysin I and packaged into granules called neurosecretory granules. The one neuron–one hormone hypothesis for the neurohypo-

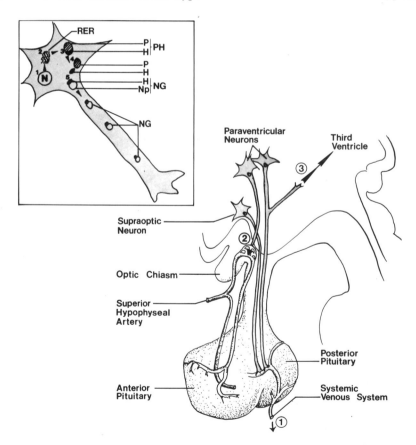

Fig. 10.2 Simplified scheme for the biosynthesis of neurohypophysial hormones. Oxytocin and vasopressin are synthesised in different neuron cell bodies (perikarya) in the hypothalamus and transported down the axon tail to the neurohypophysis. Inset shows enlargement of a neuron. The neuro-hypophysial hormone (H) is synthesised as a larger molecule (PH) by the rough endoplasmic reticulum (RER) and then cleaved off. The hormone (H) is then packaged with neurophysin (Np) to form neurosecretory granules (NG) which move down the axon tail to be stored in the neurohypophysis. Neurohypophysial hormones are secreted from the neurohypophysis into the systemic venous system 1, the hypothalamo-hypophysial portal system 2 and the third ventricle 3 (From Dawood M Y 1982 Neurohypophysial Hormones. In: Fuchs F, Klopper A (eds) Endocrinology of Pregnancy, 3rd ed, J B Lippincott & Co, Philadelphia)

physial hormones is widely accepted, although there is some tentative disagreement based on immunohistochemical studies in rats where oxytocin-positive cells are found also to be vasopressin-positive (Sokol et al, 1976). Each neurosecretory granule of oxytocin-neurophysin I contains about 6×10^{-8} mU of oxytocin (Nordmann & Morris, 1976). The neurosecretory granules are transported from the perikarya down the axon tail at a slow rate of 3 mm/hour to the axon terminal in the posterior pituitary gland (Buford & Pickering, 1973). The neurosecretory granules are released from the posterior pituitary gland in response to the appropriate stimulus.

The presence of oxytocin has also been demonstrated in the arcuate nucleus, the anterior hypothalamic nucleus, the medial pre-optic nucleus and the median eminence (George et al, 1976). It is unclear how oxytocin reaches these nuclei and whether its presence represents synthesis, storage or both.

Oxytocin is released from the neurosecretory granules by exocytosis and the membranes of the granules then fuse with the plasma membrane. Retrieval of these fused membranes from the plasmalemma into the cell is by rapid micropinocytosis (Nagasawa et al, 1970) but more recent data suggest that the membranes of the neurosecretory granules may be recaptured intact (Nordmann & Morris, 1976; Swann & Pickering, 1976). The precise role of neurophysin within the neurosecretory cell or in the release mechanism is unclear. Neurophysin may help to prevent damage to the free hormone within the cell since free oxytocin within the cell may be unfavourable to the hormone or the cell (Silverman, 1976). Oxytocin and its neurophysin (neurophysin I) appear at the same time in the circulation. The binding affinity of oxytocin to neurophysin is low and therefore they are readily dissociated after their release into the circulation. Currently oxytocin and its neurophysin are secreted into (1) the systemic circulation, (2) the third ventricle to appear in the cerebrospinal fluid (Dogterom et al, 1977), and (3) possibly into the hypothalamohypophysial portal circulation.

CONTROL OF SECRETION

The posterior lobe also has mechanisms regulating release of oxytocin and these are shown in Fig. 10.3. The peripheral stimuli known to elicit a neurohumoral reflex are stimulation of the nipple and vagina and stretching of the cervix.

In the milk-ejection reflex, stimulating the nipple triggers impulses that proceed along the peripheral thoracic nerves (T_{3-5}) and the spinal cord to the hypothalamus. This results in neuro-phyophysial release of oxytocin which then completes the reflex arc by contracting the myoepithelial cells around the alveoli and small ducts, which results in milk ejection. The reflex can be suppressed by

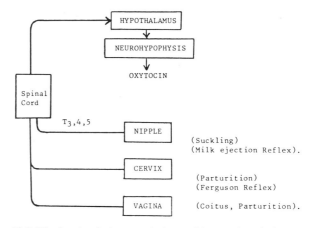

Fig. 10.3 Nipple stimulation, cervical stretching, and vaginal stimulation induce afferent neural impulses to the hypothalamus to stimulate the release of oxytocin from the neurohypophysis. Adrenergic, cholinergic, dopaminergic, opioid, and ionic mechanisms may be involved at the hypothalamo-neurohypophysial level in response to peripheral afferent stimuli

activity of the higher brain centres. Thus, although suckling elicits maternal oxytocin release, the amount released varies from individual to individual probably because of the influence of these higher centres. The rabbit releases much more oxytocin during suckling than the human does; the amount correlates significantly with the quantity of milk suckled by the litter (Fuchs et al, 1982a).

Stimulation of the cervix and vagina elicit the Ferguson reflex. Neural impulses that travel from the peripheral nerves in the cervix and vagina to the spinal cord and up the hypothalomo-neurohypophysial system cause oxytocin to be released. The circulating oxytocin then causes uterine contractions. This is best seen during the second stage of labour, when circulating oxytocin levels surge significantly in response to distension of the lower birth canal during delivery (Dawood et al, 1978b). Similarly, stretching of the cervix during pregnancy and labour, which evokes the Ferguson reflex, causes release of oxytocin and a rise in its circulating level (Dawood, 1982a). Several central mechanisms are involved in regulating the release of neurohypophysial hormones: aminergic, oncotic, opiod and hormonal (Dawood, 1982b). The aminergic mechanisms include adrenergic, cholinergic and dopaminergic pathways in the hypothalamus. Dopamine, levodopa and carbidopa inhibit spontaneous release of oxytocin from the posterior pituitary *in vitro* and *in vivo*. Thus the oxytocin in the pituitary gland is significantly increased with dopamine, levodopa and carbidopa administration. In pregnant rats, levodopa and carbidopa block oxytocin release and delay parturition (Schriefer et al, 1980). In lactating rats, the neural pathway for the reflex release of oxytocin involves both a dopaminergic and adrenergic mechanism, with the latter probably distal to the dopaminergic synapses. When injected into the cerebral ventricles, dopamine, bromocriptine, noradrenaline and phenylephrine will all produce sustained release of oxytocin in lactating rats. Catecholamine inhibitors such as the alpha adrenergic receptor antagonists, phenoxybenzamine and diethylthiocarbamate, and dopamine antagonists such as fluphenazine will block the suckling-induced release of oxytocin. Alpha adrenergic receptors are excitatory while beta adrenergic receptors are inhibitory in the milk-ejection reflex.

Adrenergic mechanisms are also involved and may potentiate the effect of osmoreceptor stimulation of oxytocin release. Suppression of alpha adrenergic receptors in the dehydrated rat causes release of oxytocin. A cholinergic component acting through nicotinic receptors is probably involved in the neural pathway controlling the suckling-induced reflex release of oxytocin in rats.

Hyperosmolality causes both oxytocin and vasopressin to be released. The plasma osmotic pressure, rather than the ionic composition is the chief determinant of which neurohypophysial hormone is released. Water deprivation and haemorrhage stimulate release of vasopressin more readily than oxytocin. The degree to which haemorrhage stimulates oxytocin secretion varies from one species to another.

Release of oxytocin depends on calcium ion concentration, probably at the internal face of the neurosecretory membranes. Both sodium (Na^+) and calcium (Ca^{2+} ion channels are important in regulating secretion of neurohypophysial hormone at the neurocellular level. Removing Na^+ inhibits and increasing Ca^{2+} uptake into neurohypophysial cells stimulates oxytocin secretion.

Endogenous peptides suppress oxytocin release tonically. However, these peptides can also enhance release of oxytocin that has been suppressed by pituitary dopamine. This is probably a disinhibitory phenomenon resulting from inhibition of dopamine. Morphine and its analogues can suppress oxytocin release in the lactating rats by an action close to the axon terminals in the posterior pituitary lobe (Clarke et al, 1979). Naloxone is able to reverse this action.

In both rat and humans, oestrogen stimulates release of oxytocin but not vasopressin. Oestrogens probably activate input from the frontal regions of the brain to the neurosecretory cells in the hypothalamo-neurohypophysial system. The rise in circulating oxytocin levels during pregnancy probably results from the rise in oestrogen levels. Progesterone suppresses neurogenically-induced oxytocin release. For example, in the goat progesterone will inhibit the release of oxytocin induced by vaginal distension. Thyrotrophin-releasing hormone stimulates secretion of both oxytocin and vasopressin in rabbits. The role of prostaglandins in regulating oxytocin release is still unclear. While maternal plasma oxytocin was found to increase during induction of labour at term with intravenous prostaglandins E_2(PGE$_2$) and F_{2a} (PGF$_{2a}$), no release of oxytocin was observed in rabbits given PGE$_2$, PGF$_{2a}$ and their 15-methyl analogues intravenously or intracerebroventricularly.

CIRCULATION AND METABOLISM

Oxytocin circulates in the blood as the free peptide since the affinity constant of neurophysin (10^6–10^7 l/mol) is too low to allow significant binding in the plasma (Pliska & Sachs, 1976). At 37°C and pH 7.4, almost no oxytocin binds to neurophysin, although the latter is also present in the circulation. Oxytocin is cleared mainly in the liver and the kidneys. The apparent volume of distribution is 305 ± 46 ml/kg (Dawood et al, 1980b) and indicates that oxytocin is distributed into both the intravascular and extravascular compartments. The half-life of oxytocin is 3–20 minutes (Fabian et al, 1969; Dawood et al, 1980b). It appears to be shorter when a higher dose of oxytocin is infused but becomes longer with lower doses of oxytocin (Fabian et al, 1969; Dawood et al, 1980b). Therefore, earlier estimates of the half-life of oxytocin using suprapharmacologic doses of oxytocin may not represent the true physiological half-life which is probably longer than generally believed. In spite of the increasing concentrations of circulating oxytocinase, the half-life of oxytocin is not significantly reduced during pregnancy. The maternal metabolic clearance rate of oxytocin at term is 19–21 ml/kg/min (Leake et al, 1980), is unaffected by pregnancy, and is similar to that found in males (Dawood et al, 1980b) and non-pregnant females (Fabian et al, 1969). In the fetal sheep, the metabolic clearance rate of oxytocin, which is 12 ml/kg/min, is similar to that of the mother (Glatz et al, 1980).

Oxytocin is excreted in the urine predominantly as biologically inactive but immunologically detectable fragments (Boyd et al, 1972). The renal clearance of oxytocin depends on both the plasma concentration of oxytocin and the volume of urine produced which suggests that the kidneys handled oxytocin in a similar way to water as opposed to solutes such as urea and creatinine.

In general, two important enzyme systems are present in the kidneys of most species: one which releases glycinamide from the C-terminals of oxytocin and occurring mainly in the rat; the other is the 'post-proline cleaving enzyme' which liberates the dipeptide Leu-Gly-NH$_2$ and is confined to certain species only (Walter, 1976). The mammary tissue, muscle, heart, uterus, hypothalamus and pituitary gland also have non-specific peptidase activity capable of degrading oxytocin. Some of the metabolites of oxytocin have been shown to have biological activity. Specifically, H-Pro-Leu-Gly-NH$_2$ inhibits secretion of melanocyte-stimulating hormone and also ameliorates the symptoms of Parkinsonism and depression (Walter, 1974).

An additional mechanism of oxytocin metabolism during pregnancy in primates is degradation by the enzyme placental oxytocinase, which is a cystine aminopeptidase produced by the placenta and which increases in concentration in the circulation with advancing gestation. This enzyme cleaves the link between the N-terminal hemicystine residue (position 1) of oxytocin and the adjacent tyrosine residue (position 2) destroying the ring structure and biological activity of the molecule (Fig. 10.1) (Tuppy, 1969). The peptide chain is further cleaved in succession up to the proline residue terminal. Degradation of oxytocin by oxytocinase may be a protective mechanism against the uterotonic effects of excessive circulating oxytocin. However, the failure of pregnancy plasma to reduce the half-life of oxytocin both *in vivo* and *in vitro* argues against a major role of oxytocinase in the metabolism of oxytocin in pregnancy (Forsling et al, 1971).

In spite of the presence of an oxytocinase in the placenta, both direct and indirect evidence of several species suggest that transplacental passage of oxytocin does not take place. In human pregnancy, the umbilical arteriovenous gradient of oxytocin can be reversed effectively when oxytocin is administered to the mother during labour (Dawood et al, 1989). In the guinea-pig (Burton et al, 1974) and the baboon (Dawood et al, 1979a), administration of oxytocin to the fetal circulation results in a rise in oxytocin concentration in the maternal circulation within a few minutes. In the sheep, oxytocin crosses the placenta (Noddle, 1964) and induces maternal uterine contraction when injected into the fetal circulation near term (Nathanielsz et al, 1973).

MECHANISM OF ACTION

Oxytocin stimulates smooth muscle contraction by a direct effect on the cell membrane. Oxytocin increases the number of normally sparse sodium gates and the frequency of electrotonic spikes in the cell membrane (Kleinhaus & Kas, 1969; Suzuki & Kuriyama, 1975). This action is probably mediated by adenosine monophosphate (AMP) and guanosine monophosphate (GMP) and is independent of prostaglandin synthesis and release from the uterus (Roberts & McCracken, 1976). At higher doses of oxytocin, partial depolarisation of the membrane occurs, and the spikes occur continuously. At still higher doses of oxytocin, there is continuous depolarisation and generation of spikes is blocked.

The action of oxytocin depends on specific cell receptors. Oxytocin receptors have been found in mammary tissues, uterus and oviduct of several species and in the human myometrium (Sterin-Borda et al, 1976; Soloff et al, 1979). The hormone is taken up only in the smooth muscle cell of the oviduct and in areas of the mammary tissue where myoepithelial cells are found (Soloff et al, 1979). Oxytocin binding activity occurs in several particulate subcellular fractions including 1000 g, 20 000 g and the 15 000 g pellets but not in the cytosol portion of the cell (Soloff, 1976). The binding of oxytocin to the myometrial receptors is increased by Mg^{2+} and Mn^{2+}, but not by Ca^{2+},

thus suggesting that Ca^{2+} which is normally essential for oxytocin-induced uterine contraction is involved in molecular events after the oxytocin-receptor interaction. The regulation of oxytocin receptors is poorly understood. In the rabbit, oestrogen induces while progesterone suppresses uterine oxytocin receptors (Nissenson et al, 1978). In the rat, oxytocin receptors are induced by oestrogen (Soloff, 1976) and are directly proportional to the ratio of oestradiol to progesterone levels in the plasma and the concentration of nuclear and cytosol oestrogen in the myometrium (Alexandrova & Soloff, 1980). In the rat, there is an abrupt rise in the myometrial concentration of oxytocin receptors just before the onset of labour (Soloff et al, 1979). However, recent findings in rats showed a lack of correlation between oxytocin receptor number and uterine tissue responsiveness to oxytocin suggesting that with oxytocin action, post-receptor mechanisms are important in determining oxytocin responsiveness (Goren et al, 1980).

Specific receptors for oxytocin and its analogues have been demonstrated in the epididymal fat cells of rats (Bonne & Cohen, 1975). These receptors modulate the 'insulin-like' effect of oxytocin which increases the oxidation of glucose to carbon dioxide in fat cells. However, oxytocin receptors of adipocytes function differently from the insulin receptors. Unlike insulin, which depresses the level of cyclic AMP by reducing adenyl cyclase, oxytocin receptors on fat cell membranes appear to have no direct connection with adenyl cyclase.

CONCENTRATION IN BLOOD AND OTHER BODY FLUIDS

During coitus

In several species, including the human, there is evidence for oxytocin release during coitus. However, it is unclear what stimuli are responsible for the oxytocin secretion. Olfactory, visual and auditory stimuli may be involved as well as stimuli arising in the vagina and cervix during coitus. In one study on human subjects, the maximum levels of oxytocin were found at the peak of orgasm in the female (Fox & Knaggs, 1969). In rabbits, plasma oxytocin levels increased in the female but not in the male following mating (Fuchs et al, 1981).

Pregnancy

Maternal oxytocin. There are only a few reported studies on oxytocin levels in the blood and/or amniotic fluid throughout pregnancy, using bioassays or radioimmunoassays (RIA) (Table 10.1). Using a specific and sensitive RIA, oxytocin can be detected in 85 per cent of the maternal plasma taken from pregnant women at 6–42 weeks gestation, while amniotic fluid has detectable

Table 10.1 Oxytocin levels in maternal blood during human pregnancy

Reference	Source of blood	Stage of pregnancy	Method of oxytocin determination	Levels of oxytocin or oxytocin-like substances*
Hawker & Robertson (1957)	Arm vein	Near term	Bioassay with extraction	1.8–85 ng/ml blood
Gonzales-Pannizza & Sica-Blanco (1957)	——	Near term	Internal tocography	20–60 pg/ml plasma
Sica-Blanco et al (1959)	——	Term	Internal tocography	20–80 pg/ml plasma
Caldeyro-Barcia & Sereno (1961)	Arm vein	Early pregnancy	Bioassay without extraction	>100 pg/ml plasma
Hawker et al (1961a)	Arm vein	Near term	Bioassay with extraction	0.4–14.0 ng/ml blood
Hawker et al (1961b)	Arm vein	Near term	Bioassay with extraction	0.24 ng/ml blood
Kumaresan et al (1974)	Arm vein (n = 280)	4–40 weeks	Radioimmunoassay without extraction	132–330 pg/ml plasma
Dawood et al (1978a,b, 1979b)	Arm vein (n = 362)	6–42 weeks	Radioimmunoassay with extraction	10.4–74.2 pg/ml plasma

* 'Oxytocin-like' refers to those assays in which the end point is uterine contraction or milk-ejection.
† Values represent the range of the means for the different weeks of gestation studied.

oxytocin levels in 90 per cent of the samples studied (Fig. 10.4). Maternal plasma oxytocin increases significantly with gestational age, rising from a mean level of 10.4 pg/ml at 8–9 weeks (IuU = 2 pg oxytocin) to 26.4 pg/ml at 37 weeks and 74.2 pg/ml at 38 weeks (Dawood et al, 1979b). The increase in maternal plasma oxytocin during pregnancy may be due to the rise in circulating oestrogen levels, since the administration of oestrogens in adult males stimulates oxytocin release

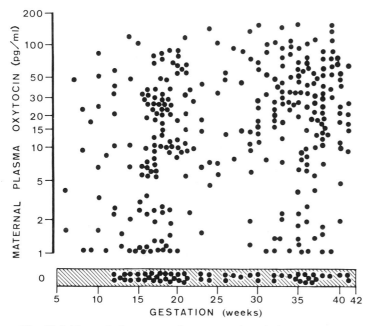

Fig. 10.4 Maternal plasma oxytocin concentrations during pregnancy (n – 362). Oxytocin is detectable in 90 per cent of the plasma samples. Note that the y ordinate is on a log scale. The mean ± (standard error) for each period of gestation is shown in triangles. Regression analysis shows there is an increase in maternal plasma oxytocin levels with advancing gestation. A significant increase in oxytocin level is observed from 38–39 weeks (From Dawood M Y et al 1979 Journal of Clinical Endocrinology and Metabolism 49: 429)

(Amico et al, 1981). During pregnancy, the maternal pituitary is the principal source of the circulating maternal oxytocin.

Amniotic fluid oxytocin concentration increases from a mean of 7.8 pg/ml at 14–15 weeks of gestation to 43.9 pg/ml at 40 weeks and 20.8 pg/ml at 41–42 weeks (Dawood et al, 1979b). Fetal urine contains oxytocin, with a mean level of 54 pg/ml and probably contributes substantially to the amniotic fluid oxytocin concentration (Dawood et al, 1978c). However, there are other sources of amniotic fluid oxytocin because the amniotic fluid to fetal urine oxytocin concentration is 2:1 in spontaneous labour. Direct diffusion of oxytocin from cord vessels is a possible source; meconium, which is rich in oxytocin (Seppala et al, 1972) contributes to amniotic fluid oxytocin under special circumstances when enhancement of uterine activity may be necessary to hasten delivery of a fetus in distress. It is evident from Table 10.1 that with bioassay, extremely high levels of oxytocin are detected, which may be partially accounted for by non-specific oxytocin-like substances; RIA measurements estimate 10 to 100 times less oxytocin in maternal blood during pregnancy. Nevertheless, even with RIA, fairly high concentrations are found by some investigators who do not use preliminary extraction of the plasma in their methods.

During labour and parturition. The available published data are summarised in Table 10.2. Coch et al (1965) found significantly higher concentrations of oxytocin in the jugular vein blood compared with peripheral venous blood. They concluded that the maternal pituitary gland releases significant amounts of oxytocin during labour. Chard et al (1970) initially found no detectable oxytocin in the maternal blood during labour, but with further studies they found measurable oxytocin in 10 per cent of the samples collected early in labour, increasing to 60 per cent as labour advanced (Gibbens & Chard, 1976). More recently, data

Table 10.2 Oxytocin concentrations in maternal blood during human labour

Reference	Stage of labour	Source blood assayed	Method of assay	Oxytocin levels
Hawker & Robertson (1957)	1st	Arm vein	Bioassay with extraction	200–2400 pg/ml blood
Caldeyro-Barcia & Sereno (1961)	1st	Arm vein	Bioassay without extraction	240 pg/ml plasma
Hawker et al (1961a)	1st	Arm vein	Bioassay with extraction	0–11 900 pg/ml blood
Hawker et at (1961a)	2nd (expulsive phase)	Arm vein	Bioassay without extraction	280 pg/ml blood
Juret et al (1961)	1st	Arm vein	Bioassay without extraction	60 000–100 000 pg/ml plasma
Coch et al (1965)	1st, 2nd, 3rd	Jugular vein	Bioassay with extraction	600–1800 pg/mlplasma
	1st, 2nd, 3rd	Arm vein	Bioassay with extraction	50–500 pg/ml plasma
Fitzpatrick & Walmsley (1965)	2nd	Arm vein	Bioassay with extraction	160–400 pg/ml plasma
Vorherr (1975)	1st, 2nd	Arm vein	Bioassay	Undetectable
Saameli (1963)	---	---	Indirect assessment using oxytocin intravenous infusion	6 pg/ml plasma
Chard et al (1970)	---	Arm vein	RIA with extraction	Detectable levels in 19%
Gibbens & Chard (1976)	1st	Arm vein	RIA with extraction	Detectable levels in up to 60%†
Bashore (1972)	1st, 2nd, 3rd	Arm vein	RIA with extraction	>40 pg/ml plasma 180 pg/ml plasma (2 cases)
Kumaresan (1974)	1st, 2nd	Arm vein	RIA without extraction	70–870 pg/ml plasma
Glick et al (1969)	1st 2nd	Arm vein	RIA with extraction	20–150 pg/ml plasma 200–400 pg/ml plasma
Dawood et al (1978a,b)	1st 2nd 3rd	Arm vein	RIA with extraction	40.3 ± 9.8 pg/ml plama* 123.9 ± 23.6 pg/ml plasma 64.5 ± 13.1 pg/ml plasma

† Oxytocin level given are 0–25 pg/ml.
* Mean ± s.e. of the mean.

from our laboratory show that maternal plasma oxytocin increases significantly from a mean level of 40.3 ± 9.8 pg/ml during the first stage of labour to 123.9 ± 23.6 pg/ml during the second stage, and declined to 64.5 ± 13.1 pg/ml during the third stage of labour (Dawood et al, 1978a,b) (Fig. 10.5). This pattern is seen both in the individual patient and in all the patients studied as a group. Thus, the release of oxytocin into the maternal circulation during the second stage is accentuated by the passage of the fetal presenting part through the cervix and the vagina via the mechanism of the Ferguson reflex (Dawood et al, 1978a,b; Coch et al, 1965).

Maternal neurohypophysial content of vasopressin and oxytocin in the sheep (Vizsolyi & Perks, 1976) and guinea-pig (Burton & Forsling, 1972) falls during pregnancy but recovers towards term with a preferential increase in oxytocin, suggesting that this is in preparation for parturition. In rats, the neurohypophysial content of both oxytocin and vasopressin falls significantly during labour, suggesting release of the hormones into the circulation (Fuchs & Saito, 1971).

Fetal oxytocin. There is a higher oxytocin concentration in umbilical cord blood samples after spontaneous onset of labour, irrespective of the mode of delivery, than in samples taken from women who are not in labour when

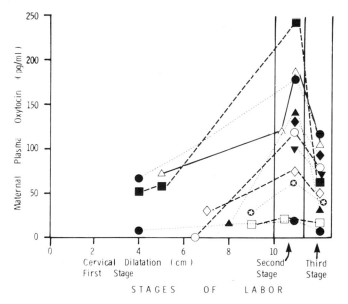

Fig. 10.5 Serial oxytocin concentrations maternal plasma in 11 women during the first, second (crowning of the fetal head), and third stages (delivery of the placenta) of normal spontaneous labour. There is a significant increase in maternal plasma oxytocin concentration from the first to the second stage of labour followed by a significant fall in the third stage of labour (Reprinted with permission from the American College of Obstetricians and Gynecologists, Obstetrics and Gynecology 51, 1978, 138)

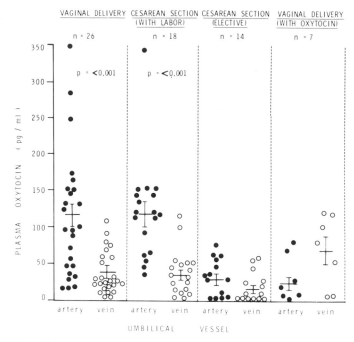

Fig. 10.6 Paired umbilical arterial and venous plasma oxytocin concentrations in women undergoing normal labour and vaginal delivery, Caesarean section with and without labour and in women given oxytocin during labour. Umbilical arterial plasma oxytocin levels are always higher than umbilical venous plasma when no oxytocin is given and are significantly higher when the women are in spontaneous labour than when they are not in labour, indicating fetal release of oxytocin in the first stage of spontaneous labour. The arteriovenous oxytocin gradient can be reversed from a fetal–maternal direction to a maternal–fetal direction when oxytocin is given. Horizontal bars represent the mean; hatched areas represent standard error of the means (Reprinted with permission from the American College of Obstetricians and Gynecologists, Obstetrics and Gynecology 52, 1978, 205)

undergoing Caesarean section (Chard et al, 1971; Dawood et al, 1978a, 1978b). Oxytocin levels were always higher in the umbilical artery than in the umbilical vein whether the women were in labour or not, so long as they were not given oxytocin, but there was a higher arteriovenous difference after the spontaneous onset of labour than before the onset of labour (Fig. 10.6) (Dawood et al, 1978c). Because the oxytocin levels are higher in the umbilical artery than the umbilical vein, the oxytocin must originate in the fetus and either be destroyed in the placenta or pass into the maternal compartment. Pressure on the fetal head is unlikely to account for the high oxytocin concentration in the umbilical artery. When intravenous or buccal oxytocin is given to stimulate uterine contractions, the oxytocin levels in the umbilical vein are higher than or similar to the levels in the umbilical artery (Dawood et al, 1978c). This demonstrates that it is possible to reverse the gradient of oxytocin toward the fetal compartment.

It is uncertain whether all the oxytocin flowing from the fetal side into the maternal compartment crosses the placenta without being inactivated by the presence of a placental oxytocinase. However, it is clear that an oxytocin

gradient can be established both from the fetus to the mother and from the mother to the fetus and that oxytocin readily crosses the placenta in the ewe (Noddle, 1964) and the baboon (Dawood et al, 1979a). The role of oxytocinase in the metabolism of oxytocin has been seriously questioned (see section on metabolism). After its transplacental passage much, if not all, of the fetal oxytocin in the umbilical artery must be readily available to stimulate the uterus.

As stated, the umbilical arteriovenous difference in oxytocin concentration is significantly higher when the woman is in established labour than when she is not (Dawood et al, 1978c). Using the arteriovenous difference in oxytocin levels, the average umbilical blood flow, and umbilical blood haematocrit values, the estimated mean secretion rates of oxytocin from the fetal to the maternal compartments have been calculated to be 2.75 mU/min (5.5 ng) when there is spontaneous labour and vaginal delivery, 3.0 mU/min (6.0 ng) in patients having Caesarean section after the onset of labour, but only 0.5 mU/min (1.0 ng) if Caesarean section is performed before the onset of labour (Table 10.3). With an estimated secretion rate of 0.5 mU/min in women who are not in labour and assuming that all the oxytocin reaches the myometrium without being degraded, only ineffectual contractions, if any, will occur until the uterine sensitivity to such doses turns on at the onset of labour (Theobald et al, 1969). However, with the secretion rate of 2.75–3.0 mU/min found after spontaneous onset of labour, effective uterine contractions will occur even if only half of this oxytocin crosses the placenta intact and reaches the myometrium, as shown by Theobald et al (1969). The amount of fetal oxytocin which is available to the mother during the first stage of labour is similar to that found in the second stage of spontaneous labour and vaginal delivery. The sudden increase in maternal plasma oxytocin observed at the second stage must be due to additional oxytocin released from the maternal neurohypophysis as demonstrated by Coch et al (1965).

Table 10.3 Estimated secretion rate of oxytocin from fetal to maternal compartment based on umbilical plasma arteriovenous difference in oxytocin concentrations (Dawood M Y et al, 1978, Obstetrics and Gynecology 52: 205)

Type of delivery	Umbilical arteriovenous difference in plasma oxytocin (mean ± s.e.) (pg/ml)	Secretion rate of oxytocin per minute (mean ± s.e.)
Spontaneous labour and vaginal delivery	73.3 ± 13.3	5.5 ± 1.0 ng (2.57 ± 0.5 mU)
Caesarean section (with labour)	81.0 ± 12.4	6.0 ± 1.0 ng (3.0 + 0.5 mU)
Elective Caesarean section (no labour)	13.8 ± 5.1	1.0 ± 0.4 ng (0.5 ± 0.2 mU)

Thus, it appears that during the first stage of spontaneous labour, fetal oxytocin plays the major role, while the maternal pituitary releases additional oxytocin to increase markedly the maternal circulating oxytocin concentration during the second stage (expulsive phase). This increase is necessary to produce the strong uterine contractions required to expel the fetus during the second stage.

Fetal urine contains oxytocin (Dawood et al, 1978c). First-voided noenatal urine has a mean oxytocin concentration of 53.8 ± 11.8 pg/ml, which is higher than in maternal urine during labour (Boyd et al, 1972). This provides further evidence for fetal participation in oxytocin release during spontaneous labour.

Little is known about the ontogeny of human neurohypophysial hormones. The concentration of oxytocin in the pituitary gland is poorly documented, whereas more is known about the situation in experimental animals. The concentration of oxytocin in the pituitary glands of 150–156 day old human fetuses was determined by bioassay to be 92–105 ng/gland (Dicker & Tyler, 1953). In a recent study using radioimmunoassay, the concentration of oxytocin in human fetal pituitary glands increased from 38.4 ng/gland at 20 weeks to 57.0 ng/gland at 32 weeks and 544 ng/gland at term (Dawood & Khan-Dawood, 1982). Therefore, it is evident that the fetal pituitary is producing oxytocin by the 20th week of pregnancy, if not earlier.

The fetal posterior pituitary gland is not only the site of storage of neurohypophysial hormones, but also synthesises vasotocin. Extracts of human fetal neurohypophysial tissue at 130–155 days gestation contain oxytocin, vasopressin, and vasotocin (Pavel, 1975). Vasotocin is also present in the fetal pineal gland in concentrations of 1.8–5.8 ng/mg tissue, but the significance of this is not understood (Legros et al, 1976).

Studies from our laboratory suggest that in human pregnancy, maternal plasma oxytocin levels are higher at term than in early pregnancy but are ineffective in activating the uterus due to insufficient uterine sensitivity (Fig. 10.7). The sensitivity of the uterus to pharmacological doses of

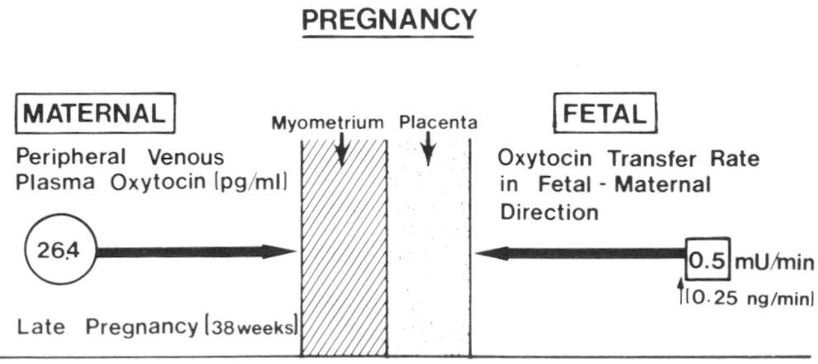

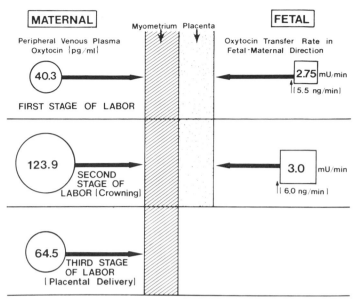

Fig. 10.8 Schematic representation of relative contribution of maternal and fetal oxytocin during spontaneous labour. During the first stage of labour, maternal plasma oxytocin levels have increased slightly compared to late pregnancy (Fig. 10.7) but fetal oxytocin levels have increased markedly, thus raising the fetal contribution of oxytocin to the myometrium during the first stage of labour. In the presence of a sensitive myometrium, such fetal and maternal oxytocin levels are capable of activating the myometrium. In the second stage of labour (crowning of the fetal head), maternal release of oxytocin contributes an important addition to the amount of oxytocin required for expulsion of the fetus and subsequent contraction of the uterus in the third stage of labour

PREGNANCY

Fig. 10.7 Schematic representation of the relative concentrations of maternal and fetal oxytocin during term pregnancy. The amount of fetal oxytocin flowing towards the placenta and uterus is insufficient to activate the myometrium. While maternal oxytocin levels are higher than in early pregnancy, an insensitive myometrium which has relatively low oxytocin receptors will not respond to the maternal oxytocin levels

oxytocin (10 mU/min or more) increases throughout pregnancy until the 36th week and remains at that level thereafter (Caldeyro-Barcia & Sereno, 1961) but, with low physiological doses of oxytocin (0.5 mU/min), the uterine sensitivity to oxytocin begins at the onset of labour (Theobald et al, 1969). With increasing uterine sensitivity which may be modulated by an increase in myometrial oxytocin receptors (Fuchs et al, 1982b), the slight increase in maternal plasma oxytocin at term is probably sufficient to activate the uterus. The increase in oxytocin is largely produced by a significant fetal infusion of oxytocin in a fetoplacental-myometrial-maternal direction during the first stage of spontaneous normal labour (Fig. 10.8). During the second stage or expulsive phase of labour, the fetal contribution of oxytocin continues as in the first stage but the marked rise in circulating maternal oxytocin levels is largely contributed by the maternal neurohypophysis, perhaps in response to the Ferguson reflex (Fig. 10.8). Of course, falling maternal oxytocin levels in the third stage of labour reflect a balance of the clearance of earlier levels and new contributions from the mother.

Lactation. Several observers have reported increased oxytocin concentrations in the maternal blood during suckling (Table 10.4). When the human infant suckles, rhythmical changes in intramammary pressure are evoked in the contralateral breast. These changes are caused by rhy-

Table 10.4 Maternal oxytocin levels during nursing in women

Refereence	Source of blood	Relationship to suckling	Method of oxytocin determination	Oxytocin level
Hawker & Robertson (1957)	Arm vein	Before suckling during suckling	Bioassay with extraction	1.4 ng/ml blood > 0.86 ng/ml blood
Hawker (1958)	Arm vein	Before suckling during suckling and 2 hrs. after suckling	Bioassay with extraction	40 pg/ml blood 100 pg/ml blood 8 pg/ml blood
Hawker et al (1961a)	Arm vein	Before suckling	Bioassay with extraction	0–8.8 ng/ml blood
Coch et al (1965)	Internal jugular vein	During suckling	Bioassay with extraction	400–600 pg/ml plasma
Coch et al (1968)	Internal jugular vein	During suckling	Bioassay with extraction and chromatography	24–50 pg/ml plasma
Fox & Knaggs (1969)	Arm vein	Before suckling During suckling	Bioassay with extraction	38 pg/ml plasma 22–244 pg/ml plasma
Weitzman et al (1980)	Arm vein	Before suckling During suckling	Radioimmunoassay with extraction	*2.2 pg/ml plasma *3.6–6.4 pg/ml plasma
Dawood et al (1981)	Arm vein	Before suckling During suckling	Radioimmunoassay with extraction	*10.8 pg/ml plasma *22.4–53.2 pg/ml plasma

* Mean values are given; statistically significant increase during suckling compared to baseline levels.

thmical contractions of the mammary myoepithelium in response to oxytocin. Release of oxytocin in response to suckling is mediated through impulses generated at the nipple and transmitted through the third, fourth, and fifth thoracic nerves via the spinal cord up to the hypothalamus to stimulate oxytocin secretion from the posterior pituitary gland (Coch et al, 1968). The release of oxytocin then completes the milk-ejection reflex.

This reflex is also responsible for the uterine contractions observed at the time of breast-feeding and often referred to as the 'afterpains'. Oxytocin levels during human lactation as determined by RIA have recently been

reported (Weitzman et al, 1980; Dawood et al, 1981). There is a significant increase in maternal plasma oxytocin levels 2 min after initiating suckling to reach maximum levels at 10 min (Fig. 10.9). There is also a simultaneous accompanying increase in plasma prolactin and thyroid stimulating hormone. It is possible that a single hypothalamic mechanism might be responsible for the release of oxytocin, prolactin, and thyrotropin during breast-feeding. The release of oxytocin during lactation may not be exclusively due to the suckling stimulus but may also include olfactory, auditory, and other stimuli. Thus, a mother who is breastfeeding may start to lactate at the sound of hearing her baby cry.

The role of oxytocin in milk-ejection is well established. In the rabbit, the rise in maternal oxytocin levels exceeds those found in women during suckling and can be correlated to the quantity of milk consumed by the litter during that particular nursing period (Fuchs et a, 1982a). In the sheep, the daily yield of milk from intact, oxytocin-treated animals but not from ovariectomised, oxytocin-treated animals is greatly increased (Fulkerson & McDowell, 1975). In the rabbit, intravenous doses of one or more units of oxytocin increases not only milk yield but also the sodium and chloride content of the milk, with a decrease in potassium and lactose and no change in fat and protein (Linzell et al, 1975). Thus, oxytocin appears to increase the permeability of the epithelium to small molecules and ions.

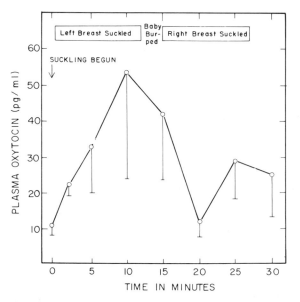

Fig. 10.9 Maternal plasma oxytocin concentrations during breastfeeding on the third to the fifth postpartum days. There is a significant increase in maternal oxytocin levels in response to suckling (From Dawood M Y et al 1981 Journal of Clinical Endocrinology and Metabolism 52: 678)

OXYTOCIN IN PATHOLOGICAL CONDITIONS

Preterm labour

Ethanol can suppress uterine activity in threatened premature human labour (Zlatnik & Fuchs, 1972). Nevertheless, it is unclear whether the alcohol acts by direct suppression of myometrial activity or by inhibiting release of neuro-hypophysial hormones or both. Evidence points to inhibition of oxytocin release because the percentage of detectable oxytocin in maternal plasma decreases significantly when alcohol is given during the advanced phase of the first stage of labour (Gibbens & Chard, 1976).

However, ethanol can also suppress prostaglandin-induced uterine activity (Karim & Sharma, 1971). There is no information on oxytocin levels or secretion in idiopathic preterm labour. Data from our laboratory indicate that there is no clearly defined oxytocin level in patients with premature labour. Mean maternal plasma oxytocin levels decline to lower levels more quickly in those patients who are successfully treated with alcohol than in those who deliver in spite of treatment. This is not altogether surprising because the uterine sensitivity to oxytocin is equally important in determining the onset of uterine contractions. Therefore, it is conceivable that the abnormality in the endocrine factor in premature labour may be a deviation from the delicate balance between oxytocin, oestrogen, and progesterone, all of which influence uterine activity either directly or indirectly by altering the sensitivity of the myometrium to oxytocin.

Maternal diabetes insipidus

In women with diabetes insipidus, labour is neither delayed nor abnormal (Hendricks, 1954), although it might be expected that the onset of labour would be delayed in such patients if the release of maternal oxytocin is crucial. An oxytocin surge found in normal pregnancy has been reported in a patient with idiopathic diabetes insipidus (Sende et al, 1976). Since this disorder limits the function of the maternal posterior pituitary gland, the increase in maternal circulating oxytocin is probably of fetal origin and may account for the ability of these patients to go into spontaneous labour. However, it should be emphasised that in patients with idiopathic diabetes insipidus, not all of the posterior pituitary gland may have been destroyed and the oxytocin reserve in most of the patients is unknown. In addition, oxytocin may continue to be produced in the paraventricular nucleus and secreted into the cerebrospinal fluid and the circulation

Dysfunctional labour

Sequential maternal plasma oxytocin concentrations appear to correlate well with the subsequent outcome of labour (Dawood et al, 1979b). Patients who have plasma oxytocin concentrations of more than 10 pg/ml throughout the second half of pregnancy ('good oxytocin secretors') develop good rhythmical uterine contractions when they go into labour and deliver vaginally without any difficulty. By contrast, those who have plasma oxytocin concentrations of less than 10 pg/ml ('poor oxytocin secretors') develop

uterine dysfunction during labour, necessitating oxytocin administration or Caesarean section.

Paraplegia

In a patient with post-traumatic paraplegia at the thoracic 4–5 level who went into spontaneous labour at term, the first stage was prolonged and maternal plasma oxytocin levels were undetectable in four out of seven samples or were low (Dawood & Fuchs, 1982). Nevertheless, the Ferguson reflex appeared intact since a surge in maternal oxytocin level was detected at crowning of the fetal head. Fetal umbilical arterial and venous levels of oxytocin were similar to those found in normal labour.

Other physiological roles of oxytocin

In addition to the various physiological and pathophysiological roles which have been described, oxytocin may have the following functions:

Central nervous system

Neurohypophysial hormones have profound effects on the learning and memory process. In this respect, the effects of vasopressin are relatively better understood than those of oxytocin. The supraoptic-neurohypophysial system is involved in the acquisition and maintenance of adaptive behaviour (Wied et al, 1977; de Wied, 1979). In rats, Bohus et al (1978) have shown that oxytocin is an amnesic neuropeptide and acts at the steps of consolidation and retrieval in the memory processes. Oxytocin might also have a behavioural effect opposite to that of vasopressin.

In vitro studies on pituitary perfusions suggest that oxytocin-stimulated luteinising hormone (LH) release and enhancement and prolongation of the LH response to gonadotrophin-releasing hormone (Dawood, 1982b). However, even in large pharmacological doses, oxytocin does not affect follicle-stimulating hormone and LH levels significantly (Dawood et al, 1980b). In supraphysiological doses, oxytocin increases the overall mitotic rate of growth hormone secreting acidophils in the rat adenohypophysis.

Insulin-like effect

Oxytocin has 'insulin-like' action on fat cells *in vitro* because, like insulin, it increases the rate at which fat cells oxidise glucose to carbon dioxide, although the mechanisms involved are different for the two hormones. Oxytocin acts through its receptors in adipocytes but is six to seven times less potent than insulin in terms of glucose oxidation (Bonne & Cohen, 1975). Nevertheless, oxytocin has no physiological effect on liver glycogen (Whitton & Hems, 1976).

Ovarian effect

Oxytocin causes contractions of the ovary, the response of which is influenced by sex hormones and, therefore, the stage of the ovarian cycle. In rats, it is interesting but so far inexplicable why oxytocin induces marked contractions of only the right ovary in late pro-oestrus but moderate contractions of both ovaries in early pro-oestrus (Sterin-Borda et al, 1976). In rabbits, oxytocin plays a role by stimulating ovarian smooth muscle to contract maximally around ovarian ovulation time to induce follicular rupture (Roca et al, 1978). Oxytocin may have a luteolytic action through an effect on uterine prostaglandin F_{2a} production in some species but the evidence is still inconclusive (Dawood, 1982b).

Cardiovascular effect

Oxytocin constricts the umbilical vessels *in vitro* (Somlyo et al, 1965) but *in vivo*, 5–10 units of oxytocin given intravenously or intra-arterially increases blood flow through the hand and forearm, decreases systolic and diastolic blood pressure, increased pulse rate and causes peripheral vasodilatation (Kitchin et al, 1959; Hendricks & Brenner, 1970). Oxytocin-induced hypotension and tachycardia are generally secondary to the peripheral vasolidation. Flattening or inversion of the T-wave of the electrocardiograph has been found in women after intravenous oxytocin (Mayes & Shearman, 1956).

A more recent study showed that given as a dilute intravenous infusion of even 80 mU, oxytocin does not significantly alter the haemodynamics of the systemic and pulmonary circulations in anaesthetised healthy adult females (Secher et al, 1978). However, if given as a bolus, 10 U oxytocin induced a drop in femoral arterial pressure of 40 per cent, systemic resistance of 59 per cent and pulmonary resistance of 44 per cent within 30 s of injection in anaesthetised healthy adult females. Thus, it is safer to give oxytocin in diluted form intravenously in women who are under anaesthesia.

Antidiuretic effects

Oxytocin has 0.5–1.0 per cent of the antidiuretic potency of vasopressin (Saunders & Munsick, 1966). A threshold dose of at least 15 mU/min of oxytocin appears to be necessary before antidiuretic responses are evoked and 45 mU/min produced maximal antidiuretic responses (Abdul-Karim & Assali, 1961). The antidiuretic effect of oxytocin is not accompanied by any change in renal blood flow or glomerular filtration rate but urinary osmolality and natriuresis is increased. Like vasopressin, oxytocin enhances water reabsorption in the distal nephron by increasing the pore size of the tubular cells.

In males

In the male, the function of oxytocin, if any, is unclear. Several studies have shown that oxytocin may affect sperm transport, possibly by an action on the smooth muscle in the seminiferous tubules, vas deferens and testicular capsule. Oxytocin infusion in rams increases sperm output rapidly, secondary to an increase in concentration in epididymal fluid (Voglmayr, 1975). In male rabbits, methallibure — an inhibitor of oxytocin release — reduces the sperm count markedly (Sharma & Hays, 1976). This effect is overcome when oxytocin is given simultaneously with methallibure, indicating that release of oxytocin during ejaculation may play a part in sperm transport. It is not known whether oxytocin is released during ejaculation. In women, oxytocin released during coitus could be responsible for the increased uterine activity experienced during orgasm which may aid sperm transport through the female genital tract.

Clinical uses of oxytocin

The most obvious use of oxytocin is related to its ability to induce uterine contractions. The clinical uses of oxytocin are summarised in Table 10.5.

Table 10.5 Clinical uses of oxytocin

Stimulation of myometrial activity (early pregnancy)
Induction of labour (preterm, term and post-term
Dysfunctional labour
Control of uterine haemorrhage
Early pregnancy (abortion, uterine curettage)
Postpartum (prophylactic, therapeutic)
Lactation difficulties (intramuscular, snuff, nasal spray).

Oxytocin levels during oxytocin administration

In main, intravenous infusion of oxytocin produces plasma oxytocin concentrations that correlate well with the dose of oxytocin given (Dawood et al, 1979b). During labour intravenous oxytocin infusion into women gave plasma concentrations of oxytocin which are related to the plasma oxytocin levels before giving the oxytocin. When buccal pitocin was given to men in doses of 400 units every 20 min, the mean level of oxytocin reached was 31.5 pg/ml (Dawood et al, 1980). It took about 20–30 min for the plasma level of oxytocin to decline by 50 per cent after stopping buccal oxytocin. In pregnant women at term or in labour, buccal oxytocin 400 units given every 20 min produced plasma levels of oxytocin that did not exceed 50 pg/ml, which is similar to maternal plasma levels found in the first stage of labour, unless the plasma level before giving the buccal oxytocin is higher than 50 pg/ml. Thus, contrary to accepted belief, administration of buccal oxytocin need not produce excessively high and non-physiological levels of plasma oxytocin. Nevertheless, the transbuccal administration of oxytocin is not widely used because of the alleged poorer control in the absorption rate.

Uterus

Oxytocin has been widely used and accepted for inducing uterine contractions of the early and late pregnant uterus and also the postpartum uterus. Oxytocin can be given subcutaneously or intramuscularly because it is rapidly absorbed to become biologically effective without causing significant cardiovascular changes. However, the intramuscular route is usually employed for the active management of the third stage of labour or after evacuation of the uterus but is currently not used to induce uterine contractions in pregnancy. For induction of labour or abortions, oxytocin is usually given as an intravenous infusion but doses of more than 5 units should never be given as an intravenous bolus injection because of the potential serious cardiovascular effects. Intravenous infusion of oxytocin should be given in a controlled titration. Uncontrolled administration of even low doses of oxytocin carry the potential hazard of uterine rupture with maternal and fetal morbidity and mortality. In the postpartum uterus, oxytocin may also be given by direct intra-myometrial injection of the uterus in the instances of severe postpartum haemorrhage with an atonic uterus. There is still a divergence of opinion on the dose of oxytocin which should be given as an intravenous oxytocin infusion for inducing or augmenting uterine contractions at or near term.

Theobald (1968) has always advocated the 'physiological oxytocin drip' and stresses that the dose of oxytocin should not exceed a concentration greater than 4–6 mU/min. In contrast, pharmacological doses of up to 137 mU oxytocin/min have been advocated by other investigators (Turnbull & Anderson, 1968). Certainly, others have found that it is rarely necessary to exceed an oxytocin dose of 5–8 mU/min and a dose of 16 mU/min should never be exceeded (Hendricks, 1963; Caldeyro-Barcia, 1964; Wood, 1969). The maternal circulating levels of oxytocin (see above) in normal spontaneous labour certainly agree with the 'physiological doses' of 4–6 mU/min recommended by Theobald (1968). Therefore, it is more prudent, physiologically, to start intravenous oxytocin infusion with a low dose of 1–2 mU increasing it slowly at regular intervals. Whatever the dose of oxytocin chosen, the patient should be carefully monitored and a physician should be available to supervise the patient while she is on the oxytocin infusion for induction of labour. In midtrimester, the uterus is more refractory and less sensitive to oxytocin. Thus, a much larger dose of oxytocin infusion is necessary to produce effective uterine contractions.

An attractive and novel method of administering intravenous infusion of oxytocin was recently described (Pavlov et al, 1978). Since the release of oxytocin is episodic

(Gibbens & Chard, 1974; Dawood et al, 1979b), the hormone was given as an intermittent oxytocin infusion (pulsed) for 1 min out of every 10. Pulsing was achieved using the Cardiff infusion system Mark III. Pavlov et al (1978) found that the induction-delivery interval was similar whether the women were given continuous oxytocin infusion or intermittent oxytocin infusion. Certainly the total dose of oxytocin required is lower with the intermittent infusion which, therefore, offers a physiological way of administering oxytocin and a potential reduction in the adverse effects of oxytocin.

Mammary gland

Decreased oxytocin secretion may lead to lactational difficulties since oxytocin is required for the milk-ejection reflex. If the synthesis and secretion of milk are not impaired, administration of oxytocin subcutaneously, intramuscularly, as a snuff or as a nasal spray can promptly elicit milk-ejection and help to establish lactation. The subcutaneous and intramuscular dose used for this is 5 U oxytocin while the dose of the solution for the nasal spray is 40 U/ml.

Side-effects of oxytocin

Overdose or inappropriate administration of oxytocin is likely to produce tumultuous labour, or hypertonic uterine activity with resulting uterine ischaemia, placental insufficiency and intra-uterine fetal asphyxia. In cases of feto-pelvic disproportion, the uterus may eventually rupture with disastrous consequences. Such undesirable side-effects can be avoided or minimised through proper, controlled and supervised administration of intravenous oxytocin infusion starting with low doses. Sometimes such side-effects may result even with low doses of oxytocin if there is uterine hypersensitivity. When such side-effects are recognised, the oxytocin infusion should be discontinued.

When given in large doses and in abundant fluid volumes deficient in electrolytes, oxytocin can cause severe water intoxication and, regretfully, such side-effects are still encountered and have been reported in a review of the literature on oxytocin for 1977–1980 (Dawood, 1982b). This complication is seen in oxytocin administration for midtrimester abortion where large doses of oxytocin are used. This complication can be avoided or minimised by appropriate use of physiological saline or Ringer's solution as the diluent for the oxytocin.

Oxytocin, if given as an intravenous bolus dose, can cause severe cardiovascular effects (see above) and sudden deaths have been reported in obstetric patients with this method of administration.

Oxytocin stimulation of labour has been associated with neonatal jaundice and the literature on this has been reviewed (Dawood, 1982b). Neonatal jaundice due to oxytocin-stimulated labour has now been shown to be due to transplacental passage of oxytocin and its action on the electrolytes and the erythrocytes of the fetus. It is now clear that the risk and severity of the neonatal jaundice is related to the total dose of oxytocin administered to the mother during labour (D'Souza et al, 1979). The fetal erythrocyte deformability has been shown to be increased by oxytocin *in vitro* in a direct dose-dependent relationship (Buchan, 1979; Singhi & Singh, 1979).

REFERENCES

Abdul-Karim R, Assali N S 1961 Renal function in human preganancy V. Effects of oxytocin on renal hemodynamics and water and electrolyte excretion. Journal of Laboratory and Clinical Medicine 57: 522–532

Acher R, Chuvet J, Olivry G 1956 Sur L'existence eventuelle d'une hormone unique neurohypophysaire. Biochimica Biophysica Acta 22: 421–427

Alexandrova M, Soloff M S 1980 Oxytocin receptors and parturition I Control of oxytocin receptors concentration in the rat myometrium at term. Endocrinology 106: 730–735

Amico J A, Seif S M, Robinson A G 1981 Oxytocin in human plasma: correlation with neurophysin and stimulation with estrogen. Journal of Clinical Endocrinology and Metabolism 52: 988–993

Bargmann W, Scharrer E 1951 The site of origin of the hormones of the posterior pituitary. American Scientist 39: 255–259

Bashore R A 1972 Studies concerning the radioimmunoassay for oxytocin. American Journal of Obstetrics and Gynecology 113: 488–496

Bohus B, Kovacs G L, de Wied D 1978 Oxytocin, vasopressin and memory: Opposite effects of consolidation and retrieval processes. Brain Research 157: 414–417

Bonne D, Cohen P 1975 Characterization of oxytocin receptors on isolated rat fat cell. European Journal of Biochemistry 56: 295–303

Boyd N R H, Jackson D B, Hollingsworth S, Forsling M L, Chard T 1972 The development of a radioimmunoassay for oxytocin: The extraction of oxytocin from urine and detemuniation of the excretion rate for exogenous and endogenous oxytocin in human urine. Journal of Endocrinology 52: 59–67

Buchan P 1979 Pathogenesis of neonatal hyperbilirubinemia after induction of labor with oxytocin. British Medical Journal 1 255–1257

Buford G D, Pickering B T 1973 Intra-axonal transport and turnover of neurophysins in the rat: A proposal for a possible origin of the minor neurophysin component. Chemical Journal 136: 1047–1052

Burton A M, Forsling M L 1972 Hormone content of the neurohypophysis in foetal, new-born and adult guinea pigs. Journal of Physiology 221: 6–7

Caldeyro-Barcia R 1964 quoted by Theobald G W 1970 The neurohypophysis and labor. In: Philipp E E, Barnes J, Newton M (eds) Scientific Foundations of Obstetrics and Gynaecology, pp 514–530. William Heinemann, London

Caldeyro-Barcia R, Sereno J A 1961 The response of the human uterus to oxytocin throughout pregnancy. In: Caldeyro-Barcia R, Heller H (eds) Oxytocin, p 177. Pergamon Press, New York

Chard T, Boyd N R H, Forsling M L, McNeilly A S, Landon J 1970 The development of radioimmunoassay for oxytocin: The extraction of oxytocin from plasma and its measurement during parturition in human and goat blood. Journal of Endocrinology 48: 223–234

Chard T, Hudson C N, Edwards C R W, Boyd N R H 1971 Release of oxytocin and vasopressin by the human foetus during labour. Nature 234: 352–354

Clarke G, Lincoln D W 1975 Evidence for a dopaminergic component in the ejection reflex of the rat. Journal of Endocrinology 67: 32–33

Coch J A, Brovetto J, Cabot H M, Fielitz C A, Caldeyro-Barcia R 1965 Oxytocin equivalent activity in the plasma of women in labor and puerperium. American Journal of Obstetrics and Gynecology 91: 10–17

Coch J A, Fielitz C, Brovetto J, Cabot H M, Coda H, Fraga H 1968 Estimation of an oxytocin-like substance in highly purified extracts from blood of puerpueral women during suckling. Journal of Endocrinology 40: 137–144

Dale H H 1906 On some physiological action of ergot. Journal of Physiology 34: 163–206

Dawood M Y 1982a Neurohypophysial Hormones. In: Fuchs F, Klopper A (eds) Endocrinology of Pregnancy, 3rd edn., J B Lippincott, Philadelphia

Dawood M Y 1982b Oxytocin, Vol II. Eden Press, Montreal

Dawood M Y, Fuchs F 1981 Maternal and fetal oxytocin levels at aprturition in a paraplegic. European Journal of Obstetrics Gynecology and Reproductive Biology 12: 1–6

Dawood M Y, Khan-Dawood F S 1982 Oxytocin (OT) Content of human fetal and newborn pituitary glands. Abstracts of the 29th Annual meeting of the Society for Gynecologic Investigation abstract #374, p 215

Dawood M Y, Raghavan K S, Pociask C 1978a Radioimmunoassay of oxytocin. Journal of Endocrinology 76: 261–270

Dawood M Y, Raghavan K S, Pociask C, Fuchs F 1978b Oxytocin in human pregnancy and parturition. Obstetrics and Gynecology 51: 138–143

Dawood M Y, Wang C F, Gupta R, Fuchs F 1978c Fetal contribution to oxytocin in human labor. Obstetrics and Gynecology 52: 205–209

Dawood M Y, Lauersen N H, Trivedi D, Ylikorkala O, Fuchs F 1979a Studies on oxytocin in the baboon during pregnancy delivery. Acta Endocrinologica 91: 704–718

Dawood M Y, Ylikorkala O, Trivedi D, Fuchs F 1979b Oxytocin in maternal circulation and amniotic fluid during pregnancy. Journal of Clinical Endocrinology and Metabolism 49: 429–434

Dawood M Y, Ylikorkala O, Fuchs F 1980a Plasma oxytocin levels and disappearance rate after buccal pitocin. American Journal of Obstetrics and Gynecology 138: 20–24

Dawood M Y, Ylikorkala O, Trivedi D, Gupta R 1980b Oxytocin levels and disappearance rate and plasma follicle-stimulating hormone and luteinizing hormone after oxytocin infusion in men. Journal of Clinical Endocrinology and Metabolism 50: 397–400

Dawood M Y, Khan-Dawood F S, Wahi R, Fuchs F 1981 Oxytocin release and plasma anterior pituitary and gonadal hormones in women during lactation. Journal of Clinical Endocrinology and Metabolism 52: 678–683

de Wied D 1979 Neuropeptides: Effects on motivation, learning and memory processes. In: Carenza L, Pancheri P, Zichella L (eds) Clinical Psychoneuroendocrinology in Reproduction, pp 15–24. Academic Press, New York

de Wied D, Bohus B, Van Ree J M, Urban I, Greidanus T B V W 1977 Neurohypophyseal hormones and behaviour. In: Moses A M, Share L (eds) Neurohypophysis, pp 201–210. r, Basel

Dicker S E, Tyler C 1953 Vasopressin and oxytocin activities of the pituitary gland of rats, guinea-pigs and cats and of human fetuses. Journal of Physiology 121: 206–214

Dierickx K, Vandesande F 1979 Immunocytochemical demonstration of separate vasopressin-neurophysin and oxytocin neurophysin neurons in the human hypothalamus. Cell and Tissue Research 196: 203–212

Dierickx K, Vandesande F, DeMey J 1976 Identification in the external region of the rat median eminence, of separate neurophysin-vasopressin and neurophysin-oxytocin containing nerve fibers. Cell and Tissue Research 168: 141–151

Dogterom J, Greidanus T B V W, Swaab D F 1977 Evidence for the release of vasopressin and oxytocin into cerebrospinal fluid: measurements in plasma and cerebrospinal fluid of intact and hypophysectomized rats. Neuroendocrinology 24: 108–118

D'Souza S W, Black P, MacFarlane T, Richards B 1979 The effects of oxytocin in induced labor on neonatal jaundice. British Journal of Obstetrics and Gynaecology 86: 133–138

du Vigneaud V, Gish D T, Katsoyannis P G, Hess G P 1958 Synthesis of the pressor antidiuretic hormone, arginine-vasopressin. Journal of American Chemical Society 80: 3355–3358

Dudley H W 1919 Some observations on the active principle of the pituitary gland. Journal of Pharmacology and Experimental Therapeutics 14: 295–312

Fabian M, Forsling M L, Jones J J, Pryor J S 1969 The clearance and antidiuretic potency of neurohypophysial hormones in man, and their plasma binding and stability. Journal of Physiology 204: 653–668

Fitzpatrick R J, Walmsley C R 1965 The release of oxytocin during parturition. In: Pinkerton J H M (ed) Advances in Oxytocin Research, pp 51–72. Pergamon Press, Oxford

Forsling M L, Boyd N R H, Chard T 1971 The dissociation of the immunological and biological activity of oxytocin: in vivo studies. In: Kirkham K E, Hunter W M (eds) Radioimmunoassay Methods, pp 549–555. Churchill Livingstone, Edinburgh

Fox C A, Knaggs G S 1969 Milk ejection activity (oxytocin) in peripheral venous blood in man during lactation and in association with coitus. nal of Endocrinology 45: 145–147

Fuchs A-R 1966 The inhibitory effect of ethanol on the release of oxytocin during parturition in the rabbit. Journal of Endocrinology 35: 125–134

Fuchs A-R, Cubile L, Dawood M Y 1981 Effects of mating on levels of oxytocin and prolactin in the plasma of male and female rabbits. Journal of Endocrinology 90: 245–253

Fuchs A-R, Dawood M Y, Cubile L 1982a Suckling induced release of oxytocin and prolactin and lactogenesis in rabbits. Endocrinology in press

Fuchs A-R, Fuchs F, Husslein P, Soloff M S, Fernstrom M J 1982b Oxytocin receptors and human parturition: A dual role for oxytocin in the initiation labor. Science 215: 1396–1398

Fuchs A-R, Saito S 1971 Pituitary oxytocin and vasopressin content of pregnant rats before and during parturition. Endocrinology 88: 574–578

Fulkerson W J, McDowell G H 1975 Artificial induction of lactation in ewes: The relative importance of oxytocin and milking stimulus. Australian Journal of Biological Science 28: 521–524

George J M 1978 Immunoreactive vasopressin and oxytocin: Concentration in individual human hypothalamic nuclei. Science 200: 342–343

George J M, Staples S, Mark P M 1976 Oxytocin content of microdissected areas of rat hypothalamus. Endocrinology 98: 1430–1433

Gibbens G L D, Chard T 1976 Observations on maternal oxytocin release during human labor and the effect of intravenous alcohol administration. American Journal of Obstetrics and Gynecology 126: 243–246

Gillespie A, Brummer H C, Chard T 1972 Oxytocin release by infused prostaglandins. British Medical Journal 1: 543–544

Glatz T H, Weitzman R E, Nathanielsz P W, Fisher D A 1980 Mebolic clearance rate and transplacental passage of oxytocin in the pregnant ewe and fetus. Endocrinology 106: 1006–1011

Glick S M, Kumaresan P, Kagan A, Wheeler M 1969 Radioimmunoassay of oxytocin. In: Margoulies M (ed) Protein and Polypeptide Hormones, pp 81–83. Excerpta Medica Foundation, Amsterdam

Goren H J, Geonzon R M, Hollenberg M D, Lederis K, Morgan D O 1980 Oxytocin Action: Lack of correlation between receptor number and tissue responsiveness. Journal of Supramolecular Structure 14: 129–138

Gonzales-Panizza V H, Sica-Blanco Y 1957 Proceedings of the second Uruguayan Congress of Obstetrics and Gynecology 2: 330

Hawker R W 1958 Oxytocin in lactating and non-lactating women. Journal of Endocrinology and bolism 18: 54–60

Hawker R W, Robertson P A 1957 Oxytocin in human female blood. Endocrinology 60: 652–657

Hawker R W, Walmsley C F, Roberts V S, Blackshaw J K, Downes J C 1961a Oxytocic activity of blood in parturition and lactating women. Journal of Clinical Endocrinology 21: 985–995

Hawker R W, Walmsley C F, Roberts V S, Blackshaw J K, Downes J C 1961b Oxytocic activity of human female blood. Endocrinology 69: 391–394

Hendricks C H 1954 The neurohypophysis in pregnancy. Obstetrical and Gynecological Survey 9: 323–341

Hendricks C 1963 quoted by Theobald G W 1970 The neurohypophysis and labour. In: Philipp E E, Barnes J, Newton M (eds) Scientific Foundations of Obstetrics and Gynaecology, pp 514–530. William Heinemann, London

Hendricks C H, Brenner W E 1970 Cardiovascular effect of oxytocic drugs used postpartum. American Journal of Obstetrics and Gynecology 108: 751–760

Juret T, Suzor R, Poly-Marchetti P 1961 quoted by Driessche R V. In: Caldeyro-Barcia R, Heller H (eds) Oxytocin, p 400. Pergamon Press, New York.

Karim S M M, Sharma S D 1971 The effect of ethyl alcohol on prostaglandin E_1 and F_{2a} induced uterine activity in pregnant women. Journal of Obstetrics and Gynaecology of the British Commonwealth 78: 251–254

Kitchin A H, Konzett H, Pickford M 1959 Comparison of effects of valyl[3]-oxytocin and syntocinon in the cardiovascular system of man. British Journal of Pharmacology 14: 567–570

Kleinhaus A L, Kas C Y 1969 Electrophysiological actions of oxytocin on the rabbit myometrium. Journal of General Physiology 53: 758–780

Konschegg A V, Schuster E 1915 Ueber die Beeinflussung der Diurese durch Hypophysenextrakte. Deutsche Medizinische Wochenschrift 41: 1091–1095

Kumaresan P, Anandarangam P B, Dianzon W, Vasicka A 1974 Plasma oxytocin levels during human preganancy and labor as determined by radioimmunoassay. American Journal of Obstetrics and Gynecology 119: 215–223

Leake R D, Weitzman R E, Fisher D A 1980 Pharmacokinetics of oxytocin in the human subject. Obstetrics and Gynecology 56: 701–704

Legros J J, Louis F, Demoulin A, Franchimont P 1976 Immunoreactive neurophysins and vasotocin in human foetal pineal glands. Journal of Endocrinology 69: 289–290

Linzell J L, Peaker M, Taylor J C 1975 The effects of prolactin and oxytocin on milk secretion and on the permeability of the mammary epithelium in the rabbit. Journal of Physiology 253: 547–563

Mayes B T, Shearman R P 1956 Experience with synthetic oxytocin: The effects on the cardiovascular system and its use for the induction of labour and control of the third stage. Journal of Obstetrics and Gynaecology of the British Commonwealth 63: 812–818

Nagasawa J, Douglas W W, Schulz R A 1970 Ultrastructural evidence of secretion by exocytosis and of 'synaptic le' formation in posterior glands. Nature 227: 407–409

Nathanietsz P W, Comline R S, Silver M 1973 Uterine activity following intravenous administration of oxytocin to the foetal sheep. Nature 243: 471–472

Nissenson R, Flouret G, Hechter O 1978 Opposing effects of estradiol and progesterone on oxytocin receptors in rabbit uterus. Proceedings of the National Academy Science 75: 2044–2048

Noddle B A 1964 Transfer of oxytocin from the maternal to the fetal circulation of the ewe. Nature 203: 414

Nordmann J J, Morris J F 1976 Membrane retrieval at neurosecretory axon endings. Nature 261: 723–725

Oliver G, Schafer E A 1895 On the physiological action of extracts of pituitary body and certain other glandular organs. Journal of Physiology 18: 277–279

Ott I, Scott J C 1910 The action of infundibulin upon the mammary secretion. Proceedings of the Society for Experimental Biology and Medicine 8: 48–49

Pavel S 1975 Vasotocin biosynthesis by neurohypophysial cells from human fetuses: Evidence for its ependymal origin. Neuroendocrinology 19: 150–159

Pavlov C, Barker G H, Rovebts A, Chamberlain G V P 1978 Pulsed oxytocin infusion in the induction of labour. British Journal of Obstetrics and Gynaecology 85: 96–100

Pliska V, Sachs H 1974 The interaction of lysine vasopressin with free and agarose-bound borne neurophysin II. European Journal of Biochemistry 41: 229–239

Roberts J S, McCracken J A 1976 Does prostaglandin F_{2a} released from the uterus by oxytocin mediate the oxytocin? Biology of Reproduction 15: 457–463

Robinson A G 1973 Isolation, assay and secretion of individual human neurophysins. Journal of Clinical Investigation 55: 360–367

Roca R A, Garofalo E G, Martino I, Piriz H, Rieppi G, Maraffi M, Ohahian C, Gadola L 1978 Effects of oxytocin antiserum and of indomethacin on LCG-induced ovulation in the rabbit. Biology of Reproduction 19: 552–557

Saameli K 1963 An indirect method for the estimation of oxytocin blood concentrations and half-life in pregnant women near term, American Journal of Obstetrics and Gynecology 85: 186–192

Sanders W G, Munsick R A 1966 Antidiuretic potency of oxytocin in women post partum. American Journal of Obstetrics and Gynecology 95: 5–11

Sawyer W H 1964 Vertebrate neurohypophysial principles. Endocrinology 75: 981–990

Schriefer J A, Lewis P R, Miller J W 1980 Effect of dopamine on length of gestation and on the release of fetal oxytocin in rats. Journal of Pharmacology and Experimental Therapeutics 212: 431–434

Seccher N J, Arnsbo P, Wallin L 1978 Hemodynamic effects of oxytocin (syntocinon) and methyl ergometrine (methergin) on the systemic and pulmonary circulations of pregnant anaesthetized women. Acta Obstetricia et Gynecologica Scandinavica 57: 97–107

Sende P, Pantelakis N, Suzuki K, Bashore R 1976 Plasma oxytocin determinations in pregnancy with diabetes insipidus. Obstetrics and Gynecology 48: 38–41

Seppala M, Aho I, Tissari A, Ruoslahti E 1972 Radioimmunoassay of oxytocin in amniotic fluid, fetal urine and meconium during late pregnancy and delivery. American Journal of Obstetrics and Gynecology 114: 788–795

Sharma O P, Hays R LA 1976 A possible role for oxytocin in sperm transport in the male rabbit. Journal of Endocrinology 68: 43–47

Sica-Blanco Y, Gonzalez-Panizza V H, Caldeyro-Barcia R 1959 Abstract of the 21st International Congress of Physiological Science, p 252

Silverman A J 1976 Ultrastructural studies on the localization of neurohypophysial hormones and their carrier proteins. Journal of Histochemistry and Cytochemistry 24: 816–827

Singhi S, Singh M 1979 Pathogenesis of oxytocin-induced neonatal hyperbilirubinemia. Archives of Diseases of Childhood 54: 400–402

Sokol H W, Zimmermann E A, Sawyer W H, Robinson A G 1976 The hypothalamic-neurohypophysial system of the rat: Localization and quantitation of neurophysin by light microic immunocytochemistry in normal rats and in Bratteboro rats deficient in vasopressin and neurophysin. Endocrinology 98: 1176–1188

Soloff M S 1976 Oxytocin receptors in the mammary gland and uterus. In: Blecher M (ed) Methods in receptor Research, Part II, p 511. Marcel Dekker Inc, New York

Soloff M S, Alexandrova M, Fernstrom M J 1979 Oxytocin receptors: triggers for parturition and lactation? Science 204: 1313–1315

Somlyo A V, Woo C Y, Somlyo A P 1965 Responses of nerve-free vessels to vasoactive amines and polypeptides. American Journal of Physiology 208: 748–753

Sterin-Borda L, Borda E, Gimeno M F, Gimeno A Z 1976 Spontaneous and prostaglandin or oxytocin induced mobility of rat ovaries isolated during different stages of the estrous cycle: effect of norepinephrine. Fertility and Sterility 27: 319–327

Suzuki H, Kuriyama H 1975 Comparison between prostaglandin E_2 and oxytocin actions on pregnant mouse myometrium. Japanese Journal of Physiology 25: 345–356

Swaab D F, Pool C W, Nijveldt F 1978 Immunofluorescence of vasopressin and oxytocin in the rat hypothalamo-neurohypophyseal system. Journal of Neural Transmission 36: 195–216

Swann R W, Pickering B T 1976 Incorporation of radioactive precursors into membrane and contents of the neurosecretory granule of the rat neurohypophysis as a method of studying their fate. Journal of Endocrinology 68: 95–108

Theobald G W 1968 Oxytocin reassessed. Obstetrical and Gynecological Survey 23: 109–131

Theobald G W 1970 The neurohypophysis and labour. In: Philip E E, Barnes J, Newton M (eds) Scientific Foundations of Obstetrics and Gynaecology, pp 514–530. William Heinemann, London

Theobald G W, Robards M F, Suter P E N 1969 Changes in myometrial sensitivity to oxytocin in man during the last six weeks of pregnancy. Journal of Obstetrics and Gynaecology of the British Commonwealth 76: 385–393

Tuppy H 1969 The influence of Enzymes on Neurohypophyseal hormones and similar peptides. Handbook of Experimental Pharmacology 23: 67

Turnbull A C, Anderson A B M 1968 Uterine Contractility and oxytocin sensitivity during human pregnancy in relation to the onset of labour. Journal of Obstetrics and Gynaecology of the British Commonwealth 75: 271–277

Vandesande F, Dierickx K, DeMey J 1975a Identification of the vasopressin-neurophysin II and the oxytocin-neurophysin I producing neurons in the bovine hypothalamus. Cell and Tissue Research 156: 189–200

Vandesande F, Dierickx K, DeMey J 1975b Immunohistochemical demonstration of oxytocin and the vasopressin-producing neurons in the magnocellular hypothalamic neurosecretory system of the cow, the rat and the Brattleboro rat. Annals of Endocrinology 36: 379–380

Vizsolyi E, Perks A M 1976 Neurohypophysial hormones in fetal life and pregnancy I. Pharmacological studies in the sheep (Ovis aries). General and Comparative Endocrinology 29: 28–40

Voglmayr J K 1975 Output of spermatozoa and fluid by the testis of the ram and its response to oxytocin. Journal of Reproduction and Fertility 43: 119–122

Vorherr H 1972 ADH and oxytocin in blood and urine of gravidas and parturients. Abstracts of the 19th Annual Meeting of the Society for Gynecologic Investigation, abstract #38

Walter R 1974 Oxytocin and other peptide hormones as prohormones. In: Hatotani N (ed) Psychoneuroendocrinology, p. 285. Karger, Basel

Walter R 1976 Partial purification and characterization of post-proline cleaving enzyme: Enzymatic inactivation of neurohypophyseal hormones by kidney preparations of various species. Biochimica et Biophysica Acta 422: 138–158

Weitzman R E, Leake R D, Rubin R T, Fisher D A 1980 The effect of nursing on neurohypophyseal hormone and prolactin secretion in human subjects. Journal of Clinical Endocrinology and Metabolism 51: 836–839

Whitton P D, Hems D A 1976 Action of vasopressin-related peptides on glycogen metabolism in the perfused rat liver. Biochemical Pharmacology 25: 405–407

Zlatnik F J, Fuchs F 1972 A controlled study of ethanol in threatened premature labor. American Journal of Obstetrics and Gynecology 112: 610–612

Physiology and pharmacology of prostacyclines and prostaglandins

INTRODUCTION

The existence of a substance or a group of substances with smooth muscle-stimulating and vasodepressor properties was described in the beginning of the 1930s. The active principle was given the name prostaglandin by von Euler, who established that the compound(s) behaved as polar fatty acids and thus belonged to a new group of naturally occurring substances. Prostaglandins are a unique group of substances, differing from the classical hormones by neither being synthesised by special types of cells nor stored in the tissues where they are formed. Furthermore, they are metabolised quickly which, to an even greater extent, applies to endoperoxides from which prostaglandins are produced. A more adequate designation for prostaglandins is local hormones or tissue hormones, which indicates partly that the majority of tissues have a capacity to syn thesise them and partly that they are mainly inactivated at the site of the synthesis. Prostaglandin breaking down enzymes are thus just as widely distributed in tissues as prostaglandin-synthetase. The concentration of prostaglandin in a given situation is, therefore, the net result of the tissue capacity to synthesise and metabolise prostaglandin.

Against this background it is not surprising that prostaglandin has engaged scientists with their interest directed towards widely separated organs and functional courses within basic as well as the clinical research. In particular the reproductive tract, the central nervous system, the circulatory system and blood, the kidneys, lungs and digestive tract have been subject to very extensive studies. These include investigation of pharmacological effects as well as the physiological and pathophysiological pathways in the organ systems involved. Therapeutic and clinical effects have also been analysed thoroughly.

At the transformation of arachidonic acid and other unsaturated fatty acid precursors to prostaglandins, labile biologically hyperactive intermediaries will appear in the form of endoperoxides. These, in turn, will be transformed to short-lived and, from a biological point of view, sometimes even more active compounds. Such a compound,

thromboxane A, with a very short half-life of approximately 30 s, will induce aggregation of blood platelets and cause vasoconstriction. During the last few years the picture has been further complicated through the finding by Vane that endoperoxides under the influence of prostacyclin synthetase in the blood vessel intima could be transformed to a previously unknown biologically active product — prostacyclin — which inhibits blood platelet aggregation and causes vasodilation.

The metabolic pathway of the arachidonic acid varies in different cells. Within certain cells, prostaglandins of the E- and F-type seem to be the major products, within others — for example blood platelets — mostly thromboxanes, and within yet another, for instance the blood vessel wall, to a great extent, prostacyclin. The appearance of these short-lived metabolites with various and often counteracting effects has led to extensive speculation regarding their importance for the maintenance of the normal aggregation of the blood platelets. The consequences of disturbances in their mutual balance for the origin of local and general thromboses, of myocardial ischemia and of angina pectoris have also been discussed.

Undoubtedly, we have at present most knowledge about the role of the prostaglandins in reproduction. In the following report the major emphasis will be within this area.

CHEMISTRY AND PHARMACOLOGY

Chemical structure

The chemical structures of the classical prostaglandins were elucidated during the late '50s and early '60s. They are all unsaturated hydroxy fatty acids with 20 carbon atoms. The characteristic structure is the prostanoic acid molecule, a cyclopentane ring with two side chains (Fig. 11.1). Depending on the number of substituents on different carbons and the structure in the five-membered ring, series of prostaglandins have been designated with letters from A to I (Bygdeman & Gréen, 1980). All pros-

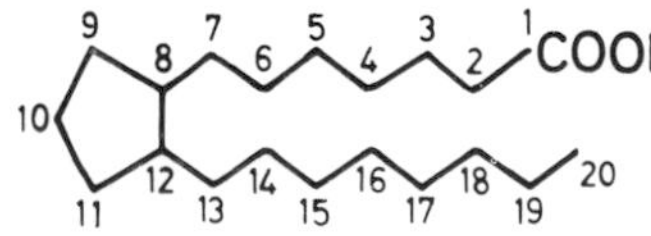

Fig 11.1 Prostanoic acid

taglandins have one or more double bonds and the number of these characterises the members of each group. They are indicated by numerical subscripts that follows the corresponding letter referring to the parent structure, e.g. E_1; E_2 and E_3. During the last decade several new groups of compounds, originating from the same unsaturated fatty acids as the classical prostaglandins, have been found in different tissues. The discovery of such biologically very active compounds as thromboxanes (Tx), prostacyclin (PG_3) and leucotrienes has initiated intense research on their possible roles in cardiovascular disease and immunological reactions. The leucotrienes have been shown to be constituents of what was known as SRS-A (slow reacting substance of anaphylaxis).

Biosynthesis

All naturally occurring prostaglandins and thromboxanes are biosynthesised from essential unsaturated fatty acids containing 20 carbon atoms. Arachidonic acid (5,8,11,14-all-*cis*-eicosatetraenoic acid) is the most important of these precursor fatty acids from a quantitative point of view. The other two precursor acids are 8,11,14-all-*cis*-eicosatrienoic and 5,8,11,14,17-all-*cis*-eicosapentaenoic acid.

Some of the presently known routes in the bioconversion of arachidonic acid are illustrated in Fig. 11.2. The first step in the route leading to the classical prostaglandins (E_2 and $F_{2\alpha}$) PGI_2 and thromboxane A_2 (TxA_2), is the formation of the cyclic endoperoxides PGG_2 and PGH_2 (only PGH_2 shown). These cyclo-oxygenase catalysed reactions are inhibited by several non-steroidal anti-inflammatory drugs (e.g. aspirin, indomethacin). The endoperoxides can be non-enzymatically transformed into PGE_2 or enzymatically into PGE_2, $PGF_{2\alpha}$, PGI_2, TxA_2 and other products (Samuelsson et al, 1975, 1978).

Bioconversion of arachidonic acid through the action of lipoxygenases may lead to formation of various hydroperoxy- and hydroxy-tetraenoic acids. Such products can also be formed non-enzymatically through auto-oxidation.

Other reactions, obviously initiated by lipoxygenase activity but involving unstable epoxide intermediates, may lead to the formation of various leucotrienes (Lt). Lt A_4 is an epoxide while Lt B_4 is a dihydroxy-eicosa-tetraenoic acid. Through the action of glutathione-S-transferase

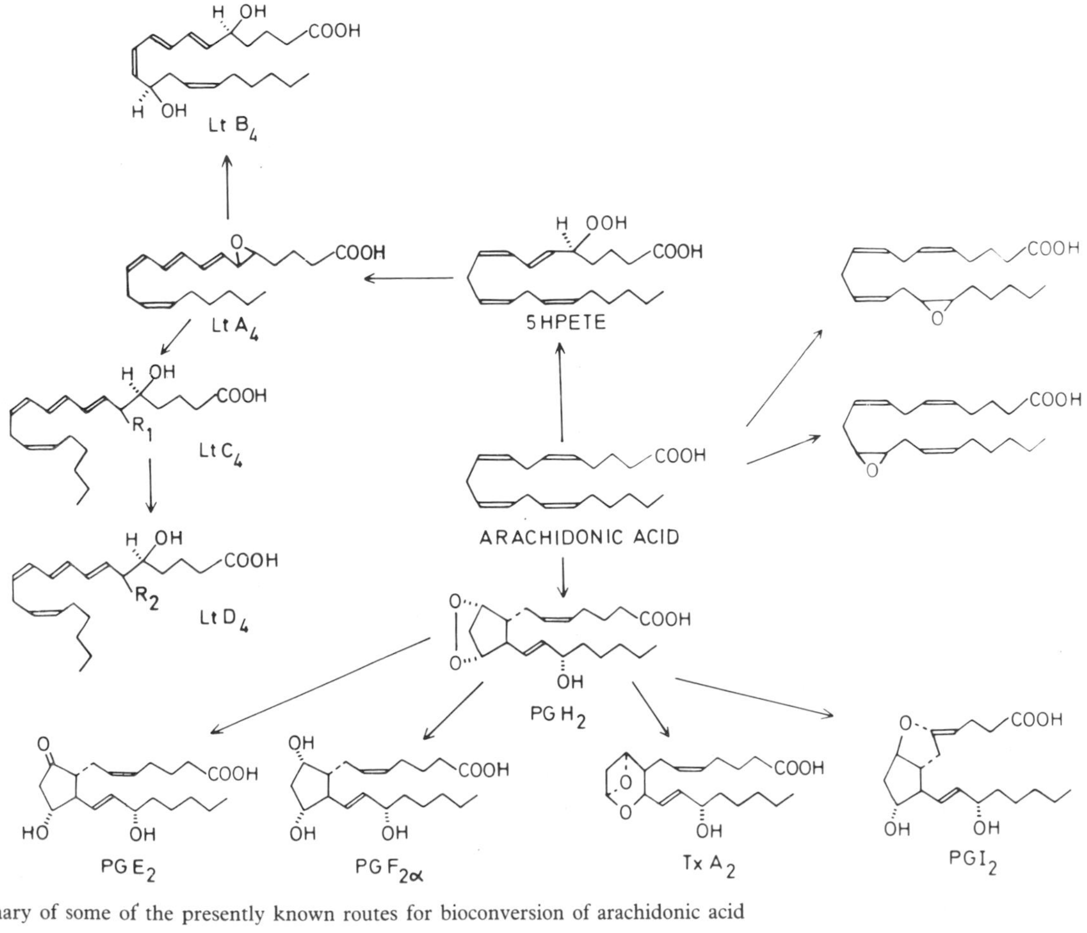

Fig 11.2 Summary of some of the presently known routes for bioconversion of arachidonic acid

glutathione is coupled to carbon 6 of Lt A_4 leading to formation of Lt C_4. Cleavage of a peptide bond in this compound by γ-glutamyl-trans-peptidase yields Lt D_4 (Samuelsson & Hammarström, 1980).

Recently, other products of arachidonic acid, which also very likely involve epoxide intermediates, have been found in incubations of microsomes from rabbit renal cortex (Oliw et al, 1981, Fig. 11.2 upper right).

Occurrence

Bioconversion of arachidonic acid can thus result in formation of a wide variety of biologically very active compounds. This has led to the concept: 'Products of the arachidonic acid cascade'. The multitude of products, some of which might be formed simultaneously in a biological system and interact with each other's formation and biological activity, indicates that the arachidonic acid cascade is a very complex phenomenon. It is of interest in this connection that non steroid inflammatory drugs inhibit formation of PGG_2 and PGH_2, while anti-inflammatory steroids inhibit the release of arachidonic acid from phospholipids, i.e. inhibit formation of all products of the arachidonic acid cascade (Hirata et al, 1980).

Formation of the endoperoxides, PGG_2 and PGH_2, and products derived therefrom, seems to be possible in almost all mammalian tissues. However, biosynthesis of TxA_2, for example, was first demonstrated in thrombocytes where it seems to be the major product formed from arachidonic acid. In many tissues small amounts of TxB_2 (a chemical degradation product of TxA_2) can be found. However, this does not necessarily mean that the tissue cells *per se* are capable of synthesising TxA_2 since thrombocytes are present in all vascularised tissues. The same is true for PGI_2 which seems to be synthesised primarily in vessel walls. Generally PGE_2 and $PGF_{2\alpha}$ stimulate smooth muscle contractions *in vivo* and *in vitro*. However, PGE compounds cause relaxation of vascular smooth muscle and therefore lower blood pressure *in vivo*. TxA_2 causes aggregation of thrombocytes and contraction of smooth muscle in vessel walls while PGI_2 has opposite effects, i.e. inhibits thrombocyte aggregation and relaxes vascular smooth muscle. It is unclear whether thromboxane and PGI_2 have a physiological function outside the mammalian circulation.

Biosynthesis of leucotrienes has so far been demonstrated in leucocytes and mast cells upon exposure to ionophore and in lung tissue. Like the classical prostaglandins, leucotrienes can also be formed from 8,11,14-eicosatrienoic acid and 5,8,11,14,17-eicosapentaenoic acid yielding leucotrienes of the 3 and 5 series (number of double bonds; e.g. LtC_3, LtC_5 etc). Leucotrienes of the C and D type are extremely potent bronchoconstrictors, up to 20 000 times more potent than histamine, and increase the permeability of microvessels. LtB_4 on the other hand has very strong chemotactic effects on leucocytes. So far

no data are available on involvement of leucotrienes in human reproductive processes.

Metabolism

Prostaglandins of the E and F type are rapidly metabolised in the human body. Blood analysis following intravenous injections of ^3H-PGE_2 revealed that 90 per cent of the compound was inactivated after 1.5 min. About 50 per cent of the radioactivity could be recovered from urine during the first 5 hours following the injection. The corresponding figure with tritium-labeled $PGF_{2\alpha}$ was 90 per cent.

The initial degradation of the primary PGs involves oxidation at C-15 by prostaglandin dehydrogenase, particularly in the lungs, followed by reduction of the 13–14 double bond and then by β- and ω-oxidation of the side chains. The wide distribution of PG dehydrogenase and $\triangle^{13}$-reductase indicates the occurrence of local metabolism at the site of synthesis. In general the metabolites of PGs are considerably less biologically active than the primary compounds (Samuelsson et al, 1975). The biologically very potent compounds PGI_2 and thromboxane A_2 are chemically labile under conditions prevailing in the human body and seem to be rapidly converted to 6-keto-$PGF_{2\alpha}$ and thromboxane B_2, respectively. These latter compounds are essentially biologically inactive. However, both TxA_2 and PGI_2 might be enzymatically attacked *in vivo* before this chemical degradation occurs. Because of the potent aggregatory effect of TxA_2 on platelets the *in vivo* metabolism is difficult to study. Isotope labelled PGI_2 has been infused in man and the structures of the major urinary metabolites have been determined (Rosenkranz et al, 1980). This study demonstrates that PGI_2 undergoes metabolic degradation similar to PGE and PGF compounds, i.e. dehydrogenation at carbon 15, reduction of the 13–14 double bond and β- and Ω-oxidation.

MALE GENITAL TRACT

Prostaglandins in seminal fluid and accessory genital glands

Human seminal fluid contains a number of different prostaglandins. These are PGE_1, PGE_2, PGE_3, $PGF_{1\alpha}$, $PGF_{2\alpha}$, 19-OH-PGE_1, 19-OH-PGE_2, 19-OH-$PGF_{1\alpha}$, and 19-OH-$PGF_{2\alpha}$ (Samuelsson, 1963; Taylor & Kelly 1974, 1975). The 8-β-isomers of the 19-hydroxy compounds seem also to be present (Taylor, 1979). The concentrations of these prostaglandins are very high in comparison with other body fluids. One ejaculate contains a total of approximately 1 mg of the different prostaglandins. The concentration varies considerably, but is approximately 60 μg/ml for the PGEs, 2.5 μg/ml for the PGFs, 300 μg/ml for the 19-OH-PGEs and 15 μg/ml for the 19-OH-PGFs (Table 11.1) (Svanborg et al, 1982; Templeton et al, 1978). Equally high concen-

Table 11.1 Prostaglandin concentration in human seminal fluid

Groups of men	Mean value (µg/ml) and range				Reference
	PGEs	PGFs	19-OH-PGEs	19-OH-PGFs	
Infertile unselected	43 (7–117) n = 17	2.6 (1.4–4.8) n = 11	260 (113–427) n = 19	17.0 (9.4–34.1) n = 10	Svanborg et al (1982)
Fertile	62 (15–144) n =10	2.8 (1.0–5.3) n = 8	326 (155–638) n = 10	14.9 (7.0–20.6) n = 8	
Fertile lit	73 (2–272) n = 22	2.1 (0.1–7.0) n = 17	267 (53–1094) n = 22	18.3 (3.0–62.0) n = 16	Templeton et al (1978)

trations of prostaglandins have also been found in semen from several non-human primates, sheep and goat, although the relation between the different compounds varies.

The human prostate, testis and seminal vesicles all contain prostaglandins of the E and F types and are also able to biosynthesise these compounds (Hamberg, 1976; Carpenter et al, 1978; Conte et al, 1980).

The main source of human seminal prostaglandins seems to be the seminal vesicles since these compounds are present in the same fraction as fructose when split ejaculates are analysed (Eliasson, 1959).

Very little is known about the factors regulating the concentration of prostaglandins in human seminal plasma. Since androgens influence the secretory properties of the seminal vesicles, it is logical to assume also an effect on prostaglandin biosynthesis and release. Sturde (1971) has also found that androgen treatment for 6–12 weeks in men results in a large increase in prostaglandin concentration measured by bioassay. A rapid increase in 19-OH-PGE production was reported by Skakkebaek et al (1976) in castrated or hypogonadal men after testosterone replacement therapy. The effect on 19-OH-PGE concentrations was more marked than that on PGE concentrations.

Prostaglandins and male fertility

The high concentration of prostaglandins in the seminal fluid of men as compared with most tissues and body fluids has led to the assumption that these compounds are intimately involved in the reproductive processes. Early results based on bioassays have shown a positive correlation between prostaglandin concentration and the ability of the couple to conceive. These results have later been confirmed by quantitative chemical methods. Human males who are infertile for no apparent reason possess significantly lower concentrations of seminal prostaglandins, especially E prostaglandins, than men of normal fertility (Bygdeman et al, 1970b; Brummer & Gillespie, 1972; Collier et al, 1975). Bygdeman et al (1970b) showed that seminal fluid from fertile men contained about 55 µg of total E prostaglandins per ml, an amount that was significantly higher than the corresponding value of 18 µg/ml in semen of men from

infertile marriages in which no other abnormalities could be detected.

A significant lower 19-OH-PGE concentration in semen from men in infertile marriages has also been reported.

Evidence for a correlation between fertility and seminal prostaglandin concentration has also been found in sheep. Following artificial insemination the fertility of the rams increased by more than 15 per cent if PGE_2 and $PGF_{2\alpha}$ were added to the diluted ram semen in such amounts that the normal PG concentration was restored (Dimov & Georgiev, 1977).

The precise mechanism by which seminal prostaglandins influence fertility is unknown. In fact, the correlation need not to be one of direct cause and effect; the infertility may be due to some other factors which also produce low prostaglandin levels in semen. If the high prostaglandin concentration in the human seminal fluid is of importance for normal fertility, at least three modes of action have been suggested. The prostaglandins may act (a) on the spermatozoa themselves; (b) on the male reproductive tract at or shortly before ejaculation; or (c) on the female reproductive tract after ejaculation.

The first possibility has found some support in the fact that certain sperm qualities may be related to the prostaglandin concentration. Sperm density correlates with the prostaglandin concentration. If the sperm concentration is high, the concentrations of PGE's and 19-OH-PGE's are low (Kelly et al, 1979; Svanborg et al, 1982b). It has also recently been found that sperm motility is correlated to the ratio between 19-OH-PGEs and 19-OH-PGFs. This ratio was significantly higher in the semen from men with sperm of normal motility than in semen where the spermatozoa had an abnormal motility (Svanborg et al, 1983).

The 19-OH-PGEs have in contrast to PGEs a marked inhibitory action on sperm respiration. When 19-OH-PGEs were incubated with washed human spermatozoa, a lowered production of labelled carbon dioxide from C-14 fructose was observed (Kelly, 1977).

That seminal prostaglandins are of importance for ejaculation is an old idea, already suggested by von Euler in the early thirties. Later studies in laboratory animals have also shown that many prostaglandins have a stimulatory effect on smooth musculature in the epididymis, vas deferens and in seminal vesicles *in vitro*. Hedquist & von Euler (1972) have suggested that classical prostaglandins, by modulating the neurotransmission in the vas deferens and in the seminal vesicles, could regulate the contractile function of the accessory sex organs. Nothing seems to be known about the functional importance of the prostaglandins in this respect in the human.

It is possible that changes in uterine contractility during intercourse may facilitate sperm transport. During sexual stimulation in the human there is a marked increase in uterine activity that changes to inhibition following female orgasm. A pressure gradient between the vagina and the uterus may be the result, favouring passive sperm transport. These changes in uterine and vaginal contractility might be caused by seminal prostaglandins but experimental evidence to support this assumption is still lacking in the human. Evidence that PGE_1, PGE_2 and $PGF_{2\alpha}$ enhance sperm migration and hence fertilisation has, however, been provided in experiments in the rabbit (Chang et al, 1973; Spilman et al, 1973).

NON-PREGNANT UTERINE AND FALLOPIAN CONTRACTILITY

Non-pregnant uterus. In vitro

A stimulatory effect of $PGF_{2\alpha}$ and $PGF_{1\alpha}$ on the myometrium and a relaxing effect of PGE_2 and PGE_1 *in vitro* were reported by Swedish investigators in the sixties (Bygdeman, 1964; Sandberg et al, 1964, 1966). These pioneer studies also revealed that PGE_1 and PGE_2 stimulated the proximal portion of the tube and relaxed the distal part of the tube and the ampulla.

Recent investigators have revealed a complex response of the myometrium to prostaglandins depending on the localisation of the fibres and the phase of the menstrual cycle. The architecture of the muscle fibres within the uterus will therefore first be classified with a stepwise dissection of the different parts. The corpus uteri is composed of three different muscle layers: a thin subperitoneal layer parallel to or in a helix along the axis of the uterus, an intermediate irregular layer, and an internal spiral-shaped layer. In the isthmic part of the uterus the muscle fibres are organised in a circular direction. In the uterotubal junction three muscles layers have been identified: an outer spiral-shaped, an intermediate circular, and an internal longitudinal layer.

The separate effect of different prostanoids on the myometrium has been studied by Wilhelmsson et al (1979–1981).

PGE₂. Administration of PGE_2 inhibits the spontaneous contractility in the intermediate and the internal layer of the corpus uteri. However, the subperitoneal myometrial fibres generally show stimulation with low doses (1 ng/ml) while higher concentrations (100 ng/ml) induce relaxation.

The isthmus uteri is essentially insensitive to PGE_2. In the utero-tubal junction PGE_2 induces a stimulatory response in the outer layer while the circular intermediate layer responds with relaxation. The internal longitudinal layer shows a complex response to PGE_2 depending upon the phase of the cycle, with stimulation around ovulation and inhibition in the other phases of the cycle.

PGF₂α. Addition of $PGF_{2\alpha}$ stimulates all layers of the corpus uteri. Similarly to PGE_2 the isthmus uteri does not respond to $PGF_{2\alpha}$. The utero-tubal junction shows a constant stimulation to $PGF_{2\alpha}$ in all layers irrespective of phase of the cycle. A mixture of $PGF_{2\alpha}$ and PGE_2 in equal concentrations causes stimulation of the corpus uteri. But when the ratio $PGE_2 : PGF_{2\alpha}$ increases to 10:1 relaxation will occur in the corpus uteri.

PGI₂. This is synthesised in the myometrium from precursors within the endometrium. Administration of PGI_2 results in an inhibitory response in all muscle fibres of the myometrium irrespective of the phase of the menstrual cycle. Similarly, the muscle layers of the utero-tubal junction also respond with inhibition to PGI_2. The efficacy of PGI_2 in relaxing the strips is estimated to be one-tenth of $PGF_{2\alpha}$.

PGH₂. Moderate doses of PGH_2 (5–100 ng/ml) elicit a stimulatory response of the myometrium. Administration of higher doses cause a biphasic response with contraction followed by subsequent relaxation. In the utero-tubal layer administration of PGH_2 results in a stimulatory response in the muscle strips of the outer spiral-shaped and the inner layer while inhibition is obtained in the intermediate layer.

TxA₂. Thromboxane is the most potent prostanoid causing stimulation of the corpus uteri and all layers of the utero-tubal junction at doses as low as 0.07 ng/ml. The thromboxane is present in the thrombocytes and it has been suggested that thromboxane in the menstrual blood may be responsible for contraction of the utero-tubal junction, thus avoiding retrograde menstruation.

Oviduct in vitro

The oviduct is separated into a circular and a longitudinal muscle layer. The transport of the ovum is believed to be mediated by muscular contractions, probably elicited by prostaglandins. The follicular fluid at ovulation contains high concentrations of prostaglandins which after the rupture of the follicle may act on the muscle layers within the oviduct, and in the mesosalpinx. An increasing effect on the tension in the ovarian ligament may also facilitate the ovum pick up.

The isthmus of the oviduct in the human has been extensively studied *in vitro* by Lindblom et al, (1978). They observed that PGE_1 and PGE_2 relax the circular muscle layer and contract the longitudinal layer. Administration of $PGF_{2\alpha}$ constantly contracts the two muscle layers in accordance with the effect on the uterus. PGI_2 has been shown to elicit a weak stimulatory response. These different responses of prostaglandins suggest an interplay on tubal function which may mediate the opening of the isthmus under a dominance of PGE_2 and locking under $PGF_{2\alpha}$ dominance.

In the ampulla the myofibrils within the mucosal folds show a stimulatory effect of $PGF_{2\alpha}$ as expected. The effect of PGE_2 on these mucosal folds is dependent upon the phase of the cycle with increased contractility around ovulation but relaxation in all other phases. It is likely that the ratio of PGE and PGF is important for normal function of the oviduct.

Non-pregnant uterus. In vivo

Regulation of non-pregnant uterine contractility

The contractility of the myometrium can be recorded by open-ended catheter, micro-balloon or micro-transducer. Characteristic contractility patterns are observed during the different phases of the cycle. In the proliferative phase the contractions are characterised by small amplitude of 10–30 mmHg, a frequency of 1–3 per min with a resting tone of 10–25 mmHg. Around the time of ovulation the tone increases to 40–60 mmHg and the frequency increases to 3–5 per min with the amplitude reduced to 5–20 mmHg. After ovulation the tone decreases to 10–30 mmHg again and the amplitude increases to 80 mmHg.

By addition of exogenous steroid hormones to postmenopausal women it has been shown that oestrogens elicit the proliferative pattern (Bengtsson & Theobald, 1966). The secretory phase pattern can similarily be evoked by the addition of progestogens. Consequently, the different patterns observed during the menstrual cycle are dependent on the steroid hormone levels. When the progesterone concentration decreases in the late secretory phase increased uterine activity during menstruation is recognised. Regular contractions with high amplitude around 100–150 mmHg appear with a basal tone around 30–50 mmHg.

Excessive endogenous synthesis of prostaglandin $F_{2\alpha}$ occurs in connection with dysmenorrhoea. A uterine hypercontractility state is recorded during menstrual cramps. Administration of a potent prostaglandin biosynthesis inhibitor reduces myometrial contractility within 50 min (Lundström et al, 1976). Obviously, the synthesis of endogenous PG can be affected rapidly thus relieving menstrual pain. The exact relationship between steroid hormones and PG synthesis is not known. It is, however, believed that PG mediates the uterine contractility following steroid hormone impulses.

Administration of PG

Intravenous administration of both PGE_2 and $PGF_{2\alpha}$ result in stimulation of the myometrium. PGE_2 is generally 2–3 times more potent than $PGF_{2\alpha}$ (50 μg, threshold dose) (Roth-Brandel et al, 1970). PGI_2 has been tested intravenously without any effect on the contractility (Wilhelmsson et al, 1981; Swahn & Lundström, 1981).

A more specific response of $PGF_{2\alpha}$ and PGE_2 is obtained when prostaglandins are injected through a thin catheter into the uterine cavity. Extensive studies have been performed by Martin & Bygdeman (1975). Their experiments revealed that the myometrium is most sensitive in the early proliferative and late secretory phases. In these periods 1 μg of PGE_2 or 2–5 μg $PGF_{2\alpha}$ will elicit a strong stimulatory response. However, around ovulation the uterus is insensitive to PGE_2 and $PGF_{2\alpha}$. Doses as high as 40–50 μg may be without effect. If the doses are increased further inhibition was found by Toppozada et al, (1974). At menstruation a complex response following PGE_2 administration is observed. Low doses of PGE_2 (2–5 μg) still stimulate contractility while higher doses (30–40 μg) relax the myometrium. $PGF_{2\alpha}$, however, invariably stimulates uterine contractility even during menstruation.

Toppozada et al (1977) reported a discrepancy between infertile women in response to PGE_2 following local administration in comparison with normally fertile women. A strong stimulatory response of the myometrium is observed in women with unexplained infertility at midcycle, while the controls respond with slight inhibition. These authors indicate that an aberrant uterine response to PGE_2 at ovulation may be an aetiologic factor in functional infertility.

PGI_2 injected locally into the uterine cavity elicits a gradual stimulation. This effect is probably not any direct effect of PGI_2 on the muscle fibres but rather a secondary effect of its strong vascular effect (Wilhelmsson et al, 1981 Swahn & Lundström, 1983).

Little is known about the in vivo effect of the other prostanoids, thromboxane and endoperoxides.

PROSTAGLANDINS AND OVARIAN FUNCTION

In laboratory animals the prostaglandins appear to be of major importance in the sequential events of ovum maturation, follicular rupture and in the life span of the corpus luteum but their role in corresponding events in the human remains to be shown.

Ovulation

In laboratory animals, the role of prostaglandins in the mechanism of ovulation is well established. Systemic or local administration of inhibitors of prostaglandin synthesis as well as intrafollicular injections of a prostaglandin F antibody inhibit ovulation (Armstrong et al, 1974). This blockade cannot be overcome by the administration of LH but is reversed by the administration of exogenous prostaglandins. The finding that indomethacin fails to prevent a spontaneous pro-oestrous LH-surge, at least in the rat, also indicates that the prostaglandins are not essential for the neuroendocrine triggering of ovulation but act at a local ovarian level. The role of prostaglandin seems to be restricted to follicular rupture since the effect of LH on ovum maturation, cyclic AMP production and proges-terone production is not influenced during the blockade of prostaglandin synthesis (Lindner et al, 1980).

The endogenous levels of $PGF_{2\alpha}$ and PGE_2 in follicular fluid show a remarkable increase as ovulation approaches, but only in those follicles which go on to ovulation (LeMaire et al, 1975).

Prostaglandin synthesis is stimulated by LH. This effect can be mimicked *in vitro* by exogenous cyclic AMP suggesting that the LH effect may be mediated by cyclic AMP. The precise mechanism by which LH and cyclic AMP influences the increase in prostaglandin is unknown. The effect of LH and cyclic AMP on prostaglandin accumu-lation does not seem to be mediated via steroid synthesis since inhibition of steroidogenesis by aminoglutethinide does not prevent the usual increase in prostaglandin synthesis in rat follicles or follicles incubated *in vitro*. LeMaire et al (1979) have suggested that LH or cyclic AMP bring about their effect on prostaglandin accumu-lation through an increase in the synthesis of a limiting enzyme in the process such as a protein kinase, an acylhy-drolase or a prostaglandin synthetase.

The mechanism by which prostaglandins stimulate follicular rupture remains unknown. It has been suggested that the accumulation of prostaglandins in follicular fluid stimulates the release of lytic enzymes in the follicular apex and its germinal epithelium resulting in a breakdown of the follicular wall. Administration of $PGF_{2\alpha}$ has also been shown to stimulate the contractility of ovarian smooth musculature. It is thus possible that the increase in $PGF_{2\alpha}$ levels in follicular fluid just before ovulation may stimulate the contractility of ovarian smooth musculature and promote the rupture of the wall of the follicles (Bjersing, 1979).

The role of prostaglandins in follicular rupture in the human is unknown. In a recent study the prostaglandin $F_{2\alpha}$ concentration was measured in ovarian follicular fluid from 34 patients in different phases of the menstrual cycle. The follicular fluid was aspirated under laparoscopy. The $PGF_{2\alpha}$ concentration increased significantly during the preovula-tory phase reaching a peak on day 14, and decreased after midcycle, very similar to the finding in animals (Darling et al, 1982).

The effect of one biosynthesis inhibitor — aspirin — on ovulation has been studied in the human. Basal body temperature, LH levels in urine, plasma progesterone and cervical mucus were followed during a control and a treat-ment cycle. No effects on the parameters mentioned above indicating inhibition of ovulation were observed. Lapa-

rotomy performed in the secretory phase excluded an entrapped ovum and follicular luteinization (Chaudhuri & Elder, 1975).

The lack of effect of aspirin makes it doubtful that pros-taglandins are involved in follicular rupture in the human but the dosage of aspirin may have been insufficient to block prostaglandin synthesis in the ovarian follicles — a parameter which was not assessed in this study. Trials with more specific and effective inhibitors of prostaglandin synthetase are necessary before final conclusions can be reached.

Regulation of the non-pregnant corpus luteum

There are considerable evidences to support the concept that in many species — e.g. sheep, cow, horse, pig, pseu-dopregnant rat, rabbit and hamster — $PGF_{2\alpha}$ formed by the endometrium is the factor which controls the life span of the functional corpus luteum. Administration of $PGF_{2\alpha}$ has an unquestionably luteolytic effect in these species resulting in a decrease in peripheral progesterone plasma levels. A pulsatile release of $PGF_{2\alpha}$ in uterine venous blood just prior to luteal regression has also been established in several animals (Kindahl et al, 1976). The very rapid inac-tivation of circulating prostaglandins seems to exclude a systemic route of supply and to favour a local mechanism for transfer of $PGF_{2\alpha}$ from the uterus to the adjacent ovary. The intimate anatomical relationship between the utero-ovarian vein and the ovarian artery and the fact that the life span of the corpus luteum is prolonged merely by separating these structure support this assumption. A countercurrent transport of ^3H-$PGF_{2\alpha}$ from the uterine vein to the ovarian artery has also been demonstrated (McCracken et al, 1973).

The factors regulating the life span of the human non-pregnant corpus luteum are mainly unknown. That $PGF_{2\alpha}$ is involved still need confirmation. However, in the human there are several events occurring that indicate that this is the case. Both PGF_2 and $PGF_{2\alpha}$ are present in the human endometrium and several studies indicate an increased synthesis towards menstruation, especially in women with dysmenorrhea (Chan & Hill, 1978; Lundström & Gréen, 1978).

If $PGF_{2\alpha}$ is involved in the corpus luteum regression one would expect an increase in the plasma concentration prior to luteal regression. Since the release of $PGF_{2\alpha}$ according to animal studies is pulsatile and of short duration blood sampling at very short intervals is a prerequisite. In two studies, at least, daily blood samples were taken from normal cycling female volunteers during the whole menstrual cycle. The concentration of 15-keto-13, 14-dihydro-$PGF_{2\alpha}$ in peripheral venous plasma was measured by radio-immunoassay. According to Kuollapis & Collins (1980) two peaks, a preovulatory one associated with a marked increase in circulating oestradiol, and a premenstrual one associated with rapidly falling levels of circulating oestradiol and progesterone, were apparent in all cycles. At least the latter peak was attributed to an increase of prostaglandin $F_{2\alpha}$ synthesis and metabolism in the endometrium. In contrast to these results, Kindahl et al (1976) found no increase in circulating levels of 15-keto-13, 14-dihydro-$PGF_{2\alpha}$ around the peri-ovulatory period or during the luteal phase.

That $PGF_{2\alpha}$ receptors have been identified in cell membranes of the human corpus luteum (Powell et al, 1974) and that there is a close anatomical relationship between the ovarian-uterine artery and the uterine veins similar to that found in animals also speaks in favour of a role of $PGF_{2\alpha}$ in regulating the life span of the corpus luteum in the human (Bendz, 1977).

The major reason against this is that administration of exogenous $PGF_{2\alpha}$ apparently does not cause the corpus luteum to regress. A transient decline in progesterone has been reported by some investigators but in most studies no significant fall in plasma progesterone could be detected (Hillier et al, 1972; Jewelewicz et al, 1972; Kajanoja et al, 1978). Even intra-uterine administration of 0.5–2.0 mg $PGF_{2\alpha}$ every second hour for 12 hours was proved ineffective in female volunteers (Lyneham et al, 1975). To overcome the possibility that the exogenously administered $PGF_{2\alpha}$ was metabolised before reaching the ovary, the compound has also been administered directly into the corpus luteum. An injection of 0.5–1.0 mg administered by this route produced a rapid and profound fall in plasma progesterone levels coinciding with the onset of uterine bleeding. The plasma levels of progesterone, however, returned to normal luteal levels before the end of the cycle (Korda et al, 1975). That a low local concentration of $PGF_{2\alpha}$ in the corpus luteum may be one reason for the lack of luteolytic effect of this compound is further substantiated by the fact that prostaglandin F analogues protected from rapid metabolic degradation have a more pronounced luteolytic effect than the parent compound (Leader at al, 1976). One possible explanation of the lack of luteolytic effect of $PGF_{2\alpha}$ in the human is that increasing amounts of $PGF_{2\alpha}$ are produced in the ovary itself at the end of the cycle saturating the receptors (Powell et al, 1974).

PREGNANT UTERUS

In vitro

One of the first observations on the effects of the prostaglandins was that they influenced the activity of human pregnant myometrium in vitro. In general, PGF compounds stimulated myometrial contractility while E prostaglandins may induce a stimulation at low dose levels but invariably reverse their effect to an inhibitory one when the dose was increased (Bygdeman, 1964). The sensitivity to $PGF_{2\alpha}$ was the same if the myometrial strips were obtained from a non-pregnant or from a mid-pregnant uterus. Brummer (1971) compared myometrial sensitivity to oxytocin and PGE_2 at mid-pregnancy and at term in vitro experiments. There was a 20-fold increase in sensitivity to oxytocin and only a 2–4-fold increase to PGE_2 with advancing pregnancy.

In vivo

Study of the pharmacological effects of the pure PGs on human uterine contractility under in vivo conditions was a natural sequential step to the earlier in vitro experiments and provided solid background for subsequent clinical trials to induce labour and abortion. In contrast to the in vitro actions, it is now established beyond doubt that both the E and F prostaglandins are potent in vivo stimulants of the human uterus at any stage of pregnancy.

The basic response of the early and mid-pregnant uterus to acute intravenous injections of the primary PGs is characterised by rapid elevation of uterine tonus that declines gradually toward the normal resting level. The increment in tone was utilised as a satisfactory parameter to evaluate the potency and to compare the dose–response relationship of various PGs. The threshold dose of a single intravenous injection at mid-prenancy is about 20 μg PGE_1, 100–200 μg $PGF_{2\alpha}$, and around 500 μg $PGF_{1\alpha}$. Separate intravenous injection of various PGs given in graded doses showed that the uterine sensitivity to PGE_1 and PGE_2 is virtually the same. The potency of PGE_1 is approximately eight times higher than $PGF_{2\alpha}$ and about 30–40 times that of $PGF_{1\alpha}$ (Bygdeman et al, 1970a).

The initial response of the early and mid-pregnant human uterus to an intravenous infusion of primary PGs generally resembles that following a single intravenous injection. However, continued administration maintains the uterine activity with the evolution of labour-like contractions as the resting pressure declines toward the preinfusion level.

If $PGF_{2\alpha}$ or PGE_2 are administered as an intravenous infusion at or near term in stepwise increasing doses, a contractility pattern developes which is indistinguishable from that of normal labour or labour induced by oxytocin. Therapeutic doses of PGE_2 or $PGF_{2\alpha}$ are significantly lower at term in comparison with those during mid-pregnancy indicating an increase in sensitivity of the myometrium during the last half of pregnancy.

If oxytocin and naturally occurring prostaglandins are compared with regard to stimulation of uterine contractility, both similarities and differences in effect can be demonstrated. As mentioned above, labours at term induced by oxytocin or by prostaglandin are very similar. On the other hand, it is well known that the non-pregnant and the early pregnant uterus are insensitive even to large doses of oxytocin. An increase in sensitivity occurs around the 20th week of gestation and there is then a progressive augmentation of the sensitivity until the 36th week after which it remains unchanged until the beginning of spontaneous labour. The situation is completely different as far as the prostaglandins are concerned. The non-pregnant uterus responds readily even to small doses of prostaglandins and the sensitivity of the uterus then remains virtually unchanged during early pregnancy and mid-pregnancy.

The effect of prostaglandins and oxytocin also differs in that the prostaglandin response has approximately three times longer duration than the oxytocin effect following single intravenous injection at mid-pregnancy (Roth-Brandel et al, 1970). If the compounds are administered extra-amniotically, oxytocin has no effect even in high doses while $PGF_{2\alpha}$ and PGE_2 administered by the same route stimulate forceful uterine contractions (Wiqvist et al, 1972). The reason for this difference is unclear but may reflect the basic difference between the compounds; oxytocin, a classical hormone, being released from an endocrine gland and carried by the circulation to its effector organ, while the classical prostaglandins are formed and act at the same place.

CLINICAL APPLICATIONS

The clinical use of prostaglandins depends mainly on the unique ability of these compounds to stimulate uterine contractility during all stages of pregnancy. The classical prostaglandins, E_2 and $F_{2\alpha}$, and various prostaglandin analogues administered by different routes are used for termination of very early pregnancy, for dilatation of the cervix before vacuum aspiration in late first trimester and early second trimester pregnancy, and for second trimester abortion. Intravenous administration of PGE_2 and $PGF_{2\alpha}$ and oral administration of PGE_2 are also used for induction of labour at or near term, and vaginal, intracervical or extra-amniotic administration of PGE_2 for ripening of the cervix prior to labour induction.

Termination of early pregnancy

While PG therapy has a recognised position in termination of second trimester pregnancies, the use of PG for menstrual regulation is still in an exploratory phase. The ultimate goal is to develop a self-administered, non-surgical procedure which could compete with vacuum aspiration. The initial trails using classical PGs were discouraging. The only effective route was intra-uterine administration and premedication was necessary to reduce the frequency of side-effects. The situation has changed, at least partly, with the availability of PG analogues. Intra-uterine administration of different analogues has been shown to be highly effective in terminating early pregnancy (Karim et al, 1977; Tagaki et al, 1977).

Encouraging progress has also been reported following vaginal administration of PG analogues. Repeated or single vaginal administration of 15-methyl-$PGF_{2\alpha}$-methyl ester has been shown to be highly effective, but even more promising seems the use of some new PGE analogues with increased stability in suppository form or in preparations for i.m. injections. To this group belong 16,16-dimethyl-trans-$\triangle^2$-PGE_1 methyl ester, 9-deoxo-16,16-dimethyl-9-methylene PGE_2 and 16-phenoxy-ω-17,18,19,20-tetranor PGE_2 methyl sulfonylamide. The two first compounds are administered vaginally, the third one by intramuscular injection.

In a comparative study all three E analogues were found to be equally effective. The frequency of complete abortion was between 92 per cent and 94 per cent. Side-effects were limited to occasional vomiting and diarrhoea in approximately 50 per cent of the patients (Bygdeman et al, 1980b, 1982). One group of patients was allowed to treat themselves at home. Prerequisites were at least one previous pregnancy and a positive attitude to home treatment. The analogue used was 9-deoxo-16,16-dimethyl-9-methylene PGE_2 which was administered vaginally twice at 6-hourly intervals. The outcome of that study, which is the first attempt of medical home abortion, was promising. The 'success rate' was even slightly higher than that found in hospital treated patients showing that selfadministration is practicable. The only problem was uterine pain. Two patients (4 per cent) experienced strong uterine pain necessitating hospital visits and an analgesic injection for alleviation (Bygdeman et al, 1981).

The clinical events following treatment are very similar following both intra-uterine and vaginal administration. Both methods result in an increase in uterine contractility followed by bleeding, which generally starts 3–6 hours after the initiation of therapy and lasts for 1–2 weeks. Clinical supervision of the patient, ultrasound examination of the uterus, as well as a decrease in the level of plasma hCG indicate that most patients abort during the first 24 hours. Minor products of conception may, however, remain in the cavity for several weeks (Mandelin, 1978). The bleeding is described by most patients as heavier than a menstrual period but is does not generally affect the haemoglobin values. Heavy blood loss occurs in less than 2 per cent of the patients.

The actual blood loss has been measured in two studies. Hamberger et al (1978) found that the average blood loss during the first 24 hours following repeated vaginal administration of 15-methyl-$PGF_{2\alpha}$ methyl ester was 37 ml. The total blood loss was 131 ml, which corresponds to that of a heavy menstruation but is greater than that generally reported for the surgical procedure. In the other study in which vaginal administration of 9-deoxo-16,16-dimethyl-9-methylene PGE_2 was used the blood loss during the entire bleeding period was 61 ml (range 21–156) (Bygdeman et al, 1983).

The abortifacient effect of prostaglandin treatment

during early pregnancy is thought to be due mainly to increased uterine activity. The fall of progesterone values after approximately 4 hours probably reflects a disruption of the implanted ovum rather than a primary luteolytic effect of the compound. The progesterone drop may facilitate the development of regular uterine contactions, but it does not appear to be necessary for the progression of the abortion process, since some patients start to bleed before the fall of the plasma progesterone concentration.

In patients who seem to abort completely, the mean plasma human chorionic gonadotrophin (hCG) concentration decreases rapidly during the day of treatment. The decrease is significant within 8 hours after the start of treatment. After 1 week the hCG concentration in plasma is 2–5 per cent of the starting value. During the second week the decrease is somewhat slower. A similar disappearance rate has been reported following interruption of early pregnancy by vacuum aspiration (Lundström et al, 1977).

There appear to be only two randomised studies of prostaglandin treatment versus surgical procedures for termination of early pregnancy. One compares intra-uterine administration of 5 mg of $PGF_{2\alpha}$ with vacuum aspiration in patients with amenorrhoea of up to 56 days; the other compares repeated vaginal administration of 16,16-dimethyl-PGE_2 with the operative procedure (Ragab & Edelman, 1976; Lundström et al, 1977). It was concluded from these studies that administration of a suitable prostaglandin by either of the two routes was as effective as vacuum aspiration for termination of early pregnancy. Both the surgical and the non-surgical method were suitable as out-patient procedures. Vacuum aspiration requires less hospital time, caused fewer gastro-intestinal side-effects, and resulted in a shorter period of bleeding.

The acceptability of vaginal prostaglandin treatment and vacuum aspiration has also been evaluated (Rosén et al, 1979). The attitudes of women towards both methods were determined before assignment to the abortion procedure, immediately after treatment and 2 weeks later. It was found that the acceptability of the method used increased throughout the study period with either method.

Dilatation of the cervix prior to vacuum aspiration

It is generally agreed that the frequency of complications following vacuum aspiration or dilatation and curettage (D & C)increases with increasing gestational age (Edelman et al, 1974).Some of these complications, e.g. cervical injury and uterine perforation, are directly related to the mechanical dilatation necessary for the procedure, especially during the late part of the first trimester and early part of the second trimester. Grimes et al (1977) have reported that if D & C is performed after the 12th week of gestation cervical injury is twice as frequent and uterine perforation more than six times as frequent as with the saline infusion technique.

Other complications, e.g. haemorrhage and incomplete evacuation of the conceptus, may possibly be related to insufficient or difficult dilatation. Increasing concern with the effects of cervical injury on long-term reproductive behaviour has also focused the interest of clinicians on methods producing gradual cervical dilatation (WHO Task Force on Sequelae of Abortion, 1979).

There are at present two methods used to achieve cervical dilatation prior to surgical evacuation of the uterus — insertion of laminaria tents and prostaglandin treatment. The main disadvantage of the clinical use of laminaria is still the risk of infection. The reported incidence of infection attributed to laminaria is between 0.8 and 2.2 per cent. Difficulties in introducing the laminaria tent may occasionally occur and transcervical migration of laminaria tents has been documented.

Several studies have shown that pre-treatment with PG analogues by noninvasive routes results in a gradual dilatation of the cervical canal (Karim & Prasad, 1979). The degree of cervical dilatation is related to the duration of treatment. A 12-hour pre-treatment period is preferable if maximum dilatation of the cervical canal is wanted. A 3-hour pre-treatment period is sufficient, however, in many patients and in the majority of the remaining ones, additional mechanical dilatation is an easy procedure (WHO Prostaglandin Task Force, 1981).

In a large multicentre study it was shown that pretreatment with 1.0 mg 15-methyl-$PGF_{2\alpha}$ methyl ester administered vaginally in comparison with placebo resulted in a significant decrease in operative blood loss and in postoperative complications (recurettage, treatment of infection and duration of bleeding). The only problem was that gastro-intestinal side-effects were more common with active suppositories than with placebo. This disadvantage seems to be almost negligible if 9-deoxo-16,16-dimethyl-9-methylene PGE_2 or 16,16-dimethyl-trans-$\triangle^2$-PGE_1 methyl ester is used instead (Prasad et al, 1978; Bygdeman et al, 1981).

Termination of second trimester pregnancy

Intra-uterine administration of $PGF_{2\alpha}$ and PGE_2 for termination of second trimester pregnancy has been used on a routine basis for several years. Whether this procedure is better than other methods in current use is difficult to evaluate since randomised studies are few. The only available ones compare intra-amniotic administration of hypertonic saline and $PGF_{2\alpha}$ (Edelman et al, 1976; WHO Prostaglandin Task Force, 1976).

These studies show that intra-amniotic administration of $PGF_{2\alpha}$ is more effective than hypertonic saline alone. The difference is reduced if $PGF_{2\alpha}$ and hypertonic saline are supplemented with intravenous infusion of oxytocin. Intra-venous oxytocin infusion is, however, inconvenient and water intoxication can occur. $PGF_{2\alpha}$ is also easier to administer than hypertonic saline since the volume to be injected is much smaller (8–10 ml compared with 200 ml).

For a number of hypothetical reasons intra-amniotic $PGF_{2\alpha}$ may also be less dangerous than saline: (1) hypernatraemia is not a risk; (2) inadvertent intravascular or intraperitoneal injection of $PGF_{2\alpha}$ appears to be less dangerous since $PGF_{2\alpha}$ is rapidly metabolised; (3) there is less tissue damage from inappropriate administration of $PGF_{2\alpha}$; and (4)consumption coagulapathies appear to be less frequent with $PGF_{2\alpha}$.

The frequency of gastrointestinal side-effects is higher following $PGF_{2\alpha}$ therapy. This is also the case for cervical laceration and cervico-vaginal fistula, especially if prostaglandin therapy is augmented with intravenous oxytocin administration. When oxytocin is used, these complications may be as frequent as 2 per cent.

The increased bleeding following abortion which has been reported by some investigators (Grimes et al, 1977) seems more likely to be due to factors such as the degree of contractility at the time of the abortion and the duration of observation before the placenta is removed than to be specifically related to prostaglandins. In practice, when hypertonic saline and classic prostaglandins are used by skilled pysicians, there are few differences in complication rates except for cervical fistulae.

Prostaglandin analogues, e.g. 15(S)15-methyl $PGF_{2\alpha}$, have been developed which are more effective and have a longer duration of action than naturally occurring prostaglandins. These compounds are more suitable than the parent compounds for single intra-amniotic injection procedures for termination of second trimester pregnancy. In a multicentre study including 1521 patients, $PGF_{2\alpha}$ (40 or 50 mg) and 15(S)15-methyl $PGF_{2\alpha}$ (2.5 mg) administered intra-amniotically were compared. Almost 95 per cent of the patients who received 15(S)15-methyl $PGF_{2\alpha}$ aborted without additional therapy. The corresponding figures for 40 and 50 mg $PGF_{2\alpha}$ were significantly lower, 81.7 and 86.6 per cent respectively (WHO Prostaglandin Task Force, 1977a).

The most important advantage of the analogues compared with other compounds presently used for termination of second trimester pregnancy is, however, that several of them, e.g. 15(S)15-methyl $PGF_{2\alpha}$ methyl ester, 16-phenoxy-ρ-17,18,19,20-tetranor PGE_2 methyl sulfonylamide, 16,16-dimethyl-trans-$\triangle^2$-PGE_2 methyl ester, and 9-deoxo-16,16-dimethyl-9-methylene PGE_2, are suitable for administration by non-invasive routes. Some of the major complications associated with second trimester abortion are due to inadvertent intravenous injection of the compound when it is administered intra-amniotically. If the vaginal or the intramuscular route is used, such complications can be avoided. These routes offer the additional advantage that the treatment is equally useful during both the early and late part of the second trimester.

The results of a multicentre study, performed by the WHO Prostaglandin Task Force, showed that repeated intramuscular injection of 15(S)15-methyl $PGF_{2\alpha}$ was an effective method to terminate second trimester preganancy. The treatment was, however, associated with a high frequency of gastrointestinal side-effects. It was therefore concluded that this method has a limited value as a primary abortion technique, but can be useful in order to finalise the abortion process when another method has failed. The frequency of gastrointestinal side effects may be reduced if the analogue 16-phenoxy-ω-17,18,19,20-tetranor PGE_2 methyl sulfonylamide is used. Karim et al (1978) have reported that approximately 90 per cent of the patients abort within 24 hours when this analogue is administered by the intramuscular route. The overall incidence of diarrhoea and vomiting was low (one episode per patient) or only slightly higher than that reported for intra-amniotic administration of hypertonic saline.

Similar progress has been achieved following vaginal administration. Vaginal administration of suppositories containing 15(S)15-methyl $PGF_{2\alpha}$ methyl ester is highly effective in terminating second trimester pregnancy. Although gastro-intestinal side-effects may be less frequent following vaginal administration of 15(S)15-methyl $PGF_{2\alpha}$ methyl ester than following intramuscular administration of the free acid of the same compound, in some patients the number of episodes of vomiting and diarrhoea remains unpleasantly high (Bygdeman et al, 1977; WHO Prostaglandin Task Force, 1977b). Vaginal administration of 9-deoxo-16,16-dimethyl-9-methylene PGE_2, an analogue which is also stable in the suppository form, is equally effective as 15(S)15-methyl $PGF_{2\alpha}$ methyl ester but the frequency of gastrointestinal side-effects is significantly lower and of the same magnitude as observed following intramuscular administration of 16-phenoxy-ω-17,18,-19,20-tetranor PGE_2 methyl sulfonylamide (Bygdeman et al, 1979).

The most effective procedure seems at present to be pretreatment with one laminaria tent for 12 hours followed by intramuscular injection of 16-phenoxy-ω-17,18,19,20-tetranor PGE_2 methyl sulfonylamide. This method is highly effective, the success rate approaching 100 per cent. The duration of labour is short (approximately 10 hours) and the frequency of gastrointestinal side-effects low or only slightly higher than that reported for hypertonic saline. Also the risk of cervical laceration seems significantly reduced (Karim et al, 1982; Bygdeman & Christensen, 1983). Table 11.2 summarises some data on non-invasive methods for termination of second trimester pregnancy. In all these studies the criteria for accepting the patients, the general management of the patients and definitions of success, complete abortion, etc have been the same. The results may therefore be more comparable than those of independent studies.

Table 11.2 Comparison of selected prostaglandin analogues administered by no-invasive routes for termination of second trimester pregnancy

Treatment	Frequency of abortion (%)	Mean No. of gastrointestinal side-effects		Duration of labour (hrs)	References
		Vomiting	Diarrhoea		
Laminaria + i.m. injection of 15-methyl PGF$_{2\alpha}$	98*	0.8	0.8	10.7	Bygdeman & Christensen (1983)
Laminaria + i.m. injection of 16-phenoxy-17,18,19,20-tetranor PGE$_2$ methyl sulfonylamide	98*	0.8	0.1	9.3	"
I.m. injection of 16-phenoxy-PGE$_2$ methyl sulfonylamide	81.3†	1.1	0.4	15.7	WHO Prostaglandin Task Force (1982)
Vaginal administration of 9-methylene PGE$_2$	83.0†	0.9	0.3	15.2	Bygdeman et al (1980a)
Vaginal administration of 15-methyl PGF$_{21}$ me-ester	80.0†	1.9	1.6	15.8	WHO Prostaglandin Task Force (1983)
Vaginal administration of 15-methyl PGF$_{2\alpha}$ methyl ester + i.m. injection of 15-me-PGF$_{2\alpha}$	93.1**	2.8	2.1	18.6	"

* Within 24 hours;   † Within 30 hours;   ** Within 36 hours.

Ripening of the cervix

The possibility of ripening the cervix at or near term is an important new therapeutic possibility for prostaglandins. An unripe cervix in late pregnancy is a bad prognostic sign, especially in the primigravida. If labour has to be induced, it may be protracted and difficult. Although the cervix ripens if given time, few, if any, obstetric indications for delivery diminish with the passage of time. The normal mechanism by which the cervix ripens before effacement and dilatation during labour is still unknown. Experimental data suggest that PGs, possible together with placental hormones, have a physiological role (Ellwood et al, 1979).

Prostaglandins, mainly PGE$_2$, have been administered orally, vaginally, into the cervical canal, or into the extra-amniotic space in clinical trials. Data indicate that extra-amniotic or intracervical administration of 0.5 mg PGE$_2$ in gel form is more effective than other routes of administration. If cervical ripening is obtained, reduced fetal and maternal complication rates will result (Ulmsten & Wingerup, 1979; Calder, 1979). The disadvantage of the therapy at present is lack of stable PG preparations.

Induction of labour

Intravenous administration of PGF$_{2\alpha}$ and PGE$_2$ has a recognised therapeutic role for induction of labour. The superiority (at most very slight) of either of these compounds over the other or over intravenous infusion of oxytocin remains a matter of controversy. The advantages and disadvantages of the three compounds were recently summarised by Thiery & Amy (1977). All three compounds are equally effective in patients with favourable prognoses for induction. PG is probably slightly superior for difficult induction and in pregnancy complicated by fetal death or anencephaly. The margin of effective dose is somewhat narrower for prostaglandin, and occasional gastrointestinal upsets and venous erythema are associated with PG therapy.

PGE$_2$ may also be given as oral tablets. The design of dose schedules in the past was dependent on clinical results. It has been shown by gas chromatography – mass spectrometry that the E metobolite reaches a peak in plasma concentration 1 hour after administration indicating that hourly administration is preferable (Bremme & Bygdeman, 1980; Bremme et al, 1980).

Oral PGE$_2$ therapy appears to be a valuable alternative to intravenous oxytocin for the induction of labour at term. The method is generally well accepted by the patient. The main advantage is the ease and simplicity of the treatment. Complications are rare, particularly in multiparous patients, with favourable prospects for induction. When combined with early amniotomy, intravenous and oral PGE$_2$ are equally effective and both procedures are more effective than intravenous oxytocin alone for labour induction.

Irregular uterine contractions may be more common during oral PGE_2 administration than during intravenous infusion of oxytocin. It is, however, equally rare with PGE_2 and oxytocin that these abnormalities, as well as hypertonus, are associated with abnormal changes in fetal heart rate. Evidence of overstimulation following oral PGE_2 is a very rare phenomenon if the dose is restricted to 1.0–1.5 mg/h (Thiery & Amy, 1978; Bremme & Bygdeman, 1980).

REFERENCES

Armstrong D T, Grinwich O L, Moon Y S, Samecnik J 1974 Inhibition of ovulation in rabbits by intrafollicular injection of indomethacin and prostaglandin F antiserum. Life Sciences 14: 129–140

Bendz A 1977 The anatomical basis for a possible countercurrent exchange mechanism in the human adnexae. Prostaglandins 13: 355–362

Bengtsson L P, Theobald G W 1966 The effects of oestrogen and gestagen on the non-pregnant human uterus. Journal of Obstetrics and Gynaecology of the British Commonwealth 73: 273–285

Bjersing L 1979 Intraovarian mechanisms of ovulation. In: Hafez E S E (ed) Human Ovulation, pp 149–157. Elsevier/North-Holland Biomedical Press

Bremme K, Bygdeman M 1980 Induction of labour by oxytoxin or prostaglandin $F_{2\alpha}$. Acta Obstetrica et Gynecological Scandinavica Suppl 92: 11–21

Bremme K, Kindahl H, Svanborg K 1980 Induction of labour by oral PGE_2 administration — evaluation of different dose schedules. Acta Obstetrica et Gynecologica Scandinavica Suppl 92: 5–10

Brummer H C 1971 Interaction of E prostaglandin and syntocinon on the pregnant human myometrium. Journal of Obstetrics and Gynaecology of the British Commonwealth 78: 305–309

Brummer H C, Gillespie A 1972 Seminal prostaglandins and fertility. Clinical Endocrinology 1: 363–368

Bygdeman M 1964 The effect of different prostaglandins on human myometrium in vitro. Acta Physiologica Scandinavica 63: Suppl 242

Bygdeman M, Gréen K, 1980 Prostaglandins and related compounds. In: Gold J J (ed) Gynecologic Endocrinology, 3rd edn, pp 801–819. Harper & Row, Hagerstown.

Bygdeman M, Christensen N 1983 Randomized comparison between laminaria and either intramuscular injection of 15-methyl $PGF_{2\alpha}$ or 16-phenoxy-ω-17,18,19,20-tetranor-PGE_2 methyl sulfonylamide. Acta Obstetrica et Gynecologica Scandinavica 62: 535–537

Bygdeman M, Kwon S U, Mukherjee T, Roth-Brandel U, Wiqvist N 1970a The effect of the prostaglandin F compounds on the contractility of the pregnant human uterus. American Journal of Obstetrics and Gynecology 106: 567–572

Bygdeman M, Fredricsson B, Svanborg K, Samuelsson K 1970b. The relation between fertility and prostaglandin content of seminal fluid in man. Fertility and Sterility 26: 622–629

Bygdeman M, Ganguli A, Kinoshita K, Lundström V, Gréen K, Bergström S 1977 Development of a vaginal suppository suitable for single administration for interruption of second trimester pregnancy. Contraception 15: 129–141

Bygdeman M, Green K, Bergström S, Bundy G, Kimball F 1979 New prostaglandin E$_2$ analogue for pregnancy termination. Lancet i: 1136

Bygdeman M. Christensen N, Gréen K, Lundström V 1980a Midtrimester abortion by vaginal administration of 9-deoxo-16,16-dimethyl-9-methylene PGE_2. Contraception 22: 153–164

Bygdeman M, Bremme K, Christensen N, Lundström V, Gréen K 1980b A comparison of two stable prostaglandin E analogues for termination of early pregnancy and for cervical dilatation. Contraception 22: 471–483

Bygman M, Christensen N, Gréen K, Zheng S 1981 Self-administration of prostaglandins for termination of early pregnancy. Contraception 24: 45–52

Bygdeman M, Christensen N, Gréen K, Zheng S, Lundström V 1983 Termination of early pregnancy — future development. Acta Obstetrica et Gynecologica Scandinavica Suppl 113: 125–129

Calder A A 1979 Prostaglandins for pre-induction ripening. In: Karim S M M (ed) Practical Applications of Prostaglandins and their Synthesis Inhibitors, pp 301–318. MTP Press Ltd, Lancaster

Carpenter M, Robinson R, Thuy L 1978 Prostaglandin metabolism by human testis. Lipids 13: 308–311

Chan W Y, Hill J C 1978 Determination of menstrual prostaglandin levels in nondysmenorrheic and dysmenorrheic subjects. Prostaglandins 15: 365–375

Chang M C, Hunt D M, Polge C 1973 Effects of prostaglandins on sperm and egg transport in the rabbit. Advances in Bioscience 9: 805–810

Chaudhuri C, Elder M G 1975 Lack of evidence for inhibition of ovulation by aspirin in women. Prostaglandins 11: 727–735

Collier J G, Flower R L, Stanton S L 1975 Seminal prostaglandins in fertile men. Fertility and Sterility 26: 868–871

Conte D, Laguzzi G, Boniforti L, Cantafora A, Di Silverio F, Latino C, Lalloni G, Mesolella V, Isidori A 1980 Prostaglandin content and metabolic activity of the human prostate. In: Crastes de Paulet A, Thaler-Dao H, Dray F (eds) Prostaglandins and Reproductive Physiology, pp 89–96. INSERM, Paris

Darling M R N, Jagee M, Elder M G 1982 Prostaglandin $F_{2\alpha}$ levels in the human ovarian follicle. Prostaglandins 23: 551–556

Dimov V, Georgiev G 1977 Ram semen prostaglandin concentration and its effect on fertility. Journal of Animal Science 44: 1050–1054

Edelman D A, Brenner W E, Mehta A C, Phillips F S, Bhatt R V, Bwiwandiwala P 1976 A comparative study of intra-amniotic saline and two prostaglandin $F_{2\alpha}$ dose schedules for midtrimester abortion. American Journal of Obstetrics and Gynecology 125: 188–195

Eliasson R 1959 Studies on prostaglandins. Acta Physiologica Scandinavica Suppl 158: 1–73

Ellwood O A, Mitchell M D, Anderson A, Turnbull A C 1979 Oestrogens, prostaglandins and cervical ripening. Lancet i: 376–377

Grimes D A, Schutz K F, Cates W, Taylor C W 1977 Midtrimester abortion by intra-amniotic prostaglandin $F_{2\alpha}$. Safer than saline? Obstetrics and Gynecology 49: 612–616

Hamberg M 1976 Biosynthesis of prostaglandin E_1 by human seminal vesicles. Lipids 11: 249–250

Hamberger L, Nilsson L, Björn-Rasmussen E, Atterfeldt P, Wiqvist N 1978 Early abortion by vaginal suppositories. Contraception 17: 183–194

Hedqvist P, von Euler U 1972 Prostaglandin induced neurotransmission feature in the field stimulated isolated vas deferens. Neuropharmacology 11: 177–187

Hillier K, Dutton A, Corker C S, Singer A, Embrey M D 1972 Plasma steroid and luteinizing hormone levels during prostaglandin $F_{2\alpha}$ administration in luteal phase of menstrual cycle. British Medical Journal 4: 333–336

Hirata F, Schiffman E, Venkatasubramanian K, Salomon D, Axelrod J 1980 A phospholipase A_2 inhibitory protein in rabbit neutrophils induced by glucocorticoids. Proceedings of the National Academy of Sciences of the United States of America 77: 2533–2536

Jewelewicz R, Cantor B, Dyrenfurth I, Warren M P, van de Wiele R L 1972 Intravenous infusion of prostaglandin $F_{2\alpha}$ in the midluteal phase of the nomal human menstrual cycle. Prostaglandins 1: 443–451

Kajanaja P, Ranta T, Seppälä M 1978 Effect of prostaglandin $F_{2\alpha}$ on ovarian and pituitary function in the midluteal phase. Prostaglandins 16: 327–332

Karim S M M, Rao B, Ratnam S S, Prasad R N V, Wong Y M, Ilancheran A 1977 Termination of early pregnancy with 16-phenoxy-ω-17,18,19,2-tetranor PGE_2 methyl sulfonylamide. Contraception 16: 377–381

Karim S M M, Chou H T, Lim A L, Yeo K C, Ratnam S S 1978 Termination of second trimester pregnancy with intramuscular administration of 16-phenoxyl-ω-17,18,19,20-tetranor- PGE₂ methyl sulfonylamide.Prostaglandins 15: 1063–1067

Karim S M M, Ratnam S S, Lim A L, Yeo K G, Choo H T 1982 Termination of second trimester pregnancy wwith laminaria and intramuscular 16-phenoxy-ω17,18,19,20-tetranor PGE₂ methyl sulfonylamide — a randomized study. Prostaglandins 23: 257–264

Kelly R W 1977 Effect of seminal prostaglandins on the metabolism of spermatozoa. Journal of Reproductive Fertility 50: 219–222

Kelly R W, Cooper I, Templeton A A 1979 Reduced prostaglandin levels in the semen of men with very high sperm concentration. Journal of Reproductive Fertility 56: 195–199

Kindahl H, Granström E, Edqvist L E, Eneroth P 1976 Prostaglandin levels in peripheral plasma during the reproduction cycle. In: Samuelsson B, Paoletti R (eds) Advances in Prostaglandin and Thromboxane Research, Vol 2, pp 667–671. Raven Press, New York

Korda A R, Shutt D A, Smith I D, Shearman R P, Lyneham R C 1975 Assessment of possible luteolytic effect of intraovarian injection of prostaglandin F₂ₐ in the human. Prostaglandins 9: 443–450

Koullapis E N, Collins W P 1980 The concentration of 13,14dihydro-15-oco-prostaglandin F₂ₐ in peripheral venous plasma throughout the normal ovarian and menstrual cycle. Acta Endocrinologica 93: 123–138

Leader A, Bygdeman M, Eneroth P, Martin N J, Wiqvist N 1976 The effect of infusion with two analogues of prostaglandin F₂ₐ on corpus luteum function. In: Samuelsson B, Paoletti R (eds) Advances in Prostaglandin and Thromboxane Research, Vol 2, pp 679–685. Raven Press, New York

LeMaire W J, Leidner R, March J M 1975 Pre- and post-ovulatory changes in the concentration of prostaglandins in rat Scaafian follicles. Prostaglandins 9: 221–229

LeMaire W J, Clark M R, Marsh J M 1979 Biochemical mechanisms of ovulation. In: Hafez E S E (ed) Human Ovulation. pp 159–176. Elsevier, Amsterdam

Lindblom B, Hamberg L, Wiqvist N 1978 Differentiated contractile effect of prostaglandins E and F on isolated circular and longitudinal smooth muscle of the human oviduct. Fertility and Sterility 11: 893–904

Lundström V, Gréen K 1978 Endogenous levels of prostaglandin F₂ₐ and its main metabolites in plasma and endometrium of normal and dysmenorrheic woman. American Journal of Obstetrics and Gynecology 130: 640–646

Lundstöm V, Gréen K, Wiqvist N 1976 Prostaglandin, indomethacin and dysmenorrhea. Prostaglandins 11: 893–904

Lundström V, Bygdeman M, Fotiou S, Gréen K, Kinoshita K 1977 Abortion in early pregnancy by vaginal administration of 16,16-dimethyl PGE₂ in comparison with vacuum aspiration. Contraception 16: 167–173

Lindner H R, Zor U, Kohen F, Bauminger S, Amsterdam A, Lahav M, Salomon Y 1980 Significance of prostaglandins on the regulation of cyclic events in the ovary and uterus. In: Samuelsson B, Ramwell P W, Paoletti R (eds) Advances in Prostaglandin and Thromboxane Research, Vol 8, pp 1371–1390. Raven Press, New York

Lyneham R C, Korda A R, Shutt D A, Smith I D, Shearman R P 1975 The effect of intrauterine prostaglandin F₂ₐ on corpus luteum function in the human. Prostaglandins 9: 431–442

Mandelin M 1978 Termination of early pregnancy by single dose of 3 mg of 15-methyl PGF₂ₐ methyl ester vaginal suppository. Prostaglandins 16: 143–152

Martin J N, Bygdeman M 1975a The effect of locally administered PGF₂ₐ on the contractility of the nonpregnant human uterus in vivo. Prostaglandins 9: 245–253

Martin J N, Bygdeman M 1975b The effect of locally administered PGE₂ on the contractility of the nonpregnant human uterus in vivo. Prostaglandins 10: 253–265

McCracken J A, Barcikowski B, Carlson J C, Gréen K, Samuelsson B 1973 The physiological role of prostaglandin F₂ₐ in corpus luteum regression. Advances in Bioscience 9: 599–624

Oliw E, Lawson J A, Brash A R, Oates J A 1981 Arachidonic acid metabolism in rabbit renal cortex. Formation of two novel dihydroxy-eicosatetraenoic acids. Journal of Biological Chemistry 256: 9924–9931

Powell W S, Hammarström S, Samuelsson B, Sjöberg B 1974

Prostaglandin F₂ₐ receptor in human corpora lutea. Lancet i: 1120

Prasad R N V, Lim C, Wong Y C, Larim S M M, Ratnam S S 1978 Vaginal administration of 16,16-dimethyl-trans-Δ²-PGE₁ methyl ester for preoperative cervical dilatation in first trimester nulliparous pregnancy. Singapore Journal of Obstetrics and Gynaecology 9: 61–71

Ragab M J, Edelman O A 1976 Early termination of pregnancy. A comparative study of intrauterine prostaglandin F₂ₐ and vacuum aspiration. Prostaglandins 11: 275–283

Rosén A S, Nystedt L, Bygdeman M, Lundström V 1979 Acceptability of a nonsurgical method to terminate very early pregnancy in comparison to vacuum aspiration. Contraception 19: 107–117

Rosenkranz B, Fischer C, Weimer K E, Froölich J C 1980 Metabolism of prostacyclin and 6-keto-prostaglandin F₁ alpha in man. Biological Chemistry 225: 10194–10198

Roth-Brandel U, Bygdeman M, Wiqvist N 1970a A comparative study of the influence of prostaglandin E₁, oxytocin and ergometrium on the pregnant human uterus. Acta Obstetrica et Gynecologica Scandinavica 49:Suppl 5: 1–7

Roth-Brandel U, Bygdeman M, Wiqvist N 1970b Effect of intravenous administration of prostaglandin E₁ and F₂ₐ on the contractility of the nonpregnant human uterus in vivo. Acta Obstetrica et Gynecologica Scandinavica 49: Suppl 5

Samuelsson B 1963 Isolation and identification of prostaglandins from human seminal plasma. Journal of Biological Chemistry 238: 3229–3234

Samuelsson B, Granström E, Gréen K, Hamberg M, Hammarström S 1975 Prostaglandins. Annual Review of Biochemistry 44: 669–695

Samuelsson B, Goldyne M, Granström E, Hamberg M, Hammarström M, Malmsten C 1978 Prostaglandins and thromboxanes, Annual Review of Biochemistry 47: 997–1029

Samuelsson B, Hammarström S 1981 Slow-reacting substances and leukotrienes (A symposium on leukotrienes, a recently discovered class of mediatros which may be involved in immediate-type hypersensitivity responses, held in London September 24, 1980). Immunology Today 2: 3–6

Sandberg F, Ingelman-Sundberg A, Rydén G 1964 The effect of prostaglandin E₁ on the human uterus and the fallopian tubes in vitro. Acta Obstetrica et Gynecologica Scandinavica 43: 95–102

Sandberg F, Ingelman-Sundberg A, Rydén G 1965 The effect of prostaglandin F₁ₐ, F₁β, F₂ₐ and F₂β on the human uterus and the fallopian tubes in vitro. Acta Obstetrica et Gynecologica Scandinavica 44: 585–594

Skakkebaek N E, Kelly R W, Cocker C S 1976 Prostaglandin concentrations in the semen of hypogonadal men during treatment with testosterone. Journal of Reproductive Fertility 47: 119–121

Spilman C H, Finn A E, Norland J F 1973 Effect of prostaglandins on sperm transport and fertilization in the rabbit. Prostaglandins 4: 57–64

Sturde H C 1971 Behaviour of sperm prostaglandins under therapy with androgen. Arzneimittel-Forschung 21: 1302–1307

Swahn M L, Lundström V 1983 The effect of prostacyclin on the myometrium in vivo. Acta Obstetrica et Gynecologica Scandinavica Suppl 113: 47–50

Svanborg, K Bygdeman M, Eneroth P, Bendvold E 1982a Quantification of prostaglandins in human seminal fluid. Prostaglandins (in press)

Svanborg K, Bendvold E, Bygdeman M, Eneroth P 1983 The relation between prostaglandins in human seminal fluid and fertility. In: Samuelsson B, Paoletti R, Ramwell P. (eds) Advances in Prostaglandin and Thromboxane Research 12: 455–459. Raven Press, New York

Tagaki S, Sakata H, Yoshida T, Nakasawa S, Fujii T L, Tominaga Y, Iwasa T, Ninagawa T, Hiroshima T, Tomida Y, Itoh K, Matsukawa R 1977 Termination of very early pregnancy by ONO-802 (16,16-dimethyl transΔ²-PGE₁ methyl ester). Prostaglandins 14: 791–798

Taylor P L 1979 The 8-iso prostaglandins: Evidence of eight components in human semen. Prostaglandins 17: 259–267

Taylor P L, Kelly R W 1975 The occurrence of 19-OH-F prostaglandins in human semen. FEBS Letters 57: 22–25

Templeton A A, Cosper I, Kelly R W 1978 Prostaglandin concentration in the semen of fertile men. Journal of Reproductive Fertility 52: 147–150

Thiery M, Amy J J 1977 Spontaneous and induced labour. Two roles for the prostaglandins. Obstetrics and Gynecology Annual 6: 127–171

Toppozada M, Graafar A, Shaala S 1974 In vivo inhibition of the human nonpregnant uterus by prostaglandin E_2. Prostaglandins 8: 401

Toppozada M, Khowessah M, Shaala S, Osman M, Rahman H A 1977 Aberrant uterine response to prostaglandin E_2 as a possible etiologic factor in functional infertility. Fertility and Sterility 28: 434–439

Ulmsten U, Wingerup L 1979 Cervical ripening induced by prostaglandin E_2 in viscous gel. Acta Obstetrica et Gynecologica Scandinavica Suppl 84: 5–21

WHO Prostaglandin Task Force 1976 Comparison of intraamniotic prostaglandin $F_{2\alpha}$ and hypertonic saline for induction of second trimester abortion. British Medical Journal 2: 1373–1376

WHO Prostaglandin Task Force 1977a Comparison of single intraamniotic injections of 15-methyl $PGF_{2\alpha}$ and prostaglandin $F_{2\alpha}$ for termination of second trimester pregnancy. American Journal of Obstetrics and Gynecology 129: 601–606

WHO Prostaglandin Task Force 1977b Repeated vaginal administration of 15-methyl-$PGF_{2\alpha}$ methyl ester for termination of pregnancy in the 13th-20th week of gestation. Contraception 16: 175–187

WHO Prostaglandin Task Force 1982 Termination of second trimester pregnancy by intramuscular injection of 16-phenoxy-ω-17,18.19,20-tetranor methyl sulfonylamide. International Journal of Gynecology and Obstetrics 20: 383–386

WHO Prostaglandin Task Force 1983 Termination of second trimester pregnancy with a long-acting vaginal pessary containing 15-methyl-$PGF_{2\alpha}$ methyl ester. International Journal of Gynecology and Obstetrics 21: 159–165

Wilhelmsson L, Lindblom B, Wiqvist N 1979 The human uterotubal junction: Contractile patterns of different smooth muscle layers and the influence of prostaglandin E_2, prostaglandin $F_{2\alpha}$ and prostaglandin I_2 in vitro. Fertility and Sterility 32: 303–307

Wilhelmsson L, Wikland M, Wiqvist N 1981 PGH_2, TxA_2 and PGI_2 have potent and differentiated actions on human uterine contractility. Prostaglandins 21: 277–286

Wiqvist N, Béguin F, Bygdeman M, Fernström I, Toppozada M 1972 Induction of abortion by extra-amniotic prostaglandin administration. Prostaglandins 1: 34–53

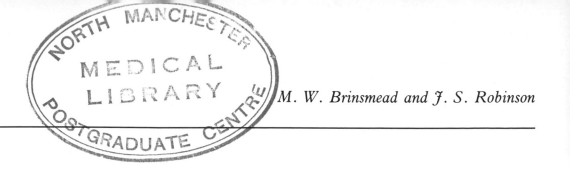

M. W. Brinsmead and J. S. Robinson

The endocrine control of fetal growth and parturition

Classical endocrinology begins with the study of those clinical and experimental situations in which a single hormone or system is deficient. The role of a particular hormone is confirmed when it is replaced and the resulting clinical condition is thereby reversed. Due largely to an impermeability of the placenta to a number of important hormones, the fetus enjoys considerable endocrine autonomy (Wolstenholme & O'Connor, 1969). This review begins with a consideration of those hormones known to be important for extra-uterine growth and assesses their possible role in the fetus. Next, the synchrony of endocrine events which result in parturition will be considered. Taken together a picture emerges of an interplay between growth and maturation which results in the successful transition of the fetus from intra-uterine life to independent existence.

FETAL GROWTH

Factors which regulate fetal growth can be broadly divided into those which are intrinsic and those which are extrinsic to the fetus. The maternal organism, by its control over supply of nutrients and oxygen, represents extrinsic constraint, and this usually operates by the regulation of uterine or uteroplacental blood flow. It is probable that such maternal factors as smoking, nutrition, hypertensive disease, chronic hypoxia and psychological stress act by this final common pathway. Chronic fetal infection and chromosomal abnormalities are examples of intrinsic factors which restrict fetal growth. At least two distinct patterns of growth retardation exist in the fetus whether assessed by morphometry at autopsy or by dynamic studies of fetal growth with ultrasound. The first is characterised by a generalised reduction in all dimensions of the fetus and this can be associated with a reduced cell number in various organs. The second category of fetal growth retardation results in a differential reduction in organ size with relative sparing of the head and brain. This chapter will develop the hypothesis that, in the face of extrinsic

constraint, the fetus will establish priorities in the distribution of available nutrients and oxygen by an alteration in its hormonal milieu. The hypothesis is supported by clinical and experimental observations in which certain hormones are missing and fetal growth retardation occurs.

Growth hormone

Growth hormone (GH) is detectable in the pituitary of the human fetus from the seventh week of gestation (Matsu-kaki et al, 1971) and is identical to that recovered from adults. Concentrations of human growth hormone (hGH) in the circulation of the fetus rise throughout the first half of pregnancy and reach a peak at about the 20th week. Thereafter, they decline steadily until term but at delivery they are still three to five times greater than basal levels in children and adults.

Grumbach, (1974) has postulated that the declining serum concentrations of hGH in the fetus during the second half of pregnancy is due to a maturation of the hypothalamic control of GH secretion and this has received support from studies in fetal sheep (Marti-Henneburg et al, 1980). Conclusions concerning the function of growth hormone in fetal life are complicated by its short half-life and rapid release from the pituitary during the stress of delivery or anaesthesia (Turner et al, 1971). There are, however, increased hGH concentrations in the cord blood of pre-term infants (Corn-blath et al, 1965), infants born to pre-eclamptic women (Laron et al, 1967), and small for dates infants (Poonai et al, 1975).

Despite the high concentrations of GH in the fetus most evidence suggests that this hormone has little influence on fetal growth. From the available clinical evidence and experimental hypophysectomy, Liggins (1974) concluded that fetuses of various species vary in their response to absence of the pituitary. Some, such as rabbits and rhesus monkeys, attain a normal size at birth while others, such as lambs and calves, show retarded growth in the absence of the pituitary. The human fetus occupies an intermediate position between these extremes: a modest reduction in growth velocity being observed in congenital malformations associated with absence or hypoplasia of the pituitary. However, the pituitary is a complex endocrine organ whose removal has other effects on such target glands as the thyroid, adrenals and gonads. It is therefore difficult to determine the role of growth hormone in those disturbances of growth which follow hypophysectomy or decapitation particularly since there have been no experiments in which growth hormone alone (or in combination with other pituitary hormones) has been replaced after such procedures.

The best evidence that growth hormone does not have an essential role in fetal life is a consideration of those children born with isolated GH deficiency. Such infants are usually of near normal birthweight but their birth length is mildly subnormal (Laron & Pertzelan, 1969) and their GH deficiency does not become clinically manifest until the post-natal age of 18 months or more (Tanner et al, 1971). Children with GH deficiency have a small head circumference at birth but catch-up growth occurs if treatment with growth hormone is started before the age of 5 years. This is accompanied by an increase in intelligence whereas untreated children remain mentally retarded (Laron & Galatzer, 1981). This suggests that GH has some role in growth and development of the brain.

A different emphasis for a role of growth hormone in brain growth is provided by experiments in rats. In this species, when GH is given to pregnant rats the offspring have a larger, more cellular brain and at maturity demonstrate superior learning abilities (Zamenof et al, 1971). This may be due to a lipolytic effect of the administered growth hormone in the dams which results in enhanced nutrition of the fetuses. However Sara et al (1979) have demonstrated that growth hormone administration to pregnant rats results in the appearance of a 'brain growth factor' in the serum of fetuses. This 'brain growth factor' may be a somatomedin.

Thyroid hormone

The thyroid of the human fetus is recognisable from the first trimester of pregnancy and is capable of synthesis of the full spectrum of iodinated products from the 10th week of gestation. Infants born with congenital hypothyroidism are usually of normal birthweight, but the role of thyroid hormones in fetal growth and development is obscured by the transplacental passage of these hormones in many species. Furthermore even so-called 'athyroitic' cretins have residual islands of thyroid tissue. The absence of the fetal pituitary does not guarantee absence of thyroid activity since the placenta produces both a chorionic thyrotrophin and thyrotrophin releasing hormones (TRH) (Mosier, 1982).

Experimental ablation of the thyroid gland in fetal animals results in differing effects in different species.

Whereas one study of thyroidectomy in fetal rabbits suggested no effect on fetal growth, other experiments in rats, guinea-pigs, sheep and monkeys suggest that the fetal thyroid has an important role in fetal body growth, lung and skeletal maturation (Thorburn, 1974; Erenberg et al, 1979; Mosier, 1982). There is also general agreement from both clinical observations and experimental studies that fetal thyroid function is necessary for normal fetal brain growth and development (Hetzel & Hay, 1979). Severe iodine deficiency, such as occurs in areas of endemic goitre, results in congenital cretinism with mental deficiency, deaf mutism, spastic diplegia and squint. This does not respond to replacement therapy with thyroid hormones or even correction of iodine deficiency in the mother if delayed until the second half of pregnancy (Pharoah et al, 1976). Fisher et al (1982) have speculated that many of the fetal effects of thyroid hormones are mediated by such growth factors as growth hormone, the somatomedins, erythropoietin, nerve growth factor and epidermal growth factor.

Insulin

Insulin acts as an anabolic hormone by stimulating cytoplasmic growth, protein, glycogen and fat synthesis. Insulin is detected in the human fetal pancreas from the end of the first trimester of pregnancy and its concentration increases progressively until, at term, it is 6-fold greater than that in the adult pancreas. Immunoreactive insulin is present in the fetal circulation from the end of the first trimester and the level remains fairly constant until term (Persson, 1981). This ontogenic pattern appears similar in all species except in the rat in which there are very high concentrations of fetal insulin just prior to delivery (Sodoyezgoffaux et al, 1981). *In vitro* studies of the fetal pancreas suggest that glucose alone is a rather poor stimulus to insulin release whereas such amino acids as arginine and leuceine are potent secretagogues (Schaeffer et al, 1973). However studies in the chronically catheterised and unstressed fetal lamb clearly indicate that insulin has a physiological role in glucose homeostasis in the fetus (Shelley et al, 1975). Transition from fetal to neonatal life, with its change from a relatively constant supply of glucose, alters the responsiveness of pancreatic beta cells to glucose and amino acids. Premature maturation of beta cell responsiveness may be induced by chronic fetal hyperglycaemia or the administration of corticosteroids to the fetus (Liggins, 1976).

Receptors for insulin are present in a variety of fetal tissues from both man and animals (Kelly et al, 1974; Sara et al, 1983). The best characterised are those in the human placenta where they are located on the brush border of the syncytiotrophoblast, a fetal tissue in direct contact with maternal blood of the intervillous space (Posner, 1974). Insulin receptors are present on erythrocytes and monocytes in the human newborn and have a greater concentration and affinity than do the same receptors in adults (Rosenfeld et al, 1979). Moreover, there is no evidence for down regulation of insulin receptors in the fetus since monocytes from infants with hyperinsulinaemia have an even higher concentration of receptors than do normal neonates (Thorsson & Hintz, 1977).

A role for insulin as a fetal growth hormone first arose from consideration of those clinical situations in which there is an excess or deficiency of fetal insulin. There is a positive correlation between infant birthweight and plasma, amniotic fluid and pancreatic concentrations of insulin (Spellacy & Buhi, 1976; Van Assche et al, 1977; Brinsmead & Liggins, 1979a; Lin et al 1981). This is even more impressive in fetal rats (Girard et al, 1976) and rabbits (Fletcher et al, 1982).

The most obvious disturbance of fetal growth associated with abnormal fetal insulin concentrations occurs in the fetus of the diabetic mother. Pederson et al (1954) formulated the hyperglycaemia-hyperinsulinism hypothesis to explain the features of these neonates. This hypothesis states that maternal hyperglycaemia results in fetal hyperglycaemia and the fetal pancreatic beta cells respond by hyperplasia and hypertrophy. This results in increased fetal insulin concentrations, an enhanced fetal utilisation of glucose and amino acids and enhanced fetal growth. The typical infant of a poorly controlled diabetic mother is large for dates, plethoric and apparently oedematous. In fact, intracellular and extracellular water is reduced in many tissues and the excess weight is due to hypertrophy and hyperplasia of many tissues. Adipose tissue, liver, heart and the adrenal gland are particularly affected by these changes (Hill, 1978). However, the fetal brain does not share this organ enlargement with maternal diabetes mellitus. This is best illustrated by experiments in which pregnant rhesus monkeys were rendered diabetic. The fetuses of such diabetic monkeys had many of the morphological changes seen in infants of diabetic women but analysis of their cerebral tissue DNA, revealed impaired brain cell growth (Cheek & Hill, 1975).

Such studies do not confirm a growth-promoting role for insulin since the growth enhancement may be due to an increased supply of such substrates as glucose, amino acids or even free fatty acids. Does insulin promote fetal growth in the presence of normal concentrations of such substrates? There is both clinical and experimental evidence which sheds light on this question. A variety of rare fetal conditions in man are associated with gigantism, visceromegaly, hyperinsulinism and neonatal hypoglycaemia. They include the Beckwith-Wiedemann Syndrome, fetopathia-diabetica, pancreatic beta cell adenoma and nesideroblastosis (Hill et al, 1980). Normal growth occurs in these children when their hyperinsulinism is treated. Chronic fetal hyperinsulinism has been studied in the rat and rhesus monkey. Picon (1967) reported that significantly larger pups are born after the daily subcutaneous

injection of insulin to near-term fetuses of pregnant rats. However, because of the high concentrations of insulin which occur normally in this species it may not be an appropriate model to study. Susa et al (1979) implanted osmotically driven minipumps, filled with insulin, into the hindlimbs of fetal rhesus monkeys between 113 and 126 days of gestation (term ≅ 160 days). This infusion resulted in concentrations of insulin which were up to 55-fold greater than that normally present in the fetus, increased fetal body weight and enlargement of liver, heart, spleen and placenta. Kidney weight and body length were unaffected and brain weight was slightly less than normal. Biochemical analysis of the liver suggested that its enlargement was due mainly to cell hyperplasia rather than hypertrophy.

Studies of insulin deficiency in the fetus produce a complementary view to those of fetal hyperinsulinism. Infants born with pancreatic agenesis are profoundly growth retarded but there is some sparing of head growth (Sherwood et al, 1974; Dodge & Laurence, 1977; Lemons et al, 1979). Intra-uterine growth retardation is a feature of transient neonatal diabetes mellitus in which there are low concentrations of insulin in the neonate (Cornblath & Schwartz, 1966). Another rare form of growth failure in childhood is due to an end organ resistance to insulin. Such children are born with the appearance of leprechauns (Donohue & Uchida, 1954). There have been few reports of attempted ablation of the fetal pancreas in experimental animals. Cheek & Hill (1975) administered a pancreatic beta cell toxin, streptozotocin, to fetal rhesus monkeys and studied them 5 weeks later at term. All but three of the animals were of normal birthweight, but examination of the pancreatic islets suggested a rapid regeneration of the pancreatic beta cells. We have administered streptozotocin to fetal lambs in mid gestation. When delivered near term, the fetuses exhibited profound growth retardation which involved total body weight, crown-rump length and limb length. The fetal kidneys and livers were very small but the brain weight was near normal and the head size measured either as length or biparietal diameter was likewise normal. These fetuses were not hypoxic but had low pancreatic insulin content, a reduced insulin response to a glucose challenge and a mild chronic hyperglycaemia (Brinsmead & Thorburn, 1982).

There is emerging evidence that insulin does not directly stimulate fetal growth but acts by the generation of insulin-like growth factors. Whilst insulin promotes cell multiplication in culture, it is only in concentrations which far exceed physiological levels and is then acting on receptors for the insulin-like growth factors (Gospodarowicz & Moran, 1976)

Somatomedins (insulin-like growth factors)

The term somatomedin was introduced in 1972 to describe

a family of related polypeptides which were believed to mediate the effects of growth hormone (somatotrophin) on skeletal growth (Daughaday et al, 1972). The existence of somatomedin was first postulated by Daughaday & Reeder (1966) who were studying the incorporation of sulphate into cartilage as a possible bioassay for growth hormone. In their studies, serum from hypophysectomised rats was ineffective in promoting sulphate uptake by cartilage *in vitro* but growth hormone, when added to the incubation, was likewise ineffective. When hypophysectomised rats were treated with growth hormone and their serum retested, it had activity which, present also in intact animals, was able to promote sulphate uptake (for reviews see Van Wyk et al, 1974; Phillips & Vassipoulou-Sellin, 1980).

Data accumulated over the ensuing years suggested that the component of serum which was responsible for sulphation activity was an insulin-like polypeptide generated predominantly in the liver. By 1978 two components of human serum with insulin-like activity had been purified and characterised. Because they were capable of supporting cell growth in culture they were re-named the insulin-like growth factors (IGF) I and II (Rindernecht & Humbel, 1976). Final substantiation of the somatomedin hypothesis did not occur until 1982 when it was shown that purified IGF I could restore growth in hypophysectomised rats (Schoenle et al, 1982).

IGF I and II have substantial primary, secondary and tertiary structural homology with proinsulin and it is considered that insulin and the IGFs have a common evolutionary ancestor (Rindernecht & Humbel, 1978). This structural homology with proinsulin has also been noted for two other polypeptides, namely relaxin and nerve growth factor. Unlike other polypeptides hormones which act rapidly and use a second messenger there is evidence that these insulin-related proteins first bind to specific receptors on the plasma membrane of their target cells and are then internalised by an endocytotic process to act as their own second messenger on a chromatin-associated receptor site in the nucleus. This event is accompanied by rapid changes in cellular metabolism and by microtubule assembly. This, in turn, results in a modulation of RNA synthesis and an expression of target cell function over a long period of time (Bradshaw & Niall, 1978).

There has been considerable interest in the possible role of IGFs in fetal growth (for review see Brinsmead & Liggins, 1979c; Sara & Hall, 1980b). An early study with a bioassay for sulphation factor demonstrated a significant, albeit statistically weak, correlation between the somatomedin activity of human cord blood and fetal weight, length and head circumferences corrected for the effect of gestational age (Gluckman & Brinsmead, 1976). This has been substantiated with a great variety of assays for somatomedin activity (D'Ercole et al, 1976; Svan et al, 1977; Ashton & Vesey, 1978; Foley et al, 1980; Falconer et al,

1981). However one difficulty in accepting a significant role for IGFs in fetal growth has been the repeated observation that, whether the somatomedins are measured by bioassay or radioimmunoassay, fetal blood contains only 10–50 per cent of the activity of that present in normal adults. This objection cannot be too strenuously upheld when it is appreciated that growing children do not achieve normal adult concentrations of IGF until the age of 6–8 years (D'Ercole et al, 1977). A relationship between IGF concentrations and the growth of normal children exists despite their paradoxically less-than-adult levels of IGF activity (Rudman et al, 1981).

It is assumed that the failure of response to IGF in the adult is a function of end organ resistance. By extrapolation therefore, the fetus may be extremely sensitive to the low concentrations of IGF present in its circulation. This possibility has been most extensively addressed by Hill et al (1981). Their studies have shown that when fetal or postnatal rat cartilage is exposed to plasma, sulphate uptake varies with age and is greatest in late fetal life. Receptors for IGF have been found in a great variety of fetal tissues including liver, lung, kidney, heart and brain (D'Ercole et al, 1976; Owens et al, 1980; Sara et al, 1981), fibroblasts (Zapf et al, 1975), chondrocytes (Zapf et al, 1978), placenta (Marshall et al, 1974; Brinsmead & Liggins, 1978; Daughaday et al, 1981a) and circulating mononuclear cells (Rosenfeld et al, 1979). In many instances the concentration and affinity of IGF receptors in the fetus are greater than those in the corresponding tissues from adults. Studies of the ontogenesis of IGF receptors in fetal sheep (Owens et al, 1980), pig (D'Ercole et al, 1976) and man (Sara et al, 1983) suggest that end organ responsiveness may be the most important component of this endocrine axis.

Hill & Milner (1981) also found that if fetal plasma is tested for sulphate uptake with cartilage from post-natal animals, low activity is found but if fetal plasma is assayed on fetal cartilage then the somatomedin activity is the same as that of adult plasma. This implies that there may be specific IGFs in fetal life which are recognised by specific fetal receptors. The question of an IGF which is unique to the fetus has been explored in man by Sara et al (1981) and Daughaday et al (1981b). Whereas IGF activity in the serum from the human fetus in mid-pregnancy is uniformly low in other assays, blood obtained at fetoscopy and studied with a radioligand assay with receptor from the brain of fetuses of similar gestation, contains IGF activity in four-fold greater concentrations than that of adults and infants born at term (Sara et al, 1981).

Daughaday et al (1981b) using a receptor purified from fetal rat placenta and IGF II as a ligand, have reported concentrations of an IGF in human newborns which are 150 per cent of those of adults. This has increased the speculation that it is IGF II which is the fetal form of IGF but this does not appear to be likely in man. The concentration of IGF II measured by specific radioimmunoassay is low in the human fetus (Zapf et al, 1981) and in our studies using a fetal receptor, which preferentially detects IGF II, we found that the concentrations of IGF in cord blood from normal neonates born spontaneously at term, is only 25 per cent of those of adults.

There is evidence from two animal sources which suggests that there may be a specific fetal IGF. Multiplication-stimulating activity (MSA), a polypeptide produced by a clone of rat liver cells in culture, is widely used as a ligand in studies of IGF receptors because of its ready availability and somatomedin-like binding properties (Nissley & Rechler, 1978). The concentration of immunoreactive MSA in the serum of fetal rats is 20–100 fold higher than those of adults (Moses et al, 1980). In this species MSA levels gradually decrease after birth at a time when another somatomedin (possibly IGF I) is rising (Sara & Hall, 1980a). Recently one of the MSA proteins has been purified and analysis of its primary structure reveals close similarity to that of human IGF II (Marquardt et al, 1981). In vitro fibroblasts from fetal rats release predominantly IGF II and fibroblasts from adult rats release predominantly IGF I. Fibroblasts from neonatal rats mimic this development switch from IGF II to IGF I in vitro (Adams et al, 1983). Longitudinal data of IGFs in fetal life are provided by studies in sheep. In this species fetal IGF I concentrations are low in early gestation, rise progressively until term, and exceed adult concentrations in the early neonatal period. In contrast fetal IGF II levels exceed adult concentrations throughout most of pregnancy and fall to low levels at the time of birth (Gluckman et al, 1983).

The IGFs are unique amongst polypeptide hormones in that they circulate in plasma bound to specific binding proteins. In normal man there are high concentrations of IGFs present in the bound form and little or no IGFs circulate free in plasma. This has resulted in considerable controversy about the in vivo activities of these polypeptides and the relevance of all hitherto used somatomedin assays which measure total IGF activity. The biological role of the carrier proteins has not been established. They may act to prolong the half-life of IGFs in plasma, reduce their rate of tissue delivery or inhibit their activity on insulin receptors (Zapf et al, 1979).

Blood from human neonates contains substantial amounts of unsaturated binding proteins for IGFs (Borsi et al, 1982) and the molecular weight distribution of IGF activity in the human fetus shows a changing pattern with increasing gestational age suggestive of an important ontogenic development of binding proteins (D'Ercole et al, 1980b). Somatomedin binding proteins have also been identified in amniotic fluid (Chochinov et al, 1977), and the cytosol of syncitium from human placenta (Deal et al, 1983). The possible regulating effect of these binding proteins on fetal IGF action and fetal growth has not been explored.

The origin of IGFs in the fetus is incompletely studied. They do not appear to be of maternal origin since placental transfer does not occur (Underwood et al, 1979). Many tissues from the fetal mouse are capable of somatomedin release when maintained in organ culture (D'Ercole et al, 1980a) and this has lead to the hypothesis that the primary action of somatomedin in the fetus might be exerted locally at its site of origin. The theoretical benefits to the fetus of the promotion and maintenance of tissue growth by local, diffusable, mitogenic factors are obvious.

The regulation of IGF activity in the fetus is also a matter for continuing speculation. Whilst in the adult animal the primary regulation is by growth hormone, nutrition, insulin, thyroxine, glucagon, glucocorticoids, sex steroids and prolactin have also been implicated (Phillips & Vassipoulou-Sellin, 1980). However it is placental lactogen which has attracted the most interest as a possible regulator of IGFs in the fetus.

Placental lactogen

There is indirect evidence suggesting that placental lactogen may stimulate IGF generation in both pregnant women and animals. Immunoreactive concentrations of IGF I in serum from women rise in the second half of pregnancy and fall rapidly after delivery (Furlanetto et al, 1978). Hypophysectomy of pregnant rats does not result in the expected fall in serum IGF activity until after the delivery of the placenta. This is ascribed to a maintaining effect from rat placental lactogen (Daughaday et al, 1979).

Placental lactogen has been largely dismissed as a significant fetal hormone. In the human fetus concentrations are generally less than 1 per cent of those in the mother (Josimovich & Archer, 1977) but this represents 10–20 ng/ml of hormone, comparable to basal levels of hGH in growing children. Human placental lactogen (hPL) when administered to pregnant rats, increases fetal body weight, glycogen, total nitrogen and triglycerides, but it lacks such effects when administered directly to the fetus (Tojo et al, 1976). Ovine placental lactogen (oPL) administered to hypophysectomised rats restores serum concentrations of somatomedin in a similar manner to oGH or hGH (Hurley et al, 1977). However, caution is necessary in the interpretation of such cross species studies since oPL has substantial somatotrophic activity whereas hPL is predominantly lactogenic.

Concentrations of placental lactogen in the ovine fetus are substantial being 8–20 per cent of maternal concentrations. They reach a peak at about 110 days of gestation and thereafter decline towards term (Chan et al, 1978a). Receptors for oPL have been identified in a number of fetal tissues, most notably the liver (Chan et al, 1978b) which may be the site of somatomedin generation. In a study carefully designed to avoid the known effects of stress, hypoxia, anaesthesia and starvation on oPL, a significant correlation between fetal concentrations of oPL and IGF (predominantly IGF II) was found in fetal sheep (Brinsmead et al, 1982). Hypophysectomy of the ovine fetus is associated with normal concentrations of oPL and IGF (Brinsmead & Liggins, 1979b). Likewise decapitation of fetal rabbits *in utero* does not affect fetal concentrations of somatomedin (Hill et al, 1979). Perhaps the best evidence for a role for placental lactogen in fetal somatomedin generation arises from a study of fibroblasts in culture. Whereas both growth hormone and placental lactogen stimulate IGF I synthesis in fibroblasts from adult rats, only placental lactogen is effective in stimulating fetal fibroblasts and IGF II is the peptide released (Adams et al, 1983). However an essential role for placental lactogen in human fetal growth can be dismissed because of the rare absence of this hormone in the serum and placenta of women who deliver a normal fetus (Nielsen et al, 1979). Genetic studies in these women confirm that there is no other protein present which is replacing placental lactogen.

Other growth factors

Epidermal growth factor (EGF) is a single chain polypeptide whose structure is unlike the insulin-related growth factors (Carpenter & Cohen, 1979). In man, it was first identified as urogastrone, a protein extracted from urine which is capable of healing gastric ulcers (Gregory, 1975). It is stored in the salivary glands of mouse and man as a high molecular weight complex. It is also found in the glands of Brunner of the human duodenum and to a much lesser extent in liver, thyroid and kidney (Thorburn et al, 1981).

EGF synthesis is regulated by testosterone, growth hormone and thyroxine. It is released from salivary glands either into the circulation or into saliva after cleavage by arginine esterase. Its release into the circulation is under α-adrenergic control and release into the saliva controlled by cholinergic stimulation. Despite a relatively high urinary output in man, EGF is present in blood only in very low concentrations (Hirata & Orth, 1979) but there is evidence that this is increased in women during pregnancy (Ances, 1973). EGF has also been detected in milk (Beardmore & Richards, 1982). EGF receptors are present in fetal mouse tissues being greatest in the amnion followed by lungs, trophoblast, limbs, yolk sac, liver, brain and heart (Nexo et al, 1980; Adamson et al 1981). The human placenta contains the richest source of EGF receptors so far identified (Hock et al, 1979).

The physiological role of EGF is unknown, but suggestions have ranged from promotion of healing in animals that lick their wounds to closure of the palate in the fetus. EGF has a wide range of actions which appear independent of its mitogenic potential. Experiments in fetal rabbits and lambs have indicated that it is capable of premature maturation of the lungs without any effect on lung or body growth (Sundell et al, 1975; Catterton et al, 1979). Other studies have suggested a complex interaction between EGF, thyroid function and adrenal maturation in the fetus (Thorburn et al, 1981). EGF, like many other growth factors, exhibits paradoxical inhibition of growth when administered in high concentrations. This is due, in part, to rapid down regulation of its receptors (Adamson et al, 1981). It is likely that most of the previously described *in vivo* experiments with EGF have used non-physiological concentrations of this hormone. This would explain its defleecing effect in fetal and adult sheep (Thorburn et al, 1981; Paranetto et al, 1982). We predict that further studies of EGF in low concentrations in the fetus at critical periods of maturation will be most exciting.

Nerve growth factor (NGF) was first identified 30 years ago as a product of a chick embryo sarcoma which promoted the outgrowth of sympathetic neurites. This protein is the best characterised and most studied of the polypeptide growth factors. However, despite a great deal of descriptive information there is no clear indication of its physiological role nor its precise mode of action (Ikeno & Guroff, 1979). Like EGF, NGF is most abundant in the submandibular glands of male mice where it exists in a large molecular weight form. Its biological activity resides in a beta subunit whose primary and tertiary structure bears substantial homology to that of proinsulin (Bradshaw, 1978).

A role for NGF in the development of the central nervous system is suggested by the effect of the administration of antibodies to NGF to neonatal and fetal rats (Gorin & Johnson, 1980; Aloe et al, 1981). This results in depletion of sympathetic and dorsal root ganglia, post-natal growth retardation, hypothermia and behavioural changes (Pearson et al, 1983).

Immunoreactive and bioactive NGF has been isolated in high yield from human placenta and amnion (Goldstein et al, 1978). There is a veno-arterial gradient for NGF in cord blood from the human neonate which further supports a placental origin for this protein (Walker et al, 1981). However, apart from a suggestion that familial dysautonomic neuropathies may result from NGF deficiency, there is no indication of the role of NGF in human development. NGF administration to rats results in a prolonged stimulation of the adrenocortical axis and a tenfold elevation in ACTH and corticosterone concentrations (Otten et al, 1979). Therefore a role for NGF in fetal maturation and parturition warrants consideration.

A great variety of other growth factors has been identified and characterised to a greater or lesser extent. Most have been studied only *in vitro* by their ability to stimulate cell growth (see Nevo & Laron, 1979; Golde, 1980; Bradshaw & Rubin, 1980 for reviews). Better characterised growth factors include fibroblast growth factor (FGF) (Gospodorowicz, 1975) and the platelet derived growth factors (PDGF) (Heldin et al, 1977). Human amniotic cells respond with mitosis to both FGF and EGF (Gospoda-rowicz et al, 1977; Chettur et al, 1978). Fetal cells, when compared to adult cells, are particularly responsive to PDGF, a phenomenon which is reminiscent of the sensitivity of fetal tissues to the insulin-like growth factors (Slayback et al, 1978).

Careful *in vitro* studies have indicated that many of the growth factors act synergistically at different stages of the cell cycle. For example, fibroblasts in the G_0 phase, first made 'competent' by transient exposure to PDGF, are then able to traverse the G_1 phase by such 'progression factors' as EGF or IGF I (Stiles et al, 1979; Clemmons & Van Wyk, 1981). Insulin enhances and hydrocortisone inhibits the stimulating effect of these growth factors. However, the effects depend on the timing of the exposure of the cells to these two hormones (De Asua et al, 1981). Such *in vitro* studies illustrate the likely complexity of the interelation between hormones and growth factors in fetal growth and maturation.

Corticosteroids

There is a variety of evidence which suggests that adrenal corticosteroids have an inhibitory effect on fetal growth. Glucocorticoids inhibit cell growth in culture (Armelin & Armelin, 1977) and this effect depends on the type of co-inducing growth factor present (De Asua et al, 1977). The administration of steroids to pregnant rats and monkeys results in delivery of a fetus with impaired body weight and cell number (Johnson et al, 1979). In one study in fetal sheep in which a twin was adrenalectomised, the experimental animals had a significantly greater weight at delivery than their intact twins (Barnes et al, 1977). Finally the administration of prednisone to pregnant women results in a significant decrease in the birthweight of their full term infants and this occurs in the absence of any serious maternal disease for which corticosteroids are normally administered (Reinisch et al, 1978). However, the hypothalamo-pituitary-adrenal axis has a significant role in fetal maturation and parturition. It is appropriate that when the fetus stops growing that its delivery should be triggered.

PARTURITION

The endocrine regulation of the growth of the fetus has been discussed in the preceeding section. It is now pertinent to pose the question — what are the signals leading to the timely delivery of the fetus? This section will concentrate on the endocrine events which may be involved in the onset of parturition. Since our knowledge of the role of the fetus in the initiation of its delivery derives largely from the elegant studies on sheep by Liggins, Thorburn and others in the last two decades, this section will begin

with an account of the initiation of parturition in ruminants. Later the endocrine events preceding parturition in man will be described.

Parturition in sheep

In the late 50s and early 60s a number of clinical syndromes associated with prolonged pregnancy in cattle and sheep were described. Those in cattle which resulted in prolongation of pregnancy to as much as 526 days (term 280 days) (Holm, 1967; Kennedy, 1971; Kennedy et al, 1975) were genetic in origin and were associated with failure of development of the anterior pituitary and adrenal cortex of the fetus. A fetal cyclopian malformation associated with prolonged pregnancy occurs in sheep grazing at high altitudes in Idaho (Binns et al, 1963). This malformation is due to ingestion of a steroidal alkaloid, 11-deoxyjervine, present in the skunk cabbage (*Veratrum californicum*) by the ewe on day 14 of pregnancy. The teratogen causes cerebral malformation in the fetus and disordered development of the hypothalamus and the pituitary leading to a complete failure of parturition. Slow growth of the fetus continues past term until the ewe eventually dies from malnutrition.

It was these observations which prompted Liggins to propose testing the effects of ablation of the fetal pituitary and adrenal glands on parturition in sheep (Comroe, 1978). If the fetal pituitary is destroyed at various stages of gestation in this species, pregnancy continues beyond term (Liggins et al, 1967). Likewise hypothalamic destruction, pituitary stalk section or adrenalectomy prevents the initiation of parturition (Liggins, 1969). A role for the pituitary and adrenal glands in parturition is supported by the increase in adrenal weight and rise in the concentration of cortisol in fetal plasma in the week before delivery (Comline & Silver, 1961; Bassett & Thorburn, 1969). Conversely premature onset of parturition occurs after infusion of adrenocorticotrophin (ACTH) or cortisol into fetal lambs (Liggins, 1968). The essential role of the pituitary-adreno-cortical axis is thus confirmed and the failure of adrenal medullary destruction or infusion of other pituitary hormones to influence the length of gestation strengthens this conclusion.

The factors responsible for the preparturient increase in the concentration of fetal cortisol have been the subject of debate because early studies demonstrated that the concentration of ACTH increased only after the rise in plasma cortisol (Rees et al, 1975b; Jones et al, 1977). However, ACTH is present in plasma in different molecular weight forms and at least five have been found in the pituitary and plasma of the fetus (Silman et al, 1979; Jones & Roebuck, 1980). The ACTH initially measured by radioimmunoassay in fetal plasma was the sum of $ACTH_{1-39}$ and higher molecular weight forms and more recent studies demonstrate that $ACTH_{1-39}$ and cortisol increase in fetal plasma at about the same time. Early in gestation the large molecular weight forms of ACTH which have low steroidogenic activity, compete with $ACTH_{1-39}$ for adrenal receptors (Jones & Roebuck, 1980). Further work is required to define the mechanism responsible for the switch by the pituitary cell to greater secretion of $ACTH_{1-39}$.

The responsiveness of the fetal adrenal to ACTH has also received attention because it changes with increasing gestation. ACTH stimulates cortisol and progesterone release early in pregnancy, but by mid-pregnancy this response is lost only to re-emerge near term (Wintour et al, 1975; Glickman & Challis, 1980). Challis and his colleagues have measured the ability of adrenal cells to produce cortisol from such different precursors as progesterone and 17α-OH progesterone. They concluded that the enzymes 17α-hydroxylase and 3β-hydroxysteroid dehydrogenase, may be partially rate-limiting in the production of cortisol until shortly before term (Challis et al, 1983).

The preparturient rise in cortisol induces changes in placental enzymes, particularly 17α-hydroxylase (Anderson et al, 1975), C_{17-20} lyase (Steele et al, 1976), and aramotase (Ash et al, 1973). These, in turn, are responsible for a switch to the secretion of unconjugated oestrogen by conversion and metabolism of progesterone. The net result is that the concentration of progesterone declines and that of oestrogen rises shortly before parturition. Withdrawal of progesterone alone (Taylor et al, 1981) or infusion of 17α-oestradiol (Currie et al, 1973) is sufficient to induce parturition in most animals. Parturition in the sheep resulting from removal of progesterone provides support for the classic progesterone block theory of Csapo (1977). Lye & Porter (1978) have shown that progesterone inhibits the sheep myometrium and blocks the action of oxytocin and prostaglandin(s). The exogenous administration of progesterone at term (Bengtsson & Schofield, 1963) fails to prevent parturition because most is metabolised to oestrogen, particularly 17β-oestradiol (Thorburn, 1979).

Since a close temporal relationship exists between utero-ovarian concentrations of unconjugated oestrogens and prostaglandin F during both induced and spontaneous parturition (Currie et al, 1973) it has been suggested that oestrogen may be the stimulus to the increased production of prostaglandin F necessary for parturition in sheep. However, Kendall et al (1977) demonstrated that parturition induced by $ACTH_{1-24}$ in ewes carrying hypophysectomised fetuses was associated with an increase in 13, 14-dihydro-15-ketoprostaglandin F (PGFM) without a concomitant rise in oestrogen. Previous studies by Mitchell et al (1976) showed that the increase in PGFM in peripheral plasma at parturition, reflects increased prostaglandin F production. Thus an increase in oestrogen may not be an essential prerequisite for either parturition or prostaglandin production. Inhibition of prostaglandin synthesis by the administration of meclofenamic acid, suggests that prostaglandins may be the final common pathway to the initiation of parturition in sheep (Mitchell & Flint, 1978)

and monkeys (Novy et al, 1974) since the normal preparturient changes in progesterone and oestrogen do not result in delivery until the suppression of prostaglandin synthesis is withdrawn.

No account of parturition would be complete without reference to the changes which occur in the cervix and which are an essential part of the process of birth. Infusion of prostaglandin $F_{2\alpha}$ into the arterial supply of the uterus or cervix results in cervical dilatation. However the success of these experiments depends on the progesterone concentration at the time of the infusion (Fitzpatrick, 1977). The compliance of the sheep cervix at parturition has been measured both *in vivo* and *in vitro*. An analysis of length/tension curves *in vitro* in conjunction with initial measurement of length allow calculation of strain, stress modulus, and break load. Each of these, except strain, was found to be lower at parturition. Fitzpatrick & Dobson (1981) suggested that hormones have a greater effect on ground substance than on collagen. Changes in modulus and stiffness can be induced by 17α-oestradiol but this is not blocked by the simultaneous infusion of meclofenamic acid. This indicates that the mechanism does not involve prostaglandins. Ellwood et al (1981) have studied the production of different prostaglandins by the cervix and suggest that prostacyclin and prostaglandin E synthesis are increased at or about the time of cervical softening. While active collagenase production is much greater if cervical tissue is collected at delivery rather than in late pregnancy, a definite link between collagenase and prostanoids has yet to be established. Cervical softening may also involve the polypeptide hormone, relaxin, but the role of this hormone in parturition in sheep has yet to be defined.

Human parturition

Recognition that the fetus is responsible for the initiation of parturition in sheep led to a re-examination of the hypothesis that the human fetus plays a similar role. Earlier investigations by Malpas (1933) of postmaturity and malformation had provided evidence that anencephaly is associated with prolonged pregnancy. Malpas (1933) drew attention to the prolongation of pregnancy associated with anencephaly and concluded: 'the onset of labour is determined by the foetus' and 'the foetal adrenal, pituitary or nervous system, perhaps in combination, are suggested as tissues possibly concerned in the actual excitation of the neuro-muscular expulsive mechanisms'. Since the combination of anencephaly and polyhydramnios was always found in the women delivering prematurely, whereas prolonged pregnancy only occurred when there was no polyhydramnios, he deduced that polyhydramnios and anencephaly appear to have opposing effects on the duration of pregnancy. Honnebier & Swaab (1973) found that 41.4 per cent, 24.1 per cent and 34.5 per cent of anencephalics without polyhydramnios deliver before 38 weeks, at term or after 42 weeks respectively. A conclusion that can be drawn from these observations is that accurate timing of parturition is lost in women whose pregnancy is complicated by anencephaly. However, the first stage of labour is not prolonged and this suggests that the initiation, not the course, of parturition is influenced by the fetal brain.

Anterior pituitary

The ACTH family of peptides has been mentioned previously but the proportions of different peptides in man differs from that of the sheep. Using techniques similar to those used for assay of the ACTH-related peptides in sheep, Silman et al (1976) have described changes in the human fetal pituitary shortly before parturition. In the fetus there is an excess of fragments of low molecular weight forms which are thought to be α-melanocyte-stimulating hormone (αMSH) and corticotrophin-like intermediate lobe peptide (CLIP). At term Silman et al (1976) reported a rapid switch to greater concentrations of $ACTH_{1-39}$, a rise in the ACTH to C-peptide ratio and suggested that this may initiate parturition.

However Tilders et al (1981) found that the substance identified by Silman et al (1976) as immunoreactive αMSH consists mostly of $ACTH_{1-13}NH_2$ (desacetyl αMSH), and this difference may be important since it has not been established which is trophic for the adrenal. Schöneshöfer & Fenner (1981) used reverse phase high-pressure liquid chromatography to examine immunoreactive ACTH extracted from human plasma and found that $ACTH_{1-39}$ is only a minor component of the immunoreactivity and that the major components are such hydrophobic substances as acetyl-$ACTH_{1-39}$. Whereas $ACTH_{1-39}$ is a potent steroidogenic substance, acetyl-$ACTH_{1-39}$ is a poor stimulator of adrenal steroids (Waller & Dixon, 1960). Barnea (1983) concluded that, not only are the cleavage reactions of the ACTH precursor molecule (proopiocortin) important, but that N-acetylation is also important. She also hypothesised that N-acetylation takes place in the human fetal pituitary and that the proportional amounts of these non-steroidogenic and steroidgenic substances vary with gestational age. This is supported by the existence of N-acetyl transferase in fetal rabbit pituitaries whose activity changes with advancing fetal age. Studies like these help to explain fetal to adult patterns of adrenal steroido-gensis and the disappearance of the fetal zone of the adrenal cortex soon after delivery. It is possible that placental ACTH (Rees et al, 1975a; Genazzani et al, 1975) may also be involved in the preparturient changes in adrenal function.

Fetal adrenal

There is an inverse correlation between adrenal weight and prolongation of pregnancy in anencephalic fetuses. Fetal adrenal hypoplasia without cerebral malformation is also associated with post maturity (O'Donohoe & Holland, 1968; Roberts & Cawdery, 1970; Fliegner et al, 1972). In contrast there is fetal adrenocortical hyperplasia in infants which die after unexplained preterm labour (Anderson et al, 1971). However, normal duration of pregnancy has occurred despite the absence of the fetal adrenal glands (Pakravan et al, 1974). Due to the inaccessability of the human fetus it has been difficult to obtain meaningful measurements of cortisol secretion by the adrenal gland. Early studies suggested that concentrations of fetal cortisol increase shortly before delivery (Murphy, 1973). However Gennser et al (1977) demonstrated that cortisol concentrations in fetal blood samples are similar if collected at elective Caesarean section, spontaneous or induced labour and they concluded that an increase in cortisol concentrations was not essential for the onset of labour. This is reinforced by failure of exogenous glucocorticoids to induce labour despite earlier reports to the contrary (Mati et al, 1973). Exogenous glucorticoids do not mimic increased fetal adrenal activity but rather suppress the fetal pituitary-adrenal axis. Thus, suppressing precursors of oestrogen synthesis prevents any increase in oestrogen concentrations in the maternal circulation (see later). Fencl et al (1980) addressed the question of adrenal function in the fetus before parturition in a different way by measuring the concentrations of corticosterone sulphate in maternal plasma. This steroid, produced by the fetal adrenal gland, is found in higher concentrations in fetal, than in maternal, plasma. It is not hydrolysed by placental sulphatase and is a poor substrate for placental 11β-hydroxysteroid dehydrogenase. Shortly before parturition increased concentrations of corticosterone sulphate appear in plasma and urine of women with no adrenals. This suggests an increase in adrenal function in the fetus which, while not necessarily initiating parturition, may have a role in preparation of the fetus for independent life, e.g. the maturation of the lung.

Oestrogen

In women oestrogen is largely fetoplacental in origin, being synthetised in the placenta by aromitisation of C_{19} precursors derived mostly from the fetal adrenal cortex (Diczfalusy & Mancuso, 1969). Maternal urinary oestrogen excretion measured several weeks or months before labour is related to the level of uterine contractility and to ultimate gestational length (Robinson & Thorburn, 1974; Anderson & Turnbull. 1969). Early excitement (Turnbull et al, 1974) over changes in the concentration of oestrogens (particularly 17β-oestradiol) which preceed parturition, has waned since oestradiol concentrations during labour are the same as those found a week earlier. However it is likely that oestrogens play a facilitatory role in the onset of parturition (Turnbull et al, 1977).

Recently, part of the Diczfalusy model of fetoplacental production of oestrogen has been questioned. Diczfalusy considered that cholesterol of maternal origin is metabolised to pregnenolone and/or progesterone in the placenta, secreted into the fetal circulation, and taken up by the fetal adrenal gland where it is metabolised to dehydroepiandrosterone sulphate. However Carr et al (1980a), suggested that less than 1 per cent of dehydroepiandrosterone sulphate produced by the adrenal gland could be derived from pregnenolone of non-adrenal origin, and that the majority begins as cholesterol in the fetal liver.

The role of cholesterol in fetal steroid biosynthesis has been investigated in adrenal glands maintained in organ culture. Low density lipoprotein stimulates steroid secretion but high density and very low density lipoprotein do not (Carr et al, 1980b; Carr & Simpson, 1980). High affinity binding sites for low density lipoproteins have been found in the fetal adrenal gland and ACTH increases this binding (Ohashi et al, 1981). Binding of low density lipoprotein to membranes prepared from the fetal zone is significantly greater than that which occurs with membranes of the neocortex (Carr et al, 1982). Within the cells of the adrenal cortex low density lipoprotein degrades to release cholesterol. Together with *de novo* synthesis (Carr & Simpson, 1980), this cholesterol is available for the biosynthesis of dehydroepiandrosterone sulphate and cortisol in the adrenal gland. The fetal liver is able to supply sufficient cholesterol to the adrenal gland to maintain steroidogenesis (Carr & Simpson, 1981, 1982).

In summary, the main pathway for oestrogen synthesis in the fetoplacental unit involves low density lipoprotein synthesis in the fetal liver, conversion to dehydroepiandrosterone sulphate in the fetal adrenal, then oestrone or oestradiol synthesis by the placenta or 16α-hydroxylation in the fetal liver followed by conversion to oestriol by the placenta.

Progesterone

An essential role for progesterone in the maintenance of pregnancy was proposed by Corner in the 1920s and strongly defended by Csapo (1977). This progesterone 'block' hypothesis was derived from species in which the corpus luteum is the major site of progesterone production. Removal of the corpus luteum in these animals leads to abortion or premature delivery unless exogenous progesterone is simultaneously given.

Declining plasma concentrations of progesterone just before the onset of labour has been reported by two groups only (Csapo et al, 1971; Turnbull et al, 1974). Turnbull et al (1974) demonstrated only a fall in the mean concentrations of plasma progesterone and progesterone 'withdrawal' does not occur in every woman before labour. Even when present, it is never as complete as that found in sheep.

Oxytocin

Oxytocin has been used in clinical practice for many years. Although it is now given intravenously on most occasions, it has been administered intramuscularly, intranasally and sublingually to induce or augment labour. It was not until sensitive radioimmunoassays were developed for oxytocin that its role in spontaneous labour began to be defined (Chard, 1973). Perhaps it came as a surprise to many obstetricians to learn that oxytocin is not the 'trigger' to spontaneous labour. Concentrations of oxytocin in maternal plasma are low and show little change before the onset of parturition but increase greatly during the expulsive phases of labour (Chard, 1977; Dawood et al, 1978; Leake et al, 1981). By demonstrating that the proportion of blood samples which contain detectable concentrations of oxytocin increase throughout the first stage of labour, Gibbens & Chard (1976) were also able to describe a pulsatile release of oxytocin into the maternal circulation.

Exogenously administered pulsed oxytocin has been successfully used to induce labour when combined with amniotomy (Pavlou et al, 1978). Induction-to-delivery and induction-to-full dilatation intervals are similar but the total dose of oxytocin required is less than when oxytocin is infused continuously. It has also been suggested that the amplitude of uterine contractions is less when pulsed oxytocin is used to induce labour (Sadone et al, 1981). It is surprising that pulsed oxytocin has not been tested more often since significantly less oxytocin may be required. One benefit of this may be a reduction in the incidence of neonatal jaundice since high concentration of oxytocin reduces red cell survival (Buchan, 1979).

During labour plasma concentrations of oxytocin and vasopressin are much higher in the fetus than the mother (Chard, 1973). Vasopressin concentrations are about tenfold higher than oxytocin concentrations. The concentrations of both peptides are much higher in the umbilical artery than vein indicating fetal secretion. Cord blood of infants delivered by elective Caesarean section contains lower concentrations of both hormones than that of infants whose mothers have been in labour. These findings prompted Chard to suggest that the posterior pituitary gland of the fetus may play a role in the onset of parturition.

Oxytocin has an important role postpartum during suckling when a rapid rise of oxytocin concentrations occurs with nipple stimulation (Weitzman et al, 1980; Lucas et al, 1980; McNeilly et al, 1983). This forms the basis of the breast stimulation test (Silverman et al, 1982) to challenge the fetus in a manner analogous to the oxytocin stress test. However, it should be noted that Leake & Buster (1981) were unable to demonstrate an increase in peripheral plasma concentrations of oxytocin with breast pumping either during pregnancy or labour. Similarly they were unable to show an increase in oxytocin concentrations with vaginal distension during pregnancy.

Prostaglandins

Prostaglandins (PG) were initially identified by von Euler because of their effects on uterine muscle but it was not until Karim (1966) reported the presence of prostaglandins E_1, E_2, $F_{1\alpha}$ and $F_{2\alpha}$ in amniotic fluid that a role for these substances in the onset and maintenance of labour was vigorously pursued. Karim & Devlin (1967) found higher concentrations of $PGF_{2\alpha}$ and $PGF_{1\alpha}$ in amniotic fluid obtained during labour than before its onset and a year later Karim et al (1968) successfully induced labour by the intravenous infusion of $PGF_{2\alpha}$. Since then many studies have described the concentrations of prostaglandins in the uterus and its contents, and in peripheral body fluids during pregnancy and parturition. Many of these studies are difficult to interpret since the collection of samples by itself generates prostaglandins. Furthermore PG metabolism by organs distal to the uterus, particularly the lung, makes samples of peripheral tissues and fluids of little value in determining the role of prostaglandins in parturition.

The concentration of PGF in amniotic fluid is higher just before the onset of labour than earlier in pregnancy (Salmon & Amy, 1973; Hibbard et al, 1974; Keirse et al, 1974). In one sense these results are valid since no significant prostaglandin synthesis occurs in amniotic fluid (Turnbull et al, 1977), but the samples in these studies were collected before and after amniotomy. Amniotic fluid obtained via an intra-uterine catheter after amniotomy contains significantly more PGF than that obtained by amniocentesis and, when allowance is made for the route of collection, there is no significant increase in PGF with increasing gestational age (Mitchell et al, 1977). Mitchell et al (1977) therefore suggested that there is local prostaglandin synthesis associated with sweeping the membranes or stretching the cervix.

Concentrations of PGE in amniotic fluid also rise before the onset of labour and Dray & Frydman (1976) propose that this prostaglandin rather than PGF may be more important in the initiation of labour. Certainly after the onset of labour there is a rapid increase in the concentrations of both prostaglandins which correlate closely with cervical dilatation (Keirse & Turnbull, 1973; Salmon & Amy, 1973; Hillier et al, 1974; Keirse et al, 1974). However whilst the concentration of 13,14-dihydro-15-keto-prostaglandin F (PGFM) rises (Turnbull et al, 1977) in amniotic fluid and in peripheral plasma during labour (Gréen et al, 1974) the concentration of the recently described metabolite of PGE, 11-deoxy-13,14-dihydro-15-keto-11β, 16ε-bicylo PGE_2, does not (Brennecke et al, 1982a).

The source of prostaglandins during labour includes decidua, myometrium and fetal membranes. From a study of hypertonic-saline-induced abortion, Gustavii (1973) demonstrated that decidual cells are readily damaged by osmotic insult whereas trophoblastic cells remain microscopically intact. Gustavii (1973) suggested that such procedures as amniotomy, sweeping the membranes from the lower uterine segment and insertion of cervical catheters act via a common mechanism which involves prostaglandin release from decidual cells. He proposed that the lysosomal membranes of decidual cells are disrupted by these procedures thereby releasing phospholipase A_2. This enzyme acts on phospholipids to release arachidonic acid for prostaglandin synthesis. The PGE and PGF thus formed causes uterine contractions which results in uterine ischaemia and further damage to lysosomal membranes. More enzyme is released and so a cycle of prostaglandin synthesis and release is established.

MacDonald and his colleagues have studied those metabolic pathways which release arachidonic acid for prostaglandin synthesis. Initially they observed that the concentrations of free fatty acids in amniotic fluid increase during labour, and that the increase in arachidonic acid was disproportionately large (MacDonald et al, 1974). They suggested that the fetal membranes are the source of this arachidonic acid and reported that arachidonic acid injected into amniotic fluid successfully induced labour. Analysis of the lipid content of the fetal membranes before and soon after the onset of labour, indicates that arachidonic acid is lost selectively from diacyl-phosphotidyle-thanolamine and phosphotidylinositol (Okita et al, 1982), and that the membranes contain an active phospholipase A_2 which exhibits a preference for that phosphatidylethaliolamine containing arachidonic acid (Okazaki et al, 1978).

Metabolism of phosphotidylinositol requires three enzymes, namely phospholipase C, diacylglycerol lipase and monoacylglycerol lipase, all of which are present in fetal membranes and decidua vera. The specific activities of phospholipase A_2 and phospholipase C increase markedly in the amnion before parturition (Sagawa et al, 1982). These enzymes are activated by calcium ions but before labour the concentration of Ca^{++} may be too low to permit their activity. Calcium ions promote the release of arachidonic acid and inhibit the recycling of the intermediate, diacyglycerol, to phosphotidyinisitol (Sagawa et al, 1982).

There is some evidence for protein inhibitors of prostaglandin synthetase and it is probable that these are activated early in pregnancy because the concentrations of prostaglandins in decidual tissue obtained at 3 to 10 weeks of gestation is lower than at any stage of the normal menstrual cycle (Maathius & Kelly, 1978). An endogenous inhibitor of prostaglandin synthesis is present in the plasma of pregnant women (Brennecke et al, 1982b) but its concentration varies little before parturition and at most, this inhibitor may play a permissive rather than an active role. Bleasdale et al (1983) have suggested that a protein inhibitor similar to lipomodulin (macrocortin) (Flower & Blackwell, 1979) is present in amniotic fluid.

Little mention has been made of other substances in the arachidonic acid cascade. Recent work suggests that prostaglandin D_2 is a major product of intra-uterine tissues. At this stage it is too early to ascribe a definitive role for this prostaglandin except to say that, together with prostacyclin (PGI_2), it may play an important role in the regulation of uterine blood flow (Clark et al, 1982). Infusion of PGI_2 reduces vasospasm and lowers blood pressure in fulminating pre-eclampsia (Fidler et al, 1980). Reports of increased concentrations of the stable metabolite of PGI_2, 6-oxoprostaglandin $F_{1\alpha}$ (Lewis et al, 1980) suggest that vasodilatation and inhibition of platelet activity may be increased in pregnancy but for a similar increase in thromboxane B_2, the stable metabolite of thromboxane A_2 which is a vasoconstrictor and actuates platelet aggregation (Ylikorkala & Viinikka, 1980).

No account of prostaglandins in human parturition would be complete without brief reference to the pharmacological induction of labour by these compounds. Many reports have confirmed that PGE and PGF can induce labour or terminate pregnancy at almost any stage of gestation. To achieve this they have been administered intravenously, intramuscularly, orally, intra- and extra-amniotically and vaginally. The local application is preferred because the side-effects are fewer but the high cost of these preparations limits their use to situations were oxytocin is less effective (Embrey, 1981). Likewise the non-steroidal anti-inflammatory group of prostaglandin synthetase inhibitors have failed to find a place in the inhibition of labour. This is because of their effects on the fetus which makes adaption to postnatal life a difficult and life threatening procedure (Manchester et al, 1976).

CONCLUSION

It is attractive to speculate that there is a common key to the regulation of both fetal growth, maturation and parturition. It makes biological sense that, in the event of severe nutritional deprivation or other adverse environment, the fetus should first respond by preserving those functions vital to its long-term survival. Brain growth is one such vital function and since this is the only organ in the fetus whose growth is apparently independent of insulin, this hormone could have a role in the distribution of available nutrients. It is of interest that insulin appears to have an inhibitory effect on fetal lung maturation because often in the event of severe fetal compromise when it is appropriate that the fetus makes preparation for a premature entry to the world, insulin concentrations are low. By its regulation of both parturition and lung maturation, cortisol therefore has a key role in the transition from fetal to extrauterine life. However it is unlikely that insulin and cortisol are only players on the stage of cell division and differentiation whose complex interrelation with other growth and maturation factors will prove most difficult to unravel.

There is a great variety of circumstantial evidence which suggests that the insulin-related growth factors are the final mediators of fetal growth whilst prostaglandins serve that role in parturition. However a delineation of the factors which regulate these hormones in the fetus has proven elusive. A consideration of animal models has served only to emphasise that different regulators are likely to operate in man. For example, there is convincing evidence in ruminants that the hypothalamo-pituitary-adrenal axis and oestrogen progesterone balance are the key to the onset of parturition but these do not appear to be as important in man. Likewise, in animals, a balance between nutrition, insulin and placental lactogen may regulate fetal insulin-like growth factors just as nutrition, insulin and growth hormone are the major regulators of extrauterine growth. However, it is clear that placental lactogen is not an essential hormone in man. It is possible that the answers to these puzzles will be found by a study of the endocrinology of a suitable primate fetus throughout its gestation. Such a search is not inappropriate when it is appreciated that the majority of perinatal loss and congenital disease arises from a disturbance of fetal growth or the inappropriate timing of parturition.

REFERENCES

Adams S O, Nissley S P, Handwerger S, Rechler M M 1983 Developmental patterns of insulin-like growth factor -I and -II synthesis and regulation in rat fibroblasts. Nature 302: 150–153

Adamson E D, Deller M J, Warsaw J B 1981 Functional EGF receptors are present on mouse embryo tissues. Nature 291: 656–659

Aloe L, Cozzani C, Calissano P, Levi-Montaccini R 1981 Somatic and behavioural postnatal effects of fetal injections of nerve growth factor antibodies in the rat. Nature 291: 413–415

Ances I G 1973 Serum concentrations of epidermal growth factor in human pregnancy. American Journal of Obstetrics and Gynecology 115: 357–362

Anderson A B M, Turnbull A C 1969, In Wolstenholme G E W,

Knight J (eds) Progesterone. Its Regulatory Effect on the Myometrium. p 106. J & A Churchill, London

Anderson A B M, Lawrence K M, Davies K, Campbell H, Turnbull A C 1971 Fetal adrenal weight and the cause of premature delivery in human pregnancy. Journal of Obstetrics and Gynaecology of the British Commonwealth 78: 481–488

Anderson A B M, Flint A P F, Turnbull A C 1975 Mechanism of action of glucocorticoids in induction of ovine parturition, effect of placental steroid metabolism. Journal of Endocrinology 66: 61–70

Armelin M C S, Armelin H A 1977 Serum and hormonal regulation of the 'resting proliferative' transition on a variant of 3T3 mouse cells. Nature 265: 148–150

Ash R W, Challis J R G, Harrison F A, Heap R B, Illingworth D V,

Perry J S Poyser N L 1973, In: Comline R S, Cross K W, Dawes G S, Nathanielsz P W (eds) Hormonal Control of Pregnancy and Parturition: a comparative analysis. Fetal and Neonatal Physiology (Sir Joseph Barcroft Symposium), pp 551–556. Cambridge University Press, Cambridge

Ashton I K, Vesey J 1978 Somatomedin activity in human cord plasma and relationship to birth size, insulin, growth hormone and prolactin. Early Human Development 2: 115–122

Barnea H 1983 Fetal pituitary and intermediate lobe function. In: MacDonald P C, Porter J eds Initiation of Parturition: prevention of prematurity. Report 4th Ross Conf Obstet Res pp 116–121. Ross Lab Columbus, Ohio

Barnes R J, Comline R S, Silver M 1977 Effects of bilateral adrenalectomy or hypophysectomy of the fetal lamb in utero. Journal of Physiology 264: 429–447

Bassett J M, Thorburn G D 1969 Fetal plasma corticosteroids and the initiation of parturition in the sheep. Journal of Endocrinology 44: 285–286

Bengtsson L P, Scholfield B M 1963 Progesterone and the accomplishment of parturition in the sheep. Journal of Reproduction and Fertility 5: 423–431

Beardmore J M, Richards R C 1982 Concentrations of epidermal growth factor in mouse milk throughout lactation. Journal of Endocrinology 96: 287–292

Binns W, James L-F, Shupe J L Everett G A 1963 A congenital cyclopian-type malformation in lambs induced by maternal ingestion of a range plant, Veratrum californicum. American Journal of Veterinary Research 24: 1164–1175

Bleasdale J E, Okazaki T, Sagawa N, Di Renzo, G C, Okita J R, Macdonald P C, Johnston J M 1983 Mobilisation of arachidonic acid for prostaglandin production. In: MacDonald P C, Porter J (eds) Initiation of Parturition: prevention of prematurity. Report 4th Ross Conf Obstet Res pp 129–137. Ross Lab, Columbus, Ohio

Borsi L, Rosenfeld R G, Liu F, Hintz R L 1982 Somatomedin peptide distribution and somatomedin-binding protein content in cord plasma: comparison to normal and hypopituitary plasma. Journal of Clinical Endocrinology and Metabolism 54: 223–228

Bradshaw R A 1978 Nerve growth factor. Annual Review of Biochemistry 47: 191–216

Bradshaw R A, Niall H D 1978 Insulin-related growth factors. Proceedings of the S E Asia and Oceania Congress of Endocrinology, Singapore, pp 358–364

Bradshaw R A, Rubin J S 1980 Polypeptide growth factors: some structural and mechanistic considerations. Journal of Supramolecular Structure and Cellular Biochemisty 14: 183–199

Brennecke S P, Bryce R L, Turnbull A C, Mitchell M D 1982a The prostaglandin synthase inhibiting activity of maternal plasma and the onset of human labour. European Journal of Obstetrics, Gynecology and Reproductive Biology 14: 81–88

Brennecke S P, Demers L M, Castle B 1982b Endogenous prostaglandin E_2 metabolite levels in the human during pregnancy as determined by a novel radioimmunoassay. Proceedings of the 1st International Austrian Prostaglandin Meeting, p 52

Brinsmead M W, Liggins G C 1978 The binding of rat liver cell multiplication-stimulating activity (MSA) to human placenta and serum proteins. Australian Journal of Experimental Biology and Medical Science 56: 527–544

Brinsmead M W, Liggins G C 1979a Somatomedin-like activity, prolactin, growth hormone and insulin in human cord blood. Australian and New Zealand Journal of Obstetrics and Gynecology 5: 130–134

Brinsmead M W, Liggins G C 1979b Serum somatomedin activity after hypophysectomy and during parturition in fetal lambs. Endocrinology 105: 297–305

Brinsmead M W, Liggins G C 1979c Somatomedins and other growth factors in fetal growth. Reviews In Perinatal Medicine 3: 203–242

Brinsmead M W, Owens P C 1982 Serum somatomedin-like activity in pregnant ewes and fetal lambs on the ontogeny of somatomedin receptors in ovine fetal liver. In: Mantell C D ed Proceedings of the Second Asia-Oceania Congress of Perinatology, pp 111–115

Brinsmead M W, Thorburn G D 1982 Effect of Streptozotocin on fetal lambs in mid-pregnancy. Australian Journal of Biological Sciences 35: 517–525

Buchan P C 1979 Pathogenesis of neonatal hyperbilirubinaemia after induction of labour with oxytocin. British Medical Journal ii: 1255–1257

Carpenter G, Cohen S 1979 Epidermal growth factor. Annual Review of Biochemistry 48: 193–216

Carr B R, Parker C R Jr, Milewich L, Porter J C, Macdonald P C, Simpson E R 1980a The role of low density, high density and very low density lipoproteins in steroidogenesis by the human fetal adrenal gland. Endocrinology 106: 1854–1860

Carr B R, Parker C R Jr, Macdonald P C, Simpson E R 1980b Metabolism of high density lipoprotein by human fetal adrenal tissue. Endocrinology 107: 1849–1854

Carr B R, Simpson E R 1980 De novo synthesis of cholesterol by the human fetal adrenal gland. Endocrinology 108: 2154–2162

Carr B R, Simpson E R 1981 Synthesis of cholesterol in the human fetus: 3-hydroxy-3-methylglutaryl coenzyme A reductase activity in liver microsomes. Journal of Clinical Endocrnology and Metabolism 53: 810–812

Carr B R, Ohashi M, Simpson E R 1982 Low density lipoprotein binding and de novo synthesis of cholesterol in the neocortex and fetal zones of the human fetal adrenal gland. Endocrinology 110: 1994–1998

Carr B R Simpson E R 1982 Cholesterol synthesis in human fetal tissues. Journal of Clinical Endocrinology and Metabolism 55: 447–452

Catterton W Z, Escobedo M B, Sexson W R, Gray M E, Sundell H W, Stahlman M T 1979 Effect of epidermal growth factor on lung maturation in fetal rabbits. Pediatric Research 13: 104–108

Challis J R G, Manchester E J, Lye S J, Patrick J E, Mitchell B F, Olson D M, Power S G A 1983 The development of the pathway for steroid synthesis. In: MacDonald P C, Porter J eds Initiation of Parturition: Prevention of prematurity. Report 4th Ross Conference of Obstetric Research, pp 11–17. Ross Lab, Columbus, Ohio

Chan J S D, Robertson H A, Friesen H G 1978a Maternal and fetal concentrations of ovine placental lactogen measured by radioimmunoassay. Endocrinology 102: 1606–1613

Chan J S D, Robertson H A, Friesen H G 1978b Distribution of binding sites for ovine placental lactogen in the sheep. Endocrinology 102: 632–640

Chard T 1973 The posterior pituitary and the induction of labour. In: Klopper A, Gardiner J (eds) Endocrine Factors in Labour, pp 61–76. Cambridge University Press, Cambridge

Chard T 1977 The posterior pituitary gland. In: Fuchs F, Klopper A (eds) Endocrinology of Pregnancy, pp 271–290. Harper & Row, New York

Cheek D B, Hill D E 1975 Changes in somatic growth after ablation of maternal or fetal pancreatic beta cells. In: Cheek D (ed) Fetal and Postnatal Cellular Growth: Hormones and Nutrition, pp 311–321. John Wiley & Sons, New York

Chettur L, Christensen E, Philip J 1978 Stimulation of amniotic fluid cells by fibroblast growth factor. Clinical Genetics 14: 223–228

Chochinov R H, Mariz I K, Hajek A S, Daughaday W H 1977 Characterization of a protein in mid-term human amniotic fluid which reacts in a somatomedin-C radioreceptor assay. Journal of Clinical Endocrinology and Metabolism 44: 902–908

Clark K E, Austin J E, Saeeds A E 1982 Effect of bisenoic prostaglandins and arachidonic acid on the uterine vasculature of pregnant sheep. American Journal of Obstetrics and Gynaecology 142: 261–268

Clemmons D R, Van Wyk J J 1981 Somatomedin-C and platelet derived growth factor stimulate human fibroblast replication. Journal of Cell Physiology 106: 361–367

Comline R S, Silver M 1961 The release of adrenaline and noradrenaline from the adrenal glands of the fetal sheep. Journal of Physiology 156: 424–444

Comroe J H 1978 Retrospectoscope: Insights into Medical Discovery p 167. Von Gehr Press, Menlo Park, California

Cornblath M, Schwartz R 1966 Transient diabetes mellitus in early infancy. In: Cornblath M, Schwartz R (eds) Disorders of Carbohydrate Metabolism in Infancy, pp 105–114. W B Saunders Co, Philadelphia

Cornblath M, Parker M L, Reisner S H, Forbes A E, Daughaday W H 1965 Secretion and metabolism of growth hormone in premature and full-term infants. Journal of Clinical Endocrinology Metabolism 25: 209–218

Csapo A I 1977 The 'see-saw' theory of parturition. In: Knight J, O'Connor M (eds) The Fetus and Birth. Ciba Foundation Symposium 47 (New Series), pp 159–195. Excerpta Medica, Amsterdam

Csapo A I, Knobil E, Van Der Molen H J, Weist W G 1971 Peripheral plasma progesterone levels during human pregnancy and labour. American Journal of Obstetrics and Gynecology 110: 630–632

Currie W B, Wong M S F, Cox R I, Thorburn G D 1973 Spontaneous or dexamethasone-induced parturition in the sheep and goat: Changes in plasma concentrations of maternal prostaglandin F and fetal oestrogen sulphate. Memoirs of the Society for Endocrinology 20: 95–118

Daughaday W H, Reeder C 1966 Synchronous activation of DNA synthesis in hypophysectomised rat cartilage by growth hormone. Journal of Laboratory and Clinical Medicine 68: 357–368

Daughaday W H, Hall K, Raben M S, Salmon W D, Van Den Brande J L, Van Wyk J J 1972 Somatomedin: proposed designation for sulphation factor. Nature 235: 107–108

Daughaday W H, Trivedi B, Kapadia M 1979 The effect of hypophysectomy on rat chorionic somatomammotropin as measured by prolactin and growth hormone radioreceptor assays: possible significance in maintenance of somatomedin generation. Endocrinology 105: 210

Daughaday W H, Mariz I K, Trivedi B 1981a A preferential binding site for insulin-like growth factor II in human and rat placental membranes. Journal of Clinical Endocrinology and Metabolism 53: 282–288

Daughaday W H, Trivedi B, Kapadia M 1981b Measurement of insulin-like growth factor II by a specific radioreceptor assay in serum of normal individuals, patients with abnormal growth hormone secretion and patients with tumor-associated hypoglycaemia. Journal of Clinical Endocrinology and Metabolism 53: 289–294

Dawood M Y, Raghavan K S, Pociask C, Fuchs F 1978 Oxytocin in human pregnancy and parturition. Obstetrics and Gynecology 51: 138–143

Deal C L, Guyda H J, Lai W H, Posner B I 1983 Ontogeny of growth factor receptors in the human fetus. Pediatric Research 16: 820–826

De Asua L J, Richmond K M Y, Otto A M 1981 Two growth factors glucocorticoid inhibition of growth promoting effects of prostaglandin $F_{2\alpha}$ on 3T3 cells. Nature 265: 450–452

De Asua L J, Richmond K M Y, Otto A M 1981 Two growth factors and two hormones regulate initiation of DNA synthesis in cultured mouse cells through different pathways of events. Proceedings of the National Academy of Sciences of the United States of America 78: 1004–1008

D'Ercole A J, Foushee D B, Underwood L E 1976 Somatomedin-C receptor ontogeny and levels in porcine fetal and human cord serum. Journal of Clinical Endocrinology and Metabolism 43: 1069–1077

D'Ercole A J, Underwood L E, Van Wyk J J 1977 Serum somatomedin-C in hypopituitarism and other disorders of growth. Journal of Pediatrics 90: 375–381

D'Ercole A J, Applethwite G T, Underwood L E 1980a Evidence that somatomedin is synthetised by multiple tissues in the fetus. Developmental Biology 75: 315–328

D'Ercole A J, Wilson D F, Underwood L E 1980b Changes in the circulating form of serum somatomedin-C during fetal life. Journal of Clinical Endocrinology and Metabolism 51: 674–676

Diczfalusy E, Mancuso S 1969 Oestrogen metabolism in pregnancy. In: Klopper A, Diczfalusy E (eds) Foetus and Placenta, pp 191–248. Blackwell Scientific Publications, Oxford

Dodge J A, Laurence K M 1977 Congenital absence of islets of Langerhans. Archives of Disease in Childhood 52: 411–413

Donohue W L, Uchida I 1954 Leprechaunism — a eupherism for a rare familial disorder. Journal of Pediatrics 45: 505–519

Dray F, Frydman R 1976 Primary prostaglandins in amniotic fluid in pregnancy and spontaneous labour. American Journal of Obstetrics and Gynecology 126: 13–19

Ellwood D A, Anderson A B M, Mitchell M D, Murphy G, Turnbull A C 1981 Prostenoids, collagenase and cervix. In: Ellwood D A, Anderson A B M (eds) The Cervix in Pregnancy and Parturition, pp 57–73, Churchill Livingstone, Edinburgh

Embrey M P 1981 Prostaglandins in human reproduction. British Medical Journal 283: 1563–1566

Erenburg A, Rhodes M L, Weinstein M M, Kennedy R L 1979 Effect of fetal thyroidectomy on ovine fetal lung maturation. Pediatric Research 13: 230–235

Falconer J, Redman C W G, Robinson J S 1981 Somatomedin-like activity in cord blood from infants of hypertensive mothers. European Journal of Obstetrics, Gynecology and Reproductive Biology 12: 151–155

Fencl M de M, Stillman R J, Cohen J, Tulchinskey D 1980 Direct evidence of sudden rise in fetal corticoids in late human pregnancy. Nature 287: 225–226

Fidler J, Bennett M J, de Swiet M, Ellis C, Lewis P J 1980 Treatment of pregnancy hypertension with prostacyclin. Lancet ii: 32–33

Fisher D A, Hoath S, Lakshmanan J 1982 The thyroid hormone effects on growth and development may be mediated by growth factors. Endocrinologia Experimentalis 16: 259–271

Fitzpatrick R J 1977 Dilatation of the uterine cervix. In: Knight J, O'Connor M eds The fetus and birth. Ciba Foundation Symposium 47 (New Series), pp 31–38, Excerpta Medica, Amsterdam

Fitzpatrick R J, Dobson H 1981 Softening of the ovine cervix at parturition. In: Ellwood D A, Anderson A B M (eds) The Cervix in Pregnancy and Parturition, pp 40–56 Churchill Livingstone, Edinburgh

Fletcher J M, Falconer J, Bassett J M 1982 The relationship of body and placental weight to plasma levels of insulin and other hormones during development in fetal rabbits. Diabetologia 23: 124–130

Fliegner J R H, Schindler I, Brown J B 1972 Low urinary oestriol excretion during pregnancy associated with placental sulphatase deficiency or congenital adrenal hypoplasia. Journal of Obstetrics and Gynaecology of the British Commonwealth 79: 810–815

Flower R J, Blackwell G J 1979 Anti-inflammatory steroids induce biosynthesis of a phospholipase A_2 inhibitor which prevents prostaglandin generation. Nature 278: 456–459

Foley T P, De Philip R, Perricelli A, Miller A 1980 Low somatomedin activity in cord serum from infants with intrauterine growth retardation. Journal of Pediatrics 96: 605–610

Furlanetto R W, Underwood L E, Van Wyk J J, Handwerger S 1978 Serum immunoreactive somatomedin C is elevated late in pregnancy. Journal of Clinical Endocrinology and Metabolism 47: 695–698

Genazzani A R, Farioli F, Hurhiman J, Fioretti P, Felber J P 1975 Immunoreactive ACTH and cortisol plasma levels during pregnancy, detection and partial purification of corticotrophin-like placental hormone: The human chorionic corticotrophin (HCC) Clinical Endocrinology 4: 1–14

Gennser G, Ohrlander S, Eneroth P 1977 Fetal cortisol and the initiation of labour. In: Knight J, O'Connor M (eds) The Fetus and birth. Ciba Foundation Symposium 47 (New Series), pp 401–420. Excerpta Medica, Amsterdam

Gibbens G L D, Chard T 1976 Observations on maternal oxytocin release during human labour and the effect of intravenous alcohol administration. American Journal of Obstetrics and Gynecology 126: 243–246

Girard J R, Rieutort M, Kervan A, Jost A 1976 Hormonal control of fetal growth with particular reference to insulin and growth hormone. In: Booth G, Bratterby L E Perinatal Medicine, pp 197–292. Almquist & Wiksell, Uppsala

Glickman J A, Challis J R G 1980 The changing response pattern of sheep fetal adrenal cells throughout the course of gestation. Endocrinology 106: 1371–1376

Gluckman P D, Brinsmead M W 1976 Somatomedin in cord blood: Relationship to gestational age and birth size. Journal of Clinical Endocrinology and Metabolism 43: 1378–1381

Gluckman P D, Butler J H 1983 Parturition related changes in insulin like growth factors -I and -II in the parinatal lamb. Journal of Endocrinology, 99: 223–232

Golde D W 1980 Growth factors. Annals of Internal Medicine 92: 650–662

Goldstein L D, Reynolds C P, Perez-Polo J R 1978 Isolation of human nerve growth factor from placental tissue. Neurochemical Research 3: 175–183

Gorin P D, Johnson E M 1980 Effects of exposure to nerve growth factor antibodies on the developing nervous system of the rat: an experimental autoimmune approach. Developmental Biology 80: 313–323

Gospodarowicz D 1975 Purification of a fibroblast growth factor from bovine pituitary. Journal of Biological Chemistry 250: 2515–2520

Gospodarowicz D, Moran J S 1976 Growth factors in mammalian cell culture. Annual Review of Biochemistry 45: 531–538

Gospodarowicz D, Moran J S, Owashi N D 1977 Effects of fibroblast growth factor and epidermal growth factor on rate of growth of amniotic fluid derived cells. Journal of Clinical Endocrinology and Metabolism 44: 651–659

Gréen K, Bygdeman M, Toppozada M, Wiqvist N 1974 The role of prostaglandin $F_{2\alpha}$ in human parturition. Endogenous plasma levels of 15-keto-13, 14-dihydroprostaglandin $F_{2\alpha}$ during labour. American Journal of Obstetrics and Gynecology 120: 25–31

Gregory H 1975 Isolation and structure of urogastrone and its relationship to epidermal growth factor. Nature 257: 325–327

Grumbach M M 1974 Growth hormone and prolactin in the human fetus. In: The Endocrine Milieu of Pregnancy, Puerperium and Childhood. Report 3rd Ross Conference on Obstetric Research, pp 68–80. Ross Labs, Colombus, Ohio

Gustavii B 1973 Studies on the mode of action of intra-amniotically and extra-amniotically injected hypertonic saline in therapeutic abortion. Acta Obstetrica and Gynecologica Scandinavica (Suppl) 25: 1–2

Heldin C H, Wasteson A, Westermank B 1977 Partial purification and characterisation of platelet factors stimulating the multiplication of normal human glial cells. Experimental Cell Research 109: 429–437

Hetzel B S, Hay I D 1979 Thyroid function, iodine nutrition and fetal brain development. Clinical Endocrinology 11: 445–460

Hibbard B M, Sharma S C, Fitzpatrick R J, Hamlett J D 1974 Prostaglandin $F_{2\alpha}$ concentrations in amniotic fluid in late pregnancy. Journal of Obstetrics and Gynaecology of the British Commonwealth 81: 35–38

Hill D E 1978 Effect of insulin on fetal growth. Seminars in Perinatology 2: 310–328

Hill D J, Davidson P, Milner R D G 1979 Retention of plasma somatomedin activity in the fetal rabbit following decapitation in utero. Journal of Endocrinology 81: 93–102

Hill D E, Boughter J M, Carlisle V L, Herzberg V L, Sziszak T J 1980 The role of insulin in fetal growth. In: Cummings I A, Funder J W, Mendlesohn F A O (eds) Endocrinology 1980. Proceedings of the VI International Congress of Endocrinology, pp 471–474. Australian Academy of Science, Canberra

Hill D J, Andrews S J, Milner R D G 1981 Cartilage response to plasma and plasma somatomedin activity in rats related to growth before and after birth. Journal of Endocrinology 90: 133–142

Hill D J, Milner R D G 1981 Somatomedins and fetal growth In: The Fetus and Independent Life. Ciba Foundation Symposium No 86, pp 124–138. Excerpta Medica, Amsterdam

Hillier K, Calder A A, Embrey M P 1974 Concentrations of prostaglandin $F_{2\alpha}$ in amniotic fluid and plasma after spontaneous and induced labours. Journal of Obstetrics and Gynaecology of the British Commonwealth 81: 257–263

Hirata Y, Orth D M 1979 Epidermal growth factor (urogastrone) in human tissues. Journal of Clinical Endocrinology and Metabolism 48: 667–674

Hock R A, Nexo E, Hollenberg M D 1979 Isolation of the human placental receptor for epidermal growth factor — urogastrone. Nature 277: 403–405

Holm L W 1967 Prolonged pregnancy. Advances in Veterinary Science and Comparative Medicine 11: 159–205

Honnebier W J, Swaab D F 1973 The influence of anencephaly upon intrauterine growth of the fetus and placenta and upon gestation length. Journal of Obstetrics and Gynaecology of the British Commonwealth 80: 577–588

Hurley T W, D'Ercole A J, Handwerger S, Underwood L E, Furlanetto R W, Fellows R E 1977 Ovine placental lactogen induces somatomedin: a possible role in fetal growth. Endocrinology 101: 1635–1638

Ikeno T, Guroff G 1979 Growth regulation by nerve growth factor. Molecular and Cellular Biochemistry 28: 67–91

Johnson J W C, Mitzner W, London W T, Palmer A E, Scott R 1979 Betamethasone and the rhesus fetus: multisystemic effects. American Journal of Obstetrics and Gynecology 133: 677–684

Jones C T, Roebuck M M 1980 ACTH peptides and development of the fetal adrenal. Journal of Steroid Biochemistry 12: 77–82

Jones C T, Boddy K, Robinson J S 1977 Changes in the concentration of adrenocorticotrophin and corticosteroid in the plasma of fetal sheep in the latter half of pregnancy and during labour. Journal of Endocrinology 72: 293–300

Josimovich J B, Archer D F 1977 The role of lactogenic hormones in the pregnant woman and fetus. American Journal of Obstetrics and Gynecology 129: 777–780

Karim S M M 1966 Identification of prostaglandins in human amniotic fluid. Journal of Obstetrics and Gynaecology of the British Commonwealth 73: 903–908

Karim S M M, Devlin J 1967 Prostaglandin content of amniotic fluid during pregnancy and labour. Journal of Obstetrics and Gynaecology of the British Commonwealth 74: 230–234

Karim S M M, Trussell R R, Patel R C, Hillier K 1968 Response of pregnant human uterus to prostaglandin $F_{2\alpha}$ — induction of labour. British Medical Journal iv: 621–623

Keirse M J N C, Turnbull A C 1973 E prostaglandins in amniotic fluid during late pregnancy and labour. Journal of Obstetrics and Gynaecology of the British Commonwealth 80: 970–973

Keirse M J N C, Flint A P F, Turnbull A C 1974 F prostglandins in amniotic fluid during pregnancy and labour. Journal of Obstetrics and Gynaecology of the British Commonwealth 81: 131–135

Kelly P A, Posner B I, Tsushima T, Friesen H G 1974 Studies on insulin, growth hormone and prolactin binding: ontogenesis, effects of sex and pregnancy. Endocrinology 95: 532–539

Kendall J Z, Challis J R G, Hart I C, Jones C T, Mitchell M D, Ritchie J W K, Robinson J S, Thorburn G D 1977 Steroid and prostaglandin concentrations in the plasma of pregnant ewes during infusion of adrenocorticotrophin or dexamethasone to intact or hypophysectomized fetuses. Journal of Endocrinology 75: 59–71

Kennedy P C 1971 Interaction of fetal disease and the onset of labour in cattle and sheep. Federation Proceedings 30: 110–113

Kennedy P C, Kendrick J W, Stormont C 1975 Adenohypophyseal aplasia, and inherited defects associated with abnormal gestation in Guernsey cattle. Cornell Veterinaria 47: 160

Laron Z, Galatzer A 1981 Effect of hGH on head circumference and IQ in isolated growth hormone deficiency. Early Human Development 5: 211–214

Laron Z, Manheimer S, Nitzman M 1967 Growth hormone, glucose and free fatty acid levels in mother and infant in normal, diabetic and toxaemic pregnancies. Archives of Disease in Childhood 42: 24–28

Laron Z, Pertzelan A 1969 Somatotrophin in antenatal and perinatal growth and development. Lancet i: 680–681

Leake R D, Buster J E 1981 The oxytocin secretory response following breast and perineal stimulation. Abstract presented at 63rd Endocrinology Society Meeting

Leake R D, Weitzman R E, Glatz T, Fisher D A 1981 Plasma oxytocin concentrations in men, non-pregnant women and pregnant women before and during spontaneous labour. Journal of Clinical Endocrinology and Metabolism 53: 730–733

Lemons J A, Ridenour R, Onsini E N 1979 Congenital absence of the pancreas and intrauterine growth retardation. Pediatrics 64: 255–257

Lewis P J, Boylan P, Friedman L A, Hensby C N, Downing I 1980 Prostacyclin in pregnancy. British Medical Journal 1: 1581–1582

Liggins G C 1968 Premature parturition after infusion of corticotrophin or cortisol into fetal lambs. Journal of Endocrinology 42: 323–329

Liggins G C 1969 The fetal role in the initiation of parturition in the ewe. In: Wolstenholme G E W, O'Connor M (eds) Fetal Autonomy. Ciba Foundation Symposium, pp 218–231. Churchill Livingstone, Edinburgh

Liggins G C 1974 The influence of the fetal hypothalamus and pituitary on growth. In: Size at Birth. Ciba Foundation Symposium, pp 165–183. Associated Scientific publishers, Amsterdam

Liggins G C 1976 Adrenocortical-related maturational events in the fetus. American Journal of Obstetrics and Gynecology 126: 931–941

Liggins G C, Kennedy P C, Holm L W 1967 Failure of initiation of parturition after electrocoagulation of the fetal pituitary gland. American Journal of Obstetrics and Gynecology 98: 1080–1086

Lin C C, Moawad A H, River P, Blix P, Abraham M, Rubinstein A H 1981 Amniotic fluid C-peptide as an index for intrauterine fetal growth. American Journal of Obstetrics and Gynecology 139: 390–395

Lucas A, Drewitt R B, Mitchell M D 1980 Breast feeding and plasma oxytocin. British Medical Journal 281: 834–835

Lye S J, Porter D G 1978 Demonstration that progesterone 'blocks' uterine activity in the ewe in vivo by direct action on the myometrium. Journal of Reproduction and Fertility 52: 87–94

Maathius J B, Kelly R W 1978 Concentrations of prostaglandin $F_{2\alpha}$ and E2 in the endometrium throughout the human menstrual cycle after the administration of clomiphene or oestrogen-progestogen pill and in early pregnancy. Journal of Endocrinology 77: 361–371

Macdonald P C, Schultz F M, Duenhoelter J H, Gant N F, Jimenez J M, Pritchard J A, Porter J C, Johnston J 1974 Initiation of human parturition. I. Mechanism of action of arachidonic acid. Obstetrics and Gynecology 44: 629–636

Malpas P 1933 Postmaturity and malformation of the fetus. Journal of Obstetrics and Gynaecology of the British Empire 40: 1046–1053

Manchester D, Margolis H S, Sheldon R E 1976 Possible association between maternal indomethacin and primary pulmonary hypertension in the newborn. American Journal of Obstetrics and Gynecology 126: 467–469

Marquardt H, Todaro G J, Henderson L E, Oroszlan S 1981 Purification and primary structure of a polypeptide with multiplication-stimulating activity from rat liver cell cultures. Journal of Biological Chemistry 256: 6859–6865

Marshall R N, Underwood L E, Voina S J, Foushee D B, Van Wyk J J 1974 Characterization of the insulin and somatomedin-C receptors in human placental cell membranes. Journal of Clinical Endocrinology and Metabolism 39: 283–292

Marti-Henneberg C, Gluckman P D, Kaplan S L, Grumbach M M 1980 Hormone ontogeny in the ovine: XI. The serotoninergic regulation of growth hormone and prolactin secretion. Journal of Clinical Endocrinology and Metabolism 107: 1273

Mati J K G, Horrobin D F, Bramley P S 1973 Induction of labour in sheep and in humans by single doses of corticosteroids. British Medical Journal 2: 149–151

Matsukaki F, Irie M, Shizume K 1971 Growth hormone in human fetal pituitary glands and cord blood. Journal of Clinical Endocrinology and Metabolism 33: 908–911

McNeilly A, Robinson I C A F, Houston M J, Howie P W 1983 Release of oxytocin and prolactin in response to suckling. British Medical Journal 286: 257–259

Mitchell M D, Flint A P F 1978 Use of meclofenamic acid to investigate the role of prostaglandin biosynthesis during induced parturition in sheep. Journal of Endocrinology 76: 101–109

Mitchell M D, Flint A P F, Turnbull A C 1976 Plasma concentration of 13, 14-dihydro-15-ketoprostaglandin F during pregnancy in sheep. Prostaglandins 11: 319–329

Mitchell M D, Keirse M J N C, Anderson A B M, Turnbull A C 1977 Evidence for a local control of prostaglandins within the pregnant human uterus. British Journal of Obsterics and Gynaecology 84: 35–38

Moses A C, Nissley S P, Short P A, Rechler M M, White R M, Knight A B, Higa O Z 1980 Increased levels of multiplication-stimulating activity, an insulin-like growth factor in fetal rat serum. Proceedings of the National Academy of Science of the United States of America 77: 3649–3653

Mosier H D 1982 Thyroid hormone. In: Daughaday W H (ed) Endocrine Control of Growth, pp 25–45 Elsevier, New York

Murphy B E P 1973 Does the human fetal adrenal play a role in parturition? American Journal of Obstetrics and Gynecology 115: 521–525

Nevo Z, Laron Z 1979 Growth factors. A review. American Journal of Diseases of Children 133: 419–428

Nexo E, Hollenberg M D, Figueroa A, Prott R M 1980 Detection of epidermal growth factor — urogastrone and its receptor during fetal mouse development. Proceedings of the National Academy of Science of the United States of America 77: 2782–2785

Nielsen P V, Pedersen H, Kampmann E M 1979 Absence of human placental lactogen in an otherwise uneventful pregnancy. American Journal of Obstetrics and Gynecology 135: 322–326

Nissley S P, Rechler M M 1978 Multiplication-stimulating activity MSA — a somatomedin-like polypeptide from cultured rat liver cells. National Cancer Institute Monographs 48: 167–178

Novy M J, Cook M J, Manaugh L 1974 Indomethacin block of normal onset of parturition in primates. American Journal of Obstetrics and Gynecology 118: 412–416

O'Donohoe D V, Holland P D J 1968 Familial congenital adrenal hypoplasia. Archives of Disease in Childhood 43: 717–723

Ohashi M, Carr B R, Simpson E R 1981 Effects of adrenocorticotrophic hormone on low density lipoprotein receptors on human fetal adrenal tissue. Endocrinology 108: 1237–1242

Okazaki T, Okita J R, Macdonald P C, Johnston J M 1978 Initiation of human parturition. X. Substrate specificity of phospholipase A_2 in human fetal membranes. American Journal of Obstetrics and Gynecology 130: 432–438

Okita J R, Macdonald P C, Johnston J M 1982 Mobilization of arachidonic acid from specific glycerophospholipids of human fetal membranes during early labour. Journal of Biological Chemistry 257: 14029–14034

Otten V, Baumann J B, Girard J 1979 Stimulation of the pituitary-adrenocortical axis by nerve growth factor. Nature 282: 413–414

Owens P C, Brinsmead M W, Waters M J, Thorburn G D 1980 Ontogenic changes in serum somatomedin-like receptor activity and tissue binding sites for multiplication stimulating activity in the ovine fetus. Biochemical and Biophysical Research Communications 96: 1812–1820

Pakravan P, Kenny F M, Depp R, Allan A C 1974 Familial congenital absence of adrenal glands: evaluation of glucocorticoid, mineralocorticoid and oestrogen metabolism in the perinatal period. Journal of Pediatrics 84: 74–78

Paranetto B A, Moore G P M, Robertson D M 1982 Plasma concentrations and urinary excretion of mouse epidermal growth factor associated with the inhibition of food consumption and wool growth in Merino wethers. Journal Endocrinology 94: 191–202

Pavlou C, Barker G H, Roberts A, Chamberlain G V P 1978 Pulsed oxytocin infusion in the induction of labour. British Journal of Obstetrics and Gynaecology 85: 96–100

Pearson J, Johnson E M, Brandeis L 1983 Effects of antibodies to nerve growth factor on intrauterine development of derivatives of cranial neural crest and placode in the guinea pig. Developmental Biology 96: 32–36

Pederson J, Bossen-Moller B, Poulsen H 1954 Blood sugar in newborn infants of diabetic mothers. Acta Endocrinologica 15: 33–52

Persson B 1981 Insulin as a growth factor in the fetus. In: Ritzen M (ed) The Biology of Normal Human Growth, pp 213–221, Raven Press, New York

Pharoah P O D, Ellis S M, Ekins R P, Williams E S 1976 Maternal thyroid function, iodine deficiency and fetal development. Clinical Endocrinology 5: 159–166

Phillips L S, Vassipoulou-Sellin R 1980 Somatomedins. Journal of the American Medical Association 302: 371–380, 438–446

Picon L 1967 Effect of insulin on growth and biochemical composition of the rat fetus. Endocrinology 81: 1419–1421

Poonai A P V, Tang K, Poonai P V 1975 Relation between glucose, insulin and growth hormone in the fetus during labour and at delivery. Obstetrics and Gynecology 45: 155–158

Posner B I 1974 Insulin receptors in human and animal placental tissue. Diabetes 23: 209–217

Rees L H, Burke C W, Chard T, Evans S, Letchworth A T 1975a Possible placental origin of ACTH in normal human pregnancy. Nature 254: 620–621

Rees L H, Jack P M B, Thomas A L, Nathanielsz P W 1975b Role of adrenocorticotrophin during parturition in sheep. Nature 253: 274–275

Reinisch J M, Simon N G, Karow W G, Gandelman R 1978 Prenatal exposure to prednisone in humans and animals retards intrauterine growth. Science 202: 436–438

Rindernecht E, Humbel R E 1976 Polypeptides with nonsuppressible insulin-like and cell-growth promoting activities in human serum: isolation, chemical characterization and some biological properties of forms I and II. Proceedings of the National Academy of Science of the United States of America 73: 2365–2369

Rindernecht E, Humbel R E 1978 Primary structure of human insulin-like growth factor II. FEBS Letters 89: 283–286

Roberts G, Cawdery J E 1970 Congenital adrenal hypoplasia. Journal of Obstetrics and Gynaecology of the British Commonwealth 77: 654–656

Robinson J S, Thorburn G D 1974 The initiation of labour. British Journal of Hospital Medicine, 6: 15–22

Rosenfeld R, Thorsson A V, Hintz R L 1979 Increased somatomedin receptor sites in newborn circulating mononuclear cells. Journal of Clinical Endocrinology and Metabolism 48: 456–461

Rudman D, Moffitt S D, Farnoff P M, Mckenzie W J, Kenny J M, Bain R P 1981 The relation between growth velocity and serum somatomedin-C concentration. Journal of Clinical Endocrinology and Metabolism 52: 622

Sadone G, Beuret T, Lewin D 1981 Déclenchement du travail par perfusion discontinue de post-hypophyse. Journal de Gynecologie, Obstetrigue et Biologie de la Reproduction 10: 857–865

Sagawa N, Okazaki T, Macdonald P C, Johnston J M 1982 Regulation of diacylglycerol metabolism and arachidonic acid release in human amniotic tissue. Journal of Biological Chemistry 257: 8158–8162

Salmon J A, Amy J J 1983 Levels of prostaglandin $F_{2\alpha}$ in amniotic fluid during pregnancy and labour. Prostaglandins 4: 523–533

Sara V R, Hall K 1980a Serum levels of IR-somatomedin A in the rat — some developmental aspects. Endocrinology 107: 622

Sara V R, Hall K 1980b Somatomedins and the fetus. Clinical Obstetrics and Gynecology 23: 765–778

Sara V R, Rutherford R, Smythe G A 1979 Influence of maternal somatostatin administration on fetal brain cell proliferation and its relationship to serum growth hormone and brain trophin activity. Hormone and Metabolic Research 4: 147

Sara V R, Hall K, Rodeck C H, Wetterberg L 1981 Human embryonic somatomedin. Proceedings of the National Academy of Science of the United States of America 78: 3175–3179

Sara V R, Hall K, Misaki M, Fryklund L, Christensen N & Wetterberg L 1983 Ontogenesis of somatomedin and insulin receptors in the human fetus. Journal of Clinical Investigation 71: 1084–1093

Schaeffer L D, Wilder M C, Williams R H 1973 Secretion and content of insulin and glucagon in human fetal pancreas slices in vitro. Proceedings of the Society for Experimental Biology and Medicine 143: 314

Schoenle E, Zapf Z, Humbel R E, Froesch E R 1982 Insulin-like growth factor I stimulates growth in hypophysectomized rats. Nature 296: 252–253

Schöneschöfer M, Fenner A 1981 ACTH immunoreactivities predominating in normal human plasma are not attributable to the human ACTH $_{1-39}$ molecule. Biochemical and Biophysical Research Communications 102: 476–483

Shelley H J, Bassett J M, Milner R D G 1975 Control of carbohydrate metabolism in the fetus and newborn. British Medical Bulletin 31: 37–43

Sherwood W C, Chance G W, Hill D E 1974 A new syndrome of familial pancreatic agenesis: role of insulin and glucagon in somatic and cell growth. Pediatric Research 8: 360

Silman R E, Chard T, Lowry P J, Smith I, Young I M 1976 Human foetal pituitary peptides and parturition. Nature 260: 716–718

Silman R E, Holland D, Chard T, Lowry A J, Hope J, Rees L H, Thomas A, Nathanielsz P W 1979 Adrenocorticotrophin-related peptides in adult and foetal sheep pituitary glands. Journal of Endocrinology 81: 19–34

Silverman F, Lustig I, Young B K 1982 Predictive value of breast stimulation. Society of Gynecological Investigation 29th Annual Meeting, Abstract 393

Slayback J R B, Cheung L W Y, Geyer R R 1978 Comparative effects of human platelet growth factor on the growth and morphology of human fetal and adult diploid fibroblast. Experimental Cell Research 110: 462–466

Sodoyezgoffaux F, Sodoyez J C, De Vos C J 1981 Evidence for placento-insular axis in the rat fetus. Diabetologia 20: 563–567

Spellacy W N, Buhi W C 1976 Glucagon, Insulin-Glucose levels in maternal and umbilical cord plasma with studies of placental transfer. Obstetrics and Gynecology 47: 291–294

Steele P A, Flint A P F, Turnbull A C 1976 Activity of steroid C-17, 20 lyase in the ovine placenta: effect of exposure to fetal glucocorticoid. Journal Endocrinology 69: 239–246

Stiles C D, Capone G T, Sher C D, Antonaides H N, Van Wyk J J, Pledger W J 1977 Dual control of cell growth by somatomedins and platelet derived growth factor. Proceedings of the National Academy of Science of the United States of America 76: 1279–1283

Sundell H, Serenius F S, Barthe P, Friedman Z, Kanarek K, Escabedo M B, Orth D N, Stahlman M T 1975 The effect of EGF on fetal lamb lung maturation. Pediatric Research 9: 271

Susa J B, McCormick K L, Widness J A, Singer D B, Oh W, Adamsons K, Schwartz R 1979 Chronic hyperinsulinaemia in the fetal rhesus monkey. Effects on fetal growth and composition. Diabetes 28: 1058–1063

Svan H, Hall K, Ritzen M, Takano K, Skottner A 1977 Somatomedin A and B in serum from neonates, their mothers and cord blood. Acta Endocrinologica 85: 636–643

Tanner J M, Whitehouse R H, Hughes P C R, Vince F P 1971 Effect of human growth hormone treatment for 7 years on growth of 100 children with growth hormone deficiency, low birthweight, inherited smallness, Turner's Syndrome and other complaints. Archives of Disease in Childhood 46: 745–781

Taylor M J, Webb R, Mitchell M, Robinson J S 1981 The effect of progesterone withdrawal during late pregnancy. Journal of Endocrinology. 92: 85–93

Thorburn, G D 1974 The role of the thyroid gland and kidneys in fetal growth. In: Ciba Foundation Symposium, Size at Birth, pp 185–200. Associated Scientific Publishers, Amsterdam

Thorburn, G D 1979 Physiology and control of parturition: Reflections on the past and ideas for the future. Animal Reproductive Science 2: 1–27

Thorburn, G D, Waters M J, Young I R, Dolling M, Buntine D, Hopkins P S 1981 Epidermal growth factor: a critical factor in fetal maturation? In: The Fetus and Independent Life, Ciba Foundation Symposium, pp 172–198. Pitman, London

Thorsson A V, Hintz R L 1977 Specific ^{125}I-somatomedin receptor on circulating human mononuclear cells. Biochemical and Biophysical Research Communication 74: 1566–1573

Tilders F J H, Parker C R, Barnea A, Porter J C 1981 The major immunoreactive α-melanocyte stimulating hormone (αMSH)-like substance found in human fetal pituitary is not αMSH but may be desacetyl αMSH (adrenocorticotrophin $_{1-13}$NH$_2$). Journal of Clinical Endoclinology and Metabolism 62: 319–323

Tojo S, Mochizuki M P L, Monikawa A, Ohga Y 1976 Biological action of human chorionic somatomammotrophin during pregnancy — its lipolytic action and fetal growth. In: Pecile A, Muller E E (eds) Growth Hormone and Related Peptides, pp 334–344. Elsevier Publishing Co, New York

Turnbull A C, Patten P T, Flint A P F, Keirse M J N C, Jeremy J Y, Anderson A B M 1974 Significant fall in progesterone and rise in oestradiol in human peripheral plasma before the onset of labour. Lancet ii 101–104

Turnbull A C, Anderson A B M, Flint A P F, Jeremy J Y, Keirse M J N C, Mitchell M D 1977 Human parturition. In: Knight J, O'Connor M (eds) Fetus and Birth, Ciba Foundation Symposium 47 New Series, pp 427–452. Excerpta Medica, Amsterdam

Turner R C, Schneeloch B, Paterson P 1971 Changes in plasma growth hormone and insulin of the human foetus following hysterectomy. Acta Endocrinologica 66: 577–586

Underwood L E, D'Ercole A J, Furlanetto R W, Handwerger S, Hurley T W 1979 Somatomedin and growth: a possible role for somatomedin-C in fetal growth. In: Giordano G, Van Wyk J J, Minuto F (eds) Somatomedins and Growth, pp 215–224. Academic Press, London

Van Assche F A, De Prins F, Aerts L, Verjans M 1977 The endocrine pancreas in small-for-dates infants. British Journal of Obstetrics and Gynaeology 84: 751–753

Van Wyk J J, Underwood L E, Hintz R L, Clemmons D R, Voina S J, Weaver R P 1974 The somatomedins: a family of insulin-like hormones under growth hormone control. Recent Progress in Hormone Research 30: 259–293

Walker P, Tarins R H, Weischsel M E, Scott S M, Fisher D A 1981 Nerve growth factor in human umbilical cord serum: demonstration of a veno-arterial gradient. Journal of Clinical Endoclinology and Metabolism 53: 218–220

Waller J P, Dixon H B F 1960 Selective acetylation of the terminal amino group of corticotrophin. Biochemical Journal 75: 320–328

Weitzman R E, Leake R D, Rubin R T, Fisher D A 1980 The effect of nursing on neurohypophyseal hormone and prolactin secretion in human subjects. Journal of Clinical Endoclinology and Metoblism 51: 836–839

Wintour E M, Brown E H & Denton D A 1975 The ontogeny and regulation of corticosteroid secretion by the ovine foetal adrenal. Acta Endocrinologica 79: 301–316

Wolstenholme C E W, O'Connor M 1969 Fetal Autonomy, Ciba Foundation Symposium. J & A Churchill, London

Ylikorkala O, Viinikka L 1980 Thromboxane A_2 in pregnancy. British Medical Journal 1: 1601–1602

Zamenof S, Van Marthens E, Gravel L 1971 Prenatal cerebral development. Effect of restricted diet — reversal by growth hormone. Science 174: 954

Zapf J, Mäder M, Waldvogel M, Schalch D S, Froesch E R 1975 Specific binding of nonsuppressible insulin-like activity to chicken embryo fibroblasts to a solubilized fibroblast receptor Archives of Biochemistry and Biophysics 168: 630–637

Zapf J, Rindernecht E, Humbel R E, Froesch E R 1978 Nonsuppressible insulin-like activity (NSILA) from human serum: recent accomplishments and their physiological implications. Metabolism 27: 1803–1828

Zapf J, Schoenle E, Jagans G, Sand I K, Grunweld J, Froesch E R 1979 Inhibition of the action of nonsuppressible insulin-like activity on isolated rat fat cells by binding to its carrier protein. Journal of Clinical Investigation 63: 1077–1084

Zapf J, Walter H, Froesch E R 1981 Radioimmunological determination of insulin-like growth factors I and II in normal subjects and in patients with growth disorders and extra pancreatic tumour hypoglycemia. Journal of Clinical Investigation 68: 1321–1330

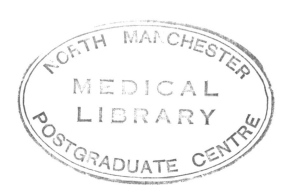

Lactation and breast feeding

Neither is woman's milk onely for young and tender infants, but also for men and women of riper years, fallen by age or sickness into compositions. Best by way I mean of nourishment for otherwise asses milk is best.

Thomas Muffett (1584)
Health's Improvements

The human female's breasts are unique organs, combining a strong psychological erotic appeal and a physical function which, until recently, was vital for the survival of the human race. In most societies the two functions are inter-linked as Erasmus Darwin noted in 1800:

'When the babe, soon after it is born into this cold world, is applied to its mother's bosom, its sense of perceiving warmth is first agreeably affected; next its sense of smell is delighted with the odor of her milk; then its taste is gratified by the flavour of it; afterward the appetites of hunger and of thirst afford pleasure by the possession of their object, and by the subsequent digestion of the aliment; and, last, the sense of touch is delighted by the softness and smoothness of the milky fountain, the source of such variety of happiness.

All these various kinds of pleasure at length become associated with the form of the mother's breast, which the infant embraces with its hands, presses with its lips, and watches with its eyes; and thus acquires more accurate ideas of the form of its mother's bosom than of the odor, flavour, and warmth which it perceives by its other senses. And hence at our mature years, when any object of vision is presented to us which by its wavy or spiral lines bears any similitude to the form of the female bosom, whether it be found in a landscape with soft gradations of raising and descending surface, or in the forms of some antique vases, or in other works of the pencil or the chisel, we feel a general glow of delight which seems to influence all our senses; and if the object be not too large we experience an attraction to embrace it with our lips as we did in our early infancy the bosom of our mothers.'

The development of the female breast under the influence of the female sex hormones at puberty is a visual sign that the woman is reaching, or has reached, reproductive capability and is sensually and sexually arousing. The development of the female breast is also an essential prerequisite for its nutritional function, that of providing milk for an infant. This is noted in the Bible in the Song of Songs in the lament: 'We have a little sister and she has no breasts. What shall we do for our sister on the day she is spoken for?'

THE DEVELOPMENT OF THE BREASTS

The human mammary glands develop from anlage in the so-called milk-ridge, a linear ectodermal thickening which extends on each side over the ventral body wall of the fetus between the bases of the limb-buds. Normally the ridge persists only in the thoracic region where epidermal thickenings occur to form the breast primordia. In the 12th week of fetal life the ectodermal thickening grows by a proliferation of its basal cells into the underlying mesenchyme to form ten to 20 buds of solid epithelial tissue. By the 15th week the buds have branched to form multiple solid cords surrounded by fatty connective tissue derived from the mesenchyme. Between the 18th and 22nd week of pregnancy the cords become canalised to form a primitive system of ducts and, at their deepest parts, further branching leads to the development of alveoli surrounded by myoepithelial cells (Fig. 13.1). What will become the nipple is, at first, a depressed hollow into which the 20 ducts open. In the perinatal period the nipple area everts by the proliferation of the underlying mesenchyme.

The breast of a neonate consists of about 20 duct systems, representing the original epidermal offshoots from the initial mammary anlage. The duct systems are intact and the alveoli functional at birth as evidenced by the temporary enlargement of the breast and the secretion of 'witches milk' in a few neonatal infants. The enlargement rapidly regresses and the breasts remain quiescent until puberty is approached, when considerable development begins under the influence of oestradiol 17-β secreted by the ovaries. As a result the ductules divide and differentiate forming lobules; there is a marked increase in alveolar formation; fat is deposited between, and surrounding, the lobular-alveolar systems and the vascularity of the developing breast increases, resulting in the thelarche. In non-primate mammals the development and differentiation of the breast duct systems at puberty depend on the effects of insulin, thyroxine and adreno-cortico-steroids, in addition to oestradiol, and these hormones may be involved in humans but evidence is lacking. The development of the

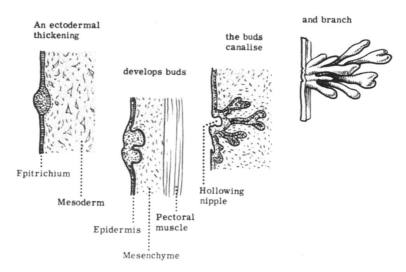

Fig. 13.1 The development of the breast in fetal life (Wendell-Smith C. P., Williams P. L. and Treadgolds 1984 Basic Human Embryology 3rd Edn London Pitman, by kind permission)

female breast to maturity continues over a period of years as described by Tanner (1962) (and see Ch. 2).

The mature female breast has been picturesquely described by Appelbaum (1970) as 'a forest consisting of ten to twenty trees all intimately bound together by interweaving vines and vegetation. Each tree is complete with its own root system and is covered by the ground.' The mature breast is dome-shaped, with the pigmented areola and nipple located at its centre. Breasts show wide variations in size and shape, due to the varying amounts of fat and the quality of the connective tissue. The skin over the breast is thin, that over the areola and nipple wrinkled. The areola contains sebaceous glands (Montgomery's tubercles) which open into its periphery. It is hairless, apart from occasional strands of lanugo hair. The size of the nipple varies, and the 15 to 20 milk ducts open into its tip. In the substance of the nipple, smooth muscle fibres are placed which contract when stimulated by temperature changes or sexual arousal. This causes the nipple to become erect.

In the non-pregnant state the ducts and lobular-alveoli are surrounded by fat, and a thicker layer covers the duct systems so that the non-pregnant breast consists largely of fatty and connective tissue (Fig. 13.2).

The alveoli form the innermost part of the duct system (the leaves of the milk tree). They are round in shape and several contiguous alveoli form an acinus. Myoepithelial cells surround each alveolus and myoepithelial cells are arranged longitudinally along the smaller ducts (Richardson, 1949, Fig. 13.3). The myoepithelial cells are intimately related to the walls of the adjacent capillaries, and are not innervated (Linzell, 1955). Their surface membranes have receptors for the posterior pituitary hormone, oxytocin, and contract strongly under its influence. In the rat, myoepithelial cells also contract following direct stimulation (Grosvenor, 1965) and may do in the

human. This is suggested by the clinical observation that breast massage (either manually or by applying hot and cold towels) leads to milk let-down, and that in some instances no detectable oxytocin (measured by a sensitive radioimmunoassay) is released in spite of adequate milk ejection (Lucas et al, 1980).

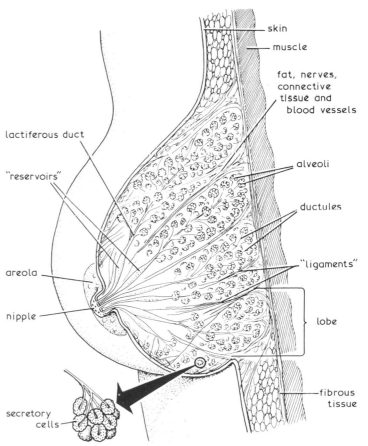

Fig. 13.2 The mature breast (Llewellyn-Jones D. 1983, Breast Feeding — How to Succeed. London, Faber, by kind permission)

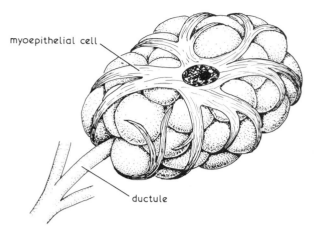

myoepithelial cell

ductule

Fig. 13.3 Myoepithelial cells (diagrammatic) (Llewellyn-Jones D. 1983 Breast Feeding — How to Succeed. London, Faber, by kind permission)

The lumen of each mammary acinus opens into the centrally located intralobular ductules (the twigs of the milk tree). The alveoli and ductules are surrounded by loose connective tissue through which capillaries pass (Fig. 13.4). The ductules combine to form small ducts,

each duct system forming a lobule (the branches of the milk tree). The lobules are surrounded by abundant dense connective tissue and adipose tissue. Groups of 30–100 lobules are arranged in lobes and their ducts enter the main lactiferous duct of the lobe (the trunk of the milk tree).

Each lobe of the breast is partially separated from the other lobes by condensations of connective tissue which form 'ligaments' in the substance of the breasts. The ligaments stretch from the fibrous tissue which underlies the breast to the thin fascial sheet underlying and attached to the skin. In this way, they maintain the breast in its fashionable, firm, conical shape.

During the menstrual cycle changes occur in the breasts. In the pre-ovulatory period, oestrogen leads to the growth of the alveoli and ductules. This growth increases in the premenstrual period, in addition, fluid is retained in the interlobular tissues, and the vascularity of the breast increases. The changes increase the size of the breasts, which may enlarge by between 7 and 44 per cent compared to their size in the early follicular phase of the menstrual cycle (Milligan et al, 1975). The sensitivity of the nipple to touch varies during the menstrual cycle, being greatest

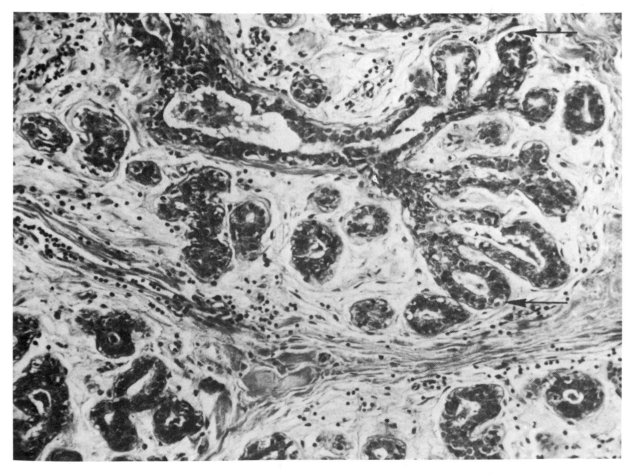

Fig. 13.4 Resting mammary gland. Portions of three lobules, the largest showing a dilated intralobular ductule lined by epithelial and myoepithelial cells (arrow). The ductule ends in a rounded alveoli to form an acinus (Salazar H., Tobon H., Josimovich J. B. 1975 In: Clinical Obstetrics and Gynaecology, Vol. 18, p. 123 Harper and Row Publishers Inc., by kind permission)

at mid-cycle and during menstruation. In pregnancy its sensitivity diminishes, but within 24 hours of childbirth, a dramatic increase in nipple sensitivity occurs (Robinson & Short, 1977).

During pregnancy, considerable growth of the glandular tissue of the breasts occurs, due to the increasing amounts of circulating oestrogen and progesterone and probably, human placental lactogen and prolactin (Josimovich, 1977; McNeilly, 1979). From early pregnancy, increased sprouting of the ducts and increased branching of the ductules and lobular development occurs, the blood vessels supplying the breast dilate, and the mammary blood flow is almost doubled. An increased amount of interstitial water is held in the breast, and additional fat is deposited between the lobules. By the 20th week of pregnancy the alveolar epithelium has changed from a two cell layer to a single layer secretory unit.

Using explants of mammary tissue of rats and mice, three hormones have been shown to be needed for the further development of the alveoli and their secretory function. These hormones are insulin, a glucocorticosteroid and a lactogenic hormone. Insulin is involved in the stimulation of the alveolar epithelial cells when they divide to form two layers. The 'daughter' cells are acted on by glucocorticosteroid and differentiate into secretory cells, which develop an extensive endoplasmic reticulum (Topper, 1976). The lactogenic hormone then acts on the secretory cells leading to the production of milk substances. In humans, two lactogenic hormones, prolactin and human placental lactogen may be involved. The latter has been demonstrated to lead to alveolar epithelial cell development in primates (Tobon et al, 1972) but no evidence of its effect on the human breast is available.

In the second half of human pregnancy the ductules proliferate and the formation of lobular-alveolar structures increases considerably, the glandular tissue increasing relative to the inter-lobular connective tissue and fat. The blood flow through the breast increases and further interstitial fluid is retained. Early in the second half of pregnancy the epithelial cells of the alveoli begin to secrete small quantities of colostrum, which pass into the ductules and may be expressed from the nipple. By the end of pregnancy each breast has become firm, full and has increased in weight by 500 to 1000 g. It has been prepared for lactation.

THE HORMONAL CONTROL OF LACTOGENESIS

The profound influence of hormones on the development of the breast has been noted; hormones are also intimately involved in the preparation of the breast for its function of producing milk for the neonate and small child. The control of milk synthesis and secretion, and its subsequent 'let-down' from the lobules to the nipple depend on a number of hormones and the inter-relating effects of these

hormones varies between mammalian species. The current concepts of the hormonal regulation of human lactation are derived, in part, from studies on humans and, in part, extrapolated from sub-primate studies.

It is generally agreed that prolactin, a peptide synthesised by specialised cells (lactotrophs) in the anterior hypophysis is the 'prime mover', inducing milk synthesis in, and secretion by, the alveolar cells of the breasts.

The synthesis and secretion of prolactin is regulated by hypothalamic dopamine which is inhibitory in its action (Tindall, 1978). A prolactin releasing factor has also been postulated, which resembles thyroid releasing hormone (TRH) in molecular character. Vorherr (1978) has shown that an injection of TRH (200–500 μg) i.v. causes a 5 to 10 fold increase in plasma prolactin levels within 20 min, and 2 hours elapses before the prolactin concentration returns to normal. However, TRH levels, although raised during pregnancy and the early puerperium, do not increase as pregnancy advances, and endogenous TRH does not appear to be involved in the reflex release of prolactin (Reichlin et al, 1976). Grandison & Guidott (1977) have suggested that prolactin release is potentiated by endorphins and these may be the transmitters within the hypothalamus which permit release of the potential prolactin releasing hormone. The prolactin molecule resembles that of human growth hormone and human placental lactogen, and has a molecular weight of 23 500. Its half-life has been estimated to between 15 and 43 min.

During pregnancy and lactation, prolactin has several properties (Josimovich, 1977).

1. It is involved (with other hormones) in preparing the alveolar epithelial cells for the secretion of milk.

2. It is the primary hormone involved in the synthesis of milk by the epithelial alveolar cells.

3. It may regulate fluid volume by an action within the amniotic sac, although this may be effected by decidual prolactin (Tomita et al, 1982).

4. It may protect the fetus against excessive loss or gain of fetal extracellular fluid, water or electrolytes.

5. In the puerperium it acts, at the hypothalamic level, to inhibit the release of gonadotrophin releasing hormone (GnRH), with the consequence that the circulating concentrations of follicle stimulating hormone (FSH) and luteinising hormone (LH) remain low. Suckling potentiates its action, either because it induces a surge of prolactin in the circulation, or facilitates the action of prolactin in some other way. The basis for the second suggestion is that in laboratory animals prolactin is ineffective in preventing LH release in the absence of a suckling stimulus (Maneckjee et al, 1978).

Prolactin secretion and release during pregnancy

During pregnancy the levels of prolactin in the blood rise in a progressive fashion in relation to the duration of pregnancy (Tyson et al, 1972; Kelly et al, 1976. The progressive rise in prolactin during pregnancy reflects an increase in the number and size of the acidophilic erythrosinophilic cells in the anterior pituitary gland (El Etreby & Gunzel, 1974). Early in the second quarter of pregnancy, large, ovoid, granular cells appear in the anterior hypophysis and are arranged as cellular cords in the centre of the pituitary alveoli. The cells, which are lactotrophic cells, appear to derive from chromophobe cells. The number of lactotrophs increases during pregnancy and by the last quarter of pregnancy they represent about 50 per cent of all acidophilic pituitary cells. During this quarter of pregnancy the hypertrophy of the lactotrophs reaches a maximum, with the development of cellular organelles and with increased granulation (especially along the plasma membranes) in the cytoplasm. Many of the cells show a variable degree of degranulation, indicating prolactin secretion.

The reason for the increased synthesis and release of prolactin is that the high circulating levels of oestrogen and progesterone inhibit the release of hypothalamic dopamine, the prolactin inhibiting factor (Tyson et al, 1975; Tindall, 1978) and, in addition, may stimulate the release of a prolactin releasing factor (PRF) which has not yet been identified. It has been suggested that TRH may be an 'alias' PRF. Although TRH releases prolactin in humans when used in pharmacological amounts (Vorherr, 1978), it does not appear to be involved in the physiological release of prolactin which follows suckling (Reinchlin et al, 1976).

Milk synthesis and secretion during pregnancy

Plasma levels of prolactin increase throughout pregnancy, reaching a maximum in the last 4 weeks but most of the prolactin fails to be bound to receptors on the alveolar epithelial cells of the breasts. The reason is not clear. One hypothesis suggests that the rising level of oestrogen and progesterone decreases the binding sites on the cell membrane of the alveolar epithelial cells and thus prevent its absorption. (Bohnet et al, 1977; Djiane & Durand, 1977). Alternatively, oestrogen may occupy the receptor binding sites. A third suggestion is that human placental lactogen (hPL) occupies the binding sites. In late pregnancy hPL levels in the blood are more than 100 times higher than those of prolactin (Robyn & Meunis, 1982). The high circulating hPL levels may be the cause of the secretion of 'milk' in the last 20 weeks of pregnancy. Alternatively, milk secretion may occur because the higher circulating concentration of prolactin overcomes the cell membrane 'block' by inducing an increase in the number of receptor binding sites, and prolactin enters the alveolar cells (Moore & Forsyth 1980). Within the cell, prolactin attaches to the Golgi apparatus (Posner, 1976) and induces RNA synthesis probably via a pathway involving prosta-

glandins and polyamines (Shiu & Friesen, 1980), which leads to the synthesis of casein, α-lactalbumin and lactose. In some mammals the effect of prolactin is facilitated by insulin and glucocorticosteroids and inhibited by progesterone in a dose dependent manner (Matusik & Rosen, 1978). The 'milk' is released into the alveolar lumen, as colostrum. Colostrum differs from mature milk in that it contains nearly four times as much protein (half of which is immunoglobin) less fat and less lactose. Its yellow colour is due to the presence of β-carotene, a precusor of vitamin A.

THE INITIATION OF LACTATION

Following childbirth, lactation ensues after an interval of 2 to 3 days, unless the mother chooses not to breast feed and is given medication to prevent lactation. The synthesis of milk in the alveolar epithelial cells, its release into the lumen of the acini and the smaller ducts, its 'let down' to the nipple and its ejection from the nipple are complex processes. Much of the information is derived from studies of lactation on sub-primate mammals, and because of species differences extrapolation to the human may not be justifiable. With this proviso, the neurohormonal control of lactation will be discussed.

Lactation starts with the synthesis of milk and its release from the alveolar epithelial cells into the lumen of an acinus (lactogenesis). The hormones required for the synthesis and secretion of milk are prolactin, growth hormone (GH), TSH (or thyroid hormones), ACTH (or glucocorticosteroids), insulin and parathyroid hormone. The relative importance of these hormones in establishing and in maintaining milk synthesis (galactopoeisis) is species dependent; but in all mammals prolactin is the major hormonal trigger.

Prolactin (PRL). With the expulsion of the placenta, the major source of oestrogen and progesterone is withdrawn and the levels of these hormones fall. By the fourth day postpartum, their levels are comparable to those found in the follicular phase of the menstrual cycle. The result of this is that the 'blockade' of prolactin binding sites (receptors) on the alveolar epithelial cells is removed and prolactin is taken up by receptors and enters the cells, to augment and magnify the changes which convert the presecretory cells into secretory cells. The changes, as shown by electromicroscopy, are (1) hyperplasia of the endoplasmic reticulum; (2) dilatation of the Golgi apparatus with the appearance of electron dense material; and (3) an increase in the microvilli of the apical surface of the epithelial cell. The evidence that the changes are related to prolactin is indirect, but is strongly suggested by the observation that similar changes are induced in the breast of pseudopregnant rabbits by the intraductal injection of ovine prolactin (Tobon & Salazar, 1975). The prolactin is bound at first to the mammary cell membrane, but enters the cell and

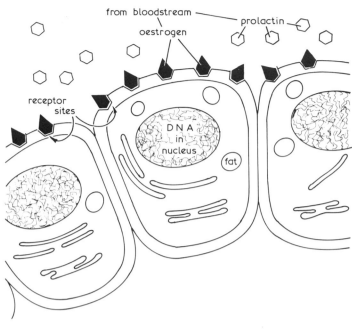

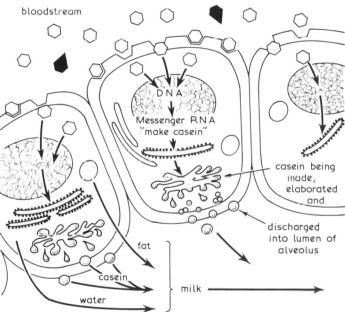

Fig. 13.5a and b Schematic representation of prolactin synthesis of casein and the secretion of milk in the alveoli of the breast (Llewellyn-Jones D. 1983 Breast Feeding — How to Succeed. London, Faber, by kind permission)

rapidly increases the formation of ribosomal RNA, transfer RNA and the RNA which causes the ribosomes to aggregate to form polysomes. Stimulated by prolactin, the alveolar cells synthesise casein and α-lactalbumin in increasing amounts, and milk is released into the lumen of the acini. (Fig. 13.5).

Growth hormone (GH). Growth hormone is galactoporetic in the goat and cow, but not in the rabbit, rat or mouse. The role of GH in human lactation is probably small, as circulating levels of GH remain unaltered throughout pregnancy (Kelly et al, 1976) and women with growth hormone-deficient dwarfism can lactate and breast feed (Rimoin et al, 1968).

Placental lactogen (HPL). Human placental lactogen has a marked immunological and structural resemblance to GH which explains why the two hormones have similar properties. During pregnancy concentrations of HPL increase in a linear manner to term, at a time when lactation is inhibited, falling abruptly after childbirth (Spellacy et al, 1966). This suggests that the role of HPL, if any, is to initiate changes in the alveoli, rather than to induce milk secretion.

ACTH and glucocorticosteroids. There is no evidence that ACTH acts on the mammary gland of any mammal, and any effect is initiated by glucocorticosteroids. In small laboratory animals injections of cortisol cause differentiation of the rough endoplasmic reticulum and the Golgi apparatus, allowing prolactin to induce milk synthesis, but there is no evidence in humans that glucocorticosteroids are involved in the initiation or maintenance of lactation.

Summary. The initiation of lactation depends on hormonally induced changes in the alveolar epithelial cells of the mammary gland. These changes may be initiated by human placental lactogen as its maximum secretion occurs in the last 10 weeks of pregnancy, when the cellular changes are maximal. Glucocorticosteroids may also be involved in the preparation of the cellular components for the impact of prolactin. Prolactin only becomes effective when its concentration is sufficiently high to 'unblock' the receptors in the cells which have been occupied by oestrogen and progesterone. In late pregnancy, milk secretion is minimal because of the sex steroid block, but once parturition has occurred, the concentration of oestrogen and progesterone fall rapidly and prolactin occupies the vacant receptor sites, initiating lactogenesis.

With the fall in the plasma concentrations of oestrogen and progesterone, which has inhibited the release of dopamine during pregnancy, it would be expected that its level would rise and suppress prolactin release. In the absence of suckling this occurs. If the mother chooses to breast feed, prolactin secretion continues because of the prolactin reflex, and galactopoeisis continues.

The prolactin reflex

Suckling stimulates sensory nerve endings which are found principally at the base of the nipple and in the inner part of the areola. The nerve impulses travel to the spinal cord and then to the preoptic area, and from there to the periventricular region of the hypothalamus, at least in the rabbit and the rat (Tindall & Knaggs, 1972). It is possible that 5-hydroxytryptamine is released and acts as a neurotransmitter inhibiting dopamine release from the medial basal hypothalamus. An alternative suggestion is that noradrenaline is involved as, in rats, suckling induces a

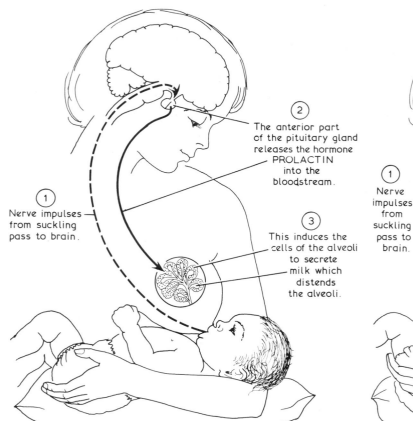

1 Nerve impulses from suckling pass to brain.

2 The anterior part of the pituitary gland releases the hormone PROLACTIN into the bloodstream.

3 This induces the cells of the alveoli to secrete milk which distends the alveoli.

Fig. 13.6 The prolactin reflex (Llewellyn-Jones D. 1983 Breast Feeding — How to Succeed. London, Faber, by kind permission)

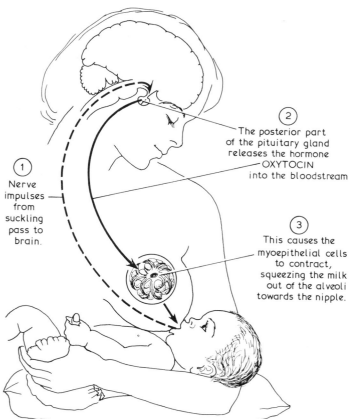

1 Nerve impulses from suckling pass to brain.

2 The posterior part of the pituitary gland releases the hormone OXYTOCIN into the bloodstream.

3 This causes the myoepithelial cells to contract, squeezing the milk out of the alveoli towards the nipple.

Fig. 13.7 The milk-ejection or let-down reflex (Llewellyn-Jones D. 1983 Breast Feeding — How to Succeed London, Faber, by kind permission)

decrease in noradrenaline in the ventromedial nucleus and the anterior hypothalamus (Moyer et al, 1979). The mechanism remains obscure, but the result is obvious. Suckling leads to a surge of prolactin which raises the prolactin level 2 to 4 fold in the first 5 to 10 min of the stimulus of breast feeding (Dawood et al, 1981) and persists for between 5 and 25 min after the baby ceases to suckle (Fig. 13.6).

The amount of prolactin released is in excess of requirements for lactation, and only that released in the first few minutes of suckling seem to be required for milk secretion. It is also likely (in the rat) that the prolactin released during one episode of suckling is used to stimulate milk secretion for the next episode: in other words, its action is delayed (Grosvenor et al, 1978).

Milk ejection

The function of prolactin is to initiate and to maintain the sequence of intracellular events which lead to the synthesis of milk and to its release into the lumen of the acini and the adjacent small ducts. These changes lead to the clinical condition of breast fullness. Unless the milk contained in the alveoli and ductules is ejected to travel along the larger ducts to reach the nipple, continued milk secretion will be suppressed as the pressure in the lumen of the alveoli rises. Milk transport (let-down) is controlled by the milk ejection reflex which is largely dependent on oxytocin release by the posterior pituitary gland (Fig. 13.7).

Oxytocin is synthesised in the cell body of neurones located in the paraventricular and supraoptic nuclei of the hypothalamus, and is transferred to the neurohypophysis via the nerve axons where it is stored. Oxytocin release is effected by several stimuli, including 'stress', pain and anaesthesia, and is inhibited by anxiety. During suckling, neural impulses from nipple stimulation pass through the thoracic nerves to the spinal cord and then to the hypothalamus to evoke the release of oxytocin from the neurohypophysis.

The nature of the transmitters involved in the neural pathway is unknown in the human, but in the rat dopaminergic and noradrenergic synapses are involved (Clarke et al, 1979). It is probable that other pathways which lead to the release of oxytocin are also involved. For example, when some mothers hear their baby crying, a feeling of 'tingling' occurs in the breasts, which resembles that felt during milk ejection, and milk may be discharged from the nipple.

Oxytocin released in response to suckling causes the contraction of the myoepithelial cells which surround each alveolus and ductule with the result that the milk is ejected into the larger ducts and the subareolar lactiferous sinuses from which it can be removed by suckling. Within 5 min of starting a breast feed, the circulating level of oxytocin in the plasma rises from a base of 10–12 pg/ml to between 20–55 pg/ml, falling as the baby's suckling diminishes, to return to the basal levels after the baby has been taken from the breast (Dawood et al, 1981).

As mentioned earlier, Grosvenor (1965) postulated that milk-ejection occurs by direct stimulation of the alveoli in the rat. This mechanism may by-pass the milk ejection reflex and may occur in humans. Lucas et al (1980) have shown in a group of ten women examined in the early puerperium (six between days 1 and 3, and four between days 6 and 10 postpartum) that oxytocin release was variable and occurred maximally late in the feed, although 90 per cent of milk flow occurs within 4 min of starting feeding (Lucas et al, 1979). They have also shown that the successful let-down of milk can occur in the absence of detectable changes to plasma oxytocin concentrations (Lucas et al, 1980).

THE MAINTENANCE OF LACTATION

Once lactation has been established, it must be maintained if the infant is to receive sufficient nutrition. Maintenance of lactation comprises two components: (1) continued adequate secretion of milk; and (2) adequate milk ejection. Of the two, the second is the more important in clinical practice and most women who claim to have 'insufficient' milk have inadequate milk ejection.

The hormonal maintenance of lactation in humans depends primarily on the continued release of prolactin in response to nipple stimulation. In other species other hormones are also involved, as evidenced by experimental studies on hypophysectomised lactating animals. Hypophysectomised rats and mice require exogenous glucocorticosteroids in addition to prolactin to continue lactation (Cowie, 1957). Goats require prolactin, growth hormone, adrenal glucocorticosteroids and tri-iodothyronine (Cowie et al, 1969). Rabbits appear to lactate if only prolactin is given (Cowie et al, 1979).

Insufficient pure prolactin is available to conduct similar experiments on large animals; however as lactation is suppressed rapidly in humans when dopamine-agonists are administered, it can be stated with reasonable confidence that prolactin is essential for continued milk secretion.

The quantity of prolactin required to maintain lactation is controversial. In earlier studies prolactin levels were found to decrease from a high of 100 μg/l in the first 4 weeks to a level lying in the higher part of the normal range

(15–25 μ/l) thereafter (Tyson, 1972; Noel et al, 1974). It has also been demonstrated that the peak incidence of suckling episodes and the peak duration of suckling were reached 4 weeks postpartum and this coincided with peak prolactin levels. After this time progressive falls occurred in the frequency and duration of suckling in the subjects studied. This was paralleled by a decline in prolactin plasma concentration, when measured 2 hours or more after a suckling episode (Howie et al, 1981). In Howie's study it was noticeable that the introduction of supplementary food ('solids') to the baby's diet led to a reduction in suckling episodes, suckling duration and plasma prolactin concentration. A baby receiving 'solids' before being put to the breast will not suckle efficiently, and will not require as many feeds at the breast. This is the probable cause of the declining prolactin levels amongst some lactating women, as it has been found that the prolactin levels decline more slowly among women who feed more than 6 times a day than in those women who feed less frequently (Delvoye et al, 1977). In societies where breast-feeding is 'on demand', and often continuous, as for example amongst rural women in Africa, the basal plasma prolactin concentrations continue to be elevated (although dropping from the 4 week postpartum peak) for at least 26 weeks and often for 52 weeks postpartum (Delvoye et al, 1976, 1978; Gross & Eastman, 1979, Howie et al, 1981). In these studies it was shown that provided the baby suckled frequently, the quantity of milk secreted did not diminish. This suggests that in humans, as in rats (Grosvenor et al, 1978) only a quantum of prolactin is required to maintain milk secretion. It can be postulated that once the receptor sites of the alveolar cells are occupied, no additional prolactin is required at that time. This supports the clinical observation that frequent (demand) feeding leads to higher milk yields than scheduled feeding. Another possibility is that as the baby becomes older, maternal-infant relationships lead to exteroceptive messages which cause periodic release of prolactin. This has been shown to occur in the rat (Mena & Grosvenor, 1972).

Whether other hormones are required to maintain lactation in humans is unclear. In one study, injections of pharmacological amounts of GH increased milk yield in hypogalactic women over controls (Lyons et al, 1968). Growth hormone is known to have intrinsic lactogenic activity in primates (Kleinberg & Todd, 1980). The relationship between adrenocorticosteroid secretion, thyroid hormone secretion and insulin release has not been studied in the human, so that their contribution to maintaining human lactation is unclear. Oestrogen in pharmacological doses inhibits lactation by occupying prolactin receptor sites in the alveoli and, in certain concentrations, by inducing dopamine release. In postpartum lactating women, the concentration of oestrogen in the plasma is low and, in physiological concentrations, oestrogens have no effect on lactation.

ENDOCRINE CHANGES DURING LACTATION

Hypothalamic gonadotrophin releasing hormone (GnRH)

In the first 7–10 days after childbirth, a bolus injection of GnRH fails to provoke a release of FSH or LH. If the woman chooses not to breast feed, an exaggerated release of FSH and LH in response to GnRH occurs between 3 and 6 weeks postpartum, which later reverts to normal (Kaye & Jaffe, 1976). In fully breast-feeding women, a normal FSH response, but a diminished LH response to GnRH occurs after 6–8 weeks of lactation (Andreassen & Tyson, 1976; Keye & Jaffe, 1976).

The release of GnRH is an indirect function of oestrogen, small amounts suppressing GnRH release (negative feedback) and a large surge causing a sudden release of GnRH (positive feedback). Baird et al (1979) have demonstrated that the injection of 1 mg oestradiol benzoate to seven lactating and seven non-lactating women, 30 and 100 days postpartum, suppressed FSH plasma levels in both groups. LH plasma levels were suppressed to a greater degree in the lactating women, at 30 and 100 days, only one showing a positive feedback at 30 days and none at 100 days. In contrast, two of the seven non-lactating women showed a positive response at 30 days, and five of the seven at 100 days. These findings suggest a reduced hypothalamic sensitivity to the positive feedback of oestrogen during lactation (Soria et al, 1976).

Gonadotrophin release during lactation

In postpartum women, lactating or not, the plasma concentrations of FSH and LH which had been low during pregnancy rise and, by 10–25 days after childbirth, lie in the normal ranges of the follicular phase of the menstrual cycle (Reyes et al, 1972; Marr et al, 1981).

The rise in FSH precedes that of LH and is greater. This is similar to the response seen in early puberty and may represent a physiological 'reawakening' of the gonadotrophs after prolonged suppression during pregnancy. Although the concentration of LH rises in lactating women, it remains in the lower part of the normal range and shows an absence of a pulsatile release. (Bohnet & Schneider, 1977) In contrast, amongst non-lactating women, LH is cyclically released by the fourth week postpartum at a time when prolactin concentrations have fallen to within the normal range (Bonnar et al, 1975).

Ovarian steroid activity during lactation

Following childbirth the high concentrations of placental oestradiol and progesterone fall rapidly and by the 7th day have reached basal levels. In non-lactating women a rise in oestradiol concentration occurs 15–25 days after childbirth, indicating a resumption of follicular development. (Bonnar et al, 1975; Rolland et al, 1975). By this time prolactin levels have fallen to within the normal range.

In lactating women the oestradiol concentrations are significantly lower than those of non-lactating women and remain low, as long as frequent suckling maintains raised prolactin levels (Baird et al, 1979). This occurs in spite of gonadotrophin levels which, as mentioned, are in the range of those found during the early follicular phase of the menstrual cycle. However, large doses of exogenous gonadotrophins (Andreasson & Tyson, 1976) or GnRH injections of sufficient magnitude to increase the release of endogenous gonadotrophin significantly, are able to stimulate ovarian follicular development and oestradiol secretion. These findings suggest that the ovary is not refractory, but has a reduced sensitivity to stimulation by gonadotrophins, possibly as gonadotrophin receptor sites are occupied by prolactin. Alternatively prolactin may alter theca granulosa cell function (McNeilly, 1979).

The findings in lactating women of (1) a reduced hypothalamic sensitivity to the positive oestrogen feedback, (2) an altered hypothalamic release of GnRH, (3) a reduced release of gonadotrophins, and (4) a reduced ovarian sensitivity to gonadotrophins, which revert to normal when suckling ceases or is reduced in frequency and prolactin levels fall to within the normal range, implicate prolactin as the main agent in lactational anovulation and amenorrhoea.

High concentrations of prolactin reduce GnRH secretion which in turn prevents LH pulsatile release, whilst permitting normal FSH release.

Prolactin may also prevent FSH (and LH) occupying receptor sites in the ovary. This would inhibit oestradiol synthesis, which in turn would prevent a positive feedback to the hypothalamus, and cause a reduced GnRH release. The frequency of suckling by inducing the prolactin reflex is the crucial behavioural factor in this sequence of endocrinological events.

THE PSYCHOSOCIAL ASPECTS OF LACTATION AND BREAST FEEDING

A woman has to make three decisions about breast feeding. The first decision is that she desires to breast feed and intends to attempt breast feeding. The second decision is that, following childbirth, she will initiate breast feeding, in other words, will suckle her baby. The third decision, which she may have to make on several occasions, is that she will continue to breast feed, despite anxieties about her baby's progress, and the conflicting advice she receives.

These decisions are inter-related, but in each different factors may influence each decision.

The decision to attempt to breast feed

When nearly all women breast fed, and families were relatively large, most girls, during childhood or adolescence, were able to see a younger brother or sister, or a cousin, being breast fed. Breast feeding was a normal event and the girl 'modelled' her behaviour on this. In the past three decades, with the decline in breast feeding and the change to smaller families, fewer girls have the opportunity to observe their mother, an aunt, or a sister breast feeding. The 'model' has largely disappeared and breast feeding is no longer seen as a normal event.

Over the same period, advertising in magazines, and on hoardings suggested that bottle feeding is beneficial for the baby and more convenient for the mother. The advertisements showed cheerful, chubby, smiling, thriving bottle fed babies cared for by well-groomed, beautiful mothers.

The anti-breast feeding influences of advertisements for bottle feeding, using a specific brand of formula milk, has had an effect on women in the developed and the developing nations. The manufacturers of baby foods claim that they stress that breast feeding is preferable, and, indeed, in most advertisements this is stated, but it tends to be obscured by the positive message that the manufacturer is emphasising, that bottle feeding is as good as breast feeding and is more convenient.

The infant food manufacturers deny that their advertising and the employment of company paid mothercraft-nurses has had any significant effect on the decline of breast feeding, but the evidence is that they have. Considerable debate, often acrimonious, has been going on since the early 1970s, and in 1981, the General Assembly of the World Health Organisation overwhelmingly approved an international code to regulate the marketing of breast milk substitutes. The code has been described by the infant food manufacturers as 'unworkable', 'unrealistic' and 'filled with defects'. How many nations will adopt and implement the code is uncertain, but its existence demonstrates that advertising of formula milk has an adverse effect on breast feeding.

The influence of the advertising campaigns of the infant food manufacturers in discouraging breast feeding has been augmented by the emphasis by advertisers and the media on the erotic nature of the breast. Women with firm, conical breasts are shown in seductive positions in advertisements which offer products as different as toothpaste and tomatoes, cigarettes and Cinzano, lingerie and laxatives, candy and cars, whisky and wild-life holidays, peanuts and petrol.

The effect of the posters on advertising hoardings, the commercials on television, or the advertisements in magazines reinforces the belief that only women who have healthy bodies, firm breasts and smiling faces will achieve success. When teenaged women contrast these beautiful models with the ageing bodies, the sagging breasts and the anxious faces of their mothers, or of relatives who are breast feeding, the belief, perhaps subliminal, begins to grow that breast feeding is old fashioned, unsexy and will destroy a woman's attractiveness to men.

This opinion is borne out by a study in the United States, of 100 women interviewed soon after childbirth. A large proportion of the women who had decided not to breast feed had made the decision because of fear of 'the loss of their figure', and consequently their attractiveness to men (Masters & Johnson, 1976). This is not purely a twentieth century anxiety. In 1682 Aphra Behn wrote that many mothers were afraid breast feeding would alter the shape of their 'pretty breasts, firm nipples, round and smooth'. And in the sixteenth century, Gnazzo wrote that many mother would 'rather pervert the nature of their children . . . than change the form of their firm, hard and round paps'.

The influences which have tended to diminish the importance of breast feeding, have not been countered by education. Most education authorities, and many school principals, feel it is neither appropriate, nor their responsibility, to discuss breast feeding when courses in human development are conducted, or permit students to watch a mother breast feed her baby, and talk with her.

The available data indicate that women who decide to breast feed are more likely: (1) to be primigravid (Boulton & Kirk, 1978); (2) to have continued school until age 18 (Martin, 1978); (3) to belong to the higher socio-economic groups as judged by the husband's or father's occupation (Kirk, 1978; Boulton & Flavel, 1978); (4) to have made their decision to breast feed before becoming pregnant (P < 0.001); (5) to have witnessed a mother breast feeding (P < 0.001); (6) to have been breast fed (P < 0.001); (7) to have thought a lot about breast feeding (P < 0.05); (8) to have attended pre-natal classes (P < 0.05) (Llewellyn-Jones, 1977).

The negative view of breast feeding could be corrected, to some extent, if information and education regarding the benefits of breast feeding was given during pregnancy. Unfortunately, many educational efforts in pregnancy are inadequate, and often given by poor communicators. Martin (1978) found in Great Britain that one-quarter of the women surveyed in 1975 had heard no mention of infant feeding at any time during attendance at ante-natal clinics, at doctors surgeries, or at ante-natal classes.

Four years later, not much improvement in the availability of ante-natal education about infant feeding had occurred. In Britain, for example, a woman doctor, Paula Bolton-Maggs wrote to the British Medical Journal in 1979 that she 'had looked forward with interest to hearing more about breast feeding during my pregnancy, since, like most doctors, I had little idea about the practicalities. I was surprised to find no interest shown in the method of feeding I might adopt when I visited GP or hospital clinics'. And, in discussing the class given by a midwife, she wrote that the midwife's advice was 'Of course breast feeding is best but if you can't, this is how to mix a bottle feed'. Dr Bolton-Maggs continued: 'The rest of the class was spent in the mechanics or artificial feeding. No doubt the midwives were strongly in favour of breast feeding, but the practical advice was mainly about bottles, partly because it is easy to demonstrate, and partly because our teachers had not had the benefit of personal experience of breast feeding'.

Skill in communication is learned, and many nurses and doctors who conduct pre-natal educational classes, are unable to explain the benefits of breast feeding, and to motivate expectant mothers to attempt to breast feed.

The lack of observation of women breast feeding, the lack of information at school about the benefits of breast feeding, and poor communication about lactation in pre-natal classes may be compounded by the attitude of the woman's husband (or the father of her child) towards breast feeding. If young women are misinformed about breast feeding, young men are even more ignorant. An investigation, in a rural area in Britain, confirmed that fathers strongly influenced the way their children were fed (Harrison, 1977). The reason for this opposition is speculative. A number of psychologists believe that some men may feel threatened by the loss of their exclusive possession of the woman's breasts, which must now be shared, in an intimate way, with the baby. Other men may fear that breast feeding will cause the woman's breast to lose their erotically arousing shape and reduce the man's sexual pleasure.

These anxieties are usually not stated openly, and the man expresses his opposition to breast feeding in devious ways, as he would be ashamed to let his real reasons be known. In such circumstances it may be impossible for a woman, who wishes to breast feed, to discuss lactation with her partner.

The decision to initiate breast feeding

The decision to initiate breast feeding depends on the desire to breast feed, augmented by encouragement in the days immediately before and immediately after childbirth. Negative influences during this period can suppress the desire, and deter the woman from initiating breast feeding. Alternatively the influences may induce a woman to initiate, but rapidly terminate, breast feeding.

It has been claimed that breast feeding is a 'confidence trick': the more confident that the woman is in her ability to breast feed, the more likely she is to succeed. Successful breast feeding depends first, on the initiation of milk secretion; second, on the continuation of milk secretion; third, on milk ejection from the alveoli to the nipple and then to the mouth of the baby; and fourth, on the ability of the baby to suckle and ingest the breast milk. As has been mentioned earlier, the initiation and the continued secretion of milk by the milk-producing cells in the alveoli of the breasts, depends mainly on the release of adequate amounts of prolactin from the pituitary gland. This is stimulated by frequent suckling and is inhibited by anxiety,

pain and by infrequent suckling. Milk ejection depends on the reflex release of oxytocin from the cells of the posterior hypophysis in response to suckling. As with the release of prolactin, oxytocin release is inhibited by infrequent suckling, by fear, by anxiety and by pain.

Unfortunately, the routines and practices adopted by some maternity hospitals have the effect of increasing a mother's anxiety and inhibiting the release of prolactin and oxytocin.

Frequent feeding is discouraged (in the misguided belief that the mother will become too tired to 'make good milk'). The duration of each feed is strictly limited to 10 min each side, 'or your nipples will become cracked'. Babies are weighed frequently to 'see if the baby is gaining weight properly', an action which may induce such anxiety that the 'let-down' reflex ceases to work properly. Although most babies are now allowed to room-in with their mother during the day, at night many babies are taken to the nursery 'so that the mother can get a good night's sleep'. In the nursery, complementary feeds may be given, either of glucose water or even of formula milk. During the day, feeding is to a strict time schedule, which is determined by hospital custom, not by the desires of the baby. Each of these practices reduces the effectiveness of the baby to initiate the prolactin reflex and the 'let-down' reflex which are essential to establish lactation.

Many of these practices currently are being modified, but are still sufficiently common for their deterrent effects on successful breast feeding to become apparent. In 1978, a report from Dundee, Scotland, showed that women who were separated from their babies at birth for 4 to 6 hours and then given the baby to feed every 2 or 4 hours, nursed their babies for a shorter time, and weaned them earlier than women whose babies were put to the breast immediately after birth and were fed 2-hourly until lactation was established, and 'on demand' from then on (Salariya et al, 1978).

The decision to continue breast feeding

Information from Australia (Boulton & Coote, 1979; Lawson et al, 1978; Llewellyn-Jones, 1977), Scandinavia (Verkasalo, 1980; Sjohn et al, 1979) the United Kingdom (Coles et al, 1978; Oakley, 1978) and the United States (Martinez & Nalezienski, 1981) shows that at least half of those women who initiate breast feeding have stopped by the time the baby is 12 weeks old.

Women give many reasons for discontinuing breast feeding. In about half, the reasons are that 'I haven't enough milk to satisfy the baby', or 'My milk didn't suit the baby', or 'The baby won't stop crying so he can't be getting enough' (West, 1980). Other reasons given, by about two-fifths of women, are that the stresses of adjusting to being a parent caused a lack of self-confidence, and anxiety, about the baby, with a resulting inhibition of the let-down reflex and breast feeding being abandoned (Sloper et al, 1977). About one-fifth of women give up breast feeding because it is painful, due to sore nipples.

In these situations, women rarely give up breast feeding without asking for help. They may discuss the problem with relatives, friends, baby-health clinic sisters, social workers, or health visitors. Less frequently they consult a doctor or a paediatrician.

All too frequently the advice they are given is conflicting and sometimes inappropriate (Box & Hart, 1975). For example a woman, who says that she has insufficient milk is often told to test weigh the baby before and after a feed. As babies take different quantities of milk in different feeds this advice is often inappropriate. Test weighing may reduce the 'let-down' reflex because of the anxiety produced by the procedure, and because the baby suckles less strongly from a woman whose milk is not flowing well (Oakley, 1978).

The advice is almost certain to lead to a reduced amount of milk produced by the mother and to the rapid discontinuation of breast feeding.

A more appropriate response would be to reassure the woman that she can produce all the milk she needs for her baby, by suckling it more often and for longer, as this will stimulate the release of prolactin and of oxytocin.

Unfortunately, the advice given by people — even trained professionals — often provokes more anxiety than no advice at all, and this leads to the decision to stop breast feeding, in many instances.

The 'nuclear' structure of the family today is an additional factor which induces many women to abandon breast feeding within the first month or two after childbirth. In Western Society in the past (and today, amongst the rural people in the developing nations), larger families, with relatives living nearby or under the same roof, meant that an experienced woman who had breast fed her baby, was always available to reassure, to advise, and to give emotional support to the new mother.

In Western Society today, where most families consist of a mother, a father and one or two children, the supportive role of readily available relatives is absent. Most relatives live some distance away, and contact is not as easy as in a village in an 'extended family'. The social support of relatives to share the burden of coping with a small baby, which seems to reject its mother and to cry constantly, is not present. The anxiety that the baby is not thriving, imposes stress on many mothers which inhibits prolactin and oxytocin release.

If a mother had an experienced relative to whom she could talk, who could reassure her and provide emotional support, the problem would be reduced. In our society such support is often unavailable, with the consequence that many women decide to give up breast feeding within a few weeks of childbirth.

A further factor leading to the decision to give up breast feeding may be the early introduction of solids into the baby's diet. Unless lactation has been fully established in hospital, the mother may experience some feeding difficulties when she returns home, and may begin supplementing breast milk with bottles of formula milk, or with solids. A survey in Sydney, in 1976–77 showed 46 per cent of the 250 mothers interviewed had started giving their baby cereal-mixes (mostly commercially prepared) within the first 2 months of life and by 3 months the percentage had risen to 69 per cent (Allen & Heywood, 1979).

If the mother gives formula milk feeds or cereals before offering her breast to the baby, he will be satiated and will not suck well. This reduces the efficiency of both the prolactin and 'let-down' reflexes, with the result that the stimulus to milk production is reduced. In addition, anxiety about the baby's health and about the mother's ability to parent the baby may inhibit the 'let-down' reflex. Breast feeding becomes unsuccessful because of a 'poor milk supply', and is abandoned.

It would seem that the availability of a community-based support and information service for breast feeding mothers, which did not give conflicting advice, would help to reduce the early cessation of breast feeding.

DRUG STIMULATION OF LACTATION

It has been observed that in a few breast feeding women, the volume of milk let-down is small, and when measurements of prolactin are made, its surge in response to suckling is not as great as expected. From this it has been argued that the relatively small amount of milk expelled is due to an inadequate prolactin secretion, rather than to a poor milk-ejection reflex. Prolactin secretion can be stimulated by blocking the dopaminergic receptors with the procainamide derivative, metoclopramide, or with sulpiride. Given orally, a single dose of metoclopramide 10 mg will increase prolactin plasma levels 3 to 8 times, and its concentration remains raised for at least 8 hours. Given in a dose of 10 mg twice or three times a day, the blood concentration of prolactin is chronically elevated for as long as metoclopramide is taken (Falachi et al, 1978; Enzman et al, 1979). Kaupilla et al (1981) in a study of 17 women with poor lactation, between the 18 and 141 days after childbirth, found that metoclopramide (10 mg three times a day) raised the prolacting levels from 19.5 ± 7.5 ng/ml to 85.5 ± 16 mg/ml. The milk yield over the period of metoclopramide administration increased from 390 ± 55 ml to 625 ± 76 ml. The medication caused no significant side effects.

Aono et al (1976) treated 66 healthy primiparous women, who were feeding six times a day for 20 min on a 3-hourly schedule, with sulpiride (50 mg twice daily) from the first postpartum day for 7 days. They compared the milk yield of these women (by test weighing and breast expression after each feed) with 64 matched controls who received a placebo. The milk yield in the sulpiride treated group on days 4 and 5 postpartum was significantly greater. Sulpiride increased prolactin levels significantly with a peak at 2 hours and raised levels for 12 hours. Aono et al also noted that at one month postpartum significantly more sulpiride treated mothers than controls were still breast feeding.

The value of sulpiride given routinely to women in the first 5 to 7 days after childbirth in initiating and maintaining lactation cannot be judged from Aono's study. In the first place the babies were fed to a schedule, not on demand; in the second place, some of the babies were given complementary feeds. Both of these behaviours reduce suckling, and hence prolactin release. But within the criteria established, sulpiride had a stimulating effect on prolactin release and hence on milk secretion.

The quantity of milk released can be increased in another way by supplementing the let-down reflex with exogenous oxytocin. Ruis et al (1981) reported a double-blind group sequential trial in which an oxytocin nasal spray was used to enhance the onset of lactation amongst 28 mothers who had given birth to a baby weighing less than 2200 g. The babies were receiving intensive neonatal care, and were unable to suckle for at least 5 days. During this time milk was removed from the mother's breasts using an Egnell pump, four times a day. Immediately before applying the pump, 1.5 iu of oxytocin was administered as a spray to each nostril, and this was repeated just before the pump was applied to the second breast. The cumulative volume of breast milk obtained between 2 and 5 days after childbirth was 3.5 times greater in those women given oxytocin.

BREAST FEEDING AND FERTILITY CONTROL

Breast feeding continues to be the most common way by which women delay a further pregnancy. Nursing influences fertility by the effect of raised circulating prolactin concentrations on gonadotrophin secretion and perhaps on an ovarian response to gonadotrophins. High prolactin levels reduce or suppress GnRH release with resulting diminished FSH and LH secretion, although the former reaches levels found in the mid follicular phase within 20 days of childbirth (Reyes et al, 1972). At this level the ovary shows no sign of activity and oestradiol levels tend to remain low. This suggests that prolactin also affects the ovary leading to an ovarian resistance, or refractory response to FSH (Zarate et al, 1972).

An alternative suggestion is that suckling itself, by ensuring a steady stream of stimuli to the hypothalamus, increases hypothalamic sensitivity to the negative feedback of ovarian sex steroids (Baird et al, 1979). This, in turn,

would inhibit the release of sufficient gonadotrophins from the anterior pituitary to induce ovulation.

If a mother nurses frequently and her baby suckles strongly, the basal level of prolactin remains elevated, with post-nursing peaks, for months. Clinical observations indicate that if a mother breast feeds, anovulation and amenorrhoea persist for up to 26 weeks after parturition compared to less than 12 weeks if the mother is not lactating (Gronin, 1978; Perez et al, 1972). These data, deriving from a time when *exclusive* breast feeding was unusual, and when supplementary feeds of 'solids' were introduced early in the neonatal period, do not necessarily indicate the effectiveness of exclusive 'demand' or 'need' nursing on fertility control. A study of !Kung women gives some indication of this. !Kung people are gatherer-hunters. !Kung mothers carry their babies in a sling and nurse frequently (four episodes of 2 min per hour, with 55 min being the maximal interval). During the night the baby lies beside the mother and feeds from her breast when he wishes, usually without waking the mother. The infant is in close proximity for the first 2 years of life, and separations are brief until the child is about $3\frac{1}{2}$ years old. The frequency of episodes of nursing diminishes in the third year of the child's life. Most !Kung nursing mothers remain amenorrhoeic for 18 months, and the interval between births is 44 months. When !Kung people settle in agricultural communities, and supplement breast feeding by giving grain and cows milk to the infant, the birth interval is reduced, mainly because of a reduced intensity of breast feeding (Kolata, 1974). In a study of 16 nursing and eight non-nursing !Kung mothers plasma levels of oestradiol and progesterone were measured. Of the 16 nursing mothers, 12 were amenorrhoeic, and four were menstruating. The oestradiol levels were 24.7 ± 6.6 pg/ml in the former and 112.3 ± 16 pg/ml in the latter. The progesterone levels were 186 ± 61 pg/ml and 2653 ± 1122 pg/ml in the latter. The non-nursing mothers had plasma levels of oestradiol 146.1 ± 7.3 pg/ml and progesterone 7553 ± 21 pg/ml in the luteal phase of the cycle. These data indicate that 'demand' nursing inhibits ovarian function in most women, and that anovulatory menstrual cycles are usual when menstruation returns.

LACTATION INHIBITION AND SUPPRESSION

Over 96 per cent of mothers are able to breast feed if they are motivated and learn to do so. The exceptions are women who have breast cancer, or are receiving anti-metabolites; women whose baby has died *in utero*, and women whose baby has a congenital defect (such as cleft palate which impairs his ability to suckle). Most mothers who choose not to breast feed to so for psychological, social, or cultural reasons rather than because breast feeding is contraindicated.

At present, in spite of a modest return to breast feeding, mainly due to the influence of lay self-help breast feeding groups, over 50 per cent of mothers request that lactation be inhibited or suppressed within the first 6 weeks after childbirth.

The sequence of hormonal events which leads to the production of milk, its secretion, its ejection and its maintenance may be interrupted at the level of the mammary alveoli, the pituitary or the hypothalamus. Lactation can be suppressed either by avoiding breast stimulation or by using hormonal methods which prevent prolactin-induced milk production by inhibiting prolactin being taken up by mammary alveolar receptors or by suppressing prolactin.

Non-hormonal methods

Breast stimulation is avoided by discontinuing breast feeding and perhaps by binding the breasts which is believed (without objective evidence) to reduce episodic nipple stimulation. The breasts are supported in an appropriate brassiere. These methods reduce or eliminate the milk-ejection reflex, and decrease the amount of prolactin released, which falls to within the normal concentration of the hormone in non-pregnant women in 4 to 14 days (Walker et al, 1975). Inhibition of the milk ejection reflex leads to distension of the alveoli which, over the course of several days, suppresses milk production, by a pressure effect; simultaneously the reduction in circulating prolactin concentration, because of the absence of the prolactin reflex, inhibits further milk synthesis. Unfortunately the breasts become congested or engorged in over 60 per cent of patients between the 3rd and the 5th days, when about half of women complain of discomfort. One woman in three complains of pain, requiring analgesics (Markin & Wolst, 1960; Morris et al, 1970, Schwartz et al, 1973).

Some workers have suggested that if fluid intake is restricted, breast congestion is less; others have claimed the fluid intake should be increased, to hasten the engorgement and so to hasten lactation suppression. A careful study by Duckman & Hubbard (1950) showed that changes in fluid intake made no significant difference to engorgement or to the severity of breast pain. In 139 women fluids were forced, in 89 women fluids were restricted, 50 women took fluids *ad lib*. Breast pain was complained of by 42.5 per cent of women and there were no inter-group differences.

Hormonal methods

Oestrogen, by occupying mammary alveolar cell membrane binding sites, or by preventing prolactin inducing the formation of receptors, inhibits or suppresses lactation, with varying degrees of success. Oestrogen in the form of diethyl stilboestrol, ethinyl oestradiol, dienoestrol and chlortrianesene, have been administered in varying doses in varying regimens, over a variable number of days with a significant reduction of engorgement and breast pain compared with placebo.

The dose appears critical: a high failure rate occurs if too little oestrogen is given (less than 4.5 mg of ethinyl oestradiol or its equivalent), whilst large doses (more than 10 mg of ethinyl oestradiol or its equivalent) are unnecessary and possibly harmful.

The results of several placebo controlled clinical trials (Newton & Newton, 1948; Markin & Wolst, 1960; MacDonald & O'Driscoll, 1965; Morris et al, 1970; Schwartz et al 1973; Utian et al, 1975; Walker et al, 1975; Nilsen et al, 1976; Dewhurst et al, 1977) showed that lactation is suppressed and painful engorged breasts are prevented in about 80 per cent of women, which is a 20 per cent improvement over placebo. However, rebound breast filling occurred in about 20 per cent of women, 7–15 days after the completion of the course.

Other workers have used the pro-oestrogen chlortrianesene (72 mg, 12 hourly for 4 days) or quinoestrol, a long acting oestrogen, in a single 2 mg or 4 mg dose, with similar results, (Grant et al, 1978). Quinoestrol increases prolactin release but inhibits its action on the alveolar cells, confirming that oestrogens act at this level rather than by suppressing prolactin release (Walker et al, 1975).

Oestrogen in large doses, given in the puerperium has caused concern about the woman's health, particularly as Daniel et al (1967) showed that there was a 10-fold increase in thromboembolism amongst non-lactating women aged 25 and over who were given diethylstilboestrol to suppress lactation compared with lactating women. In 1968, a study by Jeffcoate et al showed that inhibition of lactation by ethinyl oestradiol was associated with a 3-fold increase in thromboembolism, mainly in women over the age of 25 who had had an operative delivery. Amongst women over 35 who had an operative delivery and had lactation inhibited, the rate was 10 times higher. A third study (Stewart et al, 1969) showed that the woman's age (> 25) and delivery by Caesarean section were the significant factors for the increase in thromboembolism. The conclusion of these studies was that except for women at special risk by reason of age (especially if over 35), obesity, or past history of thromboembolism, and an operative delivery (especially Caesarean section), oestrogen therapy was acceptable to suppress lactation. However, the reports caused concern and a number of obstetricians chose other hormonal therapy (such as androgen administration), or no method at all.

Oestrogen–androgen combinations have been used by many obstetricians; the assumption being that the androgen enters the alveolar cells and occupies intracellular prolactin binding sites, and may also inhibit prolactin release (Weinstein et al, 1976). Most workers give a single injection of testosterone enanthate 360 mg and oestradiol valerate 16 mg. In reported studies this medication was no more effective than oestrogen alone in controlling breast engorgement and pain, and rebound lactation occurred in 25–45 per cent (Lo Presto & Caypinar, 1959; Markin & Wolst, 1960; Morris et al, 1970; Llewellyn-Jones & Lawrence, 1973). Other workers have prescribed oral methyl testosterone in a dose of 100–350 mg taken over a period of 6–14 days with variable results (Lass, 1942; Duffy & Cosaro, 1951; Gold et al, 1959; Biggs et al, 1978). As the total dose of androgen is equivalent to several years production of endogenous testosterone and the results not significantly superior to oestrogen or no therapy, it may be inadvisable to use the hormone, although no adverse side effects have been reported.

The anti-oestrogens, clomiphene and tamoxifen have been prescribed in three studies (Zuckerman & Carmel, 1973; Weinstein et al, 1976; Marsala et al 1978), with equivocal results. The drugs act by reducing prolactin synthesis and release, they are expensive and can be replaced by bromocriptine.

Bromocriptine, a peptide ergot alkaloid, is a long-acting dopamine agonist which mimics the action of dopamine on the pituitary lactotrophs, and at the hypothalamic level, leading to a fall in prolactin release and a reduction in plasma prolactin levels. Bromocriptine has been used successfully in lactation suppression, and in controlled trials of the drug, compared with oestrogen and placebo, has proved superior in reducing milk leakage, breast congestion, and breast discomfort. Milk leakage between days 3 and 7 is reduced to less than 10 per cent compared with a 25 per cent incidence when a placebo was used, and a 15 per cent incidence when oestrogen was administered. Breast congestion occurred in 7 per cent when bromocriptine was given compared with 45 per cent in the placebo group and 30 per cent in the oestrogen group. Breast pain occurred in 6 per cent, compared with 45 per cent in the placebo group and 25 per cent in the oestrogen group (Walker et al, 1975b).

The dose required is 2.5 mg twice daily for 14 days. In this dosage side-effects are not common. At the start of treatment some women complain of nausea but this is usually mild; later, constipation and leg cramps have been reported. Following treatment, which causes the levels of prolactin to return to normal, early ovulation may occur, and women who suppress lactation with bromocriptine should use appropriate contraceptives before resuming sexual intercourse. If they do not, pregnancy may occur and the cycle of events described in this chapter will be repeated.

REFERENCES

Allen J, Heywood P F 1979 Infant feeding practises in Sydney. 1976–77 Australian Paediatric Journal 15: 113–117
Aono T, Shioji T, Shoda T et al 1977 The initiation of human lactation and prolactin response to suckling. Journal of Clinical Endocrinology and Metabolism 44: 1101–1106
Aono T, Shioji T, Aki T, et al 1979 Augmentation of puerperal lactation by oral administration of sulpiride. Journal of Clinical Endocrinology and Metabolism 48: 478–482
Applebaum R M 1970 Management of breast feeding. Pediatric Clinics of North America 17: 203–225
Baird D T, McNeilly A S, Sawers R S, et al 1979 Failure of estrogen-induced discharge of luteinizing hormone in lactating women. Journal of Clinical Endocrinology and Metabolism 49: 500–506
Biggs J S G, Hacker N, Edwards E 1978 Bromocriptine, Methyl testosterone and placebo for inhibition of physiological lactation. Medical Journal of Australia Special supplement 23–32
Bohnet H G, Gomez F, Friesen H G 1977 Prolactin and oestrogen binding sites in the mammary gland of the lactating and non-lactating rat. Endocrinology 101: 111–1121
Bolton-Maggs P H 1979 Breast or bottle British Medical Journal 2: 371–72
Box M C O, Hart H 1975 Encouraging breast feeding Lancet ii: 1214–1216
Boulton T J C, Coote L M 1979 Nutritional studies during early childhood. Australian Paediatric Journal 15: 81–86
Boulton T J C, Flavel S E 1978 The relationship of perinatal factors to breast feeding. Australian Paediatric Journal 14: 169–173
Clarke G, Lincoln D W, Merrick L P 1979 Dopaminergic control of oxytocin release in lactating rats. Journal of Endocrinology 83: 409–420
Cronin T J 1968 Influence of lactation upon ovulation. Lancet ii: 422–424
Daniel D G, Campbell H, Turnbull A C 1967 Puerperal thromboembolism and suppression of lactation. Lancet ii: 287–289
Dawood M Y, Khan-Dawood F S, Wahi R S et al 1981 Oxytocin release and plasma anterior pituitary and gonadal hormones in women during lactation. Journal of Clinical Endocrinology and Metabolism 52: 678–683
Delvoye P, Demaegd D M, Delogne E, Desnoeck J 1977 The influence of the frequency of nursing and of previous lactation experience on serum prolactin in lactating mothers. Journal of the Biosocial Sciences 9: 447–451
Dewhurst C J, Harrison R F, Biswas S 1977 Inhibition of puerperal lactation. Acta Obstetrica et Gynecologica Scandinavica 56: 527–331
Djiane J, Durand P 1977 Prolactin-progesterone antagonism in self regulation of prolactin receptors in the mammary gland. Nature 266: 641–643
Duffy P M, Corsaro J 1941 Suppression of lactation by testosterone. Journal of the American Medical Association 116: 33–36
El Etreby M F and Gunzel P 1974 Sex hormones — effects on prolactin cells. Acta Endocrinologica (Copenhagen) 76 Suppl 189: 1–15
Falachi P, Frajese G, Sciarra F, Rocca A and Conti C 1978 Influence of hyperprolactinaemia due to metaclopramide on gonadal function in men. Clinics in Endocrinology 8: 427–432
Gold J J, Soihet S, Hankin M et al 1959 Hormone therapy to control postpartum breast manifestations. American Journal of Obstetrics and Gynecology 78: 86
Gorewit R C, Tucker H A 1979 Glucocorticoid binding in mammary tissue slices of cattle in various reproductive states. Journal Dairy Science 59: 1890–1896
Grandison L, Guidott A 1977 Regulation of prolactin release by endogenous opiates. Nature 270: 357–359
Gross B A, Eastman C J 1979 Prolactin secretion during prolonged lactational amenorrhoea. Australian and New Zealand Journal of Obstetrics and Gynaecology 19: 95–99
Grosvenor C E 1965 Contraction of lactating rat mammary gland in response to direct mechanical stimulation. American Journal of Physiology 208: 214–218
Grosvenor C E, Whitworth N, Mena F 1975 Milk secretory response of the conscious lactating rat following intravenous injection of rat prolactin. Journal of Dairy Science 58: 1803–1807
Guzman V, Toscano G, Canales E J, Zarate A Improvement of

defective lactation by using oral metoclopramide. Acta Obstetrica et Gynecologica

Harrison B M 1978 One hundred infants: how they were fed. Archives of Disease in Childhood 53: 688. Abstract from Paediatric Research Society 1978 printing

Howie P W, McNeilly A S, Houston M J, et al 1981 Effect of supplementary food on suckling patterns and ovarian activity during lactation. British Medical Journal 2: 757–759

Jeffcoate T N A, Miller J, Roos R F, Tindall V R 1968 Puerperal thromboembolism in relation to inhibition of lacatation by oestrogen therapy. British Medical Journal 4: 19–25

Josimovich, J B 1977 In: Crosignani P G, Robyn C (eds) Prolactin and Human Reproduction, p 27. Academic Press, New York

Kauppila A, Kivinen S, Ylikorkala O 1981 Metoclopramide increases prolactin release and milk secretion in puerperium without stimulating the secretion of thyrotropin and thyroid hormones. Journal of Clinical Endocrinology and Metabolism 52: 436–439

Kelly P A, Tsushima T, Shui R P C et al 1976 Lactogenic and growth hormone like activities in pregnancy as determined by radioreceptor assays. Endocrinology, 99: 765–774

Kirk T R 1978 Breast feeding and mother's education. Lancet ii: 1201–1202

Kleinberg D L, Todd J 1980 Evidence that growth Hormone is a potent lactogen in primates, Journal of Clinical Endocrinology and Metabolism 5: 1009–1013

Kolata G B 1974 Nursing frequency, gonadal function and birth spacing among !Kung Hunter-gatherers. Science 185: 932–934

Lass P M The inhibition of lactation during the purperium by methyl testosterone. American Journal of Obstetrics and Gynecology

Lawson J S, Mays C A, Oliver T I 1978 The return to breastfeeding. Medical Journal of Australia 2: 229–230

Llewellyn-Jones D, Lawrence K D 1973 A new method of inhibition of lactation. Medical Journal of Australia 2: 780–782

Llewellyn-Jones R H 1977 Psychosocial Aspects of Infant Feeding. Thesis B.Sc (Med.), University of Sydney

Linzell J L 1955 Some observations on the contractile tissue of the mammary gland. Journal of Physiology 130: 257–267

Lo Presto B, Caypinar E Y 1959 Prevention of postpartum lactation by administration of deladumone during labor. Journal of the American Medical Association 169: 130–132

Lucas A, Lucas P J, Baum J D 1979 Pattern of milk flow in breast fed infants. Lancet ii: 57–58

Lucas A, Drewett R B, Mitchell M D 1980 Breast feeding and plasma oxytocin concentrations. British Medical Journal 2: 834–35

Lyons W R, Li C H, Ahmad N, Rice-Wray E 1968 Mammotrophic effects of human hypophyseal growth hormone preparations in animals and man. Excerpta Medica International Congress Series 158: 349–363

MacDonald D, O'Driscoll K 1965 Suppression of lactation: A double-blind trial. Lancet ii: 623

Maneckjee R, Srinath B R, Moudgal N R 1976 Prolactin suppresses release of luteinising hormone during lactation in the monkey. Nature 262: 507–508

Martin J 1978 Infant Feeding. HMSO, London

Martinez G A, Nalezienski J P 1981 The recent trend in breast feeding. Pediatrics 67: 260–263

Masala A, Delitala G, Lo Dico G et al 1978 Inhibition of lactation and inhibition of prolactin release after mechanical breast stimulation in puerperal women given tamoxifen or placebo. British Journal of Obstetrics and Gynaecology 85: 134

Masters W H, Johnson V 1976 The Human Sexual Response, p 162. Little Brown and Co, Boston

Markin K E, Wolst M D 1960 A comparative controlled study of hormones used in the prevention of postpartum breast engorgement and lactation. American Journal of Obstetrics and Gynecology 80: 128–137

Marrs R P, Kletzky O A, Mishell D R 1981 Functional capacity of the gonadotrophs during pregnancy and the puerperium. American Journal of Obstetrics and Gynecology 658–661

Matusik R J, Rosen J M 1978 Prolactin induction of casein in RNA in organ culture. Journal of Biological Chemistry, 253: 2343–2347

McNeilly A S 1979 Effects of lactation on fertility. British Medical Bulletin 35: 151–154

Mena F, Grosvenor L E 1972 Effect of suckling and of exteroceptive stimulation upon prolactin release in the rat during late lactation. Journal of Endocrinology 52: 11–22

Milligan D, Drife, J O, Short R V 1975 Changes in breast volume during normal menstrual cycle and after oral contraception. British Medical Journal, 4: 494–496

Morris J A, Creasy R K, Hohe P T 1970 Inhibition of puerperal lactation. Double-blind comparison of chlorotrianisene, testosterone enanthate with estradiol valerate and placebo. Obstetrics and Gynecology 36: 107–114

Moore B P, Forsyth I A 1980 Influence of local vascularity on hormone receptors in mammary gland. Nature 77–78

Moyer J A, O'Donohue T L, Herrenkohl L R et al 1979 Effects of suckling on serum prolactin levels and catecholamine concentrations and turnover in discrete brain regions. Brain Research, 176: 125–133

Nilsen P A, Meline A B, Abildgaard U 1976 Study of the suppression of lactation. Acta Obstetrica et Gynaecologica Scandinavica 55: 39–44

Noel G L Suh H K, Frantz A G 1974 Prolactin release during nursing and breast stimulation in postpartum and non-postpartum subjects. Journal of Clinical Endocrinology and Metabolism 38: 413–423

Nutrition Ctte of the Canadian Paed. Soc. and Ctte on Nutrition of the Am. Acad of Pediatrics 1978 Breast feeding. Commentary. Pediatrics 62: 591–601

Oakley J R 1978a Increased prevalence of breast feeding British Medical Journal 2: 1435

Oakley J R 1978b Infant feeding practices, Parity and S.I.D.S. Archives of Disease in Childhood 1978b, 53: 688–689

Pasteels J L, Gausset P, Danguy A et al 1972 Morphology of the lactotropes and somatotropes of man and rhesus monkeys. Journal of Clinical Endocrinology and Metabolism 34: 959–967

Perez A, Vela P, Masnick G S, Pottern R S 1972 First ovulation after childbirth: the effect of breast feeding. American Journal of Obstetrics and Gynecology 114: 1041–1047

Posner B I 1976 Characterization and modulation of growth hormone and prolactin binding in mouse liver. Endocrinology 98: 645–654

Reichlin S, Saperstein R, Jackson I M et al 1976 Hypothalamic hormones. Annual Review of Physiology 38: 389–424

Reyes F I, Winter J S D, Faiman C 1972 Pituitary ovarian relationships during the puerperium. American Journal of Obstetrics and Gynecology 114: 589–594

Richardson K C 1949 Contractile tissues in the mammary gland with special reference to myoepithelium in the goat. Proceedings of the Royal Society of London, Series B 136: 30–45

Rimoin D L, Holzman G B, Merimee T J et al 1968 Lactation in the absence of human growth hormone. Journal of Clinical Endocrinology and Metabolism 28: 1183–1188

Robinson J, Short J V 1977 Changes in human breast sensitivity at puberty, during the menstrual cycle and at parturition. British Medical Journal 1: 1188–1191

Robyn C, Meunis S 1982 Pituitary prolactin, lactational performance and puerperal infertility. Seminars in perinatology, 6: 254–264

Ruis H, Rolland R, Doesburg W, Broaders G, Corbey R 1981 Oxytocin enhances onset of lactation amongst mothers delivering prematurely. British Medical Journal 2: 340–342

Salariya E M, Easton P C, Cater J I 1978 Duration of breast feeding after early initiation and frequent feeding. Lancet ii: 1141–1143

Schwartz D I, Evans P C, Garcia C R et al 1973 A clinical study of lactation suppression. Obstetrics and Gynecology 42: 599–606

Shiu R P C, Fiesen H G 1980 Mechanism of action of prolactin in the control of mammary gland function. Annual Review of Physiology 42: 83–96

Sjolin S, Hofvander Y, Hillervik C 1979 A prospective study of individual courses of breast feeding. Acta Paediatrica Scandinavica 68: 521–529

Sloper K S, Elsden E, Baum J D 1977 Increasing breast feeding in a community. Archives of Disease in Childhood 52: 700–702

Soria, J A, Zarate A, Canales E J, Lobos H V 1976 Effect of suckling on serum LH and FSH in nursing women. Neuroendrinology 20: 43–47

Spellacy W N, Carlson K L, Birk S A 1976 Dynamics of human

placental lactogen. American Journal of Obstetrics and Gynecology 96: 1164–1173

Stewart K S, Kerridge D F, Dennis K J 1969 Suppression of lactation. British Medical Journal 2: 249

Tanner J M 1962 Growth at Adolescence. 2nd edn. Blackwell Scientific Publications, Oxford

Tindal J S, Knaggs G S 1972 Pathways in the forebrain of the rabbit concerned with the release of prolactin. Journal of Endocrinology 52: 253–262

Tindal J S 1981 The Neuroendocrine Control of Lactation, Vol IV, pp 67–109. Academic Press, New York

Tobon H, Salazar H 1975 Ultra structure of the human mammary gland. II. Postpartum lactogenesis. Journal of Clinical Endocrinology and Metabolism 40: 834–844

Tobon H, Josimovich J B, Salazar H 1972 The ultrastructure of the mammary lactogenesis in the rabbit. Endocrinology 90: 1569–1577

Tomita K, McCoshen J A, Fernandez C S, Tyson J E 1982 Immunologic and biologic characteristics of human decidual prolactin. American Journal of Obstetrics and Gynecology 142: 420–426

Topper V J 1976 Multiple hormone interactions in the development of mammary gland in vitro. Recent Progress in Hormone Research 26: 287–303

Tyson J E, Hwang P, Guyda H, Friesen H G 1972 Studies of prolactin secretion in human pregnancy. American Journal of Obstetrics and Gynecology 113: 14–20

Tyson J E, Khojandi M, Huth J, Andreassen B 1975 The influence of prolactin secretion on human lactation. Journal of Clinical Endocrinology and Metabolism 40: 764–769

Tyson J E, Perez A, Zanartu J 1976 Human lactational response to oral thyrotropin releasing hormone. Journal of Clinical Endocrinology and Metabolism 43: 760–768

Utian W H, Begg G, Vinik A I et al 1975 Effect of bromocriptine and chlorotrianisene on inhibition of lactation and serum prolactin. A comparative double-blind study. British Journal of Obstetrics and Gynaecology 82: 755–759

Verkasalo M 1980 Recent trends in breast feeding in Southern England. Acta Paediatrica Scandinavica 69: 89–91

Vorherr M 1974 In: Larson B L (ed) The Breast: Morphology, Physiology and Lactation Academic Press, New York

Walker S, Hibbard B M, Groom G 1975 Controlled trial of bromocryptine, quinoestrol and placebo in suppression of human lactation. Lancet ii: 842–845

Weinstein D, Ben-David M, Polishuk W Z 1976 Serum prolactin and the suppression of lactation. British Journal of Obstetrics and Gynaecology 83: 679–682

West C P 1980 Factors influencing the duration of breastfeeding. Journal of Biosocial Science 12: 325–331

Zuckerman H, Carmel S 1973 The inhibition of lactation by clomiphene. British Journal of Obstetrics and Gynaecology 80: 822–823

Zarate A, Canales E S, Soria J et al 1972 Ovarian refractoriness during lactation in woman. American Journal of Obstetrics and Gynecology 112: 1130–1132

Zarate A, Villalobos E S, Canales J S et al 1976 The effect of oral administration of thyrotropin releasing hormone on lactation. Journal of Clinical Endocrinology and Metabolism 43: 301–305

Diabetes and pregnancy

This chapter attempts to analyse the scope of the diabetes–pregnancy connection and the clinical experience accumulated over the years.

In an insulin-dependent diabetic who is pregnant, a favourable metabolic environment provided by the use of insulin and depending upon the proper function of the placental-maternal unit allows the survival of a neonate which was unusual before the insulin era. The observation of an increased percentage of congenital malformations in children born from diabetic mothers even when they are treated, points to the haphazard influence of the deranged metabolism of the mother upon the developmental process of the fetus. Further specific morbidity in the surviving infant — like neonatal hyperinsulinaemia, hypoglycaemia or hypocalcaemia — indicates that functional changes brought into existence in the fetus by metabolic alterations in the mother may have an impact on the evolutionary stages in the fetus and on organic functions which may even last after birth. Normally evolutionary stages occur in an orderly sequence during development. They are related first to the mitotic activity of undifferentiated cells which proliferate; later differentiation of the cells is related to maturity which entails increase in cell size and maturation of the biochemical function of the cell including specific changes in the cell membrane and its receptors.

The sequential order of cell development modulates the velocity of fetal growth. The classical observations by Sir John Hammond on the foal size of Shetland or Shire dams when served by stallions of the other genus, confirm that factors present in the mother contribute to and regulate this velocity (Walton & Hammond, 1938). In the human, the maternal conditions which correlated positively with normal range of weight at birth were the duration of gestation, birth rank of the infants, maternal weight or maternal weight gain during pregnancy (Thomson et al, 1968).

Maternal nutriments transfered to the fetus are known to regulate the fetal growth curve within a fairly narrow margin in the human. Before 26 weeks, growth may result from cell division, increased cell size or both. Growth will be linear. After the 26th week an S-shaped pattern of growth occurs. Intra-uterine experiences may accelerate or retard this velocity and some conditions in the mother may interfere with the normal evolution of intra-uterine growth. Maternal factors of metabolic nature may have an impact on fetal development and growth at different stages. The final outcome regarding growth and maturation will depend upon the nature of the intervening factors and the time of gestation. The association of factors which both accelerate fetal growth and restrain it may further complicate the outcome.

The metabolic adaptation of the mother to pregnancy is dependent in part upon the functional integrity of the maternal endocrine pancreas. The target organ of the nutritional exchange between mother and fetus is the fetal endocrine pancreas. The structural and functional adaptation of the fetal islets also affects fetal growth and wellbeing.

Diabetes in the mother influences fetal development from conception onwards and the short and long-term consequences of this influence may not be predictable. In order to secure a healthy outcome of such pregnancies great skill and coordinated efforts of physicians, obstetricians and paediatricians are required. The association of diabetes with pregnancy may appear to be a specific clinical problem of developed countries where type I diabetes is common. But the magnitude of this metabolic problem remains to be assessed in much of the world. Four-fifths of the world population live in developing countries where the average age of the female population is under 30. The greatest problem of these pregnancies is related to the birth of small for dates infants which in some continents form 20 per cent of the total births. Follow-up of surviving infants in unfavourable conditions indicate that they are affected by neurological damage, visual defects and low intellectual quotients (Jurado-Garcia, 1978). Conditions are obviously present in mothers in the developing world which impede normal fetal growth but their biological and metabolic nature is not precisely delineated.

In these populations, where small for dates are the majority of the births and need specific intensive care for survival, large for dates are also born. The latter also create neonatal problems such as traumatic birth and respiratory distress syndrome. The fact that heavy newborns are born in populations with malnutrition indicates the overriding role of the maternal metabolic environment on development and the growth of the fetus (Habicht et al, 1974; Hoet & Krall, 1982). Moreover, the normal defence mechanisms in pregnancy associated with malnutrition are modified and both states are characterised by a greater sensitivity to infectious diseases. This higher susceptibility has been recognised for paralytic poliomyelitis, severe rubella infections and influenza, varicella, hepatitis B as well as Cocksakie B (Oleske &Minnefor, 1980). Cocksackie B virus is more destructive for the pancreatic B cell in pregnant mice and viral agents have been invoked in the cause of diabetes in susceptible human individuals (Graighead, 1977).

The association of pregnancy and diabetes may be part of the frequent morbidity seen in developing countries and it might be also population specific. In certain areas, the prevalence of diabetes outside pregnancy is higher in the female population of childbearing age than it is in males. This is even more apparent for impaired glucose tolerance in the female population of childbearing age compared to males (Zimmet et al, 1981). The reasons for having an association of diabetes and pregnancy in the developing world may be different from the developed world and the clinical aspects of the pregnancy outcome could also be different. There is a need for continuous observation and awareness of the problem of diabetes during pregnancy in any given population. This also emphasises the discrimination one has to apply when the effect of pregnancy is described in a heterogenous clinical entity like diabetes and the careful scrutiny which is demanded when analysing the effects of such heterogeneity upon pregnancy outcome.

THE EFFECT OF PREGNANCY ON THE DIABETIC MOTHER

Pregnancy in an untreated or poorly treated insulin-dependent type 1 diabetic can be disastrous. Early in pregnancy major glycosuria and ketonuria may appear; ketoacidosis may develop and if not treated adequately, the mother may die in ketoacidotic coma (Kyle, 1963). This sequence was often observed in industrialised countries before the insulin era. Pregnancy in the insulin-dependent diabetic who is poorly treated with insulin is still a major problem.

Pregnancy does not influence the long-term development of retinopathy, nephropathy or neuropathy in well controlled diabetes (Carstensen et al, 1982) even when no residual B cell function is left. Even in diabetic patients with early renal damage or background retinopathy, pregnancy as such does not produce an immediate impairment if the metabolic control is maintained close to normal indices throughout pregnancy (Mintz et al, 1978).

However, pregnancy may be associated with further deterioration in the presence of proliferative retinopathy even when the maternal blood sugars are normalised (Kitzmiller et al, 1981). Pregnancy may be contraindicated in patients with untreated proliferative retinopathy. Laser therapy will arrest the evolution of proliferative retinopathy and if used before pregnancy or early in pregnancy, it will safeguard the eye-grounds when pregnant. Laser therapy should be used before pregnancy in a diabetic with proliferative retinopathy. This also emphasises the importance of early diagnosis of diabetes in the child and the need to achieve early normalisation of the metabolic conditions when diabetes develops at childbearing age.

In diabetes with myocardial infarction, angina, or relevant ECG changes, pregnancy may be associated with a 50 per cent maternal death rate. Coronary artery bypass may aleviate the high death rate imposed by pregnancy in diabetic women with myocardial damage (Kitzmiller et al, 1982).

The association of residual insulin secretion in an insulin-dependent diabetic and the evolution of diabetic complications during pregnancy needs further assessment. The ease of control in the presence of endogenous insulin secretion has been demonstrated for non-pregnant diabetics (Binder & Faber, 1978). This important observation has been extended for the pregnant diabetic by Stangenberg et al (1982a). They indicated that endogenous insulin secretion was conducive to better control of the metabolic disturbance especially in the first and second trimester. The assessment of remaining insulin secretion with appropriate methodology such as C-peptide determination should be most valuable in clinical practice. It may help to predict the type of control which may be obtained during pregnancy. The role of islet cell antibodies and insulin antibodies on cell changes in the maternal pancreas throughout pregnancy needs further assessment.

The foregoing indicates that an insulin-dependent diabetic needs full clinical assessment before considering pregnancy. This should include a detailed clinical history of the diabetes, assessment of parameters related to renal function and lipoprotein changes (HDL especially), as well as of the presence of vascular and eye-ground complications. Measurement of residual B cell function by C-peptide determination and assay of insulin and islet cell antibodies should be undertaken.

The impact of pregnancy in a type 2 diabetic on the evolution of the disease is not easily ascertained. In this heterogenous group of patients diabetes does not have the explosive evolution seen in type 1 diabetes. Pregnancy in these patients may further impair or show up the underlying metabolic disorder but is not associated with acute episodes of ketoacidosis or obvious impairment of diabetic complications.

Therefore, pregnancy in this instance is not clearly perceived as an immediate health hazard for the mother. It may be associated with abnormal weight gain and leave the patient later with handicapping obesity or manifest diabetes, especially if the patient was not treated during pregnancy. Because of the insidious evolution of the disorder induced by the metabolic demands of pregnancy one may not be aware of the condition, resulting in its neglect.

But this questionable state of health may not be so benign as it appears. In populations with an overall prevalence of diabetes of 7 per cent, adequate screening during pregnancy shows impaired glucose tolerance or clinical diabetes in 29 per cent of women, indicating the potential for substantial underreporting. Twelve per cent remained diabetic after pregnancy (Yen, 1964). Furthermore O'Sullivan & Mahan (1980) demonstrated that 35 per cent of women with gestational diabetes became diabetic at 16 year follow-up and 20 per cent had manifest cardiovascular complications 20 years later. This was of a greater magnitude than in the control population.

The relationship of type 2 diabetes and pregnancy in the developing countries is not known but, as stated above, pregnancy might facilitate manifest diabetes in susceptible women, especially in a population with a high prevalence of diabetes. The connection might be important especially considering that more than 50 per cent of women in developing countries are of childbearing potential and that the condition, if present, may affect the short and long-term health status of the mother and her children. Awareness of the problem of diabetes and specific observations should help to solve further the high rate of maternal and perinatal mortality in developing countries where diabetes may be an unrecognised part of many short and long-term health hazards.

Effect of mother's health upon the outcome of pregnancy

Type 1 diabetes

Even before the insulin era the prime obsective was to secure not only the survival of the pregnant mother but also to ensure a successful fetal outcome. Fetal loss or neonatal death occured in 40 per cent of cases at the inception of the insulin era, after which encouraging achievements were obtained through trial and error (Kyle, 1963). The high perinatal mortality was then reduced substantially to reach the same order of magnitude seen in non-diabetic mothers when proper insulin therapy resulted in normalising the blood sugar profiles. In addition, the overall perinatal mortality in industrialised countries reached very low levels over the last decade through the improvement of general health care (Gillmer et al, 1982). The ready availability of obstetric expertise did much to achieve this goal. The survival of infants of diabetic mothers also shows this trend. These heartening and favourable results are reported by centres of excellence

where a combined approach by trained physicians, obstetricians and paediatricians together with the active participation of the mother to be and the husband achieve continuous monitoring of metabolic control and the general wellbeing of the pregnant mother.

However, in most countries only a minority of diabetic patients receive this type of medical service. The majority of diabetic pregnant women, even in developed countries are still cared for in circumstances where specialised and expert skills are not always available. Consequently fetal wellbeing may not be assured. This is apparent from the higher incidence of congenital malformations in infants where the pregnancies are supervised outside specialised centres (Pedersen & Molsted-Pedersen, 1979).

In order to compare results between centres and to give a prognosis for pregnancy outcome there needs to be uniformity in recording the maternal status including diabetic control and any complications of the disease that are present. White successfully associated the diabetic complications of the mother with the pathological features of the infant (Kitzmiller et al, 1982). In three classes — A, B and C — the fetal and neonatal risks are similar and consist of hydramnios, macrosomia with its classical consequences, and stillbirths. Traumatic births may occur also. In class A patients, the glucose intolerance is manifest after glucose loading; the fasting blood glucose remains less than 5.7 mmol/l (105 mg/dl) and the 2 hour post-prandial remains less than 6.7 mmol/l (120 mg/dl) with dietary control alone before and during pregnancy. In class B patients, insulin therapy is needed in order to achieve the above described goals, and the onset is after 20 years of age with the duration of the disease less than 10 years. Class C consists of insulin-treated patients with an age of onset between 10 and 20 years and a duration of 10–20 years. The infants of mothers from D, F and R classes have, in addition, specific characteristics such as intra-uterine growth retardation, intra-partum loss or poor neonatal survival. Class D consists of patients with diabetic nephropathy with proteinuria and class R of patients with malignant proliferative retinopathy.

The features of macrosomia in one type of patient and of small for dates with the associated perinatal problems in another type, is common when metabolic control is not well established. These neonatal features tend to fade despite the maternal diabetic complications, when optimal metabolic control is secured. Infants with congenital malformations are born in any of these classes but there is an increased probability that they will occur in the D, F and R classes.

Class T and H should be mentioned. The former comprises mothers in the post-renal transplant period where the prognosis is good for mother and child. The latter comprises mothers with coronary artery disease which is a grave risk for the mother; she may not survive pregnancy for more than six months.

In addition to the prognostic signs described by White, Pedersen (1977) has delineated those conditions associated with a poor prognosis during diabetic pregnancy. The prognostically bad signs during pregnancy (PBSP) are clinical pyelonephritis with positive urinary tract infection, associated with an acute elevation of temperature; precoma or severe acidosis with a venous bicarbonate level under 17 meq/l; pregnancy hypertension and defaulters who did not seek expert medical advice early in their pregnancy.

A further and important factor concerning the prognosis for morbidity in the newborn from a diabetic woman relates to the observation made by Stangenberg et al (1982). They studied for the first time the residual maternal B-cell secretion in insulin-dependent mothers from the first trimester of pregnancy onwards. Some mothers had an increase in their diurnal C-peptide profiles at the beginning of pregnancy without further increase with advancing pregnancy. Mothers who did not manifest this increase early in pregnancy bore infants who had the greatest neonatal complications. Neonatal symptomatic hypoglycemia, feeding problems, increased amniotic fluid volume occurred when neonates displayed an increased level of proinsulin, insulin and C-peptide in cord blood, as well as a higher birth weight. These complications occurred when the mother had no residual B cell function left.

Consequently measurement of the remaining endogenous insulin secretion in the mother may become an essential indicator for a prospective evaluation of pregnancy. The association of the presence of remaining B cell function with better fetal outcome sheds further light on previous classifications like that of White. The latter implied that early onset and long duration, which is connected with a progressive loss of B cell function is linked with increased fetal morbidity and mortality. The same holds true for the second prognostically bad signs during pregnancy of Pedersen (1977), i.e. the event of pre-coma or severe acidosis where B cell secretion should be exhausted.

In addition, the presence of insulin antibodies is associated with low or undetectable plasma levels of C-peptide implying the absence of endogenous insulin secretion in the mother and higher maternal blood glucose levels during the first part of pregnancy. In this instance, a correlation between fetal hyperinsulinism (high C-peptide levels) and respiratory disorders and hypoglycaemia has been observed. These observations imply that the lack of endogenous insulin secretion in the mother associated with the presence of insulin antibodies results in higher maternal blood sugars especially during the first and second trimester. The fetal B cell would therefore be primed early in its differentiation and maturation as well as later in its secretion of insulin. In addition, insulin antibodies cross the placenta and affect the insulin levels in the fetus which may be higher in the presence of insulin antibodies (Persson et al, 1982).

Furthermore, insulin-dependent mothers may have islet cell antibodies which may cross the placental barrier. Their role as a prognostic sign for the mother and infant has not, but should be, elucidated.

To conclude, insulin-dependent diabetic pregnant mothers (type 1 diabetes) form a heterogenous group in relation to the prognosis for the neonate. The health at birth is dependent upon the age of onset, the duration, the vascular complications of the diabetes as well as the presence in the mother's blood of antibodies against insulin and possibly islet cell antibodies. It is jeopardised further in cases of renal infection or diabetic decompensation. It is especially conditioned by the blood glucose control in the mother.

Type 2 diabetes

The type 2 diabetic mother is classified in class A of White. She has abnormal blood sugar profiles in the non-pregnant state and is not insulin dependent. If the fasting blood sugars rise to abnormal levels and insulin is needed to normalise the profiles, the patient becomes a class B patient. Some women have a normal fasting blood sugar but display abnormal post-prandial blood sugars outside as well as during pregnancy (impaired glucose tolerance as classified by WHO, 1980). Others have impaired glucose tolerance solely during pregnancy and not outside pregnancy. They have gestational diabetes or impaired glucose tolerance during pregnancy (O'Sullivan, 1963). Clinical surveys have revealed pathological events during pregnancy in relation to glucose intolerance (Hoet et al, 1960; (O'Sullivan et al, 1973; Mestman, 1980; Merkatz et al, 1980; Opperman & Camerini-Davalos, 1980).

Only a few unselected population surveys have been made of type 2 diabetes during pregnancy. They are usually carried out in populations chosen because of their high prevalence for diabetes. In Guam where the prevalence rate for type 2 diabetes is 7 per cent, 2 hour post-prandial blood glucose in excess of 8.3 mmol/l (150 mg/dl) occured in 42 per cent of the pregnant women and confirmed gestational diabetes occured in 29 per cent of the pregnant women (Yen, 1964; Kuberski & Bennett, 1980); 25 per cent remained glucose intolerant in the immediate post-partum period. In this population which has been homogeneous for more than 250 years and has a very high fertility rate, the neonatal pathology in relation to women screening positive for glucose intolerance was large for dates infants and stillbirths. In Pima Indians diabetes during pregnancy occured 40 times more frequently than in another relatively unselected subgroup and 10 times more frequently than in a selected group of the population (Pettit et al, 1980). In Pima Indians, the perinatal death rate dropped from 25 to 7 per cent from 1960–1965 to 1970–1975 (Pettit et al, 1980) and was similar in the three groups of women: the normals, those with impaired glucose tolerance and type 2 diabetics. Pregnant women in these series were treated with insulin because of high fasting blood sugar and should be classified in class B of White. This increased rate of perinatal mortality in diabetic women and the trend of lowering it with insulin treatment has been observed in previous series (Hoet et al, 1960; O'Sullivan et al, 1966). A further assessment of therapeutic results has still to be obtained.

The inter-relationship between the degree of hyperglycaemia and neonatal pathology such as excessive birth weight and the effect of insulin therapy thereupon has been noted in several series. It can be established from an epidemiological point of view in a subset of pregnant diabetics (O'Sullivan et al, 1966). In Pima Indians, the incidence of large for date infants increased with increasing glucose levels but this was not evident for the heaviest neonates or the oldest mothers (Petitt et al, 1980). The direct impact of the level of maternal blood sugar on neonatal weight in a subset of patients indicates that even in the presence of factors increasing fetal growth, intervening elements may modify this velocity. Taken together, maternal blood glucose concentration, maternal age and maternal weight have an impact on the morbidity of the pregnancy outcome. Similar reciprocal relations were found in other series of relatively unselected patients and in clinic populations where race also played a discriminating role (Merkatz et al, 1980).

The risk of developing diabetes later in life relates to the degree of blood sugar abnormality occurring late in pregnancy (O'Sullivan, 1963). An observed incidence of 7 per cent in the postpartum period, 29 per cent after 5.5 years and a cumulative incidence of 67 per cent in a North-American population at large have been reported. Pima Indian women with a glucose concentration during pregnancy of 8.8–10 mmol/l (160–179 mg/dl) have over ten times the incidence of diabetes as pregnant women with a concentration of less than 5.5 mmol/l (100 mg/dl) after 4–8 year follow-up(Petitt et al, 1980).The evolution of glucose intolerance which starts with pregnancy may be prevented by insulin treatment used during the latter part of pregnancy. This preventive effect has only been shown in a subset of patients characterised by a family history of diabetes and the birth of large for date infants (O'Sullivan & Mahan, 1980). Similarly the most frequent complication of type 2 diabetes — hypertension and E.C.G. changes — are most prevalent during a 20 year follow-up in mothers with an abnormal glucose tolerance during pregnancy not treated with insulin.

The increased perinatal mortality in Pima Indians was due in 40 per cent of the cases to congenital malformations. Just as in type 1 diabetics who have a malformation rate which is 3 to 7 times higher than in a non-diabetic population, glucose intolerance present at the inception of pregnancy may affect the early stages of an embryonic development in type 2 diabetes.

Stillbirths are also known to be increased in a type 2 diabetic population (Bennett et al, 1979). Here, also, the abnormal glucose level is predictive of the risk for stillbirth. In Nauru, a stillbirth rate of 1 per cent was observed in women who had a normal 7.7 mmol/l (<140 mg/dl) blood sugar 2 hours after 50 gm glucose load. In contrast, women with a borderline blood sugar 7.7–8.3 mmol/l (140–150 mg/dl) had a stillbirth rate of 11 per cent while women with grossly abnormal blood sugars >8.3 mmol/l (>150 mg/dl) had a rate of 10 per cent (Zimmet et al, 1981).

The loss of bimodality of glucose distribution during pregnancy in Pima Indian women 25 years and over who in the non-pregnant state display a characteristic bimodality distribution is of interest and relevance. This highlights the impact of the latter part of pregnancy on glucose homeostasis and the difficulty in determining a specific glucose level which could be regarded as a cut off value diagnostic of gestational diabetes. It is of clinical importance to recognise this difficulty as the rate of complications of pregnancy, like perinatal mortality, large for dates and toxaemia is related to the degree of glucose intolerance throughout the range of abnormality.

The majority of observations stem from communities which are conditioned by the industrialised era. No specific surveys have been reported from developing countries. However, scattered information indicates that impaired glucose tolerance might afflict the pregnant women in this area in view of some neonatal complications which are observed such as large for dates, stillbirths, congenital malformations. Obviously the major pathology is related to small for dates in the developing world.

Glucose intolerance or diabetes should not be ignored in these instances. Even in the developed world maternal diabetes was incriminated amongst the small for dates admitted to neonatal intensive care units according a large US survey in New York City (Paneth et al, 1982; Van Assche et al, 1982). Awareness and further observations are definitely warranted in order to delineate the circumstances whereby glucose intolerance could be associated with small or large for dates.

To conclude, glucose intolerance during pregnancy is associated with complications of pregnancy and subsequently an increased incidence of diabetes in the mother. A continuous range of glucose intolerance appears to influence the rates of complications of pregnancy, especially macrosomia and toxaemia and the degree of intolerance affects their severity. The rates of stillbirth and congenital malformations are associated also with glucose intolerance but they seem not to be related to its degree.

Therefore, similar glucose levels may have differing impacts on the fetus in relation to other intervening factors present in the mother or the time of gestation when they operate. In clinical medicine and obstetrics one should not be complacent about abnormal blood sugar levels during pregnancy and should be aware of the contributing hazards for the neonate and the mother.

CONGENITAL MALFORMATIONS

Even though mortality and some aspects of morbidity of the neonate have improved over the years, the congenital malformation rate has become the most important cause of pathology in infants of women with abnormal blood sugars.

The rate of congenital malformations is higher in diabetic women who are not taken care of in expert centres where a team approach is being applied. This implies that women who are not under optimal control before and at the time of conception have a haphazard evolution which unfavourably influences fetal differentiation (Pedersen & Molsted-Pedersen, 1979).

In the human, the onset of diabetes before age 25 increases the occurrence of congenital malformations (Comess et al, 1969). In one study, the duration of maternal diabetes was found relevant. In other studies, this was not noted (Bennett et al, 1979). Neither study specified the degree of control which was obtained. More congenital malformations have been observed in type 1 diabetic women with vascular disease but the presence of vasculopathy is not generally accepted as being causally related (Soler et al, 1976; Pedersen, 1977; Bennett et al, 1979). These diabetic (type 1) women are usually insulin-dependent diabetics with onset at a younger age, characterised by a long duration of the disease, with or without antibodies and having presumably no endogenous insulin. Insulin antibodies do not seem to play a role as congenital anomalies appear also in non-insulin treated diabetics albeit with a lesser frequency. Insulin antibodies should not cross the placenta before the second trimester and should therefore not be causally related to congenital malformation (Galbraith & Faulk, 1979).

The teratological factors, metabolic and others must operate before the 7th week of gestation (Mills et al, 1979). Glucose as such could be a candidate for the bone malformations and neural tubal defects; it was shown for the latter to affect neural tube unfolding *in vitro* (Deuchar, 1979). The way glucose acts is unknown. Glycosylation of protein, oxygen insufficiency and low 2.3 DPG levels are consequences of high glucose levels.

Experimental diabetes was associated with an increased risk of osseous malformations in a normal strain of small rodents (Watanabe & Ingalls, 1963; Baker et al, 1981). Appropriate insulin treatment reduced the incidence of congenital anomalies to normal (Horii et al, 1966; Baker et al, 1981; Eriksson et al, 1982). In addition, the skeletal malformations in fetuses of pregnant diabetic rats occurred if treatment with insulin was withheld specifically between day 5 and day 8 of pregnancy (Eriksson & Dahlstrom, 1982). The teratological insult must act almost directly after the implantation of the blastocyst. It still remains an enigma why all fetuses of a polythecous species are not affected in an experimental diabetic pregnancy.

Some teratological insults could be specific and have some defined organs as a target. Clinically, a virus infection like rubella affects particularly the development of the fetal heart. Congenital rubella also produces an insulinitis in the fetal endocrine pancreas where a lymphocytic infiltration occurs and diabetes may ensue (Forrest et al, 1971; Schopper et al, 1982).

Both lesions may be associated (Forrest et al, 1971). In addition, rubella has been suggested as a diabetogenic factor in subjects with predisposing histocompatible antigens (Lecompte & Gepts, 1977). A fault in the maternal immune surveillance may be a contributory factor in malformations. Insulin has been suggested to be teratogenic (Deuchar, 1979) as experimental studies have indicated that bone malformations occurred when insulin was injected into the eggs of avian embryos. In humans, insulin injected into the mother would not be responsible as it does not cross the placenta and insulin carried by insulin antibodies would not cross before the second trimester (Gillmer et al, 1982). It was also suggested that the insulin was secreted endogenously in higher quantities than normal in the fetuses of diabetic mothers (Deuchar, 1979). Insulin appears to be secreted by the fetus only after the induction of bone malformation and bones are therefore not a likely candidate. However, high insulin levels could still have a late effect on development. Insulin has been shown to arrest cartilage growth in vitro when present in supraphysiological amount (v. Bruchhausen, 1975). In addition, retardated ossification centres have been observed in infants of diabetic mothers (Pedersen & Osler, 1958).

Specific systems seem to be more vulnerable in these infants. The central nervous system as well as the cardiovascular and the genito-urinary systems are more frequently affected. The caudal regression syndrome is quite specific for infants born to diabetic mothers.

Situs inversus, anencephaly, spina bifida and rectal atresia also occur (Bennett et al, 1979). The frequency of heart anomalies and of central nervous defects seem to differ in certain diabetic populations (Farquhar, 1969). It may reflect the presence of factors of different teratological nature which are disclosed by the diabetic state.

From the present information, one might suggest that in relation to maternal diabetes, fetal heart malformations could occur in the presence of viral interference. Presentation of viral antigens by human vascular endothelial cells *in vitro* has been demonstrated (Hirschberg, 1981) and congenital heart malformation is frequent in maternal rubella infection which also produces fetal insulitis. This occurs especially in predisposed women (Forrest et al, 1971). On the other hand, the central nervous defects could be associated with a fault in maternal immune surveillance. The difficulty of proving this assertion is due to the small numbers of observations which can be made at this stage but this could explain the observed variations in diabetic populations. In any event, these different malformations form a heterogenous group and are not diabetes specific. It precludes direct determinants which are inherited and linked to genes responsible for diabetes. Why other systems like the musculo-skeletal, the sensory or the alimentary are not affected to a similar degree is not apparent.

In a type 2 diabetic population, the high risk of congenital malformation was evident when the distinction was made between diabetic and non-diabetic women, notwithstanding the degree of abnormalities of blood sugar (Bennett et al, 1979). Clinically, congenital malformations may be predicted. Growth retardation around 10–12 weeks gestation as determined by ultrasound measurements has been observed in infants who are born with congenital malformations (Fog-Pedersen & Molsted-Pedersen, 1979). The appearance of alfa-fetoprotein in high concentration in the maternal blood may herald the presence of congenital malformations which may be confirmed by ultrasound (Gillmer et al, 1982).

Epidemiological studies suggest that the pre-diabetic period in any women when metabolic disturbances have not yet developed is not associated with a higher rate of congenital anomalies of the offspring (Bennett et al, 1979).

Hypoglycaemia in the mother is not associated with an increased rate of congenital malformation, but maternal hyperglycaemia is related (Pedersen, 1977). Paternal diabetes carries no increased risk of abnormality, suggesting that genetic determinants cannot be invoked as a cause of fetal abnormality (Bennett et al, 1979).

As stated earlier, the high incidence of congenital malformations is likely to be linked with metabolic anomalies intervening early in human pregnancy. Diabetes is seldom under good control at the beginning of human pregnancy and will be further disturbed by pregnancy itself, especially when no residual B-cell function is left. Early normalisation with insulin treatment of the metabolic alteration induced by diabetes prevents the malformation. Planned pregnancies with excellent control avoid major malformations (Gillmer et al, 1982). Furthermore, an increased HbA1C at the inception of pregnancy is associated with a greater percentage of congenital anomalies although this relation could not be established at an individual level (Leslie et al, 1980; Miller et al, 1981; Gillmer et al, 1982).

Epidemiological and experimental evidence support the view that the severity of hyperglycaemia and the frequency of congenital malformations are not strictly related and that any blood sugar, having reached a critical abnormal level, is likely to be indicative of a higher risk of congenital malformations. One should not be complacent with any abnormalities in glucose tolerance which must be correctly supervised (Beard & Hoet, 1982).

THE MATERNAL-FETAL UNIT IN NORMAL AND DIABETIC PREGNANCY

The expected result of fertilisation is the birth of a normal infant. But the favourable outcome of the natural process of a pregnancy is a tribute to the biological adaptation of the mother which should proceed in an orderly fashion to avoid complications.

Some problems are related to disturbances in the anatomical contacts which are being established between the mother and the conceptus. Others are related to failure in functional interactions. The immunological acceptance of the conceptus by the mother, the maternal intermediary metabolism or the hormonal status of the maternal placental unit may be at fault. Some of these aspects are still under intensive investigation and how they relate to each other is not precisely delineated. Any disordered evolution in the immunological process or in the metabolic or hormonal balance may have pathological consequences for the neonate.

Immunological considerations

The conceptus bears antigens foreign to the maternal organism and develops in an immunologically hostile environment. The developmental progress is related to an escape of maternal immune surveillance. Initially, the trophoblast is responsible for its own survival and development. The fetus will later seek further protection to prevent rejection (Faulk & McIntyre, 1981; Faulk, 1981). Decreased immune reactivity of the mother associated with intervening processes like local mechanical barrier, blocking antibodies and soluble suppressor factors originating in the fetus are operational in the course of pregnancy (Froelich et al, 1980).

Early in pregnancy, a decrease of helper T cells occurs and is most apparent in the third trimester (Sridama et al, 1982). Auto-immune diseases are provoked by an imbalance between helper and suppressor T cells which might be reversed again during pregnancy. The subsidence of the morbid symptoms in systemic lupus erythematosus, rheumatoid arthritis and auto-immune thyroid disease has been attributed to this reversion which was induced by pregnancy. In thyroid disease during pregnancy a reduction of auto-antibodies was found. Pregnancy has occured in type 1 diabetes associated with auto-immune diseases like hyperthyroidism with macrocytic anaemia and in Addison's disease with thyroiditis and gestational diabetes (Galbraith & Faulk, 1979).

How immunological surveillance during pregnancy operates in the diabetic woman and how it affects the evolution of diabetes during pregnancy and the outcome of pregnancy is not known. The induction of the immuno-suppressive state could be related to chorionic gonadotrophin, prolactin, oestrogens, progesterone, corticoids, alfa-fetoproteins and alfa-globulin as these biological products are shown to have an immuno-depressive effect, at least in culture studies (Lawrence et al, 1980). The hormonal and immunological interdependence could still be implicated in some morbid aspects of diabetic pregnancy. Recurrent spontaneous abortion has been attributed to the failure of the maternal immune mechanisms to recognise fetal antigens of the implanted blastocyst. It occurs especially in HLA compatible couples when the mother has no easy way of recognising the features of the conceptus and does not form the appropriate blocking factors (Faulk, 1981; Taylor & Faulk, 1981). In addition, increased abortion rate and increased fetal loss have been reported in women with autoimmune diseases (Sridama et al, 1982). In type 1 diabetes where specific histocompatibility antigens are implicated, a trend to increased abortion rate has been reported (Dekaban & Baird, 1959; Kyle, 1963). This trend has been disputed at least in gestational diabetic women. The relation of this morbid event to the complex immune aspects of pregnancy warrants further exploration in type 1 diabetes and eventually also in type 2 diabetes.

Congenital malformations are frequent in infants of diabetic mothers and the role of immune factors in their occurrence should be studied. Antibodies, especially to kidney or placental antigens, have produced congenital malformations in the experimental animal (Brent, 1966). In the human fetus the antibodies which the mother produces against the incompatible antigens inherited from the father are anti-allotype antibodies of IGg origin. They cross the placental barrier at an increasingly accelerated rate during the third trimester of pregnancy (Gitlin et al, 1964) and do not seem to relate to abnormal development in the fetus with the exception of blood group incompatability causing haemolytic disease.

However, based on the concept that incomplete or chronic rejection of placental homograft could be associated with perfusion defects and hypoxia which may result in abnormal or incomplete tissue differentiation, the significance of the similarity in histocompatibility antigens in couples who have produced children with congenital abnormalities has been studied. An unexpected rate of similarity of the HLA compatibility was found between husbands and wives who have either produced children with neural tubal defects or experienced abnormal pregnancies in other ways (Faulk, 1981). This may explain why some studies showed an increased percentage of neural tubal defects in the general population and even more in the diabetic one. This is apparent in the series reported by Farquhar (1969) who found a higher rate of anencephaly in the Scottish diabetic women than in other parts of the world and invoked racial aspects or consanguineous marriages which would suggest similar histocompatibility antigens in husband and wife. A similar observation was made in the parents of infants with epidermolysis bullosa lethalis (Faulk, 1981; Stricklin et al, 1982).

Immune factors could be related to structural and/or functional changes in the endocrine pancreas of the mother or in the fetus. Islet cell antibodies or insulin antibodies together with other immunological determinants or mitogenic elements could be instrumental in the development of the hyperplasia of the B cells and the hypertrophy of the maternal islets. However, the normal adaptive changes during a normal pregnancy occur without apparent immune feature like an eosinophilic infiltration, which has never been observed in the normal maternal pancreas (Van Assche et al, 1982). The islet changes seem to be induced rather by hormonal and metabolic factors and not by immune alterations at least in the normal mother.

Islet cell antibodies have been reported in women with abnormal glucose tolerance during pregnancy some of whom became overt diabetics in the year following pregnancy (Steel et al, 1980). The islet cell antibody formation was strongly associated with DR3 and DR4 patients studied because of gestational diabetes (Rubinstein et al, 1981). In one case of diabetes (type 1) with Addison's disease, islet cell antibodies were detected in the infant's blood but they disappeared without apparent damage (Gamlen et al, 1977). However, a preferential lysis of pancreatic B cells in vitro has been induced by islet cell surface antibodies (Dobersen & Scharff, 1982). The role of these antibodies for the mother and the neonate needs further evaluation. Furthermore, transplacental passage of maternal anti-insulin antibodies and of insulin immune complexes occur in insulin treated pregnancy (Tamas et al, 1975; Bauman & Yalow 1981; di Mario et al, 1981). Both types of antibodies are of Ig origin, would cross the placenta and should have an effect on the fetal pancreas only in the second trimester.

The endocrine pancreas of infants of diabetic mothers shows in addition to hyperplasia of the B cells and hypertrophy of the islets an eosinophilic infiltration in the intra and/or peri-islet stroma in 25–65 per cent of cases. The intra-islet eosinophilic infiltration which may be observed if the mothers are insulin treated could be related to immunological reactions to the transferred insulin antibodies or insulin immune complexes. The eosinophilic infiltration in the stroma around the islet is specific for the fetus of the diabetic mother even untreated with insulin. No eosinophilic infiltrations are observed in infants with Rh incompatibility or the small for dates of diabetic mothers when hyperplasia is absent (Van Assche et al, 1982). The peri-insular stromal infiltration has no numerical relation either with the islet hypertrophy or multiplication of B cells (Silvermann, 1963).

An exudate of eosinophilic and neutrophilic leukocytes surrounding the islets appears a few hours after the administration of anti-insulin serum in the animal. Repeated injection may lead to a more chronic insulinitis which is also associated with B-cell hyperplasia (Lecompte & Gepts, 1977). This observation has been compared to the lesions seen in the pancreas of infants of diabetic mothers where fibrosis has also been observed in the neonatal period (Hultquist & Olding, 1975). The eosinophils have a putative role in clearing immune complexes and their presence points to an autoimmune process (Fauci et al, 1982). An enhanced sensitivity to viral infection is associated with an increased proliferation of B cells in the animal (Graighead, 1977). Striking lesions of insulinitis with lymphocytic infiltration have been seen in the endocrine pancreas of infants who became diabetic and who were born to mothers with a rubella infection during pregnancy (Forrest et al, 1971; Menser et al, 1978). The development of immune type of reaction and the production of eosinophils are conditioned by T lymphocytes (Fauci et al, 1982) which are relatively quiescent in the normal neonate while the suppressor cells seem to exert their specific action throughout fetal life (Palacios & Anderson, 1982; Anderson, 1982). When depletion of T lymphocytes occurs, the production of eosinophils is impeded at least in the adult. No specific data on lymphocyte function are available for infants of diabetic mothers but T helper cells might be stimulated precociously in the fetus of the diabetic mother. The thymic involution which is a feature of the macrosomic fetus with B-cell hyperplasia could be instrumental in this chain of events (Galbraigth & Faulk, 1979). In addition, the role of associated virus infections in this type of pathology has been suggested to occur in man (Schopper et al, 1982). The presence and the type of HLA-DR on human endothelial cells in the pancreas and not on endocrine cell surfaces may be relevant.

The endothelial cells can also replace macrophages in stimulating allogenic lymphocytes as accessory cells in mitogenic stimulation of T-cell activation and in presenting antigen for sensitised T cells in vitro. The latter may also occur with viral antigen presentation (Alejandro et al, 1982). These associations with viral diseases could be relevant in small for dates born in developing countries where neonatal diabetes is not infrequently encountered (Hoet & Krall, 1982). How the immunological reaction during fetal life relates to pathology in neonatal or later in life needs further clarification. The presence and the type of distribution of eosinophils in the human neonatal pancreas emphasises the immunological reaction in the fetus and neonate. The latter reaction may be induced by a virus transmitted by the mother in specifically prone subjects or related to auto-immunity or both.

Other histological, ultrastructural and enzymatic reactions of a possible immunological nature have also been described in the placenta in infection by P. Falciparum Malaria and malnutrition in addition to diabetes (Galbraight & Faulk, 1979). The two former conditions are associated with modifications of an immunological nature. Deposition of immunoglobulins and complement has been

observed, for example, in the placenta of normotensive insulin treated diabetes and in systematic lupus erythematosus. Both conditions share similar histo-compatibility antigens and the observed lesions may suggest an immunological relationship (Kitzmiller et al, 1981).

In conclusion, immunological adaptation is an essential feature of the process of maternal tolerance to pregnancy as an allogenic graft.

The failure of the immunological recognition of pregnancy by the mother could result in immune reactions which may affect the spontaneous abortion rate and be responsible for congenital malformations. An immune reaction may also involve the placenta and specifically the fetal endocrine pancreas during a diabetic pregnancy. Infants of diabetic mothers form therefore an heterogenous group from an immunological point of view.

Hormonal and metabolic adaptation

The first cleavage of the fertilised ovum occurs 36 hours after fertilisation and implantation of the blastocyst occurs 6 days later. The latter process is dependent on a delicate balance between oestrogens and progesterone whereby a minute dose of oestrogens is an absolute requirement as shown experimentally in the rat. Implantation occurs close to a maternal capillary. The trophoblast signals its presence to the mother and hPL is isolated from the placenta around 21 days after ovulation. It appears in the maternal blood around 40 days. But increased oestrogen secretion early in pregnancy with effects on carbohydrate, lipid and amino-acid metabolism soon leads to an accretion of new tissues in the feto-placental unit and in the mother. The two processes become rapidly interdependent. It is not known if this timely process is different in the diabetic.

The woman early in pregnancy displays a lower basal blood sugar than in the non-pregnant state, an increased hypoglycaemic effect of administered insulin, an increased glucose disappearance rate and an augmented tissue glycogen storage in liver, adipose tissue and muscles (Kalkhoff et al, 1979).

The facilitation of insulin action is thought to be related to the role of the oestrogen and progesterone balance early in pregnancy. How oestrogens act is not known but they are shown to increase the permeability of tight junctions at least in the gallbladder (Coleman et al, 1982). If this effect was a general feature of the hormone, it would facilitate B cell permeability and explain its increased sensitivity to secretagogues.

Glucose is not readily disposed of with advancing pregnancy whether tested by an intravenous or oral load. The glucose disappearance rate is slower and a relative insensitivity to the glucose lowering effect of exogenous insulin appears late in pregnancy. The same holds true for endogenous insulin as more insulin is secreted without inducing hypoglycaemia during a challenge with glucose or after a meal in the third trimester of pregnancy (Kalkhoff et al, 1979). Glucose is a major metabolic substrate for the growing fetus, although not the only one (Freinkel & Metzger, 1979). It crosses the placenta by facilitated diffusion (Page et al, 1981) and the fetal blood glucose concentrations parallel those of the mother, whether the latter are basal levels, post-prandial or acute injection of glucose. A materno-fetal gradient is maintained in normal animal pregnancy (Bassett & Jones, 1976; Silver. 1976; de Gasparo & Hoet, 1971).

In pregnancy special attention has been paid to the metabolism of lactate in the fetus, both in the lamb and human (Sparks et al, 1982). Glucose is the main although not the sole precursor of lactate which is also available in the presence of normal oxygen concentration. Lactate produced by the uterus and placenta is distributed asymetrically in the lamb with the greatest proportion being delivered to the fetus where it could be an important source of energy at least for specific organs (Sparks et al, 1982). Transfer from the fetus to the mother in the ovine is minimal while it appears more bidirectional in the primate. Following oxygen lack, lactate accumulates more rapidly in hyperglycaemic than in normoglycaemic fetal lambs (Shelley et al, 1975). Lactate metabolism is a sensitive indicator of pathological conditions related to oxygen deficiency in the fetus (Sparks et al, 1982).

Fasting also leads to a lower plasma glucose concentration in the last part of pregnancy than in the non-pregnant state (Freinkel & Metzger, 1979). This is attributed to an accelerated use of glucose which is constantly drawn by the fetus, while it is distributed in a larger volume in the maternal compartment. It is increasingly produced endogenously by the mother and the flow of glucose to the fetus is estimated to be 5 mg/kg/min (Kalhan & Adam, 1980). The glucose production after an overnight fast in pregnancy is obtained by gluconeogenesis which leads to a lower plasma gluconeogenic amino acid concentration like alanine. The amino acids are also further reduced by continuous extraction through an active transport mechanism in order to benefit the cellular growth of the fetus. In addition, any associated rise of ketone bodies in the mother suppresses the release by skeletal muscles of gluconeogenic amino acids such as alanine (Felig et al, 1972). The fasting state in late pregnancy therefore induces a substrate deficiency: glucose as well as amino acids are drawn by the fetus while the maternal skeletal muscles are still able to retain their nitrogen stores.

The lipid changes reflect the catabolic tendency. The free fatty acids, after decreasing in early pregnancy, tend to increase in late pregnancy. Ketone bodies behave similarly. The metabolism of adipose tissue is geared to increase fat mobilisation which prevents the adipocyte from increasing further in size and facilitates the depletion of the triglyceride stores with advancing pregnancy. It may even lead to a collapse of fat cells and an arrest of lipolysis. The

increasing FFA levels, with a rapid turnover rate having a half time of 2–3 min, ensure a major supply of energy for the cardiac and skeletal muscles while diverting glucose and other non-lipid nutrients to other tissues including the fetus. FFA is used further by the liver which produces triglycerides and ketone bodies. They are also transferred in a minor fashion to the fetus and are used by the fetal liver for energy and lipogenesis. This chain of events during fasting in late pregnancy has been described as an accelerated starvation (Metzger & Freinkel, 1979).

Still in the fasting state, a progressive increase of very low density lipoprotein without compositional changes is noticeable. In relative terms, the LDL and HDL in contrast to the VLDL contain more triglycerides, less cholesterol and slightly fewer phospholipids during pregnancy (Warth et al, 1975). On an absolute basis HDL cholesterol is unchanged or may even be increased. The essential fatty acids as well as cholesterol are required by the fetus for structural development and by the placenta for hormone precursors. The phospholipid moeity also changes during pregnancy with an increase in sphyngomyelin, lecithin and phosphadyl ethanolamine with a decrease in lysolecithin. The changes appear to be induced by oestrogens but their role is unknown.

The fed state is associated with metabolic modifications in the latter part of pregnancy which are directed again to storage of energy and to the provision of a constant availability of nutrients for fetal development. The diurnal profiles of plasma glucose levels with normal feeding display pre-prandial values which are lower and post-prandial ones which are higher than in the non-pregnant state. The insulin secretion mirrors this with enhanced insulin and C-peptide levels when glucose peaks are prolonged and glucose dips are deeper throughout the last part of pregnancy (Metzger & Freinkel, 1979).

In practice, the maximum post-prandial glucose concentration in normal women in the last part of pregnancy reaches 6.5 mM/l with the lowest values of 3.5 mM/l. Diurnal profiles of circulating amino acids following ingestion of mixed meals increase from lower pregnancy levels to smaller increments post-prandially in late pregnancy when compared with the non-pregnant state. The return to the basal level is also more rapid during pregnancy. The swift excursion of amino-acids during pregnancy indicates their greater disposition during this time. The lack of acute changes in amino acids levels following exogenous insulin during pregnancy indicates a differential sensitivity of tissues to the insulin which is imposed by the pregnant state (Stangenberg et al, 1981). It leaves the amino acids available for the developing fetus to whom they are actively transported against a concentration gradient. Diurnal changes of lipids are also characteristic of pregnancy. Plasma FFA and 3-hydroxybutyrate are rather suppressed after a meal and triglycerides are increased in the pre-and post-prandial phase. The ketone bodies, aceto-acetate and

3-hydroxybutyrate are transported from the mother to the fetus in a gradient of 2 to 1 at term in the human (Gillmer et al, 1982). They have been shown to be metabolised by the fetal brain already at the early part of gestation (Adam et al, 1975).

Maternal metabolic adaptation as it occurs when pregnancy proceeds is dependent upon fine tuning which may be easily disturbed. This is further exemplified by the elevation of FFA and 3-hydroxybutyrate following 16 or 18 hours fast which are distinctly higher in the last trimester of pregnancy than in the non-pregnant state (Metzger & Ravnikar, 1982).

The physiological resistance to insulin which is needed in late normal pregnancy to direct the nutrients to the fetus has been attributed to decreased insulin sensitivity due to a reduction of the number of insulin receptors. The increased plasma concentrations of HPL, progesterone, oestrogens and cortisol, in addition to the effect of hyper-alimentation which is characteristic for pregnancy, have been postulated to induce alterations in the insulin receptor (Beck-Nielsen et al, 1979).

These factors have also been suggested to act at the post-receptor level. The changes in insulin receptors during pregnancy might be due also to alterations in pathways of insulin action distal to the insulin receptors and do not seem to be primarily involved in insulin resistance during pregnancy (Pedersen et al, 1981).

How the metabolism of the mothers in food-deprived conditions adapts during pregnancy is not known. How chronic infections add to the probable failure of metabolic adaptation remains unknown also. But the low birthweight (< 2.5 kg) and the increased overall infant mortality in developing countries could be part of the damaging consequences of metabolic inadaptation in the absence of regular and efficacious feeding habits. However, even an appropriate protein supplementation in a caloric and energy deprived population only increased the mean birthweight within a narrow margin of ± 200 g indicating how the mother must be under the influence of metabolic constrains during pregnancy which are imposed by other factors such as chronic infection (Habicht et al, 1974).

GESTATIONAL DIABETES

Although the definition of gestational diabetes may differ among authors, a satisfactory comparative study has been carried out by Gillmer & Persson (1979) who analysed the diurnal insulin levels in relation to different metabolic parameters. They showed the concordance of abnormal glucose profiles with the pathological results of the oral glucose tolerance curve. This study was carried out in the third trimester on 24 normal and 13 chemical diabetics. The latter were proven to be gestational diabetics because their infants displayed the stigma of infants of diabetic mothers having an increased glucose disposal rate at birth. A further study indicated also a strong correlation between the abnormal glucose profiles and the glucose disappearance after an IV load in the mother. The normal pregnant woman had an insulin secretion calculated on the basis of the total insulin area under the curve which correlated well with the diurnal glucose level. The lean pregnant women with chemical diabetes do not display this correlation. The chemical diabetic women were characterised during pregnancy therefore by a reduced insulin secretion. They also showed elevated free fatty acid levels.

Overweight women with chemical diabetes during pregnancy and treated with a diet restricted in calories and carbohydrates displayed an exaggerated insulin response which was still inadequate to maintain normoglycemia. Free fatty acids, glycerol and 3-hydroxybutyrate profiles tended to be higher as would be expected in the presence of inadequate insulin effect. In overweight women with chemical diabetes during pregnancy, triglycerides during a diurnal profile were elevated above normal. The profiles of glucose, triglycerides and branch chain amino-acids (leucine, isoleucine and valine) deviated even more from normal when the fasting blood glucose exceeded 5.8 mM (105 mg/dl) in gestational diabetes than when the blood sugar was below 5.8 mM (Metzger et al, 1980). Cholesterol and lipoprotein lipid levels in the fasting state at different times of gestation are not dramatically changed in chemical diabetics although a trend to lower HDL-cholesterol was noted (Knopp et al, 1980). The severity of the abnormality of the different metabolic parameters is compatible with an insulinopenia albeit the latter was not absolute. Type 1 insulin-dependent pregnant diabetics may display residual B function which may be a feature also in non-pregnant type 1 diabetics (Persson et al, 1982). The residual B-cell function, although reduced, is reflected by substantial C-peptide levels during daily profiles. This does affect the trend of the metabolic adaptation of the mother to pregnancy. It is associated with the maintenance of a stable glucose profile close to normal, especially during the first and second trimester of pregnancy. The glucose profiles were markedly unstable when the patient was deprived of residual B-cell function. During the third trimester, the glucose profiles were stable and comparable in both groups of patients with or without endogenous secretion. During each trimester the profiles of 3-hydroxy-butyrate tended to be higher in the patients without residual B-cell function (Persson et al, 1982).

The data although not uniform indicate that the severity of the metabolic changes during pregnancy especially blood sugar, FFA and 3-hydroxybutyrate levels are closely related to a graded insulinopenia. In gestational diabetes the latter would tend to appear especially in the third trimester while in insulin-dependent diabetics they are already substantially disturbed in the first and second trimesters and become relatively less so in the third. The perturbation should be greatest in the third trimester when insulin resistance is the greatest but the patients are usually better treated by that time. The significance of these changes in relation to the persistence of residual B cell function also manifests itself in the morbidity of the neonates even though the number of the insulin-dependent type 1 diabetics studied in this way is still limited.

The infants of mothers without B-cell function and with unstable metabolic profiles in the first and second trimester and stable ones in the third had higher amniotic fluid C-peptide values, increased infant skinfold thickness and more neonatal complications like hypoglycaemia, hyper-bilirubenia and feeding problems (Stangenberg et al, 1982a, b; Persson et al, 1982). This observation emphasises the importance of the residual B-cell function and the pre-eminence of the degree of control which is needed in the first and second trimester in order to secure the birth of an infant without morbid symptoms which are related to a precociously challenged fetal metabolic homeostasis. A close to normal control in the third trimester is not enough when associated with poor control in the first and second. Definite influences act upon the maturation process of the fetus and induce functional consequences which will manifest themselves later. A specific case in point is the evident change in neonates who even in the presence of similar blood sugars in the third trimester had a higher insulin secretion at birth when their endocrine pancreas has been precociously stimulated by unstable metabolic profiles in the mother during the first and second trimester. This unfavourable evolution of the fetus might be responsible for further short and possibly long-term morbidity in the neonate (Stangenberg et al, 1982a, b; Persson et al 1982).

The maternal endocrine pancreas

The metabolic adaptation to the varying needs of the different stages of the pregnancy is related to an appropriate bi-hormonal secretion of the maternal endocrine pancreas. During pregnancy insulin secretion predominates and glucagon secretion revealed greater than normal suppression when challenged (Freinkel et al, 1979). Experimental data suggest that combined oestradiol and progesterone might be responsible for the bi-hormonal adaptation of the maternal endocrine pancreas. This functional adaptation is consistent with the histological and ultra-structural observations of the islet of Langerhans observed in normal pregnant animals which display a hightened activity (Van Assche et al, 1982). Likewise, the pancreases from 15 pregnant women were studied by Rosenlöcher (1932) and an additional five by Van Assche & Aerts (1979). The B-cell hyperplasia and the islet hypertrophy are apparent at the end of pregnancy and are associated with an increase in size and number of blood vessels which is concentrated in the endocrine tissue of the pancreas. These features suggest an enhanced blood flow with an increased absolute number of glucagon A cells but no further biological or histological information is available concerning the gut glucagon cells during pregnancy. The insulin/glucagon cell ratio remains in favour of the insulin cells. This is consistent with the bi-hormonal secretory adaptation to pregnancy which in turn would favour the insulin effect on retention and storage of dietary nutrients (Freinkel et al, 1979).

In human pregnancy, the structural changes in the islets related to the hyperplasia of B cells and to some extent of A cells are not seen before the 20th week. (Van Assche et al, 1982).

One is tempted to compare these observations with the findings of Ogilvie (1964) who noted in obese subjects with a normal glucose tolerance an increase in the islet tissue and the size of the islets which are respectively 56 per cent and 65 per cent greater in the obese than in the normal. Hyperinsulinism is also a characteristic of the obese subject. The structural changes in the endocrine pancreas of the pregnant female occur in the course of the accretion of new maternal tissue and prevail when the total weight gain is the greatest. At 20 weeks an average of 50 per cent of the pregnancy weight seems to be gained (Pitkin, 1980). This weight gain is associated with hyperinsulinism and also with a moderate induction of insulin resistance seen at the latter part of pregnancy and which has been compared to the changes specific for obesity (Beck-Nielsen et al, 1979).

Up to mid-pregnancy normal pregnant women have unchanged fasting insulin levels and only display hyper-insulinaemia after a glucose infusion. After mid-pregnancy, from week 26 onwards, the pregnant women show insulin levels which are doubled in the fasting state and trebled in response to a glucose infusion (Lind et al, 1979). At the inception of pregnancy the B cells seem not to proliferate and acquire only a greater sensitivity to a challenge; later, after mid-pregnancy the B cells increase in number and the islet size is augmented. This is related to a greater than normal insulin level, fasting as well as after a challenge (Saudek et al, 1975).

In the human, the fasting glucagon levels are lower in mid-pregnancy with an increase of up to 50 per cent at the end of pregnancy (Kuhl & Horst, 1976).

Glucagon levels during an oral glucose tolerance show greater suppression at mid-pregnancy than in the non-pregnant state. The suppression is greatest in late pregnancy. In obesity similar changes in glucagon level had an upward trend before rather than after weight reduction and swift glucagon suppression occurs during a glucose tolerance (Sherwin et al, 1976).

The structural and functional adaptive changes tend to be similar in obesity and in late pregnancy when weight gain has occurred. Observations in animals could be relevant in this regard. In the rat, the total amount of endocrine tissue increases at mid-pregnancy and the structural changes parallel the functional modifications (Van Assche & Aerts, 1975, 1979).

At the end of pregnancy (day 20) the increased secretion of insulin and the volume density of the B cells per total rat pancreas was nearly trebled whereas the number of B cells per islets was doubled. The increased percentage of light B granules and the increased volume of the mitochondria indicate an increased secretory capacity of the individual B cell although not of the A cell. In addition, the distribution of the PP and glucagon cells which is unequal between the head and the tail tends to disappear and the number of somatostatin cells to diminish at the end of a normal pregnancy in the rat (Van Assche & Aerts, 1975, 1979). Before the 10th day of pregnancy an increased islet cell size is also observed but the structural changes show an increase of intra-and extra-cellular water as well as the vascularity of the endocrine pancreas (Van Assche & Marynissen, 1982, personal communication). This could be related to a greater influx of nutrients per cell and would fit with the enhanced although moderate secretory capacity of the B cell in early pregnancy. Hormonal influences could be influential here as oestrogen and chorionic gonadotrophin may induce a greater sensitivity to secretagogues (Malaisse et al, 1969). The islet changes throughout pregnancy in the rat and presumably in the human are not determined (or induced) by an identified single event.

Gastrointestinal modifications due to pregnancy must also be considered. They may influence the insulin secretory response of the endocrine pancreas as the latter is conditioned by the quality and the composition of the food consumed by the rat in the non-pregnant (Tejning, 1947) or the pregnant state (Blazquez & Lopez Quijada, 1970). The daily intake of food increases 20 per cent during pregnancy in the rat. Withholding this additional food is associated with a reduction of the secretory activity of the B cells normally seen in pregnancy and adding carbohydrates specifically restores the sensitivity (Howell et al, 1973). Several hormonal and nutritional changes occur during pregnancy which may interact to produce increased gastrointestinal growth and secretion. The weight, mucosal volume and peptic and parietal cell population of the stroma increase steadily during pregnancy to a maximum before the greatest increase in food intake (Van Assche et al, 1982). In addition, active transport of glucose across the intestine increases during pregnancy (Llarade et al, 1966).

It is possible therefore that the growth of the endocrine pancreas during pregnancy may be a consequence of a more rapid entry of nutrients into the blood circulation following a meal, as the command of the insulin secretory response is regulated by gastrointestinal hormones. Other hormonal changes like increasing prolactin levels have also been related to the nutritional state in the pregnant rat (Reusens et al, 1976, 1979). The study of the adaptation of the A–B cell couple during pregnancy demands therefore that it be integrated with the adjustment of the entero-insular axis.

Histological data on the endocrine pancreas of gestational diabetics are not available. However, Ogilvie (1964) noted in adult onset diabetes, often related to obesity, a reduced mean weight of islet tissue and also a mean weight of B cells. Three factors contributed to the noted reduction: the weight of the pancreas, number of islets per gram of pancreas and proportion of B to A cells. The mitogenic factors which should operate here were not effective anymore. Comparing the structural changes in the endocrine pancreas of the pregnant women with the obese, it is interesting to speculate on the inability of the B cells to proliferate when pregnancy needs are pressing. Around 28–32 weeks, gestational diabetes may become apparent which could be related to this inability to proliferate. This suggestive interpretation is possibly confirmed in the animal. Rats with experimental diabetes and rats of the second generation born from diabetic mothers, which in both conditions were normoglycaemic before pregnancy, became glucose intolerant at the end of pregnancy and did not exhibit the normal hyperplasia and hypertrophy of the islets (Aerts & Van Assche, 1979). Again this is only a manifestation in late pregnancy. More needs to be learned from histological and ultrastructural analysis of the maternal pancreas throughout pregnancy.

Placenta and fetal supply line

The hormonal and metabolic derangements which occur in a diabetic pregnancy are assumed to have a profound influence on the maturation and growth of the placenta. Both gross as well as structural anomalies of chorionic villi, stroma and vasculature have been described in placentae of diabetic patients. The nature and the frequency of the placental lesions differ between published reports; as emphasised by Fox (1978), the placental lesions seen in diabetic pregnancy are not unique to this condition. They may also be present in non-diabetic pregnancy. The lack of concordance among authors is a consequence of different conditions and lack of standardisation. First various techniques for the preparation of tissue material have been employed while comparable criteria for the selection of tissue specimens as regards their location in the placenta is not evident. Marked regional variations in villous morphology are known to exist.

The state of health of the mother also influences the histological features of the placenta. Severe diabetic angiopathy in the mother, hypertension and pre-eclampsia or acute and chronic infections may induce lesions in the placenta (Emmrich et al, 1975). In addition, the quality of diabetic control throughout pregnancy may induce further morbid structural changes in the placenta.

In a diabetic patient without severe angiopathy, the placenta together with the umbilical cord is characteristically enlarged. Heavier than normal, it should be compared to the small and light placenta with extensive and intensive infarction which is seen frequently in growth retardation and is typical of mothers with severe angiopathy (White class D F R). The increase in placental mass, associated with high birthweight as seen in diabetic women who are free of vascular complications, is due to the proliferation of cytotrophoblast and syncytiotrophoblast as reflected in increased DNA content and cell numbers (Winnick & Noble, 1967). Immature villi and villi with syncytial knots are more frequent in diabetes than in non-diabetic matched controls. This reflection of immaturity may be compatible with a more active growth than normal.

The excessive growth of the placenta as well as of the fetus may be the consequence of fetal hyperinsulinism (Adamsons & Myers, 1975; Susa et al, 1979). Planimetric studies of well defined cotyledons in the placenta from insulin-dependent diabetic patients without pregnancy complications such as hypertension or pre-eclampsia have shown an increased branching of chorionic villi which may account for a 25 per cent increase in placental area of exchange (Teasdale, 1981; Bjork & Persson, 1982). A further increase in feto-maternal exchange may be brought about by structural lesions such as vasculo-syncytial membranes (i.e. a segment of the villus where the fetal capillary is covered by a very thin syncytium only) and syncytial knots which tend to move the fetal and maternal circulations closer together. The increase in the frequency of syncytial vascular membranes, of syncitial knots and of villous areas as calculated by planimetric measurements is related to the increased instability of maternal blood glucose control in the first two trimesters of pregnancy (Bjork & Persson, 1982). In addition, syncytial knots and vasculo-syncytial membranes are formed rapidly during hypoxia as shown by *in vitro* studies using human chorionic villi (Tominanga & Page, 1966; Fox & Page, 1970).

The functional significance of these placental changes which tend to increase the areas of exchange between mother and fetus may represent a compensatory response to chorionic tissue hypoxia (Bjork & Persson, 1982; Bjork et al, 1982). Poor diabetic control may be responsible for hypoxia since blood oxygen release would be impaired as a consequence of elevated maternal HbAlC and/or of altered concentration of red blood cell 2,3 diphosphogly-cerate (2–3 DPG). The suggestion that hypoxia exists at the fetal and placental levels is supported further by the recent demonstration of significantly decreased arterial oxygen saturation and arterial oxygen tension in non smoking insulin dependent diabetic women during the last trimester of pregnancy (Madsen & Ditzel, 1982). The arterial oxygen saturation decreased with increasing HbAlC levels and although the 2–3 DPG concentration in red cells was increased the 2–3 DPG induced change in oxygen affinity was impaired (Madsen & Ditzel, 1982). The possibility that the fetus of the diabetic may suffer chronic hypoxia has

long been recognised (Berglund & Zetterström, 1954). Polycythaemia and increased extra-medullary erythropoi-esis are prominent findings in the newborn of diabetic mothers. Elevated plasma levels of erythropoeitin have also been demonstrated in the offspring (Widness et al, 1981). The foregoing hypoxia-compensating responses in the fetus may result from impaired oxygen supply from the mother. In addition, fetal hypoxia may also be a direct consequence of the fetal hyperinsulinism and/or hyperglycaemia as suggested from experimental studies in the fetal rhesus monkey and the fetal lamb (Widness et al, 1981; Philipps et al, 1981, 1982).

The association of fetal hyperglycemia with a decreased fetal oxygen content (Philipps et al, 1982) is consistent with the reduced margins with which the fetus of the diabetic mother has to survive the intra-uterine ordeal. This becomes further apparent in the greater rise in plasma lactate and decline in pH in the hyperglycaemia rather than in the normoglycaemic fetal lamb during exposure to hypoxia (Shelley et al, 1975). To what extent hypergly-caemia in the fetus of a poorly controlled diabetic and its consequential impaired tolerance to oxygen lack may explain abnormalities in fetal breathing movements as well as sudden intra-uterine death in late pregnancy remains speculative. Available clinical and experimental data point to the importance of the maternal metabolic control which may influence significantly the fetal supply line of nutrients as well as of oxygen. The maternal metabolic control modulates the perinatal outcome and especially the rate of stillbirths (Persson et al, 1978). Although a greater placental exchange area in the diabetic may be regarded as a compensatory response to anoxia, it is not obvious that this leads to an improved maternal–fetal exchange. An increased branching of chorionic villi could threaten further the fetal supply line by reducing the intervillous space and alter the blood flow pattern. Indeed measurement of the uteroplacental blood index in pregnant diabetics using 113 m indium as a tracer revealed a 35–45 per cent reduc-tion of placental blood index compared to values in non-diabetic controls (Nylund et al, 1982). This reduction of placental blood flow index could be attributed to a decreased volume in the intervillous space. The oxygen reserve represented by the blood content (or volume) in the intervillous space corresponds normally to a fetal need of 1–1.5 min and thus may be easily reduced. Hypoxia in the fetus would therefore be induced at the maternal side by the reduced availability of oxygen in the red blood cell, in the placenta by reduced placental blood flow index and in the fetus by chronic low fetal oxygen tension. Even if the latter is induced by chronic fetal hyperinsulinism, as shown experimentally, the features of profound growth promoting effects due to these excessive fetal insulin level may still be present. The experimental observation in the chronically insulin injected fetus implies that augmented fetal growth may occur without concommitant elevation of maternal substrate levels in blood (Susa et al, 1979). It means that fetal hyperinsulinism *per se* may induce an excessive transfer of nutrients from the mother to the fetus. Nesidioblastosis of the pancreas is a condition in the human showing an association of excessive fetal size and hyperinsulinism without evidence of any disturbance of maternal metabolism (Aynsley-Green et al, 1981).

In pregnancy complicated by diabetes, the fetal supply line may vary considerably. At one extreme, a markedly increased availability of nutrients to the fetus leads to accelerated fetal growth as is seen in patients with short duration of diabetes (White's class A–B and in patients with gestational diabetes). These large for dates infants whose birthweight and length exceeds the 90th percentile or + 2 s.d. above the mean normal for gestational age and sex are distinguishable by a typical plethoric appearance at birth. They display a disharmonious body composition with increased amounts of body protein, glycogen and fat with a selective organomegaly mainly affecting adipose tissue, heart, liver and adrenals. This tendency to be both heavier and larger than average for their period of gestation is clinically not manifest until after the 28th week of gestation (Cardell, 1953). The role of the enhanced stimulation of the fetal pancreas in this regard will be discussed later. Among the greatest clinical hazards for the large for dates neonate is unrecognised cephalo-pelvic disproportion leading to protracted labour and delivery with possible shoulder dystocia. More severe birth trauma may prevail as well as asphyxia.

At the other end of the clinical spectrum, a markedly reduced supply line in the mother may lead to fetal growth retardation. Diabetic mothers with severe diabetic angiopathy show this feature frequently (Van Assche et al, 1982). If the pregnancy is also complicated by hypertension and/or pre-eclampsia specific spiral artery lesions produce a further decrease of utero-placental blood flow and hence an impaired maturation and growth of the fetus (Bjork et al, 1982). In this condition, the small for date (SFD) whose weight is below the 10th percentile or below 2 s.d. of the mean of normal for gestational age and sex, features reduced energy stores of fat and glycogen and diminished numbers and sizes of cells in many organs. Body weight is often more affected than body length and head circumference. These neonates have diminished subcutaneous tissue, the skin is wrinkled with a poor turgor and they have an anxious appearance. The nutritionally deprived SFD fetus or infant runs an increased risk of developing fetal distress, asphyxia and post-partum hypoglycaemia which is not due to high insulin levels but is rather a consequence of their low hepatic glycogen.

However, the majority of the offspring of diabetic mothers who were insulin treated display a fetal growth pattern in between those two extremes represented by the large for dates and the small for dates. In a series of 217 infants of diabetic mothers collected between 1969 and 1976, 36 per cent were large for dates, 4.1 per cent small for dates and 60 per cent were infants with an appropriate size at birth (Lemons, 1981).

It is suggested that a factor or factors which are growth restraining operate in the maternal-placental unit. The regulation of substrate concentrations in maternal blood may influence the supply line to the fetus. Thus the tendency to increased birthweight in infants of diabetic mothers tends to decrease with the intensity of treatment during pregnancy and the infant's appearance at birth normalises. The relation between the fetal supply line is further illustrated by a significant correlation between maternal glucose level during the last trimester and both the total skinfold thickness and the mean gluteal adipose cell diameters of the newborn (Whitelaw, 1977; Persson et al, 1979). The increase of fetal adipose tissue mass with increasing maternal hyperglycaemia is in accord with the hypothesis that fetal hyperglycaemia and hyperinsulinism enhance triglyceride synthesis within the adipose tissue. The fetal endocrine pancreas is therefore a prime target in the maternal-placental supply line.

The Fetal Endocrine Pancreas

One of the principal targets of the placental-fetal supply line remains the fetal endocrine pancreas. In macrosomic infants the pancreatic weight is not often reported although Neaye (1965) calculated it to be 110 per cent of the normals. The endocrine pancreatic status of the infants of diabetic mothers has been fully described. The most typical aspects of the fetal pancreas in these infants are hyperplasia of the insulin producing B cells and the hypertrophy of the islets (Dubreuil & Anderodias, 1920; Van Assche, 1970; Hultquist, 1971). Furthermore the islets have a pronounced vasculature (Van Assche & Aerts, 1975; Van Assche et al, 1982). No other maternal condition induces these changes in the fetal pancreas. The structural adaptation of the fetal islets can however precede overt diabetes in the mother (Van Beeck, 1939; Woolf & Jackson, 1957).

An intact hypothalamo-hypophyseal system is also necessary for the occurrence of B-cell hyperplasia; only those anencephalics with a functional hypothalamo-hypophyseal system born to diabetic mothers display B-cell hyperplasia and an increased insulin level in the cord blood. Only these anencephalics had a tendency to be macrosomic in relation to their gestational age (Van Assche et al, 1979; Hoet, 1969).

An important and characteristic feature of the infant of the diabetic mother is also the structural association between adrenal enlargement and hyperplasia of the pancreatic islets (Naeye, 1965). Definite enlargement of the fetal adrenal has been recorded which reflected especially an increase in the cortical fetal zone. In newborns with intra-uterine growth retardation born to diabetic mothers, islet cell hypertrophy and B cell hyperplasia may still be present but to a much lesser extent than in large neonates (Van Assche et al, 1982). In the underweight infant, the adrenal fetal cortex was also reduced in weight, in number of cells and in the cytoplasm of individual cells. The permanent cortex exhibited parallel but less significant features (Naeye, 1965). Fetuses and newborns with intra-uterine growth retardation born to non-diabetic mothers are characterised by a marked hypoplasia of the insulin producing B cells which occurs both in the human and in the experimental animal (Van Assche et al, 1977; De Prins & Van Assche, 1982, personal communication).

Information is scarce about the development of the insular tissue of normal fetuses born to normal mothers. The endocrine population and the proportion of endocrine tissue in the pancreas changes markedly in early life. In the embryo the pancreatic polypeptide containing cells become evident from week 10 of gestation and are located mainly in the ventral primordium which becomes the posterior part of the head of the pancreas (Stefan et al, 1982). The glucagon rich lobe where the somatostatin cells are also concentrated is dorsally derived and is constituted by the anterior part of the head, the isthmus, the body and the tail of the pancreas. All endocrine cells are not solely concentrated in the fetal islets; they are also dispersed in clusters in the endocrine pancreas (Rahier et al, 1981). Islets in offspring of diabetic mothers are apparently more enlarged in the tail portion of the pancreas and are least in the posterior part of the head of the organ. The number of B cells is increased especially in the dorsal lobe or tail of the pancreas together with an increased number of PP cells (Van Assche et al, 1982). The structural changes of the fetal endocrine pancreas early in diabetic pregnancy are not frequently reported but they have important implications.

In vitro experiments indicate an increased insulin release by 11 weeks of gestation by fetal pancreas of infants born to decompensated diabetic mothers. The *in vitro* response of the fetal pancreas was modulated by the metabolic control of the mother. A normal *in vitro* insulin response was obtained in infants born from mothers with tight metabolic control early in pregnancy. From the available data it becomes apparent that the fetal insular pancreatic tissue already undergoes early structural changes and seeks a functional adaptation to the maternal surfeit before 16 weeks gestation (Reiher et al, 1982). These changes reflect functional alterations which induce an enhanced secretion of insulin; the role of insulin as a growth promoting factor has been emphasised by the late Jorgen Pedersen as long ago as 1954. Fetal growth is modulated by genetic determinants, sufficient and qualified nutrients, an adequate line of supply and hormones which could be of maternal or fetal origin.

Insulin is regarded as an essential growth promoting hormone in the fetus (de Gasparo & Hoet, 1971; Persson, 1981). Its anabolic effect is well recognised in the adult.

High fetal insulin levels associated with hyperplasia and hypertrophy of the fetal islets are related to the surfeit which the macrosomic infant of a diabetic mother has to endure (Thomas et al, 1967, Naeye, 1965).

As one would expect in classical endocrinology, infants born without the endocrine pancreas exhibit the opposite clinical picture (Hill, 1979). Emaciation, dehydration, hyperglycaemia, if not recognised, are the classical features, often ending in early death.

In a normal fetus, the differentiated B cells are capable of synthesising and storing insulin and its precursor proinsulin from the 10th week of gestation. At 11 weeks, the pancreas contains an amount similar to the adult (2 units). It contains 3 to 6 times more with advancing pregnancy. Insulin is present in the human fetal plasma around the same time and is found in amniotic fluid from the 17th week.

Insulin present in the fetal compartment is considered on good grounds to be of fetal origin. The compiled value of normal plasma insulin levels at birth is $\pm 10\ \mu U/ml$. An increase of insulin levels after stimulation has been demonstrated before birth but an adult type of biphasic insulin release in a normal neonate under glucose stimulation is unlikely. The biphasic insulin release at birth is a characteristic feature of the infant of the diabetic mother who will dispose of the glucose much more readily than the normal. The time at which this excessive insulin is being secreted and when it acquires the excessive anabolic and lipogenic action remains a matter of debate (Wellman & Volk, 1977; Van Assche et al, 1982).

Much information is also forthcoming from animal experiments. In normal animals with a short gestational period like the rat, the B cell exhibits its proliferation in the last quarter of pregnancy; in animals with a longer gestational period such as the monkey, the B cell develops at mid-pregnancy (Chi, 1978, Erickson et al, 1980). The pancreatic insular changes in fetuses born from experimental mild diabetic animals parallels the structural evolution seen in large for date infants (Van Assche et al, 1982; Remacle et al, 1982). In experimental diabetic pregnancy with decompensated diabetes the structural changes relate to those observed in small for dates (Ericksson et al, 1980; Van Assche et al, 1977, 1982).

Experimental *in vitro* data suggest also that amino acids stimulate the endocrine cells of fetal rat endocrine pancreas before the first half of pregnancy. Glucose would be the major stimulatory factor of B-cell proliferation in the second half of pregnancy when it is more sensitive to lower levels than in the adult (Milner, 1979; Swenne, 1982). The fetal insular pancreatic tissue seems also to have a greater pool of proliferating B cell capable of reentering the replication cycle than the adult (Swenne 1982).

Human and experimental data indicate that structural changes occurring early in fetal life eventuate on an undifferentiated endocrine pancreatic cell. Later, the proliferative capacities of the B cells which respond early to stimulating nutriments from the mother would result in fetal insulin levels higher than normal. The biological effect of the stimulation might not be directly apparent. The latter is also dependent upon the advent of insulin receptors and their affinity is under study (Kaplan et al, 1979). In the latter part of pregnancy, even in the presence of high insulin levels the 'down regulation' of insulin receptors is not seen in the newborn of the diabetic mother. While this could be attributed to immaturity in the receptor system it could still enhance further the effect of insulin, promoting the storage of energy reserves in the form of glycogen and fat. Normalisation of the blood sugar of the mother also normalises the insulin receptor features in the newborn (Kaplan et al, 1979).

Fetal size and both plasma insulin and C-peptide levels are significantly interrelated at the latter part of a diabetic gestation especially if the diabetes has been of short duration. Neonatal size is also correlated with the endocrine mass and the latter with B-cell volume (Naeye, 1965). The tendency to become heavier and longer than average for the gestational age becomes more manifest after the 28th week of gestation. This is also applicable to the placenta and the umbilical cord. The growth promoting effect of insulin on selective organs could also be related to its interaction with other growth stimulating peptides some of which might be specific for the fetus (Sara et al, 1980, 1981; Fletcher et al, 1982).

In addition, the total skin fold thickness and the mean gluteal adipose cell diameter of the newborn correlate with the glucose values of the last trimester of pregnancy (Whitelaw, 1977; Persson et al, 1978). Hence the importance of the normalisation of the maternal blood sugar throughout pregnancy in order to prevent the structural changes of the fetal pancreas in the early part of pregnancy and a lipogenic action of the elevated circulating insulin in the presence of high glucose levels, specifically in the latter part of pregnancy.

In small for dates born to diabetic mothers with vascular complications or in growth retardated pups born to severe ketotic diabetic rats degranulation of the B cells is a common finding (Van Assche et al, 1982). The pancreatic insulin content and the blood insulin levels in these fetuses and neonates are also decreased. The severe growth retardation seems to begin at approximately 28th and 30th week. The same occurs in infants who later develop transient diabetes. These structural and functional features could result from a delayed maturation of the B cell; whether overstimulation leads to exhaustion has still to be demonstrated. The foregoing indicates that the fetal B cells undergo structural and functional changes which may be related to the whole spectrum of the abnormal features from the large to the small for dates born to diabetic mothers.

The quality of maternal control effects the fetal-placental supply line and plays a decisive role in fetal survival. It also influences the infant's size at birth, large for dates as well as small for dates. Both types will have their own clinical characteristics. Macrosomic infants of diabetic mothers with poorly regulated diabetes feature delayed functional maturation of organ functions. This implies that the expected correlation between gestational age and functional ability is no longer apparent, a fact that is best illustrated by the incidence of respiratory distress syndrome which is almost six times higher in infants of diabetic mothers than in infants of non-diabetic mothers of comparable gestational age and mode of delivery.

It has been hypothesised that delayed pulmonary maturity with impaired production of surfactant might be directly related to fetal hyperinsulinism. A great number of recent reports also demonstrate a markedly lower incidence of RDS as well as an overall lower rate of morbidity in offspring of diabetic mothers who have been subjected to a strict diabetic control during pregnancy. These data as well as experimental results tend to support the idea that fetal hyperglycaemia and/or fetal hyperinsulinism are closely related to the occurence of fetal and neonatal complications such as macrosomia (Susa et al, 1979; Pedersen, 1977; Sosenko et al, 1979), selective organomegaly (Hirschfeld et al, 1979; Wolfe & Way, 1977; Whitelaw, 1977; Breitweser et al, 1980), respiratory distress (Smith et al, 1975; Stubbs & Stubbs, 1978; Hallman & Teramo, 1979), hypoglycaemia (Persson, 1975; Phelps et al, 1978; Sosenko et al, 1979, Heding et al, 1980), polycythemia and increased erythropoiesis (Naeye, 1965; Widness et al, 1981), hyperbilirubinaemia (Stevenson et al, 1979; Peevy et al, 1980) and delayed functional maturation of the gastro-intestinal tract (Davis & Campbell, 1974; Davis et al, 1974).

The future of the infant of diabetic mothers

From previous evidence it is apparent that many organs may be affected including parathyroid adenoma, ovarian cyts and fibrosis of testicular tissue (Naeye, 1965). In view of the striking changes in the fetal endocrine pancreas, the possibility of diabetes in the progeny has to be taken into consideration. In insulin-dependent diabetics, with whom are associated an increase in the HLA-DRw3 and DRw4 distribution, the infants are liable to inherit partly similar genetic distribution. To become diabetic, they need in addition an environmental trigger. For non-insulin dependent diabetics, the infants are more likely to inherit the diabetic trend which may become apparent only later in life. No follow-up of children is known at the present which differentiates between these two groups. The incidence of juvenile diabetes or diabetes occurring at a young age in children of diabetic mothers at large varies between 0.5 and 1.0 per cent for a follow-up between 1 and 26 years according different series. Based on data concerning 464 children of diabetic mothers the calculated risk of becoming diabetic at the age of 25 years is also 1.5 per cent (Gillmer et al, 1982). In these series, the control of the mother was not taken into account. However, diabetes has been found especially in children of diabetic mothers with a White class D. In addition, fibrosis in the endocrine pancreas of infants of diabetic mothers dying at 3 and 6 months of age has been found (Hultquist & Olding, 1975). The peri-insular and intra-insular infiltration of lymphocytes or eosinophils should also be of concern. These considerations led us to analyse the diabetic trend in second and third generation rats born to mothers with streptozotocin induced diabetes (Aerts & Van Assche, 1979).

The findings indicated a loss of glucose tolerance during a stressful situation like a pregnancy which was associated with structural changes in the endocrine pancreas indicating a loss of adaptative compensation.

In vitro observations indicate also that the proliferating pool of B cells in pups born from severe diabetic mothers is strikingly reduced (Swenne, 1982). Other studies show that the proliferation remains increased for at least 48 hours *in vivo* and for 7 days *in vitro* for pups born from moderately diabetic rats (Remacle et al, 1982). The clinical and experimental data suggest an earmarking of the fetal endocrine pancreas which may be related to the metabolic state of the mother. How this make up of the endocrine pancreas together with the other already known factors such as histocompatible antigens, islet cell antibodies and genetic trend for diabetes affects the future of the infant of diabetic mother awaits further investigation. The foregoing indicates that a genetic heterogeneity exists (Simpson, 1979). One should however not be complacent about the changes in the fetal endocrine pancreas as they may be influenced by medical intervention in the mother and the inheritence of an appropriate insulin secretory function might eventually be better secured.

MONITORING OF A DIABETIC PREGNANCY

Medical surveillance

The aim of medical treatment during a diabetic pregnancy is foremost the prevention of keto-acidosis possibly induced by pregnancy itself. This will safeguard the mother's and fetus's health. It is also of paramount importance to prevent the occurrence of diabetic complications in the mother even though proliferative retinopathy and cardio-vascular disease remain susceptible to aggravation even when normal metabolic control during pregnancy is achieved.

The outcome of pregnancy should include a perinatal mortality and neonatal morbidity comparable or lower than the levels observed in the non diabetic population. The prevention of short and possibly long-term morbidity of the infant later in life should also be taken

into consideration. In order to achieve this multifaceted goal during pregnancy, specific anti-diabetic therapy should be applied and the efficacy of the therapy should be measured as a function of the pregnancy outcome.

The normalisation of the glucose profile by appropriate insulin therapy in insulin-dependent diabetics has demonstrated over the years an unprecendented lowering of the perinatal mortality and morbidity in any of the White classes or in any situation where the prognosis might be jeopardized by diabetic or non-diabetic complications as described by Pedersen. The efficacy of proper insulin therapy is clearly demonstrated also when the metabolic profiles in the mother and in the neonate are analyzed (Gillmer et al, 1982). Besides efficient insulin therapy, a team approach is advocated by specialised centres in order to obtain a favourable outcome of these pregnancies. Despite this, there is a need for dissimenation of knowledge and we know better than we did which therapeutic measures to advocate. This is essential because the majority of the pregnant diabetic women type 1, type 2 and gestational diabetics are cared for at primary health care level in many countries. In non insulin-dependent diabetics, the assesment of the efficacy of any therapeutic regimen requires careful analysis.

In populations with a high prevalence of diabetes and a high fertility rate, the assessment of therapeutic efficacy might be forthcoming. But, when diabetes has a rather low prevalence or when the fertility rate is low, the screening and the diagnostic procedures to be applied as well as the therapy to be instituted are a matter of debate (Hadden, 1980). The present investigations confirm that the differentiation, maturation and functional adaptation of the fetus are very sensitive to the glucose profiles in the mother. This sensitivity may engender specific morbidity in the fetus. Characteristic endpoints besides perinatal mortality should still be sought. One approach could be to screen all pregnant women for glucose intolerance, but this is rarely feasible. Several programmes have been suggested taking into account the cost benefit diagnostic yield together with a satisfactory specificity (Hoet & Baird, 1979). But very few screening programmes which have been proposed are based using as endpoint the sensitivity of fetal insulin secretion related to the crude fetal outcome (i.e. perinatal mortality or birthweight) or the diabetic future of the pregnant women over the years. Administrative recommendations like the ones proposed by the WHO Non Communicable Disease Ad Hoc Committee (1980) are not concerned with issues like fetal adaptation and remain therefore remarkably hazardous for the fetus or the neonate. These screening criteria for blood sugar propose higher levels than those which are recommended as levels for good control outside, and definitely during pregnancy. These epidemiological recommendations have introduced an inconsistent clinical situation.

In pregnancy, specific conditions prevail where maternal

measurements including the mean diurnal glucose concentrations and various indices that may be derived from an oral GTT correlate well with neonatal glucose concentrations (Gillmer & Persson, 1979). The handling of glucose by the neonate and his insulin levels may form a rational basis for delineating the normal and abnormal glucose tolerance of the mother. This has been the basis used to define a dividing line after a 50 g dose of oral glucose, giving 1 and 2 hours plasma glucose values of 9.2 and 6.7 mmol/l respectively.

The American Diabetes Association Workshop Conference on Gestational Diabetes (Report of Workshop Chairmen, 1980) recommended retention of the criteria established by O'Sullivan & Mahan (1973) and which have been the basis of an analysis of pregnancy outcome, perinatal morbidity like birthweight and overt diabetes as well as diabetes complications in the mother later in life. They recommend administration of 100 g of glucose and determination of venous plasma glucose values which should meet or exceed two of the following levels as verified by the Somogyi Nelson Method:

Fasting : 5.8 mmol/l
1 hour : 10.6 mmol/l
2 hours : 9.2 mmol/l
3 hours : 8:1 mmol/l

The treatment advocated during pregnancy in a diabetic type 2 or in a woman with an impaired glucose tolerance curve before and during pregnancy is diet and insulin.

In gestational diabetes diet is usually favoured but insulin is frequently advocated. The assessment of the result of these therapeutic regimens remains under study.

The consideration related to the diagnostic criteria and the therapeutic regimen should not be forgotten or discarded as the ratio of gestational diabetics to established diabetics is 4 : 1. This indicates that physicians and obstetricians are confronted with the challenging clinical situation of diagnosis and therapy more often in a diabetic susceptible population than in established diabetes. Regardless of the present low level of perinatal mortality in Western Countries, one cannot afford to overlook the small but significant added risk of perinatal mortality amongst gestational diabetics. Congenital malformations may not be apparent as the metabolic imbalance occurs rather after the 28th week and usually in women over 25 years but other pregnancy problems may arise like hydramnios, overweight infant with traumatic delivery, stillbirth or small for dates. In one study, 25 per cent of the infants of gestational diabetic did experience some morbidity including hypoglycaemia, hypocalcaemia and/or hyperbilirubinaemia (Persson, 1981).

The evolution to overt diabetes in the mother later in life related to glucose tolerance changes during pregnancy has been reported. Prevention of diabetes and its inherent cardio-vascular morbidity by insulin and dietary therapy during pregnancy has been suggested after 20 years of

recurrent screening. This unique observation should not be discarded lightly. Glycosylated haemoglobin (HbA_1C) may be able to reflect glucose intolerance up to 3 months previously but it appears at the present not to be the exclusive reliable parameter to diagnose gestational diabetes early. One may deplore not having more accurate and fixed parameters which may form a basis for taking diagnostic and therapeutic measures in pregnant women. Even the bimodal distribution of blood sugars characterising a diabetic population outside of pregnancy disappears when the women become pregnant (Pettitt et al, 1980). It is however not astonishing to be confronted with this type of situation if one considers that pregnancy is a highly demanding biological process involving a constant change in the structure and function of the maternal endocrine pancreas. Further studies on the maternal endocrine pancreas are needed and may give further insight in the adaptive metabolic changes which may help us in our diagnostic and therapeutic approach.

In conclusion, to screen for carbohydrate intolerance in pregnancy is mandatory and should be performed at the latest at 28th week. A simple screen will alert the obstetrician, physician and paediatrician to patients who are likely to present diabetes-related problems on the basis of past obstetric and clinical history, obesity and clinical examination; the family history also contributes. It may help to identify women susceptible to the development of diabetes or associated complications later in life.

Medical care

Diet

Eating patterns may trigger the onset of diabetes (type 2) and influence its evolution, especially when they lead to obesity. Frequency of meals and eating patterns modulate the metabolic homeostasis in normal pregnancy (Metzger & Ravnikar, 1982).

Even without significant weight change, reduction of carbohydrate intake lowers the blood glucose levels in non-pregnant subjects. The degree of refinement of the carbohydrate consumed influences the excursions in blood glucose and insulin levels. The present recommendations for diabetes highlight a restriction of energy intake which should aim at maintaining an ideal body weight with the provision of 45–50 per cent of this intake being unrefined carbohydrates (Gillmer et al, 1982). In normal pregnancy, the needed energy intake is approximately 300 ml of milk above a 'good' nutrition. In developed countries, concern is expressed that high energy diets may predispose to excessive maternal weight gain which may engender obstetric complications. Clinical studies have indicated that caloric restriction including carbohydrate reduction may have improved some aspects of pregnancy outcome in specific population studies (Gillmer et al, 1982).

In the pregnant diabetic (type 1, type 2 or gestational) who is of normal weight to start with the weight gain pattern should be comparable to that in non-diabetic pregnant woman. Similar nutritional standards have to be applied for the pregnant diabetic with a normal weight as for the normal pregnant woman who is not diabetic: no under-feeding to avoid ketonuria and no excess food intake because insulin is being used. The feeding patterns should also aim at an even distribution during the day. The body weight gain should be assessed regularly. An increase in cell body mass is favoured and a protein intake of 1.3 g/kg is recommended while 45 per cent of calories should be in the form of unrefined carbohydrates which means approximately a 200 g allowance a day. The mean total gain by term is 11 kg for normals (Pitkin, 1980).

Gillmer & Persson (1979) prescribe an individual diet based on energy expenditure with an average amount of calories from carbohydrate, fat and protein to be respectively of 45, 27 and 28 per cent. During the last trimester, at least 1600 kcal is proposed daily. The average blood sugar levels and other metabolic parameters including ketone bodies are maintained close to a normal range in insulin-dependent diabetics.

In obese non insulin-dependent diabetics or in gestational obese diabetics caloric restriction demands special consideration. Comparison has been made in obese pregnant mothers between unrestricted and restricted food intake (1800–2000 calories with 150–180 g carbohydrates). Weight gain was less in the dieted obese women (6.0 kg) than in any other group (12 kg). There was no striking effect of dieting on birthweight in the neonates of this sample of subjects (Borberg et al, 1980). Obese women had fatter neonates than the normal or thin women regardless of diet. The insulin levels, basal or after a challenge, were higher in obese than in normal pregnant women. They were lower in the dieted obese than in the obese not on diet.

Glucose tolerance remained unchanged in both groups. These observations indicate that hormonal adaptation imposed by pregnancy can be modulated by changing the food intake in obese pregnant women. It is tempting to relate this to the islet cell hyperplasia which occurs normally during the latter part of pregnancy and which can be prevented when extra feeding is withheld — at least in the pregnant rat as discussed earlier.

The observation that gestational diabetes may be attributed to the failure of insulin secretion to increase in response to the demands of pregnancy, suggests that caloric restrictions may be the appropriate measures in the initial management of mild diabetes at least at the end of pregnancy. However, in view of the fatness of the infants delivered by both the obese and dieted women (Borberg et al, 1980), it remains relevant to consider insulin therapy especially when diabetes or impaired glucose tolerance arise at the beginning of pregnancy. The neonate is very sensitive to minor glucose changes in the mother. Even in the offspring of mothers with mild glucose intolerance according to O'Sullivan & Mahan's criteria, islet function at birth was identical to the islet reaction when the mother had a severe form of diabetes (Ogata et al, 1980).

Also post-receptor changes have been demonstrated in obese subjects outside of pregnancy, changes that may be normalised with insulin (Scarlett et al, 1982). It is not known if this occurs in pregnancy but this observation could be a further basis for insulin therapy during pregnancy. A potential cause for concern related to caloric restriction during pregnancy is the possible harmful consequences of elevated ketone levels (Berendes, 1975). Other studies have refuted this assertion (Naeye 1979). Careful metabolic observations regarding, for example, fasting 3-hydroxybutyrate concentration did not support the initial observations (Gillmer & Persson, 1979). No psychopathological alterations are currently reported in children of well compensated diabetic mothers (Gillmer et al, 1982).

Insulin therapy

Non insulin-dependent diabetics. In non insulin-dependent diabetics, insulin has been advocated at the inception of the diagnosis especially if made before pregnancy. This appears to be necessary because high fasting blood glucose levels in the mother have been related to high C-peptide levels in the amniotic fluid indicating an excessive fetal insulin secretion which may be related to fetal morbidity (Ogata et al, 1980).

The management of gestational diabetes remains a matter of concern (Report of workshop chairmen, 1980). In a population with low prevalence of diabetes and with low fertility rate, medical intervention is thought to be generally unnecessary by some authors, provided good antenatal supervision is available (Hadden, 1980). However, treatment with diet and insulin in the latter part of pregnancy has been shown to reduce fetal loss and birthweight (O'Sullivan & Mahan, 1980). Regression analysis did not allow differentiation of insulin versus diet in that long-term and unique study. A striking result of insulin therapy has been the reduction of the neonatal weight in another study (Opperman & Camerini-Davalos, 1980). Medical intervention with insulin has been advocated also in high risk groups which should be defined by their past obstetric history (Hoet et al, 1960; Gabbe, 1980; Gyves et al, 1980; Hoet, 1980).

The lowest perinatal loss rate has been observed when, in addition to dietary measures, insulin was used if the 2 hour post-prandial blood glucose was higher than 6.7 mmol/l. The subjects are cared for on an ambulatory basis with careful medical and obstetric monitoring (Gyves et al, 1980). The insulin regimen at the time of its institution is not always well defined in the different reported studies. Single dose insulin is advocated when the fasting glucose remains within normal limits. Occasionally, insulin is administered in this instance at lunch time to avoid midmorning hypoglycaemia. Twice daily administration might be needed if the fasting blood glucose levels are above normal. The risk of nocturnal hypoglycaemia has to be considered as well as the need for increasing the total amount given when pregnancy advances. Roversi et al (1980) have been using three or more daily administrations of highly purified insulin with the intent to have maximal tolerated insulin dose. Excellent fetal outcome has been obtained in the diabetics of all White classes or in gestational diabetics although a trend of birthweights lower than normal has created some concern (Beard, 1979). The regimen of a maximal tolerated dose requires multiple daily injections and may not confer any specific advantage in the gestational diabetic or in the mild form of diabetes during pregnancy (class A) over the now well accepted once or twice administered insulin under proper home glucose monitoring. The advantage of the method advocated by Roversi is the use of very purified insulin. The insulin used during pregnancy should be characterised as being the least antigenic. Antigenecity remains a feature of all the insulin preparations presently available but to a varying degree. Protamine zinc may be an additional factor in this regard. However, the antibody formation to insulin could be related more to a genetic disposition of the subject rather than to the potential antigenecity of the insulin used (Bodansky et al, 1982). The total dosage used daily during pregnancy ranges from 10 to 228 units (Gyves et al, 1980).

Insulin-Dependent Diabetes. In these subjects normalisation of the glucose profile should be obtained. In the first half of this century, perinatal mortality in the insulin-dependent diabetic pregnant woman was already known to increase in relation to decrease in the degree of medical and obstetric care which was graded as complete, partial or non-existing supervision (Lawrence & Oakley, 1942). The consequences of excellent control which can now be monitored on an ambulatory basis are striking and override the clinical results of even good or moderate control. This excellent control should be achieved throughout pregnancy, inception included. The residual B-cell function during pregnancy is important as it confers better control especially during the first and second trimester of pregnancy. This observation concerning the importance of the residual B-cell function in non-pregnant individuals has been further confirmed during pregnancy when metabolic parameters have been analysed meticulously during the three trimesters. It highlights the essential role of the endocrine function of the maternal pancreas during pregnancy with regard of fetal outcome. (Persson et al, 1982).

High motivation in the patient and her husband as well as home monitoring are essential factors which determine the feasibility of achieving excellent control.

The mixture of insulin which is advocated consists of soluble short-acting and long-acting insulin twice a day. Occasionally a small dose of long-acting insulin has to be given before retiring in order to have a close to normal fasting blood glucose levels. (Jovanovic & Peterson, 1982). Other regimens are also used, for example a background insoluble zinc insulin of long duration, in association with soluble insulin administration before each meal, which yield satisfactory results. The use of HbAlC is advocated as an added parameter for evaluating control and compliance but it cannot be used for prospective equilibration. More recently, insulin has been administered throughout the day by a mechanical pump to normalise blood sugar and the other metabolic parameters. Excellent results occur with this procedure, but it remains experimental except in brittle pregnant diabetics. The use of mechanical devices is costly, requires close monitoring and compliance and does not prevent the occurrence of dramatic hypoglycemia (Gillmer & Persson, 1982).

A major consideration related to insulin administration is antibody formation in the mother. Further studies are needed to determine if they have a deleterious effect upon residual B-cell function in the mother and if so how this may affect control and outcome of the pregnancy. In addition, insulin antibodies cross the placenta and as mentioned earlier, affect fetal insulin secretion with functional hypertrophied and hyperplastic islets of Langerhans. No eosinophilic infiltration is observed in the fetal endocrine pancreas if the mother's blood sugar has been normalised with insulin (Van Assche et al, 1982). Human insulin or dephenylated insulin is currently used in pregnancy with the object of avoiding antibody formation. This later objective has not been realised; systematic information is not available as yet to determine the functional and structural consequences of antibodies against human insulin in the human neonate. The strict control of diabetes intrapartum is important as the normalisation of the maternal blood sugar reduces the incidence of hypoglycaemia in the infant in whom an Apgar of at least 7 might be expected (Persson, 1975). The intravenous administration of glucose and insulin during the period of labour should deliver 1.8–2 units of soluble insulin per hour after a loading dose of 0.02–0.05 units per kg given in a bolus. The bolus may not be given if less than 40 units daily are used to achieve normal glucose levels throughout the latter part of pregnancy. The glucose administration should also be precisely monitored i.e. about 12 g/h in a 5 per cent solution. This reflects the amount of energy consumed during the process of labour and delivery.

Obstetrical care

Diabetes and pregnancy are a challenge for the obstetrician even when correct medical care tending to achieve normal blood sugars throughout pregnancy has made the task of the obstetrician and the neonatologist much easier. Nevertheless obstetric care and neonatal care remain essential.

Modern treatment begins prior to conception in the known diabetic. The mother, the husband and the general practitioner have to be instructed how perfect diabetic control must be achieved. There should be a full explanation on the risks of diabetes in pregnancy and how these risks can be reduced. The severity of diabetes and the presence of vascular, retinal and renal complications must be verified before conception. Contraception should ideally be continued until optimum diabetic control is achieved, when pregnancy should be initiated. The woman should be taught to take her basal body temperature in order to know the exact date of conception.

At the inception of pregnancy, combined diabetic and obstetric care must be instituted. Early in pregnancy true gestational age must be confirmed by clinical and ultrasonic means. Early ultrasonic screening of the fetus has shown that these fetuses in early pregnancy are on average smaller than normal and it is postulated that an insufficiently corrected metabolic homeostasis before conception and in the early weeks of pregnancy results in an environment unfavourable for normal embryonic development, leading not only to early retarded growth but also, on occasions, to congenital malformations (Pedersen & Molsted-Pedersen, 1979; Sutherland et al, 1981). It is not yet clear if amniocentesis for chromosome analysis and alpha-fetoprotein determination should to be performed in each diabetic pregnancy (Van Assche et al, 1982).

During the subsequent course of pregnancy careful assessment of fetal growth must be sought using clinical (fundus height) and ultrasonic methods (i.e. biparietal diameter, cross-sectional body area). Early detection of overgrowth or retardation of the fetus is important. Some severe congenital malformations may also be detected. At each antenatal visit careful screening for complications such as pregnancy-induced hypertension, maternal infections and hydramnios remain important goals.

During the last trimester of pregnancy fetal well being has to be assessed continuously. Home monitoring of blood glucose has reduced the need to take the pregnant diabetic into the antenatal ward from 32 weeks onwards. However, fetal surveillance needs constant obstetric supervision.

Fetal wellbeing can be assessed by the evaluation of fetal movements, by antenatal heart rate recording, by oestriol determination in urine or in blood and by plasma hPL concentrations. Patients with class A diabetes who have no obstetric complications are allowed to go close to term (38–39 weeks).

For the insulin-dependent diabetic woman it is generally accepted that fetal pulmonary maturity should be assessed prior to planned delivery by the measurement of the L:S ratio; in diabetics, it is suggested that the ratio is ideally 4 in order to be certain that hyaline membrane disease with surfactant deficiencies and transient tachypnoea may be avoided. Induction of labour should be performed as late as possible in pregnancy but prior to 39 weeks, provided that fetal well being and fetoplacental function remain normal. The interval between the rupture of membranes and delivery of the baby must not be more than 24 hours; fetal heart rate monitoring is necessary throughout labour. There must be a strict control of maternal blood sugar preferably with insulin and glucose infusion as stated earlier.

The expertise of a neonatologist is necessary when the decision is made to induce and particularly at the time of delivery.

Neonatal care

Newborn infants of diabetic mothers have long since been classified as high risk babies. It must be emphasised that they constitute a very heterogeneous group not only with regard to factors such as maternal age, weight, parity and acute complications during pregnancy but most important with respect to the degree of diabetic angiopathy and quality of diabetic control before and throughout pregnancy.

The pattern of changes in fuel homeostasis and energy metabolism which accompanies the transition from intra-uterine to extra-uterine existence may be modified greatly by the degree of functional immaturity and adaptation as well as the nutritional status at birth. This is especially evident among large for dates and small for dates infants of diabetic mothers who are at increased risk of developing asphyxia around birth and neonatal hypoglycaemia.

The outlook for intact survival of infants of diabetic mothers has improved markedly over recent years in specialised centres where a team approach calling for expert centralisation has been applied. The outlook remains less satisfactory outside these centers. Even in most developed countries 75 per cent of these high risk pregnancies are cared for in non-specialised centres where there is insufficient awareness of the specific health care required by pregnant diabetics.

In any event, neonatal complications still occur in about 50 per cent of infants of insulin-dependent diabetic mothers and approximately 25 per cent of infants of gestational diabetic mothers (Gillmer et al, 1982). The type of neonatal morbidity which occurs include asphyxia, cardiorespiratory problems, hypoglycaemia (i.e. < 1.1 mmol/l in low birthweight infants less than 2.5 kg and below 1.7 mmol/l in infants more than 2.5 kg). Electrolyte disturbances including hypocalcaemia (< 1.8 mmol/l), polycythaemia (venous hematocrit > 60 per cent) hyperbilirubinaemia and feeding problems (feeding by nasogastric route or significant amounts of gastric residue) are frequent events. Before discussing in more detail the management of some of these complications it is necessary to summarise specific features which should be considered in the routine care of the newborn of a diabetic mother. Ideally the delivery should be planned and great effort should be made to keep the maternal blood glucose levels within the physiological range (5–6 mmol/l) in the hours prior to and during delivery. The risk of developing neonatal hypoglycaemia and in the case of hypoxia or asphyxia the risk of severe lactic acidosis is consequently reduced. A paediatrician experienced in resuscitation of the newborn should be present whether delivery is vaginal or by Caesarian section. As soon as the infant is born, the following systematic points of action are mandatory:

1. Early clamping of the cord, i.e. within 30 s of delivery.
2. Evaluate vital signs, i.e. Apgar score at 1 and 5 min.
3. Clear oropharynx and nose of mucus. Later empty the stomach; be aware that stimulation of the pharynx with the catheter may lead to reflex brady-chardia and apnoea.
4. Avoid heat loss, keep neonate warm, transfer to incubator prewarmed to 34 °C.
5. Perform a preliminary physical examination to detect major congenital malformation.
6. Monitor heart, respiratory rate, color, motor behaviour at least during the first 24 hours after birth.
7. Start early feeding, preferably breast milk at 4–6 hours after delivery. Aim at full caloric intake (125 kcal/kg/24 h) at 5 days, devided in 6–8 feeds a day.
8. Promote early infant-parent relationship (bonding).

The neonate is usually best cared for in a specialised neonatal unit and interference should be minimal. The new born should be allowed to recover and normalise his body temperature and metabolic acidosis should be eliminated. In order to recognise some neonatal complications, haemoglobin, haematocrit (venous), blood glucose, calcium (venous) and bilirubin should be determined.

The most remarkable change in morbidity which has occurred over the last decade is the dramatic fall in respiratory distress due to hyaline membrane disease or pulmonary surfactant deficiency. The improvement is probably the result of strict control of maternal diabetes during pregnancy.

A less severe respiratory complication is transient tachypnea which is due to the lack of another surfactant-phophatidyl-glycerol. Other conditions associated with cyanosis and rapid respiratory movement which must be considered include pneumothorax, diaphragmatic hernia, cardiac malformation, polycythaemia and hypoglycaemia. Therefore, whenever the infant's respiratory rate is increase and/or cyanosis is present, blood gases, blood glucose and hematocrit should be determinated. X-ray of lungs and heart as well as ECG should be performed.

Cardiomegaly in the absence of congenital heart disease without symptoms or associated with either transient or more protracted symptoms may occur in 30–50 per cent of infants of diabetic mothers.

Electrocardiographic studies have shown hypertrophy of the ventricular walls and in particular the intra-ventricular system and abnormalities in the transitional circulation (Gutgesell, 1976; Wolfe et al, 1977; Hirschfeld et al, 1979).

These hypertrophic changes of the heart seem to be related to fetal hyperinsulinism. This view is supported by an association between cardiomegaly, ECG abnormalities and elevated plasma C-peptide levels at birth (Freyschuss et al, 1982). Symptoms of cardio-respiratory distress in this condition do not respond favourably to treatment with digitalis and diuretics. They should not be used unless it can be shown that myocardial contraction is depressed. The use of beta blocking agents has been favoured with successful results together with early clamping of the umbilical cord which should be performed to avoid unnecessary overload of the circulation. As previously discussed extramedullary hematopoesis and polycythemia are characteristic findings in the child of insulin-dependent mothers. Haematocrit values exceeding 60 per cent are often associated with hyperviscosity, sludging of the erythrocytes and hence impaired perfusion of various organs. The hyperviscosity syndrome is characterised by plethora, cardio-respiratory distress and neurological symptoms. This condition is favourably influenced by phlebotomy or modified exchange transfusion. This treatment should be considered whenever the central haematocrit exceeds 70 per cent in view also of the fact the offspring of insulin dependent mothers more commonly develop renal vein thrombosis than infants of non-diabetic mothers.

Metabolic maladjustment to hypoglycaemia also remains a feature. Despite the fact that most infants of diabetic mothers, excluding the small for dates infants, have larger stores of both glycogen in the liver and elsewhere, as well as triglycerides in adipose tissue, they seem to be unable adequately to mobilise substrates from these stores particularly during the first post-natal hours. During this time period plasma concentrations of glucose, free fatty acids (FFA) and ketone bodies are suppressed. The hepatic glucose production rate is decreased. The infants have an increased ability to dispose of intravenously administered glucose. All these metabolic alterations are transient and more likely the consequences of fetal and subsequent neonatal hyperinsulinism. Symptomatic neonatal hypoglycaemia (i.e. presenting symptoms and signs such as respiratory distress, cyanosis, jitteriness, convulsions, etc) is treated with glucose administered intravenously (0.5–1.0 g glucose/kg body weight) followed by continuous glucose infusion (4–8 mg/kg body weight/min) in order to avoid reactive hypoglycemia. The growth retarded infant of the diabetic mother is also liable to develop hypoglycaemia because of reduced energy stores of both glycogen and fat together with an impaired capacity for gluconeogenesis.

Available evidence suggests that neonatal hypoglycaemia can be prevented in most infants of diabetic mothers by strict control of maternal blood glucose throughout pregnancy and around birth, by the initiation of early feeding and by avoiding heat loss.

In 1974 Davis and co-workers described a clinical syndrome which they designated the neonatal left colon syndrome (micro-colon) and which seemed to be a more frequent neonatal complication in infants of insulin-dependent mothers than in other newborn infants. The clinical features associated with this condition are failure to pass meconium, abdominal distention and bile-stained vomitus. Contrast radiography shows a markedly diminished calibre of the left colon from the splenic flexure, a picture similar to that of Hirchsprung's disease of the newborn. The symptoms of lower intestinal obstruction are usually of short duration and may even be absent in some infants who only exhibit the typical radiographical finding (Davis et al, 1974). Ganglion cells of a proposed immature appearance have been described in the intermyenteric plexus of the left colon (Davis & Campbell, 1974) but others have not found this abnormality. The reason for this apparently delayed functional maturation of the gastrointestinal tract in infants of insulin-dependent mothers is unclear. The presence of this condition in the offspring of diabetic mothers may be causally related to both the increased frequency of polyhydramnios in diabetic pregnancy and to the increased incidence of feeding problems in the newborn. This speculation is partly supported by the recent observation of an association between large amniotic fluid volumes and feeding problems in the newborn in diabetic pregnancy (Stangenberg et al, 1982b). In the experimental animal with mild diabetes a marked delay in structural maturation of the gastrointestinal tract occurs affecting especially the brush border cells (Reusens et al, 1982). In addition, the immaturity of the autonomic nervous system may affect the gastrointestinal tract and might be responsible for some of the features of perinatal morbidity (de Gasparo et al, 1978).

REFERENCES

Adam P A, Raiha N, Rahiala E L, Kekomaki M 1975 Oxydation of glucose and D-B-OH-Butyrate by the early human fetal brain. Acta Pediatrica Scandinavica 64: 17–24

Adamsons K, Myers R 1975 Circulation in the intervillous space; Obstetrical consideration. In: Gruenwald P (ed) Fetal Deprivation in the Placenta and its Maternal Supply line, pp 158–177. MTP, Lancaster

Aerts L, Van Assche F A 1979 Is gestational Diabetes an acquired condition? Journal of Developmental Physiology 1: 219–225

Alejandro R, Shienvold F L, Vaerewyck Hajek S, Ryan U, Miller J, Mintz D H 1982 Immunocytochemical localization of HLA-DR in human islets of Langerhans. Diabetes 31: Suppl 4: 17–22

Anderson U 1982 Ontogenic development of human lymphocyte functions. Thesis, Karolinska Institute, Stockholm

Aynsley-Green S, Polak J M, Bloom S R, Cough M H, Keeling J, Ashcroft S J H, Turner R C, Baum J D 1981 Nesidioblastosis of the pancreas: definition of the syndrome and the management of the severe neonatal hyperinsulinaemic hypoglycaemia. Archives of Diseases Childhood 56: 496–508

Baker L, Egler J M, Klein S H, Goldman A S 1981 Meticulous control of diabetes during organogenesis prevents congenital lumbo sacral defects in rats. Diabetes 30: 955–959

Bassett J M, Jones C T 1976 Fetal glucose metabolism, In: Beard R W, Nathanielz P W (eds) Fetal Physiology and Medicine. The Basis of Perinatology, pp 158–172. W B Saunders, London

Bauman W A, Yalow R S 1981 Transplacental passage of insulin complexed to antibody. Proceedings of the National Academy of Sciences. 78: 4588–4593

Beard R W 1979 Blood sugar levels in pregnancy, In: Pregnancy Metabolism, Diabetes and the Fetus, p 312. Ciba Foundation Symposium. Excerpta Medica, Amsterdam

Beard R W, Hoet J J 1982 Is gestational diabetes a clinical entity? Diabetologia, 23: 307–312

Beck-Nielsen H, Kuhl C, Pedersen O, Bjerre-Christensen C, Nielsen T T, Klebe J G 1979 Decreased insulin binding to monocytes from normal pregnant women. Journal of Clinical Endocrinology and Metabolism 49: 810–814

Bennett P H, Webner C, Miller M 1979 Congenital anomalies and the diabetic and prediabetic pregnancy. In: Pregnancy Metabolism, Diabetes and the Fetus, pp 207–218. Ciba Foundation Symposium. Excerpta Medica, Amsterdam

Berendes H W 1975 Effect of maternal acetonuria on IQ of offspring In: Camerini-Davalos R A, Cole H S (eds) Early Diabetes in Early Life, pp 349–352. Academic Press, New York

Berglund G, Zetterström R 1954 Infants of diabetic mothers. In:Foetal Hypoxia in Maternal Diabetes. Acta Paediatrica Scandinavica 43: 368–373

Binder C, Faber O K 1978 Residual B-cell function and its metabolic consequences. Diabetes 27: Suppl 1: 226–229

Bjork O, Persson B 1984 Villous structure in different parts of the cotyledon in placentas of insulin dependent diabetic women: a morphometric study. Acta Obstetrica Gynecologica Scandinavica 63: 37–43

Bjork O, Persson B, Stangenberg M, Vaclavinkova V 1984 Spiral artery lesions in relation to metabolic control in diabetes mellitus. Acta Obstetrica et Gynecologica Scandinavica 63: 123–127

Blasquez E, Lopez-Quijada C 1970 The effect of high protein diet on plasma glucose concentration, insulin sensitivity and plasma insulin in rats. Journal of Endocrinology 46: 445–451

Bodansky H J, Cudworth A G, Drury P L, Kohner E M 1982 Risk factors associated with severe proliferative retinopathy in insulin dependent diabetes mellitus. Diabetes Care 5: 97–104

Borberg C, Gillmer M D G, Brunner E J, Gunn P J, Oakley N W, Beard R W 1980 Obesity in pregnancy: the effect of dietary advice. Diabetes Care 5: 476–481

Breitweser J A, Meyer R A, Sperling M A, Tsang R C Kaplan S 1980 Cardiac septal hypertrophy in hyperinsulinemic infants. Journal of Pediatrics 96: 535–539

Brent R L 1966 Immunological aspects of developmental biology. Advances in Teratology 1: 81–129

v. Bruchhausen F 1975 Action of insulin on some other organs and on differentiation In: Hasselblatt A, v. Brucchausen F (eds) Insulin 2, pp 435–495. Springer Verlag, Berlin

Cardell B S 1953 The infants of diabetic mothers: a morphological study. Journal of Obstetrics and Gynaecology of the British Commonwealth 60: 834–853

Carstensen L L, Frost–Larsen K, Fugleberg S, Nerup J 1982 Does pregnancy influence the prognosis of uncomplicated insulin dependent diabetes mellitus? Diabetes Care 5: 1–5

Coleman C, Elias E, Iqbal S, Hickey A 1982 Oestrogen-induced cholestasis may be due to increased permeability to tight junctions. Biochemical Society Transactions 10: 222–223

Comess L J, Bennett P M, Burch T A, Miller M 1969 Congenital anomalies and diabetes in Pima Indians of Arizona. Diabetes 18: 471–477

Davis W S, Campbell J B 1974 Neonatal left colon syndrome occurence in asymptomatic infants of diabetic mothers. American Journal of Diseases in Children 129: 1024–1027

Davis W J, Allen R P, Favara B E, Stovis T L 1974 Neonatal small colon syndrome. American Journal Roentgenology, Radium Therapy and Nuclear Medicine 120: 322–329

Dekabah A, Baird R 1959 The outcome of pregnancy in diabetic women. Journal of Pediatries 55: 563–569

Deuchar E M 1979 Experimental evidence relating fetal anomalies to diabetes In: Sutherland H, Stowers J (eds) Carbohydrate Metabolism in Pregnancy and the Newborn, pp 247–263. Springer Verlag, New York

Dobersen M J, Scharff 1982 Preferential lysis of pancreatic B cells by islet cell surface antibodies. Diabetes 31: 459–462

Dubreuil G et Anderodias J 1920 Ilôts de Langerhans géants chez un nouveau-né issu de mére glycosurique. Comptes Rendus Société Biologique (Paris) 20: 1940–1941

Emmrich P, Godel E, Amendt P, Muller G 1975 Schwangerschaft bei Diabetikerinnen mit Diabetischer Angiopathie-Klinische Ergebnisse in Korrelation zur Morphologischen Befunden an der Plazenta. Zentral blatt fuer Gynaekologie 97: 875

Ericksson U, Dahlstrom E 1982 Diabetes in pregnancy: congenital malformations in the rat. Effects of maternal hyperglycemic episodes in early gestation. Diabetologia 23: 165–166 (Abst)

Ericksson U, Andersson A, Efendic S, Elde R, Hellerstrom C 1980 Diabetes in Pregnancy: effects on the foetal and newborn rat with particular regard to bodyweight, serum insulin concentration and pancreatic contents of insulin, glucagon and somatostatin. Acta Endocrinologica 94: 354–364

Ericksson U, Dahlstrom E, Larsson S, Hellerstrom C 1982 Increased incidence of congenital malformations in the offspring of diabetic rats and their prevention by maternal insulin therapy. Diabetes 31: 1–6

Farquhar J 1969 Prognosis for babies born to diabetic mothers in Edinburgh. Archives of Disease in Childhood 44: 36–44

Fauci A S, Harley J B, Roberts W C, Ferrans V J, Gralnick H R, Bjornson B H 1982 The idiopathic hypereosinophilic syndrome. Annals of Internal Medicine 97: 78–92

Faulk W P 1981 Human trophoblast antigens: role in normal and abnormal pregnancies. Bulletin Académie Royale de Médecine de Belgique 136: 379–388

Faulk W P, McIntyre J A 1981 Trophoblast survival transplantation 32: 1–5

Felig P, Kim Y J, Lynch V, Hendler R 1972 Amino-acid metabolism during starvation in human pregnancy. Journal of Clinical Investigation 51: 1195–1202

Fletcher J M, Flaconer J, Bassett J M 1982 The relationship of body and placental weight to plasma levels of insulin and other hormones during development in fetal rabbits. Diabetologia 23: 124–130

Fog-Pedersen J, Molsted-Pedersen L 1979 Early growth retardation in diabetic pregnancy. British Medical Journal 1: 18–19

Forrest J M, Menser M A, Burgess J A 1971 High Frequency of diabetes mellitus in young adults with congenital rubella. Lancet ii: 332–334

Fox H 1978 The development and structure of the placenta In: Major Problems in Pathology, Vol 7, p 1. W B Saunders, London

Fox H, Path M C 1970 Effect of hypoxia on trophoblast in organ culture: a morphologic and autoradiographic study. American Journal of Obstetrics and Gynecology 107: 1058–1064

Freinkel N, Metzger B E 1979 Pregnancy as a tissue culture experience: the critical implications of maternal metabolism for foetal development In: Pregnancy Metabolism, Diabetes and the Fetus, Ciba Foundation Symposium 63, pp 3–23. Excerpta Medica, Amsterdam

Freinkel N, Phelps R L, Metzger B E 1979 Intermediary metabolism during normal pregnancy In: Sutherland H M, Stowers J M (eds) Carbohydrate Metabolism in Pregnancy and the Newborn, pp 1–31. Springer Verlag, Berlin

Freyschuss U, Gentz, G, Noack G and Persson B 1982 Circulatory adaptation in newborn infants of strictly controlled diabetic mothers. Acta Pediatrica Scandinavica 71: 209–215

Froelich C J, Goodwin J S, Bankhurst A D, Williams R C 1980 Pregnancy, a temporary fetal graft of suppressor cells in autoimmune disease? American Journal of Medicine 69: 329–331

Gabbe S T 1980 Effects of identifying a high risk population. Diabetes Care 5: 486–488

Galbraight R M, Faulk W P 1979 Immunological considerations of the materno-fetal relationship in diabetes mellitus In: Merkatz I R, Adam P A J (eds) The Diabetic Pregnancy a Perinatal Perspective, pp 111–121. Grune and Stratton, New York

Gamlen T R, Aynsley-Green A, Irvine W J, Mc Callum C J 1977 Immunological studies in the neonate of a mother with Addison's disease and diabetes mellitus. Clinical and Experimental Immunology 28: 192–195

de Gasparo M, Hoet J J 1971 Normal and abnormal foetal weightgain In: Rodriguez R R, Valance-Owen J (eds) Diabetes, Proceedings of the 7th Congress of the International Diabetes Federation, pp 667–677. Excerpta Medica, Amsledam

de Gasparo M, de Herdt P, Hoet J J 1978 Effect of maternal carbohydrate intolerance on the development of the autonomic innervation of the fetal rat pancreas In: Camerini-Davalos R A, Hanover B (eds) Treatment of Early Diabetes, pp 115–122. Plenum Press, New York

Gillmer M D G, Persson B 1979 Metabolism during normal and diabetic pregnancy and its effect on neonatal outcome In: Pregnancy Metabolism, Diabetes and the Fetus, Ciba Foundation Symposium 63, pp 93–121. Excerpta Medica, Amsterdam

Gillmer M D G, Oakley N W, Persson B 1982 Diabetes Mellitus and the Fetus In: Beard R W, Nathanielz P W (eds) Fetal Physiology and Medicine, 2nd edn, W B Saunders, London

Gitlin D, Kumate J, Urrusti J, Morales C 1964 The selectivity of the human placenta in the transfer of plasma proteins from mother to fetus. Journal of Clinical Investigation 43: 1938–1951

Graighead J E 1977 Viral diabetes. In: Volk B W, Wellmann K F (eds) The Diabetic Pancreas, pp 467–489. Plenum Press, New York

Gutgesell H P, Hullins C E, Gilette P C, Speek M, Rudolph A J, McNamara D G 1976 Transient hypertrophic subaortic stenosis in infants of diabetic mothers. Journal of Paediatrics 89: 120–125

Gyves M T, Schulman P K, Merkatz I R 1980 Results of individualized intervention in gestational diabetes, Diabetes Care 3: 495–498

Habicht J P, Lechtig A, Yarbrough C H, Klein R E 1974 Maternal nutrition, birthweight and infant mortality In: Size at Birth, Ciba Foundation Symposium, pp 354–377. Associated Sci Pub

Hadden D R 1980 Screening for abnormalities of carbohydrate metabolism in pregnancy 1966–1977: the Belfast experience. Diabetes Care 3: 440–446

Hallman H, Teramo K 1979 Amniotic fluid phospholipid profile as predictor of fetal maturity in diabctic prcgnancies. Obstetrics and Gynecology 54: 703–707

Heding L G, Persson B and Stangenberg M 1980 B-cell function in newborn infants of diabetic mothers. Diabetologia 19: 427–432

Hill D E 1979 Effect of Insulin on fetal growth In: Merkatz I R, Adam P A J (eds) The Diabetic Pregnancy: a Perinatal Perspective, pp 155–165. Grune and Stratton, New York

Hirschberg H 1981 Presentation of viral antigens by human vascular endothelial cells in vitro. Human Immunology 2: 235–246

Hirschfeld S S, Fanaroff A A, Merkatz I R 1979 Cardio-vascular abnormalities in infants of diabetic mothers In: Merkatz I R, Adam P (eds). The Diabetic Pregnancy: A perinatal Perspective pp 249–260. Grune and Stratton, New York

Hoet J J 1969 Normal and abnormal foetal weightgain In: Foetal Autonomy, Ciba Symposium, pp 186–213. Churchill, London

Hoet J J Effects of interventions in gestational diabetes. Diabetes Care 3: 497–498

Hoet J J 1982 Health care for the younger generation of South East Asia. International Diabetes Federation Bulletin 27: 8–9.

Hoet J J, Beard R W 1979 Clinical perspectives in the care of the pregnant diabetic patient In: Pregnancy Metabolism, Diabetes and the Fetus, Ciba Foundation Symposium 63, pp 283–300. Excerpta Medica, Amsterdam

Hoet J J, Krall L P 1982 Healthcare in developing countries. International Diabetes Federation Bulletin, in press

Hoet J P, Gommers A, Hoet J J 1960 Causes of congenital malformations: Role of prediabetes and hypothyroidism In: Congenital Malformations, Ciba Foundation Symposium, pp 219–235. Boston, Little, Brown

Horii K, Watanbee G, Ingalls T H 1966 Experimental diabetes in pregnant mice. Prevention of congenital malformation in offspring by insulin. Diabetes 15: 194–204

Howell S L, Green I C, Montague W 1973 A possible role of adenyl-cyclase in the long-term dietary regulation of insulin secretion of rat islets of Langerhans. Biochemical Journal 136: 343–349

Hultquist G T 1971 Morphology of the endocrine organs in infants of diabetic mothers. In: Rodriguez R R, Valance-Owen J (eds) Diabetes Mellitus, pp 686–684. Excerpta Medica, Amsterdam

Hultquist G T, Olding L 1975 Pancreatic islet fibrosis in young infants of diabetic mothers. Lancet ii: 1015–1016

Jovanovic L, Peterson C M 1982 Optimal insulin delivery for the pregnant diabetic patient. Diabetes Care 5: 24–37

Jurado-Garcia E 1978 Perinatal care in Mexico In: Aladejem S, Brown A K, Sureau C (eds) Clinical Perinatology, pp. 560–575

Kalhan C, Adam P A J 1980 Quantitative estimation of systemic glucose production in normal and diabetic pregnancy. Diabetes Care 3: 410–415

Kalkhoff R K, Kissebah A H, Kim H J 1979 Carbohydrate and lipid metabolism during normal pregnancy: relationship to gestational hormone action In: Merkatz I R, Adam P A J (eds) The Diabetic Pregnancy: a Perinatal Perspective, pp 3–21. Grune & Stratton, New York

Kaplan S A, Neufeld N D, Lippe B M, Barrett C T 1979 Maternal diabetes and the development of the insulin receptors In: Merkatz I R, Adam P A J (eds) The Diabetic Pregnancy: a Perinatal Perspective, pp 169–174. Grune & Stratton, New York

Kitzmiller J L, Aiello L, Kaldany A, Younger M D 1981 Diabetic vascular disease complicating pregnancy. Clinical Obstetrics and Gynecology 24: 107–123

Kitzmiller J L, Cloherty J P, Graham C A 1982 Management of Diabetes and Pregnancy. In: Kozak G P (ed) Clinical Diabetes Mellitus, pp 203–214. W B Saunders, Philadelphia

Knopp R H, Chapman M, Bergelin R, Wahl P W, Warth M R, Irvine S 1980 Relationships of lipoprotein lipids to mild fasting hyperglycaemia and diabetes in pregnancy. Diabetes Care 3: 416–420

Kuberski T T, Bennett P H 1980 Diabetes mellitus as an emerging health problem on Guam. Diabetes Care 3: 235–241

Kuhl C, Holst J J 1976 Plasma glucagon and insulin: glucagon ratio in gestational diabetes. Diabetes 25: 16–23

Kyle G C 1963 Diabetes and pregnancy. Annals of Internal Medicine 59: Suppl 3: 1–82

Llarralde J, Fernandez-Otero P, Gonzalez M 1966 Increased active transport of glucose through the intestine during pregnancy. Nature 209: 1356–1357

Lawrence R D, Oakley W 1942 Pregnancy and diabetes. Quarterly Journal of Medicine 11: 45

Lawrence R, Church J A, Richards W, Borzy M 1980 Immunological mechanisms in the maintainance of pregnancy. Annals of Allergy 44: 166–173

Lecompte P M, Gepts W 1977 The pathology of Juvenile diabetes In: Volk B W, Wellmann K F (eds) The Diabetic Pancreas, pp 325–363. Balliére Tindall, London

Lemons J A, Vargas P, Delaney J J 1981 Infant of the diabetic mothers: review of 225 cases. Obstetrics and Gynecology 57: 187–192

Leslie R D G, Pyke D A, John P N, Withel J M 1980 Haemoglobin AIC in diabetic pregnancy. Lancet ii: 958–959

Lind T, Burne J M, Kuhl C 1979 Metabolic changes in pregnancy relevant to diabetes In: Sutherland H W, Stowers J M (eds) Carbohydrate Metabolism in Pregnancy and the Newborn 1978, pp 32–46. Springer Verlag, Berlin

Madsen H, Ditzel J 1982 Changes in red bloodcell oxygen transport in diabetic pregnancy. American Journal of Obstetrics and Gynecology 143: 421–424

Malaisse W J, Malaisse-Lagae F, Picard C, Flament-Durant J 1969 Effect of pregnancy and chorionic growth hormone upon insulin secretion, Endocrinology 84: 41–44

Di Mario U, Andreani D, Lavicoli M, Gargiulo P, Galfo C, Musacchio N, Falucca F 1982 Humoral Immunity in Pregnant Diabetic Patients: Islet cell antibodies and immune complexes. Diabetologia 23: 164 (Abst)

Menser M A, Forrest J M, Bransby R D 1978 Rubella infection and diabetes mellitus. Lancet i: 58–60

Merkatz I R, Duchon M A, Yamashita T S, Houser H B 1980 A pilot community-based screening program for gestational diabetes. Diabetes Care 3: 453–457

Mestman J H 1980 Outcome of diabetes screening in pregnancy and perinatal morbidity in infants of mothers with mild impairment of glucose tolerance. Diabetes Care 3: 447–452

Metzger B E, Freinkel N 1979 Effects of Diabetes mellitus on endocrinologic and metabolic adaptations of gestation In: Merkatz I R, Adam P A J (eds) The Diabetic Pregnancy: A Perinatal Perspective, pp 23–34. Grune and Stratton, New York

Metzger B E, Ravnikar V 1982 'Accelerated starvation' and the skipped breakfast in late normal pregnancy. Lancet: i: 588–592

Metzger B E, Phelps R L, Freinkel N, Navickas I E 1980 Effects of gestational diabetes on diurnal profiles of plasma glucose, lipids and individual amino-acids. Diabetes Care 3: 402–409

Miller E, Hare J W, Cloherty J P, Gleason R E, Soeldner J S, Kitzmiller J L 1981 Elevated maternal Hemoglobin AlC in early pregnancy and major congenital anomalies in infants of diabetic mothers. New England Journal of Medicine 304: 1331–1334

Mills J L, Baker L, Goldman A S 1979 Malformations in infants of diabetic mothers occur before the seventh gestational week: implications for treatment. Diabetes 28: 292–293

Milner R D G 1979 Amino-acids and B cell growth in structure and function In: Merkatz I R, Adam P A J (eds) The Diabetic Pregnancy: A Perinatal Perspective, pp 145–154. Grune & Stratton, New York

Mintz D H, Skyler J S, Chez R A 1978 Diabetes mellitus and pregnancy. Diabetes Care 1: 49–63

Naeye R l 1965 Infants of diabetic mothers: quantitative morphologic study. Pediatrics 35: 980–989

Naeye R L 1979 Outcome of diabetic pregnancies. In: Pregnancy Metabolism, Diabetes and the Fetus, Ciba Foundation Symposium pp 227–254. Excerpta Medica, Amsterdam

Nylund L, Lunell N O, Lewander R, Persson B, Sarby B, Thornstrom S 1982 Utero-placental bloodflow in diabetic pregnancy. Measurement with indium 113 m and a computor-linked gamma camera. American Journal of Obstetrics and Gynecology 144: 298–302

Ogata E S, Freinkel N, Metzger B E Phelps R L, Depp R, Boehm J J, Dooley S L 1980 Perinatal islet function in gestational diabetes: assessment by cord plasma C. peptide and amniotic fluid insulin. Diabetes Care 3: 425–429

Ogilvie R F 1964 The endocrine pancreas in human and experimental diabetes In: The Aetiology of Diabetes Mellitus and its Complications, Ciba Foundation Colloquia on Endocrinology Vol. 15, pp 49–66. Churchill London

Oleske J M, Minnefor A B 1980 Viral and chlamydial infections In: Grieco M H (ed) Infections in the Abnormal Host, pp 382–405. Yorke Medical Books, USA

Oppermann W, Camerini-Davalos R A 1980 Early diabetes during pregnancy. Diabetes Care 3: 465–467

O'Sullivan J B 1963 Gestational diabetes: unsuspected asymptomatic diabetes in pregnancy. New England Journal of Medicine 264: 1082–1085

O'Sullivan J B, Mahan L M, Charles D, Dandrow R V 1973 Screening criteria for high risk gestational diabetic patients. American Journal of Obstetrics and Gynecology 116: 895–899

O'Sullivan J B, Mahan C M 1980 Insulin treatment and high risk groups. Diabetes Care 3: 482–485

O'Sullivan J B Gellis S S, Dandrow R W, Tenney B O 1966 The potential diabetic and her treatment in pregnancy, Obstetrics and Gynecology 27: 683–689

Page E W, Villee C A, Villee D B 1981 Human Reproduction, Essentials of Reproductive and Perinatal Medicine, 3rd ed, W B Saunders, Philadelphia

Palacios R, Anderson U 1982. Autologous mixed lymphocyte reaction in human cord blood lymphocytes: decreased generation of Helper and cytotoxic T cell functions and increased proliferative response and induction of Suppressor T cells. Cellular Immunology 66: 88–98

Paneth N, Kiely J L, Wallenstein S, Marcus M, Parter J, Susser M 1982 Newborn intensive care and neonatal mortality in low-birthweight infants: a population study. New England Journal of Medicine 307: 149–155

Pedersen J 1977 The Pregnant Diabetic and her Newborn. Munksgaard, Copenhagen

Pedersen J, Osler M 1958 Development of ossification centres in infants of diabetic mothers. Acta Endocrinologica 29: 467–469

Pedersen J, Molsted-Pedersen L 1979 Congenital malformations: the possible role of diabetes care outside pregnancy. In:

Pregnancy Metabolism, Diabetes and the Fetus, Ciba Foundation Symposium, pp 265–271. Excerpta Medica, Amsterdam

Pedersen O, Beck-Nielsen H, Klebe J G 1981 Insulin receptors in the pregnant diabetic and her newborn. Journal of Clinical Endocrinology and Metabolism 53: 1160–1166

Peevy K J, Landaw S A, Gross S J 1980 Hyperbilirubinemia in infants of diabetic mothers. Journal of Paediatrics 66: 417–419

Persson B 1975 Glucose tolerance in the newborn In: Sutherland H W, Stowers J H (eds) Carbohydrate Metabolism in Pregnancy and Newborn, pp 106–126. Churchill Livingstone, Edinburgh

Persson B 1981 Insulin as growth factor in the fetus In: The Biology of Normal Human Growth, pp 213–221. Raven Press, New York

Persson B, Gentz J, Lunell N O 1978 Diabetes in pregnancy In: Scarpelli E M, Cosmi E V (eds) Reviews in Perinatal Medicine, Vol 2, pp 1–55. Raven Press, New York

Persson B, Gentz J, Stangenberg M 1979 Neonatal problems In: Sutherland H W, Stowers j M (eds) Carbohydrate Metabolism in Pregnancy and the Newborn, pp 376–391. Springer-Verlag, Berlin

Persson B, Heding L, Lunell N O, Pschera H, Stangenberg M, Wager J 1982 Fetal Beta-cell function in diabetic pregnancy. American Journal of Obstetrics and Gynecology (in press)

Pettitt D J, Knowler W C, Baird H R, Bennett P H 1980 Gestational diabetes: infant and maternal complications of pregnancy in relation to third trimester glucose tolerance in the Pima Indians. Diabetes Care 3: 458–464

Phelps R L, Freinkel N, Rubenstein R H, Kuzuya H, Metzger B E, Boehm J J, Molsted-Pedersen L 1978 Carbohydrate metabolism in pregnancy, XV Plasma C. peptide during intravenous glucose tolerance in neonate from normal and insulin-treated diabetic mothers. Journal of Clinical Endocrinology and Metabolism 46: 61–68

Philipps A S, Dubin J W, Raye J R 1981 Fetal metabolic response to endogenous insulin release.American Journal of Obstetrics and Gynecology 139: 441–445

Philipps A F, Widness J A, Garcia J F, Raye J R, Schwartz R 1982 Erythropoietin elevation in the chronically hyperglycemic fetal lamb. Proceedings of the Society of Experimental Biology and Medicine 170: 42–47

Pitkin R M 1980 Nutritional requirements in normal pregnancy. Diabetes Care 3: 472–475

Rahier J, Wallon J, Henquin J C 1981 Cell population in the endocrine pancreas of human neonates and infants. Diabetologia 20: 540 546

Reiher H, Fuhrmann K, Besch W, Hahn von Dorsche H, Noalk S, Hahn H J 1982 Different insulin secretion of pancreas from fetuses of diabetic and non-diabetic patients in vitro. Diabetologia 23: 195

Remacle C, Reusens-Billen B, Daniline J, Hoet J J 1982 Cell proliferation in islets of fetuses and neonates from normal and diabetic mothers. Diabetes 31: Suppl 2: 160(a)

Report of Workshop Chairmen, Summary and Recommendations 1980. Diabetes Care 3: 499–501

Reusens B, Hoet J J, Kuhn E R 1976 Prolactin and glucose levels in fetal and maternal rat plasma. I R C S Medicine 4: 325–326

Reusens B, Kuhn E R, Hoet J J 1979 Fetal plasma prolctin levels and fetal growth in relation to maternal C B 154 in the rat. General and Comparative Endocrinology 39: 118–120

Rosenlocher K 1932 Die Veränderungen des Pankreas in der Schwangerschaft bei Mensch und Tier. Archiv für Gynäkologie 151: 567

Roversi G D, Gargiulo M, Nicolini U, Ferrazzi E, Pedretti E, Gruft L, Tronconi G 1980 Maximum tolerated insulin therapy in gestational diabetes. Diabetes Care 3: 489–494

Rubinstein P, Walker M, Krassner J, Carrier C, Carpenter C, Doberson M J et al 1981 HLA antigens and islet cell antibodies in gestational diabetes. Human Immunology 3: 271–275

Sara V R, Hall K, Wetterberg L 1980 Growth hormone dependent polypeptides and the brain In: de Wied D, van Keep P A (eds) Hormones and the Brain, pp 63–72. M T P, Lancaster

Sara V R, Hall K, Rodeck C H, Wetterberg L 1981 Human embryonic somatomedin. Proceedings of the National Academy of Sciences 78: 3175–3179

Saudek C D, Finkowski M, Knopp R H 1975 Plasma glucagon and insulin in rat pregnancy. Journal of Clinical Investigation 55: 180–187

Scarlett J A, Gray R S, Griffin J, Olefsky J M, Kolterman O G 1982 Insulin Treatment reverses the Insulin Resistance of Type II Diabetes Mellitus. Diabetes Care 5: 353–363

Schopper K, Matter L, Flueler U, Werder E 1982 Diabetes Mellitus, endocrine antibodies and prenatal rubella infection. Lancet ii: 159

Shelley H J, Bassett J M, Milner R D G 1975 Carbohydrate metabolism. British Medical Bulletin 31: 37–43

Sherwin R S 1976 Hyperglucagonemia and blood glucose regulation in normal obese and diabetic subjects. New England Journal of Medicine 294: 494

Silver M 1976 Fetal energy metabolism In: Beard R W, Nathanielz P W (eds) Fetal Physiology and Medicine: The Basis of Perinatology, pp 173–193. W B Saunders, London

Silverman J L 1963 Eosinophilic infiltration in the pancreas of infants of diabetic mothers. A clinico-pathological study. Diabetes 12: 528–534

Simpson J L 1979 Genetics of Diabetes Mellitus and anomalies in offspring of diabetic mothers In: Merkatz I R, Adam P A J (ed) The Diabetic Pregnancy. A perinatal Perspective, pp 235–248. Grune Stratton, London

Smith B T, Grond C J P, Robert M F, Avery M E 1975 Insulin antagonism of cortisol action on lecithin synthesis by cultured fetal lung cells. Journal of Pediatrics 87: 953–955

Soler N G, Walsch C H, Malins J M 1976 Congenital malformations in infants of diabetic mothers. Quarterly Journal of Medicine 45: 303–313

Sosenko I R, Kitzmiller G L, Loo S W, Blix p, Rubenstein A H, Gabbay K H 1979 The infant of the diabetic mother: correlation of increased cord C. peptide levels with macrosomia and hypoglycaemia. New England Journal of Medicine 301: 859–862

Sparks J W, Hay W W, Bonds D, Meschia G, Battaglia F C 1982 Simultaneous measurements of lactate turnover rate and umbilical lactate uptake in the fetal lamb. Journal of Clinical Investigation 70: 170–192

Sridama V, Pacini F, Yang S L, Moawad A, Reilly M, Degroet J L 1982 Decreased levels of Helper T cells: a possible cause of immuno-deficiency in pregnancy. New England Journal of Medicine 307: 352–356

Stangenberg M, Persson M, Fredholm B B, Lindblad B S n, Stange L 1981 Insulin induced hypoglycaemia in diabetic women during late pregnancy and one year post-partum. British Journal of Obstetrics and Gynaecology 88. 619–627

Stangenberg M, Persson B, Fredholm B B, Lunell N O 1982a Profiles of intermediary metabolites in insulin dependent pregnant diabetic women with or without endogenous insulin production. Diabetes Care, 15: 409–413

Stangenberg M, Persson B, Vaclaninkova M 1982b Amniotic fluid volumes and concentrations of C. peptide in diabetic pregnancies. British Journal of Obstetrics and Gynaecology 89: 536–542

Steel J M, Irvine W J, Clarke B F 1980 The significance of pancreatic islet cell antibody and abnormal glucose tolerance during pregnancy. Journal of Clinical and Laboratory Immunology 4: 83–85

Stefan Y, Grasso S, Perrelet A, Orci L 1982 The pancreatic polyppeptide rich lobe in human pancreas: definitive identification of its derivation from the ventral pancreatic primordium. Diabetologia 23: 141–142

Stevenson D, Bartoletti S, Ostrander C R, Johnson J D 1979 Pulmonary excretion of carbone monoxide in the human infant as an index of bilirubin production. II. Infants of Diabetic Mothers. Journal of Pediatrics 94: 956–958

Stricklin G P, Welgus H G, Bauer E A 1982 Human skin collagenase in recessive dystrophic epidermolysis bullosa. Purification of a mutant enzyme from fibroblast. Journal of Clinical Investigation 69: 1373–1382

Stubbs W A, Stubbs S H 1978 Hyperinsulinism, diabetes mellitus and respiratory distress of the newborn, a common link? Lancet i: 308–309

Susa J B, Mc Cormick K L, Widness J A, Singer D B, Oh W, Adamsons K, Schwartz R 1979 Chronic hyperinsulinemia in the fetal Rhesus monkey. Effects of fetal growth and composition. Diabetes 28: 1058–1063

Sutherland H W, Pedersen J S, Molsted-Pedersen L 1981 Treatment of diabetic pregnancy: special reference to fetal growth In: Van Assche

F A, Robertson W P (eds) Fetal growth retardation, pp 197–207. Churchill Livingstone, Ediburgh

Swenne I 1982 Regulation of growth of the pancreatic B-cell: an experimental study in the rat, Acta Universitatis Upsaliensis. Abstracts of Uppsala Dissertations from the Faculty of Medicine 414, pp 1–33

Tamas G, Bekefi D, Gaal O 1975 Insulin antibodies in diabetic pregnancies. Lancet i: 521

Taylor C, Faulk W P 1981 Prevention of recurrent abortion with leukocyte transfusions. Lancet ii: 68–70

Teasdale F 1981 Histomorphometry of the placenta of the diabetic woman: classification of diabetes mellitus. Placenta 2: 241–252

Tejning S 1947 Dietary factors and quantitative morphology of the islets of Langerhans. Acta Medica Scandinavica Suppl 198: 1–154

Thomas K, de Gasparo M, Hoet J J 1967 Insulin levels in the umbilical vein and in the umbilical artery of newborns of normal and gestational diabetic mothers. Diabetologia 3: 299–304

Thomson A M, Billewicz W Z, Hytten F E 1968 The assessment of fetal growth. Journal of Obstetrics and Gynaecology of the British Commonwealth 75: 903–916

Tominanga T, Page E 1966 Accomodation of the human placenta to hypoxia, American Journal of Obstetrics and Gynecology 94: 679–691

Van Assche F A 1970 The fetal endocrine pancreas, a quantitative morphologic approach. Thesis, Katholieke Universiteit Leuven, Belgium

Van Assche F A, Aerts L 1975 Light and election microscopic study of the endocrine pancreas during normal pregnancy and diabetic pregnancy. Diabetologia ii: 381–389

Van Assche F A, Aerts L 1979 The maternal endocrine pancreas. In: Sutherland H W, Stowers J M (ed) Carbohydrate Metabolism in Pregnancy and the Newborn 1978, pp 115–131. Springer Verlag, Berlin

Van Assche F A, De Prins F, Aerts L, Verjasen M 1977 The endocrine pancreas in small for dates infants. British Journal of Obstetrics and Gynaecology 84: 751–753

Van Assche F A, Hoet J J, Jack P 1982 The endocrine pancreas of the pregnant mother, fetus and newborn In: Beard R W, Nathanielz P W (eds) Fetal Physiology and Medicine. W B Saunders, New York

Van Beek C 1939 Kan men aan een doodgeborene de diagnose diabetes mellitus der moeder stellen. Nederlands Tijdschrift voor Geneeskunde 83: 5973

Walton A, Hammond J 1938 The maternal effects on growth and conformation in Shire horse-Shetland pony crosses. Proceedings of the Royal Society of Medicine B 125: 311–335

Warth M R, Arky R A, Knopp R H 1975 Lipid metabolism in pregnancy III Altered lipid composition in intermediate, very low and high-density lipoprotein fractions. Journal of Clinical Endocrinology and Metabolism 41: 649–655

Watanabee G, Ingalls T H 1963 Congenital malformations in the offspring of alloxan diabetic mice. Diabetes 12: 66–72

Wellman K F, Volk B W 1977 The islets of infants of diabetic mothers In: Volk B W, Wellman K F (eds) The Diabetic Pancreas, pp 365–380. Plenum Press, New York

Whitelaw A 1977 Subcutaneous fat in newborn infants of diabetic mothers: an indication of quality of diabetic control. Lancet i: 15–18

WHO Expert Committee on Diabetes Mellitus, Second Report, 1980. Technical report series 646, Geneva

Widness J A, Susa J B, Garcia J F, Singer D B, Seghal P, Oh W, Schwartz R H C 1981 Increased erythropoiesis and elevated erythropoietin in infants born to diabetic mothers and in the hyperinsulinic Rhesus fetus. Journal of Clinical Investigation 67: 637–642

Winnick M, Noble A. 1967 Cellular growth in human placenta. II Diabetes mellitus. Journal of Pediatrics 72: 216–219

Wolfe R R, Way G L 1977 Cardiomyopathies in infants of diabetic mothers. Johns Hopkins Medical Journal 144: 177–180

Woolf N, Jackson W P U 1957 Maternal prediabetes and the foetal pancreas. Journal of Pathology and Bacteriology 74: 223–226

Yen S S C 1964 Abnormal carbohydrate metabolism and pregnancy: a study among pregnant Guamanian women. American Journal of Obstetrics and Gynecology 90: 468–473

Zimmet P, Taylor R, King H, Geddes W, Pargeter K 1981 The impact of modernization on the health of a Pacific nation. The Kiribati diabetes and cardio-vascular survey, pp 1–18. Australian Development Assistance Bureau, Melbourne

The thyroid and parathyroid glands in pregnancy

MATERNAL THYROID PHYSIOLOGY

The clinical impression presented by many women during pregnancy is one of mild hyperthyroidism. Bright-eyed with a warm moist skin and abundant energy, many pregnant women also have a raised pulse rate and sometimes palpitations. There may be heat intolerance and emotional lability, and laboratory tests can reveal an increased basal metabolic rate (Burrow, 1972) and raised level of protein-bound iodine (Heinemann et al 1948). If a goitre is present this almost always enlarges due to increased urinary loss of iodide although there is little evidence of increased thyrotrophic activity. In order, therefore, to appreciate the changes caused by hyperthyroidism during pregnancy it is essential to have a clear idea of normal maternal thyroid physiology and it should be admitted at once that there are considerable gaps in our knowledge, and in some areas frank disagreement, for example, over the role and nature of the placental thyrotrophins. Whether or not a normal woman is mildly hypermetabolic during pregnancy is largely a philosophical question as absolute standards are difficult to define; various physiological changes occur although the levels of free (unbound) thyroid hormones do not appear to increase.

Basal metabolic rate (BMR)

The elevation of the BMR in pregnancy has been carefully investigated, and is largely accounted for by the increase in oxygen demand by the fetus, enlarged uterus and maternal heart (Burwell 1954). Clearly therefore the BMR is no indicator of hyperthyroidism in the second or third trimesters.

Thyroid hormone levels

It has long been known that the protein bound iodine (PBI) level in the serum is raised during pregnancy. Radio-immunoassay of the total serum thyroxine (T4) concentration shows this to be similarly raised, and tri-iodo-thyronine (T3) slightly less so. These changes were eventually explained by Dowling et al (1956) and in 1960 when with Freinkel & Ingbar he showed that the level of thyroxine-binding-globulin (TBG) in the blood was elevated, thus providing increased binding sites for circulating thyroid hormones (Dowling et al, 1960). The reason for this elevated TBG, which is manufactured in the liver, is the raised oestrogen level in pregnancy, and similar changes are seen in women taking exogenous oestrogens such as the contraceptive pill. Although a raised TBG and total serum T4 might account for the clinical pattern of the mild hypermetabolic state seen in pregnancy, free (unbound) levels of thyroid hormones appear unchanged and both the volume of distribution and the fractional turnover of all thyroxine are decreased when measured using injected radio-iodine labelled T4. When corrected for the increase in maternal surface area during pregnancy, the net T4 turnover and hormonal requirements are in fact unchanged compared with the non-pregnant state (Dowling et al, 1967).

Thyroid enlargement

Where goitre is endemic, it is usual for the thyroid to increase in size during pregnancy (Crooks et al, 1964), and Halnan (1958) demonstrated that this was accompanied by an increased uptake of radioactive iodine in the thyroid and also, more importantly, by an increased clearance of urinary iodide (Crooks et al, 1967). Iodide clearance by the renal tubules is increased in the presence of oestrogens and probably accounts both for the so-called puberty goitre and for the prevalence of thyroid enlargement during pregnancy.

Thyrotrophins (TSH)

There are conflicting reports as to whether TSH is raised in the normal woman during pregnancy. If there is an increase in TSH, it is probably confined to the early part of pregnancy and some of these reported findings have been questioned (Malkasian & Mayberry, 1970). TSH can be measured by radio-immunoassay or bioassay and the results of these two very different techniques do not always correspond.

A more sensitive measure of TSH in pregnancy is the TSH response to thyrotrophin-releasing hormone (TRH) which is brisk in the euthyroid patient but absent in hyperthyroidism. Burrow et al (1975) studied the TSH response to TRH at various stages during pregnancy and compared these with non-pregnant controls and with women receiving oral contraceptives. In essence, the women who were 16–20 weeks pregnant had a greater TSH response than either the non-pregnant controls or those women in the 6–12 week period of pregnancy. Women on oral contraceptives had a response similar to the 16–20 weeks pregnant group. This increased TSH responsiveness is difficult to explain; it may reflect the enlarged TBG pool in pregnancy with its increased binding capacity for thyroid hormones or may be due to oestrogen induced TSH increase. The presence of increased TSH responsiveness is further evidence against increased thyroid activity *per se*, since a minimal rise in circulating thyroid hormones usually decreases the responsiveness to TSH.

Placental TSH

In 1965 Hennen introduced the possibility of a new factor which might explain some of the unusual laboratory findings in thyroid function during pregnancy. He showed that the normal placenta contained a thyroid stimulator and recent work suggests there may be more than one. On the one hand there is human chorionic gonadotrophin (hCG) which on a molecular basis has about 1/4000 the effectiveness of pituitary TSH (Hershman & Starnes, 1971; Hershman, 1972), and on the other hand there is the possibility of a specific human chorionic thyrotrophin (hCT) which has been shown to occur in quantities exceeding those of TSH in the pituitary itself and has about 60 per cent of its effectiveness (Tojo et al, 1973). By 1972 Hershman in Los Angeles had shown that there were large quantities of this hCT in hydatidiform mole and also in choriocarcinoma (see also the next section, on hydatidiform mole).

The clinical assessment of hyperthyroidism is notoriously difficult even with the most careful scoring indices and therefore it is not surprising that some observers (such as Hershman himself) have recorded a frequent association of hyperthyroidism with hydatidiform mole while others, like Galton et al (1971), have commented that most of their patients with this condition were euthyroid. Valerie Galton has had exceptional experience in this field, with access to patients not only in the United States and Mexico but from Japan as well; her work suggests that much of the increased TSH activity noted in the past is related to the contribution of hCG which has TSH-like activity but which does not

usually produce clinical hyperthyroidism. It is interesting that patients with multiple pregnancies also have high levels of hCG in their blood, sometimes as high as those seen in hydatidiform mole, but their thyroid function remains normal.

Hydatidiform mole

In 1972 Hershman reviewed thyroid function in patients with benign and malignant trophoblastic tumours and reported 37 with increased thyroid function but without clear clinical evidence of hyperthyroidism; however, eight patients with hydatidiform mole had clinical hyperthyroidism and five with choriocarcinoma also showed evidence of this.

The thyrotrophin in hydatidiform moles has been extracted, purified and identified. This molar TSH (or hMT, human molar thyrotrophin) has a longer duration of action than pituitary TSH, in the mouse bioassay. A further problem is that high levels of human chorionic gonadotrophin (hCG) have also been produced by these tumours and this, too, is a weak thyroid stimulator. It has been suggested that hMT may in fact be hCG or a precursor for hCG. Such enormous quantities of hCG are produced by a hydatidiform mole that the concentration is capable of causing significant thyroid stimulation even including clinical hyperthyroidism.

Thyroid tests in pregnancy

Radioactive iodine must never be used to test thyroid function in a pregnant woman since after 10–12 weeks the isotope is concentrated significantly in the fetal thyroid (Fisher & Dussault, 1974), and after that in amounts much greater than in the maternal thyroid (Fisher et al, 1970). Thus the risks of inducing malignant change in the child's thyroid at some later date must be quite high, and other radionuclides, e.g. ^{99m}Tc, should also be avoided.

The laboratory tests which can safely be used are summarised in Table 15.1 where the results obtained in pregnancy are compared with those in non-pregnant women. There is no golden rule for the interpretation of these tests and due allowance must be made for such factors as iodine deficiency, iodine excess or the taking of various medicines which have an effect on thyroid metabolism (De Visscher & Burger, 1980).

Biochemical assessment of the pregnant woman's thyroid status is complicated by her high TBG levels which produce a corresponding increase in total circulating thyroid hormone levels. Measurement of the total serum T4, the most widely available test of thyroid function, is thus misleadingly high in pregnancy.

Metabolically active (free, unbound) T4 constitutes less than 0.05 per cent of the total serum T4 and assays for this free component are now available. In the free thyroxine

Table 15.1 Thyroid Function Tests in Pregnancy

Test	Normal Range in Women	Euthyroid	Pregnant women Hyperthyroid	Hypothyroid
T4 (nmol/l)	60–128	Raised	Raised	Normal or low
T3 (nmol/l)	1.2–2.8	Raised	Raised	Normal or low
T3 resin uptake	Depends on laboratory	Low	Normal or raised	Low
Free T4 index	technique	Normal	Raised	Low
Free T4 (nmol/l)	12–36	Normal	Raised	Low
Free T3 (pmol/l)	6–12	Normal	Raised	Normal or low
TSH (μu/ml)	0.5–6	Normal	Low	Raised
TSH in TRH test (μu/ml)	8–30	Normal	Low	Raised

index the degree of saturation of TBG binding sites is determined by the T3 resin uptake test. The patient's serum sample is incubated with a known quantity of radioiodine-labelled T3 and any excess labelled T3, which is not immediately bound to the patient's TBG, is absorbed onto an ion-exchange resin and measured directly, the result being expressed as a percentage of the initial dose. This figure is then divided by the mean value determined for a normal population studied by the same laboratory to give the T3 resin uptake (RT3U) which is multiplied by the total serum T4 to give the free thyroxine index:

$$FT4I = \frac{patient's\ RT3U}{mean\ normal\ RT3U} \times total\ serum\ T4$$

A high resin uptake value indicates increased saturation of TBG and therefore a higher fraction of the total serum T4 must be unbound, confirming hyperthyroidism. Values obviously vary between laboratories but a normal RT3U result is around 25–35 per cent. In pregnancy the increased TBG level results in a lower saturation, usually less than 25 per cent.

The free triiodothyronine index (FT3I) is the product of the T3 resin uptake test and the total serum T3. It can be useful in distinguishing thyrotoxicosis when the FT4I is borderline, and is of course raised in T3-toxicosis.

Serum TSH concentrations (usually less than 5 mU/l) can be measured precisely by radio-immunoassay and, as already discussed, are usually in the non-pregnant range though there may be a small rise in the first trimester. Subclinical (latent) hypothyroidism may cause elevation of the TSH while other tests of thyroid function are still normal. Serial determination of TSH levels is a useful way of monitoring thyroxine dosage in hypothyroidism as adequate treatment suppresses TSH to within the normal range.

Serum thyroid auto-antibodies, to thyroglobulin or microsomes, are occasionally detected in pregnancy and in the euthyroid woman may herald the development of auto-immune hypothyroidism or hyperthyroidism later in pregnancy, or even during the puerperium. A previous history, or family history, of thyroid disease therefore makes this test advisable. It is now being recognised that a fall in the level of antibodies in pregnancy may herald a transient attack of hyperthyroidism postpartum which then gradually leads into hypothyroidism.

FETAL AND NEONATAL THYROID PHYSIOLOGY

The development of neonatal thyroid function

The evolution of the fetal thyroid gland and its eventual independent functioning have been as intensively studied as maternal thyroid physiology. The first signs of thyroid tissue develop about the 15th day of fetal life and during the next 2 weeks the gland migrates from the foramen caecum at the base of the tongue down to its final site just below and adjoining the thyroid cartilage. By 32 days there are two lobes, and some rapidly dividing cells begin to have the appearance of follicles; a little intracellular colloid is evident between 10 and 12 weeks (Shepard, 1967). Studies with radioactive iodine, which for the most part have been carried out on women about to undergo therapeutic abortion, have confirmed that the fetal thyroid can concentrate the isotope at this time, with organic binding and the first synthesis of iodinated thyronines (Hodges et al, 1955; Evans et al, 1967). At about 12 weeks there is also evidence of TSH in the pituitary (Fisher, 1973) so that by the end of the first trimester the pituitary-thyroid axis is already present and apparently capable of function.

Is the fetal hypothalamo-pituitary-thyroid system developing and functioning independently of the mother's hormonal climate by this stage? It appears likely that the fetus is indeed independent because the placenta is essentially impermeable to TSH (Jost & Picon, 1970), T4 (Osorio & Myant 1960) and T3 (Fisher et al, 1973) in the human as well as in most experimental animals; there is also no correlation between maternal and fetal concentrations of T4, T3 or TSH at any time during pregnancy. The levels of T4 and TSH in fetal blood only reach significant levels by 18 to 20 weeks, after which they show an abrupt rise. Normal levels are only recorded by about the middle of the second trimester, and these are confirmed by the similar pattern of appearance of FSH, LH and hCG in the fetus (Fisher, 1975).

Following the sudden rise in fetal T4 and TSH around 20 weeks, from 22 to 26 weeks the fetal TSH continues to rise until it exceeds the maternal level. This appears to be due to a concurrent increase in TBG levels, stimulated by placental oestrogens in the fetus. Around this time there is histological evidence of maturation of the hypothalamus and of the hypothalamo-pituitary portal blood system in the pituitary stalk. These changes would allow central neural stimuli to be transmitted to the pituitary and presumably levels of thyrotrophin-releasing hormone (TRH) must be similarly elevated. Naturally much of the research in this field has been done, perforce, in animals, particularly the sheep and rat; species differences must be borne in mind and the results not extrapolated uncritically to the human. Indeed the newborn rat is probably only at the level of development of the human fetus during the third trimester, and many of the changes which occur *in utero* in man are mirrored by those in the newborn rat during its first few days of independent life.

It is important to point out at this stage that whereas TSH, T4 and T3 do not pass through the human placenta, iodides and most of the anti-thyroid medicines in current use do so freely. This explains some of the problems encountered when hyperthyroidism is being treated in the mother.

Probably the most important fact to emerge in recent studies of the human fetus and neonate is the presence of high levels of reverse T3 (rT3) in the blood (Chopra et al, 1975). This is a normal fetal constituent at this period and is produced as a result of the metabolism of thyroxine in the peripheral tissues of the infant. Since rT3 has practically no metabolic action it is surprising that the concentration of normal T3 in the fetus is so much lower than in the adult. The higher level of rT3 in the cord blood of the neonate than in maternal blood, with T3 being lower than in the mother, offers a useful method of diagnosing infant hypothyroidism, the importance of which will be discussed later in this chapter. At the same time the determination of rT3 in amniotic fluid offers the possibility of diagnosing fetal hypothyroidism during pregnancy by amniotic puncture. Whether or not the amniotic fluid also offers a route for the treatment of the hypothyroid fetus is at present purely conjectural.

The maturation of nervous tissue in the fetus

The need for normal levels of thyroid hormone to ensure development of the fetal brain has been known for over 100 years, and indeed it has been recorded from ancient times that where goitre is severely endemic there will be found a certain number of cretins who show retarded growth of the brain and body. The word cretin is often used wrongly and the Oxford English Dictionary states that it comes from the Swiss patois and means a Christian, i.e. a 'human creature' as distinguished from the brutes: the sense here is that these beings are really human despite their physical and mental deformity. Thus, sporadic congenital hypothyroidism should not be described as cretinism and the more recent use of 'cretin' as slang is another good reason for reserving it for the endemic condition. The development of the fetal brain is peculiarly sensitive to the action of T4 and T3, demonstrating more clearly than any other tissue the effects of hypothyroidism, and for this reason has been

thoroughly investigated. The review by Brasel in the Kroc Foundation Symposium on Perinatal Thyroid Physiology and Disease is an excellent source of information in this field (Brasel & Boyd, 1975). Since it is difficult to obtain human tissue to study, much of our information comes from animal work and again it is unwise to extrapolate these findings to man. In severe hypothyroidism in the fetus the axones are poorly myelinated and the neurones display inadequate dendritic arborisation so that only a few synapses develop normally. Recent work on the rat cerebellum by Nunez (Francon et al, 1977) showed that microtubule assembly was abnormal and this was due, not to the amount of tubulin itself, but to lack of a substance required for its assembly, the so-called 'tau' factor (Weingarten et al, 1975). Since thyroid hormones are necessary for this factor, especially during the first weeks of post-natal life in the rat, normal nerve growth is limited in experimental hypothyroidism.

One of the main techniques used to assess brain development has been the accurate measurement of brain DNA concentration, which is a good measure of cell density and therefore cell size (Balázs, 1972). In hypothyroidism both the total cell mass and the proper differentiation of individual neural units is reduced. These prenatal changes, if followed by severe untreated hypothyroidism for some time after birth, can result in irreversible damage to brain growth. Perhaps the most important lesson from these observations is that systematic screening for congenital hypothyroidism should be adopted universally.

Hypothyroidism in the fetal and neonatal period may also result from an abnormality in embryological development of the thyroid gland. The lingual thyroid, the partially undescended thyroid and athyreosis are often associated, with stunting of stature and inadequate secretion of thyroid hormones. To these anomalies must be added those inherited or inborn errors of thyroid hormone synthesis; all these conditions produce infantile hypothyroidism, screening tests for which are discussed later in this chapter.

Neonatal development

Studies on the development of the human neonate in conditions of hypothyroidism are conspicuous for their scarcity, and for this reason much of our knowledge is derived from the experimental rat. It has already been pointed out that the newborn rat develops more like the human fetus during the third trimester, and therefore too close a comparison of the animal model with the human should not be made.

It appears that in the rat the secretion of hormones by the hypothalamus, pituitary and thyroid begins at approximately the same time, and all three organs mature together. According to Dussault (1975), peak values for TRH coincide well with the serum T4 levels and it is not difficult to compare these rat findings with those in the human. At human birth the level of T3 is almost undetectable but rises swiftly within hours of delivery (Chopra et al, 1975). At this time rT3 levels are already high. In the latter part of pregnancy the fetal T4 levels normally exceed those of the mother, as already indicated, and it is tempting to suggest that the improvement in symptoms occasionally reported in hypothyroid mothers during the latter part of pregnancy may be due to the transplacental transfer of fetal thyroid hormones to the mother (Montgomery, 1979).

The effect of maternal hypothyroidism on fetal development has been investigated by a number of workers, especially Graham & Blizzard (1973), and Stanbury & Kroc (1972). Evelyn Man (Man et al, 1971) studied the IQ of children (mainly 4–7 years old) born of hypothyroid mothers not adequately treated in pregnancy; the scores of subsequent children, born from treated pregnancies, were significantly better.

The question as to whether thyroid medication of mothers who are grossly hypothyroid has an effect on subsequent fetal development has been answered in part by the field studies in which grossly iodine-deficient women were injected with iodised poppy seed oil (Lipiodol) and their subsequent pregnancies monitored. For example, in Western New Guinea which contains an area of extreme endemic goitre, Adams et al (1968) found a high incidence of goitre and associated defects, including mental deficiency, motor abnormalities, deafness and deaf mutism. According to the time in pregnancy when the iodised oil was given they concluded that 'damage to the defectives is done in the early months of pregnancy, and may at least be due in part to maternal hypothyroidism'.

Neonatal hormone levels

In recent years a great deal of research has been directed to the changes in the level of thyroid hormones in the newborn baby (Ginsberg et al, 1978). At birth there is a rapid rise in the neonatal TSH and this is accompanied by a marked increase in serum T3 followed later by a rise in T4. The levels of free T3 and free T4 are correspondingly elevated, and these produce the characteristic metabolic changes. It is not yet clear why high levels of rT3 are seen in the neonate, nor why they fall subsequently, changes which appear independent of T3 concentrations. Presumably two different systems de-iodinate the iodo-thyronines but the reason for this is not known.

Screening the newborn for hypothyroidism

There are many possible causes of hypothyroidism in infancy: agenesis or dysgenesis of the thyroid gland, inborn errors of thyroid metabolism, ingestion by the mother of goitrogenic drugs (especially the anti-thyroid preparations and iodides), and not least endemic goitre. No matter what the cause, it is important that the infant should be treated as early as possible and this has led to the introduction of screening methods which can detect hypothyroidism in the first days of life.

Most screening techniques rely on a sample of cord or heel prick blood, which is dried on filter paper and sent to a central laboratory where it can be analysed (Dussault & Laberge, 1973). If cord blood is used the timing of the sample is of course crucial since the changes which have been reported above in the level of the various constituents are most marked in the first 24 hours. Therefore a sample of heel capillary blood taken at 5–10 days and preferably repeated at 6 weeks provides a maximum of information, since there is minimal transfer of T4, T3 and TSH through the placenta and a rapid rise in TSH in the neonate. T3 levels do not faithfully represent thyroid status so that estimation of T4 and TSH are most informative, the 6-week sample being timed to follow the levelling off of TSH. Reverse T3 is virtually absent in congenital hypothyroidism (Burger et al, 1976). Results vary from centre to centre but approximately one child in every 4000 live births is likely to show a lowered level of thyroid hormones and immediate treatment can be instigated. Transplacental passage of blocking antibodies is a recognised but very rare cause of neonatal hypothyroidism.

Neonatal thyrotoxicosis

Hyperthyroidism is rare in the newborn and often the mother is similarly affected, or has had Graves' disease in the past (Hollingsworth & Mabry, 1975). The presence of a high titre of thyroid stimulating immuno-globulins (TSI) in both fetus and mother is one of the strongest arguments in support of the view that TSI's are of importance in the aetiology of Graves' disease (Munro, 1977).

There is a close relationship between the level of TSIs in the fetus and in the mother during the last trimester of pregnancy, and high maternal levels may help to predict Graves's disease in the baby. In a highly selected group of 96 pregnancies, Munro encountered no fewer than 12 examples of neonatal thyrotoxicosis, many of the mothers having a history of previous babies with the syndrome. Occasionally, a hyperthyroid neonate has a euthyroid mother, but then there is often a tell-tale scar on the mother's neck where the disease has previously been treated, or a history of Graves' disease responsive to anti-thyroid drugs.

The syndrome in the newborn is not usually difficult to control and responds well to propranolol and either carbimazole or propylthiouracil. The TSIs do not remain for many weeks in the infant's blood and spontaneous recovery is thus the rule. More rarely the hyperthyroidism persists and requires treatment in the growing child. The accompanying exophthalmos frequently fails to regress, and if control is not careful the child may show more rapid growth than normal. There is usually a strong history of Graves' disease in such patients. General consensus now recommends surgical treatment in children with severe hyperthyroidism as soon as they are of school age and certainly before puberty. Severe hyperthyroidism in a child can be defined as that which is difficult to control medically and, as such, interferes with normal schooling.

HYPERTHYROIDISM IN PREGNANCY

Although women with severe hyperthyroidism are unlikely to become pregnant, those with mild or moderate over-activity of the thyroid gland frequently do so. It is then necessary to control the hyperthyroidism — since there is no specific cure — in order to safeguard the health of the mother and to maintain optimal conditions for the normal development of the fetus. The problems of diagnosis, both clinical and laboratory, have already been discussed and we are therefore now concerned solely with treatment.

The use of radioactive iodine is absolutely contraindicated during pregnancy because of the risks of radiation to the fetal thyroid and the subsequent development of thyroid cancer. The choice therefore lies between anti-thyroid drug therapy and surgery; there are those who plead eloquently for each of these lines of treatment. In the hands of a skilled thyroid surgeon who frequently performs subtotal thyroidectomy there is no doubt that this operation provides almost instantaneous relief of thyrotoxicosis with a minimum of risk. On the other hand it is equally possible for a physician to control the condition successfully with anti-thyroid drugs in such a way that the woman is delivered of a normal full-term fetus. What then are the advantages and disadvantages of these two modes of therapy?

Anti-thyroid therapy

Propylthiouracil (PTU), carbimazole and methimazole can all be used to control hyperthyroidism. PTU not only restricts T4 synthesis but also blocks the peripheral conversion of T4 to T3. All three drugs freely cross the placenta and if given in excess will produce a goitre in the fetus since it too will be producing TSH during the second and third trimesters. Some clinicians have used Fraser's technique (Fraser & Wilkinson, 1953), so successful in non-pregnant women, of adding thyroxine to the anti-thyroid drug and thus blocking overactivity of the thyroid gland but ensuring a normal circulating level of thyroid hormone. In pregnancy T4 does not cross the placenta and therefore with high doses of anti-thyroid substance the fetal thyroid will be blocked. In the early days of anti-thyroid therapy it was not unusual in the obstetric ward to see a woman with well-controlled hyperthyroidism delivered of a baby with a fair-sized goitre. Almost always the thyroid enlarge-

ment would disappear spontaneously in the early weeks of life and it is not difficult to treat the baby's hypothyroidism, which resolves when the residual drugs have been metabolised. No difference has been detected in IQ or development between children whose mothers received anti-thyroid drugs throughout pregnancy and their non-exposed siblings, in various studies. Nor have specific malformations been noted in the offspring of mothers treated with PTU and carbimazole. Methimazole, to which carbimazole is converted in vivo, has been rarely associated with aplasia of the skin of the scalp in the baby at birth (McCarroll et al, 1976).

In patients with severe hyperthyroidism, the use of the beta-adrenergic blocking agents, especially propranolol, is particularly valuable and no harm has been reported from its short-term use in low dosage in the pregnant hyperthyroid mother. However the chronic use of propranolol during pregnancy, or use in high dosage (240 mg/day) in the management of phaeochromocytoma during pregnancy, has been reported as causing intra-uterine growth retardation, hypoglycaemia and bradycardia, producing small for dates infants with a small placenta (Lowe et al, 1976; Goluboff et al, 1974).

β-agonists often used to treat premature labour must never be given to women who are or have been thyrotoxic because of maternal and fetal risks.

Iodides are the traditional way of controlling hyperthyroidism, although their effectiveness may not be long-lived. In a small proportion of patients the chronic use of the iodide may result in goitre formation and has been reported as causing a fetal goitre sufficiently large to asphyxiate the infant at birth (Ayromlooi, 1972). Preparations containing iodide should therefore not be used at all throughout pregnancy.

The secret of successful management of the hyperthyroid pregnant woman is regular adjustment of the dose of the drug to the patient's clinical and laboratory status so that the hyperthyroidism is controlled with a minimum of therapy. In the postpartum period, however, there are two potential hazards.

In the first place all the anti-thyroid drugs are not only secreted in the mother's milk but some of them are concentrated there so that if the baby is breast fed it will receive a considerable dose of the anti-thyroid agent and this is most undesirable. Propylthiouracil offends least in this respect. The baby must therefore be weaned and the mother's milk-flow dried up as conveniently and comfortably as possible for her. The other problem is that most patients with hyperthyroidism in pregnancy become less toxic and there is a tendency for the disease to flare up in the postpartum period; the mother must therefore be kept under close observation for some months after childbirth. Finally the thyrotoxic woman who wishes to become pregnant may also be treated by the use of anti-thyroid drugs but must inform her physician as soon as she believes she is pregnant, so that management can be changed as necessary.

Thyroidectomy

There are many excellent reports in the literature of considerable series of pregnant women who have had their hyperthyroidism treated by subtotal thyroidectomy during the second trimester with the delivery of a normal healthy fetus at term, for example that of Hawe & Francis (1962) and Holt et al (1970). However in recent years this form of therapy has rather fallen into desuetude, probably for two reasons. On the one hand there has been increasing skill in the management of the disease using anti-thyroid drugs, especially since the risks of damaging the fetal thyroid by overdosing the mother have been realised (Selenkow, 1972). Secondly the skills of the surgeon in performing thyroidectomy for hyperthyroidism have been diminished by the success and availability of radioactive iodine for treating this disease, which is the commonest form of treatment in most countries except the United Kingdom.

The advantages of subtotal thyroidectomy during the second trimester lie in rendering the patient euthyroid almost immediately with little risk of anoxaemia to the fetus during anaesthesia, and there is little or no risk of abortion by this stage. Thirdly the mother will be able to breast feed her baby if she so wishes as she will no longer require anti-thyroid drugs which would otherwise be excreted in her milk. The psychological effects of thyroidectomy in hyperthyroidism should not be underestimated and patients who have been controlled on one occasion with anti-thyroid drugs and on another occasion by thyroidectomy are known to volunteer that the latter technique has much to commend it. In skilled hands the chances of damage to the parathyroids or recurrent laryngeal nerves is minimal. In addition, thyroidectomy is the only form of treatment which permanently reduces the levels of human thyroid stimulating immunoglobulins although there is some reduction during carbimazole therapy and a transient fall after [131]I.

Thyroid crisis

Thyroid crisis (otherwise known as thyroid storm) is very rare in pregnancy. Most women affected were known to be thyrotoxic either during or before the pregnancy and did not receive anti-thyroid therapy when pregnant. The crisis is usually characterised by restlessness, dehydration, tachycardia and hyperpyrexia. The exhausted mother is at risk of losing her baby either spontaneously or during Caesarean section. Heart failure may complicate the thyrotoxicosis, especially if there is pre-existing mitral stenosis (Howe & Francis, 1961).

Adequate hydration is essential, and the fever may respond to tepid sponging, though chlorpromazine may also be necessary. An early reduction in thyroid hormone secretion is secured with aqueous potassium iodide (0.1–0.5 ml/day) given orally or intravenously; the drug is discontinued once control is achieved. Propylthiouracil (up to 150 mg 4 times a day) produces a slower but more prolonged reduction in circulating thyroid hormone concentrations, and is maintained when iodine treatment has been discontinued. Propranolol in modest dosage and for a few weeks only is probably safe in pregnancy, and provides effective beta-blockade against the peripheral effects of thyroxine, particularly the restlessness and tachycardia.

HYPOTHYROIDISM IN PREGNANCY

Severely myxoedematous women rarely become pregnant, and are at risk of spontaneous abortion and stillbirth. Lesser degrees of hypothyroidism in pregnancy may be suspected from excessive fatigue, suggestive facies (a dry skin, pallor and excessive weight gain) and slow relaxing reflexes. The diagnosis must be confirmed biochemically and is characterised by a low serum thyroxine, T3 and free thyroxine index in the face of a raised TSH level (Table 15.1). In mild cases the T3 is often normal. Adequate treatment with thyroxine (0.1–0.2 mg/day) restores all these hormone levels to the normal range, and biochemical monitoring should continue throughout pregnancy and also during the puerperium.

THYROID CANCER AND PREGNANCY

The development of carcinoma of the thyroid in pregnancy is very rare but the presence of palpable nodules in the neck should raise suspicion of the diagnosis and the patient should be submitted to surgery during the second trimester. One of the authors has seen a solitary nodule in the thyroid gland increase considerably in size during pregnancy and then shrink in the puerperium; when removed, because the mother contemplated a further pregnancy, the nodule was found to be a well-differentiated papillary carcinoma.

A previous history of carcinoma of the thyroid is not a contraindication to pregnancy and the survey by Rosvoll & Winship (1965) showed that pregnancy did not adversely affect the prognosis of patients with treated thyroid cancer. Any woman who has been treated surgically for either papillary or well-differentiated follicular carcinoma of the thyroid and who is taking suppressive thyroxine treatment should be advised to continue this during pregnancy; if there is any increase in the size of the remnant of the thyroid gland, the dose should be increased. Blood samples should be taken for TSH estimation to allow adjustment of the dose of thyroxine until adequate suppression of TSH is achieved. Montgomery (1979) records ten patients who previously had excision of thyroid carcinomas, who subsequently bore 13 children between them without loss.

THE PARATHYROID GLANDS

It is not surprising that there are so many gaps in our knowledge of calcium metabolism and the function of the parathyroid glands in pregnancy and the neonate since it is only recently that accurate measurements of serum calcium have become generally available in many hospitals as a result of the introduction of the auto-analyser. Biochemical screening with this device has revealed hyperparathyroidism as one of the commonest endocrine diseases, being detected in about one in every 1000 adults in the UK and USA. Many of these patients with a mildly raised serum calcium, usually due to a tiny adenoma in one parathyroid gland, are asymptomatic and it is still a matter for debate whether they should undergo operation to remove the adenoma. As to fetal parathyroid function, most of our knowledge is derived from animal studies and there is not a great deal of this. Virtually the only abnormality of parathyroid function to be recorded in the neonate is manifested as tetany in the newborn and this may be a useful diagnostic clue to unrecognised hyperparathyroidism in the mother. However, hyperparathyroidism does occur extremely rarely in the neonatal period.

Physiology of the parathyroid glands in pregnancy

The full-term fetus contains between 25 and 30 g of calcium which are obtained from the mother via the placenta mainly during the third trimester. Thus the mother's calcium metabolism undergoes widespread and profound changes during pregnancy and these are reflected in the hormonal changes during pregnancy which accompany them (Pitkin, 1975). In the first place the additional calcium which must be absorbed from the diet is obtained by a rise in the level of 1,25 dihydroxycholecalciferol which is a metabolite of vitamin D produced during its transit through the liver and the kidney, as first described by DeLuca (1973). The mother's supply of vitamin D comes largely from the effect of sunlight on the skin and from the diet. It is significant that vegetarian diets are particularly low in their content of vitamin D in many countries.

Another source of calcium from the mother is from mobilisation of her own stores in the skeleton. This is brought about primarily by parathyroid hormone which induces subperiosteal resorption of bone. Thus it is not surprising that the maternal level of parathyroid hormone has been reported as rising in the latter half of pregnancy and not falling completely until the end of lactation, since a supply of calcium is also required for the milk flow. It is believed that the rise in 1,25 dihydroxycholecalciferol together with increased calcium absorption from the gut is responsible for the transfer of the necessary calcium to the developing fetus. In healthy women there are conflicting reports on whether or not the level of PTH rises in pregnancy but on balance it seems unnecessary that it should, on an adequate European style diet.

How then does the mother protect her skeleton from this calcium loss? Whitehead et al (1981) from King's College Hospital and Hammersmith Hospital in London studied a group of healthy volunteers throughout pregnancy and lactation, and found a significant rise in their calcitonin levels. It was necessary to concentrate the levels of the hormone before radio-immunoassay since they are extremely low in women. These workers suggest that an important function of calcitonin is the protection of the healthy maternal skeleton from excessive subperiosteal resorption. The raised level of calcitonin during lactation would also support such a proposition.

Hyperparathyroidism in pregnancy

Hyperparathyroidism is very rare in pregnancy and when Ludwig (1962) reviewed the literature he could only report 40 pregnancies in 21 mothers with primary hyperparathyroidism and they showed a complication rate of 50 per cent. Delmonico et al (1976) found the complication rate to be 80 per cent in the 13 patients whom they described. Since Petit & Clark (1947) described their successful removal of a parathyroid adenoma during pregnancy there have only been a further 13 similar cases (including one of the authors') described in the literature and it is satisfactory to report that in all of these patients complications have been remarkably few. In 1979 three patients were reported from Hammersmith Hospital who had hyperparathyroidism in pregnancy upon whom one of the authors had operated (Salem & Taylor 1979).

The first patient was transferred to the hospital extremely ill with emaciation, thirst, nausea and skeletal pains. She had been delivered 2 weeks previously by Caesarean section at full term for a transverse lie. Relevant investigations were as follows: serum calcium 3.8 mmol/l (normal 2.15–2.65); serum phosphorus 1.1 mmol/l (normal 0.8–1.4); total proteins 66 g/l (normal 65–80); alkaline phosphatase 1155 i.u./l (normal 30–130); serum magnesium 0.3 mmol/l (normal 0.8–1.2). X-rays of her hands showed marked subperiosteal erosions, bone resorption and early cyst formation and X-ray of the skull showed a classic 'pepper-pot' effect.

An attempt to control her hypercalcaemia was made using calcitonin intravenously, a fluid diuresis and oral phosphates. Her magnesium deficiency was also corrected. However, despite good rehydration, the calcium level could not be controlled and on the third day after admission surgical exploration of the neck was performed. A parathyroid adenoma $3 \times 2.5 \times 2$ cm was removed from the lower right position. Postoperative recovery was complicated by hypocalcaemia which was controlled with calcium gluconate i.v. and she received oral calcium and vitamin D for a further 2 months. Her recovery was complete and she remains normocalcaemic. In 1978 she had a normal pregnancy and delivery with no complications.

The second patient had had three previous miscarriages and her recent pregnancy had been complicated by a threatened abortion at 11 weeks. The baby was born prematurely at 35 weeks. Three days postpartum the baby developed tetany and this was shown to be due to hypocalcaemia. Investigation of the mother showed a normal serum calcium and phosphorus level and a raised alkaline phosphatase. She was thought to have mild osteomalacia due to an inadequate intake of vitamin D during her pregnancy, and she was treated with a short course of the vitamin.

Two months after completing this course her serum calcium level had risen to 2.8 mmol/l (normal 2.15–2.65) and her serum phosphorus was at the lower limit of normal. The results of other biochemical estimations were normal. The serum parathyroid hormone (PTH) level was 1.1 μg/l (normal <0.75). A diagnosis of primary hyperparathyroidism was made and, at operation, a small parathyroid tumour ($0.5 \times 0.4 \times 0.2$ cm) was removed from the left upper position. The patient made a satisfactory recovery and her serum calcium remains in the normal range.

The third patient had had two normal pregnancies in the previous eleven years. During 1976 and 1977 she had had several attacks of renal colic and was eventually investigated and found to have hypercalciuria and mild hypercalcaemia (Ca^{++} 2.7 mmol/l) thought to be due to mild hyperparathyroidism. The serum calcium levels were controlled at that time by dietary measures alone. However, when she became pregnant it was felt that she should have surgical treatment for the hyperparathyroidism and at 22 weeks gestation she had an adenoma of the parathyroid ($1.5 \times 0.7 \times 0.5$ cm) removed from the left lower position. Apart from a little temporary hypocalcaemia which was treated with oral calcium supplements she made an uneventful recovery. She continued on oral calcium for the rest of her pregnancy and had a normal delivery at full term of a healthy female baby. There were no neonatal complications.

These three patients illustrate most of the features of this rare condition and also underline the fact that removal of the parathyroid adenoma provides a virtual cure. It is important to monitor the level of serum calcium in the mother daily after operation since hypocalcaemia is common and tetany may develop. Adequate hydration is essential and the addition of calciferol 500 units daily will enable the patient to obtain from her diet the calcium she requires. If, however, tetany occurs it is wise to infuse a dilute solution of calcium and this is best managed by adding 10 ml of 10 per cent calcium gluconate to a unit of saline and administering this slowly intravenously. Rapid injection of calcium solutions can cause flushing, headache and even in extreme circumstances cardiac arrest.

Neonatal hypoparathyroidism

This rare abnormality of parathyroid function in the newborn presents as tetany and the usual cause of this is hyperparathyroidism in the mother. Thus, if it occurs, the mother's serum calcium should immediately be estimated and should be repeated on a number of days since the level regularly rises and falls in HPT. The presence of neonatal tetany is often the first indication that the mother has hyperparathyroidism.

Calcium ions can move freely across the placenta but the parathyroid hormone does not cross from mother to fetus (Northrop et al, 1977) so a raised calcium level in the mother will pass through the placenta to the fetus (Wagner et al, 1964) and this can in its turn suppress the secretion of parathyroid hormone by the fetal parathyroids (Bruce & Strong, 1955).

Levels of parathyroid hormone in the neonate may vary from laboratory to laboratory and it is helpful to know the normal for the particular technique which is being used. In addition it should be remembered that mothers may show an elevated level of parathyroid hormone during the latter part of pregnancy, possibly due to inadequate calcium in the diet and lack of sun, and it has been proposed by Bakwin (1937) that the fall in the circulating calcium which is recorded soon after birth in the baby is due to underactivity of the parathyroid glands which could be related to the hyperactivity of the maternal parathyroids in pregnancy.

Tetany due to hypoparathyroidism in the newborn is usually shortlived as the parathyroid glands recover their normal function spontaneously. If, however, tetany is severe it should be treated with intravenous calcium gluconate and oral 1-alpha-hydroxy-vitamin D3.

Neonatal hyperparathyroidism

This, the rarest of all the endocrine abnormalities to be dealt with here, is appropriately last. Only sixteen cases have been described in the literature and we have experience of one more (Lynn, 1982, personal communication). The condition was first reported by Pratt et al (1947) and is a serious and life-threatening disorder which affects the neonate in the first few days of life and sometimes even *in utero*. The baby often appears normal at birth but rapidly develops hypotonia and feeds poorly, has constipation and fails to thrive. If unrecognised or left untreated the hypercalcaemia reaches extreme levels of 6 mmol/l or more. The skeleton is soon involved with widespread demineralisation of the bones and, as a result, a common complication is rib fractures. Respiratory distress follows and is the commonest cause of death (Thompson et al, 1978). The condition may be familial but no connection has been discovered with the multiple endocrine neoplasia syndromes.

Marx et al (1982) first drew attention to an association between neonatal severe primary hyperparathyroidism and familial hypocalciuric hypercalcaemia. This variety of raised serum calcium presents as a familial abnormality with no detectable changes in the parathyroid glands and no increased excretion of calcium in the urine which is typical of HPT. It appears that the parathyroid glands in familial hypercalcaemic hypocalciuria are less sensitive than normal to the concentration of serum ionised calcium

(Thorgeirsson et al, 1981) and this would provide a possible explanation for neonatal hyperparathyroidism if the newborn inherited an extreme form of this insensitivity to its circulating calcium level. At the present time treatment is best managed by radical subtotal parathyroidectomy; even as little as half of one gland can regenerate and cause a return of the disease (Thompson et al, 1978). Alternatively total parathyroidectomy with replacement therapy of 1-alpha-hydroxy-vitamin D3 and calcium is equally successful and there is evidence from a single case (Lynn, 1982, personal communication) of normal calcium homeostasis returning after one year and further replacement therapy being unnecessary.

REFERENCES

Adams D D, Kennedy T H, Choufoer J C, Querido A 1968 Endemic goiter in Western New Guinea. III. Thyroid-stimulating activity of serum from severely iodine-deficient people. Journal of Clinical Endocrinology 28: 685–692
Ayromlooi J 1972 Congenital goiter due to maternal ingestion of iodine. Obstetrics and Gynecology 39: 818–822
Bakwin H 1937 Pathogenesis of tetany of the newborn. American Journal of Diseases of Children 54: 1211–1226
Balázs R 1972 Effects of hormones and nutrition on brain development. Advances in Experimental Medicine and Biology 30: 385–415
Brasel J A, Boyd D B 1975 Influence of thyroid hormones on fetal brain growth and development. In: Fisher D A, Burrow G N (eds) Perinatal Thyroid Physiology and Disease, Kroc Foundation Symposia Vol 3 pp 59–71, Raven Press, New York
Bruce J, Strong J A 1955 Maternal hyperparathyroidism and parathyroid deficiency in the child. Quarterly Journal of Medicine 24: 307–319
Burger A, Buerer T, Sizonenko P, Lacourt G 1976 Reverse T3 in screening for neonatal hypothyroidism. Lancet ii: 39–40
Burrow G N 1972 The Thyroid Gland in Pregnancy. W B Saunders, Philadelphia
Burrow G N, Polackwich R, Donabedion R 1975 The hypothalamic-pituitary-thyroid axis in normal pregnancy. In: Fisher D A, Burrow G N (eds) Perinatal Thyroid Physiology and Disease, Kroc Foundation Symposia Series Vol 3, pp 1–10. Raven Press, New York
Burwell C S 1954 Circulatory adjustments to pregnancy. Bulletin of the Johns Hopkins Hospital 95: 115–129
Chopra I J, Sack J, Fisher D A 1975 Circulatory 3,3,5-triiodothyronine (reverse T3) in the human newborn. Journal of Clinical Investigation 55: 1137–1141
Crooks J, Aboul-Khair S A, Turnbull A C, Hytten F E 1964 The incidence of goitre during pregnancy. Lancet ii: 334–336
Crooks J, Tulloch M I, Turnbull A C, Davidsson D, Skulason T, Snaedal G 1967 Comparative incidence of goitre in pregnancy in Ireland and Scotland. Lancet ii: 625–627
Delmonico F L, Neer R M, Cosini A B et al 1976 Hyperparathyroidism in pregnancy. American Journal of Surgery 131: 328–337
DeLuca H F 1973 The kidney as an endocrine organ for the production of 1,25 dihydroxyvitamin D3, a calcium mobilizing hormone. New England Journal of Medicine 289: 359–365
Dowling J T, Freinkel N, Ingbar S H 1956 Thyroxine-binding by sera of pregnant women, newborn infants, and women with spontaneous abortion. Journal of Clinical Investigation 35: 1263–1276
Dowling J T, Freinkel N, Ingbar S H 1960 The effect of estrogens upon the peripheral metabolism of thyroxine. Journal of Clinical Investigation 39: 1119–1130
Dowling J T, Appleton W G, Nicoloff J 1967 Thyroxine turnover

during human pregnancy. Journal of Clinical Endocrinology and Metabolism 27: 1749–1750
Dussault J H 1975 Development of the hypothalamic-pituitary-thymic axis in the neonatal rat. In: Fisher D A, Burrow G N (eds) Perinatal Thyroid Physiology and Disease, Kroc Foundation Symposia Vol 3. Raven Press, New York
Dussault J H, Laberge C 1973 Dosage de la thyroxine (T4) par methode radioimmunologique dans l'eluat de sang seche: Nouvelle methode de depistage de l'hypothyroide neonatale. Union Medical de Canada 102: 2062–2064
Evans T C, Kretzchmer R M, Hodges R E, Song C W 1967 Radioiodine uptake studies of the human fetal thyroid. Journal of Nuclear Medicine 8: 157–165
Fisher D A 1973 Fetal maternal thyroid relationships. International Congress Series No 273, pp 1045–1050. Excerpta Medica, Amsterdam
Fisher D A 1975 Thyroid function in the fetus. In: Fisher D A, Burrow G N (eds) Perinatal Thyroid Physiology and Disease. Kroc Foundation Symposia Vol 3, pp 21–32. Raven Press, New York
Fisher D A, Dussault J H 1974 Development of the mammalian thyroid gland. In: Handbook of Physiology, Section 7 Endocrinology Vol III Thyroid, pp 21–38. American Physiological Society Washington
Fisher D A, Hobel C J, Garza R, Pierce C A 1970 Thyroid function in the pre-term fetus. Pediatrics 46: 208–216
Fisher D A, Dussault J H, Hobel C J, Lam R W 1973 Serum and thyroid gland triiodothyronine in the human fetus. Journal of Clinical Endocrinology and Metabolism 36: 397–400
Francon J, Fellous A, Lennon A M, Nunez J 1977 Is thyroxine a regulatory signal for neurotubule assembly during brain development? Nature 266: 188–190
Fraser T R, Wilkinson M 1953 Simplified method of drug treatment for thyrotoxicosis using a uniform dosage of methyl thiouracil and added thyroxine. British Medical Journal 1: 481–484
Galton V A, Ingbar S H, Jiminez-Fonseca J et al 1971 Alterations in thyroid hormone economy in patients with hydatidiform mole. Journal of Clinical Investigation 50: 1345–1354
Ginsberg J, Walfish P G, Chopra I G 1978 Cord blood reverse T3 in normal, premature, euthyroid, low T4 and hypothyroid newborns. Journal of Endocrinological Investigation 1: 73–77
Goluboff I G, Sisson J C, Hamburger J I 1974 Hyperthyroidism associated with pregnancy. Obstetrics and Gynecology 44: 107–116
Graham G C, Blizzard R M 1973 Thyroid hormonal studies in severely malnourished Peruvian infants and small children. In: Gardner L I, Amacher P (eds) Endocrine Aspects of Malnutrition, Marasmus, Kwashiorkor and Psychosocial Deprivation, pp 205–219. Kroc Foundation, Santa Ynez, California
Halnan K E 1958 The radioiodine uptake of the human thyroid in pregnancy. Clinical Science 17: 281–290

Hawe P, Francis H H 1962 Pregnancy and thyrotoxicosis. British Medical Journal 2: 817–822

Heinemann M, Johnson C E, Man E B 1948 Serum precipitable iodine concentrations during pregnancy. Journal of Clinical Investigation 27: 91–97

Hennen G 1965 Detection and study of human-chorionic-thyroid-stimulating factor. Archives of Internal Physiology and Biochemistry 73: 689–695

Hershman J M 1972 Hyperthyroidism induced by trophoblastic thyrotropin. Mayo Clinic Proceedings 47: 913–918

Hershman J M, Starnes W R 1971 Placental content and characterisation of human chorionic thyrotrophin. Journal of Clinical Endocrinology and Metabolism 32: 52–58

Hodges R E, Evans T G, Bradbury J T, Keettel W C 1955 The accumulation of radioactive iodine by human fetal thyroid. Journal of Clinical Endocrinology and Metabolism 15: 661–667

Hollingsworth D R, Mabry C C 1975 Congenital Graves Disease In: Fisher D A, Burrow G N (eds) Perinatal Thyroid Physiology and Disease. Kroc Foundation Symposia Vol 3, pp 163–183. Raven Press, New York

Holt W A, Talbert L M, Thomas C G et al 1970 Hyperthyroidism during pregnancy. Obstetrics and Gynecology 36: 779–785

Howe P, Francis H H 1961 Pregnancy and thyrotoxicosis. British Medical Journal 2: 817–822

Jost A, Picon L 1970 Hormonal control of fetal development and metabolism. In: Advances in Metabolic Disorders, Vol 4, pp 123–184. Academic Press, New York

Lowe D C, Hadden D R, Montgomery D A D, Weaver J A 1976 Propranolol as sole therapy for thyrotoxicosis; long-term follow up. In: Thyroid Research, Proceedings of the Seventh International Thyroid Conference, Boston 1975, pp 429–433. Excerpta Medica, Amsterdam

Ludwig G D 1962 Hyperparathyroidism in relation to pregnancy. New England Journal of Medicine 267: 637–642

Malkasian C D, Mayberry W E 1970 Serum total and free thyroxine and thyrotropin in normal and pregnant women, neonates, and women receiving progestogens. American Journal of Obstetrics and Gynecology 108: 1234–1238

Man E B, Holden R H, Jones W S 1971 Thyroid function in human pregnancy, VII. Development and retardation of 4 year old progeny of euthyroid and of hypothyroxinemic women. American Journal of Obstetrics and Gynecology 109: 12–19

Marx S J, Attie M F, Spiegel A M, Levine M A, Lasker R D, Fox M 1982 An association between neonatal severe primary hyperparathyroidism and familial hypocalciuric hypercalcaemia in three kindreds. New England Journal of Medicine 306: 257–264

McCarroll A M, Hutchinson M, McAuley R, Montgomery D A D 1976 Long term assessment of children exposed in utero to carbimazole. Archives of Disease in Childhood 51: 532–536

Montgomery D A D 1979 Thyroid disease in pregnancy. Ulster Medical Journal 1: 69–82

Munro D S 1977 Autoimmunity and the thyroid gland. Proceedings of the Royal Society of Medicine 70: 855–857

Northrop G, Misenhimer H R, Becker F O 1977 Failure of parathyroid hormone to cross the non-human primate placenta. American Journal of Obstetrics and Gynecology 129: 449–453

Osorio C, Myant N B 1960 Thyroid hormones in pregnancy. British Medical Bulletin 16: 159–164

Petit D W, Clark R L 1947 Hyperparathyroidism and pregnancy American Journal of Surgery 74: 860–866

Pitkin R M 1975 Calcium metabolism in pregnancy: a review. American Journal of Obstetrics and Gynecology 121: 724–737

Pratt E L, Geren B B, Neuhauser E B D 1947 Hypercalcaemia and idiopathic hyperplasia of the parathyroid glands in an infant. Journal of Pediatrics 30: 388–99

Rosvoll R V, Winship T 1965 Thyroid carcinoma and pregnancy. Surgery, Gynecology and Obstetrics 121: 1039–1042

Salem R, Taylor S 1979 Hyperparathyroidism in pregnancy. British Journal of Surgery 66: 648–650

Selenkow H A 1972 Antithyroid-thyroid therapy of thyrotoxicosis during pregnancy. Obstetrics and Gynecology 40: 117–121

Shepard T H 1967 Onset of function in the human fetal thyroid: Biochemical and autoradiographic studies from organ culture. Journal of Clinical Endocrinology and Metabolism 27: 945–958

Stanbury J R, Kroc R L 1972 Human development and the thyroid gland: relation to endemic cretinism. In: Advances in Experimental Medicine and Biology, Vol. 30, Plenum Press, New York

Stevenson J C, Hillyard C J, MacIntyre I 1979 A physiological action for calcitonin: protection of the maternal skeleton. Lancet ii: 769–770

Thompson N W, Carpenter L C, Kessler D L, Nishiyama R H 1978 Hereditary neonatal hyperparathyroidism. Archives of Surgery 113: 100–103

Thorgeirsson U, Casta J, Marx S J 1981 The parathyroid glands in familial hypocalciuric hypercalcaemia. Human Pathology 12: 229–237

Tojo S, Kanazawa S, Nakamura A, Kitagachi S, Mochizuki M 1973 Human chorionic TSH (hCTSH, hCT) during normal or molar pregnancy. Endocrinology Japan 20: 505–515

De Visscher M, Burger A 1980 Evaluation of Thyroid Function in the Thyroid Gland, pp 169–214. Raven Press, New York

Wagner G, Transbol I, Melchior J C 1964 Hyperparathyroidism and pregnancy. Acta Endocrinologica 47: 549–564

Weingarten M D, Lockwood A H, Hwo S Y, Kirschner M W 1975 A protein factor essential for microtubule assembly. Proceedings of the National Academy of Science USA 72: 1858–1862

Whitehead M, Lane G, Young O, Campbell S, Abeyasekera G, Hillyard C A, MacIntyre I, Phang K G, Stevenson J C 1981 Interrelations of calcium-regulating hormones during normal pregnancy. British Medical Journal 2: 10–12

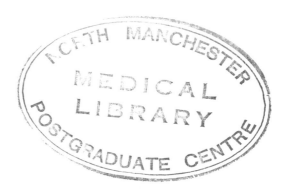

Diseases of the adrenal cortex and medulla in pregnancy: anterior and posterior pituitary deficiency

EFFECTS OF PREGNANCY ON ADRENAL HORMONE ASSAYS

Plasma cortisol levels rise progressively through pregnancy, falling back to normal within a week of delivery (Martin & Mills, 1958; Schteingart, 1967; Wintour et al, 1978). This change is accounted for by an oestrogen induced rise in transcortin, an increase exceeding that induced by oestradiol administration (Doe et al, 1969). Free cortisol levels have been variously reported as normal by Booth et al (1961) or slightly elevated by Burke & Roulet (1970) and cortisol production rate as unchanged (Migeon et al, 1963) or slightly raised (Cope & Black, 1959).

The diurnal variation in plasma cortisol level is qualitatively similar to that of non-pregnant women and men with the difference between high and low levels noted by Burke & Roulet (1970) to be diminished late in pregnancy. Normal pulsatile secretion is observed.

Plasma cortisosterone becomes significantly elevated by 12 weeks, increasing towards term, while 11-deoxycorticosterone (DOC) and 11-desoxycortisol rise earlier, the former to a proportionately greater degree than other corticosteroids (Wintour et al, 1978). Plasma aldosterone rises progressively from the 12th week to the 28th week becoming significantly elevated by the 20th week and remains so until term (Wintour et al, 1978). It is likely that whatever the cause of the aldosterone increase, normal physiological regulation is still intact since mineralocorticoid lowers and sodium restriction increases plasma aldosterone levels in pregnancy. Plasma renin activity rises and is positively correlated with rising aldosterone levels. Plasma renin concentration increases to peak values in the first trimester, falling towards term. Much of the increase in renin concentration in early pregnancy is due to the presence of biologically inactive renin, active renin concentration rising in parallel with plasma renin activity. Angiotensin II increases early, the rise persisting throughout pregnancy. Within 2 weeks of delivery, levels of plasma renin concentration, angiotensin II and aldosterone are back to normal but renin substrate remains elevated for 2 months. These relationships between plasma renin activity, concentration and substrate, angiotensin II and plasma aldosterone have been reviewed by Symonds (1981).

The explanation for the increased activity of the renin angiotensin aldosterone system in pregnancy is unclear. It may be a response to the natriuretic effect of progesterone or to the substrate stimulant effect of oestrogen, the former being more likely since renin concentration is also increased.

Carr et al (1981) have reported that although plasma ACTH rises as pregnancy progresses, levels in pregnancy are lower than those of non-pregnant women. The diurnal rhythm of ACTH secretion is preserved, being most evident in the third trimester, secretory spikes also being noted in this report.

Urinary cortisol excretion measured as urinary 17-hydroxy corticosteroids remains within the normal range although mean values rise slightly as pregnancy progresses (Martin & Mills, 1958). Luttrell & Steinbeck (1977) in longitudinal studies, noted raised levels of cortisol glucosiduronate in some of the women followed through pregnancy. Burke & Roulet (1970) studying women late in pregnancy noted elevated urinary free cortisol in all subjects. These observations may reflect a rise in plasma free cortisol which could also account for the lower plasma ACTH levels in pregnancy noted by Carr et al (1981). Urine aldosterone also rises progressively from late in the first trimester to ten times normal levels late in pregnancy (Lamminausta & Erkkola, 1977).

Pregnancy does not appear to influence the measurement of catecholamines or their metabolites in blood or urine nor to call for modification in interpretation of the results of such measurements in the diagnosis of phaeochromocytoma.

DIAGNOSIS OF ADRENAL DISEASE IN PREGNANCY

The progressive increase in plasma cortisol during pregnancy due to increased cortisol binding globulin demands careful appraisal of this estimate and of the results of suppression and stimulation tests in the evaluation of adrenal function. Studies of diurnal rhythm remain reliable however since this phenomenon is unaffected although the difference between morning and evening levels diminishes late in pregnancy (Burke & Roulet, 1970). Urine cortisol metabolites (17 OHCS) and urine free cortisol measurements are useful screening tests bearing in mind the fact that some elevation above the normal non pregnancy range may occur, particularly late in pregnancy (Burke & Roulet, 1970). It would be prudent for laboratories to establish their own normal ranges.

The measurement of plasma cortisol and ACTH and of urine cortisol in the basal state and following dexamethasone and metyrapone can be used as in the non-pregnant state to establish the differential diagnosis of the cause of Cushing's syndrome. The ACTH stimulation test can also be used as in the non pregnant state to establish the diagnosis of primary adrenal failure.

If the clinical diagnosis of aldosterone producing adenoma is suspected during pregnancy because of hypertension and hypokalaemia, alkalosis and tetany, and plasma renin activity is suppressed, confirmation can be made by the conventional studies of potassium, renin and aldosterone levels during salt restriction, salt loading, and mineralocorticoid administration. Alterations from the basal state follow the same patterns as those in the non-pregnant woman.

Since pregnancy does not affect the measurement of levels of catecholamines or their metabolites, standard diagnostic criteria apply in suspected cases of phaeochromocytoma.

Giving careful consideration to the extent of radiation exposure in the individual case and with the use of modern techniques of catheter placement for venous sampling to localise tumours and the use of limited abdominal CT scanning, radiology in conjunction with ultrasound adds a new dimension, as yet rarely explored, to the diagnosis of adrenal tumours in pregnancy.

PRIMARY ALDOSTERONISM IN PREGNANCY

Two cases of primary aldosteronism associated with pregnancy have been reported by Gordon & Tunny (1982) with a review of seven other case reports. Hypertension is not invariably present, serum potassium not always low nor plasma renin activity suppressed, probably reflecting the balance between excess aldosterone secreted by the tumour and the raised progesterone level which opposes its action. Thus the progesterone rise of pregnancy may prevent the development of classic features of primary hyperaldosteronism, so that these features appear after delivery. Where aldosterone secretion is very high the protection afforded by progesterone is overcome and hypertension and hypo-

kalaemia may emerge along with renin suppression. The high DOC levels of pregnancy may further complicate the manifestations of hyperaldosteronism since they could have an additive effect or conceivably suppress aldosterone secretion.

PHAEOCHROMOCYTOMA IN PREGNANCY

In a major literature review of phaeochromocytoma in pregnancy, Schenker & Chowers (1971) reported 43 maternal deaths in 89 women undergoing 112 pregnancies. In 22 patients, the diagnosis was made during pregnancy, four of these patients died; in 32, the diagnosis was made after delivery, four of these patients dying from the consequences of phaeochromocytoma and in the remaining 35 patients, the diagnosis was made postmortem. None of these patients was treated by modern pharmacological methods including alpha blockade. In another review of 42 patients where antepartum diagnosis was made, the picture was changed dramatically with the introduction of alpha blockade (Burgess, 1979). Maternal mortality was abolished in all 16 alpha blocked patients (being 9 per cent in 22 unblocked patients). Fetal loss was reduced by this treatment from 75 per cent to 17 per cent where the diagnosis was made in the first or second trimester and from 42 per cent to zero where phaeochromocytoma was recognised in the third trimester.

The symptoms of phaeochromocytoma are not influenced by pregnancy and in the classical setting of paroxysmal hypertension with associated headaches, palpitation and sweating, it is not difficult to recognise. The diagnosis should also be considered where, presumably due to changes in pressure on the tumour, high blood pressure falls to normal or low levels on change from the recumbent to the upright posture or hypertension appears on palpation of the uterus in identifying the fetal position. In all reports of cases undiagnosed at the time of maternal or fetal death, a feature is made of the fact that retrospectively the diagnosis could have been made had symptoms been interpreted correctly. Severe pre-eclampsia, essential hypertension, shock and death antepartum or after delivery have all been described in the clinical profiles of unrecognised instances of phaeochromocytoma in pregnancy. Sprague et al (1972) suggested that in the presence of sustained hypertension and presumed pre-eclampsia the occurrence of minimal proteinuria and oedema calls for consideration of phaeochromocytoma as an alternative cause.

It is of interest that maternal symptoms of catechol excess similar to those seen in phaeochromocytoma have been observed in patients whose fetuses developed neuroblastoma (Voûte et al, 1970; Pochedly, 1976).

Following the diagnosis of phaeochromocytoma alternative treatment programmes have been proposed (Burgess,

1979; Schenker & Granat, 1982) although medical therapy with alpha blockade is the mainstay. This seems safe for the fetus and enables extended medical treatment during pregnancy. No reports of alpha blockade usage extend beyond 8 weeks duration, thus the effects on the fetus of very long-term treatment are unknown. Such medical management with delayed delivery by Caesarean section in cases recognised early in pregnancy has not been reported often, but appears safe (Leak et al, 1977; Burgess, 1979; Schenker & Granat, 1982). They have also advocated vaginal delivery in blocked patients with tumour resection deferred to a later time. However in some instances, where this regimen has been followed, tumour compression during labour has caused catechol release resulting in marked exacerbation of clinical features, maternal medical difficulty and fetal death (Schenker & Granat, 1982).

The optimal timing of surgery is not clear from the literature. In general, if the diagnosis is made early in pregnancy and the tumour localised, provided optimal blood pressure and volume control can be achieved, tumour excision can be undertaken safely in the second trimester. A few cases have been so managed with low maternal mortality but with poor fetal survival. Where the diagnosis is made later in pregnancy, combined Caesarean section and tumour excision has been widely practised under andrenergic blockade without maternal mortality and with low fetal hazard. In many case reports, localisation has not been made or attempted, search for the tumour being deferred until Caesarean section. In some instances the tumour has not been found, being removed at a second operation after postpartum localisation by conventional means.

CUSHING'S SYNDROME IN PREGNANCY

The coincidence of untreated Cushing's syndrome and pregnancy is rare. Grimes et al (1973) reported the association of Cushing's disease and pregnancy in a patient who was delivered of a live infant at term, the mother having undergone right adrenal resection for adenoma at 16 weeks, being maintained on cortisone during the remainder of her pregnancy. With this case report, a literature review of 26 pregnancies in 21 patients was made. In that total experience, 17 (63 per cent) of the 27 infants survived, the fetal loss being accounted for by six abortions (22 per cent), three still births (11 per cent) and one neonatal death (4 per cent). Of these 21 patients, three underwent bilateral total adrenalectomy and two, unilateral adrenalectomy during pregnancy. The infants of all these patients survived.

No single explanation for the high fetal mortality is apparent but several possibilities exist. Glucose intolerance has been commonly observed in the case histories of women who suffered fetal loss. The coexistent hyperten-

sion could also be a significant factor. Although fetal adrenal suppression may not occur in women taking large steroid doses in pregnancy (Bongiovanni & McPadden, 1960), in one report of Cushing's disease in pregnancy (Kreines & De Vaux, 1971) evidence is presented that transient adrenal insufficiency occurred in a surviving infant. In an account of two further patients with untreated Cushing's syndrome (Kreines et al, 1964) where the babies were stillborn, the fetal adrenals were atrophic suggesting that fetal adrenal suppression had occurred. It is possible that the unremitting secretion from an adrenal tumour or bilaterally hyperplastic glands have a greater suppressant effect on the fetal pituitary adrenal axis than that of intermittent maternal steroid dosage. Although animal studies have suggested that congenital fetal abnormality might be a clinical problem in pregnancies where maternal adrenal cortical steroid excess co-existed, this has not been borne out in studies of women taking pharmacological doses of steroid while pregnant (Bongiovanni & McPadden, 1960; Yaekel et al, 1966), nor in case reports of women pregnant while suffering from untreated Cushing's syndrome.

The onset or exacerbation of Cushing's syndrome in pregnancy has been reported by Calodney et al (1971) and remission associated with termination of pregnancy by Kreines et al (1964) and Calodney et al (1971). While these fluctuations in the clinical expression of adrenal cortical excess could be coincident with pregnancy, and due to the well known cyclic nature of the disease in some patients, the association of these changes with pregnancy and its termination seem significant in the cases reported. No currently known effect of pregnancy on ACTH or cortisol secretion, their regulation or their peripheral actions, explains these reported effects of pregnancy on the course of Cushing's syndrome.

Not one of the many modalities of treatment of Cushing's syndrome seems uniquely suitable for the management of the pregnant patient. Where the clinical manifestations are florid and require urgent control, in our opinion surgical resection of the adrenal hormone source remains the method of choice as it is in the non-pregnant state. Evaluation of the severity of hypertension, protein catabolism, the dangers of infection and diabetes, all maternal and fetal hazards, will influence this decision. It is implicit that an accurate diagnosis of cause be made before attempting adrenal surgery.

There is no contraindication to pituitary irradiation where urgent control of the disease is not required and pituitary surgery can be safely performed in pregnancy (Martin & Taft, 1972).

In a report by Gormley et al (1982) metyrapone in doses up to 2 g daily was used successfully from the 29th week to delivery at the 37th week. There were no fetal problems although maternal oestriol was reduced. These authors noted that as there is evidence of transplacental transfer of metyrapone (in experimental animals) caution should be exercised in the use of inhibitors of cortisol synthesis since the fetal adrenal has such an important role particularly at the time of delivery. Cyproheptadine (Kasperlek-Zaluska et al, 1980) has also been effectively used in pregnancy as an inhibitor of ACTH secretion without adverse maternal or fetal effects.

ADRENAL INSUFFICIENCY AND PREGNANCY

The reports of Fitzpatrick (1922), Knowlton et al (1949) and Brent (1950) documented the high maternal and fetal mortality where pregnancy was associated with Addison's disease in the pre-cortisone era. These early reports did not suggest that there was any change in the course of adrenal insufficiency during pregnancy. With the advent of desoxy-corticosterone fluid replacement and antibiotics, some pregnancies were successfully carried to term with the delivery of infants who behaved normally and mothers who lactated. The dramatic change following the introduction of cortisone is illustrated by the early reports of Hunt & McConahey (1953) and Hendon & Melick (1955) showing no fetal or maternal mortality in all seven pregnancies described. Today, pregnancy in a women with adrenal insufficiency, adequately steroid replaced, should be normal. Untreated women with adrenal insufficiency have reduced fertility which becomes normal with replacement therapy.

In developed Western countries bilateral adrenal insufficiency is almost always due to autoimmune adrenalitis. Tuberculous destruction of the adrenal gland is still a common cause of the condition in countries where this disease is prevalent. The clinical features of Addison's disease are well known and the cardinal signs of postural hypotension and pigmentation are usually associated with weight loss, tiredness, anorexia and vomiting. These are the same in the pregnant and non-pregnant state. Pregnant women with Addison's disease usually have known and treated pre-existing disease. However the condition may be recognised during pregnancy or the purperium and so require urgent treatment. In the literature (Brent, 1950) and in our own experience women have presented with collapse during the stress of delivery, clinical evidence of Addison's disease being present on review of the preceding clinical course. Addison's disease presenting as maternal collapse in the purperium has been reported by McGill (1971); we have had similar experiences. The placenta possesses an active 11-β-dehydrogenase (Murphy et al, 1974) but does not synthesise cortisol which could protect the mother in late pregnancy. The possibility of transfer of fetal corticosteroids to the maternal circulation has been raised and there is evidence that this occurs. However it is uncertain whether the amounts which cross the placenta are sufficient to have a significant maternal effect (Taft, 1972; Le Febre, 1976; Chatteraj et al, 1976; Cawood et al, 1976).

Normal maintenance therapy with cortisone acetate 25–50 mg/day or hydrocortisone 20–40 mg/day plus fludrocortisone 0.1 mg/day, commonly remains unchanged throughout pregnancy. It has been observed both by ourselves and by Schenker & Luttwak (1970) that some women require additional salt-retaining hormone during the second and third trimesters to avoid postural hypotension. The explanation of this is not clear although the natriuretic effect of high progesterone levels has been implicated. It is usually only necessary to increase fludrocortisone slightly and to be aware of the possible side-effects of fluid retention and oedema. The value of plasma renin activity measurement as a guide to minerocorticoid replacement is limited by the pregnancy induced rise in this parameter. Greater experience by individual laboratories in this unusual clinical situation should increase the usefulness of the estimation.

The course of pregnancy is usually uneventful and the method and timing of delivery in women with adrenal insufficiency should be determined entirely by obstetric considerations. It is usual to give an injection of 100 mg hydrocortisone when labour commences and repeated 12 hourly if necessary where delivery is delayed, in order to avoid stress-related adrenal insufficiency. Similarly, hydrocortisone will be needed to cover intercurrent infection, anaesthesia and any operative procedure.

Pre-eclampsia had been reported in Addison's disease before the use of corticosteroid replacement and in treated women has the same characteristics as normal pregnancy (Moses et al, 1959). The demonstration that there was no increased production of either aldosterone or hydroxysteroids during pregnancy in women who have previously undergone bilateral adrenalectomy (Baulieu et al, 1957; Moses et al, 1959; Christy & Jailer, 1959) discredited the theory that pre-eclampsia was due to corticosteroid or salt-retaining hormones produced from the placenta. Similarly, there is no evidence that the course of adrenal insufficiency is improved by placental hormone production in pregnancy.

The early observation by Osler (1967) that the infants born to mothers with Addison's disease were smaller than average has been disputed by Hilden & Rannike (1971) and it seems that the birthweight is normal for gestation.

Immuno-fluorescent adrenal autoantibodies are detected in the majority of women with autoimmune Addison's disease (Blizzard et al, 1967; Irvine et al, 1967). Like other maternal autoantibodies these readily cross the placental barrier and are detected in cord blood. They behave as passive antibodies and become undetectable in the infant's plasma by the age of 6–12 months (Nerup, 1974; Gawler et al, 1977). Baum & Chantler (1968) described neonatal hypoglycaemia with inappropriately high plasma insulin in an infant with the appearance of the child of a diabetic mother born to a woman with Addison's disease whose glucose tolerance was normal immediately postpartum. Although adrenal and parietal cell antibodies were present in maternal and cord blood, pancreatic islet cell antibodies were not looked for. It is recognised that multiple auto-immune endocrinopathy may occur in one individual (Turkington & Lebovitz, 1967; Irvine et al, 1968). Insulin-dependent (type 1) diabetes (Francisco & Rocca, 1966; Gawler et al, 1977) and autoimmune thyroid disease (Graves' disease or Hashimoto's thyroiditis) (Poonai et al, 1977) have been described in pregnancy associated with Addison's disease. Even in the absence of clinically recog-nised disease it is possible for maternal antibodies to be present and potentially to cause effects in the neonate. Future careful study of these women and their babies will be required to clarify this possibility although in general there appeared to be no common neonatal complications in the infants of mothers with autoimmune adrenal insufficiency.

Lactation appears to be normal in women with adrenal insufficiency and there is no reason to discourage breast feeding whilst the mother is maintained on normal steroid replacement. Irvine et al (1968) described premature ovarian failure due to steroid-specific autoantibodies in association with Addison's disease. Its prevalence however is uncertain. In our experience women with Addison's disease have normal reproductive lives.

The management of pregnancy in women after bilateral adrenalectomy for Cushing's syndrome or other reasons is no different to that for primary adrenal insufficiency (Moses et al, 1959; Bergman et al, 1960; Schenker & Luttwak, 1970). We have not found the need to modify steroid replacement in such patients. In some, hyperten-sion which has persisted from the previous condition may require standard additional therapy. Data are not currently adequate to determine whether the neonatal course of the infants of these patients is different from those infants born to mothers with autoimmune adrenalitis.

In all women with adrenal insufficiency, episodes of vomiting or dehydration from any cause or intercurrent severe infection during pregnancy will require urgent treat-ment. In addition to the increased corticosteroids used in a conventional manner in such circumstances, intravenous therapy must be considered so as to avoid the placental insufficiency associated with the maternal hypotension. Antibiotics should be given early and in full doses as appropriate.

PITUITARY DEFICIENCY IN PREGNANCY

Anterior pituitary deficiency

In this section the effects of partial or complete hypo-pituitarism in pregnancy are described and management discussed. The course and management of pituitary tumours in pregnancy are dealt with elsewhere in this book. Attention is drawn to the entity of lymphocytic hypophysitis as an apparent autoimmune disease occurring in pregnancy or postpartum (Asa et al, 1981, Ch. 25).

Pregnancy may occur spontaneously in women with partial anterior pituitary deficiency particularly if appro-priate replacement hormone is given. Otherwise ovulation induction may be required as described in Chapter 27. Once pregnancy has been achieved, normal replacement requirements should not alter except that additional corti-costeroids will be required in the same circumstances as for women with adrenal insufficiency. Bromocriptine if used to induce pregnancy will usually be discontinued as described elsewhere in this volume (Ch. 26).

Reports of pregnancy by Taft (1972), Bowers & Jubiz (1974) and Grime & Brooks (1980) in pre-existing hypo-pituitarism or after hypophysectomy during pregnancy by Martin & Taft (1972) indicate that with adequate hormone replacement the course of pregnancy and the onset of labour are normal. This is in accord with the evidence that neither oxytocin nor anti-diuretic hormone from the pos-terior pituitary or median eminance of the hypothalamus are necessary for the initiation or normal progression of labour (Chard, 1972). No specific neonatal problems have been described and although lactation is normally absent it may occur spontaneously if there is a continuing secretion of prolactin by the original lesion (unpublished observation).

Diabetes insipidus

Anti-diuretic hormone deficiency implying a lesion in the median hypothalamus or supraoptic nucleus causing diabetes insipidus may occur with or without total or partial anterior pituitary deficiency. In the latter circum-stance which most commonly follows surgery for pituitary tumour and very rarely postpartum haemorrhage, the features of diabetes insipidus depend on the presence of a basal secretion of corticosteroid hormones to promote normal free-water clearance. In the case report of Van der Wildt et al (1980) the onset of diabetes insipidus in pregnancy was the first sign of a pituitary tumour but this sequence is very rare.

As in the non-pregnant state, anti-diuretic replacement therapy is used in the treatment of diabetes insipidus for the patient's comfort and convenience, and also for protec-tion from the risks of unexpected fluid restriction. The intranasal preparations (1-deamino-8-arginine vasopressin, DDAVP) and lysine-vasopressin have largely replaced the use of either aqueous or oily pitressin injection for routine care. Other drugs such as chlorpropamide and carbima-zepine have a facilitating effect on the action of anti-diuretic hormone and may be very effective in symptomatic control of partial diabetes insipidus. Chlorthiazide or other similar diuretics have also been shown to be useful, presumably by reducing free-water clearance, although their mode of action in this regard is not entirely clear. The management of diabetes insipidus, where it co-exists with anterior pituitary deficiency, is as described for the isolated deficiency, care being taken to ensure corticosteroid replacement should such be required.

The clinical effect of diabetes insipidus on pregnancy and *vice versa* were well described some years ago by Blotner & Kunkel (1942) and Hendricks (1954). The symptoms of thirst and polyuria do not change consistently during pregnancy. Individual case reports have described exacerbation, improvement or no change in fluid requirements and although these variations may be due to different degrees of ADH deficiency, no clear explanation has emerged (Hendricks, 1954; Moldavsky & Griffin, 1968; Oravec & Licardus, 1972; Hime & Richardson, 1978; Phelan et al, 1978). As Hendricks (1954) clearly pointed out, the situation may be confused by the occurrence of psychogenic polydipsia or other conditions of pregnancy which affect fluid balance. It is thus essential, if the diagnosis of diabetes insipidus has not been clearly established, to verify the diagnosis by the use of either a controlled water deprivation test with the measure of plasma and urine osmolality or the infusion or hypertonic saline. This procedure has not been followed in some cases and throws doubt on the entity described by Aguilo et al (1969) as pseudo-diabetes insipidus in pregnancy.

The management of pregnancy in diabetes insipidus is not different from normal. It has been clearly shown by both bioassay (Hawker et al, 1967; Chau et al, 1969) and immunoassay (Sende et al, 1976) that oxytocin levels are normal in isolated diabetes insipidus and clinical observation confirms that labour and lactation occur normally (Blotner & Kunkel, 1942; Hendricks, 1954; Hime & Richardson, 1978; Phelan et al, 1978). Possible complications due to a hypertrophied bladder and dilated ureters causing obstruction as described by Hendricks (1954) appear very rare.

The use of ADH replacement preparations such as pitressin and more recently DDAVP (Burrow et al, 1981) are unlikely to induce premature labour as they do not contain oxytocin. However, in excess dose, side-effects of smooth muscle contraction are well recognised and uterine irritability in the late stages of pregnancy has been described (Oravec & Licardus, 1972). It is thus prudent to continue normal replacement therapy throughout pregnancy and labour avoiding excessive dosage. Although no specific contraindications to the use of chlorpropamide and carbamezapine exist in pregnancy there are no reports of their use throughout pregnancy in this circumstance. No specific neonatal problems in association with diabetes insipidus have been recorded. Familial diabetes insipidus is not usually manifest in the neonatal period and does not commonly become apparent till the age of 2–5 years (Martin, 1959).

Nephrogenic diabetes insipidus

This is due to impairment of tubular response to normal ADH levels and can be associated with impairment of renal function as the defective tubular function may be due to chronic pyelonephritis or other renal pathology. In this circumstance renal function must be taken into account in the management of pregnancy. The more common causes are either congenital isolated nephrogenic diabetes insipidus or chronic therapy with lithium salts for the treatment of manic depression or other psychiatric disorders. In all forms of nephrogenic diabetes insipidus chlorthiazide 0.5 g twice daily is the most useful drug to reduce fluid turnover. Potassium replacement may be required. No specific changes in pregnancy have been recorded in the presence of nephrogenic diabetes insipidus but few reports have been made (Burstein & Chen, 1970; Mizrahi et al, 1979).

In both pituitary and nephrogenic diabetes insipidus water and electrolyte balance are maintained normally provided the thirst centre is intact and there is free access to water. Deliberate or inadvertent water restriction can produce rapid dehydration and hyperosmolality in untreated diabetes insipidus.

REFERENCES

Aguilo F, Vega L, Haddock L, Rodriguez O 1969 Diabetes insipidus syndrome in hypopituitarism of pregnancy. Acta Endocrinologica 60 (Supple 137): 1–32

Asa S L, Bilbao J M, Kovacs K, Josse R G, Kreines K 1981 Lymphocytic hypophysitis of pregnancy resulting in hypopituitarism — a distinct clinico-pathologic entity. Annals of Internal Medicine 95: 166–171

Baulieu E, deVigan M, Bricaire H, Jayle M 1957 Lack of plasma cortisol and urinary aldosterone in a pregnant woman with Addison's disease. Journal of Clinical Endocrinology and Metabolism 17: 1478–1482

Baum J D, Chantler C 1968 Hyperinsulinemic child of mother with Addison's disease. Journal of the Royal Society of Medicine 61: 1261–1262

Bergman P, Ekman H, Hakansson B, Sjogren B 1960 Adrenalectomy during pregnancy with the appearance of pre-eclampsia at term in a case of Cushing's syndrome. Acta Endocrinologica 35: 294–298

Blizzard R M, Chee D, Davis W 1967 The incidence of adrenal and other antibodies in the sera of patients with idiopathic adrenal insufficiency (Addison's disease). Clinical and Experimental Immunology 2: 19–30

Blotner H, Kunkel P 1942 Diabetes insipidus and pregnancy. New England Journal of Medicine 227: 287–292

Bongiovanni A M, McPadden A I 1960 Steroids during pregnancy and possible fetal consequences. Fertility and Sterility 11: 181–186

Booth M, Dixon P F, Gray C H, Greenway J M 1961 Protein binding of cortisol in health and pregnancy. Journal of Endocrinology 23: 25–35

Bowers J H, Jubiz W 1974 Pregnancy in a patient with hormone deficiency. Archives of Internal Medicine 133: 312–314

Brent F 1950 Addison's disease and pregnancy. American Journal of Surgery 79: 645–652

Burgess G E 1979 Alpha blockade and surgical interaction of phaeochromocytoma in pregnancy. Obstetrics and Gynecology 53: 266–270

Burke C W, Roulet F 1970 Increased exposure of tissues to cortisol in late pregnancy. British Medical Journal 1: 657–659

Burrow G N, Wassenaar W, Robertson G L, Sehl H 1981 DDAVP treatment of diabetes insipidus during pregnancy and the postpartum period. Acta Endocrinologica 97: 223–225

Burstein P, Chen C 1970 Diabetes insipidus nephrogenic type, complicating pregnancy. American Journal of Obstetrics and Gynecology 108: 1292–1293

Calodney L, Eaton R P, Black W, Cohn F 1973 Exacerbation of Cushing's syndrome during pregnancy. Report of a case. Journal of Clinical Endocrinology and Metabolism 36: 81–86

Carr B R, Parker C R Jr, Madden J D, McDonald C P, Porter J C 1981 Maternal plasma adrenocorticotrophin and cortisol relationships throughout human pregnancy. American Journal of Obstetrics and Gynecology 139: 416–422

Cawood M L, Heys R F, Oakey R E 1976 Corticosteroid production by the human fetus: evidence from analysis of urine from women pregnant with normal or anencephalic fetus. Journal of Endocrinology 70: 117–126

Chard T 1972 The posterior pituitary in human and animal parturition. Journal of Reproduction and Fertility, Suppl 16: 121–138

Chattaraj S C, Turner A, Pinkus J, Charles D 1976 The significance of urinary free cortisol and progesterone in normal and anencephalic pregnancy. American Journal of Obstetrics and Gynecology 124: 848–853

Chau S S, Fitzpatrick R J, Jamiesson B 1969 Diabetes insipidus and parturition. Journal of Obstetrics and Gynecology of British Commonwealth 76: 444–450

Christy N P, Jailer J W 1959 Failure to demonstrate hydrocortisone and aldosterone during pregnancy in Addison's disease. Journal of Clinical Endocrinology and Metabolism 19: 263–266

Cope C L, Black E G 1959 The hydrocortisone production in late pregnancy. Journal of Obstetrics and Gynaecology of the British Empire 66: 404–408

Fitzpatrick G 1922 Addison's disease complicating pregnancy, labour or the puerperium. Surgery, Gynecology and Obstetrics 35: 72–76

Francisco F R, Rocca L 1966 Diabete, maladie d'Addison et grossesse. Diabete 14: 115–117

Gawler T R, Aynsley-Green A, Irvine W J, McCallum C J 1977 Immunological studies in the neonate of a mother with Addison's disease and diabetes mellitus. Clinical and Experimental Immunology 28: 192–195

Grimes H G, Brooks M H 1980 Pregnancy in Sheehan's syndrome. Report of a case and review. Obstetrical and Gynecological Survey 35: 481–488

Grimes E M, Fayez I A, Miller G L 1973 Cushing's syndrome and pregnancy. Obstetrics and Gynecology 42: 550–559

Gordon R D, Tunney J T 1982 Aldosterone-producing-adenoma (A-P-A): effect of pregnancy. Mineralocorticoids in Essential and Secondary Hypertension. Supplement to Clinical and Experimental Hypertension In press

Gormley M J J, Hadden D R, Kennedy T L, Montgomery G A, Murnaghan G A, Sheridan B 1982 Cushing's syndrome in pregnancy treatment with metyrapone. Clinical Endocrinology 16: 203–293

Hawker R W, North W G, Colbert I C 1967 Oxytocin blood levels in two cases of diabetes insipidus. Journal of Obstetrics and Gynecology of the British Commonwealth 74: 430–431

Hendon J R, Melick R A 1955 Pregnancy in Addison's disease. Journal of the Kentucky State Medical Association 53: 141–143

Hendricks C H 1954 The neurohypophysis in pregnancy. Obstetrical and Gynecological Survey 9: 323–341

Hilden J, Rannike F 1971 On birth weight and gestation period in infants born to mothers with Addison's disease. Danish Medical Bulletin 18: 62–65

Hime M C, Richardson J A 1978 Diabetes insipidus and pregnancy. Obstetrical and Gynecological Survey 33: 375–379

Hunt A B, McConahey W M 1953 Pregnancy associated with diseases of the adrenal glands. American Journal of Obstetrics and Gynecology 66: 970–987

Irvine W J, Stewart A G, Scarth L 1967 A clinical and immunological study of adrenocortical insufficiency (Addison's disease). Clinical and Experimental Immunology 2: 31–69

Irvine W J, Chan M W, Scarth L, Kolb F O, Hartog M, Bayliss R, Drury M 1968 Immunological aspects of premature ovarian failure associated with idiopathic Addison's disease. Lancet ii: 883–887

Kasperlik-Zaluska A, Migdalske B, Hartwig W, Wilczynska J, Marianowski L, Stopinska-Gluszka U, Lozinska D 1980 Two pregnancies in a woman with Cushing's syndrome treated with cyproheptadine. British Journal of Obstetrics and Gynecology 87: 1171–1173

Knowlton A I, Mudge G H, Jailer J W 1949 Pregnancy in Addison's disease. Journal of Clinical Endocrinology and Metabolism 9: 514–528

Kreines K, De Vaux W D 1971 Neonatal adrenal insufficiency associated with maternal Cushing's syndrome. Pediatrics 47: 516–519

Kreines K, Perin E, Salzer R 1964 Pregnancy in Cushing's syndrome. Journal of Clinical Endocrinology and Metabolism 24: 75–79

Lamminausta R, Erkkola R 1977 Renin-angiotensin-aldosterone system and sodium in normal pregnancy: a longitudinal study. Acta Obstetrica et Gynecologica Scandinavica 56: 221–225

Leak D, Carroll J J, Robinson D C, Ashworth E J 1977 Management of phaeochromocytoma during pregnancy. Obstetrical and Gynecological Survey 37: 583–585

LeFebvre Y, Marier R, Amyo T, Bilodeau R, Hotte R, Raynault P, Durocher J, Lanthier A 1976 Maternal, fetal and intra-amniotic hormonal and biologic changes resulting from a single dose of hydrocortisone injected in the intra-amniotic compartment. American Journal of Obstetrics and Gynecology 125: 609–612

Luttrell B M, Steinbeck A W 1977 Urinary excretion of cortisol and cortisone glucosiduronates in pregnancy. Medical Journal of Australia 1: 552

McGill I G 1971 Addison's disease presenting as a crisis in the puerperium. British Medical Journal 2: 566

Martin F I R 1959 Familial diabetes insipidus. Quarterly Journal of Medicine 28: 573–582

Martin D J, Mills I H 1958 The effects of pregnancy on adrenal steroid metabolism. Clinical Science 17: 137–146

Martin F I R, Taft P 1972 Hypophysectomy for diabetic retinopathy during pregnancy. Diabetes 21: 972–975

Migneon C J, Green O C, Exkert J P 1963 Study of adrenocortical function in obesity. Metabolism 12: 718–739

Mizrahi E M, Hobbs J F, Goldsmith D I 1979 Nephrogenic diabetes insipidus in transplacental lithium intoxication. Journal of Paediatrics 94: 493–495

Moldavsky L F, Giffin M 1968 Diabetes insipidus in pregnancy. American Journal of Obstetrics and Gynecology 100: 878–879

Moses A M, Lobotsky J, Lloyd C W 1959 The occurrence of pre-eclampsia in a bilaterally adrenalectomized woman. Journal of Clinical Endocrinology and Metabolism 19: 987–994

Murphy B, Clark S, Donald I, Pinsky M, Vedady D 1974 Conversion of maternal cortisol to cortisone during placental transfer to human fetus. American Journal of Obstetrics and Gynecology 118: 538–541

Nerup J 1974 Addison's disease — serological studies. Acta Endocrinologica 76: 142–158

Osler M 1967 Pregnancy and endocrine disorders. Incidence and obstetrical considerations. Acta Obstetrica et Gynecologica Scandinavica, Suppl 10, 46: 49–57

Oravel D, Lichardus B 1972 Management of diabetes insipidus in pregnancy. British Medical Journal 4: 114–115

Phelan J P, Guay A T, Newman C 1978 Diabetes insipidus in pregnancy. American Journal of Obstetrics and Gynecology 130: 365–366

Pochedly C 1976 Neuroblastoma. Publishing Sciences Group, Acton, Massachussetts

Poonai A, Jelercic F, Pop-Lazic B 1977 Pregnancy with diabetes mellitus, Addison's disease and hypothyroidism. Obstetrics and Gynecology, Suppl 1, 49: 86–88

Schenker J G, Luttwak E 1970 Pregnancy and delivery after bilateral adrenalectomy for phaeochromocytoma. Journal of Obstetrics and Gynecology of British Commonwealth 77: 1031–1035

Schenker J G, Chowers I 1971 Phaeochromocytoma and pregnancy. Review of 89 cases. Obstetrical and Gynecological Survey 26: 739–747

Schenker J G, Granat M 1982 Phaeochromocytoma and pregnancy — an updated appraisal. Australian and New Zealand Journal of Obstetrics and Gynecology 22: 1–10

Schteingart D E 1967 Adrenal function in disease and pregnancy. Clinics in Obstetrics and Gynecology 10: 85–105

Sende P, Pantelakis N, Suzuki K, Bashare R 1976 Plasma oxytocin determination in pregnancy with diabetes insipidus. Obstetrics and Gynecology, Suppl 1, 48: 38–41

Sprague A D, Thelin T J, Dilts P V 1972 Phaeochromocytoma associated with pregnancy. Obstetrics and Gynecology 39: 887–891

Symonds E M 1981 The renin-angiotensin system in pregnancy. Obstetrics and Gynecology Annual 10: 45–65

Taft P 1972 Endocrine disease in pregnancy. Medical Journal of Australia 1: 868–874

Turkington R W, Lebovitz H E 1967 Extra-adrenal endocrine deficiencies in Addison's disease. American Journal of Medicine 43: 499–507

Van der Wildt B, Drayer J, Eskes T 1980 Diabetes insipidus in pregnancy as a first sign of a craniopharyngioma. European Journal of Obstetrics and Gynecology 10: 269–274

Voûte P A, Waldman S K, van Putten W J 1970 Congenital neuroblastoma. Symptoms in the mother during pregnancy. Clinical Pediatric Journal 9: 206

Wintour E M, Coghlan J P, Oddie C J, Scoggins B A, Walters W A W 1978 A sequential study of adrenocorticosteroid level in human pregnancy. Clinical and Experimental Pharmacology and Physiology 5: 399–403

Yackel D B, Kempers R D, McConahey W M 1966 Adrenocorticosteroid therapy in pregnancy. American Journal of Obstetrics and Gynecology 96: 985–981

Intersexuality

INTRODUCTION

The last decade has seen substantial progress in our understanding of normal sexual differentiation. This chapter will begin with a summary of those events, will look at genetic and endocrine control and then classify the various types of human intersexuality. Finally, a clinical approach to the differential diagnosis and management of these patients will be presented. However, no details of surgical technique will be given. The writer has discussed much of this material elsewhere (Shearman, 1979, 1981, 1982).

NORMAL SEXUAL DIFFERENTIATION

At fertilisation the ovum and sperm contain the haploid number of chromosomes — in the human ovum 22 autosomes plus an X chromosome, in the sperm 22 autosomes with either an X or Y chromosome. This union will normally result in a conceptus with 46 chromosomes; a female with 44 autosomes and XX sex-chromosomes (46, XX) or a male with a similar number of autosomes and XY sex-chromosomes (46, XY). Thus will be determined *chromosomal sex*.

Despite this initial chromosomal directive the early embryo is morphologically sexually indifferent, with Wolffian and Müllerian ducts and an undifferentiated gonadal ridge. The first objective sign of sexual differentiation is the development from the gonadal ridge of the embryonic testis or ovary, the former evoked by XY, the latter by XX sex-chromosome complement. Thus will be determined *gonadal sex* (primary sex determination).

In the normal female fetus, Wolffian structures will atrophy, the Müllerian ducts will develop into uterus, Fallopian tubes and upper vagina, while the cloaca assumes normal female characteristics. In the normal male, the Müllerian structures will regress and the Wolffian ducts will develop into vas deferens, seminal vesicles and epididymis. Concurrently, the cloaca will masculinise, with the development of penis, penile urethra and scrotum. Thus

will be determined *internal genital* and *external genital* sex (secondary sex determination). The *sex of rearing* will be based on inspection of the external genitals. It has been widely held that this simply made decision will provide the major component in the child's psychosexual orientation (Money, 1968a). As will be discussed below, a few vital chinks have been found in this armourial orthodoxy.

Although not the same as sex of rearing and poorly understood, it is not unreasonable to introduce the concept of *brain sex*.

We have then, to deal with five sorts of sex — chromosomal, gonadal, internal genital, external genital or body sex (phenotype), sex of rearing and perhaps brain sex.

A simple explanation of all this would be to say that beyond the chromosomal level the ovary is responsible for female differentiation and the testis for masculine development. The sequences are, however, more fascinating and capable of almost infinite variety.

ENDOCRINOLOGY AND CYTOGENETICS

General principles

There is no way that any clinician will ever understand the problems of intersexuality without a thorough grasp of the mechanisms controlling normal sexual differentiation *in utero*.

In the human species — unlike, for example, birds — the male is heterogametic. Male chromosomal sex is determined at the moment of conception by an XY heterogametic complement, female chromosomal sex by the XX homogametic complement.

The early embryo is sexually bipotential. Before the sixth week, the gonadal ridge is morphologically undifferentiated irrespective of chromosomal sex. While the testis begins to emerge structurally after the seventh week, ovarian development is not apparent until the thirteenth week. It is almost a tautology to say that the gonadal ridge differentiates into an ovary in response to XX chromosomes and into a testis if the chromosomal complement is

XY, at least in species like the human where the male is heterogametic. Far more important is the question 'Why?'

It remains to be determined just what in the XX make-up dictates ovarian differentiation. For example, if a fetus with Turner's syndrome and 45,X karyotype aborts, which the vast majority do, the ovarian tissue contains many ova (Singh & Carr, 1966). Later, in the majority of patients, all that can be found is ovarian stroma without any hint of an ovum. How the second X maintains these follicles is unknown but it is important to note that one X, unaccompanied except for a normal cohort of autosomes, is enough to induce ovarian development at a fetal level. Wachtel (1979) has raised the question of whether or not there is an ovary inducing molecule. Although this is an attractive hypothesis, at the moment there is no evidence that such a discrete molecule exists.

Ohno (1967) suggested that the Y chromosome had multiple copies of a gene which was essential for the development of the heterogametic sex. In 1973, Jost and his colleagues predicted that the Y chromosome must contain an organiser substance to cause testicular differentiation. It is now clear that an important component of this organiser substance is the histocompatibility-Y (H-Y) antigen which will be discussed in more detail below. Reverting to the time of embryonic sexual indifference, at this stage not only is the gonadal ridge undifferentiated, but neither the Müllerian and Wolffian ducts, nor the cloaca give any morphological clue to the ultimate sexual destiny of the embryo. It is only after the testis develops that the Müllerian ducts regress and the Wolffian ducts differentiate while the cloaca shows penile development with a penile urethra and labio-scrotal fusion. If Dr Pangloss ruled a perfect world, it could be said that the ovary caused female differentiation at an internal and external genital level and that the testis did the same for the male. In a technical and intellectual *tour de force* in the late 1940's and 1950's, Jost showed that this was not so.

'In the same way pure mathematical speculation allowed C. J. Adams and Le Verrier to predict the existence of Neptune, although the planet was only seen later that year, Jost concluded that the results of his surgical experiments in rabbit fetuses could be explained only by the existence of a distinct morphogenetic secretion responsible for the regression of Müllerian ducts in male fetuses' (Josso et al, 1977).

Jost (1953) developed what was then a unique amalgam of technique and intuitive reasoning in 1953. He resolved the formidable technical problem of removing the gonadal ridge from fetal rabbits before the state of sexual differentiation and noted that all the litter when delivered at term were apparent females, irrespective of chromosomal sex. Their cloacal differentiation was feminine. Wolffian ducts had regressed, while Müllerian ducts had developed into Fallopian tubes, uterus and upper vagina. These newborn, of course, had no gonads.

The crucial factor emerging from these experiments was that at a fetal and infantile level, female internal and external genital sex are the neutral or asexual norm, not requiring an ovary for guidance. The corollary was that a testis was essential to transform this neutral imperative into a normal male at both the internal and external genital levels.

Jost then entered the heady realm of theoretical biology. He theorised as follows:

1. The presence of a testis was necessary to inhibit the otherwise inexorable development of Müllerian ducts.

2. Concurrently it caused evolution of Wolffian structures, and at the same time,

3. Transformed the 'neutral' cloaca into that of the male infant.

4. The testicular secretion responsible for the first of these was different from the second and third.

Experiments of nature, time and scientific endeavour have shown Jost to be correct, absolutely. de Grandmaison would have been proud of this latter day French example of 'L'attaque á outrance' (Horne, 1977). Fortunately, Jost's philosophy has held together rather better than that of de Grandmaison and his disciples.

These proposals might be best discussed in sequence.

Ovarian induction. The female equivalent of the male H-Y antigen has not been found and it seems likely that a single determinant does not exist. While a single X will induce fetal development of the ovary, including transmigration of germ cells, the second X chromosome is usually necessary for ovarian maintenance. In the classic case of Turner's syndrome there is no second sex chromosome at all but in other cases either deficiency of the X short arm (Xp) or the X long arm (Xq) is associated with ovarian failure. Determinants for ovarian maintenance are, therefore, located on both Xp and Xq, although the precise region on Xq is uncertain (Simpson & Lebeau, 1981). Determinants for stature are closely related in site to those for ovarian maintenance on Xq but at a different site from ovarian determinants on Xp. The gospel that two more or less intact X chromosomes are essential for ovarian maintenance is shaken severely by well documented cases of pregnancy in non-mosaic 45, X individuals. Ten such patients have been reported (Wray et al, 1981).

H-Y antigen. Eichwald & Silmser (1955) showed a sex-related incidence of skin graft rejection in inbred mice. The antigenic basis of this was demonstrated by Goldberg et al (1971). In 1975, Wachtel et al showed that the responsible histocompatibility antigen was on the Y chromosome. This is now called the histocompatibility-Y (H-Y) antigen.

This antigen seemed to be responsible for the critical induction of the testis, critical because on this testicular induction depends the consequent cascade of events affecting the Müllerian and Wolffian ducts and the cloaca. In 1978, Ohno indicated that 'if H-Y antigen is not expressed, XY individuals develop as females' while acknowledging that 'the primary sex determining role played by the Y is indeed confined to testicular organisation'. Further support for the role of the H-Y antigen in testicular induction was forthcoming when it was found in some XX individuals bearing testes, for example some true hermaphrodites and the very uncommon XX male (de la Chapell et al, 1978). No doubt George Orwell would have been delighted to note that the XX male syndrome is very common in pigs; it is much less common but nevertheless well documented in the human. These men have azoospermic testes and carry the H-Y antigen. They have no germ cells, so it seems likely that while the H-Y antigen is a male determining substance, it cannot be 'the sole male determining factor on the Y chromosome, since it does not appear to account for germ cell sex' (Short, 1979). In the Steel mutant mouse the germinal ridge remains unpopulated with primordial germ cells. In the male, sex cord formation always takes place, further evidence that sex cord development is H-Y dependent but germ cell migration H-Y independent (McCoshen, 1982). The H-Y antigen is also probably responsible for hilus cell development (Meade et al, 1981). The quite extraordinary potency of the antigen is shown by its ability to induce bovine XX embryonic gonads to form seminiferous and rete tubules and tunica albuginea (Ohno et al, 1979).

The beautiful simplicity of this proposal has been disturbed by further work from Wachtel and his colleagues (Dorus et al, 1977). The antigen has been found in patients with 46, XY pure gonadal agenesis (an XY female). These potentially disturbing and conflicting problems have been discussed by Jones et al (1979). In fact, Ohno had anticipated these problems when in 1978 he went on to suggest that the capacity to express the H-Y antigen related not only to its presence but also to the ability of specific receptors to bind the antigen. This philosophy has been expanded by Muller et al (1979) and Wachtel (1979).

It is important to grasp the concept that the H-Y receptors are found only in the gonads, so that the effects of the H-Y antigen on sexual differentiation must, presumably, be mediated by its primary effect on testicular differentiation. It is also important to note that something beyond the H-Y antigen is essential for the incorporation of the vital germ cells into an otherwise normal testis. Just as man may not live by bread alone, so something more than the H-Y antigen is needed to arouse the gonadal ridge to its true testicular potential; but at least a start has been made.

Anti-Müllerian factor (AMF). Jost's theories, mentioned above, had important support from a classic experiment of nature — what used to be called the virilising male intersex. These infants, born with equivocal but usually substantially virilised external genitals are found to have a male karyotype, morphologically and steroidogenically normal testes but completely normal uterus, Fallopian tubes and upper vagina. Under these circumstances the absence of some factor that would normally have

suppressed the Müllerian ducts had to be invoked. The first step in proof, as distinct from speculation, was the development by Picon (1969) of an *in vitro* method to test anti-Müllerian activity. Using Jost's theories and Picon's techniques, Josso (1977) has summarised the work she has done.

The responsible substance has been shown to have a predominantly local action. The original designation of 'anti-Müllerian hormone' (AMH) may therefore not be entirely appropriate for etymological purists and it is more frequently now called anti-Müllerian factor (AMF). In the rat, guinea-pig and pig, AMF activity precedes the appearance of the Leydig (interstitial) cells. The same precedence is seen in the human where AMF appears in the fetus of 20 mm crown rump (CR) length and Leydig cells appear at the 30 mm CR length. The development of AMF activity is synchronous with the development of the seminiferous tubule. In all species studied, including the human, this activity declines but is still detectable at birth. Donahoe et al (1977) provided good evidence that the

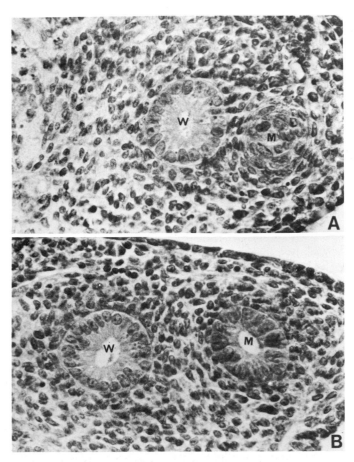

Fig. 17.1 A. A 14.5-day-old fetal rat reproductive tract exposed for 3 days to partially purified 'fetal' incubation medium incubated overnight with immunoglobulins isolated from control rabbit serum. Müllerian duct (M) has disappeared, Wolffian duct (W) is normal. B. Same experiment performed with immunoglobulins isolated from serum of rabbit immunised against 'fetal antigen'. Müllerian duct (M) is normal (Reproduced with permission: Picard et al 1978)

human infantile testis produces AMF until the age of 2 years, although activity is much greater during the first year than the second. The site of production is almost certainly the Sertoli cell. Functionally it is unrelated to the H-Y antigen and structurally unrelated to testosterone. AMF is a macromolecule. Picard et al (1978) showed that it is a glycoprotein with a molecular weight of either 124 000 daltons (density gradient sendimentation) or 250 000 daltons (gel filtration). Physiologically the activity of this 'hormone' is local (Fig. 17.1), not systemic and is seen of its centripetal best in the true hermaphrodite where the side bearing the testis shows complete Müllerian inhibition while the ovarian side develops a Fallopian tube and hemi-uterus. The developmental disparity in a true hermaphrodite with a lateral ovotestis and a contra-lateral ovary is shown in Fig. 17.2.

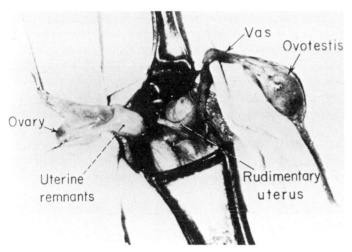

Fig. 17.2 Intra-operative photograph in a newborn true hermaphrodite showing ipsilateral localised action of Müllerian inhibiting substance. The Müllerian duct has regressed on the side of the ovotestis where there is only a vas. The Müllerian duct is preserved on the side of the ovary, i.e. there is a fallopian tube and uterus (Reproduced with permission: Donahoe et al, 1977)

Wolffian evocation. Jost (1953) showed that while testosterone implants had no effect on Müllerian development, there was Wolffian differentiation and virilisation of the cloaca. Similarly, the curious antiandrogen, cyproterone acetate, when administered to the male fetus has no effect on Müllerian inhibition but does prevent differentiation of Wolffian ducts and concurrently produces 'males' with ambiguous external genitalia (Neumann et al, 1970).

There is no doubt then that AMF inhibits Müllerian ducts and that a different substance evokes Wolffian ducts and masculinises the cloaca. The time sequence of testosterone secretion by the human fetus described by Ambramovich & Rowe (1973) and confirmed by Diez D'Aux & Murphy (1974) fits a dual role of Wolffian evocation and cloacal masculinisation. Figure 17.3 shows the testicular concentration of testosterone, androstenedione and dehydroepiandrosterone from the sixth to the 19th week of

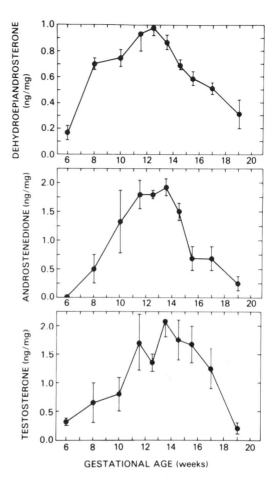

Fig. 17.3 Steroid concentrations of human testis 6th–19th week of gestation (Reproduced with permission: Tapanainen et al, 1981)

pregnancy. However, many clinical syndromes cannot be explained by stating simply that testosterone causes these two events. Nor does it explain why a female infant exposed to the androgenic assault of congenital adrenal hyperplasia *in utero* has no development of Wolffian ducts but variable, sometimes almost complete virilisation of the cloaca. Testosterone is effective, *de novo*, in the evocation of Wolffian derived structures (Imperato-McGinley & Peterson, 1976). The timing must be critical. In the crucible of nature, the Wolffian ducts are exposed to testosterone as soon as the Leydig cells differentiate. In the aberrations of nature seen in congenital adrenal hyperplasia, Wolffian inhibition has already occurred before the cloaca is stirred by the late but powerful call of ectopic androgens. So another important principle is that physiological testosterone production in the male fetus evokes a Wolffian reponse and induces masculine external genitals, while the pathological female intersex is exposed too late for the androgenic stimulation to affect the former but in ample time to modify, albeit usually incompletely, the latter. At no time of embryogenesis will androgens affect the Müllerian ducts.

Cloacal transformation. The adreno-genital syndrome or

congenital adrenal hyperplasia (CAH) has long been known for its association in the affected female with normal Müllerian structures, vestigial Wolffian ducts and degrees of virilism of the external genitals up to and including a complete penile urethra. The data of Ambramovich referred to before, indicate that fetal testosterone is sufficient to explain Wolffian evocation and masculinisation of the cloaca. More than this is required to etch the fine details within the broad outline of normal embryology. Apart from CAH, the clues are provided by two additional conditions — that of testicular feminisation and the familial male hermaphrodites from the Dominican Republic. In the first of these (Morris, 1953), an XY male, bearing testes, is born with the phenotype of a female but is found to have a short vagina of cloacal origin — the lower third — but no Müllerian or Wolffian ducts. At puberty they feminise despite the production of normal male levels of testosterone and dihydrotestosterone (DHT), the latter converted from the former by a 5α-reductase. The second (Peterson et al, 1977; Wilson et al, 1981) also lack Müllerin ducts, have normally differentiated Wolffian structures but are partially virilised at an external genital level — an enlarged clitoris, bifid scrotum and urogenital sinus. There is no evidence of prostatic development. At puberty the larynx and muscles masculinise while the phallus and bifid scrotum flourish. The testes if previously undescended, often descend. The testes are histologically normal and the post-pubertal male has normal levels of testosterone — sometimes even above the normal range and low levels of DHT.

The experimental road that explains these caprices of nature has been long and hard. In 1973, Bardin and his colleagues summarised their extensive data showing that the testicular feminisation syndrome was due to a lack of androgen receptors in all target tissue that would bind and, therefore, recognise testosterone, behaving as though there was no testosterone (Bardin et al, 1973). On the other hand, the second group can bind androgens in the target area — the urogenital sinus, urogenital tubercle, urogenital folds and Wolffian ducts, but had a relative deficiency of 5-α-reductase to convert testosterone into DHT. At a fetal level, the latter is the biological executive in this area, testosterone being something of an office boy. Since, at a fetal level, the Wolffian ducts respond to testosterone alone they develop normally. Because of the relative deficiency (but not absolute absence) of the 5-α-reductase, specific RNA synthesis in the cloacal area and in the prostatic utricle is inadequate. There is incomplete masculinisation of the external genitals (Wilson et al, 1981).

Physiologically, androgen cytosol and nuclear receptors vary, dependent on the ambient androgen exposure. At times of high androgen levels (the newborn, puberty and postpubertal males) the receptor is predominantly nuclear whereas at other stages it is predominantly in the cytosol (Fichman et al, 1981). More subtle defects in androgen receptors may lead to other familial types of cloacal dif-

ferentiation previously classified under the eponyms of Lubbs and Reifenstein, amongst others (see below). Receptor deficiencies are usually familial. Finally, a variety of enzymatic defects in the transformation of cholesterol to testosterone may reduce the amount of androgen available to affect these changes (Wilson et al, 1981).

Cloacal differentiation is therefore dependent on four phenomena; first on the ability of the testis to produce testosterone; secondly on the ability of the target organs to bind androgens. If the target cells lack this receptor, testosterone passes like a stranger in the night and neutral, female absolutism reigns supreme, producing the syndrome of testicular feminism; thirdly on a 5-α-reductase to convert the testosterone to the more biologically potent form, at least in this region in the fetus, of dihydrotestosterone; fourthly qualitative defects in the receptor or post receptor/complex deficiencies may impede the normal androgen response. In essence, the Wolffian duct responds to the call of testosterone alone; the fetal cloaca needs testosterone if it is able to recognise it, but having made its acquaintance can only respond maximally by converting testosterone in situ to DHT and binding this normally to a receptor. Clinically, absence of testicular androgens or lack of the specific receptors will result in the development of a female vulva and failure of the Wolffian ducts to develop. Relative lack of specific androgen receptors or late exposure of the cloaca to other androgens will result in variable and usually incomplete masculinisation of the cloaca.

In summary the important concepts of sexual differentiation are that:

1. XX is usually needed for normal ovarian development and maintenance, although rarely a single X will suffice.

2. The H-Y antigen complex probably evokes the testis, as long as there are specific receptors. However, it will not, by itself, induce germ cell colonisation of the gonad.

3. In the absence of a gonad, female development is the neutral or asexual norm.

4. The Sertoli cells of the testis produce anti-Müllerian factor. A male intersex lacking AMF will have a uterus, tubes and vagina.

5. Fetal testosterone evokes Wolffian structures but has not effect on Müllerian ducts.

6. Fetal testosterone will virilise the cloaca if it is bound to the target cells and can be converted to and bound as DHT.

7. A relative deficiency of 5-α-reductase will impair the cloacal response to testosterone, but will not affect Wolffian evocation, the latter being dependent on testosterone without the need for conversion.

8. Abnormal or ectopic androgen stimuli, depending on timing and biological potency, may cause variable, even almost complete masculinisation of the female cloaca but never affect Müllerian development in a chromosomal and

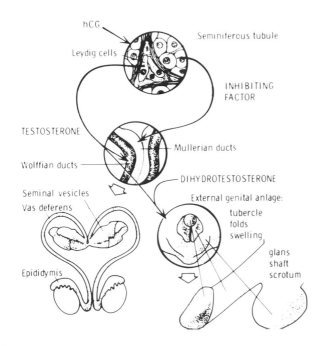

Fig. 17.4 Schematic representation of the three hormones necessary for development of the male phenotype — testosterone and Müllerian inhibiting factor from the testes, and dihydrotestosterone from the periphery (Reproduced with permission: Imperato-McGinley & Peterson, 1976)

gonadal female. In these clinical syndromes the androgenic stimulus arrives too late to switch on the Wolffian ducts.

These steps are shown schematically in Fig. 17.4 and 17.5. A more global view is seen in Fig. 17.6.

Sex of rearing? Sexual differentiation of the brain. This writer is not competent to discuss the emotional determinants of psychosexual orientation. There is very good evidence that the 'sex' of the brain in many species can be modified by exposure to various steroids in the neonatal period — for example, female hamsters will develop a male type running pattern, female rats develop a non-cyclic male pattern of gonadotrophin release with polycystic ovaries. On the other hand, a fetal ewe exposed to testosterone *in*

utero will develop a male type of sexual behaviour. This chapter, however, is about humans. How do we see *homo* compared with the rodent or ovine species? The only honest answer is 'rather obscurely'. In many ways the brain may be seen to represent a classical terminal non-replicative structure which in most species completes development (in the numerical cellular sense) *in utero* but in the human this goes on for several months after birth (Freinkel & Metzger, 1979). It is often believed that the human hypothalamus undergoes sexual differentiation *in utero* and cannot be modified by androgenic exposure in the immediate post-partum period. However, if this was so, then in the commonest human clinical condition of aberrant androgen exposure of the female fetus (congenital adrenal hyperplasia), the hypothalamus of such a female should be masculinised. In practice, while this may rarely occur (Jones, 1979), most girls with CAH treated early have substantially normal reproductive development and behaviour. The exposure of the brain to androgens post-natally may be of critical importance in the differentiation of the human both endocrinologically and behaviourally. The data of Forest et al (1976) show the pattern of testosterone in the normal human male infant (Fig. 17.7). It will be noted that at birth the male fetus is exposed to substantially higher concentrations of testosterone than the female. This is due presumably to the effects of human chorionic gonadotrophin (hCG) on the fetal Leydig cells. After the expected neonatal fall there is then a prolonged rise from the 30th to the 60th day of extra-uterine life reaching levels not seen again until adolescence. Perhaps it is this neonatal exposure that imprints the potential for male pattern of non-cyclic hypothalamic function on the newborn human male infant. Perhaps, also, it may imprint behavioural patterns. It is of interest to note that children with a 5-α-reductase deficiency, while usually brought up as girls, will in many instances become behaviourally masculine after puberty (Imperato-McGinley et al, 1979). It is not meant to make life any more difficult than it should be to indicate that in the male, testosterone becomes effective in the

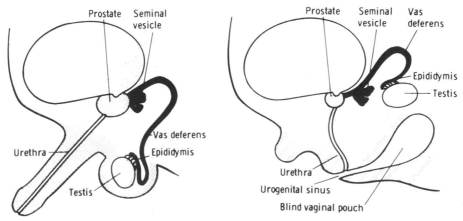

Fig. 17.5 Illustration of the hypothesis for the role of testosterone and dehydrotestosterone in sexual differentiation in *in utero*. Dark stippled area = testosterone-dependent. Light stippled area = dehydrotestosterone-dependent (Reproduced with permission: Imperato-McGinley & Peterson, 1976)

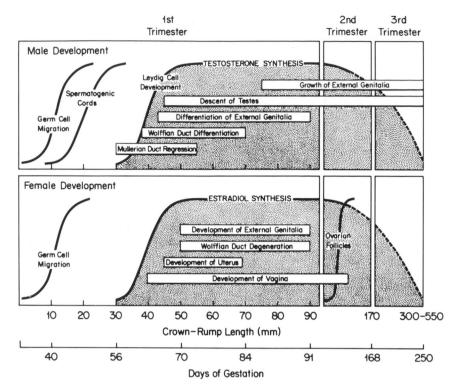

Fig. 17.6 Sexual differentiation (Reproduced with permission: Wilson et al, 1981)

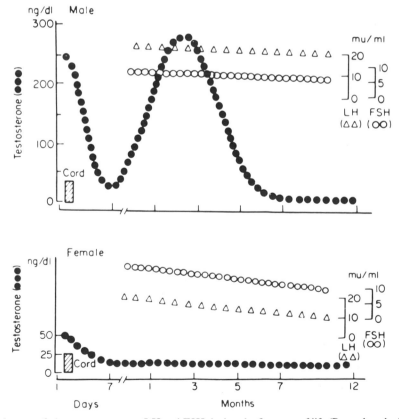

Fig. 17.7 Diagram illustrating changes of plasma testosterone, LH and FSH during the first year of life (Reproduced with permission: Forest et al, 1976)

hypothalamus after aromatisation to oestradiol 17β (Naftolin et al, 1975), although some doubts have been expressed about the relevance of this to the human (Martini, 1982). Since DHT cannot be aromatised to an oestrogen and these individuals produce normal or high normal amounts of testosterone, the Naftolin hypothesis fits this clinical circumstance.

In the state of present knowledge it is impossible to unravel the multiple threads of sexual differentiation of the brain, but it is increasingly difficult to accept that the sex of rearing is the only determinant in psychosexual orientation.

ABNORMAL SEXUAL DIFFERENTIATION

Any definition should be finite but it is difficult to find a definition that meets all the demands of intersexuality. A working definition is that an intersex is an individual where there is conflict between chromosomal sex, gonadal sex, internal genital sex and external genital (phenotypic) sex (Shearman, 1981).

CLASSIFICATION OF INTERSEX

It is impossible to draw up a classification that suits every reader. The classification used in this chapter has been evolved over many years but the writer is still fully conscious of its imperfections (Table 17.1). Overlap here is unavoidable. Some true hermaphrodites have chromosomal abnormalities and others have the H-Y antigen on their X chromosome, but since their claim to uniqueness lies in their dual gonads they are classified here at that level. Similarly, infants lacking anti-Müllerian factor are classified in the gonadal level, even though the cloacal appearances indicate that they must certainly have partial end organ resistance as well. Clinically there is very substantial overlap in some of the various syndromes of defective androgen synthesis receptors but since those classified are capable of endocrinological differentiation, this has been used as the basis for that section of Table 17.1.

Chromosomal level

Abnormalities of sex chromosomes may consist of sex chromosome deletion or addition. This chromosomal polymorphy may arise during meiosis, when each cell of the conceptus will be similarly affected, or after conception during mitosis, when two or more stem lines will arise, giving chromosomal mosaicism. In addition, it is now evident that at several genetic loci, the H-Y antigen complex is also of importance in inducing various types of intersex. In addition to its expression on the Y chromo-

Table 17.1 Classification of intersexes

Chromosomal level
  Turner's Syndrome, Turner Mosaic and other X deletions
  Triple X female
  Klinefelter's Syndrome
  XYYmale
  45,X/46,XY (mixed gonadal dysgenesis)

Aberrations of H-Y antigen

Gonadal level
  True hermaphrodite
  True gonadal agenesis
  Absent anti-Müllerian factor
  Embryonic androgen deficiency
    (a) Leydig cell hypoplasia
    (b) Enzymatic defects in testosterone synthesis

End organ resistance
  Defective androgen receptors
    (a) Testicular feminisation
    (b) Reifenstein's (and other eponymic) Syndromes, incomplete testicular feminisation
  5-α-reductase deficiency
  Post-receptor resistance

Female intersexuality
  Progressive:
    Congenital adrenal hyperplasia
  Non-progressive:
    (a) Maternal androgens
    (b) Exogenous progestins
    (c) Danazol
    (d) Spontaneous

some other loci appear to be X linked and also to exist on autosomes (Wilson et al, 1981).

Turner's syndrome. First described by Turner (1938) the syndrome included short stature, sexual infantilism, cubitus valgus, shortening of the fourth metacarpal and webbing of the neck. The nipples are widely spaced and pectus cavum is commonly present. Congenital cardiac lesions, particularly coarctation of the aorta may also be noted. The diagnosis may be made rarely in the neonatal period by the presence of peripheral oedema.

Most patients are chromatin negative and their karyotype is 45,X. Some individuals will be 45,X/46,XX mosaics while others will have deletion of either the short or long arm of the X chromosomes. Since streak gonads are found whether the p or q arm of the X chromosome is deleted, it seems that each arm contains more than one gonadal determinant (Bercue & Schulman, 1980; Simpson & Lebeau, 1981).

As would be expected, in the absence of Sertoli cells, Müllerian development is normal with uterus, tubes and vagina (however, rarely, coincidental concurrence of Turner syndrome with utero-vaginal agenesis has been described), while in the absence of Leydig cells the vulva and lower vagina are completely feminine.

Most embryos with a 45,X karyotype will abort and unlike trisomic conceptions, monosomy X is associated with young maternal age (Warburton et al, 1980).

Triple X female. This syndrome was first described by Jacobs et al (1959) and may never reach the level of clinical consciousness. Some of these women have oligomenorrhoea and/or a premature menopause but many have normal fertility. Mental retardation is more common than in females blessed with only two X chromosomes.

Klinefelter's syndrome. The original syndrome described by Klinefelter et al (1942) included atrophy of the seminiferous tubules, azoospermia, gynaecomastia and eunuch-oidism; the last two features are by no means constant. Mental retardation is more common than in other males. The testes are uniformly small, usually less than 5 ml in volume, buccal smears are chromatin positive and the commonest karyotype is 47,XXY. Less frequently, more complex karyotypes of 48,XXXY or mosaicism of 46, XY/47,XXY are present. These men usually cross the path of a gynaecologist as the azoospermic male partner of an infertile marriage. The subject has been fully reviewed by Paulsen et al (1968).

XYY male. The first group of these men described were significantly taller than average, with variable intelligence, their clinical spectrum being dominated by violent anti-social behaviour. Although it is clear that this pattern may occur with an XYY karyotype, it is now evident that some apparently normal men have the same chromosomal aberration.

45, X/46, XY (mixed gonadal dysgenesis). This syndrome may present at birth with an infant displaying equivocal genitals — usually clitoral hypertrophy and variable degrees of labio-scrotal fusion. Less frequently, the infant may be phenotypically female and develop slight clitoral hypertrophy at puberty. Less often, it would be an acci-dental diagnosis when investigating what is clinically a 'typical' case of Turner's syndrome or true gonadal agenesis (Shearman, 1968; Gantt et al, 1980).

In the patients I have seen with this syndrome, internal genital sex has been feminine and one of them was of normal height. In the much larger experience of 15 patients described by Gantt et al (1980) uterine and fallopian tube development was also normal but short stature was very common. The most frequent mode of presentation was delayed puberty.

The gonadal area shows wide variability ranging from bilateral 'streaks' to unilateral testicular tissue (abdominal, inguinal or scrotal). About 25 per cent of these individuals will have dysgenetic tumours (Schellhas 1974).

Aberrations of H-Y antigen

The XX male. These men tend to be shorter in stature than normal and have small azoospermic testes (de la Chapell et al, 1978). Although somewhat similar in appear-ance to a man with Klinefelter's syndrome they usually have a micro penis, gynaecomastia is common, the voice remains unbroken and facial hair remains immature. They

have high levels of LH and FSH, low levels of testosterone that may or may not increase on hCG stimulation (Perez-Palacios et al, 1981; Schweikert et al, 1982). The import-ance of the H-Y antigen is shown by the fact that a group of these XX males have been found to be H-Y antigen positive and the mothers of these XX males also expressed the H-Y antigen in varying degrees. It is not clear whether the H-Y antigen has been translocated on to an autosome or on to one of the X chromosomes.

The XY female. It would be convenient if all 'female' individuals with an XY karyotype could be discussed within this one group (Dewhurst & Spence, 1977). The genetics of this complex problem have been discussed in detail by Wachtel (1979), who not unexpectedly tries with great skill to attribute the complexities of the clinical syndromes to absence of the H-Y antigen, absence of H-Y antigen receptors or partial deletion of H-Y genes. However, there is still insufficient information about H-Y antigenicity in many types of XY females to consider them all in detail in this particular section. For that reason, this part of the chapter will deal with principles and some of the details will be discussed in other sections below.

In clinical terms the classification proposed by Cleary et al (1977) is easier to understand. The clinical syndrome will be determined by whether the potential testis never develops (embryonic failure), fails after Müllerian inhibi-tion has become effective (mid-fetal) or after the 20th week of pregnancy when complete masculine differentiation will have occurred. In the first of these, failure of the testis to develop at all will leave the model of Jost's rabbits where the Wolffian ducts will regress, and the Müllerian ducts will develop into Fallopian tubes, uterus and upper vagina. Because of the absence of testicular androgens, the cloaca will maintain its neutral feminine asexual norm. The clinical presentation of these individuals is usually with primary amenorrhoea and sexual infantilism and they can only be distinguished from true gonadal agenesis (see below) by their chromosomal structures. Because of the increased incidence of dysgenetic tumour of the streak gonads in these individuals, the karyotype is of great importance in clinical management. Some of these patients are H-Y negative and it is easy to understand why there is no gonadal development under these circumstances. Many of them, however, are H-Y positive and it is in this group that Wachtel invokes the absence of the gonadal receptor for the H-Y antigen.

Failure of the testis to develop beyond embryonic func-tion (mid-fetal failure) will lead to inhibition of the Müllerian ducts by AMF and some ambiguity of the external genitals. In these individuals, apart from an XY karyotype and streak gonads there are no Müllerian nor Wolffian ducts, the clitoris may be slightly enlarged and there will be varying degrees of labio-scrotal fusion with either an absent or rudimentary vagina.

Failure of the testes at a later stage in pregnancy,

previously called bilateral anorchia, cause the birth of a male with normal external genital sex, development of Wolffian structures but no detectable testicular tissue. Because of this they do not masculinise at the time of normal puberty. It must be assumed that the testis has been functional to cause Müllerian inhibition, Wolffian evocation and masculinisation of the cloaca, but that for reasons that are currently unknown, the testis then undergoes complete disintegration.

Gonadal level

True hermaphrodite. For this diagnosis to be reached, true testicular tissue and ovarian tissue must be present — not just stroma — but both primordial follicles and seminiferous tubules. External genital sex and internal genital sex vary widely, the former as a rule being predominantly male, while a uterus is usually present. Gonadal elements may be lateral — a testis on one side and an ovary on the other; unilateral — a testis or ovary and an ovatestis on the other; or bilateral with an ovatestis on each side.

The commonest chromosomal structure of these individuals is 46,XX but XX/XXY mosaics have been described. The rarest karyotype is 46,XY and has been seen in one of our own patients (Shearman et al, 1964). True hermaphroditism appears to be disproportionately common among the Bantu and van Niekerk (1976) analyses 340 cases in the published literature and 27 of his own, a uniquely large experience. While the presence of the H-Y antigen in either reduced quantities or in mosaic form may explain the presence of testicular and ovarian tissue in XX true hermaphrodites, there is to date, no acceptable explanation for the presence of ovarian tissue in true hermaphrodites with a 46,XY constitution. For those who wish to read further about this fascinating but rare problem, the book by Jones & Scott (1971) can be recommended as a classic.

Traditionally, the management of these individuals has been to readjust the external genitals to correlate with the sex of rearing. However, it should be noted that some of these true hermaphrodites are happily bisexual and at least three of them have born children without prior medical intervention (Tegenkamp et al, 1979), while ovulation has been induced using pituitary gonadotrophins in one true hermaphrodite with a male phenotype (Perez-Palacios et al, 1981b). There are no published reports of a true hermaphrodite having sired a child.

True gonadal agenesis. This condition is also called pure gonadal dysgenesis and one form has already been mentioned under the XY female. The condition is characterised by the complete absence of germinal tissue, female external and internal genital sex and absence of other congenital malformations. The karyotype may be 46, XX or 46,XY.

Although absence of the H-Y antigen explains some of these patients with 46,XY karyotype, it does not explain the absent gonad in those who are antigen positive, nor its absence in those with a 46,XX karyotype. They do, however, provide another justification for the reversed anthropomorphism of Jost's findings in rabbits to the human. The usual presentation is of primary amenorrhoea and sexual infantilism in an individual of normal or slightly increased height. The initial differentiation should lie between true gonadal agenesis and hypogonadotrophic hypogonadism, the distinction being readily made by an adequate study of gonadotrophin levels. Because of the risk of dysgenetic tumour in the XY individual, determination of the karyotype is mandatory.

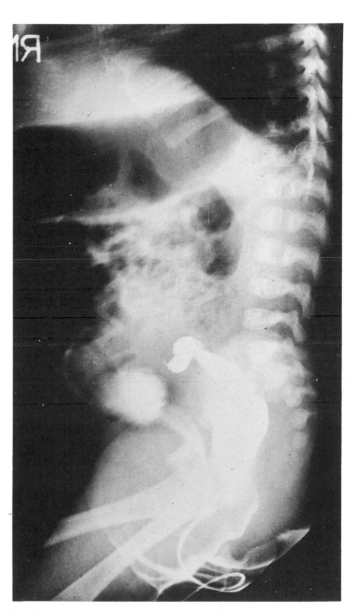

Fig. 17.8 X-ray study of a neonatal intersex. The child was a chromosomal and gonadal male whose testes did not produce anti-Müllerian factor. The bladder is shown anteriorly and the vagina and uterus posteriorly (Reproduced with permission: Shearman, 1968)

Absent anti-Müllerian factor. These children had been previously classified as virilising male intersexes (Shearman 1968, 1981). These children are eloquent testimony to the multi-faceted inducer role of the testis. At birth the clitoris is enlarged with variable degrees of labio-scrotal fusion and a urogenital sinus. Identical external genitals may be seen in other forms of intersexuality. Radiological studies will show a normal vagina, uterus and Fallopian tubes (Fig. 17.8). Bilateral testes are present usually in the ovarian fossa but sometimes in the inguinal region and the karyotype is 46,XY. While the testicular tissue is morphologically identical to that of a normal male of the same age (Fig. 17.9). and is able to produce testosterone, it cannot produce anti-Müllerian factor. Left untreated, these children will undergo further virilism at puberty.

Because of the incomplete masculinisation of the external genitals, in addition to postulating complete absence of anti-Müllerian factor, it is necessary to invoke partial end organ resistance, either of the 5α-reductase type, or receptor complex deficiency.

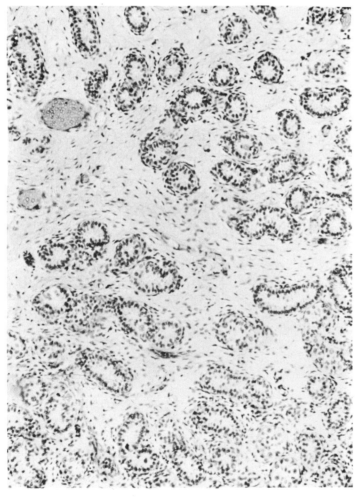

Fig. 17.9 Testis removed at the age of 3 months from the patient whose radiological findings are shown in Fig. 17.8

Embryonic androgen deficiency

Leydig cell hypoplasia. This is an uncommon condition, described by Berthezene et al (1976) and Brown et al (1978). The patient will present as a phenotypic female and reach the clinical arena when they present with primary amenorrhoea and sexual infantilism. Sexual hair is scanty, there may be slight labial fusion and a short blind vagina. Müllerian structures are completely inhibited, but the epididymis and vas deferens are present. Testes which may be abdominal or in the inguinal region show seminiferous tubules with some spermatogonia and either notably inconspicuous or completely absent Leydig cells. Unlike the complexities of the XY female, the embryology of this type of intersexuality is quite straightforward — no Leydig cells, no testosterone, no Wolffian evocation and minimal or no masculinisation of the cloaca. As would be expected with Sertoli cells, Müllerian inhibition is complete. If only life were so simple! Schwartz et al (1981) have now described a further patient who at birth had ambiguous genitalia and cryptorchidism and, when investigated as an infant, no endocrinological or morphological evidence of Leydig cells. However, because of the partial masculinisation of the external genitals in the last patient and the finding of epididymis and vas deferens in all three it must be assumed that there had been some degree of androgen production during the first trimester of pregnancy.

Enzymatic defects in testosterone synthesis. Five separate genetic defects have been identified which interfere with the transformation of cholesterol to testosterone — 20, 22 — desmolase, 3-β-hydroxysteroid dehydrogenase, 17-α-hydroxylase, 17, 20 — desmolase and 17-β-hydroxysteroid dehydrogenase (Wilson et al, 1981).

The commonest group of genetically determined enzymatic defects in steroid synthesis are those relating to 21 and 11 hydroxylase deficiency causing adrenal hyperplasia and in those specific patients genital tract abnormalities are secondary to abnormal androgen production from the adrenal cortex. Some types of adrenal hyperplasia will have deficiencies common to both the adrenal cortex and the gonads. Unlike the common forms of adrenal hyperplasia, in these defects some of the affected males will develop as phenotypic women with complete failure of virilization of the Wolffian ducts and external female genitalia. In none of the individuals bearing testes are Müllerian ducts developed. This is discussed in much more detail in Chapter 18.

END-ORGAN RESISTANCE

Defective androgen receptors

Complete testicular feminisation. The syndrome was first documented properly by Morris in 1953. It is unusual for the condition to be diagnosed in the neonate, as on routine examination the baby appears completely feminine. With the increasing use of diagnostic amniocentesis, not surprisingly, cases have now been described of a 46,XY karyotype determined by amniotic fluid cell culture culminating in the birth of an apparent female with this syndrome. Occasionally, the presence of an inguinal hernia in childhood containing a testis will suggest the diagnosis, but the majority of patients present at puberty with primary amenorrhoea. The characteristic clinical picture is that of a female of normal height with well developed breasts but scanty or absent axillary and pubic hair. The vulva is completely feminine but the vagina is short and 'blind', the uterus and tubes absent. Bilateral testes may be found in the inguinal canal or, more commonly, in the 'ovarian fossa'.

Testicular tissue removed from the postpubertal patient shows tubules lined with immature germ cells and Sertoli cells, while Leydig cells appear disproportionately common (Fig. 17.10).

The karyotype is 46,XY and since the condition is familial, it is not uncommon to see 'sisters' with the same condition.

The testes are hormonally competent both *in utero* and after puberty. Müllerian inhibition is complete, the feature being one of end organ resistance to testosterone due to absence of the cytosol androgen receptors in the target organ (Bardin et al, 1973).

Reinfenstein's (and other eponymic syndromes), incomplete testicular feminisation. These conditions include in addition to that detailed by Reinfenstein those described by Rosewater, Gibert, Dreyfus, and Lubbs (Wilson et al, 1981). A wide spectrum of disorders are seen ranging from gynaecomastia and azoospermia to the presence of the pseudovagina. The most common presentation is that of a male neonate with perineoscrotal hypospadias. Cryptorchidism is common and the testes are usually small but contain apparently normal Leydig cells. Psychosexually most of the subjects are male. Endocrinologically postpubertal individuals have high levels of testosterone, LH and oestradiol and have many endocrinological similarities to the testicular feminisation syndrome. All of these conditions show a quantitative defect in androgen receptors (Wilson et al, 1981), not dissimilar to that found in what has been called the 'incomplete testicular feminisation syndrome' (Medina et al, 1981). Relative deficiency of androgen receptors may be responsible for some cases of simple hypospadias (Svensson & Snochowski, 1979).

5-α-reductase deficiency. The best documented group with this syndrome is seen in the several publications by

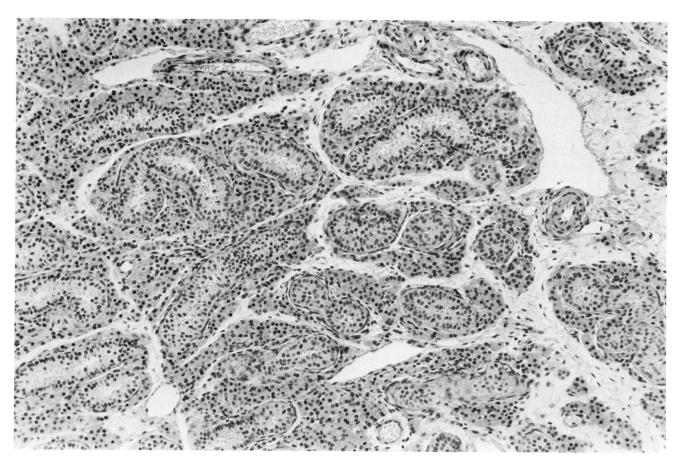

Fig. 17.10 Section of testis removed from an 18-year-old patient with testicular feminism

Peterson and Imperato-McGinley (Peterson et al, 1977; Imperato-McGinley et al, 1979). At birth these children have a markedly bifid scrotum that appears labia-like. There is a clitoris-like phallus and a urogenital sinus with a blind vaginal pouch. The testes may be in the abdomen, in the inguinal canal or scrotum. Müllerian structures are completely inhibited and Wolffian ducts normally developed. After puberty plasma testosterone levels reach those of a normal male and the subjects virilise rapidly with deepening of the voice and rapid muscular development. The phallus grows, the scrotum becomes rugose and pigmented while in most individuals the testes descend into the scrotum if they are not already there. There is no gynaecomastia. The subjects have erections and there is an ejaculate from the urethral orifice on the perineum. As mentioned above, although frequently reared as girls, these individuals often become behaviourally masculine after puberty. There is currently no acceptable explanation for the greater degree of virilism seen at puberty in these individuals when compared with that seen during embryogenesis.

In the familial types, the deficiency in 5-α-reductase is believed to be due to the homozygous state of an autosomal recessive gene that is manifest clinically only in males. In the patients that I have seen with this condition family size was small and the condition appeared to be sporadic. The external genitals of such an individual first seen at the time of an inappropriate puberty are shown in Fig. 17.11.

Post-receptor resistance. These rare conditions are still not fully characterised (Amrhein et al, 1977). The clinical appearance can be identical with that of the complete testicular feminising syndrome ranging through the incomplete forms of that syndrome to appearances very similar to the Reifenstein syndrome. However, these individuals have normal levels of 5-α-reductase, normal androgen receptors and normal androgen production. The androgen receptor is not thermolabile and it is possible that the defects may involve the intranuclear processing of the hormone-receptor complex (Wilson et al, 1981).

Female intersexuality

Progressive — congenital adrenal hyperplaseia: (adrenogenital syndrome). This condition has been mentioned briefly above and is covered very fully in Chapter 18. To save unnecessary reduplication it will not be considered further here except to reiterate that depending on the enzyme defects there may be inappropriate virilisation of the external genitals of the female infant (in the most common form) or apparent female external genital development of a chromosomal and gonadal male (very uncommon forms).

Non-progressive. These individuals are female at a chromosomal, gonadal and internal genital level. At birth external genital sex is equivocal, resembling the sex seen in common forms of congenital adrenal hyperplasia. There

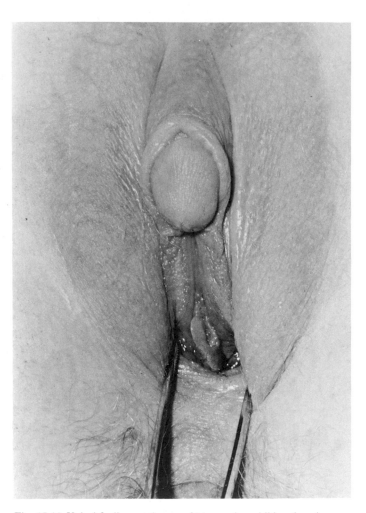

Fig. 17.11 Vulval findings at the age of 14 years in a child undergoing masculinising puberty. The enlarged clitoris and normal urethral opening are visible. This appearance is assumed to be due to a partial reductase deficiency (Reproduced with permission: Shearman, 1981)

is usually clitoral enlargement with or without some degree of labio-scrotal fusion. However, there is no further progress of the virilism at any time. As might be expected, this condition is related to exposure of an otherwise normal female fetus to an abnormal androgenic stimulus *in utero*.

This stimulus may be endogenous or exogenous. The classic example of the former is the case described by Brentnall (1945) of a woman who developed virilism during pregnancy from what ultimately proved to be an arrhenoblastoma. The female infant had labio-scrotal fusion, clitoral hypertrophy and a urogenital sinus.

The exogenous stimulus may very rarely be testosterone although there is no good reason why this should ever be given to a woman in pregnancy. In the 1950s and 60s when synthetic progestins were widely used for the treatment of threatened or recurrent abortion, this type of intersexuality was often seen and has been described fully by Grumbach et al (1959). Not unexpectedly, the same type of abnormality has now been described in a female infant whose mother took Danazol (the 2, 3-d-isoxazole derivative of 17-α-ethinyltestosterone) described by Duck & Katayama (1981). Very rarely the condition appears to arise spontaneously in women who have received no therapy and where there is no evidence of ectopic androgen production by the mother (Wilkins, 1960).

As in the external genital virilism of congenital adrenal hyperplasia, internal genital sex is never affected.

DIFFERENTIAL DIAGNOSIS AND TREATMENT

It should be apparent that the problem of intersexuality may declare itself at the time of birth because of ambiguous external genitalia, during childhood because of precocious heterosexual puberty of during adolescence, because the type of puberty is inappropriate to the sex of rearing or because puberty does not occur. It should also be apparent that some types of intersexuality (e.g. the XYY male or the triple-X female) may pass from birth to death without ever clouding the clinical horizon.

The major urgency of differential diagnosis lies with those cases presenting at birth. Any obstetrician, at any time, may be confronted with a newborn baby whose sex cannot be assigned with certainty on simple inspection. As discussed previously (Shearman, 1981) the management of the problem begins at this point when the mother asks, 'is it a boy or a girl?'

It is clinically indefensible to say 'I think it's a girl — or a boy'. Both immediately and in long-term management it is far better to indicate that ambiguity exists that will be resolved rapidly by further study. The problems inherent in this unfortunate clinical situation have been nicely discussed by Money (1968a, b).

Until fairly recently it was assumed that the decision of crucial importance was the assignment of the sex of rearing and that this should be done as rapidly as possible. The guidelines laid down by Money were: 'There are two good sex assignment rules to follow.

This first is: do not assign a new born hermaphrodite to the sex for which it cannot by surgery be made coitally adequate. This rule applies regardless of genetic or gonadal sex and also of hormonal sex, which can be controlled pharmacologically. The rule applies chiefly to male hermaphrodites with a clitoro-penis which cannot be properly masculinised but in whom an artificial vagina can be successfully constructed. The second rule is: do not impose a sex reassignment on older hermaphrodite children and adults if psychologically it would be equivalent to an announcement that you yourself should be reassigned' (Money, 1968b).

Of great importance here is one's attitude to the impact that sex of rearing has on gender identity. Until the second half of the 1970s it was widely assumed that the sex of rearing was of paramount importance in gender identity

and that this became firmly imprinted in the child's mind by the age of 2.5 or 3 years. Any effort to change gender role after this time was said to be fraught with disaster. Experience with the familial male intersexes due to 5-α-reductase deficiency has caused second thoughts about this (Greene et al, 1978; Imperato-McGinley et al, 1979). There is ample evidence that in these individuals and in some true hermaphrodites, a musculinising puberty will bring with it a complete reversal in gender role and sexual behaviour. I have seen several children with apparent 5-α-reductase deficiency or absent anti-Müllerian factor and one true hermaphrodite who have begun to virilise at puberty because the diagnosis was not established until that age. In none of these children have I been impressed that there is gender reversal.

Until there is better evidence to the contrary I believe that Money's dicta are correct. When one looks at a child with clitoral hypertrophy, a urogenital sinus and some degree of labio-scrotal fusion the technicalities of fashioning a penis and penile urethra are overwhelmingly difficult whereas the fashioning of an artificial vagina is, relatively speaking, much more simple.

Although this attitude may need revision in the next few years, in the newborn it still seems good advice to assign the sex of rearing to the sex that can be made coitally adequate.

When presented with this problem in the neonate the requisite investigations will be chromosome studies, urinary and plasma hormone assays, radiography and occasionally exploratory laparotomy. Where exploratory laparotomy is done there should be facilities for frozen section of biopsied gonads. In children with severe adrenal hyperplasia, evidence of salt loss may make treatment mandatory before hormonal confirmation of the diagnosis is reached. Installation of gastrographin into the urogenital sinus will be invaluable in determining the internal genital sex.

When corrective surgery of the external genitals is required, this should as a rule be undertaken before the child is old enough to notice her difference from other girls. The operation most frequently indicated is clitoridectomy and this should be done before the age of 2 or 3 years. Exploratory laparotomy will usually only be indicated in male intersexes or where true hermaphroditism is suspected. A good working rule is that a male (XY) intersex showing virilism at birth will virilise at puberty. If the assigned sex is female, the testes should be excised long before puberty.

The construction of an artificial vagina, where indicated, should usually be deferred until somatic growth has been completed. The methods of vaginal reconstruction are discussed more fully in Chapter 24, but it might be noted that whereas the simple procedure using graduated dilators gives remarkably good results in girls with otherwise uncomplicated utero-vaginal agenesis, a procedure of the

MacIndoe type is often needed in intersexes lacking a vagina. The only other surgery required will be removal of streaks in XY females because of the 25 per cent chance of developing a dysgenetic tumour. Orchidectomy in girls with testicular feminism after puberty has been achieved is also indicated because of the lesser but still measurable risk of developing a seminoma. The use of corticosteroids in children with adrenal hyperplasia is discussed in Chapter 18.

Those children born without gonads, or where testes have been removed duriing childhood, will obviously need hormonal replacement therapy to achieve a normal puberty. This should be initiated with very small doses of oestrogens so that the girl will be accustomed to these without undue breast soreness or nausea. Many XY females seem to be remarkably resistant to the mammary effects of exogenous oestrogens; in these circumstances augmentation mammoplasty has a place in the cosmetic and emotional management of the patient. It should be stressed that when oestrogens are used in an intersex who has a uterus, prolonged treatment with oestrogens alone increases substantially the risk of endometrial carcinoma. Cyclic progestins should always be given with the oestrogens. Details of hormone replacement therapy are given in Chapter 24.

Acknowledgement

I am grateful to have permission to reproduce here some material from Shearman (1979, 1982).

REFERENCES

Abramovich D R, Rowe P 1973 Fetal plasma testosterone levels at mid-pregnancy and at term: relationship to fetal sex. Journal of endocrinology 56: 621–622
Amrhein J A, Klingensmith G, Walsh P C, McKusick V A, Midgeon C J 1977 Partial androgen insensitivity. The Reifenstein syndrome revisited. New England Journal of Medicine 297: 350–356
Bardin C W, Bullock L P, Sherins R H, Mowszowicz I, Blackburn W R 1973 Androgen metabolism and mechanism of action in male pseudohermaphroditism: a study of testicular feminization. Recent Progress in Hormone Research 29: 65–109
Bercue B B, Schulman J D 1980 Genetics of abnormalities of sexual differentiation and female reproductive failure. Obstetric and Gynecological Survey 35: 1–11
Berthezene F M G, Forest M G, Grimbaud J A, Mornex R 1976 Leydig-cell agenesis. A cause of male pseudo-hermaphroditism New England Journal of Medicine 295: 969–972
Brentnall C P 1945 Case of arrhenoblastoma complicating pregnancy. Journal of Obstetrics and Gynaecology of the British Empire 52: 235–240
Brown D M, Markland C, Dehner L P 1978 Leydig cell hypoplasia: a cause of male psedohermaphroditism. Journal of Endocrinology 46: 1–7
De la Chapell A, Koo G C, Wachtel S S 1978 Recessive sex determining genes in human XX male syndrome. Cell 15: 837–842
Cleary R E, Caras J, Rosenfeld R L, Young P C M 1977 Endocrine and metabolic studies in a patient with male pseudohermaphroditism and true agonadism. American Journal of Obstetrics and Gynecology 128: 862–827
Dewhurst C J, Spence J E H 1977 The XY female. British Journal of Hospital Medicine 498–506
Diez D'Aux R C, Murphy B E P 1974 Androgens in the human fetus. Journal of Steroid Beiochemistry 5: 207–210
Donahoe P K, Ito Y, Morikawa Y, Hendren W H 1977 Mullerian inhibiting substance in human testes after birth. Journal of Pediatric Surgery 12: 323–330
Dorus E, Ambrose A P, Koo C G, Wachtel S S 1977 Clinical pathologic and genetic findines in a case of 46,XY, pure gonadal dysgenesis (Swyer's syndrome). II. Presence of H-Y antigen. American Journal of Obstetrics and Gynecology 127: 829–831
Duck S C, Katayama K P 1981 Danazol may cause female pseudohermaphroditism. Fertility and Sterility 35: 230–231
Eichwald E J, Silmser C R 1955 Skin communication. Transplantation Bulletin 2: 148–149
Fichman K R, Nyberg L M, Buznovszky P, Brown T R, Walsh P C 1981 The ontogeny of the androgen receptor in human foreskin. Journal of Clinical Endocrinology and Metabolism 52: 919–923
Forest M G, De Peretti E, Bertrand J 1976 Hypothalamic-pituitary-gonadal relationships in man from birth to puberty. Clinical Endocrinology 5: 551–569

Freinkel N, Metzger B E 1979 Pregnancy as a tissue culture experience: the critical implications of maternal metabolism for fetal development. In: Pregnancy Metabolism, Diabetes and the Fetus. Ciba Foundation Symposium No 63, pp 3–23. Excerpta Medica, Amsterdam
Gantt P A, Byrd J R, Greenblatt R B, McDonough P G 1980 A clinical and cytogenetic study of fifteen patients with 45,X/46,XY gonadal dysgenesis. Fertility and Sterility 34: 216–221
Goldberg E H, Boyse E A, Bennett D, Scheid M, Carswell E A 1971 Serological demonstration of H-Y (male) antigen on mouse sperm. Nature 232: 478–480
Greene S A, Symes E, Brook C G D 1978 5α-reductase deficiency causing male pseudohermaphroditism. Archives of Diseases of Childhood 53: 751–753
Grumbach M M, du Charme J R, Moloshok R E 1959 On the fetal masculinizing action of certain oral progestins. Journal of Clinical Endocrinology 19: 1369–1380
Horne A 1977 The Price of Glory. Verdun, 1916, p 11. Macmillan, London
Imperato-McGinley J, Peterson R E 1976 1976 Male pseudohermaphroditism: the complexities of male phenotype development. American Journal of Medicine 61: 251–272
Imperato-McGinley J, Peterson R E, Gautier T, Sturla E 1979 Androgens and the evolution of male-gender identity among male pseudo hermaphrodites with 5α-reductase deficiency. New England Journal of Medicine 300: 1233–1237
Jacobs P A, Baikie A G, Court Brown W M, MacGregor T N, Maclean N, Harnden D G 1959 The evidence for the existence of the human 'super female'. Lancet ii: 423–425
Jones H W 1979 A long look at the adrenogenital syndrome. Johns Hopkins Medical Journal 145: 143–149
Jones H W, Scott W W 1971 Hermaphroditism, genital anomalies and related endocrine disorders, 2nd edn. Williams & Wilkins, Baltimore
Jones H W, Rary J M, Rock J A, Cummings D 1979 The role of the H-Y antigen in human sexual development. Johns Hopkins Medical Journal 145: 33–43
Josso N, Picard J-Y, Tran D 1977 The anti-Mullerian hormone. Recent Progress in Hormone Research 33: 117–167
Jost A 1953 Problems of fetal endocrinology: the gonadal and hypophyseal hormones. Recent Progress in Hormone Research 8: 379–418
Jost A, Vigier B, Prepin J, Perchelle J P 1973 Studies on sex differentiation in mammals. Recent Progress in Hormone Research 29: 1–41
Klinefelter H F, Reifenstein E C Jnr., Albright F J 1942 Syndrome characterised by gynecomastia, aspermatogenesis without a-leydigism, and increased excretion of follicle stimulating hormone. Journal of Clinical Endocrinology 2: 615–627

Koike S K, Jimbo T, Mizuno M, Sakamoto S 1981 Studies on Mullerian Inhibitors in rats and pigsby semi quantitative bioassay. Asia-Oceania Journal of Obstetrics and Gynaecology 7: 259–271

McCoshen J A 1982 In vivo sex differentiation of congeneic germinal cell aplastic gonads. American Journal of Obstetrics and Gynecology 142: 83–88

Martini L 1982 The 5α-reductase of testosterone in neuroendocrine structures. Biochemical and physiological implications. Endocrine Reviews 3: 1–25

Meade K W, Wachtel S S, Davis J R, Lightner E S 1981 H-Y antigen in XO/x, iso(X) mosaic Turner syndrome. Obstetrics and Gynecology 57: 594–599

Medina M, Chavez B, Perez-Palacios G 1981 Defective androgen action at the cellular level in the androgen resistance syndromes. I. Differences between the complete and incomplete testicular feminization syndromes. Journal of Clinical Endocrinology and Metabolism 53: 1243–1246

Money J 1968a Sex Errors of the Body. Johns Hopkins Press, Baltimore

Money J 1968b Hermaphroditism and pseudohermaphroditism. In: J J Gold (ed) Gynecologic Endocrinology, pp 449–464. Hoeber New York

Morris J M 1953 Syndrome of testicular feminization in male pseudohermaphrodites. American Journal of Obstetrics and Gynecology 65: 1192–1211

Muller U, Wolf U, Siebers J-W, Gunther E 1979 Evidence for a gonad-specific receptor for H-Y antigen: binding of exogenous H-Y antigen to gonadal cells is independent of β2-microglobulin. Cell 17: 331–335

Naftolin F, Ryan K J, Davies I J, Reddy V V, Flores F, Petro Z, Kuhn M, White R J, Takaoka Y, Wolin L 1975 The formation of estrogens by central neuro endocrine tissues. Recent Progress in Hormone Research 31: 295–315

Van Nierkerk W A 1976 True hermaproditism. An analytic review with a report of 3 new cases. American Journal of Obstetrics and Gynaecology 126: 890–907

Neumann F, Von Berswordt-Wallrabe R, Elger W, Steinbeck H, Hehn J D, Kramer M 1970 Aspects of androgen-dependent-events as studied by anti-androgens. Recent Progress in Hormone Research 26: 337–405

Ohno S 1967 Sex Chromosome and Sex Linked Genes. Springer, Berlin

Ohno S 1978 The role of the H-Y antigen in primary sex determination. Journal of the American Medical Association 239: 217–220

Ohno S, Nagai Y, Ciccarese S, Iwata H 1979 Testis-organizing H-Y antigen and the primary sex-determining mechanism in mammals. Recent Progress in Hormone Research 35: 449–470

Paulsen C A, Gordon D L, Carpenter R W, Gandy H M, Drucker W D 1968 Klinefelter's syndrome and its variants: a hormonal and chromosomal study. Recent Progress in Hormone Research 24: 321–353

Perez-Palacios G, Medina M, Ullao-Aguirre a, Chavex B A, Villareal G, Dutrem M T, Cahill L T, Wachtel S 1981a Gonadotrophin dynamics in XX males. Journal of Clinical Endocrinology and Metabolism 53: 254–257

Perez-Palacios G, Carneuale A, Escobar N, Villareal G, Fernandez del C C, Medina M 1981b Induction of ovulation in a true hermaphrodite with male phenotype. Journal of Clinical Endocrinology and Metabolism 52: 1257–1259

Peterson R E, Imperato-McGinley J, Gautier T, Sturla E 1977 Male pseudo hermaphroditism due to steroid 5α-reductase deficiency. American Journal of Medicine 62: 170–179

Picard J-V, Tran D, Josso N 1978 Biosynthesis of labelled anti-Mullerian hormone by fetal testes: evidence for the glycoprotein nature of the hormone and for its disulfide-bonded structure. Molecular and Cellular Endocrinology 12: 17–30

Picon R 1969 Action due testicule foetal sur le development in vetro des canaux de Muller chez le rat. Archives d'Anatomie Microscopique et de Morphologie Experimentale, Paris 58: 1–19

Schellhas H F 1974 Malignant potential of the dysgenetic gonad. Obstetrics and Gynecology 44: 198–309

Schwartz M, Imperato-McGinley J, Peterson R E, Cooper G, Morris P L, MacGillivray M, Henslie T 1981 Male pseudohermaphroditism secondary to an abnormality in Leydig cell differentiation. Journal of Clinical Endocrinology and Metabolism 53: 123–127

Schweikert H U, Weisback L, Leyendecker G, Schwinger E, Wartenberg H, Kruck F 1982 Clinical, endocrinological and cytological characterization of two 46,XX males. Journal of Clinical Endocrinology and Metabolism 54: 745–752

Shearman R P, 1968 A physiological approach to the differential diagnosis and treatment of primary amenorrhoea. Journal of Obstetrics and Gynaecology of the British Commonwealth 75: 1101–1107

Shearman R P 1979 Endocrinology of the feto-maternal unit. In: Shearman R P (ed) Human Reproductive Physiology. 2nd edn, ch 4, pp 97–126. Blackwell Scientific Publications, Oxford

Shearman R P 1981 The intersexes. In: Dewhurst C J (ed) Integrated Obstetrics and Gynaecology for Postgraduates. 3rd edn, Ch 4, pp 37–48. Blackwell Scientific Publications, Oxford

Shearman R P 1982 Intersexuality. In: Beumont P J V, Burrows G D (eds) Handbook of Psychiatry and Endocrinology, Ch 12, pp 325–354. Elsevier, Amsterdam

Shearman R P, Singh S, Lee C W G, Hudson B, Ilbery P L T 1964 Clinical, hormonal and cytogenetic findings in a true hermaphrodite. Journal of Obstetrics and Gynaecology of the British Commonwealth 71: 627–633

Short R V 1979 Sex determination and differentiation. British Medical Bulletin 35: 121–127

Simpson J L, Lebeau M M 1981 Gonadal and statural determinants on the X chromosome and their relationship to in vitro studies showing prolonged cell cycles in 45,X; 46,Xdel(X) (p11); 46,Xdel(X) (q13); and 46,X, del(X) (q22) fibroblasts. American Journal of Obstetrics and Gynecology 141: 930–938

Singh S, Carr D H 1966 The anatomy and histology of XO human embryos and fetuses. Anatomical Record 155: 369–383

Svensson J, Snochowski M 1979 Androgen receptor levels in preputial skin from boys with hypospadias. Journal of Clinical Endocrinology 49: 340–345

Tapanainen J, Kellokumpu-Leehten P, Pelliniemi L, Huhtaniemi I 1981 Age-related changes in endogenous steroids of human fetal testis during early and mid pregnancy. Journal of Clinical Endocrinology and Metabolism 52: 98–102

Tegenkamp T R, Brazell J W, Tegenkamp I, Labidi F 1979 Pregnancy without benefit of reconstructive surgery in a bisexually active true hermaphrodite. American Journal of Obstetrics and Gynecology 135: 427–428

Turner H H 1938 Syndrome of infantilism, congenital webbed neck and cubitus valgus. Endocrinology 23: 566–574

Wachtel S S 1979 The genetics of intersexuality: Clinical and theoretic perspectives. Obstetrics and Gynecology 54: 671–685

Wachtel S S, Ohno S, Koo G C, Boyse E A 1975 Possible role for H-Y antigen in the primary determination of sex. Nature 257: 235–236

Warburton D, Kline J, Stein Z, Susser M 1980 Monosomy X: a chromosomal anomaly associated with young maternal age. Lancet i: 167–169

Wilkins L 1960 Masculinization of the female fetus due to the use of synthetic progrestogens during pregnancy. Acta Endocrinologica 35: (Suppl 51) 671

Wilson J D, Griffin J E, George F W, Leshin M 1981 The role of gonadal steroids in sexual differentiation. Recent Progress in Hormone Research 37: 1–33

Wray H L, Freeman M V R, Ming P-M L 1981 Pregnancy in the Turner syndrome with only 45,X chromosomal constitution. Fertility and Sterility 35: 509–514

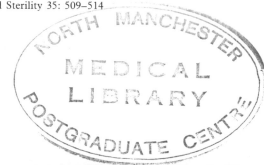

Congenital adrenal hyperplasia

HISTORICAL PERSPECTIVE

It was only by the discovery in 1950 that cortisone successfully arrested the process of virilisation that the adrenogenital syndrome (congenital adrenal hyperplasia-CAH) became clearly understood. For example, in 1937, Young, in his classic book, 'Genital Abnormalities, Hermaphroditism and Related Adrenal Disturbances,' described patients with the adrenogenital syndrome under at least three separate headings. Actually, it was Creccio in 1865 who first clearly described the abnormality although Creccio himself, in the description, did not recognise the association of the adrenal enlargement with the clinical picture. Creccio's exposition is a model of pathological description and is one of the classical descriptions of a disease.

In June of 1820, a woman in Naples gave birth to an infant who was identified by the midwife as a female and she was given the name of Josephine. However, the family was never completely happy about this decision and at the age of 4, Josephine was taken by the family to a surgeon who declared that the patient was a male with testicles in the abdomen. The child was, therefore, put into male attire and the name shortened from Josephine to Joseph. This caused considerable consternation in the neighborhood. At the age of 12, he became a valet in the home of a wealthy Neopolitan family. At 18 years of age, Joseph had the voice of a man and a rapidly increasing beard and, according to Creccio's account, began to have adventures with women. Actually, this reassured the father who had noticed the absence of nocturnal emissions and was concerned about the real sex of his child. The following year, his employers found it necessary to change his service because of his relations with the chambermaid. In the meantime, Joseph contracted a venereal disease twice and this too reassured his father. At the age of 25, he fell in love with another maid, young and gentle, 'qui lui rendait passion pour passion.' Presents were exchanged and Joseph was requested to produce his birth certificate. When he discovered that he had been pronounced at birth to be a female, he procrastinated. In the meantime, his fiance had become

intimate with a new lover, 'but Joseph conducted himself with dignity.' Having been foiled in his matrimonial intentions, he strayed and became a drunkard and braggart of his numerous amorous conquests. He smoked continually, turned against religion, wished to destroy the images of the saints and constantly frequented cabarets where it is said he excelled in telling obscene stories. He died at the age of 43 years.

The autopsy revealed the following data. His height was 156 cm (Fig. 18.1). The circumference of his neck was

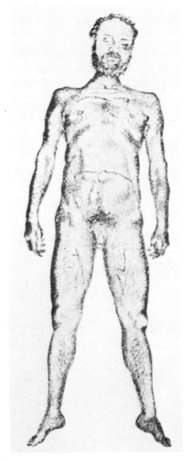

Fig. 18.1 Joseph Martzo of Naples. A sketch made post-mortem

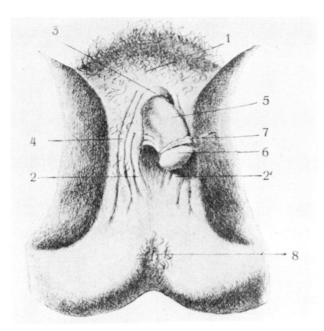

Fig. 18.2 Joseph Martzo. A sketch of the external genitalia

38 cm. His chest was 65 cm. The circumference around the iliac crest was 69 cm. The arms, hands and feet were quite small. The penis was 6 cm in length. It is said that it measured at least 10 cm on erection. The urinary meatus was at the base of the penis. There was no scrotum nor were any testicles palpable (Fig. 18.2). The prostate did not present any anomaly.

On opening the abdomen, a normal uterus and tubes surprisingly were discovered. The ovaries were found in the normal position, were elongated and smooth (Fig. 18.3). They showed no traces of corpora lutea and no

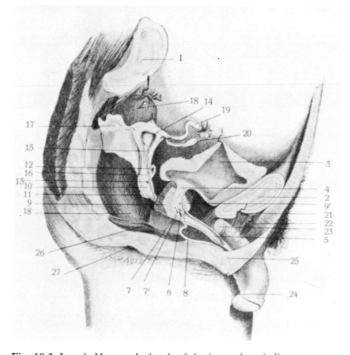

Fig. 18.3 Joseph Martzo. A sketch of the internal genitalia

irregularities. Microscopically, the ovaries did not show any abnormalities, nor did any of the other tissues of the female generative tract so examined. The vagina opened into the urethra and measured 6.5 cm in length and 4 cm in circumference. The communication with the urethra was in the form of a valvule situated next to the prostatic portion. On each side was an opening which simulated the ejaculatory ducts into which a probe could be passed for a short distance. The adrenals were almost as large as the kidneys which were normal in size.

As stated above, Creccio did not understand the relation between the enlarged adrenals and the other findings in his case, nor did those who came after him.

This is quite evident as this macabre story was repeated some 85 years later.

In 1905 in Baltimore, there was a child whose external genitalia was so deformed that its sexual identity was a matter of considerable uncertainty. Nevertheless, he was considered to be a male and Robert was selected for his name. He was legally recorded as a boy and, of course, given male attire and toys. There seemed no problem with this decision in view of the fact that Robert's early growth and development were extra-ordinarily good and, although he was slight, his physical strength and aggressiveness, if not his skill, dominated the activities of the children in the neighborhood. When Robert was a little over 11 years of age, his parents decided that further consultation was required because of his deformed genitalia which had caused so much anxiety at birth. Therefore, Robert was taken to the Out-Patient Department of the Johns Hopkins Hospital for this purpose. He was directed to the Department of Urology where eventually he came under the care of Dr Hugh Hampton Young, the then Professor of Urology. A diagnosis of hypospadius and cryptorchidism was made. Nevertheless, Dr Young and his staff noted certain unusual features about the patient. In spite of all this, there was considerable surprise at the laparotomy when there was encountered by the resident surgeon, a uterus, two fallopian tubes, and two structures which had the appearance more of ovaries than of testes. The confusion about the diagnosis and the proper procedure is clearly revealed by the operation which was selected. This consisted of the removal of the right tube and ovary and nothing more. Histological examination of the removed structures revealed that what was removed was, in fact, just that, a Fallopian tube and an ovary.

Dr Young clearly revealed the thinking of the era when he told Robert's parents that microscopical examination of the gonad, the structure which, by the criteria then in vogue rendered the ultimate decision of sexual identity, had proven that their child was a girl. Therefore, according to Dr Young, it was appropriate that the sex of rearing should be changed from a male to a female.

The parents could scarcely believe their ears and fled from the hospital one block east to the priest of St Andrews parish. This cleric, who was quite familiar with Robert, shared the view of the family and supposed that some mistake surely had been made. The family, with the support of the priest, rejected Dr Young's advice and thereby anticipated later psychosexual studies which indicated the inadvisability of changing a sex of rearing at the time of puberty. In the end, however, Dr Young relented to the extent that he allowed his resident urologist to attempt to form more masculine external genitalia by constructing a urethra. Incidently, the results of this surgery were entirely unsatisfactory.

Robert was unaware of all the family discussions and was discharged from the hospital to continue his role as a male. As an adult, he was short and rather slight but in the business world, was successful for he became the proprietor of a small gasoline filling station not very far from the Johns Hopkins Hospital.

Robert was entirely male in his orientation and activities and, like his predecessor Joseph, became the constant companion of a young woman in his neighbourhood. Eventually, they decided to be married, and Robert and the girl consulted their parish priest to arrange for the wedding ceremony. As chance would have it, the priest they consulted was the same priest who had been consulted by the family some years before at the time Dr Young discovered that Robert had ovaries. The priest was uncertain what to do but eventually told Robert that he was aware of the fact that there were some genital abnormalities and that he, the priest, would be glad to perform the wedding ceremony if Robert could secure a certificate confirming that there was no physical impairment to his marriage.

Robert was in no way concerned about this requirement for in truth he had already demonstrated to himself and to his partner that he was sexually competent. He, therefore, applied to the hospital for such a certificate. He once again came under the care of Dr Young who, of course, remembered the incidence of several years before.

Dr Young was uncertain as to what to do, and his curiosity led him to re-admit Robert to the hospital for further examination (Fig. 18.4, 18.5). On the occasion of this admission, cystoscopy was carried out. Dr Young was able to introduce the tip of the cystoscope into the urogenital sinus and into the vagina where he identified the cervix which, of course, had been there all along. Dr Young again revealed thinking of this era for he refused to give Robert the certificate certifying to his masculinity. The record did not reveal whether Dr Young indicated that Robert should change his sex of rearing at that time.

Within a few days, Robert was brought to the emergency room of the hospital. He was unconscious and anuric for he had taken a large dose of bichloride of mercury, a method of suicide in vogue at that time. Hospitalised and unconscious and unable to complain, he was born not to the urological ward but to the third floor of the women's

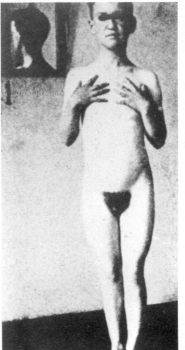
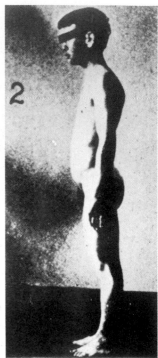
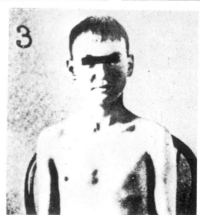

Fig. 18.4 Patient R. S. A photograph taken in 1915 when he was 11 years of age

clinic where, by the sex of his gonad, he belonged and where, as a student, the senior author of this paper had the opportunity to observe the tragedy that was intersexuality.

Robert died without regaining consciousness and the then Professor of Pathology, Dr William MacCallum, himself performed the autopsy. In spite of Creccio's careful pathological description, the pathological findings of this disorder were not widely known and the autopsy was attended by a large number of observers.

As in the case of Creccio, MacCallum verified the presence of a normal uterus, absence of one tube and ovary, which had been previously removed, but the presence of the opposite normal tube and ovary (Fig. 18.6). Again, the main anatomical changes were noted to be in the adrenals which were huge and were described as exactly as in Joseph's case as being as large as his kidneys which were normal in size for kidneys (Fig. 18.7).

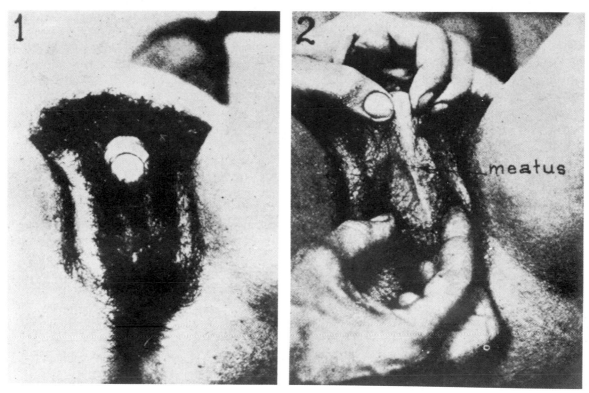

Fig. 18.5 Patient R. S. A photograph of the external genitalia taken in 1915 when he was 11 years of age

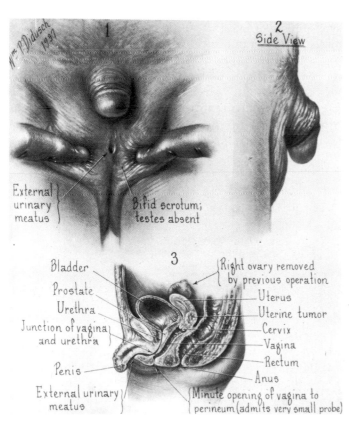

Fig. 18.6 Patient R. S. Age 31. A sketch of the external and internal genitalia made post-mortem

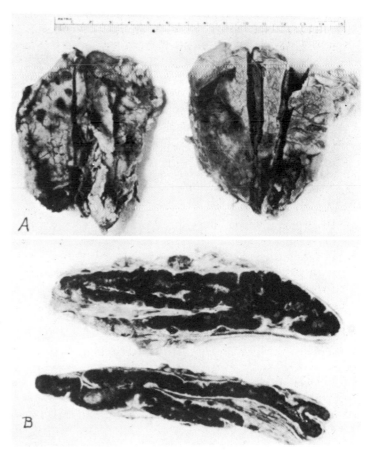

Fig. 18.7 Patient R. S. A photograph of the adrenal glands at autopsy

Thus, although the anatomical findings of this disorder had been described, first by Creccio, then by MacCallum and by others, they were not widely known. Furthermore, the psychosexual orientation of these patients was not at all understood and the danger of attempting to make the psychosexual orientation conform to the anatomical structure of the gonad was by no means appreciated.

It was into this environment that Lawson Wilkins stepped when he began his study of the adrenogenital syndrome. The revelation that cortisone could reverse the relentless progress of the virilisation in these cases provided an opportunity for John Money and others to study the psychosexual orientation of such individuals and required development of appropriate surgical procedures to reconstruct the male genitalia to conform to the female sex which, with cortisone therapy, obviously became the most appropriate rearing for these individuals.

ENZYMATIC VARIATIONS

From cholesterol to △5-pregnenolone to cortisol, there are at least five major enzymatic steps (Fig. 18.8). A deficiency at any one of these steps interferes with the normal production of cortisol. This is the basic deficiency in the syndrome of adrenal hyperplasia. However, there are several variations depending on precisely which step is deficient. Examples have been recorded of deficiencies at each of the five major steps. By far, the most common defect is in hydroxylation at the 21 position. However, as with many enzymatic defects, there seems to be a spectrum of deficiency so that there is a spectrum of clinically distinguishable situations in the female resulting from a deficiency at the 21 position. In the historical section are two examples of the simple virilising form of the disease and

its relentless virilisation. Under circumstances which are even now not clear, the virilising form of the disorder may be associated with serious sodium loss, the so-called 'salt losing form' of the disorder which can be fatal and in its full blown form, was universally fatal until it was recognised that cortisone treatment was useful. At the other end of the spectrum are examples of females with minor or, indeed, no congenital abnormalities due to virilisation but who have oligomenorrhea, perhaps some hirsutism and usually infertility and who seem to have a mild defect at the 21 position. This mild defect is also correctable by appropriate doses of cortisone. C-21 deficiencies are by no means sex limited. Males also may be affected with an entirely different clinical spectrum as will be noted below.

The second most common defect is the 11β-hydroxylase defect encountered mostly in females associated with minor or no deformities of the external genitalia associated with some oligomenorrhea and hirsutism but characterised principally by hypertension. This is an extremely important group to recognise as early recognition of the cause of the hypertension and its treatment with cortisone can result in the reversal of this undesirable and, indeed, potentially fatal manifestation.

The defects due to 17α-hydroxylation are far less common still and result in most bizarre clinical manifestations as these patients are unable to synthesise either androgens or oestrogens. The result is that sex identification is difficult in the male. The failure to be able to synthesise androgens results in female genitalia in genetic males. Thus, broadly considered, congenital adrenal hyperplasia can result in misdiagnosis of sex either way.

The 3β-ol-dehydrogenase defect, which is required for the conversion of △5-pregnenolone to progesterone is likewise unusual and usually fatal although some mild cases have recently been recognised. An enzymatic defect

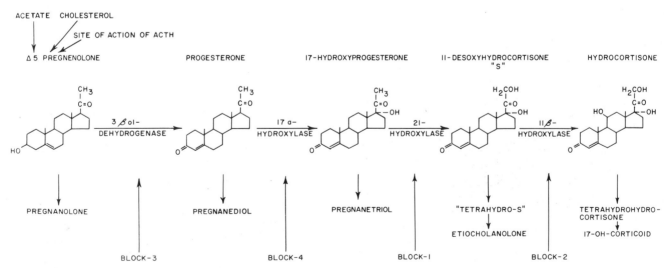

Fig. 18.8 The enzymatic steps in the biosynthesis of cortisol with a localisation of the various defects causing congenital virilising adrenal hyperplasia

between cholesterol and $\triangle$5-pregnenolone is a very rare disorder and fortunately so because it is uniformly fatal. It was described by Prader years ago under the heading of lipoid adrenal hyperplasia.

Thus, broadly considered, adrenal hyperplasia covers a wide spectrum of disorders. However, from a practical point of view, when one speaks of congenital virilising adrenal hyperplasia, one is thinking of a defect at the 21 position, for about 95 per cent of all individuals affected with adrenal hyperplasia have a defect at the 21 position. This is the best understood and this chapter will concern itself principally with defects at the C-21 position, but for completeness, defects at the other positions will be included.

C-21 Hydroxylase deficiency in the female

Clinical considerations

If the diagnosis of *simple virilising adrenal hyperplasia* is not made in infancy, an unfortunate series of events occurs. Because the adrenals secrete an abnormally large amount of virilising steroid hormone, even during embryonic life,

such infants are born with abnormal genitalia. The details of the defects of the genitalia will be described later, but in the fully developed case, there is fusion of the scroto-labial folds and in unusual instances, there is formation of a penile urethra. The clitoris is greatly enlarged so that it may be mistaken for a penis and sexual identification at birth is not always easy. There are, to be sure, no gonads palpable within the fused scroto-labial folds and their absence has sometimes given rise to the mistaken diagnosis of male cryptorchidism. In most cases, there is a single meatus below the tip of the phallus, usually in the perineum or at the junction of the perineum with the phallus, and the vagina, as well as the urethra, enter this persistent urogenital sinus in a rather consistent fashion as will be detailed further on.

During infancy, provided there are no serious electrolyte disturbances, these children, if untreated, grow at a rate greater than normal so that for a time they generally exceed the average in both height and in weight. However, this accelerated growth results in early epiphyscal closure so that full adult growth may be obtained by the age of 10 years, or even earlier. This results in adults who are shorter than average (Fig. 18.9, 18.10, 18.11).

At an early age, the process of virilisation begins. Pubic hair may appear at the age of 2 years, and rarely earlier, but most often somewhat later. This is followed by the development of axillary hair and finally the appearance of

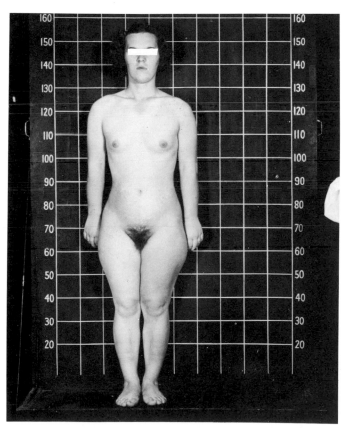

Fig. 18.9 A patient with congenital virilising adrenal hyperplasia at 17 years of age. She had received no cortisone therapy until she was 16 and she exhibits the features of untreated patients. She is short in stature with extremities that are relatively short for the length of the torso. The feminisation she exhibits in the photograph is the result of 8 months treatment with cortisone

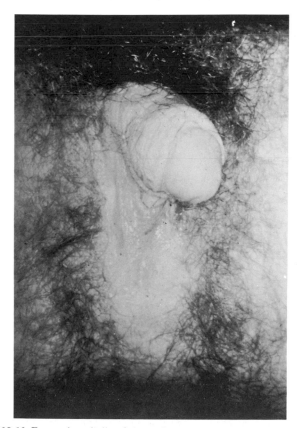

Fig. 18.10 External genitalia of the patient shown in Fig. 18.9

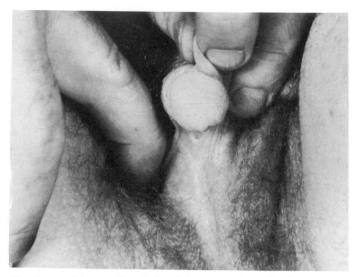

Fig. 18.11 The external genitalia of the patient shown in Fig. 18.9. The phallus is elevated to illustrate the fusion of the scroto-labial folds with an external meatus along the shaft of the phallus

body hair and a beard which is often troublesome enough to require shaving. Acne may develop. Puberty never appears. There is no breast development. Menstruation does not occur.

During this entire process, the intermediate metabolites prior to the enzyme block are greatly elevated as is the urinary 17-ketosteroid excretion in the urine.

The course of events described above has not been observed since the disorder has been understood and the ability has been at hand to make the diagnosis in infancy and to use cortisone or one of its analogues for therapy. Nevertheless, it is important for the student and practitioner to understand the consequences of failure of therapy for even now treatment is often less than ideal, especially during infancy and childhood when oral medication is the

mode of therapy and when the motivation to take the medication may be less than ideal on the part of the child or her parents. To prevent the events described above, continuous therapy, which is increased with advancing age, must be carried out conscientiously during the adolescent and adult period. If this is not done, problems of height and reproduction will be the undesirable consequence.

Individuals with virilising hyperplasia may have the complicating syndrome of electrolyte imbalance, the so-called *salt losing type of adrenal hyperplasia*. In infancy, this is manifest by vomiting, progressive loss of weight, dehydration, and unless recognised promptly, often by death. Such episodes are, in fact, a form of Addisonian crisis. The condition is sometimes misdiagnosed with dire consequences. The characteristic findings are an exceedingly low serum sodium and a high potassium value. Any serum sodium below normal must be regarded with suspicion and any value below 120 mEq/l requires energetic therapy. Serum potassium may be elevated prior to the sodium deficiency. Treatment may result in the dangerous level of 11 mEq/l apparently due to a shift of potassium into the extracellular fluid caused by only a modest decrease in potassium urinary excretion.

It can be estimated that approximately one-half of all infants affected with defects at the C-21 position have the salt losing type of hyperplasia.

In the event the patient proves to have the complicating salt losing variety of the disorder, therapy will be required with desoxycorticosterone in addition to cortisol as will be described in detail in the section on therapy.

Pathological changes

Adrenal. Interest in the endocrinological changes associated with CAH has overshadowed interest in the patho-

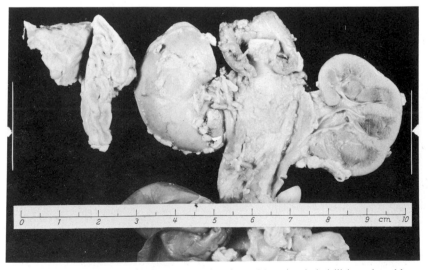

Fig. 8.12 An autopsy specimen of the kidneys and adrenals of an untreated patient with congenital virilising adrenal hyperplasia who died of Addisonian crisis at the age of 3 weeks. Notice the size of the adrenals in comparison to the kidneys

logical anatomy of the disorder. Nevertheless, a knowledge of the pathological changes provides an exquisite understanding of the disorder.

The pathological changes in the adrenal gland were completely reviewed by Jones & Jones (1954), based on a study of 15 specimens from female pseudohermaphrodites. Due to the advent of cortisone therapy in 1950, there has been little opportunity for further study of the untreated adrenal.

The adrenals in all cases were greatly enlarged over the normal size for the age (Fig. 18.12). The largest adrenal glands weighed 80 and 90 g, respectively, compared to a normal adult weight of about 5 g. (These were the adrenals of Robert referred to in the section on historical perspective.) Grossly, the outer layers of the normal cortex are yellow and the inner, or reticular, layer is thin and light brown. In these cases, the pathologist at the time of autopsy, uniformly described the fresh adrenals as being composed of an outer pale or white zone in addition to a darker brown or reddish inner zone.

Microscopically, all cases showed some degree of hyperplasia of the reticular zone of the cortex. In general, the degree of hyperplasia seemed to increase with age. It was most easily seen in adults where upward of 90 per cent of the cortex was occupied by reticularis, compared to a normal adult composition of from one-quarter to one-third of the cortical width (Fig. 18.13, 18.14). An estimation of the degree of reticular hyperplasia in infancy and childhood depends upon a comparison of the gland in question with the expected reticular width for the age. According to Blackman (1946) and in agreement with other studies, the fetal reticular zone normally disappears by the end of the

first month of post-natal life. The adult reticular zone, lying next to the fascicular zone and composed of cells smaller and with darker nuclei than those of the fetal reticular zone (haematoxylin and eosin), first appears as a thin layer at about 1 week of age. This layer gradually enlarges and becomes pigmented, until it occupies its adult proportion of one-quarter to one-third of the cortical width at puberty. In infant hermaphrodites, there was great hyperplasia of the adult reticular zone and in all instances, this zone occupied well over half the cortex, even in a patient who died at the age of 7 days. The hyperplasia of adult reticularis was, therefore, very great when compared with the expected reticular development at the corresponding age.

The fetal reticularis did not participate in the hyperplastic process. Fetal reticularis was present in five patients under 5 months of age, but was less noticeable with increasing age until at the age of 5 months, it was scarcely present.

In addition to reticular hyperplasia, the glands under discussion exhibited other abnormalities. In four young infants who died and in a gland removed surgically from a patient age 5 months, the glomerular layer, which is concerned with electrolyte metabolism, was practically absent, although in two instances a few cells apparently belonging to the glomerulosa could be seen within the fibrous capsule. In other glands the glomerulosa seemed normally formed or actually hyperplastic. In an adult 29 years old, the glomerular layer was about 30 cells deep compared to a normal depth of about five. In eight instances, there was considered to be some degree of glomerular hyperplasia. It may be significant that the four

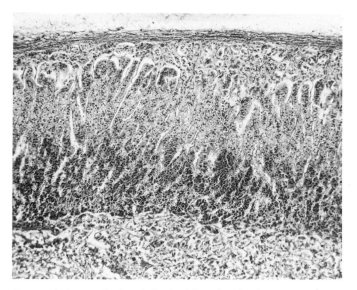

Fig. 18.13 A normal adrenal clearly delineating the three zones: the zona reticularis above, the zona fasciculata, and the zona reticularis below (H & E, × 56)

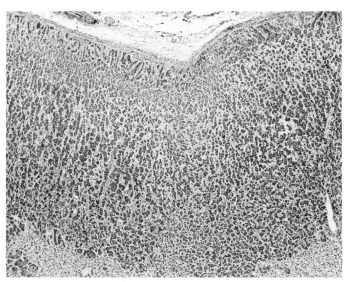

Fig. 18.14 Photomicrograph of case R. S. An untreated patient with congenital virilising adrenal hyperplasia. Note the great hyperplasia of zona reticularis and the difficulty of identifying the zona fasciculata (H & E, × 30)

infants with deficient glomerulosa died in Addisonian crisis and the child 5 months old, who had an adrenalectomy exhibited serious electrolyte imbalance.

The fascicular zone also exhibited marked variation. There was recognisable fasciculata in all instances. In all adults, it was no more than ten cells thick, compared to a normal thickness of 30 to 50 cells and in some areas it was absent. This variation in fasciculata in different areas of the same gland was characteristic for the majority of specimens. The fasciculata normally contains spongy, vacuolated cytoplasm when studied in the routine haematoxylin and eosin section. In the cases under discussion, the fasciculata was mainly composed of cells which exhibited homogeneous eosinophilic non-vacuolated cytoplasm. The fasciculata seemed to become less prominent with increasing age. It is interesting that in two instances in glands from patients who presented a slightly less severe form of the abnormality, the fasciculata approached normal and contained cells with more prominent vacuolisation.

The studies with the formalin fixed material for lipid seemed most significant. Normally, the reticularis contains very little lipid. The fasciculata contains abundant lipid and the glomerulosa contains less. In the hyperplastic glands, there was substantial lipid in the reticularis of five of seven specimens. The fetal reticularis, where present,

also reacted positively, as is normal. The lipid was acetone soluable (Figs. 18.15–18.18).

The absence of lipid from the fasciculata together with

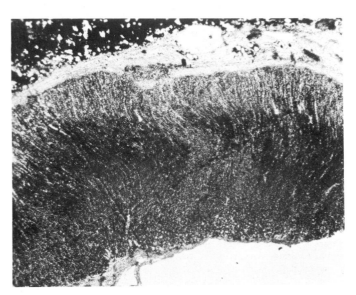

Fig. 18.16 The adrenals of a patient with untreated congenital virilising hyperplasia. Stained with Sudan black B to show the absence of lipid in the zona fasciculata and the heavy deposition of lipid in the zona reticularis. (Sudan black B, × 30)

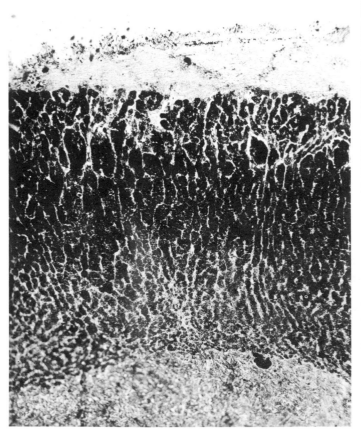

Fig. 18.15 A normal adrenal stained with Sudan black B to show the heavy lipid content of the zona fasciculata (Sudan black B, × 57)

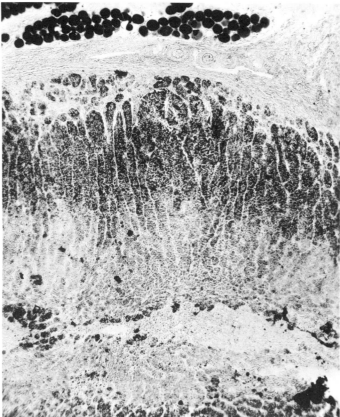

Fig. 18.17 A normal adrenal stained with Sudan III. Note the heavy lipid content of the zona fasciculata and the absence of lipid in the zona reticularis (Sudan III, × 5)

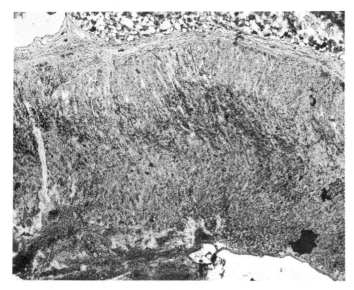

Fig. 18.18 The adrenals of a patient with untreated congenital virilising adrenal hyperplasia stained with Sudan III. Note the absence of lipid in the zona fasciculata and the deposition of more than normal lipid in the zona reticularis. (Sudan III, × 30)

its anatomical deformity may be of considerable importance in view of the probability that this layer is concerned with the production of the glucocorticoids. It is entirely likely that this abnormality of the fasciculata is the fundamental pathological change in this syndrome and that all other changes pathologically and endocrinologically and, therefore, clinically are the result of this fascicular abnormality.

One may summarise the adrenal changes by noting that the great adrenal enlargement seems to be due principally to a reticular hyperplasia and that this hyperplasia in untreated patients apparently becomes more marked with increasing age. In some instances, the glomerulosa seems to participate in the hyperplasia, although in four glands of patients with fatal electrolyte depletion, the glomerulosa was absent. The fasciculata was greatly diminished in amount or entirely absent. Lipid studies showed absence of fascicular and glomerular lipid, contrary to the normal situation, while there was an abnormally strong lipid reaction in the reticularis in five of the seven cases studied (Fig. 18.19).

Ovary. In view of the absence of menstruation in untreated patients, the ovaries of these patients are of considerable interest. Ovarian tissue or sections were studied in 17 untreated patients and reported by Jones & Jones (1954). In infants, the ovaries showed no recognisable change from normal. There were abundant primordial follicles, some of which had developed to become macroscopically visible, but none were greater than 4 mm in diameter. A few antrum follicles were seen. Atretic follicles were also noted. The ovarian stroma was normally sparse. The ovary in older untreated hermaphrodites became increasingly abnormal. In the teenage individuals, there

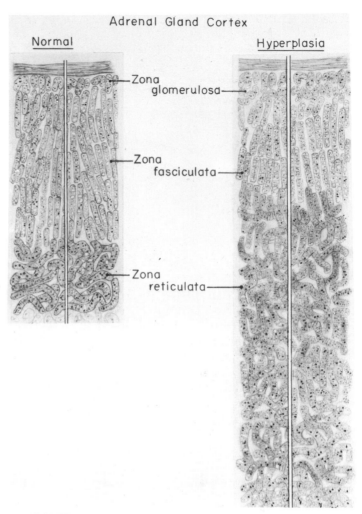

Adrenal Gland Cortex

Normal — Hyperplasia

— Zona glomerulosa —

— Zona fasciculata —

— Zona reticulata —

Fig. 18.19 The normal and hyperplastic adrenal glands illustrating the changes associated with congenital virilising adrenal hyperplasia

were also primordial, developing and antrum follicles, but there was no sign of recent or previous ovulation. The ovaries of two hermaphrodites, 29 and 32 years old, were greatly abnormal, age considered. There were no primordial follicles and no developing or atretic follicles. The ovarian cortex consisted entirely of stroma (Fig. 18.20). In one of these ovaries, there were a few structures suggesting very old corpora albicantia in spite of the absence of a history of any menstrual bleeding. There was no sign of luteinisation about the developing or atretic follicles in any case of marked hermaphroditism. In two patients showing a less severe degree of the abnormality, there was some luteinisation. It is interesting that it was in these latter two cases that the adrenal sections contained some normal fasciculata.

The ovarian changes may be summarised by stating that in infants, children and teenagers, there seemed to be normal follicular development to the antrum stage but no evidence of ovulation. As the hermaphrodites aged, there was less and less follicular activity and a disappearance of primordial follicles. It should be noted that this disappear-

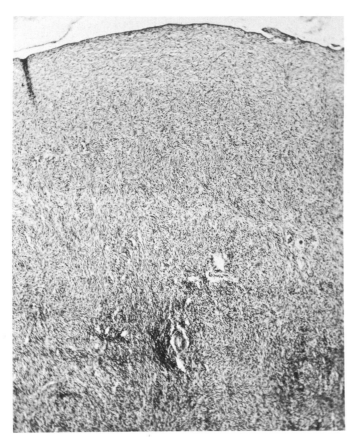

Fig. 18.20 Ovary of a 29-year-old untreated patient with congenital virilising adrenal hyperplasia. Note the relative sparcity of germ cells (H & E, × 48)

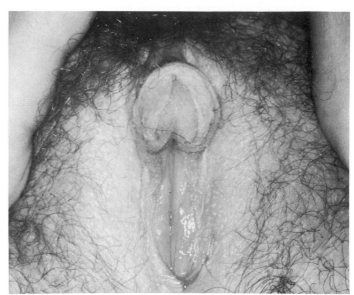

Fig. 18.21 An external genitalia of an adult with a relatively mild form of congenital virilising adrenal hyperplasia. Note the enlargement of the clitoris and relatively little or no fusion of the scroto-labial folds

ance must not be as complete as it seemed to be microscopically, as cortisone therapy, even in adults, usually results in ovulatory menstruation after a treatment period of 4–6 months.

Developmental anomalies of the genitalia

The study of a relatively large number of cases of female hermaphroditism due to congenital adrenal hyperplasia, has indicated that the Wolffian ducts atrophy in the usual manner. Furthermore, the Müllerian derivatives are uniformly present in an undeveloped state. There are, however, serious anomalies of the urogenital sinus derivatives.

The description about to be made of the anomalies which arise from these structures is based upon a study of

over 300 hermaphrodites with congenital adrenal hyperplasia and somewhat fewer cases of a less severe form of the anomaly in patients with primary amenorrhoea who virilised at puberty. Women, who at first glance appear normal, may exhibit very mild forms of congenital adrenal hyperplasia and have minor anomalies of the external genitalia, such as an enlarged clitoris (Fig. 18.21). The description is made in some detail because of the important surgical anatomical considerations involved in the reconstruction of these abnormal genitalia.

The phallus is composed of two lateral corpora cavernosa, but the corpus cavernosum urethrae is normally absent. The external urinary meatus is most often located at the base of the phallus. However, an occasional case may be seen where the urethra does extend to the end of the clitoris. The glans penis and the prepuce are present and indistinguishable from these structures as developed in the male. The scroto-labial folds are characteristically fused in the midline, giving a scrotal-like appearance with a median perineal raphe, although they seldom enlarge to normal scrotal size. No gonads are palpable within the scroto-labial folds. In circumstances where the anomaly is not so severe, as in patients with post-natal virilisation, the fusion of the scroto-labial folds is not so complete and by gentle retraction, it is often possible to locate not only the normally

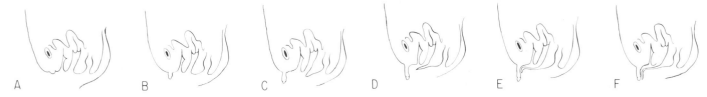

Fig. 18.22 Progressive stages of virilisation of the external genitalia in congenital virilising adrenal hyperplasia. A = normal; B–E = progressive stages of virilisation; F = complete masculinisation of external genitalia of a female patient

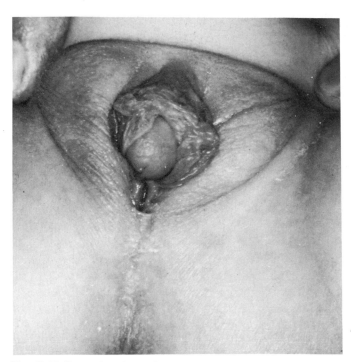

Fig. 18.23 External genitalia of a patient with CAH with a type B deformity of the external genitalia as illustrated in Fig. 18.22

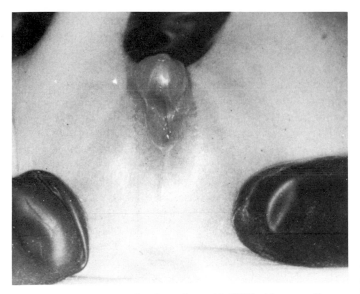

Fig. 18.24 External genitalia of a patient with CAH with a type C deformity of the external genitalia as illustrated in Fig. 18.22

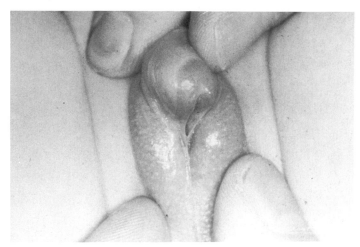

Fig. 18.25 External genitalia of a patient with CAH with a type D deformity of the external genitalia as illustrated in Fig. 18.22

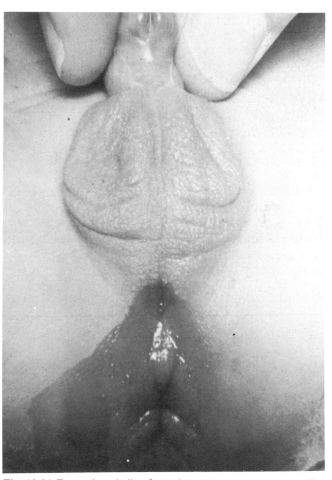

Fig. 18.26 External genitalia of a patient with CAH with a type E deformity of the external genitalia as illustrated in Fig. 18.22

located external urinary meatus, but the orifice of the vagina. These various degrees of fusion form a continuous series of abnormalities (Figs. 18.22, 18.23, 18.24, 18.25, 18.26, 18.27).

An occasional case is encountered where no communication can be found between the urogenital sinus and the vagina. Careful endoscopic examination has shown that in no case has the vagina communicated with that portion of the urogenital sinus which gives rise to the female urethra in the case of a female or the prostatic urethra in the case of a male. The vaginal communication was always in relation to the caudal urogenital sinus derivatives so that the sphincter mechanism is fortunately not involved and the anomalous communication is with that portion of the sinus yielding the vaginal vestibule in the female and the

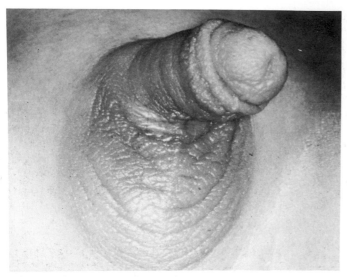

Fig. 18.27 External genitalia of a patient with CAH with a type F deformity of the external genitalia as illustrated in Fig. 18.22

membranous urethra in the male. From the point of view of the gynaecologist, it is much clearer to speak of the vagina and (female) urethra as entering a persistent urogenital sinus rather than to speak of the vagina as entering the (membranous male) urethra.

Endocrinological findings

A deficiency in 21-hydroxylase enzyme leads to decreased conversion of 17α-hydroxyprogesterone to desoxycortisol and thus, to a decrease in cortisol production (Fig. 18.8). The diminished cortisol production causes an increase in ACTH which leads to an increased production of 17α-hydroxyprogesterone, and 17α-hydroxypregnenolone and an increased conversion of these compounds to adrenal androgens. The 17α-hydroxyprogesterone is increased 10–400 fold in the untreated patient making its determination the most useful diagnostic test for the 21-hydrox-

ylase defect (Hughes & Winters, 1976, 1977). In normal newborns, the plasma 17α-hydroxyprogesterone is elevated during the first 24–36 hours of life. It is also elevated in some stressed or ill newborns; thus, the collection of blood for 17α-hydroxyprogesterone determination should be delayed until the second day of life in a female with ambiguous genitalia, or in a male infant from an affected family. Pregnanetriol is the urinary excretory product of 17α-hydroxyprogesterone and has been used in the past as a diagnostic marker for the disorder.

ACTH should be elevated in the untreated patient; however, it is not consistently elevated and does not differentiate between the various adrenal enzyme defects. ACTH determinations do not appear to be useful in either the initial diagnosis or in the continuing management of patients with congenital adrenal hyperplasia (Fukushima et al, 1975; Smith et al, 1980; La Franchi, 1980). All of the adrenal androgens, △4-androstenedione, dehydroepiandrosterone (DHEA) and testosterone, are increased in the untreated patient. Elevated serum androgen levels are not diagnostic of the disorder, but may be extremely useful to follow as indicators of appropriate therapy. Increased androstenedione and DHEA lead to an increased excretion of urinary 17-kestosteroids which, in the past, has been used in diagnosis and to follow adequacy of therapy.

With initiation of hydrocortisone therapy, 17α-hydroxyprogesterone, androstenedione, DHEA, and testosterone levels return to normal. Therapy may be monitored with plasma 17α-hydroxyprogesterone levels which should remain below 200 ng/dl. In the prepubertal child and the adult female, androstenedione or testosterone are also useful indicators of hormonal control (Korth-Schutz, 1978). In the pubertal or adult male, androstenedione continues to be a sensitive indicator of adrenal hyperfunction.

In two-thirds of patients with the 21-hydroxylase defect, the synthesis of aldosterone is also impaired (Fig. 18.28).

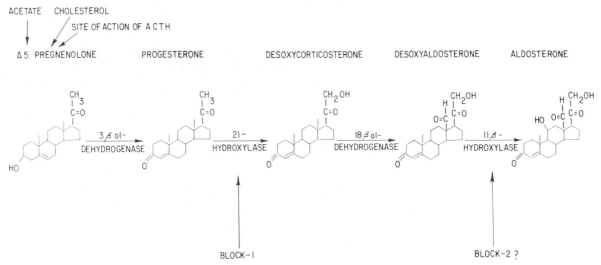

Fig. 18.28 Enzymatic steps in the biosynthetic pathway of aldosterone

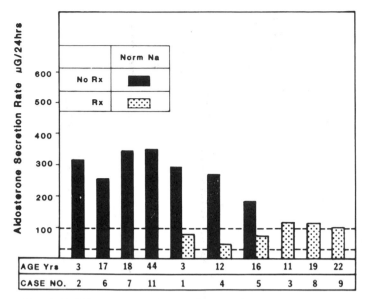

Fig. 18.29 Aldosterone secretion rate in ten patients with the simple virilising form of CAH. All patients were on a normal sodium diet and were either untreated or had been treated for at least 7 days. The shaded area represents the range of variation of aldosterone secretion rate in six normal adults on a normal sodium diet. When patients were untreated the secretion rates were greater than normal whereas they came to be within the normal range after 1 week of treatment (Reproduced from Journal of Clinical Investigation, 1965, 44, 1505–1513, by copyright permission of the American Society for Clinical Investigation)

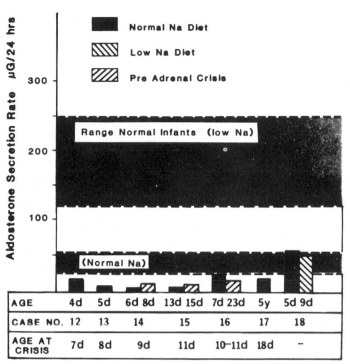

Fig. 18.30 Aldosterone secretion rate inpatients with the salt-losing form of congenital adrenal hyperplasia. The seven patients presented in this figure had no therapy and were receiving a normal sodium diet at the time of the study. A second study was carried out on patients 14, 15 and 16 just before an adrenal crisis and on patient 18 went on a low-dodium diet. The patients are arranged according to the severity of their salt-losing tendency as determined by their age at the time of the first spontaneous adrenal crisis. Patient 18 did not go into crisis even when on a low sodium diet for 4 days (Reproduced from Journal of Clinical 1965, 44, 1505–1513, by copyright permission of the American Society for Clinical Investigation)

If unrecognised, symptomatic aldosterone deficiency may develop with hyperkalaemia, hyponatermia, dehydration, and secondary hypotension. While patients with a complete defect in 21-hydroxylation have a depletion of total body sodium at birth, serum sodium is usually preserved within the normal range for 5–10 days (Loras et al, 1970). Aldosterone secretory rates in these patients are below normal and do not increase with sodium depletion; in contrast, patients with incomplete 21-hydroxylase defect have an elevated aldosterone secretory rate prior to cortisol therapy consistent with a hyperfunctioning adrenal gland (Figs. 18.29 and 18.30). (Kowarski et al, 1965). Plasma renin activity is elevated in patients with aldosterone deficiency and may aid in the diagnosis of the complete form of the disorder prior to a severe salt wasting crisis. Additionally, plasma renin activity is useful in assessing adequacy of mineralocorticoid therapy on a chronic basis (Hughes, 1976; Rosler, 1977).

Genetic aspects

Congenital virilising adrenal hyperplasia is due to a defective gene coding for the 21-hydroxylase enzyme. The disorder is inherited in an autosomal recessive manner. Original studies in 1956 by Childs et al, calculated a rough incidence in the state of Maryland for affected children as 1:67 000 live births. This suggested a gene frequency, or the heterozygous state, of 1:129 normal individuals. More recent studies, (Prader et al, 1962; Qazi & Thompson, 1972; Werder et al, 1980; Murtaza et al, 1980), all working among predominantly caucasian population, suggest an incidence of 1:12 000 to 13 000 live births. The studies by Prader et al (1962, 1980) surveyed the population of Switzerland and found an overall incidence of 1:15 472 for affected children with the 21-hydroxylase deficiency. The incidence calculated from the number of females recognised is 1:12 098; this incidence figure is thought to more accurately reflect the true incidence since the disorder is more likely to be recognised in affected females than in the male. In several of the cantons of Switzerland, the incidence was as high as 1:7000 live births. The overall data from Switzerland give a gene frequency of 1:56. A similar retrospective study from Wales (Murtaza et al, 1980) and from Canada (Qazi et al, 1972) also found a calculated gene frequency of approximately 1:55 for the combined frequency of simple virilising and the salt-losing variety of the disorder. The studies from Wales, Canada and Switzerland found that two-thirds of the affected children had the salt-losing form of the disorder. Hirschfeld & Meshman (1969) in a population of Alaskan Eskimos found a remarkable incidence of 1:490 giving a gene frequency of about

1: 11. In round numbers in the Caucasian population, it may not be too inaccurate to think in terms of a gene frequency of 1:60 for the combined simple and salt-losing form of the disorder.

As with all autosomal recessive disorders, affected children of unaffected heterozygous parents appear in the ratio of one affected to three unaffected individuals. Of the three non-affected individuals, two will be heterozygous carriers. Therefore, the answer to the parents of an affected child as to the possibility of a second affected child is that there is a 1 in 4 possibility and that this possibility stays the same no matter how many children the parents have. There seems to be no predilection for sex.

Much work has been done attempting to identify heterozygous carriers for the disorder. At the present time, the best available technique seems to be that proposed by Gutai et al (1977). The test involves the administration under basal conditions of an intravenous bolus of 1.0 mg of synthetic 1–24 ACTH (cortrosyn) and the determination of plasma progesterone and 17-hydroxyprogesterone at 30, 45, and 60 min intervals following the ACTH administration. The combined rate of increased progesterone and 17-hydroxyprogesterone in heterozygotes exceeds by 2 s.d. the values of the control group. However, Gutai et al (1977) in the initial publication point out that there was about a 30 per cent false identification rate among obligate heterozygotes. Subsequent workers have confirmed this finding. Thus, the cortrosyn challenge test is very useful, if it is positive but has a false negative rate.

Dupont et al (1977) first reported that the gene responsible for the 21-hydroxylase deficiency was closely linked to the HLA complex. The HLA complex is known to be located on the short arm of chromosome 6. Webb et al. (1980) provided cytogenetic evidence for locating the gene for CAH on chromosome 6. Subsequent to DuPont's discovery, several other groups have confirmed this finding and applied it to a determination of the carrier status. For example, Bias et al (1981) did HLA and other typing as well as ACTH stimulation in seven families. The carrier status correlated with the appropriate HLA haplotype in all offspring with two exceptions which were thought to be due to intra-HLA recombination. The present evidence seems to indicate that the 21-hydroxylase deficiency gene is very closely linked to the HLA-B locus.

The HLA data speak to the question of whether one or more genes are involved in the simple virilising and salt-losing forms of the disorder. In view of the fact that the HLA linkage seems to be the same regardless of whether the patient is affected with the salt-loosing form of the disorder or not suggests that the locus is the same and that if the genes are different, there may well be an allelic series. If this were the case, one could expect a minimum of three genetic forms of congenital adrenal hyperplasia; that is, a salt-losing homozygote, a non-salt-losing homozygote, and cases with both a salt-losing and a non-salt-losing gene.

Phenotypically, therefore, one might predict that the salt losing cases would be of at least two types, a severe homozygous type and a milder heterozygous type.

Brautbar et al (1979) determined that there was no linkage between HLA and congenital adrenal hyperplasia due to the 11β-hydroxylase deficiency.

The relationship of HLA, if any, to the other forms of adrenal hyperplasia has apparently not been determined.

Prenatal diagnosis

In special circumstances, the prenatal diagnosis of congenital adrenal hyperplasia may be indicated. In view of the reasonably satisfactory therapy of the condition, amniocentesis is certainly not indicated as a routine even when there is a known risk for the disorder. On the other hand an affected parent or a prospective parent who has intimate knowledge of the disorder may wish to know whether a fetus is affected, even with the option of abortion.

Nagamani et al, (1978) reported the use of elevated amniotic fluid 17α-hydroxyprogesterone levels for this purpose. While the endocrinological determination of an affected fetus *in utero* is possible, the use of HLA haplotyping gives reassuring confirmatory evidence. A number of workers have utilised this technique. For example, Forrest et al (1981) determined amniotic fluid levels of 17-hydroxyprogesterone and testosterone in 17 pregnancies at risk for congenital adrenal hyperplasia and compared these results to 75 normal controls. The fetus was predicted to be unaffected in 12 cases on the findings of normal levels of both 17-hydroxyprogesterone and testosterone. HLA typing confirmed normality in the 12 cases revealing, however, five carriers, five homozygous normal individuals, and two indeterminant. Three fetuses were predicted to be congenital adrenal hyperplasia affected on unambiguously high levels of 17-hydroxyprogesterone and testosterone. The HLA typing was in agreement. The diagnosis was confirmed in two abortuses and one female newborn by physical and hormonal studies.

However, in two cases, the levels of 17-hydroxyprogesterone and testosterone were normal, but the HLA genotypes were identical to siblings affected with congenital adrenal hyperplasia. The normal physical and hormonal findings in the two aborted fetuses seemed to exclude the virilising form of adrenal hyperplasia. It was thought that the discrepancy in the HLA genotyping was on the basis of recombination.

It is clear from the above study that for the best results, both the HLA genotyping and the amniotic fluid levels of hydroxyprogesterone and testosterone would be the best method for prenatal detection.

Pathogenesis

The critical effect of the enzymatic defect in congenital adrenal hyperplasia is the inability to synthesise cortisol. There is a see-saw homeostatic relationship between cortisol and pituitary ACTH whereby ACTH is suppressed by increase of cortisol administration or production and ACTH is increased in the absence of such negative feedback from cortisol. Therefore, in affected individuals, there is a great increase in ACTH production. The adrenal responds the only way it can: by excess secretion of that part of the adrenal which is competent to respond; namely, the zona reticularis which has as its primary function the production of the sex steroids, both oestrogen and androgen. Not only does this portion of the adrenal respond with increased production but is stimulated to respond by hyperplasia so that the number of cells is greater as noted in the section on pathology. An affected individual may actually have adrenal cortisol production which is in the normal range. However, this is obtained only by a very large excess of ACTH secretion. The products of the zona reticularis are overwhelmingly androgenic and, therefore, virilise the external genitalia during embryonic life. The feedback on the hypothalamus suppresses the pituitary gonadotrophins. The principal agent in this action is probably the excess oestrogen from the zona reticularis. In any case, in the fully affected individual, the pituitary gonadotrophins do not increase at the expected time of puberty with the result that the untreated patient does not have pubertal changes nor does menstruation occur. Therapy with cortisol reverses all these changes by suppressing the excess pituitary ACTH with the result that the excess output of the oestrogen and androgen from the zona reticularis is decreased and, therefore, the negative feedback on the pituitary gonadotrophin is removed so that pubertal changes and menstruation will occur in properly treated individuals.

Less clear is the interrelationships between aldosterone production and the salt-losing form of the disorder. It has been demonstrated in the simple virilising form of the disorder that there seems to be excess aldosterone secretion. This apparently has no biological effect for reasons which even now are not entirely clear. In the salt-losing form of the disorder, the aldosterone production is deficient. This is somewhat puzzling because, in the biosynthetic pathway to cortisol, 21-hydroxylation has as a substrate 17-hydroxyprogesterone. On the other hand, in the biosynthetic pathway to aldosterone, 17-hydroxylation is not required and 21-hydroxylation occurs with progesterone as a substrate. This would imply the non-specificity of the substrate for the 21-hydroxylase enzymatic defect. This seems to be an exception to the general rule of one enzyme–one substrate.

As mentioned in the section on the genetics of this disorder, it may well be that the various forms of adrenal hyperplasia are due to genes of an allelic series so that the gene defect in the salt-losing form may be somewhat different from the gene for the simple virilising form. As will be mentioned under therapy for the salt-losing form of the disorder, treatment with cortisone does not completely replace the deficiency and supplementary therapy, first with desoxycorticosterone acetate and subsequently with fludrocortisone acetate is required for homeostasis.

The question of whether there are multiple or a single 21-hydroxylase defect in hyperplasia has been studied by a number of investigators in a variety of ways. For example, West et al (1979) measured the activity of the 21-hydroxylase or hydroxylases by sampling the plasma 17-hydroxyprogesterone and cortisol levels simultaneously at frequent intervals throughout the day in two patients with the simple virilising form of hyperplasia and in three patients with the salt-losing form. Plasma progesterone and corticosteroid concentrations were also measured on the same blood samples as an index to progesterone 21-hydroxylase activity in the corticosterone biosynthetic pathway. During periods of maximal adrenal secretory activity, it was found that plasma 17-hydroxyprogesterone concentrations were markedly elevated in all patients while cortisol levels were either low normal in the non-salt losers or low in the salt losers. At the same time, plasma progesterone and corticosteroid concentrations were normal or elevated in both forms of hyperplasia. The authors interpreted these results as being in favour of a multiple enzyme deficiency in the pathogenesis of adrenal hyperplasia.

Psychological aspects

The case histories of the two individuals detailed in the section on historical perspective underline the importance of the psychological aspect of individuals affected with adrenal hyperplasia.

In the contemporary setting, a misdiagnosis of sex is extremely unlikely so that there is little chance that it will be necessary to deal with the psychological problems in an adult who has been reared in an inappropriate gender. Thus, in the contemporary setting, it is unlikely that the patient will have problems with psychosexual orientation provided treatment is instituted early endocrinologically and surgically and those dealing with the patient are understanding and oriented about problems of sexual development. Thus, it is of importance that the parents, grandparents, or others, who might deal with an infant with anomalies of the external genitalia be made to understand that this represents no innate imprinting of a contrary sex but rather is a developmental defect which can be corrected by appropriate surgery and which will have no long-term deleterious effects.

Such has not always been the case. When cortisone first became available as therapy in the 1950s, many individuals

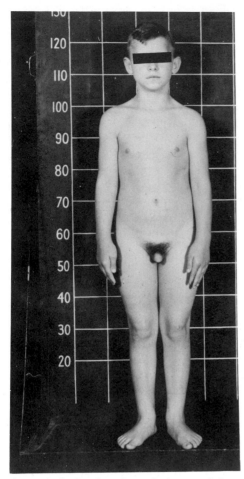

Fig. 18.31 A genetically female patient raised as a male because of a mistaken diagnosis of the genetic sex at birth

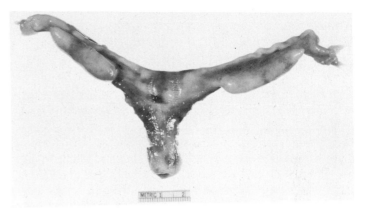

Fig. 18.33 The uterus, tubes and ovaries of the patient shown in Fig. 18.31

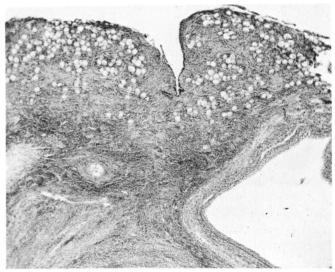

Fig. 18.34 The ovaries of the patient shown in Fig. 18.31. Note the large number of primary follicles in this individual operated upon prior to the age of puberty

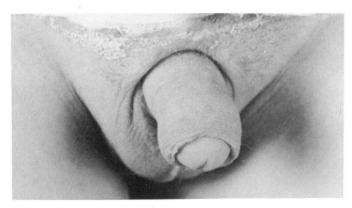

Fig. 18.32 The external genitalia of the patient shown in Fig. 18.31

at all stages had the opportunity to be treated. Some of these had been reared in an inappropriate sex (Fig. 18.31, 18.32, 18.33, 18.34). There was, therefore, an extraordinary opportunity to study those factors which influence gender role and John Money et al (1955), Anka Ehrhardt et al (1968) and others in a series of studies were able to elucidate those factors which were most important in forming the gender role of not only these patients but of

normal individuals. Money et al (1955) found that gender role and outlook as man or boy, girl or woman, was found to be in agreement with the sex of rearing in a very high percentage of patients and was not to be automatically or instinctively determined by genetic consideration, gonads or hormones. However, Ehrhardt et al (1968) found that among girls with the adrenogenital syndrome who were treated early, such patients, in comparison with suitable controls, showed a much higher interest in masculine associated clothing and toy preference and very little interest in feminine associated clothing and toys. In general, the patients considered themselves and were considered tomboys. Their tomboyism, however, did not exclude a concept of eventual romance, marriage, and motherhood. These authors raised the question of whether the tomboyish traits were a product of their early androgenisation *in utero* perhaps as a result of action of the androgens on the hypophysis or related areas of the brain. A critical point, of historical interest in the 1980s, was the effect of the age of operation on the ultimate psychosexual orientation of the individuals. This was studied by Lewis et al (1970), and it was found that it was best to do reconstructive surgery prior to the initiation of memory, i.e. prior to about 18 months of age, but that surgery could be done at a later date provided, and only provided, that suitable counselling was carried out principally with the parents so that they understood and did not impart to the child any discordance as to the sexual orientation and any discordance with regard to the desired psychosexual orientation.

In summary, the present evidence indicates that there is no need to be concerned about the psychosexual orientation of a patient affected with congenital adrenal hyperplasia provided reconstructive surgery to external genitalia is carried out prior to 18 months of age and provided that the parents and others who may be closely associated with the patient are suitably counselled so that they understand that the abnormalities of the external genitalia are a developmental defect which is easily corrected by surgery and does not represent a basic uncorrectable expression of sexuality. On the other hand, the subsequent studies of Lewis demonstrated that surgery could be carried out at a later time provided that intensive counselling bordering on psychotherapy be carried out, not only with the patient, but by those in contact with her.

An interesting sidelight of the psychological studies of patients with virilising hyperplasia was the observation first made by Money & Lewis (1966) that affected individuals often had an IQ somewhat higher than might be expected. In the Money & Lewis original study for example, 60 per cent of the patients had IQs above 110 whereas only 25 per cent would be expected to have such a value. These workers suggested that this unexpected finding might be explained by the exposure of the individual during intra-uterine life and later to the abnormal steroids.

This matter has been studied by other workers. Wentzel et al (1978) confirmed the fact that IQ measurements in patients with congenital adrenal hyperplasia were significantly higher than normal. However, they also noted that there was no difference between the IQ of affected patients and their unaffected siblings but not of the parents. They therefore, concluded that it was neither the pre- nor postnatal androgen exposure or a genetic linkage that could be responsible for the increased IQ in congenital adrenal hyperplasia. They thought that the explanation was most likely due to methodological factors such as the application of outdated standards to IQ tests of a subsequent generation.

Endocrinological treatment

As in the two case histories initially presented, the female newborn almost always presents with ambiguity of the external genitalia. The birth of such an infant should be considered an emergency with the goal of appropriate gender assignment as soon as possible with as little untoward psychological trauma to the family as possible. Happily, recognition of the relative frequency of the adrenogenital syndrome is now the rule rather than the exception and appropriate gender assignment is usually suspected in the delivery suite and confirmed within hours after birth.

When an infant with ambiguous genitalia is born, the initial examination in the delivery room can frequently provide enough information to suggest the appropriate sex assignment. The presenting abnormalities of the clitoris and urogenital sinus are discussed elsewhere (Developmental Anomalies) and, as noted, may vary from mild enlargement of the clitoris without significant posterior fusion to complete fusion of the labio-scrotal folds with a penile urethra and a phallus enlarged to the size found in a normal newborn male. It is important to note that in the female pseudo-hermaphrodite, gonads will not be palpable in the labio-scrotal folds. Thus, a female gender assignment may be suspected, if, on careful examination of the infant, gonads cannot be identified. A rectal examination in female pseudo-hermaphrodites, will reveal an infantile cervix.

It is frequently helpful at this point to reassure the parents that the newborn is a healthy baby, but that the baby does have a birth abnormality of the external genitalia and further evaluation will be necessary to determine the exact aetiology of the problem. If the physical examination is most consistent with a female gender, one can share that information with the parents, suggest that the newborn is a girl and that an adrenal abnormality is the most usual cause for the present genital abnormality. Further studies and/or consultations may be undertaken to confirm the diagnosis.

The most helpful initial tests are the examination of buccal cells for Barr bodies, and pelvic ultrasonography or vaginogram. Ultrasonography of the pelvis is helpful to reveal a normal uterus if a cervix cannot be appreciated on physical examination. One can perform a cystovaginogram to confirm the presence of the uterus; however, excessive manipulation in the newborn may result in significant infection (i.e. cystitis, pyelonephritis). Thus, one wants to exercise caution in these radiographical studies. Chromosomal analysis from a bone marrow aspirate can be available within 24 hours; however, because of the invasiveness of the procedure, it is not generally recommended.

Once the diagnosis of the female pseudo-hermaphrodite has been made, 21-hydroxylase deficiency is far and away the most likely aetiology. A presumptive diagnosis can be made and the parents informed of this diagnosis and the need for further tests to confirm it. The most definitive test is a serum 17α-hydroxyprogesterone level which is best done on the infant (Fig. 18.35). Although cord blood may be used, a high false negative rate has been reported by Pang et al (1979) when using cord blood. In many places, the 17α-hydroxyprogesterone determination may require 7–10 days for completion while a 24-hour urinary 17-ketos-

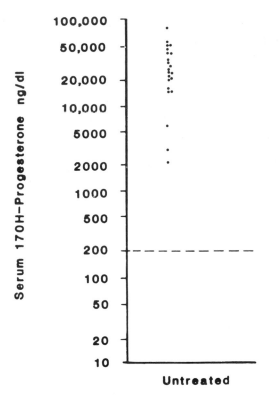

Fig. 18.35 Serum 17-OHP levels in CAH infants less than 3 years of age before cortisol therapy. The broken line indicates the upper limit of normal used in this study (Hughes & Winter, 1978)

teroid is generally available within 2 or 3 days. While the urine is much more cumbersome to collect, it may give prompt preliminary confirmation of the diagnosis. A 24-hour urinary pregnanetriol may be measured on the same urine collection (Wilkins, 1965).

Ideally, by 24–72 hours of life, a presumptive diagnosis may be made and the necessary confirming laboratory tests collected. Once this has been accomplished, specific therapy may be initiated. The goal of medical therapy is to provide adequate glucocorticoid levels and to suppress abnormal adrenal androgen production. In the infant with salt wasting, one has the added goal of adequate mineralocorticoid action for normal water and salt metabolism. If these goals are accomplished, children with 21-hydroxylase deficiency may expect to grow and develop normally.

Hydrocortisone suspension is the treatment of choice for the infant and the young child because of the flexibility of dosage available. The initial therapy recommended by Migeon (1968) is 30–50 mg/m²/day given as an oral preparation divided into 8 hour doses. The initial high dose of cortisol is designed to achieve rapid ACTH suppression in expectation of decreasing the size of the hyperplastic adrenal glands. Two weeks after initiation of therapy, the dose is decreased to 20–25 mg/m²/day, again divided into 8 hour doses. Hughes (1982) has recommended successful therapy of prepubertal children with 10–20 mg/m²/day. In our experience, many prepubertal children may be managed quite nicely on this lower dosage. The lower dose

has the benefit of avoiding excessive glucocorticoid treatment with its attendant poor growth (Rappaport et al, 1973; Laron & Pertzelan, 1968.; Brook et al, 1974).

Prior to the availability of a reliable oral hydrocortisone suspension, hydrocortisone was given intramuscularly once every 3 days in a dose of 37.5 mg/m²/dose. An occasional patient may benefit from this parenteral therapy if compliance with oral medication is not reliable.

Throughout childhood, the glucocorticoid requirement increases with increasing body size, but remains 10–25 mg/m²/day. As puberty supervenes, the glucocorticoid requirement may increase from the lower range of 10 mg/m²/day towards the upper range of 25 mg/m²/day.

To assess adequacy of therapy, many biochemical parameters have been recommended. Historically, 24-hour urinary 17-ketosteroids and pregnanetriol excretion have been used (Wilkins, 1965). More recently, plasma 17α-hydroxyprogesterone has been suggested as the best steroid to evaluate therapy (Hughes & Winter, 1976). However, there may be marked diurnal variation in 17α-hydroxyprogesterone (Meyer et al, 1977), and it may be more responsive to acute stresses (Frish et al, 1981) than adrenal androgens. Many centres now use both 17α-hydroxyprogesterone and simultaneous androstenedione or testosterone levels to follow therapy. Korth-Schutz et al (1978) demonstrated nicely the advantages of androstenedione in all patients and the usefulness of testosterone in prepubertal patients and older females. Most investigators now attempt to maintain 17α-hydroxyprogesterone, androstenedione, and testosterone within the normal range for age while carefully observing for signs of hypercortisolism. If attention is given to appropriate mineralocorticoid therapy, as discussed below, excellent metabolic control can be achieved.

The salt-losing syndrome

Although infants with the salt-wasting form of the disorder have a depletion of total body sodium at birth, their sodium and potassium levels are usually normal during the first 5–7 days of life. Daily determination of electrolytes from 3 days to 10 days of age may be necessary for confirmation of aldosterone deficiency. An increased plasma renin activity may suggest salt wasting prior to the development of abnormal serum electrolytes. If by day 10 of life the electrolytes remain normal, one may wish to measure the plasma renin activity as a final confirmation of normal mineralocorticoid production.

If the salt-wasting variety is diagnosed by a rising serum potassium, a falling serum sodium and an increasing renin activity, mineralocorticoid therapy is indicated. Parenteral therapy with 1 mg of desoxycorticosterone every 24 hours is indicated for the ill infant with an unreliable gastrointestinal tract. The majority of infants may be treated orally with 9α-fludrocortisol in a dose of 0.1–0.2 mg per day.

Here also, if compliance with oral medication is unreliable, long-term therapy with desoxycorticosterone (DOCA) pellets may be used. The pellets are implanted under the skin, usually in the scapular region. Two 125 mg pellets will usually provide adequate mineralo-corticoid action for 6–9 months, although plasma renin activity may rise within 1–2 months (Kennan et al, 1982). Several authors have pointed out the dangers of hypertension with excessive mineralo-corticoid therapy (Vasquez & Kenny, 1972; Kirkland et al, 1973). If DOCA pellets are implanted, blood pressure determinations in the immediate post-operative period are necessary to judge the appropriateness of the dose selected. Children receiving mineralo-corticoids require blood pressure monitoring as part of each follow-up visit.

The importance of mineralo-corticoid therapy for adequate suppression of ACTH, thus suppression of adrenal androgen production, has been pointed out by Hughes & Winter (1976) and confirmed by other investigators (Rasler et al, 1977; Jansen et al, 1981). This work suggests that the individual with persistent salt wasting exhibits persistent adrenal hyperfunction and excessive adrenal androgen production despite adequate or excessive glucocorticoid therapy. If mineralo-corticoid therapy is increased in these patients, excessive adrenal androgen production ceases and the glucocorticoid dose may be decreased. These studies suggest that some patients without overt salt wasting may be improved by the addition of 9α-fludrocortisol to their regime.

Previous reports suggest that mineralocorticoid therapy may be discontinued after infancy (News, 1974). More recent data documents the continuing need for mineralo-corticoid therapy (Hughes et al, 1979; Jansen et al, 1981; Keenan et al, 1982). These data combined with the data demonstrating excessive adrenal androgen production when inadequate mineralo-corticoid therapy is given, strongly suggest that in the female adequate mineralo-corticoid therapy is essential throughout life. Adequacy of mineralo-corticoid therapy may be estimated by assessment of plasma renin activity. Normal values in children engaged in usual activities range from 2.7–7.0 ng/ml/h (Dechaux et al, 1982) and values within this range can be accepted as indicative of good control.

Late diagnosis of the simple virilising variety

A few patients without salt wasting have genital abnormalities which are so mild at birth that the diagnosis is delayed until further virilisation occurs. In the untreated patient, pubic hair usually appears between 1 year and 6 years of age. Usually, this is accompanied with noted clitoral enlargement and an excessive growth rate.

The diagnosis may be established in the same manner as it is in the infant, although other virilising conditions should be considered. Once the diagnosis is established,

hydrocortisone is given in a dose of 20–25 mg/m²/day divided into 8 hour doses, as it is given for the child diagnosed at birth. Assessment of adequacy of therapy is similar to that for patients diagnosed in infancy.

In children with the simple virilising form of the disorder who are not recognised until later in childhood, adrenal androgen production causes advancement in bone maturation which may result ultimately in short stature, even with adequate treatment (Brook et al, 1974). Several authors do report some success in enhancing growth in these patients by using greater doses of hydrocortisone (Rappaport et al, 1973; Bongiovanni et al, 1973). Dosages between 30 and 45 mg/m²/day seemed predominently to reduce bone maturation while allowing some linear growth.

Long term prognosis of the simple virilising variety

Prior to the availability of cortisone therapy, the majority of patients with the salt-losing syndrome died in early infancy. Those patients who survived infancy, experienced rapid growth and progressive virilisation in childhood, short stature and lack of feminine secondary sexual development in adolescence, as well as virilism and infertility in adulthood. With the advent of cortisone therapy, it was anticipated that these children would lead a normal life unhampered by virilisation. A generation of children have now received the benefits of cortisone therapy for the 21-hydroxylase deficiency. We can now look back and evaluate, not only survival, but quality of life. Several studies have now been completed to attempt to answer the question: Can women with the 21-hydroxylase deficiency achieve (1) normal adult height; (2) timely development of female pubertal changes; (3) normal fertility; and (4) normal psychosexual orientation?

Early studies suggested that despite prompt initiation of cortisone therapy, patients with congenital adrenal hyperplasia do not achieve normal adult height (Bergstrand, 1966; Hamilton, 1972). Rappaport et al (1973) reported that a normal growth velocity could be achieved with a hydrocortisone dose of 15–36 mg/m²/day ($\bar{x}$ dose = 25 ± 0.9 mg/m²/day), while excessive glucocorticoid therapy, especially in infancy, was associated with a diminished growth rate. Several long-term follow-up studies (Brook et al, 1974; Klingensmith et al, 1977; Kirkland et al, 1978) have reported the achievement of normal adult heights in early-treated patients. The mean adult height of female patients treated prior to 6 years of age was 157.4 ± 7.4 cm (25th percentile) in the series from Johns Hopkins (Klingensmith et al, 1977) and 162.5 ± 5.2 cm (40th percentile) in the series from Baylor College of Medicine in patients treated prior to 3 years of age (Kirkland et al, 1978). The mean United States adult female height is 164.8 ± 5.9 cm (Hamill et al, 1977). Other investigators have reported no influence of treatment on final height in females (Styne et al, 1977). The reasons for the discrepancy in findings of these reports remain unclear.

Development of secondary sexual characteristics in early-treated patients appears to occur within the normal time frame (Jones & Verkauf, 1971; Giddick & Hammand, 1975; Klingensmith et al, 1977). Although the mean age for pubarche occurs slightly earlier than the normal mean, thelarche occurs at the expected time. The mean age of menarche may be delayed even in early-treated patients but generally occurs within the normal range in the well-treated patient. If thelarche is delayed, or if menarche fails to occur, undertreatment is usually the cause. In the series reported by Klingensmith et al (1977), 75 per cent of patients with delayed sexual development or menstrual abnormalities, failed to take their medication regularly. The high incidence of poor compliance stresses the need for continuing medical education and motivation of the older child and teenager.

Fertility was evaluated in 22 patients in the series reported by Klingensmith et al (1977). Four patients were over 20 years of age when hydrocortisone therapy became available; none of these patients become pregnant. Ten of the remaining 18 patients successfully achieved pregnancy. Fifteen pregnancies resulting in ten live births were reported. Two of the 15 pregnancies were electively terminated in the first trimester and there were three spontaneous abortions in three separate patients. Pregnancy and delivery were tolerated well, although all patients reported have been delivered by Caesarian section. No alteration in glucocorticoid dosages were required during pregnancy, and intravenous hydrocortisone was given during labour and delivery as for any other surgical procedure. The glucocorticoid preparation for seven of ten successful pregnancies was either cortisone acetate in a mean dose of 35.8 mg/m²/day, or prednisone given as 6–7 mg/m²/day. The range of 17-ketosteroids at the onset of pregnancy was 2.5–5.3 mg/24 hours indicating little adrenal androgen production. The majority of the young women studied were first treated with cortisone between 6 and 20 years of age. It is anticipated that fertility rates will be as good, or better, in the young women who are diagnosed and begun on therapy earlier in life.

We are now in the midst of the 'second generation' of patients with congenital adrenal hyperplasia who have had the benefit of hydrocortisone and mineral-corticoid therapy. The documented ability to achieve normal height, sexual development and fertility in the majority of patients places the burden upon the physician to attain these goals. Kirkland et al (1978) as well as others (Bailey et al, 1978; Hendricks et al, 1982) suggest that clinical evaluations three or four times per year are required to achieve satisfactory growth in the child; one would anticipate that similar close follow-up is necessary for normal pubertal development, and normal reproductive function.

To attain the best long-term results, growth velocity and sexual maturation should be evaluated at every follow-up visit. Blood determinations of 17α-hydroxyprogesterone and/or adrenal androgens, or urinary 17-ketosteroids and pregnanetriol should be studied two to four times per year and assessment of skeletal maturity evaluated yearly until growth is completed. Under- or over-treatment with glucocorticoids may be corrected promptly using these measurements at frequent intervals. Education and counselling must be provided frequently so that informed and willing compliance with the treatment regime occurs.

With care and attention, patients with this once life-threatening and disfiguring disorder can expect to become normal, healthy adults with healthy children.

Surgical treatment

In the reconstruction of the masculinised external genitalia toward feminine lines, the surgical anatomy is of considerable importance. This is especially true with respect to the site of communication of the vagina with the urogenital sinus. This point is discussed above and it will suffice here to recall that study on many cases has shown that the vaginal communication is almost always in relation to the caudal urogenital sinus derivatives. This means that the vagina communicates with that portion of the urogenital sinus which, in a male, gives rise to the membranous portion of the male urethra and which, in the female, becomes the vaginal vestibule. It is almost never in communication with the portion of the urogenital sinus which becomes the prostatic urethra in the male, i.e. the entire urethra in the female. This is of considerable surgical importance for it means that the anomalously persistent urogenital sinus may be boldly incised to the vaginal communication without fear of disturbing the urinary sphincter. Such an anatomical finding tallies with the clinical observation that hermaphrodites with anomalies of the external genitalia, as a rule, do not have problems of urinary continence (Fig. 18.36).

However, Hendren & Crawford (1969) identified a few patients in whom the vagina entered the urogenital sinus in that portion from which the posterior urethra is derived. While we recognise this variation in the point of junction, it remains our opinion that the communication is seldom sufficiently posterior to be concerned about urinary continence.

It is our belief that the reconstruction operation is best carried out before 18 months of age. The key to the operation is the identification of the vagina, and if by sounding this can be identified soon after birth, the operation may be conveniently done at any time. In any case, the operation cannot be satisfactorily completed until the vagina can be identified. The objective is to complete the procedure at a time when the structures are of a size to permit ease of handling and yet prior to the age when the anomalies may prove embarassing. If the patient is first seen at an

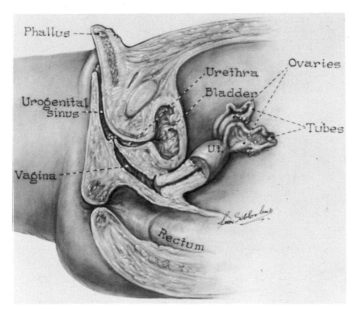

Fig. 18.36 The sagittal view of a genetic female patient with CAH This patient has a type C defect of the external genitalia but the relationship of the vagina to the urinary tract is basically the same regardless of the degree of masculinisation of the external genitalia

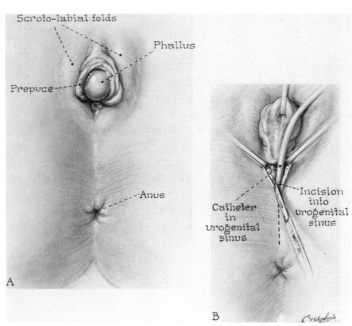

Fig. 18.37 The genitalia of a patient with masculinised genitalia due to CAH. B. The first incision in the reconstruction of the external genitalia

older age, the operation may be carried out at any time. There is no reason to delay operation until puberty and there are many advantages from a psychological point of view to proceed as early as possible.

The basic operation

In patients with adrenal hyperplasia, reconstruction of the external genitalia will be the only operation performed in the average case.

When the operation is carried out at the ideal age, the structures are so small that it is impossible to introduce a finger into the urogenital sinus, so that all tissues must be handled throughout the operation by means of small and delicate tissue forceps. It is also necessary to have available small haemostatic forceps and tiny scissors. Fine suture material like #00000 synthetic suture on an atraumatic needle is used throughout.

As a preliminary to the operation, the urogenital sinus may be thoroughly investigated with a small McCarthy panendoscope to determine accurately the position and size of the vaginal communication. If sound or catheter can be easily introduced into the meatus of the urogenital sinus and into the vagina, the endoscopy may be omitted. Special care is needed not to introduce the sound into the urethra, for the urogenital sinus is incised on the instrument to within 2 or 3 cm of the anus; if the sound is in the urethra by mistake, there is danger of incising the latter structure (Fig. 18.37). After the urogenital sinus has been incised, the urethral orifice may be discovered in the normal position for the female urinary meatus. A small catheter may then be introduced through the urinary meatus

purposes of identification throughout the remainder of the operation. In order to attach the edges of the vagina to the skin, it is usually necessary to free the vagina posteriorly and laterally to secure sufficient mobilisation to have these structures meet without tension (Fig. 18.38). It is unnecessary to free the vagina anteriorly, as this would require its separation from the urethra and sufficient mobilisation can ordinarily be obtained by lateral and posterior dissection. When sufficient freedom has been secured, the edges of the vagina may be secured to the skin with interrupted stitches of #00000 suture on an atraumatic reverse cutting

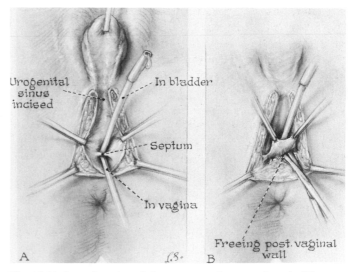

Fig. 18.38 A continuation of the reconstructive operation. A. The urogenital sinus has been opened and the external meatus of the urethra has been revealed. B. Freeing the posterior and lateral aspects of the vagina in order to bring that comfortably to the skin area

needle. In an infant, four or five such stitches around the edge of the vagina are usually sufficient. The edges of the incised sinus membrane may then be sutured to the skin anteriorly, as shown in the illustration. An umbilical tape or a small sponge impregnated with Vaseline may be introduced in the vagina to assure its patency (Figs 18.39 and 18.40).

Attention is directed to the enlarged clitoris. This may be simply amputated with the fashioning of a non-functioning cosmetic clitoris (Figs 18.41 and 18.42). This technique was used for years. Several children so treated now have normal adult sexual function proving that the technique can still be useful.

However, a technique has become available which gives a somewhat better cosmetic result. This attempts to preserve a shell of the glans on a pedicle flap. The shaft of the clitoris is sub-totally resected and the stumps reanastomosed (Figs 18.43 and 18.44). The nerve supply to the glans is severed during this procedure so that sensation in the glans is diminished. However, sexual function seems to be satisfactory.

Rajfer et al (1982) have suggested a dorsal approach to the sub-total resection of the corpora. This has the advantage of preserving the ventral nerve supply and should preserve sensation in the glans. While this is theoretically desirable and can be recommended for suitable cases, as mentioned above, lack of clitoral sensation does not seem to be an important point in the later erotic behaviour of patients treated by procedures which sever the dorsal nerves to the glans.

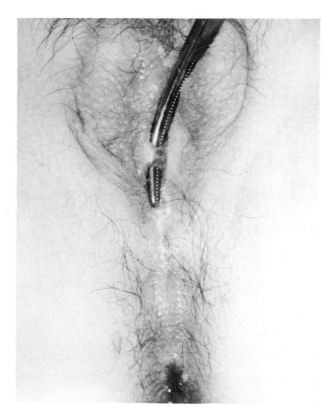

Fig. 18.40 A post-operative adhesion from the consequence of not packing apart the fresh incisions of the external genitalia

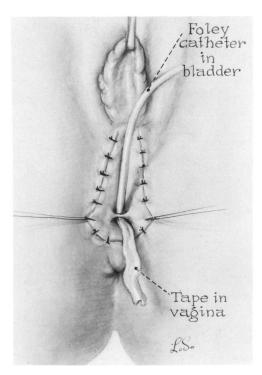

Fig. 18.39 Completion of the first step in the reconstruction of the external genitalia

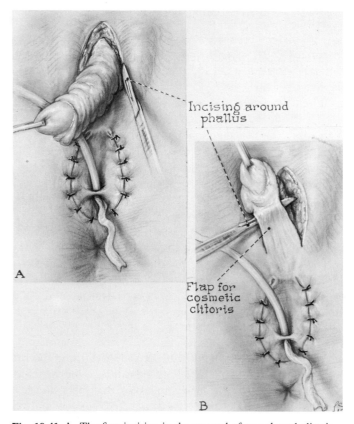

Fig. 18.41 A. The first incision in the removal of an enlarged clitoris. B. The development of the posterior flap for the cosmetic clitoris

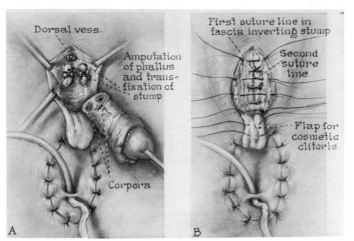

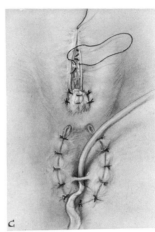

Fig. 18.42 A. The removal of the clitoris. A. The first steps in the closure of the incision. C. The completion of the operation with the formation of a cosmetic clitoris by folding the posterior flap

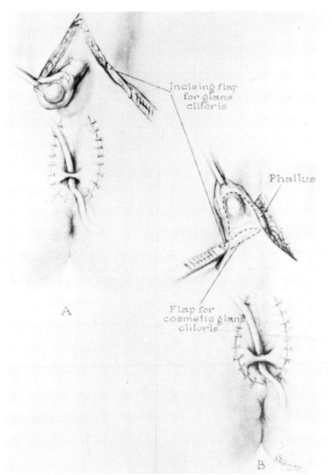

Fig. 18.43 An improved method for removing part of the clitoris. A. Note the broad base of the flap. This is required to support the circulation for the portion of the glans which is to be preserved. B. A further development of the pedicle flap containing the tip of the glans

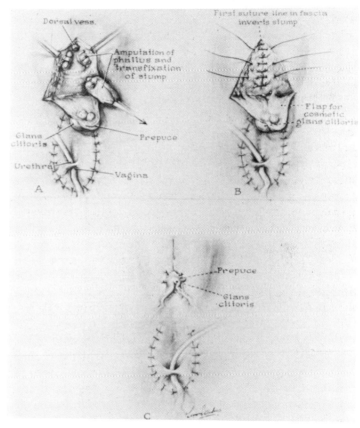

Fig. 18.44 A. The resection of the shaft of the enlarged phallus. B. Partial closure of the defect before replacing the flap. C. The flap has now been sutured into place

The indwelling catheter may be left in place for a few days until the oedema of the surrounding structures has subsided. This is particularly useful in children with metabolic disorders where accurate urine collection is desirable. A pressure dressing for 24 hours is useful.

Operations for minor deformities. In a very few patients with the adrenogenital syndrome, the clitoral enlargement is primarily the result of growth of the prepuce with little or no enlargement of the corpora or glans. This may be true regardless of the degree of fusion of the scroto-labial folds. In such a circumstance, the fleshy clitoris may be removed without disturbing the corpora or glans by a butterfly incision, drawing together the defect from side to side by interrupted stitches (Fig. 18.45).

Operation when the vaginal orifice is difficult to locate. As previously mentioned, identification and catheterisation or

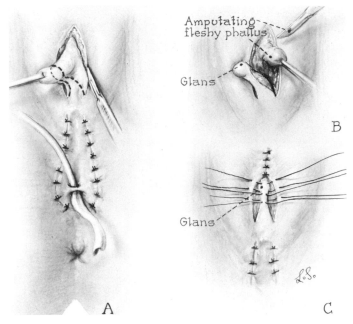

Fig. 18.45 An operation for the removal of a redundant prepuce. A. The limits of the incision. B. The amputation of the prepuce. C. The completion of the operation

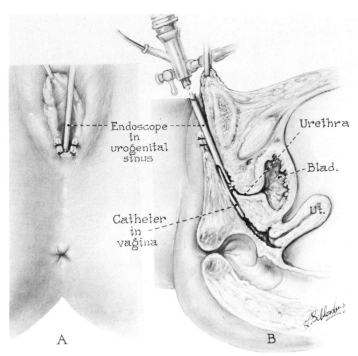

Fig. 18.46 The use of the endoscope with a small ureteral catheter to identify a vaginal orifice which otherwise cannot be seen. A. The partial opening of the urogenital sinus to allow the introduction of a larger size panendoscope. B. A diagram of the use of the catheter. The catheter may enter the vagina even though it may not be visualised through the endoscope

sounding of the vaginal orifice preoperatively is the key to a successful one-stage procedure. It is very seldom that it can be found at operation if it has not been previously identified. However, if it cannot be located by sounding, it can sometimes be seen be endoscopy; often the reverse is the case and it can be sounded but not seen. When sounding and vision both fail, immediately prior to surgery, it is well worth attempting to introduce a small (No. 4 or 5) ureteral catheter into the vagina by blindly probing through the endoscope along the posterior wall of the urogenital sinus. Sometimes, when worked successfully, this finds the orifice. If so, the catheter can be left within the vagina as a guide to the surgical exposure of the area (Figs 18.46 and 18.47). In the event that the vaginal orifice cannot be located by any of these manoeuvres, a planned two-stage operation may be indicated. At the first stage, the objective would be to obtain cosmetically female genitalia by removing the clitoris and partially incising the urogenital sinus without exteriorising the vagina. The exteriorisation of the vagina may conveniently be postponed until a later date when identification of the vaginal orifice by sounding becomes possible.

Operation when the vagina is imperforate. Very, very rarely (only three times in about 300 operations, in personal experience) the vagina does not communicate with the urogenital sinus (Fig. 18.48). This is, perhaps, not astonishing, as the point of communication of the vagina with the urogenital sinus is homologous with the hymenal area and very rarely in an otherwise normal female the hymen is imperforate. For such a circumstance, we have found it helpful to pass a sound downward from above to

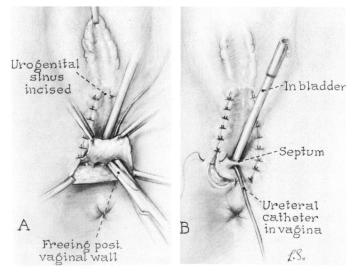

Fig. 18.47 The operation with the ureteral catheter in place. A. The development of the posterior wall of the vagina. B. The completion of the operation. The ureteral catheter may be removed at this point

identify the vagina in the perineum. With such a guide, the edges of the vaginal epithelium can be located and sutured to the skin (Fig. 18.49). Until the uterus enlarges somewhat from its infantile state, the cavity is not large enough to accommodate even a uterine sound. Therefore, if such an operation is contemplated, it should not be done until

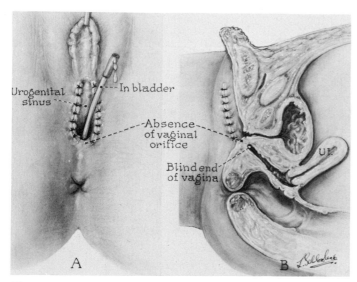

Fig. 18.48 An imperforate hymen in a patient with congenital adrenal hyperplasia. A. A partial opening of the urogenital sinus in order to give an acceptable cosmetic appearance to the genitalia. B. The vagina cannot be exteriorised at this point because the opening does not exist

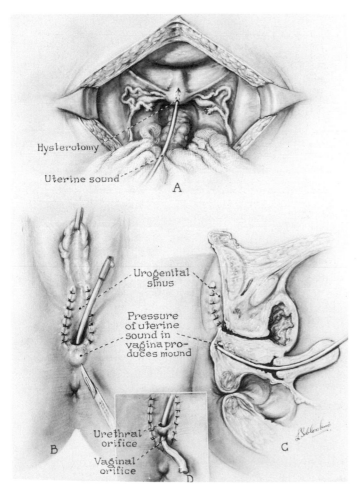

Fig. 18.49 A manoeuvre to identify the vagina where there is no communication with the vagina to the urogenital sinus. A. A uterine sound passed through the fundus at laparotomy. B. The mound in the vagina produced by the uterine sound passing through the uterus into the vagina. C. A sagittal diagram of that situation

there is palpable enlargement of the uterus at the onset of puberty.

Operation with a posterior flap. Sometimes it is difficult, especially in patients with copious subcutaneous fat, to approximate the vagina with the skin, particularly posteriorly. When such a situation is anticipated, the flap technique originally advocated by Fortunoff et al (1964) has been used successfully (Figs 18.50 and 18.51).

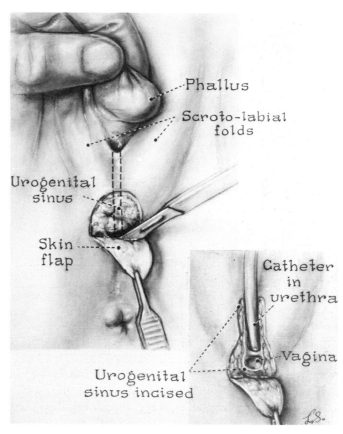

Fig. 18.50 A method of using a skin flap posteriorly to bridge the gap between the vagina and the skin

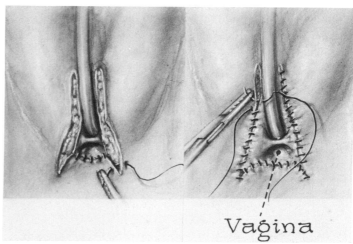

Fig. 18.51 Further steps in the procedure shown in Fig. 18.50

Results of operations

The results of the application of these procedures in patients with virilising adrenal hyperplasia were reviewed by Jones & Verkauf (1970). Subsequent clinical experience would tend to substantiate these findings.

The complete operation (cosmetic correction and exteriorisation of the vagina) cannot always be carried out and for various good reasons, it may be important to construct cosmetically female genitalia even though the vagina cannot be exteriorised in the initial operation. However, including patients younger than 18 months of age, the complete operation has been done in by far the majority of cases (Table 18.1).

Table 18.1 Initial operation on genitalia at Johns Hopkins Hospital in 84 females with congenital adrenal hyperplasia reared as females

Operation[a]*	Number of patients
Clitorectomy	7
Circumcision	11
Clitorectomy + exteriorisation of urogenital sinus	9
Clitorectomy + exteriorisation of vagina	52
Excision of clitoral stump + exteriorisation of vagina	1
Partial clitorectomy, transplantation of glans clitoris + exteriorisation of vagina	1
Circumcision + exteriorisation of vagina	4
Exteriorisation of vagina†	9
Total	84

* [a]Cosmetic reduction in size of labia also done in four cases.
[b]Six of these had previous clitorectomy at another hospital.

In 84 patients with congenital adrenal hyperplasia, the success of the operative procedure was evaluated by determining the number of patients requiring reoperation in relation to the age at which surgery was done. This review showed that as long as the vagina could be identified, the complete operation could be carried out successfully regardless of age (Table 18.2). It should also be noted that the severity of the deformity had no relation to the end results.

Secondary operations. Secondary operations upon the vaginal outlet may be required. This is the case if the basic operation is deliberately done in two stages for whatever reason. This may be indicated if the vaginal orifice is not readily identifiable and it seems desirable to construct

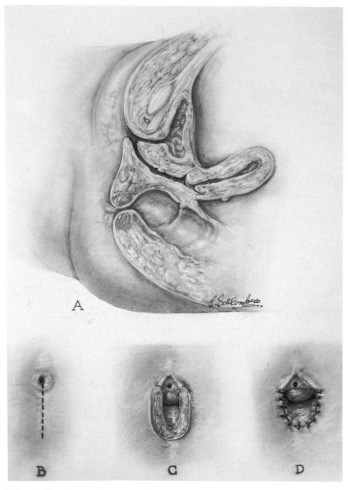

Fig. 18.52 A secondary operation on the external genitalia when the vagina has not been satisfactorily exteriorised at the first procedure. A. A sagittal view of the situation. B, C and D. Further steps in the procedure which consist simply of carrying the posterior incision further posteriorly and suturing the edges of the exteriorised vagina to the skin

cosmetically acceptable female genitalia at a very early age. Under this circumstance, the clitoroplasty can be done in the newborn period and the vagina exteriorised at a much later date.

However, even when the complete operation is attempted at an early age, the vagina is sometimes not satisfactorily exteriorised. The principal difficulty here is failure to carry the midline incision far enough posteriorly. This requires a second procedure which, in essence completes the first one by continuing the midline incision far enough posteriorly (Fig. 18.52).

Table 18.2 Relationship of success of operation to pre-operative identification of vagina

Vagina identified	Successful completion of initial operation	Reoperation necessary	Unsuccessful completion of initial operation	Reoperation necessary
Yes (65)	64	4	1	1
No (11)	3	0	8	8
No information (2)	2	0	0	0

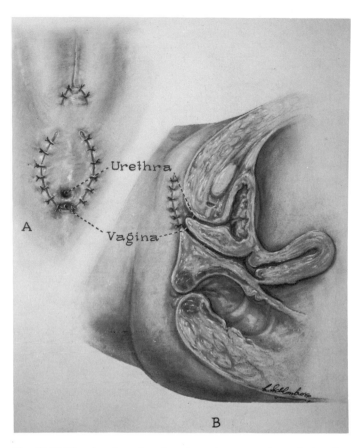

Fig. 18.53 The situation when there is contracture at the vaginal outlet.
A. The original operation which satisfactorily exteriorised the vagina.
B. A sagittal view of that situation

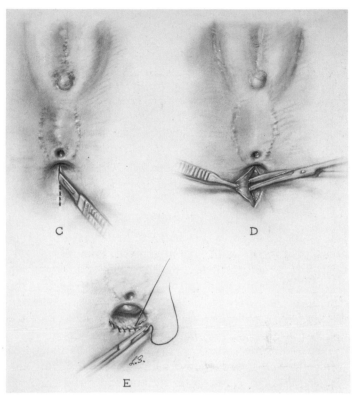

Fig. 18.54 The situation when there is secondary contracture at the vaginal outlet. C. Reopening of the vagina by an operation which is essentially the same as shown in Fig. 18.52 for extending the posterior incision. D. Freeing the vagina. E. The suturing of the vagina to the skin with the sutures in the opposite direction from the incision to enlarge the outlet

At other times, there may be contraction at the vaginal outlet even if the operation is done adequately in the first instance. The vaginal orifice may be enlarged by making an incision in the midline and closing it at 90 degrees to the original axis of the incision (Figs 18.53 and 18.54). These procedures can be done on an out-patient basis.

Attenuated C-21 hydroxylase deficiency in the female

As early as 1954, Jones & Jones suggested that some young women with hirsutism and menstrual irregularities may have a mild 21-hydroxylase defect. Attempts to prove this hypothesis using urinary 17-ketosteroid or pregnanetriol determinations were unsatisfactory. Recently, Rosenwaks et al (1979) demonstrated abnormal basal 17-hydroxyprogesterone levels and an abnormal response to ACTH in two women with post-pubertal hirsutism, menstrual irregularities, and normal external genitalia. These women proved the existence of an attenuated form of CVAH. The case histories of these young women are indistinguishable from those of patients with polycystic ovarian disease. The differentiating finding is the elevated basal 17-hydroxyprogesterone level and the abnormal response to ACTH. The basal 17-hydroxyprogesterone levels may be in the range

found in classical 21-hydroxylase deficiency as is their response to ACTH.

Family studies by Migeon et al (1980) and Chrousos et al (1982) have shown that the parents of patients with attenuated 21-hydroxylase deficiency respond to ACTH in a manner identical to that of obligate heterozygotes for the classical 21-hydroxylase deficiency (Table 18.3) using criteria described by Gutai (1977). These family studies prove that the attenuated form of the 21-hydroxylase defect is a genetically determined defect in 21-hydroxylation rather than an acquired deficiency. The onset of symptoms after puberty may be related to normal adrenal maturation at puberty which is associated with a 4-fold increase in the activity of the adrenal enzyme 17-desmolase (Schiebinger et al, 1981). The enzyme converts 17-hydroxyprogesterone to androstenedione and, thus, may be responsible for the increasing symptomatology during adolescence. At this time, the attenuated form of 21-hydroxylase deficiency accounts for 6–12 per cent of patients presenting with hirsutism and menstrual irregularities (Chrousos et al, 1982).

In family studies of patients with classic 21-hydroxylase defect, including patients with salt wasting, New et al (1981) have also reported finding patients with attenuated

Table 18.3   Results of i.v. ACTH stimulation test in a family with attenuated 21-hydroxylase defect. The sum of the rate of increased in 17-OHP and P differentiates normals from heterozygotes. A rate of increase greater than 6.5 ng/dl/min is characteristic of the heterozygote state (4e)

Subject	17-OPH (ng/dl)		P (ng/dl)		Sum of differences (ng/dl)	Rate (ng/dl/min)
	Base line	30 min	Base line	30 min		
Father	33	346	38	95	370	12.3
Mother	56	585	24	81	536	18.0
Brother	102	150	26	68	90	3.0
Sister	117	287	41	77	205	6.8
Patient	666	8300	48	351	7937	264

17-OHP = 17-Hydroxyprogesterone; P = progesterone

CVAH. Additionally, they have identified clinically normal family members with biochemical findings identical to those of patients with the attenuated form of the 21-hydroxylase defect. They have termed this condition 'cryptic' 21-hydroxylase deficiency. They suggest that the dehydroepiandrosterone:androstenedione ratio following ACTH infusion is the best method to identify these individuals.

Genetic studies indicate that patients with the attenuated form of the 21-hydroxylase defect are not unusual heterozygotes, but are homozygotes for an abnormal 21-hydroxylase gene (Migeon et al, 1980; Laron et al, 1980; Levine et al, 1981). The difference in the clinical expression of the attenuated and cryptic forms of the disorder is unclear, but may be due to modifying genes affecting androgen action, or androgen metabolism. Furthermore, HLA antigens and genetic markers demonstrate that the attenuated/cryptic gene is associated with the same HLA antigens and markers that are associated with the classic 21-hydroxylase deficient gene (Pollack et al, 1981). This suggests that these genes are allelic mutations for 21-hydroxylase deficiency.

For many years, it has been suggested that the salt-wasting form of classical 21-hydroxylase deficiency is a more complete form of the defect than is the simple virilising disorder. With the discovery of the attenuated gene, it has been proposed that the varying phenotype is a result of a variable genotype (Migeon et al, 1980). One proposal for the varying genotypes and phenotypes now recognised within the 21-hydroxylase defect is illustrated in Table 18.4.

Much work remains to be done to determine further the

Table 18.4   Allelic genotypes and their associated clinical results in the 21-hydroxylase deficiency

Genotype	Phenotype
Normal/normal	Unaffected: normal
Classic CAH/normal	Unaffected: hetrozygote
Attenuated CAH/normal	Unaffected: hetrozygote
Classic CAH/classic CAH	Affected: salt loser
Classic CAH/attenuated CAH	Affected: simple virilised, late onset, or cryptic
Attenuated CAH/attenuated CAH	Affected: late onset or cryptic

genotypic variations in the 21-hydroxylase defect. The attenuated disorder and the cryptic form are fascinating variations of a well-known enzymatic defect and are quite helpful in demonstrating genotypic variations in enzymatic abnormalities.

C-21 hydroxylase deficiency in the male

As noted in the section on genetics, a deficiency in the 21-hydroxylase enzyme is an autosomal recessive disorder and should affect females and males equally. A decreased number of affected males compared to females in large series (Murtzaza et al, 1980) suggests an increase in infant mortality for undiagnosed males with the salt-wasting form of the disorder. The male infant with the 21-hydroxylase deficiency has no anatomical abnormality at birth to call attention to his disorder; therefore, the initial presentation in the male is dependent on the presence or absence of the salt-wasting syndrome. Those infants with the salt-wasting form of the disorder frequently present *in extremis* at 1–3 weeks of age with profound electrolyte abnormalities and shock from dehydration. Sepsis or pyloric stenosis are commonly thought to be the aetiology for the infant's illness until the electrolyte determinations are evaluated. Laboratory results show a hyponatraemic dehydration with marked hyperkalemia (Table 18.5).

In most instances, resuscitation with a glucose containing normal saline solution provides prompt improvement. In some cases, therapy to decrease acutely the serum potassium is necessary. Treatment with both glucocorticoid and mineralocorticoid may be given to stabilise the patient without compromising the diagnosis. In the severely ill infant, 17α-hydroxyprogesterone levels

Table 18.5   Routine laboratory findings in salt-wasting 21-OH deficiency in ten male patients

	Mean	Range
Age at diagnosis	2.7	1–5
Serum sodium (me/l)	112	98–133
Serum potassium (me/l)	8.0	6.7–10.0
Blood area nitrogen (mg/dl)	39	26–54

will remain elevated into the diagnostic range for 24–72 hours after the initiation of the therapy. The diagnosis, as in the female, can be made with a serum 17α-hydroxyprogesterone determination as well as a 24 hour urinary 17-ketosteriod and pregnanetriol measurement.

The males with the simple virilising form of the 21-hydroxylase enzyme defect present with isosexual pseudo-precocious puberty. As in the untreated female, pubarche occurs between 1 and 6 years of age. Penile enlargement occurs at the same time. As a rule, the testicles remain small and soft during childhood as excessive adrenal androgens produce the masculinisation. The diagnosis of 21-hydroxylase deficiency in these patients is established as discussed above. As in females who present later in childhood, other virilising disorders need to be ruled out.

Medical therapy in males with 21-hydroxylase deficiency is identical to that for females. As in the later diagnosed females, assessment of plasma renin activity should be made to determine the need for mineralocorticoid therapy and one should not rely on the absence of history of severe salt-wasting episodes to rule out mineralocorticoid deficiency.

Long term follow-up of males with the 21-hydroxylase deficiency indicates that a normal growth velocity and a normal adult height is attainable in 75 per cent of patients (Kirkland et al, 1978; Duck, 1980), although, as in the studies in the females, conflicting reports exist (Styne et al, 1977; Viban et al, 1978). Urban et al (1978) studied male sexual development and fertility in 20 patients. Of the 20 patients, two had never received hydrocortisone therapy, three had been off therapy for 7–15 years, and 15 had been continuously on treatment. Seventeen patients were examined and found to have normal examinations including normal testicular volume and consistency regardless of status of glucocorticoid replacement at the time of examination. Normal LH values were reported for all 18 patients evaluated and normal FSH values in all but 3 patients. All of the patients had normal testosterone levels. All 20 patients were evaluated for fertility. Fifteen of the 20 had fathered children, three of the remaining five patients had a normal semen analysis. One patient with abnormal sperm motility (3 per cent) was a heavy drug abuser; the other patient, an 18 year old, had a decreased sperm count (15.5×10^6) despite normal testosterone and gonadotrophin levels and a normal physical examination. It is of interest to note that five of the 15 patients with normal fertility had either never received hydrocortisone therapy or had been treated only during childhood.

From the studies available it would appear that the male patients with the 21-hydroxylase deficiency can live a normal life with a normal height expectancy and normal fertility. It is still unresolved whether or not the male individual needs continuous therapy since fertility appears to be unaffected by the status of glucocorticoid therapy. A report of an adrenal cortical tumour in a 60-year-old female patient with untreated CAH (Van Seters et al, 1981) raises the question of malignant potential in patients with continuously stimulated adrenal glands and, therefore, suggests that therapy may be warranted in these individuals. However, the incidence of tumours in patients with untreated CAH is unclear and, therefore, firm recommendation cannot be made at this time.

C-17α hydroxylase deficiency

17α-Hydroxylation is required in the biosynthetic pathway from cholesterol to cortisol (Fig. 18.8). Defects in this enzymatic pathway properly belong under the rubric of adrenal hyperplasia as any defect in the synthesis of cortisol results in hyperplasia of the zona reticularis of the adrenal. However, individuals with this disorder in no way resemble patients with classical virilising adrenal hyperplasia due to the C-21 hydroxylation defect. This is a rare disorder. At the time of the report of Jones et al (1982) of an affected male, only 11 such cases had appeared in the literature. Patients with 17α-hydroxylase deficiency usually present with lack of pubertal development and hypertension (Fig. 18.55). The external genitalia of male patients appear entirely female or quite ambiguous (Figs 18.56 and 18.57).

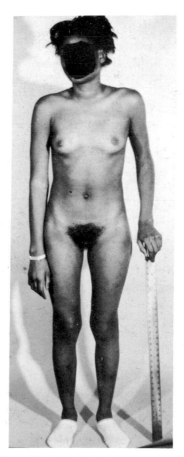

Fig. 18.55 A patient with the 17-α-hydroxylase deficiency. Notice the modest, but spontaneous, breast development

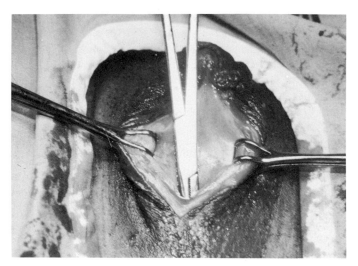

Fig. 18.56 The external genitalia prior to the first operative procedure on them

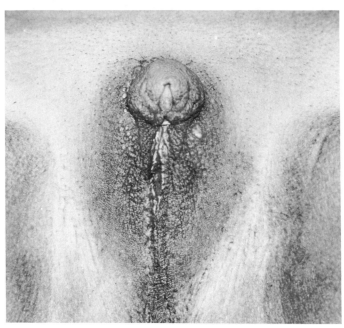

Fig. 18.57 The external genitalia just prior to the operation to create a vagina

Defective steroidogenesis results in inadequate conversion of progesterone to 17-hydroxyprogesterone and of pregnenolone to 17-hydroxyprognenolone. Consequently, there is not only inadequate cortisol production, but inadequate androgen production. Among 46,XY patients with testes, this is responsible for inadequately virilised external genitalia. However, there seems to be a wide spectrum in the appearance of the genitalia. Some might be quite feminine with a relatively deep vagina presumably of utriculovaginal origin as seen in patients with the androgen insensitivity syndrome or there may be almost complete fusion of the scroto-labial folds with total inhibition of vaginal development. Phallic development is always limited whereas the Müllerian structures are uniformly totally inhibited by the anti-Müllerian hormone produced by the testes.

Because cortisol synthesis is compromised by the enzymatic defect in the synthetic pathway, adrenocorticotropin hormone (ACTH) secretion is markedly increased. As the mineralo-corticoid pathway does not require 17-hydroxylation, the excess ACTH results in excessive production of 11-deoxycroticosterone and corticosterone, but not aldosterone. As 11-deoxycorticosterone and corticosterone are potent mineralo-corticoids, their increased secretion explains the hypertension that occurs among patients with the 17α-hydroxylase deficiency.

The diagnosis may be made by determining the various steroid intermediates in the blood serum. Plasma levels of progesterone, 11-deoxycorticosterone and corticosterone will be elevated as expected for the steroid precursors prior to the 17α-hydroxylase step.

Treatment with cortisone will usually lower the blood pressure although in patients with long-standing hypertension, the result is often not spectacular.

Reconstructive surgery of the external genitalia will be required as appropriate (Fig. 18.58). As mentioned above, the external genitalia of these patients are sometimes

entirely feminine, but in others, there will be fusion of the scroto-labial folds and either no or a very short vagina.

An inguinal hernia has been a common finding in 46,XY patients with this disorder.

Symptomatology of 46,XX patients is quite different. The enzyme 17-hydroxylase is necessary for oestrogen

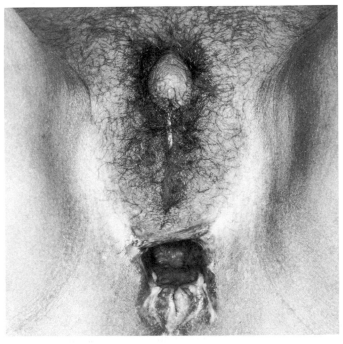

Fig. 18.58 The external genitalia a few weeks after the construction of a vagina. The cosmetic appearance after a vagina has been created in what is essentially a male perineum with no spontaneous vaginal development is never completely ideal

synthesis. As with the 46,XY patients, among 46,XX patients there will be excess synthesis of deoxycorticosterone and corticosterone so that hypertension results. Oestrogen lack results in primary amenorrhoea and absence of sexual maturation. Because there is no negative feedback by oestrogen on the pituitary, elevated values of follicle stimulating hormone are found. This results in persistent and repeated ovarian enlargement so that infarction and twisting the ovaries has been not uncommon in the cases that have been reported.

Suppressive therapy with cortisone or one of its analogues and oestrogens have lowered the blood pressure and produced feminisation in most patients although as mentioned with the males in patients who have had elevated blood pressure of long standing, therapy is usually less than completely satisfactory.

C-11 hydroxylase deficiency

The 11β-hydroxylation is the final step in the synthesis of cortisol (Fig. 18.8); it is also required in the synthesis of aldosterone (Fig. 18.28). Deficiencies in this enzyme are second in frequency to the 21-hydroxylase enzyme. One study in Switzerland of the prevalence of this disorder found approximately one case per 300 000 population (Werder et al, 1980). This suggests 5 per cent of patients

with congenital adrenal hyperplasia will have the 11β-hydroxylase defect. Extrapolation from reports from Johns Hopkins (Klingensmith et al, 1977; Urban et al, 1978) suggests that the 11β-hydroxylase defect occurs with a frequency of 2.6 per cent of patients with CAH in that clinic. As in the 21-hydroxylase defect, isolated populations have been reported with higher instances (Porter et al, 1977). The 11β-hydroxylase defect also is inherited in an autosomal recessive manner. Contrary to the 21-hydroxylase defect, it does not appear to be linked to the HLA loci and detection of the heterozygote by hormonal studies is unsatisfactory (Pang et al, 1980). Prenatal diagnosis of the disorder from amniotic fluid and maternal urinary steroids may be possible (Rosler et al, 1979).

A defect in 11β-hydroxylation (Fig. 18.59) results in a decreased cortisol production with a concomitant increase in ACTH. As in the 21 hydroxylase defect, the increase of ACTH causes an excessive production of adrenal androgens, especially Δ4-androstenedione (Levine et al, 1980; Cathelinean, 1980). Additionally, excessive quantities of deoxycorticosterone are produced resulting in hypertension in most, but not in all, patients (Cathelinean, 1980). The clinical presentation of these patients is similar to that of males and females with the simple virilisation form of the 21-hydroxylase defect with the added finding of hypertension. The hypertension is usually quite marked (150/100

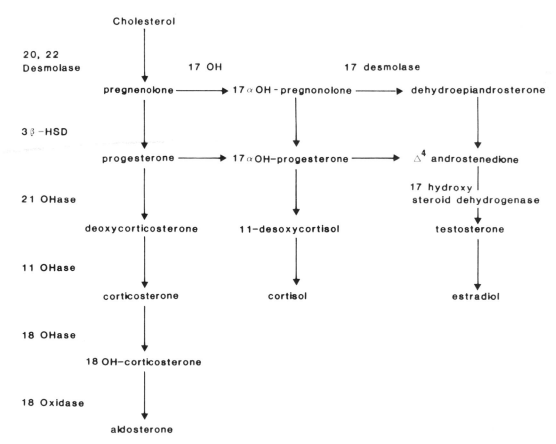

Fig. 18.59 Comprehensive schema of intermediate metabolites from cholesterol to aldosterone, cortisol and oestradiol

to 290/200) and if undetected until later life may be refractdry to therapy. It can lead to all of the complications of hypertension of other aetiologies.

The diagnosis is established by finding elevated plasma levels of 11-desoxycortisol and DOC, low plasma cortisol, and elevated 17-hydroxycorticoids (tetrahydro-11-deoxy-cortisol) and 17-ketosteroids. If hypertension is present, the diagnosis is not usually puzzling; however, in the newborn at least one case of 11β-hydroxylase deficiency was difficult to distinguish from the 21-hydroxylase defect (Holcombe et al, 1980). In this case, the urinary steroid pattern was identical to a group of infants with 21-hydroxylase deficiency and the infant exhibited marked salt wasting, also consistent with that diagnosis. Presumably, in these cases plasma determination of 11-deoxycortisol, 17α-hydroxyprogesterone and DOC would differentiate these enzymatic defects.

Treatment and continuing management are similar to that for the 21-hydroxylase defect. Hydrocortisone is given in doses sufficient to suppress 11-deoxycortisol and DOC into the normal range. Large series of patients have not been evaluated to establish the optimal dose of hydrocortisone, but a dose of 15–25 mg/m²/day is satisfactory in most patients. Several reports (Levine et al, 1980; Halcombe et al, 1980) confirm abnormal aldosterone synthesis following glucocorticoid therapy suggesting the theoretical need for mineralo-corticoid therapy in this disorder once DOC is suppressed. However, most patients seem to do well on glucocorticoid replacement alone. Surgical correction of the virilised external genitalia is the same as in the more common 21-hydroxylase defect.

The few patients with this disorder included in long-term follow-up studies (Klingensmith et al, 1977; Urban et al, 1978) suggested they also have an excellent prognosis for normal growth, sexual development, fertility, and life expentancy if the hypertension is controlled.

As in the 21-hydroxylase defect, an attenuated form of the 11β-hydroxylase defect has been reported which presents post-pubertally (Cathelineau et al, 1980). These patients present with hirsutism, menstrual irregularities, and variable degrees of hypertension. An ACTH stimulation test, as in the 21-hydroxylase defect, may be necessary to confirm the diagnosis. In the attenuated 11β-hydroxylase defect, 11-deoxycortisol and DOC will be the most diagnostic steroids after ACTH stimulation, with 11-deoxycortisol values above 5 mg/dl and DOC values 2–20 times normal.

C-3-β-hydroxysteroid dehydrogenase deficiency

A deficiency in 3-β-hydroxysteroid dehydrogenase leads to a decreased production in all classes of adrenal steroids (Fig. 18.59). The decrease in cortisol production triggers an increased ACTH secretion followed by an increased production of pregnenolone and 17α-hydroxypregneno-lone. The increased 17α-hydroxypregnenolone is converted to dehydroepiandrosterone, which cannot be converted to more potent adrenal androgens.

This is an extremely rare condition first reported by Bongiovani in 1962, and estimated to occur in 1:500 000 live births. Since the initial report only a handful of patients with the complete form of the disorder have been reported who have survived the newborn period.

Newborns present with ambiguous genitalia and salt wasting secondary to a deficient aldosterone production. Both males and females will have ambiguous genitalia; the females are virilised by the increased dehydroepiandrosterone levels, and the males are inadequately virilised secondary to inadequate circulating testosterone levels. In a female infant, the 3-β-hydroxysteroid dehydrogenase defect must be distinguished from the more common 21-hydroxylase defect. In 3-β-hydroxysteroid dehydrogenase deficiency, the 17α-hydroxypregnenolone is decreased contrary to the increased values found in 21-hydroxylase deficiency, pregnenolone and dehydroepiandrosterone levels are increased while androstenedione and testosterone are decreased. Urinary determination of pregnanetriol is not helpful to distinguish between the two defects, but a distinctive urinary steroidal pattern can be detected using gas-liquid chromatography (Bongiovani, 1980).

Medical management of patients with 3-hydroxysteroid dehydrogenase defect is identical to that for patients with the salt-losing form of the 21-hydroxylase defect. The long-term outcome is greatly influenced by the presence of the enzymatic defect in the gonad as well as the adrenal (Zachmann, 1979; Martin et al, 1980).

It is now recognised that an attenuated form of this defect also exists. Female patients present with post-pubertal hirsutism and menstrual irregularities, including primary amenorrhea (Rosenfield, 1980). A plasma 17α-hydroxypregnenolone determination appears to exhibit the most striking abnormality with values 50–150 times normal (15 000–50 000 ng/nl vs 200–300 ng/dl). Dehydroepiandrosterone determinations are more readily available and are suggested as the best screening test for this disorder in the patient with hirsutism and menstrual irregularities (Bongiovani, 1980). The ratios of 17α-hydroxypregnenolone to 17α-progesterone, and dehydroepiandrosterone to androstenedione are increased 3–10 fold compared to normal controls. This difference is accentuated by ACTH infusion. During ACTH infusion the Δ5-compounds, i.e. pregnenolone and dehydroepiandrosterone, rise, while the steroids distal to the enzymatic defect, i.e. Δ4-compounds, show little change. These patients also exhibit mildy abnormal aldosterone production and increased plasma renin activity.

Therapy with a glucocorticoid and 9α-fludrocortisol is indicated and prevents further virilisation. Menses have become more regular with some ovulatory menses reported (Rosenfield et al, 1980; Bongiovani, 1980). The recognition of the attenuated 3-β-hydroxysteroid dehydrogenase defect is too recent to estimate the frequency of this disorder among patients with hirsutism and menstrual irregularities. Thus, much work remains to be done in defining the frequency of this disorder and determining the success of therapy.

Lipoid adrenal hyperplasia

Congenital adrenal lipoid hyperplasia, or Prader's disease, is characterised by severe adrenocorticol insufficiency.

None of the patients reported have survived; all have massively enlarged lipid-laden adrenal glands (Prader & Siebermann, 1957). Markedly diminished cholesterol side-chain cleavage enzyme activity has been demonstrated in adrenal tissue from a patient with this disorder. With the inability to convert cholesterol to pregnenolone, one would anticipate a diminished production of all adrenal steroids. Male infants described have had completely feminine external genitalia indicating the enzyme deficiency is present in the gonads as well as the adrenal.

REFERENCES

Bailey C C, Komrower G M, Palmer M 1978 Management of congenital adrenal hyperplasia. Urinary steroid estmation — review of their value. Archives of Disease in Childhood 53: 132

Bergstrand C G 1966 Growth in congenital adrenal hyperplasia. Acta Paediatrica Scandinavica 55: 463

Bias W B, Urban M D, Migeon C J, Shu S H, Lee P A 1981 Intra-HLA recombinations localizing the 21-hydroxylase deficiency gene within the HLA complex. Human Immunology 2: 139

Blackman S S Jr 1964 Concerning the function and origin of the reticular zone of the adrenal cortex. Bulletin of the Johns Hopkins Hospital 78: 180

Bongiovani A M 1962 The adrenogenital syndrome with deficiency of 3β-hydroxysteroid dehydrogenase. Journal of Clinical Investigation 41: 2086

Bongiovani A M 1980 Urinary steroidal pattern of infants with congenital adrenal hyperplasia due to 3β-hydroxysteroid dehyrogenase deficiency. Journal of Steroid Biochemistry 13: 809

Bongiovani A M 1981 Acquired adrenal hyperplasia: with special reference to 3β-hydroxysteroid dehydrogenase. Fertility and Sterility 35: 599

Bongiovani A M, Moshang T Jr, Parks J S 1973 Maturational deceleration after treatment of congenital adrenal hyperplasia. Helvetica Paediatrica Acta 28: 127

Brautbar C, Rosler A, Landau H, Cohen T, Nelken D, Cohen T, Levine C, Sack J, Benderli A, Moses S, Lieberman E, Dupont B, Levine L S, New M I 1979 No linkage between HLA and congenital adrenal hyperplasia due to 11βhydroxylase deficiency. New England Journal of Medicine 300: 205

Brook C G D, Zachmann M, Prader A, Murset G 1974 Experience with long-term therapy in congenital adrenal hyperplasia. Journal of Pediatrics 85: 12

Cathelineau G, Brerault J L, Fiet J, Julien R, Dreux C, Canivet J 1980 Adrenocortical 11-βhydroxylation defect in adult women with postmenarchial onset of symptoms. Journal of Clinical Endocrinology and Metabolism 51: 287

Childs B, Grumbach M M, Van Wyk J J 1956 Virilizing adrenal hyperplasia: a genetic male hormonal study. Journal of Clinical Investigation 35: 213

Chrousos G P, Loriaux D L, Mann D L, Cutter G B 1982 Late onset 21-hydroxylase deficiency mimicking idiopathic hirsutism or polycystic ovarian disease. Annals of Internal Medicine 96: 143

Crecchio L 1865 Annals of Hygiene 25: 178

Dechaux M, Broyer G, Lenoir G, Limal J M, Sachs C. 1982 Nyctohemeral rhythm of plasma renin activity and plasma aldosterone in children. Pediatric Research 16: 354

Duck S C 1980 Acceptable linear growth in congenital adrenal hyperplasia. Journal of Pediatrics 97: 93

Dupont B, Smithwick E M, Oberfield S E, Lee T D, Levine L S 1977 Close genetic linkage between HLA and congenital adrenal hyperplasia (21 hydroxylase deficiency). Lancet ii: 1309

Erhardt A A, Evers K, Money J 1968 Influence of androgen and some aspects of sexually dimorphic behavior in women with the late treated adrenogenital syndrome. John Hopkins Medical Journal 123: 115

Forrest M G, Betuel H, Couillin P, Boue A 1981 Prenatal diagnosis of congenital adrenal hyperplasia due to 21-hydroxylase deficiency by steroid analysis in the amniotic fluid of mid pregnancy: Comparison with HLA typing in seventeen pregnancies at risk for CAH. Prenatal Diagnosis 1: 197

Fortunoff S, Lattimer J K, Edson M 1964 Vaginoplasty techniqe for female pseudohermaphrodites. Surgery, Gnecology and Obstetrics 188: 545

Frish H, Parth K, Schober E, Swoboda W 1981 Circadian patterns of plasma cortisol, 17-hydroxyprogesterone and testosterone in congenital adrenal hyperplasia. Archives of Disease in Childhood 56: 208

Fukushima D K, Finkelstein J W, Yoshida K, Boyar R M, Hellman L 1975 Pituitary-adrenal activity in untreated congenital adrenal hyperplasia. Journal of Clinical Endocrinology and Metabolism 40: 1

Guati J P, Kowarski A A, Migeon C J 1977 The detection of the heterozygous carrier for congenital virilizing adrenal hyperplasia. Journal of Pediatrics 90: 924

Hamill P W, Drizd T A, Johnson C L, Reed R B, Roche 1977 NCHS Growth Curves for children birth — 18 years, Series II. Date from the National Health Survey No 165. DHEW publication No (PHS) 78-1650 National Centre for Health Statistics, Hyattsville, Maryland

Hamilton W 1972 Congenital adrenal hyperplasia. Clinics in Endocrinology and Metabolism 1: 503

Hendren W H, Crawford J D 1969 Adrenogenital syndrome: the anatomy of the anomaly and its repair — some new concepts. Journal of Pediatric Surgery 4: 49

Hendricks S A, Lippe B M, Kaplan S A, Lavin N, Mayes D M 1982 Urinary and serum steroid concentrations in the management of congenital adrenal hyperplasia. American Journal of Diseases of Children 136: 229

Hirshfeld A J, Fleshman J K 1969 An unusually high incidence of salt-losing congenital adrenal hyperplasia in the Alaskan eskimo. Journal of Pediatrics 75: 492

Holcombe J H, Keenan B S, Nichols B L, Kirkland R T, Clayton G W 1980 Neonatal salt loss in the hypertensive form of congenital adrenal hyperplasia. Pediatrics 65: 777

Hughes I A 1982 Congenital and acquired disorders of the adrenal cortex. Clinics in Endocrinology and Metabolism 11: 89

Highes I A, Wilton A, Lole C A, Gray O P 1979 Continuing need for mineralocorticoid therepy in salt-losing congenital adrenal hyperplasia. Archives of Disease in Childhood 54: 350

Hughes I A, Winter J S D 1976 The application of a serum 17OH-progesterone radioimmunoassay to the diagnosis and management of congenital adrenal hyperplasia. Journal of Pediatrics 88: 766

Hughes I A, Winter J S D 1977 17-α-hydroxyprogesterone and plasma renin activity in congenital adrenal hyperplasia. In: Lee P A, Plotnick L P, Kowarski A A, Migeon C J (eds) Congenital Adrenal Hyperplasia p. 141. University Park Press, London

Jansen M, Wit J M, Van Den B, Rande J L 1981 Reinstitution of mineralocorticoid therapy in congenital adrenal hyperplasia. Effects on control and growth. Acta Paediatrica Scandinavica 70: 229

Jones H W Jr, Jones G S 1954 The gynecological aspects of adrenal hyperplasia and allied disorders. Americal Journal of Obstetrics and Gynecology 68: 13

Jones H W Jr, Verkauf B S 1970 Surgical treatment in congenital adrenal hyperplasia — age at operation and other prognostic factors. Obstetrics and Gynecology 36: 1

Jones H W Jr, Verkauf B S 1971 Congenital adrenal hyperplasia: age at menarche and related events at puberty. American Journal of Obstetrics and Gynecology 109: 292

Jones H W Jr, Lee P, Rock J A, Migeon C J 1982 A genetic male with 17-α-hydroxylase deficiency. Obstetrics and Gynecology 59: 254

Keenan B S, Holcomber J H, Wilson D P, Kirkland R T, Potts E, Clayton G W 1982 Plasma renin activity and the response to sodium depletion in salt-losing congenital adrenal hyperplasia. Pediatric Research 16: 118

Kirkland J L, Kirkland R T, Librik L, Clayton G W 1973 Iatrogenic hypertension in children with congenital adrenal hyperplasia. Journal of Pediatrics 83: 687

Kirkland R T, Keenan B S, Holcombe, Kirkland J L, Clayton G W 1978 The effect of therapy on mature height in congenital adrenal hyperplasia. Journal of Clinical Endocrinology and Metabolism 47: 1320

Klingensmith G J, Garcia S C, Jones H W Jr, Migeon C J, Blizzard R M 1977 Glucocorticoid treatment of girls with congenital adrenal hyperplasia: effects on height, sexual maturation and fertility. Journal of Pediatrics 90: 996

Korth-Schutz S, Virdis R, Saenger P, Chow D M, Levine L S, New M I 1978 Serum androgens as a continuing index of adequacy of treatment of congenital adrenal hyperplasia. Journal of Clinical Endocrinology and Metabolism 46: 452

Kowarski A A, Finklestein J W, Spaulding J S, Holman G H, Migeon C J 1965 Aldosterone secretion rate in congenital adrenal hyperplasia. A discussion of the theories on the pathogenesis of the salt-losing from of the syndrome. Journal of Clinical Investigation 44: 1505

La Franchi S 1980 Plasma adrenocorticotropin hormone in congenital adrenal hyperplasia. Importance in long-term management. American Journal of Diseases of Children 134: 72

Laron Z, Pertzelan A 1968 The comparative effect of 6-α-methylprednisolone and hydrocortisone on linear growth of children with congenital adrenal virilism and Addison's disease. Journal of Pediatrics 73: 774

Laron Z, Pollack M S, Zamir R, Roitman A, Dickerman Z, Levine L S, Lorenzen F, O'Neill C J, Pang S, New M I, Dupont B 1980 Late onset 21-hydroxylase deficiency and HLA in the Ashkenazi population: a new allele at the 21-hydroxylase locus. Human Immunology 1: 55

Levine L S, Rauh W, Gottesdiener K, Chow D, Guncaler P, Rapaport R, Pang S, Schneider B, New M I 1980 New Studies of the 11-β-hydroxylase enzymes in the hypertensive form of congenital adrenal hyperplasia. Journal of Clinical Endocrinology and Metabolism 50: 258

Levine L S, Dupont B, Lorenzen F, Pang S, Pollack M, Overfield S E, Kohn B, Lerner A, Cacciari E, Mantero F, Cassio A, Scaroni C, Chiumello G, Rondanini G F, Gargantini L, Giovannelli G, Virdis R, Bartolotta E, Migliori C, Pintor C, Tato L, Barboni F, New M I 1981 Genetic and hormonal characterization of cryptic 21-hydroxylase deficiency. Journal of Clinical Endocrinology and Metabolism 53: 1193

Lewis V G, Erhrhardt A A, Money J 1970 Genital surgery in girls with the adrenogenital syndrome subsequent psychological developments. Obstetrics and Gynecology 36: 11

Loras B, Haour F, Bertrant J 1970 Exchangeable sodium and aldosterone secretion in children with congenital adrenal hyperplasia due to 21-hydroxylase deficiency. Pediatric Research 4: 145

Martin F, Perheentupa J, Adlercreutz H 1980 Plasma and urinary androgens and oestrogens in a pubertal boy with 3β-hydroxysteroid dehydrogenase deficiency. Journal of Steroid Biochemistry 13: 197

Meyer W J III, Gutai J P, Keenan B S, Davis G R, Kowarski A A, Migeon C M 1977 A chronological approach to the treatment of congenital adrenal hyperplasia. In: Lee P A, Plotnick L P, Kowarski A A, Migeon C J (eds) Congenital Adrenal Hyperplasia p 203. University Park Press, London

Migeon C J 1968 Updating of the treatment of congenital adrenal hyperplasia. Journal of Pediatrics 78: 805

Migeon C J, Rosenwaks Z, Lee P, Urban M, Bias W 1980 The attenuated form of congenital adrenal hyperplasia as an allelic form of 21-hydroxylase deficiency. Journal of Clinical Endocrinology and Metabolism 51: 647

Money J, Hampson J G, Hampson J L 1955 An examination of some basic sexual concepts: the evidence of human hermaphroditism. Bulletin of the John Hopkins Hospital 97: 301

Money J, Lewis V 1966 I Q genetics and accelerated growth: adrenogenital syndrome. Bulletin of Johns Hopkins Hospital 118: 365

Murtaza L, Sibert J R, Hughes I, Balfour I C 1980 Congenital adrenal hyperplasia — a clinical and genetic survey. Archives of Disease in Childhood 55: 622

Nagamani M, McDonough P G, Ellegood J O, Mahesh V B 1978 Maternal and amniotic fluid 17-α-hydroxyprogesterone levels during pregnancy: diagnosis of congenital adrenal hyperplasia in utero. American Journal of Obstetrics and Gynecology 130: 781

New M I, Dupont B, Pollack M S, Levine L S 1981 The biochemical basis for genotyping 21-hydroxylase deficiency. Human Genetics 58: 123

Newns G H 1974 Congenital adrenal hyperplasia. Archives of Disease in Childhood 49:

Pang S, Levine L S, Chow D M, Faiman C, New M I 1979 Serum androgen concentrations in neonates and young infants with congenital adrenal hyperplasia due to 21-hydroxylase deficiency. Clinical endocrinology 11: 575

Pang S, Levine L S, Lorenzen F, Chow D, Pollack M, Dupont B, Genel M, New M I 1980 Hormonal studies in obligate heterozygotes and siblings of patients with 11-β-hydroxylase deficiency congenital adrenal hyperplasia. Journal of Clinical Endocrinology and Metabolism 50: 586

Pollack M S, Levine L S, O'Neill G J, Pang S, Lorenzen F, Kohn B, Rondanini G F, Chiumello G, New M I, Dupont B 1981 HLA linkage and B14, DRI, BFS haplotype association with the genes for late onset and cryptic 21-hydroxylase deficiency. American Journal of Human Genetics 33: 540

Porter B, Finzi E, Leiberman E, Moses S 1977 The syndrome of congenital adrenal hyperplasia in Israel. Pediatrics 6: 100

Prader A, Siebermann R E 1957 Nebennieren in suffizienz bei kongenitafer lipoidhyperplasia der nebenneieren. Helvetica Paediatrica Acta 12: 569

Prader A, Anders G J P A, Habich J 1962 Zur genetik des kongenitalen adrenogenitalen syndrome. Helvetica Paediatrica Acta 17: 271

Qazi Q H, Thompson M W 1972 Incidence of salt-losing form of congenital virilizing adrenal hyperplasia. Archives of Disease in Childhood 47: 302

Rajfer J, Ehrlich R M, Goodwin W E 1982 Reduction clitoroplasty via ventral approach. Journal of Urology (in Press)

Rappaport R, Bouthreuil E, Marti-Henneberg C, Basmaciogullari A 1973 Linear growth rate, bone maturation and growth hormone secretion in prepubertal children with congenital adrenal hyperplasia. Acta Paediatric Scandinavica 62: 513

Riddick D H, Hammond C B 1975 Long-term steroid therapy in patients with adrenogenital syndrome. Obstetrics and Gynecology 45: 15

Rosenfield R, Rich B, Wolfsdorf J, Casorla F, Parks J, Bongiovanni A, Wu C, Shackleton C 1980 Pubertal presentation of congenital △5-3β-hydroxysteroid dehydrogenase deficiency. Journal of Clinical Endocrinology and Metabolism 51: 345

Rosenwaks A, Lee P A, Jones G S, Migeon C J, Wentz A C 1979 An attenuated form of congenital virilizing adrenal hyperplasia. Journal of Clinical Endocrinology and Metabolism 49: 335

Rosler A, Levine L S, Schneider B, Novogroder M, New M I 1977 The interrelationship of sodium balance, plasma renin activity and ACTH in congenital adrenal hyperplasia. Journal of Clinical Endocrinology and Metabolism 45: 500

Rosler A, Leiberman E, Rosenmann A, Ben-Uzilio R, Weidenfeld J 1979 Prenatal diagnosis of 11-β-hydroxylase deficiency congenital adrenal hyperplasia. Journal of Clinical Endocrinology and Metabolism 49: 546

Schiebinger R J, Albertson B D, Cassorla F G, Bowyer D W, Geelhoed G W, Cutler G B Jr, Loriaux D L 1981 The developmental changes in plasma adrenal androgens during infancy and adrenarche are associated with changing activities of adrenal microsomal 17-hydroxylase and 17, 20-demolase. Journal of Clinical Investigation 67: 1177

Smith R, Donald R A, Espiner, Glatthaar C, Abbot G, Scandrett M 1980 The effect of different treatment regimens on hormonal profiles in congenital adrenal hyperplasia. Journal of Clinical Endocrinology and Metabolism 51: 230

Styne D M, Richards G E, Bell J J, Conte F A, Morishima A, Kaplan S L, Grumback M M 1977 Growth patterns in congenital adrenal hyperplasia: correlation of glucocorticoid therapy with stature. In: Lee P A, Plotnick L P, Kowarski A A, Migeon C J (eds) Congenital adrenal hyperplasia, p. 247. University Park Press, London

Urban M D, Lee P A, Migeon C J 1978 Adult height and fertility in men with congenital virilizing adrenal hyperplasia. New England Journal of Medicine 299: 1392

Van Seters A P, Vam Aalderen W, Moolenaar A J, Garsiro M C B, Van Roon R, Backer E T 1981 Adrenalcortical tumor in untreated congenital adrenocortical hyperplasia associated with inadequate ACTH suppressibility. Clinical Endocrinology 14: 325

Vazquesz A M, Kenny F M 1972 Hypertension secondary to excessive desoxycorticosterone implants or 9-α-fluorocortisol in salt-losing congenital adrenal hyperplasia. Journal of Pediatrics 81: 549

Webb T, Mackintosh P, Wells L J 1980 cytogenetic evidence for the localization of the gene for congenital adrenal hyperplasia. Clinical Genetics 17: 349

Wentzel U, Schneider M, Zachman M, Knorr-Murset G, Wever A, Prader A 1978 Intelligence of patients with congenital adrenal hyperplasia due to 21-hydroxylase deficiency their parents and unaffected siblings. Helvetica Paediatrica Acta 33: 11

Werder E A, Siebenmann R E, Knorr M, Urset G, Zimmerman A, Sizonenko P C, Theintz P, Girard J, Zachmann M, Prader A 1980 The incidence of congenital adrenal hyperplasia in Switzerland — a survey of patients born in 1960 to 1974. Helvetica Paediatrica Acta 35: 5

West C D, Athcheson J V, Stanchfield J B, Rallison M L, Chavre V J, Tyler F H 1979 Multiple or single 21hydroxylase in congenital adrenal hyperplasia? Journal of Steroid Biochemistry 11: 1413

Wilkins L 1965 The Diagnosis and Treatment of Endocrine Disorders in Childhood and Adolescence, 3rd edn, p. 360. Thomas, Springfield, Illinois

Wilkins L, Lewis R A, Klein R, Rosemberg E 1950 The suppression of androgen secretion by cortisone in a case of congenital adrenal hyperplasia. Bulletin of the Johns Hopkins Hospital 87: 249

Young H H 1937 Genital anomalies. Hermaphroditism and Related Adrenal Diseases. Williams & Wilkins Company, Baltimore

Zachmann M 1979 3β-hydroxysteroid dehydrogenase deficiency. Hormone Rearch 11: 292

Precocious puberty in the female

When the physical features of puberty make their appearances significantly earlier than the times indicated in Chapter 2, puberty may be regarded as precocious. This is a disturbing condition for the parents of a child so affected and, whether investigation shows that a serious cause is present or not, very careful management is required.

AETIOLOGY

A number of pathological processes may give rise to precocious puberty, but it must be admitted at the outset that the largest group of girls with these features do not have any abnormality at all; they are then described as examples of constitutional precocious puberty. We can only assume that in these children the hypothalamus and pituitary have escaped from the usual state of inhibition which characterises childhood at an unusually early age without there being any evident cause for this. Rayner (1981) comments that assessment of a large number of reported cases shows 80 per cent of affected girls to be examples of constitutional precocity.

Probably the second most likely cause of precocious puberty is the presence of some intracranial lesion such as previous meningitis or encephalitis, a small space occupying lesion such as a ventricular hamartoma (Schmidt et al, 1958; Sherwin et al, 1972) or a pineal tumour (Kitay, 1954) or other cerebral tumour which seems to have triggered off premature hypothalamic/pituitary activity. A possibly related cause to this is a condition known as the McCune/Albright syndrome (McCune & Bruch, 1957; Albright et al, 1937). In this disorder there are wide-spread cystic bony changes — it is called polyostotic fibrous dysplasia — and it is also associated with abnormal function of a number of endocrine glands, notably the hypothalamus, pituitary, thyroid and parathyroid. There are other curious features of this syndrome such as the appearance of areas of light brown skin pigmentation — cafe au lait spots, as they are called — although the precise inter-

relationship between these various features and precocious puberty is imperfectly understood.

In the conditions so far considered it will be seen that the precocious puberty changes are of hypothalamic/pituitary origin. The same changes may arise for an entirely different reason without the involvement of hypothalamic/pituitary activity. This occurs when there is a feminising ovarian tumour present which is producing sufficient oestrogen to bring about the changes of secondary sexual development and vaginal bleeding. Various histological forms of tumour may be encountered which will be considered presently. In an attempt to distinguish hypothalamic/pituitary puberty from that due to an ovarian tumour, the latter has sometimes been labelled 'precocious pseudo-puberty', although perhaps 'precocious sexual development' would be a better description. One other possible explanation for secondary sexual development and vaginal bleeding in a little girl must be considered. This is the accidental ingestion of an oestrogenic preparation of some kind. The child may have taken some of her mother's supply of combined oral contraceptive pills which she has mistaken for sweets and such an exogenous cause should be kept in mind. Rarely other causes of precocious sexual development may be found which are set out in Table 19.1.

Table 19.1 Aetiology of precocious puberty

Constitutional	
Neurological:	cerebral tumors, hydrocephalus, cysts, meningitis, encephalitis, polyostotic fibrous dysplasia, neurofibromatosis, tuberose sclerosis, etc.
Adrenal tumours	
Ovarian tumours	
Gonadotrophin-secreting tumours:	chorionepithelioma, hepatoblastoma
Others:	hypothyroidism, exogenous oestrogens

CLINICAL FEATURES

The clinical features of precocious puberty will vary depending upon its cause.

In constitutional precocious puberty (Fig. 19.1), the

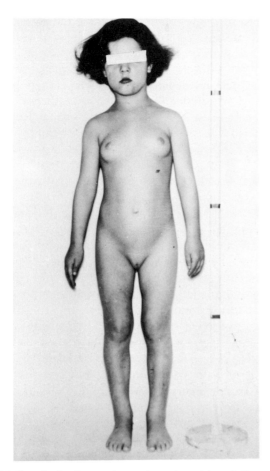

Fig. 19.1 Constitutional precocious puberty in a girl aged 4½ years (Courtesy of Professor R. S. Illingworth and Balliere Tindall)

changes of puberty occur in more or less their usual order at an unusually early age. It is customary therefore for such an affected child to show breast development and a growth spurt first, followed soon afterwards by the presence of sexual hair and lastly by menstruation; since the order of events in normal puberty varies, however, there is a variation in this form of precocious puberty also. What is usually a striking feature, however, is the increased growth in height of such an affected child which, in combination with the visible signs of secondary sexual development, give her the appearance of being much older than she really is. The physical features here described are not always progressive. It seems evident that from time to time precocious sexual changes can be transitory and after several weeks, or perhaps a little longer, full remission takes place. Grant (1980) found such complete remission to occur in six patients who had shown signs of secondary sexual development before the age of 6 years out of a total of 32 girls with precocious sexual features who were investigated.

In cerebral precocious puberty a similar pattern can usually be discerned. The only direct evidence suggesting that there may be a cerebral cause for the condition will be in those children where there is a chronic neurological

fault such as hydrocephalus, previous encephalitis or evident mental retardation. Such cases are comparatively uncommon however, and a cerebral cause for the precocity must be excluded by investigation.

There are usually characteristic clinical features in the McCune-Albright syndrome. One of the most important of these, from the clinican's point of view, is that vaginal bleeding may occur at an unusually early stage in the disease and may indeed be the first sign of abnormality. Heller et al (1978) found vaginal bleeding to be the first abnormal feature in seven out of nine patients with the McCune-Albright syndrome; by contrast in 15 cases of constitutional precocious puberty such bleeding was the first sign only once. The cafe au lait spots on the body surface are a most striking clinical feature indicating the diagnosis of polyostotic fibrous dysplasia. These are often quite large and very irregular in shape as can be seen from Fig. 19.2 and they are light brown in colour. The back, face, shoulders and neck are the areas most commonly affected although the spots may appear elsewhere also; they may be evident at birth even though the other features of puberty do not appear for some time. These spots are not always evident upon those areas of skin normally exposed even at a clinical examination and it is advisable to remove all the child's clothes and to examine the entire skin surface (Dewhurst, 1980). Other glandular dysfunctions may sometimes be seen as well; moreover a particularly distressing aspect of the syndrome is the tendency to fractures in the affected bones which can be frequent and widespread in patients who are markedly affected.

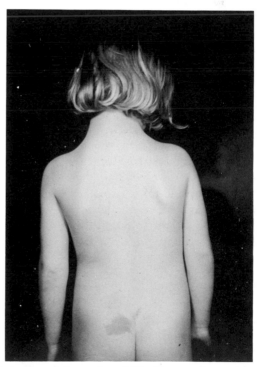

Fig. 19.2 A cafe au lait spot in a child with precocious puberty due to the McCune-Albright Syndrome

Apart from the obvious signs of secondary sexual development which result from the premature stimulation of the ovary from whatever cause, another result, upon which considerable emphasis must be placed, is the possibility of cyst formation in the ovary. These cysts are follicular in type and, although many are comparatively small, some may reach a sufficient size to be felt on abdominal examination and certainly on rectal examination. It will immediately be apparent here that this is not an easy clinical feature to assess since such an ovarian mass may *result* from premature ovarian stimulation in, for example, constitutional precocious puberty, or may *cause* it if the tumour in question is a new growth. More will be said about this matter later when treatment is dealt with more fully.

The possibility that a child with precocious puberty changes may have a feminising ovarian tumour is obviously an important matter. It must be stressed that these feminising tumours are rare and that constitutional precocious puberty, cerebral precocious puberty and the McCune-Albright syndrome are all more common. The features which particularly suggest that a feminising new growth may be present are, of course, the palpation of a pelvic swelling first and foremost; granulosa cell tumours and other feminising ovarian tumours are generally sufficently large to be palpated without difficulty and even if the tumour is not evident on abdominal palpation, bimanual rectal examination will usually disclose its presence. Other features which suggest that a new growth is responsible may be the occurrence of vaginal bleeding at a very early stage before the other features of secondary sexual development are pronounced (although this also may be evident in patients with the McCune-Albright syndrome) and the lack of pronounced bone growth which would make the child obviously taller than her chronological age. It must be stressed, however, that these features are variable and seldom can a firm clinical diagnosis be arrived at. On very rare occasions there may also be evidence of precocious androgenic activity (Dewhurst & Folinsbee, 1980). The granulosa/theca group of tumours are capable of producing both oestrogens and androgens (Nokes et al, 1959; Ryan, 1979) although the clinical features resulting from stimulation by the former are much more common. Heterosexual puberty changes would more strongly suggest the presence of an adrenal tumour, which, although rarely associated solely with feminisation, is more often found in girls who are becoming masculinised.

Investigations

Further investigation is necessary in almost all children showing precocious sexual changes. Only if the appearance of secondary sexual development were fractionally early and clinical examination entirely negative, may these investigations be omitted. Since, as already indicated, FSH, LH oestrogens and androgens are all detectable at an early age by modern methods of assay, and since the normal ranges are wide, measurement of these substances is less helpful than one would imagine. The mere detection of FSH and LH does not, of itself, indicate any abnormality since both may be evident in the normal child who is prepubertal. If an LH-RH stimulation test is indertaken then a response characteristic of early or mid-puberty, such as has already been described, may be obtained which, would be evidence in favour of the condition being hypothalamic/pituitary origin. An assay of oestrogen may or may not be helpful; sometimes very high levels are obtained which strongly suggest the possibility of a feminising ovarian tumour, although this is not an invariable finding (Rayner, 1981). Grant (1980) has reviewed endocrine patterns in precocious puberty. Whatever the cause of the condition is is likely that a vaginal smear will show the presence of oestrogen activity.

X-ray examination may be helpful in a variety of ways. An X-ray of the hand and wrist should be undertaken to form an estimate of the bone age. In patients with precocious puberty of cerebral or constitutional origin; the bone age is often greatly advanced (Fig. 19.3); if a feminising tumour is to blame the advance in bone age, if present at all, is often much smaller. A survey of the bony skeleton, including the long bones, should be undertaken to look for evidence of the McCune-Albright syndrome. Various changes may be observed; there may be rarifaction which gives rise to pseudocyst formation and these lesions are characteristically evident in some bones and absent in others. Bone overgrowth, notably in the base of the skull, is sometimes evident: this may cause pressure on the optic formina and lead to proptosis (Benedict, 1962). A disorder giving similar appearances is hyperparathyroidism although in this condition the changes are generalised throughout the body whilst in the McCune-Albright syndrome localised affected areas are more common (Rasmussen, 1974). An X-ray of the skull should also be undertaken; abnormalities of the sella turcica or calcification above the sella may suggest an intracranial fault.

If the patient is a very young child the likelihood of an intracranial cause for the condition is greater and further investigation may be required. A CT scan should be undertaken to eliminate a dangerous space occupying lesion and if this facility is not available, consideration should be given, in consultation with a paediatrician, to ventriculography being performed.

An investigation which is proving more valuable in girls with a variety of possible gynaecological conditions is an ultrasound scan. This may clearly show the presence of an ovarian swelling and variations in the picture over a number of weeks may give some indication as to the nature of the swelling. As already indicated, there are occasional examples of transient ovarian activity giving rise to some sign of secondary sexual development and perhaps even vaginal bleeding after which the features retrogress. The

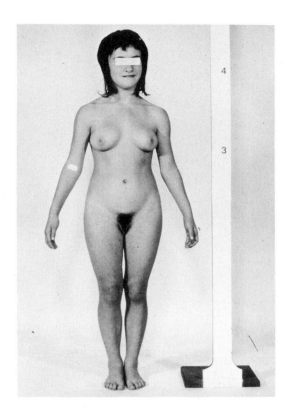

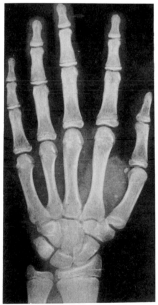 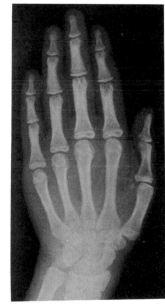

Fig. 19.3 (a) A child aged 7 years with consititional precocious puberty. (b) Advanced bone age in the child shown in Fig. 19.3a. On the left is shown the radiological appearance of the hand and wrist of a normal child aged 13; on the right is shown the X-ray of the patient comparable with age 13 (by kind permission of Marcel Dekker and Co.)

presence of a small follicular ovarian cyst which shrinks over a period of several weeks may then be evident upon ultrasound scanning. Alternatively the characteristics of the impedence to the passage of the sound waves may suggest that the tumour is a new growth when surgical exploration of the pelvis is likely to be indicated.

TREATMENT

The care of a little girl with precocious puberty usually falls ,to the paediatrician in collaboration with an endocrinologist, family doctor, social workers, school teachers, etc. The gynaecologist also sometimes has a part to play and this may be a very important one; generally a pelvic swelling will have been felt or its presence suspected and the gynaecologist is asked for an opinion as to its nature and management.

There are a number of important aspects to the management of a patient with precocious puberty. One obvious risk, of course, is that the child may be the victim of sexual assault and may even become pregnant. In a number of instances precocious pregnancies at a very early age have been reported. The striking example is that of Lina Medina, who had a Caesarean section when $5\frac{1}{2}$ years old, but there have been other pregnancies in children aged 6, 7, 8 and 9 years (Sickel, 1946). One patient (Furtado, 1947) from Brazil was delivered of twins when she was 7 years of age. These very early pregnancies have been reviewed by Dewhurst (1963, 1981).

The risk that this may happen is one reason why attempts have been made to inhibit premature hypothalamic pituitary activity and bring the process of precocious puberty temporarily to an end. Two drugs have been used for this purpose — medroxyprogesterone acetate (Provera) and cyproterone acetate (Androcur). Provera has been used in doses of 100–200 mg intramuscularly every 2–4 weeks to bring about hypothalamic suppression. Under this regime of management regression of many of the signs of secondary sexual development is evident and there is cessation of menstruation, but the treatment is less satisfactory in inhibiting bone growth (Kaplan et al, 1968). It is desirable to slow down this advanced bone growth if possible since it will result in the patient being initially taller than her class mates, but the early fusion which will occur in the epiphyses will result in her ultimate stature being shorter than that of most girls undergoing puberty at the correct time. The ultimate affect of Provera in preventing short stature has been disappointing. A further disadvantage is that the drug has sometimes caused adrenocortical suppression (Sedeghi-Nejad et al, 1971) whilst when the drug is ultimately stopped hypothalamic/pituitary activity has remained depressed for a period of time in some cases. If this treatment is contemplated a paediatric endocrinologist should be closely involved.

The alternative is to use the antiandrogen substance, cyproterone acetate (Neumann & Hamada, 1964) which has become more popular in the management of precocious puberty in Europe in recent years. Oral treatment has been given with doses of 70–150 mg/m² per day (Kauli et al, 1976) and good results on the regression of breast development, etc. have been reported. It is doubtful however, if this drug is much more effective in inhibiting early bone growth than medroxyprogetserone acetate. Werder et al (1974) were unable to demonstrate an effect on the ultimate height. Bossi et al (1973) and Kauli et al (1976), however, claimed that there was a beneficial effect on linear growth and delay in bone maturation provided the drug was used before children had attained a bone age of 11 years. It certainly cannot be said without question that there will be a valuable growth effect if cyproterone acetate is to be used although the drug does control the other signs of secondary sexual development well and there are further benefits. There appears to be reduction in aggressive behaviour and less masturbation after its use and it is relatively free from side-effects. Occasionally however, fatigue is evident, perhaps as a result of adrenocortical suppression (Leading article, 1981). Rayner (1981) regards it as the drug of choice in early puberty at the present time.

Mention should be made of the importance of the social management of a child with precocious puberty. There are often behavioural problems, and educational problems since it is easy to believe such a child to be older an more mature than she really is. The co-operation of parents, social workers, teachers and the family doctor is of great value in proper management.

When a definitive pelvic swelling has been felt or a size-able lower abdominal mass is clearly evident, a gynaecologist should be consulted for operation is usually necessary. It has already been mentioned, and must be stressed again, that such a mass may be a feminising ovarian tumour *causing* precocious sexual development, or it may be a follicular cyst *resulting* from the premature stimulation of the ovary. Operation will then be necessary and with the abdomen open it must be determined which of these two is present since the management is quite different.

The characteristics of a simple follicular cyst are well known to gynaecologists. These cysts are thin-walled and the fact that they contain serous fluid is generally easily identified. At one point it is usually possible to distinguish a condensation of normal ovarian tissue. Sometimes such cysts are bilateral. If such are the findings it is imperative that as much normal ovarian tissue as possible be preserved. The cyst should be excised by the standard procedure of ovarian cystectomy.

When excision of a follicular cyst has been carried out by the procedure of cystectomy the physical signs of precocious puberty have, in a number of instances, retrogressed (Jolly, 1955). This does not happen in the majority, however, and it now seems likely that in those where retrogression has been evident this would have happened in any event even if the cyst had not been removed, the cases probably being examples of transient precocity as already outlined.

The appearance of a granulosa/theca cell tumour is somewhat different. These tumours are predonimantly solid although it will be evident when their cut surface is examined that they are composed of a mixture of solid and

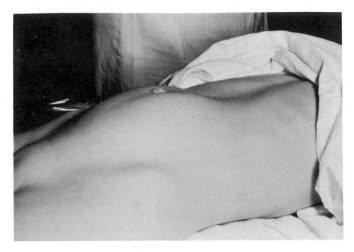

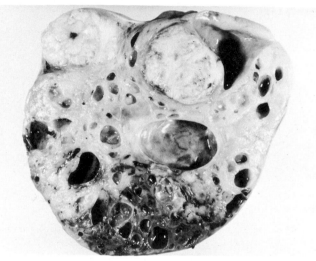

Fig. 19.4 (a) The abdominal appearances in a child with precocious puberty due to the presence of a granulosa cell tumour which is seen in cut section in Fig. 19.4b

cystic areas and haemorrhage is often a striking feature (Fig. 19.4). Normal ovarian tissue cannot be clearly identified at any site. The tumours are generally unilateral and the appearances do not resemble the follicular cyst described above.

Management of a granulosa/theca cell tumour in a little girl does not call for radical measures although usually the complete removal of the ovary on the affected side is necessary. These tumours are, at least in theory, malignant (Fox & Langley, 1974) although the degree of malignancy is low and the prognosis with unilateral removal is good. Unilateral salpingo-oophorectomy, or better still, unilateral oophorectomy, if the ovary can be readily removed *in toto* without damaging the tube, is all that is required unless there are clear signs that an extension of a malignant process has already taken place. Should there be such evidence of obvious malignancy then there will scarcely be any alternative to total hysterectomy and bilateral salpingo-oophorectomy with perhaps deep X-ray treatment later. Although the likelihood of having to do a procedure of this nature is small it is generally wise to inform the parents of this possibility before the operation is undertaken and to obtain their permission to do it. I have, on one occasion, encountered a patient from whom a granulosa cell tumour had been enucleated, in the manner of an ovarian cystectomy, at the age of 6, the ovary then being reconstituted. Two years later the tumour recurred on the same side although with no evidence of further spread. This indicates the essentially low grade of malignancy in such tumours but indicates also that anything less than oophorectomy on the affected side is probably inadequate.

Under what circumstances might it not be appropriate to open the abdomen in a child in whom the presence of a pelvic swelling seemed highly likely? It may be unnecessary to operate if the pelvic swelling concerned was initially a small one, felt only with difficulty but confirmed by ultrasound, in which regression was demonstrated by subsequent ultrasonic scans over the next few weeks. In these circumstances it would seem probable that the cyst in question was the result of premature ovarian stimulation and was retrogressing.

Reference has already been made to children who show transient sings of secondary sexual development with perhaps menstruation and then these signs begin to retrogress. In a number of such patients there appears to be small ovarian cyst formation, perhaps producing sufficient oestrogen to stimulate secondary sexual development, but then the cyst shrinks so that further treatment is unnecessary.

Another circumstance in which a palpable swelling need not necessarily be explored immediately might be if there was clear evidence, for example, that the patient had the McCune-Albright syndrome. Cyst formation in the ovary is sometimes encountered in this disorder and can readily be assumed to be of the follicular or possibly the lutein variety. Huffman (1981) records that when material has been excised from the ovary in this syndrome it has generally shown evidence of follicular growth without ovulation. On one occasion, however, I saw obvious luteinisation in the walls of an ovarian cyst removed from a child only a few months of age with the McCune-Albright syndrome. It may be mentioned here also that there is some evidence that the youngest mother in the world — Lina Medina of Peru — who was delivered by Caesarean section when she was 5½ years old, may have suffered from this syndrome (Editorial Comment, 1961)

PARTIAL FORMS OF PRECOCIOUS PUBERTY

Occasionally one may see a young patient with only one precocious physical sign of puberty. This may be pubic hair only (premature pubarche or adrenarche, Fig. 19.5), breast development only (precocious thelarche, Fig. 19.6), or menstruation only (precocious menarche, Fig. 19.7).

We do not understand why such isolated manifestations of puberty occur. It has been postulated that they arise because of unusual sensitivity of one or other end organ to the very low levels of circulating oestrogens — or in the case of premature pubarche, androgens — in the child. They may, of course, be the first manifestation of true precocious puberty and this is where their clinical importance lies. Such a child should be examined and investigated in a manner closely similar to what has been described in the foregoing section. If the condition is truly a single manifestation of precocity no unusual physical features will be evident. Even hormone assay will, in most instances, demonstrate levels which are appropriate for the child's

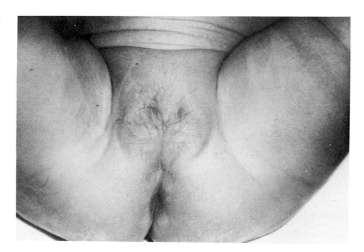

Fig. 19.5 Premature pubarche in a child aged 1½ years

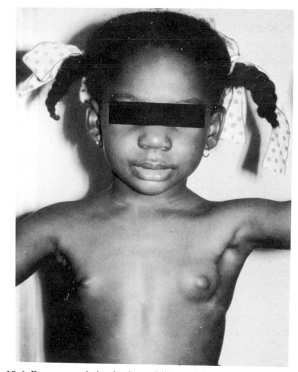

Fig. 19.6 Premature thelarche in a child aged 5 years

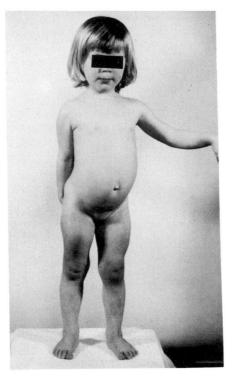

Fig. 19.7 Premature menarche in a child aged 1½ years who had been having periodic 'menstruation' for almost 12 months at more or less regular intervals. Note the absence of secondary sexual development

chronological age whilst bone age will similarly correspond. In the case of premature pubarche, however, Sizonenko (1978) showed seven girls so affected to have a generally taller stature, a slightly advanced bone age and a slightly raised plasma DHEA and DHEA sulphate. Despite these changes the menarche occurred at the normal age of 13 which corresponded closely to that of other girls from the same area.

In girls with precocious thelarche one breast may become enlarged before the other when, as already stressed, there is a real risk of unwise surgery being performed to carry out a biopsy. Even when both breasts show some enlargement there may well be fluctuation in the condition from time to time. Caprano et al (1971) have reviewed this condition well.

The most potentially serious of these isolated manifestations of precocity is vaginal bleeding. A child who has no signs of secondary sexual development but who bleeds per vaginam may have one of several possible abnormalities to explain this symptom. The most serious risk is that she may have a malignant genital tract tumour, probably in the vagina or cervix. There may be a foreign body in the vagina giving rise to a blood stained discharge; she may have precocious puberty as already discussed, or she may have one of a variety of vulval lesions such as a prolapsed urethra, condylomata accuminata or lichen sclerosus which has bled following scratching (Heller et al, 1978). So important is it to exclude a malignant vaginal or cervical tumour that an examination under anaesthesia should be undertaken at an early stage. If this examination is negative and no pelvic swelling can be palpated the bleeding may be the first manifestation of the McCune-Albright syndrome so an X-ray of the long bones would be necessary. It should be remembered that such a child might have had access to an exogenous source of oestrogen which have given rise to the symptom.

Reassurance can only be given to the parents when all the other possible causes of these symptoms have been investigated and excluded. Careful follow-up is essential if only that we may learn more about the natural history of this disorder. In a number of instances (Heller et al, 1979) the symptom of vaginal bleeding has disappeared after months or years and the menarche has eventually occurred at more or less the proper time.

The behaviour or one child reported in detail by Heller et al (1979) casts serious doubt upon the suggestion that these symptoms arise because of unusual sensitivity of the end organ to very low oestrogen levels. The child's mother was able to predict when the episodes of vaginal bleeding were due because of the irritable behaviour of her little daughter as occurs in the number of women with premenstrual tension.

REFERENCES

Albright F, Butler A M, Hampton A O et al 1937 Syndrome characterised by osteitis fibrosa disseminata, areas of pigmentation and endocrine dysfunction with precocious puberty in females, report of five cases. New England Journal of Medicine 216: 727

Benedict P 1962 Endocrine Features in Albright's syndrome (fibrous dysplasia of bone). Metabolism 11: 30

Bossi E, Zurbrugg R P, Joss E E 1973 Improvement of adult height prognosis in precocious puberty by Cyproterone acetate. Acta Paediatrica Scandinavica 62: 405

Caprano V J, Bayonet-Rivera N P, Aceto T, MacGillivray M 1971 Premature Thelarche. Obstetric and Gynaecological Survey 26: 2

Dewhurst C J 1963 Gynaecological Disorders of Infants and Children. Cassell & Co. London

Dewhurst Sir John 1980 Precocious Puberty. In: Practical Pediatric and Adolescent Gynecology, Ch 6, p 118. Marcel Dekker, New York

Dewhurst Sir John 1981 Childhood and Adolescent Pregnancies. In: Huffman J W, Dewhurst Sir John, Capraro V J (eds) The

Gynecology of Childhood and Adolescence, Ch 24, p 560. W B Saunders, Philadelphia

Editorial Comment 1961 Obstetric and Gynaecological Survey 16: 242

Folinsbee C D, Smith P A and Dewhurst Sir John 1981 Iso and heterosexual precocity associated with an ovarian granulosa/theca cell tumour. Journal of Obstetrics and Gynaecology 1: 257

Furtado A H 1947 Gravidez Precoce. Revista Ginecologia e d'Obstetricia (Rio de Janeiro) 1: 439

Grant D B 1980 Variations in the clinical and endocrine patterns of female precocious puberty. Serono Symposium No 36 In: E Cacciari, A Prader (eds) Pathophysiology of Puberty, p 175. London

Heller M E, Savage M O, Dewhurst J 1978 Vaginal bleeding in childhood: A review of 51 patients. British Journal of Obstetrics and Gynaecology 85: 721

Heller M E, Dewhurst C J, Grant D B 1979 Premature menarche without other evidence of precocious puberty. Archives of Disease in Childhood 54: 472

Huffman J W 1981 The Gynecology of Childhood and Adolescence. W B Saunders, Philadelphia

Jolly H 1955 Sexual Precocity. C C Thomas, Springfield, Illinois

Kaplan S A, Ling S M, Irani N G 1968 Idiopathic isosexual precocity. Therapy with medroxy progesterone. American Journal of Diseases of Children 116: 591

Kauli R, Pertzelam A, Prager-Lewin R 1976 Cyproterone acetate in treatment of precocious puberty. Archives of Disease in Childhood 51: 202

Kitay J I 1954 Pineal lesions and precocious puberty: A review. Journal of Clinical Endocrinology 14: 622

McCune D J, Bruch H 1937 Osteodystrophia fibrosa: Report of a case in which the condition was combined with precocious puberty, pathological pigmentation of the skin and hyperthyroidism, with a review of the literature. American Journal of Diseases of Children 54: 806

Neumann F, Hamada H 1964 Intrauterine feminisierung mannlicher rattenfeten durch das stark gestagen wirksame 6-chlor-A-1.2 methylen-17 alfa-hydroxyprogesterone-acetate. Symposum der Deutschen Gesellschaft fur Endokrinologie, p 301. Springer, Berlin

Rasmussen H 1974 Parathyroid hormone, calcitonin and the calciferols. In: Williams R (ed) Textbook of Endocrinology, 5th edn. W B Saunders, Philadelphia

Rayner P H W 1981 Early Puberty. In: Brook G D (ed) Clinical Paediatric Endocrinology, Ch. 13, p. 224. Blackwell Scientific Publications, Oxford

Schmidt E, Hallevorden J, Spatz H 1958 Die Entstehung der Hamartome am Hypothalamus mit und ohne Pubertas praecox. Deutsche Zeitschrift fur Nervenheilkunde 177: 235

Seckel H P G 1946 Precocious sexual development in children. Medical Clinics of North America 30: 183

Sedeghi-Nejad A, Kaplan S L, Grumbach M M 1971 The effect of medroxyprogesterone acetate on adrenocortical function in children with precocious puberty. Journal of Pediatrics 78: 616

Sherwin R P, Grassi J E, Sommers S C 1962 Hamartomatous malformation of the posterolateral hypothalamus. Laboratory Investigation 11: 89

Sizonenko P C 1978 Delayed Puberty: Adrenal: IV International Symposium on Pediatric and Adolescent Gynaecology, Florence, p 35

Werder A, Murset G, Zachmann M et al 1974 Treatment of precocious puberty with Cyproterone acetate. Pediatric Research 8: 248

Polycystic ovarian disease

HISTORICAL BACKGROUND

Sclerocystic changes in the human ovary were clearly described by Chereau in 1845, and wedge resection of such ovaries was being practiced in Europe before 1897 by Gusserow, Martin, Wiedow, Zweifel, and others. In the United States, Findley described wedge resection for 'cystic degeneration' of the ovary as early as 1904. Occasional reports continued to appear over the years. In 1935 this gross anatomical abnormality was related by Stein & Leventhal to a clinical syndrome consisting of 'menstrual irregularity featuring amenorrhea, a history of sterility, masculine type hirsutism, and less consistently, retarded breast development and obesity.' The delineation of a putative syndrome and especially the report of benefits produced by wedge resection made polycystic ovarian disease (PCOD) a happy hunting ground for theorists, whose speculations were not encumbered by too many facts, and for surgeons, who were understandably delighted with a disorder that responded to a straightforward operative approach.

In the last two decades, clinical re-evaluation of PCOD and evolution of our knowledge of hypothalamic-pituitary-ovarian relationships have shed new light on this fascinating disorder.

GENETIC ASPECTS

Early anecdotal reports of abnormal karyotypes in patients with polycystic ovarian disease were not confirmed by subsequent studies. However, one investigation using the newer banding techniques (Parker et al, 1980) found 5 of 15 patients to have pseudodiploidy with trisomy 14 present in 2–4 per cent of the cells — a high incidence which is extremely rare in the general population.

Several investigators (Cooper et al, 1968; Givens et al, 1971; McDonough et al, 1972) have observed familial patterns. In one study of 18 families (Cooper et al, 1968) the findings were compatible with autosomal dominant transmission. However, X-linked transmission cannot be ruled out (Givens et al, 1971). The variety of operative findings — ranging from a small cystic ovary on one side with a streak ovary on the other to Turner phenotypes with polycystic ovaries, or to mosaicism such as 46, XX/45, X or 46, XX/46, XXq — are consistent with the variability of X-linked disorders in general. It is perhaps relevant that the nymphomaniac cow syndrome is X-linked, and that a relationship between faulty X-chromosomes and increased follicular atresia is well established.

Twins with polycystic ovaries and a normal sibling have been reported. (McDonough et al, 1977) All three had elevated urinary pregnanetriol levels. In two families characterised by women who had polycystic ovarian disease, three of the men had low testosterone values and high LH/FSH ratios (Givens et al, 1971).

The relationship of 3β-ol-dehydrogenase deficiency in some patients with PCOD (Axelrod et al, 1965; Lorber et al, 1978) to the wider spectrum of individuals with this enzyme deficiency remains to be clarified.

ANATOMICAL PATHOLOGY

At first, some gynaecologists believed the gross and microscopic appearance of the polycystic ovary of adult women to be unique and characteristic. Enlarged pearly-white sclerosed gonads with numerous subcapsular cysts identified the condition. However, polycystic ovaries are found with high frequency in other situations. They were noted in fetuses, infants and children by pathologists of the nineteenth century. In 1963, Merrill observed that the highest incidence in children was at the age of 2, when 80 per cent of ovaries had gross cysts, and half showed luteinisation and thecal hyperplasia. The latter findings were even more common in prepubertal and adolescent ovaries. While hyperplastic and/or atretic changes of the follicles are not unexpected in the menarcheal years with their immature pattern of gonadotrophin secretion, the findings in infants and children (excluding neonates in whom maternal gonadotrophins can be expected to have residual effects) are surprising and still unexplained. According to Merrill, the ovaries of girls aged 10 to 15 'demonstrated all of the morphological features described as characteristic of the polycystic ovary syndrome,' and ten of 15 such ovaries even showed cortical fibrosis. From a morphological point, therefore, it may be exceedingly difficult to distinguish an adolescent ovary which will eventually produce the symptomatology of polycystic ovarian disease from one which will not. While the origin of PCOD is evidently difficult to study prospectively, it is not clear why so little retrospective work has been done to delineate early signs and symptoms which might given an insight into the evolution of this disorder.

The morphological appearance of adult ovaries in 'classical' polycystic ovarian disease was accepted by Morris & Scully (1958) as consisting of bilateral enlargement and a thickening of the tunica albuginia. Although primary and secondary follicles are present in normal number, the ovarian cortex is filled with subcapsular follicular cysts representing antral follicles at different stages of atresia.

In 1960, Roberts & Haines described a variety of histological patterns in 'Stein-Leventhal' patients leading them to question the existence of a single syndrome. The gross morphological heterogeneity of polycystic ovaries was also appreciated by Smith et al (1965) who reported normal appearing ovaries in 40 per cent of their patients with PCO syndrome, and no thickening of the tunica in 46 per cent of those who did manifest gross ovarian enlargement. The existence of unilateral polycystic ovaries in patients presenting with a clinical course consistent with PCOD has also been documented. (Delahunt et al, 1975). More recently, Govan & Black (1981) reported on 40 patients with primary oligomenorrhea, most of whom were obese and hirsute. Tissue was collected for evaluation through wedge resection (in ten patients) or ovarian biopsy. Uniformly, the ovaries were bilaterally enlarged, showed a smooth, white cut surface and numerous subcapsular cystic follicles ranging from 6 to 10 mm in diameter. This is striking, since the normal follicle expands up to 20–25 mm in diameter prior to ovulation. The surface epithelium of the ovary is typically 3–4 cells thick. In contrast, the surface of the polycystic ovary is hypertrophic, containing multiple fibrous bands throughout the cortex running parallel to the ovarian surface. Primordial follicles embedded in this fibrous stroma showed evidence of oocyte degeneration (pycnosis and reduced cytoplasmic/nuclear ratios). In addition to the general cortical fibrosis, there was also fibrous replacement of the ovarian stroma with a corresponding reduction in normal stromal tissue. Thus, there appears to be an inverse correlation between the degree of cortical fibrous tissue and the number of normal-appearing follicles. (Govan & Black, 1981) A comparison of 45 polycystic and normal ovaries by electron microscopy revealed the capsular thickening to be ordinary fibroplasia with collagen fibrils forming the microarchitecture. (Green & Goldzieher, 1965) Although the pre-ovulatory follicle in a normal ovary is surrounded by multiple layers of theca cells, thecal hyperplasia occurs in the majority of follicles in PCO patients. Since the cell membrane of theca cells has abundant LH receptors, the elevated serum LH concentrations (Berger et al, 1975; DeVane et al, 1975; Rebar et al, 1976) commonly found in PCO patients may be directly related to the elevated peripheral steroid concentrations. Evidence for this was provided by Erickson et al, (1979) who found that theca tissue explanted from polycystic ovaries preferentially secretes androstenedione in response to LH stimulation. On the other hand, Wilson et al (1979) reported that theca cells either from polycystic or normal ovaries show a similar capacity to secrete androgens. McNatty et al (1980) evaluated thecal tissue derived from a 15-year-old girl with hyperandrogenism, probably resulting from a PCO-like syndrome, and found that it secreted more androgen on a per unit mass basis than theca removed from either healthy or atretic follicles in patients with normal ovaries. Thecal tissues from hyperandrogenic ovaries produced 2–5 times more androstenedione than normal ovaries and four times as much testosterone as was produced in vitro by normal thecal tissue.

Govan & Black (1981) noted premature luteinisation of the granulosa cells of PCO follicles. Further, these granulosa-luteal cells showed many pycnotic changes, suggesting disruption of cell growth and maturation. The cells were vacuolated and positive to histochemical stains for lipids. Stains were also positive for lipid globules of various sizes in the PCO follicles. In addition, histochemical staining for 3β-ol-dehydrogenase was found to be positive in most PCO follicles, suggesting active steroidogenesis. Another feature typical of PCO is the increased prevalence of Call-Exner bodies within the follicle complex. Although these androgen formations are found in the follicles of pregnant women, they are scarce during normal folliculogenesis. Thus, although cystic follicles are found throughout the polycystic ovary, there is, in general, a limitation of follicular growth manifested primarily by a decrease in granulosa cell proliferation and by early luteinisation. The decreased number of follicles at various stages of growth and atresia, together with hypertrophy and hyperplasia of the epithelial components, suggest the picture of an organ undergoing chronic stimulation.

Although the general appearance of the polycystic ovary is that of a disrupted state of folliculogenesis, this is not always the case. Corpora lutea are found in 20 per cent of polycystic ovaries (Goldzieher & Axelrod, 1963). Although Baird et al (1977) found evidence of ovulation as suggested by a significant rise in serum progesterone levels, most morphological descriptions of PCO report a smooth cortical surface lacking the usual ovulatory stigma. When taken together, these observations suggest that, whereas gener-

Table 20.1 Steroids in human follicular fluid

Follicles	Oestradiol	Progesterone	17-OH Prog	DHEA	Androstenedione
Follicular phase of cycle					
Early follicular phase	38–440	66–130	—	—	50–113
Mid-follicular phase 8 mm diam.	1100–2600	250	—	—	320–745
8 mm diam.	200	100	—	—	
Late follicular phase 8 mm diam.	1800–2400	1300	—	—	120–676
8 mm diam.	300	250	—	—	
Polycystic ovarian syndrome	20	70–130	20–390	—	25–1960
Pre-ovulatory phase of cycle					
Ovulatory	616–3700	7000–18 000	1100–6300	2–7	21–107
Non-ovulatory	9–98	3–227	27–714	60–388	213–2169

alised luteinization may occur, evidence of corpus luteum formation and follicular rupture is uncommon in polycystic ovaries.

Short & London in 1961 determined the steroid content of follicular fluid in polycystic ovaries and found high concentrations of androstenedione, whereas the level of oestradiol corresponded to that of normal midfollicular phase ovaries (Table 20.1). An analysis of steroid hormone concentrations in cyst fluid from polycystic ovaries indicates that cystic fluid is rich in androgen, especially androstenedione and testosterone, while containing little oestrogen or progesterone. In some cysts, there is an excess of 17-hydroxyprogesterone and dehydroepiandrosterone, but little oestrogen, progesterone, or androstenedione. (Edwards, 1980). The typical patterns of polycystic ovarian syndrome suggest difficulty in the conversion of androgens to oestrogens or more rarely, conversion of pregnenolone to progesterone and 17-hydroxyprogesterone. These enzymic conversions require the presence of aromatase and 3β-ol-dehydrogenase, respectively. It has been suggested that cyst fluid steroid concentrations may affect the surrounding gonadal tissue. However, concentrations of androgen-binding protein as high as those of plasma have been found in this fluid (Vigersky & Lorlaux 1976) indicating that much of the potential biological activity has been neutralised.

Polycystic changes of a somewhat different type have been observed in various forms of adrenocortical hyperfunction (Kim et al, 1979). The gross ovarian changes associated with corticosteroid overproduction, as in Cushing's syndrome, differ from those of the classic sclerocystic ovary, since the ovaries in Cushing's syndrome are generally of normal or subnormal size, capsular fibrosis is patchy and variable, and subcortical cysts are rare. Theca cell hyperplasia or luteinisation have not been observed. Furthermore, the number of primordial follicles appears to be diminished rather than increased.

Sclerocystic ovarian changes are also seen in congenital adrenal hyperplasia. This is not unexpected, since increased gonadrotrophin output (in some way related to intense pituitary ACTH secretion) has been found in such cases (Stevens & Goldzieher, 1968).

Polycystic ovarian changes have been reported in association with adrenocortical or ovarian tumours. (Givens et al, 1975; Babaknia et al, 1976) In fact, ovarian tumours of all types are reported to occur in association with polycystic ovarian disease with a frequency ranging from 4.6 per cent to 20 per cent. (Babaknia et al, 1976). This is a strong argument for laparoscopic visualisation of suspected PCOD, especially if ultrasonography indicates ovarian enlargement. Involvement of the stroma, especially that of the medullary region of the ovary, is unequivocal. Although gross histological changes such as stromal hyperplasia and luteinisation are not found consistently, the steroidogenic potential of the stroma (particularly with respect to androgen biosynthesis) has been demonstrated conclusively by *in vitro* techniques. It is currently a matter of debate whether ovarian hyperthecosis and PCOD are separate entities or merely different manifestations of the same disorder. Certainly, many of the clinical and morphological festures are similar (Givens et al, 1971; Aiman et al, 1978). There has even been reported a case of bilateral PCOD with unilateral hyperthecosis (Farber et al, 1978) where the latter was shown, by venous catheterisation, to be the chief source of testosterone and androstenedione. Stroma from hyperandrogenic ovaries produced 49 to 150 times more testosterone per unit mass *in vitro* than the stroma from normal ovaries (McNatty et al, 1980). Since the entire stromal mass exceeds the total mass of thecal tissue by 5000-fold in a normal patient, it seems probable that the stromal compartment of hyperandrogenic ovaries is a major source of the androgens found the follicle as well as in peripheral blood. It is difficult, then, to determine the source of androgens in PCO patients since both antral follicles and stromal tissue contain cells capable of androgen secretion in response to LH stimulation.

The analogies which may be drawn between the stromal cells of the human ovary (Mossman et al, 1964) and the 'interstitial gland' of animal ovaries provide fertile ground for speculation. One unconfirmed study (Nebel et al, 1971) described 'coelomic mesotheliumlike cells' in the stroma of polycystic ovaries and suggested that these cells might possess a primordium in common with adrenocortical cells, thus accounting for ovarian adrenocortical-like activities such as ll-hydroxylation. It is well known that the ovaries of certain rodents, such as the 13-lined ground squirrel, possess the capability of taking on adrenocortical functions. Relevant to this question is a slide shown to us by Dr John Woodruff of Johns Hopkins University School of Medicine in which a perfect mini-adrenal with all three zones intact was embedded within human ovarian stroma. It is apparently not a unique finding (Symonds & Driscoll, 1973).

SYMPTOMATOLOGY

Searching for patients with sclerocystic ovaries on the basis of infertility, amenorrhoea, and hirsutism artificially predetermines the symptomatology associated with the anatomical changes. It is essential to study the prevalence of polycystic ovaries under other circumstances. In one series of 12 160 unselected gynaecological laporatomies, (Vara & Niemineva, 1951) a 1.4 per cent frequency of polycystic ovaries was observed. In large groups of infertile women, prevalences of 0.6 per cent to 4.3 per cent have been noted (Breteche, 1952; McGoogan, 1954). In 740 consecutive autopsies (including an unspecified number of children and old women), bilateral polycystic ovaries were found in 3.5 per cent (Sommers & Wadman, 1956). Evidently the gross anatomical lesion is fairly common. Widespread use of the laparoscope will undoubtedly change our perceptions still further. Clearly, the archaic 'syndrome' of Stein and Leventhal identified only a small and empirically selected fraction of the much larger population of patients who actually have polycystic ovarian disease. Adherence to this set of clinical criteria deprived many women of the benefit of appropriate medical or surgical therapy.

Since the gross anatomical lesion of sclerocystic ovarian disease is relatively common, it is necessary to re-examine the frequency of relevant signs and symptoms in the inherently biased set of patients who have been surgically explored. In 1962 a comprehensive review of published cases of surgically proven polycystic disease (Goldzieher & Green, 1962) found the frequencies for the major clinical features as summarized in Table 20.2 Amenorrhoea was present in only about 50 per cent of cases, infertility in 74 per cent, hirsutism in 69 per cent, and obesity in 41 per cent. In some recent series (Yen et al, 1976) the incidence of obesity prior to menarche has been as high as 90 per cent. In contrast to the usual clinical impression, cyclic menses occurred in 12 per cent and evidence of ovulation (such as dysmenorrhoea, biphasic basal body temperature curves, or visualisation of a corpus luteum) in nearly one-quarter of the patients. Thus, the allegedly characteristic signs and symptoms are not found with sufficient consistency to justify the designation of a syndrome. Similar conclusions have been reported by others: Netter et al (1961) remarked with Gallic hyperbole that this was 'a

Table 20.2 Symptomatology associated with surgically proven cases of PCOD. Summary of findings in 1079 cases published in 187 references

Symptom	Usable no. of cases	Incidence Mean (%)	Incidence Range (%)
Obesity	600	41	16–49
Hirsutism	819	69	17–83
Virilisation	431	21	0–28
Cyclic menses	395	12	7–28
Functional bleeding	547	29	6–25
Amenorrhea	640	51	15–77
Dysmenorrhea	75	23	—
Biphasic basal body temperature	238	15	12–40
Corpus luteum at operation	391	22	0–71
Infertility	596	74	35–94

(From: Goldzieher J W: Polycystic ovarian Disease. Fertility Sterility 35: 371 1981. Reproduced with the permission of the publisher, The American Fertility Society)

fugitive syndrome with limits less well defined than those of the Sahara or Sudan.'

Very little is known of the true frequency of symptoms associated with polycystic ovarian disease. Certain recognised symptoms, such as the post-menarcheal onset of oligo-amenorrhoea, hirsutism, and infertility, suggest to the gynaecologist the possibility of this disorder; the frequency of these symptoms will have a positive bias, since more patients with PCOD with these symptoms will be identified than patients with the disorder but without these symptoms. A modern retrospective study of the symptomatology of *all* patients in whom laparotomies (for whatever reason) reveal these gross anatomical changes in the ovary is clearly needed. The possibility of PCOD should be kept in mind in all cases of anovulation and even of persistent menstrual disturbances which appear at or shortly after menarche.

The detection of enlarged ovaries by palpation or ultrasonography is not essential to the diagnosis. Cases with ovaries of normal size or even unilateral (Vejlsted & Albrechtsen, 1976) enlargement are known. There is even a case of bilateral PCOD with unilateral hyperthecosis (Farber et al, 1981). A study of 301 patients with PCOD (Smith et al, 1965) found 68 patients who had a thickened ovarian tunica albuginea and clinical symptoms including hirsutism, menstrual disturbances, and obesity; 45 had enlarged ovaries and 23 had normal-sized ovaries. The symptomatology and clinical response to therapy of the two groups were indistinguishable. In 59 patients with a normal (i.e. non-sclerotic) tunica albuginea, there was again no difference in symptomatology or clinical response between those with enlarged ovaries and those with normalised ovaries. Interestingly, however, hirsutism was almost always absent in patients with a normal tunica, a fact consistent with the concept that ovarian sclerosis is related to excessive (local) androgen levels.

Another group of investigators (Raj et al, 1977) came to different conclusions. They separated their cases into those in whom ovary enlargement was relatively small (i.e. less than twice normal size) and those in whom the enlargement was greater. Of their 100 cases, 67 fell into the former group, but this picture is somewhat clouded by the fact that 19 of the patients had undergone wedge resection prior to these studies. It is also difficult to ascertain whether the claim of an association of normal plasma LH levels with relatively small ovaries was supported by a later compendium (Raj et al, 1978). In any event, the larger ovaries were reported to be associated with significantly less hirsutism (82 per cent versus 100 per cent), although there was no difference in testosterone levels; with more infertility (64 per cent versus 35 per cent); and with fewer elevated levels of urinary 17-ketosteroids; and a substantially better response to clomiphene in terms of ovulation (91 per cent versus 75 per cent) and conception (51 per cent versus 25 per cent). The small ovary group was thought to have predominantly adrenal hyperandrogenism and was treated accordingly. Other investigators (Givens et al, 1976; Valkov & Dokumov 1977; Rebar et al, 1978). Have failed to find any relation between ovarian size and plasma LH level. Indeed, LH values are very variable (see below), and many studies have failed to obtain a sufficient number of samples over a sufficient period of time to make a valid assessment of the prevailing level. Hyperprolactinaemia is not uncommon in PCOD (Futterweit & Krieger, 1979; Falaschi et al, 1980; Shapiro, 1981). In one series of 12 patients with PCOD (Jaffee et al, 1978) five had abnormally elevated serum prolactin levels without galactorrhoea. Basal and stimulated levels of steroid and pituitary hormones were no different from those of normoprolactinemic women, and none of them had abnormal tomograms. However, another study showed that 12 of 13 patients with elevated prolactin also had elevated LH/FSH ratios whereas only six of 12 normoprolactinemic PCOD cases showed this feature. Those with an elevated LH/FSH ratio (whether eu- or hyper-prolactinaemic) were hyper-responders to a TRH test (Corenblum & Taylor, 1982). In another series, (Wortsman & Hirschowitz 1980) six of 21 patients with PCOD were reported to have hyperprolactinaemia with or without galactorrhoea; three had abnormal sellas. In three other PCOD patients with abnormal sellas (Futterweit & Krieger, 1979) the usual endocrine disorders were absent: testosterone and LH levels were not elevated, there was no withdrawal bleeding after progesterone administration, and both clomiphene and wedge resection failed to restore cyclic ovulatory function even after surgical removal of a pituitary adenoma in two instances.

Since 1974 a number of patients with acanthosis nigricans, marked insulin resistance due to alteration in insulin-receptor interaction, virilism and polycystic ovaries (either enlarged or normal-sized) have been reported. Most of the women have been Negro, and were relatively free of

episodes of ketoacidosis; moreover, the glucose intolerance had a remarkable tendency to remit (Kahn et al, 1976). In one instance (Cole & Kitabchi 1978) insulin resistance was reversed with a combination type oral contraceptive. In another case of PCOD with galactorrhoea, pituitary microsurgery was followed by normalisation of glucose tolerance in the absence of any weight changes (Shapiro, 1981). A comparison of eight patients with PCOD and six obese control subjects (Borghen et al, 1980) showed a significant correlation between basal plasma insulin and androgen (testosterone, androstenedione) levels. There was also a positive correlation between the increased insulin response to an oral glucose load and the plasma testosterone level in the PCOD group. There was no elevation of growth hormone and no difference in plasma cortisol level to account for the difference between the two groups. Moreover, the insulin resistance in PCOD does not appear to be related to the obesity itself (Kaplan et al, 1982). This is a new and as yet unexplored aspect of polycystic ovarian disease.

LABORATORY EVALUATION

Endocrine studies of PCOD serve three purposes: (1) to differentiate women with oligomenorrhoea, with or without hirsutism, into various aetiologic and therapeutic categories; (2) to establish the endocrine pathogenesis of the disorder in a particular individual or in a particular group of subjects selected for study; and (3) to test for the existence of occult neoplasms in women with hirsutism.

The most direct approach is catheterisation of the ovarian and adrenal venous drainage (Kirschner & Jacobs 1972; Wajchenberg et al, 1981). This technology has provided fundamental information (Fig. 20.1a & b), and has confirmed the major role of androstenedione and testosterone overproduction by the ovary, together with additional overproduction by the adrenal in a substantial minority of cases. Laatikainen et al (1980) found ovarian venous oestradiol levels similar to the normal follicular phase; theca cell hyperplasia correlated best with elevated ovarian vein androgens. There are hazards as well as inaccuracies associated with this procedure (Wentz et al, 1976). There is a 5 per cent or greater complication rate in adrenal vein catheterisations, including occasional haemorrhagic destruction or infarction of the adrenal. In any event, the hazards of the procedure — at least in some hands — raise questions about its justification in benign conditions such as PCOD. On another level, there is an inherent error due to the complex and diffuse venous drainage of the adrenal, and an analogous problem with the ovarian circulation. Calculations of total ovarian or adrenal steroid secretion on the basis of such sampling are subject to large errors, particularly in the case of the adrenal, which additionally is operating under stress, and secretes

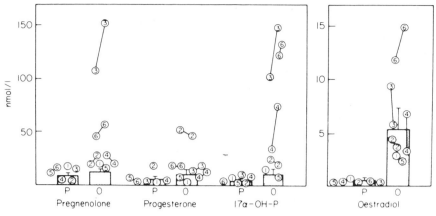

Fig. 20.1a Peripheral (P) and ovarian (O) venous plasma levels of androgens in patients with polycystic ovaries

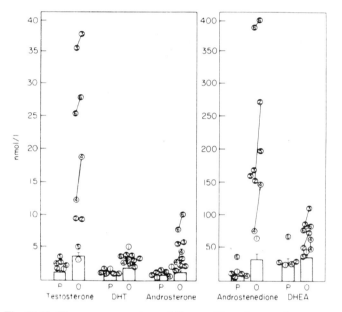

Fig. 20.1b Plasma concentrations of C_{21} steroids and oestradiol, as in Fig. 20.1a (reprinted with permission from Laatikainen et al, 1980)

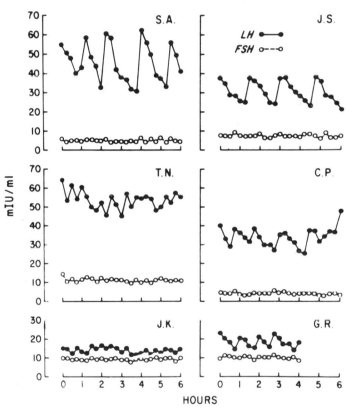

Fig. 20.2 Representative patterns of plasma gonadotropins in PCOD. Note absence of FSH pulsations in contrast to LH (reprinted with permission from Rebar et al, 1976)

in an episodic manner. Catheterisation is a valuable investigative tool when used with judgement in skilled hands. It may still have a place among the methods used to localise a suspected neoplasm although it is hardly a casually recommended diagnostic procedure, especially since computerised axial tomographic scanning and ultrasonography have added a new dimension to tumour localisation.

At one time it was believed that precise, sensitive, specific radioimmunoassays to measure steroid and protein hormones would quickly elucidate the endocrine mechanisms in PCOD. In fact, the answers continue to be elusive and interpretation of the data is far more difficult than was anticipated. For example, there has been a good deal of difference in reports of the LH/FSH levels in PCOD. Most investigators have reported exaggerated pulsations and/or persistently high LH levels and relatively or absolutely reduced levels of FSH, resulting in an elevated LH/FSH ratio (Fig. 20.2). Others (Berger et al, 1975; Vejlsted &

Albrechtsen, 1976) have classified cases of PCOD into those with elevated or with normal levels of LH. Some of this confusion undoubtedly originates in the fact that the hormones were measured in the plasma once daily or less often. However, plasma concentrations of LH and FSH as well as gonadal steroid hormones such as testosterone oscillate in cycles ranging from a few minutes to 1 hour or more. The amplitude of these oscillations is substantial, and a sample taken at a zenith or a nadir by random chance might suggest entirely different views of the disorder. The importance of multiple sampling for obtaining meaningful estimates of prevailing ('average') plasma levels cannot be overemphasised. A mathematical analysis of testosterone, FSH, and LH oscillations in men (Goldzieher et al, 1976) suggested that three blood samples, taken at 15–20 min intervals for steroids or at 60 min intervals for gonadotrophins and *averaged by pooling the blood samples in one test tube*, yields a more reliable average value than do single or dual samples. This simple and cost-effective modification is helpful for studies of gonadotrophins and androgens; one may also use radioimmunoassay of *urinary* FSH and LH, since the integrated output represented by the first morning urine sample, calculated per gram of creatinine, correlates well with the 24 hour output. The problem of the pulsation of corticoid hormones is also solved by the use of urinary 17-hydroxycorticosteroid measurement expressed as milligrams *per gram of creatinine*. Rapid multiple sampling does not, of course, take into account slow diurnal rhythms or the rhythms associated with the menstrual cycle itself. Another technical point also merits discussion: the notion of determining hormonal changes in a normal cycle and using these as a 'control' for subsequent manipulations or observations. Although the literature abounds with beautiful illustrations of steroid and gonadotropic rhythms in a 'normal cycle' based on averaging numbers of cycles, these illustrations often bear little resemblance to the events in a single cycle. There is considerable variability between cycles in the same individual and ten-fold variability in the hormonal levels of cycles between different individuals (Johansson et al, 1971).

The measurement of plasma androgens and their correlation with clinical hirsutism (Deutsch et al, 1978) is a complex subject. The blood production rate of testosterone correlates well with hirsutism, but it is not a procedure suitable for routine diagnostic use. The inadequate correlation of *total* plasma testosterone with hirsutism is explained only in part by the inadequacy of conventional sampling techniques. Another factor is the level of non-protein-bound (i.e. biologically active) testosterone, which is influenced by the concentration of sex hormone-binding globulin. This substance itself is subject to diminished synthesis under the influence of androgens (Duignam et al, 1975) or certain synthetic progestins and therefore acts as an internal feedback loop augmenting the potency of a given level of plasma testosterone. Earlier methods for measurement of free testosterone were cumbersome (e.g. equilibrium dialysis), but it has been demonstrated that the testosterone concentration in saliva correlates highly with unbound plasma testosterone and therefore provides a most convenient index (Smith et al, 1979b). Additionally, the ratio of plasma testosterone to SHBG concentration has been found to have a better correlation with hirsutism than the level of T alone (Mathur et al, 1981).

Measurement of androstenedione is probably just as important as the measurement of testosterone (Deutsch et al, 1978) and important pathophysiological insights are often gained when androstenedione levels are altered by diagnostic or therapeutic procedures. Although dihydrotestosterone is biologically the most active androgen and probably the one that interacts with cutaneous androgen receptors, measurement of this steroid has not added much of clinical utility. Some investigators measure a group of biologically active 17β-hydroxy C_{19} steroids as a more comprehensive index of androgenic exposure. The role of DHEA sulfate measurement is discussed on page 413. Recently, the 3α, 17β,-diol glucuronide metabolite of androstenedione has been reported to be a reliable marker of 'androgenicity' in the peripheral blood of hirsute patients (apparently none of them with PCOD) (Horton et al, 1982).

Similar technical questions arise with regard to the relative merits of measuring oestradiol and oestrone individually or as 'total oestrogen.' In special investigations of the steroid pathophysiology of PCOD this dual measurement may be valuable, but for clinical purposes it is probably superfluous. The problem of protein-bound versus free oestrogen may also have to be considered. These issues have important biological implications but a critical evaluation in a well-designed clinical setting has yet to be carried out.

The steroids of interest in polycystic ovarian disease have multiple sources of origin: ovarian, adrenal, and peripheral. Androstenedione entering the blood stream of a normal woman is derived approximately equally from ovaries and adrenals. The peripheral conversion of androstenedione to testosterone normally accounts for one-half to two-thirds of testosterone production; a minor contribution arises from peripheral conversion of dehydroepiandrosterone (DHEA), and the remainder represents ovarian secretion. Peripheral conversion of androstenedione to oestrone also accounts for the relatively normal or occasionally elevated plasma levels of this steroid. Since androstenedione production may be increased five-fold or more in PCOD, even a normal rate of conversion (approximately 1 per cent) may yield 150 to 200 µg of oestrone. This partly explains the old paradox of a hypothesised defect in ovarian aromatisation in the face of normal plasma oestrogen levels. It is evident that the prevailing plasma levels or rate of urinary metabolite excretion rarely pinpoint the site of abnormal secretory activity (except in the case of DHEA sulphate), nor do they mirror the concentration at a site of action — e.g. the ovarian follicle. As a consequence, various manoeuvres have been developed to suppress or stimulate one or the other hormone source and to infer from the results something about the pathogenesis of the disorder. We and others (Farber et al, 1978) have repeatedly pointed out the inherent fallacies in these procedures.

It is a general clinical impression that the one-third of hirsute women who are eumenorrhoeic (Abraham et al, 1976) are likely to have hyperandrogenism primarily of adrenal origin, whereas the two-thirds who are oligo-amenorrhoeic (such as patients with PCOD) are likely to have an ovarian source of androgens with or without an added adrenal component. Plasma steroid measurements discriminate these two groups of women less successfully than one would expect. The 17-hydroxyprogesterone level was found to be elevated in 90 per cent of the women in both groups, and responded equally to stimulation with chorionic gonadotrophin (hCG) or suppression with dexamethasone (DXM). DHEA levels and responses were similar; the frequency of elevated testosterone and androstenedione levels was the same, as was the response to hCG; only the suppressibility with DXM was less in the oligo-amenorrhoeic group. Paradoxically, suppressibility of DHEA sulphate, a steroid essentially of adrenal origin, was less in the oligo-amenorrhoeic women than in the eumenorrhoeic subjects (Abraham et al, 1975). Hirsute oligo-menorrhoeic women with laparoscopically normal ovaries may respond to hCG or DXM as expected of PCOD rather than like adrenal hyperplasias (Lisse et al, 1980). Nevertheless, some investigators maintain confidence in tests using prolonged suppression with corticosteroids (with and without stimulation with hCG) and suppression with oestrogens or contraceptive steroid combinations.

Let us first examine DXM suppression, which presumes to alter adrenal function without affecting ovarian dynamics. One investigator (Abraham et al, 1976) has progressively recommended longer and longer treatment to increase the merits of this procedure. By contrast, Steinberger et al (1982) have studied the prognostic value of the effect of a 1 mg dose of DXM given at midnight on the next morning plasma testosterone in a group of 106 consecutive hirsute patients. Higher LH/FSH ratios were found in the group that did not respond with a normal (27–33 per cent) fall in plasma testosterone. This group also did not show as good a response to chronic prednisone therapy as the other hirsute subjects, although exceptions were observed. In patients with PCOD sudivided into those with normal sized or enlarged ovaries, the effect of DXM was the same except for somewhat lesser suppression of plasma testosterone, androstenedione, and 17-hydroxyprogesterone in the latter group (Lachelin et al, 1979). Others have shown that DXM suppresses urinary and plasma levels of LH as well as FSH, androstenedione, and testosterone in patients with elevated plasma LH levels. However, in subjects with normal levels of LH, DXM *increased* LH, androstenedione and testosterone, and *decreased* FSH (Givens et al 1975).

There is considerable evidence that DXM has effects other than those on the adrenal. The follicular phase is lengthened in normal women given DXM even though no changes in oestrogens or LH are observed. Goldzieher et al have shown in rats, baboons, and humans that corticosteroids affect gonadotrophins and are even able to inhibit the LH surge in the face of a rapidly rising plasma oestrogen level (Cunningham et al, 1978). The most direct evidence stems from ovarian vein catheterisation, with which it has been shown that the administration of DXM decreased ovarian vein androgens (Kirschner & Jacobs 1971; Wajchenberg et al 1981). Thus, although DXM suppression may be of value in discriminating ready suppression from resistance to suppression (with the careful inferences that have been drawn by Steinberger et al (1982) from such data), it cannot be regarded as a maneuver uniquely measuring an index of adrenal cortical function.

Metopyrone, a drug which indirectly stimulates adrenal activity via the hypothalamus and is therefore a test of this system, has its own disadvantages. The administration of metopyrone increases plasma oestradiol and LH when given during the follicular phase of normal cycles. (Givens et al, 1976a) Moreover, this compound is known to block part of the aromatising system (19-hydroxylation) in the hamster adrenal; whether it affects human ovarian enzymes similarly is not known. Thus this agent, too, is not without gonadal impact.

Stimulation of the adrenal with ACTH, usually in large doses, has been carried out in attempts to assess the adrenal androgen contribution. There are several assumptions involved which must be examined. Recent studies showing that there is synchrony of the episodic secretion of adrenal steroids such as cortisol and DHEA have tended to imply that *all* adrenal secretory products are under parallel and equivalent control. That this is not the case was pointed out by Gallagher and others decades ago; it also is evident in Cushing's syndrome without masculinisation, in adrenal hyperplasia producing virilism without glucocorticoid effects, and in adrenal hypertension and virilisation with minimal impairment of corticoid dynamics. Episodic adrenal secretion does not tell the whole story; in fact, it neglects the level of the tonic stimulus, which may be altered without being detected by customary methods for measuring ACTH. There are, in fact, animal studies which suggest that continuous low-level ACTH stimulation can produce qualitative changes in the mix of secreted adrenal hormones. Studies of cell cultures from normal and polycystic ovaries (Wilson et al, 1979) have recently suggested that ACTH may exert a stimulatory effect on theca cells. Finally, ACTH administration affects LH levels (Givens et al, 1976b). It is evident, therefore, that interactions between the gonadotrophic and corticotrophic regulatory systems exist, and this raises problems of interpretation in terms of adrenal versus ovarian origin of the observed changes.

The use of drugs which suppress ovarian function presents similar problems. Contraceptive steroids are known to decrease adrenal activity, and plasma androgens are diminished in the long-term in ovariectomised women given these agents. The effects of oestrogens on the adrenal cortex have been documented in a long series of animal experiments (for citations see Goldzieher, 1968). Suppression of gonadotrophin secretion by long-acting GnRH agonists is a promising approach to achieving a reversible 'medical oophorectomy' (Chang et al, 1982).

Ovarian stimulatory procedures meet similar obstacles: clomiphene has adrenal effects (Givens et al, 1976b), the use of hCG is not without its problems, and the response of the ovary to manipulation of the pituitary by GnRH is extremely complex. Since 1945, when Reifenstein and his colleagues suggested that hCG influences the adrenal, there have been scattered reports of various circumstances in which this phenomenon was presumed to occur (Goldzieher, 1968; Koritnik et al, 1980) entirely aside from clear-cut cases of adrenal neoplasms sensitive to hCG stimulation and oestrogen suppression. (It may be pointed out that there are also cases of ACTH-responsive ovarian and testicular tumours (Vasquez et al, 1982) Indeed, by 1975 some investigators (Abraham et al, 1975) concluded that the hCG test was of no value, as similar results were obtained in regularly cycling women and in oligomenorrhoeic women with hirsutism.

PATHOPHYSIOLOGY

Hypothalamic-pituitary relationships

Since chronic anovulation and disordered LH/FSH secretion (i.e. an elevated LH/FSH ratio) appear to be fundamental features of PCOD, it is evident that the hypothalamic-pituitary system must play an important role in the pathogenesis of this disorder; indeed, many investigators believe that the nidus of the events which result in PCOD is to be found in this locality.

In attempting to explore the origin of the increased LH/FSH ratio, the prevailing steroid environment is a logical place to begin. Unfortunately, the data are conflicting. The LH level has been found to correlate directly (Mortimer et al, 1978) or inversely (Duignan et al, 1975) with plasma testosterone, or the response of LH to gonadotrophin-releasing hormone (GnRH) has been correlated directly with the testosterone level (Legros et al, 1975). Some investigators have found a correlation of plasma LH with the level of oestradiol (Patson et al, 1975; Katz et al, 1978), unbound oestradiol (Lobo et al, 1981) or oestrone and oestradiol (DeVane et al, 1975), or oestrone but not oestradiol (Kandeel et al, 1978), or not the the oestrogen level at all. Changing oestrogen levels may account for a decrease in LH which was seen when 'pure' FSH was given to clomiphene-resistant subjects (Schoemaker et al, 1978). This question is further complicated by a report (Lobo et al 1982) that the ratio of bioassay to radioimmunoassay values of LH was increased in ten of 18 subjects with PCOD, suggesting qualitative alteration of LH in some cases.

The relationship between suprahypothalamic inputs, the

hypothalamic area which secretes GnRH, and the anterior pituitary is an exceedingly complex one. Quigley et al (1981) studied the response of LH to inhibition by dopamine in eight cases of PCOD and concluded that there was an enhanced sensitivity. However, this may simply have been due to the initially elevated LH levels, for the same kind of enhanced sensitivity is seen at the time of the LH surge. Studies with naloxone, an opioid antagonist, (Blankstein et al, 1982) have been interpreted as uncovering the inhibitory action of an endogenous opiod pathway upon hypothalamic GnRH secretion, an effect perhaps mediated by an interaction with dopamine. In any event, both European and American investigators have observed that opioid antagonists increase the frequency and amplitude of LH pulses (Groffman et al, 1981; Robert et al, 1981). The role of endogenous opioids in the exaggerated pulsatile pattern of LH in PCOD remains to be explored. Givens et al (1980) have observed that obese hyperandrogenic, oligoamenorrhoeic women (two of them with PCOD) had elevated levels of beta endorphin and beta lipotrophin.

The concept of negative and positive feedback loops on hypothalamus and pituitary that are regulated by gonadal steroids has also been further complicated by evidence that compounds other than these classic regulators exists: for example, 'inhibin'-like material in ovarian follicular fluid which suppressed serum FSH levels (Marder et al, 1977) or 'gonadocrinins' from the same source that stimulate gonadotrophin secretion (Ying & Guillemin, 1980). Prolactin (Dorrington & Gore-Longton, 1982), GnRH itself and other 'growth factors' (Mondschein & Schomber, 1981) or other intrafollicular proteins (diZerega et al, 1982) might inhibit local FSH action (Jones & Hsueh, 1982). This domain may well hold surprises which will fundamentally alter our concepts of the hypothalamic-pituitary-gonadal regulatory system. Among the unresolved problems is the apparent ability of the pituitary gonadotrophe to secrete FSH and LH in a non-simultaneous and non-parallel fashion, even though there appears to be only one hypothalamic gonadotrophin-releasing polypeptide. Differential effects produced by progesterone or oestrone (Chang & Jaffe, 1978; Chang et al, 1982) may be one explanation (Resko et al, 1981).

The necessity for the GnRH stimulus to be pulsatile has been well documented. In adult women, LH pulses in the follicular phase of the cycle occur at 1–2 hour intervals; in the luteal phase the frequency may be lower but the amplitude of the pulses is higher. In patients with PCOD the amplitude and/or frequency of LH pulses are substantially increased (Baird et al, 1977; Rebar et al, 1976; Wentz et al, 1976) (see Fig. 20.2), but there is great day-to-day variation in these characteristics as well as in the resulting 'average' level. Of particular interest is the character of the FSH output, which remains in the normal or subnormal range, shows much less pulsation, and does not appear to correlate with LH dynamics. One study with a long-acting analogue of GnRH (Vierhapper et al, 1979) found that the response of LH to GnRH differs in males and females. Women with hyperandrogenic states (adrenal adenoma, congenital adrenal hyperplasia, idiopathic hirsutism) still had the female pattern of response, suggesting that androgen levels *per se* were not responsible for the observed sex difference. When GnRH became available for clinical investigation, it was hoped that this specific pituitary stimulant would answer many questions regarding the role of pituitary versus hypothalamus in a variety of endocrine disorders. Unfortunately, GnRH has been less helpful in differential diagnosis than was expected. In general, the response of plasma LH to a bolus or a brief infusion of GnRH correlates quite well with the basal level of LH; thus the dynamic test often provides little additional information. This has proved to be the case in PCOD. Although some investigators (Zarate et al, 1973; Valkov & Dokumov, 1977) have found the response of LH to GnRH to be similar to that found during the follicular phase of normal women while others (Duignan et al, 1975) have found the FSH response to be similar to that of normal women but the LH response to be very variable, most (Katz & Carr, 1976; Patton et al, 1975; Aono et al, 1979; Vierhapper et al, 1979) found an exaggerated response when basal LH levels were high and a relatively normal response when basal levels were normal. In one study of the biphasic pattern of LH release (Mortimer et al, 1979) the readily releasable 'first pool' of gonadotrophin appeared to be augmented in PCOD.

The response to GnRH has been used to explore the sensitivity and capacity of the gonadotrophin-releasing mechanism in the context of the steroidal environment, especially with respect to prevailing oestrogen and androgen levels. The normal menstrual cycle already illustrates the changing response of the pituitary gonadotrophe to alterations in the oestrogen level. The influence of oestrogen on LH secretion is extremely complex, and is not very well understood. It is at least triphasic: (Hagino & Goldzieher, 1970) very small doses (e.g. 10 μg of ethinyloestradiol orally to a human subject) are stimulatory; larger infused doses such as 10–132 μg of oestradiol/hour (Gual et al, 1975; Rebar et al, 1978) are inhibitory (with a subsequent rebound), and very large doses (such as 20 mg of Premarin intravenously) are stimulatory (Aono et al, 1979). In addition, one must specify whether the response under examination is instantaneous (i.e. minutes), slow (hours), or delayed (days); the response to a single exposure may be quite different from the response to daily administration over days or weeks (Goldzieher et al, 1975) and the oestrogen level antecedent to the experiment may be critical (Rebar et al, 1978). With the variety of protocols that have been used in normals and PCOD (for a review of older studies, see Shaw et al, 1975),it is possible to arrive only at very general inferences. Most investigators have

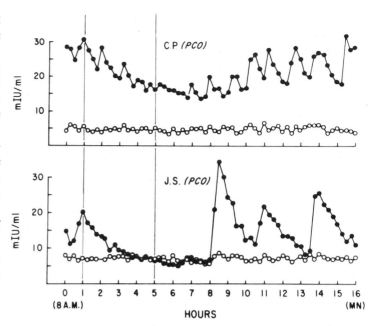

Fig. 20.3 Effect of infusion of oestradiol at 50 μg/h on plasma gonadotropins in PCOD (reprinted with permission from Rebar et al, 1978)

concluded that the immediate negative and positive feedback responses of LH to oestrogenic stimuli in PCOD are comparable to those of normal women (Baird et al, 1977). The results are most convincing when oestrogen stimuli within the physiological range are used (Fig. 20.3). An LH surge subsequent to the administration of 1 mg of oestradiol benzoate was observed in 15 to 19 women with PCOD, and an FSH surge in eight of these 15 — a response somewhat greater than expected. Those who did not respond to this stimulus also did not respond to clomiphene (Shaw et al, 1975). The response to intravenous Premarin was also found to be normal (Aono et al, 1979). On the other hand, one study of the effects of oestradiol benzoate on the response to GnRH yielded unusual results: (Kandeel et al, 1978) PCOD generally showed less augmentation of the GnRH response by oestrogen than did the controls (the opposite conclusion has been reached by other investigators (Rebar et al, 1978)). However, one set of these patients with PCOD had a greater response to GnRH given 92 hours after oestrogen administration than at 44 hours: these women had a good response to clomiphene. In the other women who had higher basal levels of LH at the start, the response to GnRH at 44 hours after oestrogen was greater than that at 92 hours, and these women had a relatively poor response to clomiphene (Kandeel et al, 1978).

Some experiments where a positive feedback response to oestrogen was not found, were performed before there was an appreciation of the role of prolactin and the value of bromocriptine (Aono et al, 1979).

It is well known that oestrogen affects LH and FSH plasma levels differentially. Chang et al (1982) studied FSH and LH in normals given oestrone in the follicular phase and in PCOD subjects injected with this steroid for periods up to 14 days, attaining a level 2–3 times the physiological one. There was no change in gonadotropoins or in response to GnRH in the normals. In PCOD, the LH level and the response to GnRH were also unaffected, but there was a progressive *decline* in FSH. This suggested to them an explanation for the relatively diminished levels of FSH in some cases of PCOD, but supporting clinical evidence was not provided. Studies of pituitary inhibition by high-dose oral contraceptives point to a more profound origin of the abnormal LH/FSH ratio (Givens et al, 1974). There was a curious delay of some days in the response of plasma LH (both in spiking activity and average concentration) to treatment with oral contraceptives, whereas FSH levels tended to decrease promptly. The full effect was reached only after approximately 3 weeks of therapy. A high degree of correlation (r = 0.97) was observed between the changing levels of LH and testosterone or androstenedione. The correlation persisted even after medication was discontinued, which suggests (at least in the seven women studied) that androgen production was under LH control (i.e. presumably ovarian in origin). Rebound of plasma gonadotrophin was immediate, whether after one cycle or after 1 year of therapy; FSH rebounded sooner than LH. In other circumstances it has also been shown that long-term suppression is not progressive and rebound is prompt (Goldzieher et al, 1970). Of particular interest was the observation that the abnormal LH/FSH ratio present before treatment persisted even during suppression of the pituitary by the contraceptive steroids. This observation appears to raise some question about the role of androgens (which were reduced by 60 per cent to 75 per cent in these cases) in the genesis of the disordered LH/FSH ratio.

Progesterone, whose absence in PCOD is given insufficient consideration, has profound effects on the hypothalamic-pituitary system and indirectly also on the effects of oestrogen upon this system. Suprachiasmatic lesions in rats dissociate the response to progesterone administration: the release of LH by progesterone is blocked, whereas the release of FSH is not (Bishop et al, 1972). Since the localisation of gonadotrophin regulation in the rat hypothalamus differs from that in primates (e.g. lesions which interrupt cyclic oestrous activity in rats do not affect cyclicity in rhesus monkeys or baboons), the clinical importance of this observation remains undefined. However, in the late follicular phase of the normal human cycle small increases in plasma progesterone augment the release of LH and probably that of FSH, and modulate the effect of GnRH as well (Chang & Jaffe, 1978). Timing is critically important: if progesterone appears after the increase in the oestrogen level begins, the LH surge is accelerated and an FSH surge is augmented; if the progesterone increase is too early, the gonadotrophin surge is blocked (March et al, 1979). An adequate level of oestrogen is also essential, for in patients with PCOD with low plasma oestradiol levels

an injection of progesterone has no effect, whereas with follicular levels of oestradiol the gonadotrophin surge can be induced by progesterone, to be followed by a luteal phase (Belisle, 1979). The same phenomenon is also found in PCOD: the oestrogen-induced augmentation of the response to GnRH is further augmented by the administration of progesterone (Shaw et al, 1976). It is clear that the absence of progesterone from the steroidal milieu of PCOD is an important factor; however, its exact role in the pathophysiology of the disease, as well as its role in the abnormal LH/FSH ratio, has not been clarified. It is noteworthy that induction of ovulation (by whatever means) in PCOD is often followed by a normalisation of the LH/FSH ratio for some period of time.

Androgens are also known to influence the ovulatory mechanism. In model experiments with rodents (Hagino & Goldzieher, 1975), testosterone has been shown to raise the electrical threshold of the medial preoptic area of the hypothalamus, to decrease the rate of release and synthesis of FSH during the ovulatory surge, and to reduce the storage and the rate of release of LH; there was also some suggestion of direct target-organ (i.e. ovarian) effect. Clinically, a prolongation of the follicular phase and an abbreviation of the luteal phase have correlated with hyperandrogenism and can be reversed by corticosteroid therapy which suppresses the hyperandrogenism (Rodriguez-Rigau et al, 1979; Smith et al 1979). Some investigators have inferred that androgens are important in the pathogenesis of PCOD by inhibiting the response to GnRH; (Duignan et al, 1975); certainly the high correlation between LH and plasma androgen level is an important observation.

The role of corticosteroids in the regulation of gonadotrophin secretion has not been explored intensively. An increase in urinary LH excretion during treatment with corticosteroids was observed several decades ago (for a review see Goldzieher, 1968). An increase in FSH excretion by women with PCOD receiving corticosteroids has been documented (Butt et al, 1963). This latter finding assumes increasing significance in explaining the therapeutic effect of these agents (see below). It is interesting that the administration of metopyrone, which decreases plasma cortisol levels by blocking one or more of the adrenal ll-hydroxylases, is associated with an increase in plasma and urinary LH levels (Givens et al, 1976). The administration of certain synthetic corticosteroids can produce antiovulatory effects (for review see Cunningham et al, 1978) if triamcinolone acetonide is given on the first day of the cycle, an increasing oestrogen level cannot induce the usual gonadotrophin surge. The interaction of prolactin and gonadotrophin secretion is well known, but this subject is beyond the scope of this chapter. However, the common occurrence of hyperprolactinaemia in PCOD indicates that malfunction of this system may be important in certain instances. A hyper-response of prolactin to haloperidol has

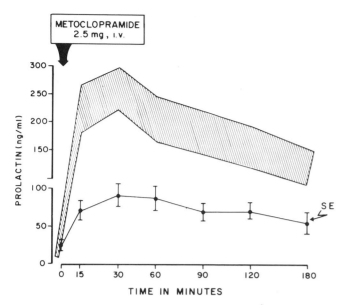

Fig. 20.4 Response of plasma prolactin to an intravenous bolus of metoclopramide in PCOD. The normal response is shown by the hatched area (reprinted with permission from Alger et al, 1980)

been reported in both normo- and hyperprolactinaemic pCOD; whether this is due to elevated oestrogen levels, as Falaschi et al (1980) believe, remains to be demonstrated. Alger et al (1980) have observed a blunted response to an intravenous bolus of metoclopramide in nine patients with PCOD, suggesting that, even with normal prolactin levels, the dopaminergic control of prolactin secretion may be disturbed (Fig. 20.4).

The differential regulation of LH and FSH levels is one of the important and poorly understood areas of gonadotrophin dynamics, and further developments in this field may be critical to an understanding of one of the characteristic (and very possibly, pathogenetic) features of polycystic ovarian disease.

Ovarian steroidogenesis

In the 1960s the steroidogenic activity of the polycystic ovary was examined by studies of the steroid content of ovarian cyst fluid and by *in vitro* incubations of sliced or minced ovarian tissue with radioactive substrates (Axelrod & Goldzieher, 1961, 1962). Both of these approaches indicated a deficiency of aromatisation and as excess production of androgens such as androstenedione. One study (Axelrod et al, 1965) also described a case of deficiency of Δ^5-3β-HSD in ovarian as well as adrenal tissue. These findings precipitated a lively controversy. Some questioned the interpretation of steroid concentrations in cyst fluid, and indeed it was some time before it was demonstrated that leakage of steroids from follicular fluid was extremely slow (Giorgi et al, 1969) and that the data yielded a useful insight into the follicular microenvironment (Kemeter et al, 1979). Others thought that the notion of an aromatase

deficiency had to imply a total genetic defect similar to classic 21-hydroxylase deficiency. Finally, some investigators believed that the excess androgen production resulted from increased tissue mass rather than from malfunction of some cell types. In order to appreciate the recent studies of polycystic ovarian tissue, it is first necessary to examine the function of the normal follicle and stroma up to the stage of the pre-ovulatory oestrogen surge.

While limited data are now available from studies of human follicles, an extensive literature describes studies employing the hypophysectomised immature female rat (HIFR) to elucidate the relative roles of granulosa and theca cells response to LH and FSH stimulation (received in Richards, 1978). According to current theories on the mechanisms of protein hormone action, (Richards & Midgley, 1976) membrane receptors are required for the direct action of gonadotrophic hormones on their respective target cells. In preantral follicles, membrane receptors for LH are located on thecal and other types of interstitial cells outside the lamina basalis, while FSH receptors appear confined to the granulosa cells within the lamina basalis.

Following hypophysectomy, ovaries contain predominantly small preantral follicles. When oestradiol is administered most of these follicles increase in size by granulosa cell proliferation and antrum formation. With oestradiol and FSH stimulation, granulosa cells acquire LH receptors (Zeleznik et al, 1974; Amsterdam et al, 1975). When oestradiol is administered alone to HIFR, granulosa cell FSH receptor concentrations remain unchanged with an overall decrease in LH receptor number, suggesting that the enhanced responsiveness of oestradiol-primed follicles to gonadotrophins may not simply be related to an increase in the number of granulosa cell gonadotrophin receptors *per se* (Louvet & Vaitukaitis, 1976). Thus, FSH more than oestradiol appears to increase granulosa cell FSH receptors in a dose and time related fashion. In the presence of both FSH and oestrogen, a significant enhancement of granulosa cell LH receptors has been reported, suggesting a synergism between these two hormones may be required for preovulatory follicle maturation (Zeleznik et al, 1974). What are the effects of LH on follicular development, especially the FSH oestradiol mediated acquisition of granulosa cell LH receptors? Recent studies, (Richards & Midgley, 1976; Rao et al, 1977) have shown that LH-induced luteinisation and progesterone secretion by antral follicles diminish both LH and FSH receptor concentration. Granulosa cell luteinisation has also been associated with the loss of adenyl cyclase activity, an intermediary step in LH and FSH action (Hunzicker-Dunn & Birnbaumer, 1976). When HIFR were challenged with FSH and then FSH/hCG, an increase in granulosa cell LH receptor content occurred. Following additional FSH and hCG treatment, a prolonged increase in LH receptor content accompanied the appearance of large antral follicles. In contrast, hCG given alone to oestradiol-primed rats did not increase LH receptors;

and in addition, the follicles appeared morphologically atretic (Richards, 1974; Harman et al, 1975). Thus, LH/hCG appears to act directly on granulosa cells, but only when the granulosa cells have first been exposed to oestradiol and FSH. Moreover, an ovulatory dose of LH or hCG given prior to appropriate granulosa cell maturation may not have the desired effect on sequential granulosa cell maturation but rather lead to the disruption of pre-ovulatory growth and ovulation.

In summary, the process of pre-ovulatory follicular maturation requires both steroid and protein hormones. Oestradiol or FSH by themselves appear to act on granulosa cells to increase their own receptor number, whereas FSH following oestradiol exposure induces the formation of large preantral follicles whose granulosa cells contain both FSH and LH receptors. Further, LH acts synergistically in oestradiol-primed preantral follicles to enhance FSH stimulation of LH receptor. Only then can LH act on these pre-ovulatory follicles to bring about luteinisation evidenced by reduced oestradiol, FSH and LH receptors and the development of progesterone secretion. Therefore, the initiation of follicular oestrogen production and the ability of granulosa cells to respond to oestrogen appears to determine whether a follicle can undergo successful pre-ovulatory maturation or becomes atretic. In addition to gonadotrophins, a variety of non-steroidal regulators of folliculogenesis have been identified in follicular fluid including inhibitors and stimulators of granulosa cell maturation and luteinisation (Ledwitz-Rigby et al, 1977) oocyte maturation inhibitor, and follicle stimulating hormone (Tsafrir & Channing, 1975) receptor binding inhibitor (Reichert & Abou-Issa, 1977; Darga & Reichert, 1978). Further, a widely studied substance referred to as inhibin or folliculostatin, which acts by regulating FSH secretion independently of LH, has been reported in bovine, (DeJong & Sharp, 1976) porcine, (Marder et al, 1977; Schwartz & Channing, 1977; Welschen et al, 1977) and human follicular fluid, (Chari et al, 1981) as well as in the medium of rat granulosa cell cultures (Erickson & Hsueh, 1978). These substances have been reviewed elsewhere (Channing et al, 1982, Franchimont & Channing, 1981). These observations suggest that, in addition to the intra-follicular steroidal mileau, a variety on non-steroidal compounds, perhaps secretory products of the granulosa cells, contribute to the regulation of folliculogenesis.

The human preantral follicle is similarly influenced by its endocrine environment, including that produced by the stroma (Ross & Lipsett, 1978). As in the case of the rat, oestrogen synergised by FSH stimulates granulosa cell proliferation (Goldenberg et al, 1972). By the time of menstruation, the largest of the ripening follicles with a full complement of granulosa cells is already 4 mm in size. Thus it has increased some 80 times in diameter and now contains approximately 10^6 granulosa cells. During the early follicular phase, FSH and low concentrations of oestrogen are present in the antral fluid of a large proportion of small antral follicles. The oestrogen induces FSH receptors, (Richards & Midgley, 1976) and FSH in turn stimulates further FSH receptor formation if ample substrate in the form of androstenedione is present (Moon et al, 1978; McNatty et al, 1979; Brailly et al, 1981). More than 90 per cent of antral follicles over 1 mm diameter have already begun to undergo some atretic changes. The microenvironment of these follicles (i.e. whether it is androgen- or oestrogen-dominant) undoubtedly influences its fate, and this may be observed in vitro (Schbreiber et al, 1976; Ross & Lipsett, 1978; Bomsel-Helmreich et al, 1979; McNatty et al, 1980). Aromatisation may be a central regulator of follicular maturation, and inhibition of aromatisation may suppress continued follicle maturation to ovulatory status (Moon et al, 1978; McNatty et al, 1979; Hillier et al, 1979; Leung & Armstrong, 1980). It is noteworthy that the intrafollicular concentrations of steroids and gonadotrophins correlate better with mitotic and biosynthetic activities of the granulosa cells than do plasma hormone levels (McNatty et al, 1979). The entry of significant quantities of LH into the follicle (how was it kept out up to this point?) inhibits further mitosis, and together with prolactin initiates the secretion of increasing amounts of progesterone (McNatty et al, 1975; McNatty & Sawers, 1975; Sanyal et al, 1974) and luteinisation of the cells. The dominant follicle arises from the ovary secreting less progesterone (diZerega et al, 1982) and requires continued FSH secretion for its support (diZerega et al, 1982).

In the theca, the production of androstenedione and the conversion of some of it to 5α-reduced metabolites increases with increasing follicular size. The granulosa cells also produce 5α-reduced androgens. These compounds may be of importance in that they appear to inhibit granulosa cell aromatase (Hillier et al, 1979). The theca, while primarily an androgen producer, also has the capacity to produce oestrogen, and this is found to increase as cells from progressively more mature follicles are studied. In atretic follicles the theca remains endocrinologically active but loses its ability to aromatise (McNatty et al, 1979; McNatty et al, 1980).

The function of the stroma depends on the gonadotrophic environment, and the presence of LH is associated with decreased in vitro aromatase activity (McNatty et al, 1979b). During these events, most of the antral follicles are undergoing atresia. They continued to synthesise androstenedione, but they lose their aromatase activity and thus have a lowered capacity to synthesise oestrogen. Apparently this activity cannot be recovered, and it is associated with a loss of the ability of the granulosa cells to undergo mitosis. Later, they are unable in tissue culture to transform into the progesterone-secreting state (McNatty & Sawers, 1975). On the one hand, the process of atresia is enhanced by androgens, which antagonise oestrogen-induced follicular development (Louvet et al, 1975). On the other, androgens synergise with FSH, which tends to oppose atresia (Nimrod & Lindner, 1976). Premature exposure of a follicle to LH (either endogenously or by parenteral injection) (Tamada & Matsomoto, 1969; Williams & Hodgen, 1980) produces atresia of the dominant follicle. Prolactin may also play a role: if the plasma prolactin level exceeds 100 ng/ml, the intrafollicular prolactin concentration also rises, and this is associated with a decrease in the number of granulosa cells as well as of the intrafollicular concentration of oestradiol and FSH (McNatty, 1979). If hyperprolactinaemia is induced in women by administration of metoclopramide at the beginning of the cycle, multiple small (2–6 mm) follicles develop but fail to grow, and in many instances there is no selection of a dominant follicle. In some instances this disturbed follicular growth is nevertheless associated with normal plasma progesterone levels — possibly an iatrogenic analogue of the luteinised unruptured follicle (Kauppila et al, 1982).

Thus, although ovarian tissues (Goldzieher & Axelrod, 1969) as well as granulosa cells, theca cells, and stromal cells (McNatty et al, 1979a) have the capacity to biosynthesise progesterone, androstenedione, testosterone, dihydrotestosterone, oestrone, and oestradiol in vitro, the actual steroidogenic patterns of these cell types differ. The role of various hormones in stimulating or inhibiting biosynthetic pathways in the preovulatory granulosa and theca is shown in Fig. 20.5. Subsequently, LH stimulates the enzyme systems converting cholesterol to pregnenolone, progesterone to 17α-hydroxyprogesterone, and 17α-hydroxyprogesterone to androgens (Makris & Ryan, 1980). It is also at this point that prostaglandins may affect steroid biosynthesis by blocking the ability of LH to activate the adenyl cyclase system (McNatty et al, 1975).

When cultured cells are obtained from polycystic ovaries, it has been found (Wilson et al, 1979) that cells from midantral (4–7 mm) follicles of both normal and polycystic ovaries show essentially no difference in steroid biosynthetic potential. Although these cells have little aromatase activity even when androstenedione is added as substrate, they can aromatise when appropriately stimulated by FSH (Erickson et al, 1979).

In follicles from PCO patients with a high LH:FSH ratio, there were fewer LH receptors (though of normal affinity) than are found in normal pre-ovulatory follicles (Rajaniemi et al, 1980). Th elevated LH may have caused down-regulation and loss of receptors, as has been shown in the case of hCG therapy. In larger (8–15 mm) follicles, one can observe a dose-dependent increase in the production of oestrogen from androgen even without FSH treatment (however, follicles over 8 mm in size are much more likely to have significant endogenous levels of FSH). Theca cells from both normal and polycystic ovaries were also found to be alike (Wilson et al, 1979) producing primarily androstenedione and very little oestrone. The pattern was merely amplified by FSH/LH (Pergonal). On the other hand, cultured medullary tissue from polycystic ovaries may show more androgen production than cultures from normal ovaries, especially if hyperthecosis is present.

These studies underscore the vital role of FSH and the possibility that FSH deficiency underlies the development of aromatase deficiency. Clinical studies are confirmatory, in that a sharp increase in oestrogen levels and subsequent ovulation can be induced in patients with PCOD (Taymor et al, 1972; Bertrand et al, 1976) with the use of pure FSH. From the vantage point of the 1980s, it is seen that the studies of 20 years ago were correct in focusing on the defect in aromatase. The role of the various cell types in steroid synthesis in normal and atretic follicles, as well as the critical role of FSH, put these findings into a contemporary perspective.

Other enzymatic disturbances in polycystic ovaries have also been reported. Concurrent Δ⁵-3β-HSD deficiency in both adrenal and polycystic ovarian tissue was reported in 1965 (Axelrod et al, 1965). The likelihood that this might be a genetic enzyme deficiency is strengthened by the report of a similar deficiency in the testes of a subject with the Δ⁵-3β-HSD deficiency form of congenital adrenal hyperplasia (Schneider et al, 1975). Others (Gyory et al, 1975) have found similar evidence in ovarian tissue from PCOD, and clinical studies in hirsute amenorrhoeic women (Lorber et al, 1978; Gibson et al, 1980; Laatikainen et al, 1980; Goebelsmann, 1981) have shown a relative increase in plasma levels of DHEA or its sulfate, pregnenolone and 17-hydroxypregnenolone. This excess appeared to be derived from both adrenals and ovaries, again suggesting a concurrent abnormality, sometimes of a subtle nature.

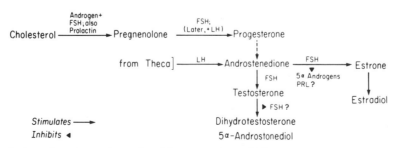

Fig. 20.5 Biosynthetic activities in the cultured granulosa cells of the pre-ovulatory follicle (modified from Dorrington & Armstrong, 1979)

Measurement of DHEA sulphate is a screening test for this condition. The occult form may require the demonstration of hyperresponsiveness to ACTH and/or hCG. Adult cases of congenital adrenal hyperplasia due to incomplete 21-hydroxylase deficiency may resemble PCOD clinically (Lobo & Goebelsmann, 1981). High levels of 17-hydroxy-progesterone or a hyperresponse of this steroid to ACTH stimulation will identify the condition.

Incubations of mitochondria obtained from polycystic ovaries (Maschler et al, 1976) with radioactive steroids were found to demonstrate 11β-hydroxylase activity with C_{21}-hydroxy compounds. This finding identifies the origin of 11-ketopregnanetriol found in the urine of some patients with PCOD. How this biosynthetic potential, considered typical of adrenal cells, has come to be activated in mitochondria from polycystic ovaries is a challenging question for future research.

In view of the popularity of ovarian wedge resection at one time, it is remarkable how little information there is regarding the short-term and long-term hormonal consequences of this procedure. A study of two cases with frequent measurements during the intra- and postoperative period (Katz et al, 1978) (Fig. 20.6) showed an immediate and dramatic decrease in plasma oestrogen to approximately one-quarter of the prevailing level. It was already evident after the first ovary was wedged; by contrast, the plasma testosterone level did not decline until 6–24 hours later (this fall in testosterone appears to be a fairly consistent observation in other reports). In the first postoperative week the elevated LH/FSH ratio declined from 2.3 to 0.3 and pulsatile gonadotrophic activity increased; spontaneous ovulation occurred in both cases within 1 month and conception within 4 months. In another case, (Mahesh et al, 1978) wedging resulted in a decline of plasma oestradiol, progesterone, 17-hydroxyprogesterone,

androstenedione and dehydroepiandrosterone in the postoperative week, whereas FSH and the elevated levels of LH and testosterone were unchanged. Subsequently a gradual decline in LH levels and a slow increase in oestradiol levels presaged the events of a normal ovulatory cycle. Following this ovulation, the LH/FSH ratio became normal. A series of ten patients studied preoperatively and 10 days postoperative (Valkov & Dokumov, 1977) showed no change in plasma oestradiol levels but a 40 per cent decline in testosterone after surgery; moreover the elevated LH level and its exaggerated response to GnRH also disappeared.

Eight clomiphene-resistant patients with PCOD presented a somewhat different picture (Judd et al, 1976). Wedging caused a prompt decline in plasma oestrone and oestradiol, reaching a nadir on the 3rd postoperative day. The elevated LH levels were unaffected until ovulatory gonadotrophin surges occurred 13–25 days postoperatively. In the women who did not ovulate there was a transient decrease in LH levels which reached a nadir on the 16th day and then returned to preoperative levels. Significant decreases in testosterone and androstenedione occurred immediately after surgery; androstenedione returned to preoperative levels whereas the testosterone concentration eventually leveled off below the pretreatment value regardless of whether the subject ovulated or not. Tanaka et al (1978) are the only investigators to report a consistent decline of elevated gonadotrophins after wedging; however 82 per cent of their patients ovulated postoperatively. In hyperthecosis, the substantial bilateral testosterone secretion was normalised for at least 6 months by surgical reduction of the stromal tissue (Belisle et al, 1981).

If one can draw any conclusions from this limited experience, it is that the dramatic effect of surgical intervention, first on the circulating oestrogen and then on the

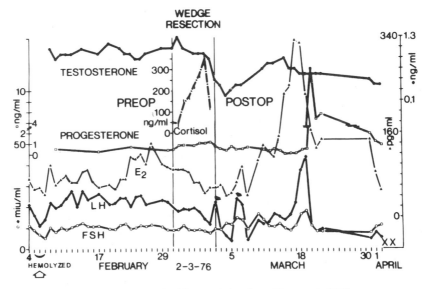

Fig. 20.6 Acute hormonal effects of wedge resection (reprinted with permission from Katz et al, 1978)

androgen levels, affects the hypothalamic-pituitary system, which is seen to be relatively responsive in many cases. The failure to see consistent changes in the LH/FSH ratio requires further study, probably with more frequent sampling. In any event, the normalisation of the LH/FSH ratio in some cases, especially after the first successful ovulation, speaks strongly for the reactive nature of this disorder and suggests that lowered oestrogen levels, post-ovulatory progesterone levels, and decreased androgen exposure may be involved in this process.

The important role or progesterone is emphasised by a study (Beslisle, 1979) of its effect in normal women, castrated women, and women with polycystic ovaries. In the presence of follicular phase levels of plasma oestradiol, a low, transient pulse of progesterone was consistently shown to elicit prolactin and LH surges, followed by a deficient or moderately satisfactory luteal phase.

Our knowledge of the status of biochemical abnormalities in PCOD following pregnancies and/or wedge resection is evidently quite fragmentary and also needs amplification. There is some evidence for a persistent decrease in testosterone production (for citations, see Kandeel et al, 1978). A study of the androgen status of 12 subjects who had become menstrually normal was carried out 6–18 months postoperatively (Vejlsted & Albrechtsen, 1976); it revealed no significant changes in 17-ketosteroid excretion, a persistent stimulatory effect of hCG on ovarian androgens, and no effect on the rate of hair growth, even though plasma testosterone levels were decreased by 32 per cent.

The adrenal factor

Involvement of the adrenal in PCOD has been recognised since 1937, when Broster observed concurrent adrenal and ovarian hyperplasia during surgery. Similar conclusions were drawn from numerous dynamic studies involving adrenal suppression with DXM or stimulation with ACTH. Selective hyper-responsiveness of adrenal androgens in comparison with corticosteroid production was inferred several decades ago from the response of urinary steroid excretion to ACTH administration. The response of a broad spectrum of adrenal steroids in plasma to a bolus of ACTH has suggested that abnormalities in adrenal biosynthesis, particularly in the activities of Δ^5-3 β-HSD and 11β-hydroxylase, are common in patients with hyperandrogenism, including those with PCOD. (Goldzieher et al, 1976; Gibson et al, 1980) Another possibility, purely speculative, is the existence of factor(s) which selectively stimulate adrenal androgen production. Recently it was reported (Parker & Odell, 1977) that a bovine pituitary extract differed from ACTH in producing hypersecretion of androstenedione and DHA compared to cortisol, in both dogs and sheep.

Whether corticotrophin releasing factor and vasopressin have qualitatively similar effects on ACTH release, and whether they play any role in the corticosteroid/androgen profile of adrenal secretion is another interesting speculation. The sensitivity and capacity of the adrenal response in PCOD has been studied carefully. In one investigation (Lachelin et al, 1979) the circadian rhythm of adrenal steroids was found to be intact, and minimal pulses of $ACTH_{1-24}$ produced similar responses in normal subjects and patients with PCOD. However, with maximal-response infusions over several hours, the subjects with PCOD showed a greater increase in plasma DHEA, progesterone, 17-hydroxyprogesterone and 17-hydroxy-pregnenolone, but subnormal response of androstenedione, testosterone, and androstanediol. These results differ from an earlier study (Givens et al, 1975a) in which hirsute women were first suppressed with a small dose of DXM to inhibit basal secretion and then stimulated with a minimal dose of 0.5 unit of $ACTH_{1-39}$. Half of these women had an exaggerated diurnal variation of androstenedione, and nine out of 17 had an exaggerated response to the ACTH pulse. Some also had an exaggerated response of 17-hydroxyprogesterone, again suggesting a mild, compensated defect in 21-hydroxylase activity. On the basis of this study, the investigators inferred that 47 per cent of the 19 women had ACTH-independent hyperandrogenism, 6 per cent had purely ACTH-dependent hyperandrogenism, and 47 per cent had a mixed adrenal-ovarian disorder.

It is interesting to compare these results with data from direct catheterisation of the venous supply. Direct sampling has demonstrated secretion of androstenedione, testosterone, and DHEA by adrenal and ovary. In 13 women (only two of whom were shown to have PCOD) (Kirschner & Jacobs, 1971) the major source of androstenedione and testosterone was the ovaries in nine and both ovaries and adrenals in four. In eight other PCO patients, (Wajchenberg et al, 1981) there was exclusively adrenal secretion of testosterone and/or androstenedione in two, combined adrenal/ovarian secretion in three and an ovarian source in three. Subsequent investigations have reinforced the conclusion that a significant percentage of patients with PCOD have isolated or concurrent adrenal hyperandrogenism. This is also reflected in the results of metopyrone administration: in normal subjects there is no increase in urinary oestrogens, but when it is given to patients with PCOD, there is a 60–100 per cent increase in urinary oestrogens, presumably derived from aromatisation of the increased adrenal androstenedione output. In some patients with PCOD other adrenal steroids such as cortisol also show an excessive response to ACTH; interestingly, this has been reported to decrease after wedge resection. This would suggest that pituitary-ovarian dynamics are capable of influencing the pituitary-adrenal relationship. In fact, there are many sites of action where ovarian steroids can influence the adrenal axis; conversely,

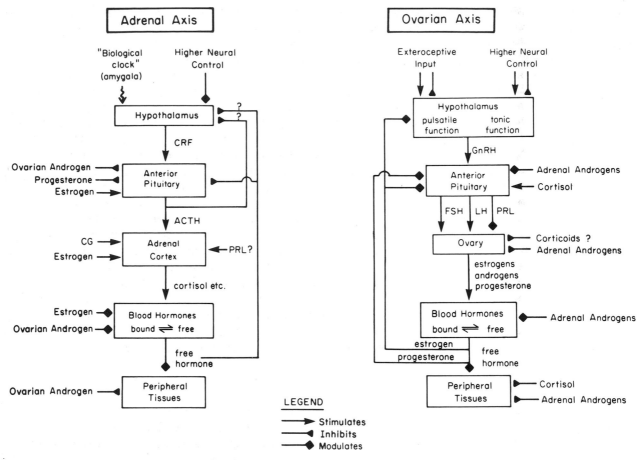

Fig. 20.7 Schematic diagram of adrenal/ovarian interplay.

there are many sites where adrenal steroids can influence the gonadal axis (Fig. 20.7).

The role of the adrenal in the pathogenesis of PCOD has been emphasised by one group of investigators (Yen et al, 1976) who pointed to the frequent onset of hirsutism and obesity prior to or about the time of menarche, along with the well-known occurrence of persistent oligomenorrhoea from the outset. Adrenal androgen secretion is an early and important phase ('adrenarche') of the pubertal process. In fact, in congenital adrenal hyperplasia, elevated ACTH secretion is probably responsible (by way of excessive adrenal androgen levels) for a premature onset of the sleep-associated secretion of LH (Boyer et al, 1973) and eventually with persistently elevated plasma LH (Stevens & Goldzieher, 1968). Thus it has been postulated that adrenal hyperfunction at the time of adrenarche may be responsible for the obesity and hirsutism, and that peripheral metabolism of increased adrenal androgens results in increased oestrogen levels, which initiate the vicious circle of persistently elevated LH levels, increased follicular atresia, increased ovarian androgen levels, and decreased ovarian oestrogen secretion that is characteristic of PCOD. The androgen overproduction may be the result of a compensated enzymatic deficiency, as pointed out above. On the

other hand, exogenous obesity in prepubertal girls may itself increase plasma levels of pregnenolone, DHEA, androstenedione and prolactin, implying that obesity may advance maturation of adrenal function, especially of the Δ^5 pathway, while gonadal secretion of oestrogen is impaired (Valkov & Dokumov, 1977). As far as we know, no one has looked for premature adrenarche in the children of women with PCOD.

ANIMAL MODELS

Progress in understanding the mechanism of PCOD would accelerate if an appropriate animal model were available. One must ask the question: what features of the clinical disorder constitute the essential parts of the complex? Although it is clearly a matter of judgment, in our view the basic necessities would be: (1) a multicystic ovary which shows evidence of chronic stimulation, continuing follicular growth, atresia and cystic degeneration; (2) a disruption of menstrual or oestrous regularity; (3) evidence of gonadotrophic disturbances in the form of a persistent elevation of LH levels and/or a disproportionately high LH/FSH ratio; (4) disturbance of ovarian oestrogen synthesis, in the sense that an excessive amount of androgen is produced in proportion to the amount of oestrogen (however, this is a secondary criterion, as the disorders of the ovary appear to be induced by gonadotrophic disturbances which in turn induce enzyme defects; those defects which appear to be genetic are not an invariable feature of the clinical disorder); and (5) if possible, evidence that the experimental situation also induces adrenal hyperfunction or malfunction.

The genetically X-linked 'nymphomaniac' cow (Garm, 1949) studied several decades ago by Gassner, is an interesting if somewhat inconvenient model which deserves renewed attention.

Many years ago, Leathem and his colleagues succeeded in producing massive cystic ovaries in rodents by rendering them hypothyroid and administering chorionic gonadotrophin. However, there are no data regarding the endogenous gonadotrophic milieu of this preparation, and there appeared to be *augmented* aromatisation of androstenedione.

Polycystic ovaries develop in rats brought into persistent oestrus by exposure to constant illumination. Plasma levels of LH are unchanged or only slightly elevated, but the prooestrous LH surge disappears even though ovulation may continue to occur for a time. FSH levels are normal or slightly elevated. Both FSH and LH levels increase after castration in the usual way. The LH pulse seen in ovariectomised animals given oestradiol benzoate is not observed in such animals under constant light, suggesting involvement of the hypothalamus (Mennin & Gorski, 1975). However, the positive feedback induced by progesterone is not disturbed. As far as we know, no recent studies of steroidogenesis in ovaries in persistent oestrus have been carried out nor have the effects of clomiphene or corticosteroids been examined. Adrenal function has not been evaluated. One of us (JWG) has tried to reproduce PCOD in primates by putting them under constant illumination, but the baboons disobligingly continued to cycle as before.

Polycystic ovaries also result from neonatal androgenisation. In the normal female rat, a surge of FSH at 10–15 days of age is thought to be essential for the development of the first crop of follicles. Prior administration of testosterone propionate blocks the expected surge; subsequently there is a lower level of FSH and LH does not show the normal pubertal rise. FSH levels in adult androgenised females are similar to those in normal animals and LH levels, if anything, are slightly depressed. The facilitatory action of oestrogen or progesterone, alone or in combination, is abolished, and this may be the major functional defect in these animals. However, these animals also have greatly stimulated mammary glands suggesting elevated prolactin levels. The ovaries display a defect in aromatisation in that substantial amounts of androgen, but no oestrogen, are produced during *in vitro* incubation with precursors (Goldzieher & Axelrod, 1963). Interestingly,

both neonatal steroid treatment and hypothalamic lesions which produce persistent oestrus also cause adrenal hypertrophy.

Another type of polycystic ovary has been produced in rats by the administration of DHEA starting at 27 days of age (Mahesh, 1980). This model is interesting in that the condition regresses after cessation of the treatment. The treatment produces a low level of LH, slightly elevated FSH, and markedly elevated prolactin. The conversion of DHEA to oestrogen was a prerequisite for the various effects observed. Nothing has been reported about effects on the adrenal.

In these and in other studies in rodents, the question of species differences becomes important, because the rat, in contrast to man, requires both LH and prolactin for ovulation and maintenance of the corpus luteum. Thus the utility of rodent models remains speculative. It is of interest, however, that a single injection of oestradiol valerate in the adult rat (Brawer et al, 1978) can produce histological degenerative changes in the arcuate nucleus along with persistent oestrus, elevated LH and normal FSH levels, and small polyfollicular ovaries.

THERAPY

Medical management

Pragmatically, the medical management of PCOD can be divided into two categories — that for women who do *not* wish to become pregnant immediately and that for women who do.

It is quite clear that surgery (wedge resection) has no place in the management of women who do not wish to conceive immediately. The treatment of choice is an oral contraceptive of a potency sufficient to reduce LH to the normal level or below (Givens et al, 1974). In general, this implies the use of an agent containing 80 μg of ethynyl oestrogen or more for several cycles, to be followed by a preparation containing 50 μg of oestrogen. Oral contraceptives with an even lower oestrogen content do not produce a profound depression of LH within the first few cycles of treatment. It has been claimed (Raj et al, 1981) that even a 30 μg oestrogen oral contraceptive will reduce free testosterone to normal levels (largely by increasing SHBG), but the equally important effect on LH levels was not ascertained. The use of contraceptive steroids under these circumstances has a number of therapeutic benefits: (1) the excessive LH production is normalised; (2) overstimulation of the ovaries ceases and consequently there is a decrease in the rate of follicular atresia and cyst formation, lessening of stromal hyperplasia and hyperstimulation, and lessening of ovarian androgen production; (3) the decrease in plasma androgen levels lessens the acne, seborrhoea, hirsutism, weight gain and other more subtle effects. The oestrogens in the contraceptive increase the plasma level of sex hormone binding globulin, especially if one of the more oestrogenic combinations is used; this further decreases the biological activity of the plasma androgens; (4) oestrogens inhibit the enzyme which converts testosterone to the more active 5α-dihydrotestosterone in the skin; (5) the contraceptive steroids have an indirect inhibitory effect on the adrenal and lessen the androgenic output from this source; and (6) the contraceptive steroids ensure an appropriate stimulus to the endometrium and cyclic shedding, thus serving as prophylaxis against endometrial hyperplasia and neoplasia. Whether this would also decrease the incidence of ovarian neoplasma is unknown, but long-term oral contraceptive users are reported to have half the usual incidence of ovarian cancers. There is some concern about so-called post-pill amenorrhoea and the possibility that contraceptive steroid therapy will worsen an already disturbed hypothalamus. This notion is based on the observation that women treated for oligomenorrhoea with contraceptive steroids may have a recurrence of their symptomatology or show prolonged amenorrhoea after ending such therapy. What is not taken into account in this line of thought is the natural evolution of the primary disorder — the way it would have progressed if no treatment at all had been given. There are no clinical data which adequately evaluate the difference between the eventual course of oligomenorrhoea treated with contraceptive steroids or with other modalities. Consequently no firm conclusions can be drawn until appropriate clinical trials have been performed. In the absence of such information, and in view of the clear cut benefits which have been enumerated, contraceptive steroid treatment represents the optimal approach at the present time.

Other methods of gonadotrophic suppression have also been advocated (Hirschowitz et al, 1968; Frolich et al, 1980; Wortsman & Hirschowitz, 1980). Large doses of injectable medroxyprogesterone acetate (Depo-Provera, 400–600 mg twice monthly) reduced plasma LH and testosterone levels significantly and produced substantial improvement of hirsutism. An increase in plasma prolactin levels and some aggravation of galactorrhoea were observed. Ovarian shrinkage persisted for up to 2 years, LH and testosterone relapsed partially after about a year, at which time galactorrhoea disappeared and prolactin fell to about 50 per cent of baseline values. The disadvantages of this therapy are the same as when it is used for contraceptive purposes: complete disruption of menstrual regularity, mild weight gain, a small increase in the incidence of headache, and a long delay in the elimination of the tissue deposits of the microcrystalline steroid. As long as these limitations are understood, the safety of such injections (however at a lower dose) is documented by 15 years of use as a contraceptive by millions of women.

Implants of oestradiol (100 mg every 6 months) have been studied in a few patients with PCOD (Gambrell, 1976) and have been found to reduce ovarian size and halt the progression of hirsutism. Progestogen therapy was required to prevent irregular bleeding or hypermenorrhoea. Since it is necessary to use progestational therapy in addition to the implants in this regimen, it appears to have little clinical appeal and runs the risks associated with continuous oestrogen exposure if the progestin therapy happens not to be adequately pursued.

Outside the USA, cyproterone acetate, a progestin closely related to medroxyprogesterone or megestrol, has been widely and successfully used an an antiandrogen in acne and hirsutism. Its active metabolite, the 15-hydroxy derivative, appears to have even better attributes. It will have an obvious role in the management of PCOD. Spironolactone (100–200 mg daily) has been suggested as an antiandrogen (Boisselle & Tremblay, 1979). In addition to this effect, which is probably through competition for androgen receptors of the hair follicles, it appears to decrease urinary ketosteroid excretion and testosterone production. These treatments are discussed in detail in Chapter 21.

The occurrence of hyperprolactinaemia (with or without galactorrhoea) in PCOD is now well established. This clearly indicates a role for bromocriptine after appropriate diagnostic investigation. In some instances, doses as large as 20 mg/day produced good results, allegedly without side-effects (Blum et al, 1981). In normoprolactinaemic patients, the drug may work as an androgen synthesis inhibitor. Another potent agent reported to be of value is cimetidine at the rather large, costly dose of 1500 mg/day (Vigersky et al, 1980) presumably through its action as an androgen receptor blocker.

In older women who are no longer interested in fertility and in whom prolonged suppressive therapy is inconvenient or inadvisable, surgical extirpation of the ovaries (and uterus) is a valuable option, especially in view of the increased incidence of endometrial and ovarian neoplasia in PCOD. The advantages of this option are apparent; any residual androgen production from the adrenals should be amenable to suppression with minimal doses of corticosteroids. The need for appropriate oestrogen replacement therapy goes without saying.

Neoplasia is a generally underemphasised complication of PCOD. One group of 97 young women with endometrial hyperplasia (25 per cent of them also had PCOD) was followed for up to 14 years (Chamlian & Taylor, 1970) and 14 per cent developed endometrial carcinoma. Of approximately 70 such cases reported to date (Fechner & Kaufman, 1974; Katz & Carr, 1976; McDonald et al, 1977) only four were poorly differentiated, and the vast majority have been stage 0 or stage 1. In fact, there were proportionately fewer stage II lesions than in a large series of endometrial carcinomas not associated with ovarian lesions and the 5- and 10-year survival rates in PCOD cases were significantly higher. The incidence of nulliparity and of a second primary malignancy were similar in the series with and without concomitant ovarian abnormalities, but obesity, hypertension, and diabetes (more common than usual in both series) were even more prevalent among the patients with associated ovarian disease (McArthur et al, 1958). Conservative therapy with progestational compounds in large doses has been recommended in selected cases (Grattarola, 1969; Fechner & Kaufman, 1974; Eddy, 1978). As early as 1948 Novak & Dubledje pointed out that certain benign lesions of the endometrium may simulate adenocarcinoma. This issue, both in general and in respect to cases associated with PCOD, merits intensive review.

For therapy when fertility is desired, the use of corticosteroids has been recommended for many years, even though the dual action of these agents (adrenal-inhibiting and gonadotrophin stimulating) has not been generally recognised. Correction of the hyperandrogenic state has substantial benefits on menstrual regularity, indicating once again the effects of androgen on the function of the hypothalamic-pituitary gonadal mechanism. In a very large series (Smith et al, 1979), significant prolongation of the follicular phase and shortening of the luteal phase were found to be associated with clinical hyperandrogenism and elevated plasma testosterone levels; the implications for menstrual irregularity and relative infertility are evident. The use of 5–10 mg prednisone daily initiated ovulatory activity in five of 14 amenorrhoeic hirsute patients and in ten of 11 anovulatory patients (Rodriguez-Rigau et al, 1979) a maximal effect was achieved within 2 months. These findings, substantiated by plasma testosterone monitoring, confirm earlier studies (Smith et al, 1965) in which return of ovulation and conception rates in patients with PCOD treated with corticosteroids equalled those obtained with wedge resection. Only one series which used cortisone rather than synthetic corticosteroids reported negative results. Present concepts of pituitary-adrenal dynamics indicate that a given dose of corticosteroid is more effective in its ACTH-suppressive effect if given at night. Concern regarding the long-term effects such therapy appears to be unwarranted. It must be kept in mind that the adrenals being treated are hyperactive and hyper-responsive, and are simply kept in leash by this treatment. This cannot be equated with the suppressive and hypotrophic effects of corticosteroid therapy (especially of large doses) to which *normal* adrenals are subjected in the course of anti-inflammatory, immunosuppressive, or other medical therapy.

The induction of ovulatory surges and luteal phases of more or less adequate length by a single injection of progesterone (Belisle, 1979) suggests a therapeutic modality which has not been explored: the use of intravaginal or injected progesterone (on a more prolonged basis) or of other non-pituitary-inhibiting progestins in patients with PCOD with adequate oestrogen levels. Both from a practical and from an investigative point of view,

data from such clinical trials would be of considerable interest.

The administration of clomiphene or its active isomer is an established, important modality for patients who are interested in conception; it is not advised as a method for repetitive production of menstrual cycles. Reports of success have reached as high as 87 per cent ovulations and 43 per cent pregnancies in a substantial number of selected patients. A 1967 summary stated that 359 of 436 patients with 'Stein-Leventhal syndrome' ovulated after one course of treatment and 58 more (an aggregate of 95 per cent) responded to further therapy (Johnson, 1967). Recently 91 per cent of a series of 55 patients with PCOD treated for infertility ovulated and 51 per cent conceived (Raj et al, 1977) In another series, 68 per cent of women who had failed to respond to wedge resection ovulated with clomiphene and half became pregnant. Failure to respond to wedge resection or to corticosteroid therapy is no contra-indication for a trial of clomiphene, and *vice versa*.

Many 'ovulatory' cycles induced by clomiphene have a luteal phase defect as shown by relatively low levels of plasma progesterone and an abbreviated post-ovulatory interval (Bertrand et al, 1976). These findings are consistent with the benefits of LH (as chorionic gonadotrophin) given to those patients in whom clomiphene alone appears to be unsuccessful. The role of intrafollicular FSH deficiency in the atresia of follicles suggests that properly timed administration of preparations high in FSH might also have advantages. A recent summary (Wang & Gemzell, 1980) of 77 cycles of treatment with human menopausal gonadotrophin and hCG in 41 clomiphene-unresponsive patients with PCOD yielded a 66 per cent conception rate, a 24 per cent abortion rate, 36 per cent multiple pregnancies and three instances of severe hyper-stimulation syndrome. Another series (Kemmann et al, 1981) of 62 cycles in 24 patients yielded a 58 per cent pregnancy rate with an average of 2.4 treatment cycles per pregnancy. There were seven singletons, five twins and three abortions, with no complications. Kamrava et al (1982) have used 'pure' FSH from the NIH in two clomiphene-hCG failure patients, and obtained ovulations with 80 Iu/day given for 4 weeks. Interestingly, there was an erratic *decline* in LH preceding the ovulatory LH surge.

Under all circumstances the hypersensitivity of the polycystic ovary to gonadotrophic stimuli must be kept in mind, and a conservative, monitored approach used to minimise hyperstimulative complications. (see Ch. 27)

Early experiments with GnRH or its superagonists failed to take into account paradoxical effects of these peptides and the need for pulsatile administration. Recent experiments with variations in pulse amplitude and frequency are actually reported to have *produced* polycystic ovaries of some sort. In any event, investigations of the effect of such pulsatile administration on the gonadotrophin pattern of PCOD and the ovarian consequences thereof have not as yet been reported. Shutting down gonadotrophin secretion by continued use of a long-acting GnRH may have therapeutic potential under special circumstances.

Wedge resection

The effectiveness of the therapeutic approach was first thought to result from removal of the fibrous ovarian capsule which allegedly interfered with extrusion of the ovum. Various surgical procedures, some of them rather drastic, were developed on this basis. A number of observations cast doubt upon this hypothesis: for example, removal of one ovary without touching the other was reported to restore cyclic menses (the single published instance of this in the older literature has not been confirmed in three subsequent cases). Even the minor trauma of laparoscopic biopsy in six women unresponsive to clomiphene and hCG (McNatty et al, 1979c) appears to have initiated menses and resulted in conception without further treatment (a placebo effect?). Early reports on the efficacy of wedge resection were generally enthusiastic, but a review of worldwide results reported up to 1962 (Table 20.3) yielded conception rates ranging from 89 per cent down to only 13 per cent, and normalisation of cycles from 95 per cent to 13 per cent) (Goldzieher & Green, 1962). Improvement of hirsutism was generally poor, with positive results in less than 20 per cent. A recent report has summarised the 10-year follow up of 90 consecutive wedge resections in the Johns Hopkins Hospital experience (Adashi et al, 1981). Overall, 91 per cent ovulated, but only 68 per cent did so regularly; their conception rate was

60 per cent. Among the 26 per cent who were oligoovulators the pregnancy rate was only 29 per cent. The life table cumulative probability of conception was 73 per cent, the monthly fecundability rate 1.34 per cent. (A suitable mathematical approach to pregnancy rates in such series has been described recently by Guzick et al (1981)). The number of clomid failures in this series is not clear, but an additional consideration was the 23 per cent of concomitant tuboperitoneal adhesive disease discovered at surgery; when present, this halved the pregnancy rate. The effect of post-wedge resection adhesive disease could not be evaluated.

Numerous investigators have found no relationship between the response to surgery and the size of the ovaries, the urinary steroid excretion, (Vejlsted & Albrechtsen, 1976) or to any other laboratory parameter. However, it is now clear that a surgical failure does not imply a poor prognosis for medical therapy, and vice versa.

Post-operative relapse is not uncommon. By 1968 warnings were sounded regarding post-operative adhesions and their role in post-wedge infertility. Ovarian atrophy as well as periovarian and peritubal adhesions were reported (Toaff et al, 1976). In a series of 173 wedge resections (Buttram & Vaquero, 1975) there were 34 patients in whom endoscopy or laparotomy was justified 1 year or more after the wedge resection: all were found to have adhesions. Among this number were 12 who had conceived in the first year after surgery and who were subsequently infertile. Some evaluation of long-term results was possible from this large series. Of these 173 patients, 6.3 per cent showed no improvement of their menstrual cyclicity at all; in 31.8 per cent the improvement was temporary. Only 42.6 per cent of those desiring pregnancy conceived, and all conceptions took place within the first year, thus emphasising the transitory nature of some of the benefits of wedge resection.

Microsurgical techniques are now being used at wedge resection, and at least in experimental animals (Eddy et al, 1980) the decrease in adhesive disease is highly promising. When combined with procedures shown to be of benefit in the surgical treatment of endometriosis, (Buttram, 1979) these advances suggest that the option of wedge resection the in management of PCOD needs to be re-evaluated.

Table 20.3 Results of wedge resection, from the literature prior to 1962. Summary of findings in 1097 cases published in 187 references (from Goldzieher & Green 1962)

Symptom	Usable no. of cases	Frequency	
		Mean (%)	Range (%)
Regular cycles	447	80	6–95
Pregnancy	640	63	13–89
Decreased hirsutism	205	16	0–18

REFERENCES

Abraham G E, Chakmakjian Z H, Buster J E 1975 Ovarian and adrenal contribution to peripheral androgens in hirsute women. Obstetrics and Gynecology 46: 169–173

Abraham G E, Maroulis G , Buster J E, Chang R J, Marshall J R 1976 Effect of dexamethasone on serum cortisol and androgen levels in hirsute patients. Obstetrics and Gynecology 47: 395–402

Adashi E Y, Rock J A, Guzick D, Wentz A C, Jones G S, Jones H W Jr 1981 Fertility following bilateral ovarian wedge resection: a critical analysis of 90 consecutive cases of the polycystic ovary syndrome. Fertility Sterility 36: 320–325

Aiman J, Edman C D, Worley R J, Vellios F, MacDonald P C 1978

Androgen and estrogen formation in women with ovarian hyperthecosis. Obstetrics and Gynecology 51: 1–9

Alger M, Vazquez-Matute L, Mason M, Canales E, Zarate A 1980 Polycystic ovarian disease associated with hyperprolactinemia and defective metoclopramide response. Fertility and Sterility 34: 70–71

Amsterdam A, Koch Y, Lieberman M E, Lindner H R 1975 Distribution of binding sites for human chorionic gonadotropin in the preovulatory follicle of the rat. Journal of Cell Biology 67: 894–900

Aono T, Miyake A, Shioji T, Yasuda M, Koike K, Kurachi K 1979 Restoration of oestrogen positive feedback effect on LH release by bromocryptine in hyperprolactinaemic patients with galactorrhoea-amenorrhoea. Acta Endocrinologica 91: 591–600

Aono T, Miyazaki M, Miyake A, Kinugasa T, Kurachi K, Matsumoto K 1977 Responses of serum gonadotropins to LH-releasing hormone and oestrogens in Japanese women with polycystic ovaries. Acta Endocrinologica 85: 840–849

Axelrod L R, Goldzieher J W 1961 Enzymic inadequacies of human polycystic ovaries. Archives Biochemistry Biophysics 95: 547–548

Axelrod L R, Goldzieher J W 1962 The polycystic ovary. III. Steroid biosynthesis in normal and polycystic ovarian tissue. Journal of Clinical Endocrinology Metabolism 22: 431–440

Axelrod L R, Goldzieher J W, Ross S D 1965 Concurrent 3β-hydroxysteroid dehydrogenase deficiency in adrenal and sclerocystic ovary. Acta Endocrinologica 48: 392–412

Babaknia A, Calfopoulos P, Jones H W Jr 1976 The Stein-Leventhal syndrome and coincidental ovarian tumors. Obstetrics and Gynecology 47: 223–224

Baird D T, Corker C S, Davidson D W, Hunter W M, Michie E A, Van Look P F A 1977 Pituitary-ovarian relationships in polycystic ovary syndrome. Journal of Clinical Endocrinology Metabolism 45: 798–809

Belisle S 1979 Early and late hormonal changes following progesterone injection to patients with secondary amenorrhea. Fertility Sterility 32: 414–419

Belisle S, Lehoux J G, Benard B, Ainmelk Y 1981 Ovarian hyperthecosis: in vivo and in vitro correlations of the androgen profile. Obstetrics and Gynecology 57: 70S

Berger M J, Taymor M L, Patton W C 1975 Gonadotropin levels and secretory patterns in patients with typical and atypical polycystic ovarian disease. Fertility Sterility 26: 619–626

Bertrand P V, Butt W R, Crooke A C, Sutaria U D 1976 Analysis of variables in treatment of anovulation with human gonadotrophins. Endocrinologie Experimentale (Bratislava) 10: 271–282

Bishop W, Kalra P S, Fawcett C P, Krulich L, McCann S M, 1972 The effects of hypothalamic lesions on the release of gonadotropins and prolactin in response to estrogen and progesterone treatment in female rats. Endocrinology 91: 1404–1410

Bjersing J 1979 Intraovarian mechanisms of ovulation. Human Ovulation 3: 149–157

Blankstein J, Reyes F I, Winter J S D, Faiman C 1981 Endorphins and the regulation of the human menstrual cycle. Clinical Endocrinology 14: 287–294

Blum I, Bruthis S, Kaufman H 1981 Clinical evaluation of the effects of combined treatment with bromocryptine and spironolactone in two women with the polycystic ovary syndrome. Fertility and Sterility 35: 629–633

Boisselle A, Tremblay R R 1979 New therapeutic approach to the hirsute patient. Fertility and Sterility 32: 276–279

Bomsel-Helmreich O, Marik J, Hulka J F, Papiernik E 1979 Preovulatory morphology and steroid content of follicles. Human Ovulation 3: 121–132

Boyer R M, Finkelstein J W, David R, Roffwarg H, Kapen S, Weitzman E D, Hellman L 1973 Twenty-four hour patterns of plasma luteinizing hormone and follicle stimulating hormone in sexual precocity. New England Journal of Medicine 289: 282–286

Brailly S, Gougeon A, Milgrom E, Bomsel-Helmreich O, Papiernik E 1981 Androgens and progestins in the human ovarian follicle: differences in the evolution of preovulatory, healthy nonovulatory, and atretic follicles. Journal of Clinical Endocrinology Metabolism 53: 128–134

Brawer J R, Naftolin F, Martin J, Sonnenschein C 1978 Effects of a single injection of estradiol valerate on the hypothalamic arcuate nucleus and on reproductive function in the female rat. Endocrinology 103: 501–512

Breteche J 1952 Kystes ovariques et ovarites sclero-cystique dans la sterilite. Bulletin Federation Gynecologie and Obstetrique Francaise 4: 149–153

Burghen G A, Givens J R, Kitabchi A E 1980 Correlation of hyperandrogenism with hyperinsulinism in polycystic ovarian disease. Journal of Clinical Endocrinology Metabolism 50: 113–116

Butt W R, Crooke A C, Cunningham F J, Palmer R 1963 the effect of dexamethasone on the excretion of oestriol and follicle-stimulating

hormone in patients with Stein-Leventhal syndrome. Journal of Endocrinology 26: 303–304

Buttram V C Jr 1979 Surgical treatment of endometriosis in the infertile female: a modified approach. Fertility Sterility 32: 635–640

Buttram V C Jr. Vaquero C 1975 Post-ovarian wedge resection adhesive disease. Fertility Sterility 26: 874–876

Chamlian D L, Taylor H B 1970 Endometrial hyperplasia in young women. Obstetrics and Gynecology 36: 659–666

Chang R J, Jaffe R B 1978 Progesterone effects on gonadotropin release in women pretreated with estradiol. Journal of Clinical Endocrinology Metabolism 47: 119–125

Chang J, Laufer L, Meldrum D, DeFazio J, Lu J 1982 Sex steroid secretion in polycystic ovarian disease following ovarian suppression by a long-acting GnRH agonist. Program of Meeting, Endocrine Society, San Francisco, Abstract #642, p 240

Chang R J, Mandel F P, Lu J K H, Judd H L 1982 Enhanced disparity of gonadotropin secretion by estrone in women with polycystic ovarian disease. Journal of Clinical Endocrinology Metabolism 54: 490–494

Channing C P, Anderson L D, Hoover D J, Kolena J, Osteen K G, Pomerantz S H, Tarrabe K 1982 The role of nonsteroidal regulators in the control of oocyte and follicle maturation. Recent Progress in Hormone Research 38: 331–408

Chari S, Aumuller G, Daume E, Strum G, Hopkinson C 1981 The effects of human follicular fluid inhibin on the morphology of the ovary of the immature rat. Archives of Gynecology 230: 239–245

Cole C, Kitabchi A E 1978 Remission of insulin resistance (IR) with Orthonovum in a patient with polycystic ovarian disease and acanthosis nigricans (PCOD-AN). Clinical Research 26: 412A

Cooper H E, Spellacy W N, Prem K A, Cohen W D 1968 Hereditary factors in the Stein-Leventhal syndrome. American Journal of Obstetrics and Gynecology 100: 371 387

Corenblum B, Taylor P J 1982 An investigation of the hyperprolactinemic/polycystic ovary syndrome. Fertility and Sterility 137: 292–293

Cunningham G R, Goldzieher J W, de la Pena A, Oliver M 1978 The mechanism of ovulation inhibition by triamcinolone acetonide. Journal of Clinical Endocrinology Metabolism 46: 8–14

Darga N C, Reichert L E 1978 Some properties of the interaction of follicle stimulating hormone with bovine granulosa cells and its inhibition by follicular fluid. Biology of Reproduction 19: 235–241

DeJong F H, Sharpe R M 1976 Evidence for inhibin-like activity in bovine follicular fluid. Nature 263: 71–72

Delahunt J W, Clements R V, Ramsay I D, Newton J, Collins W P, Landon J 1975 The monocystic ovary syndrome. British Medical Journal 4: 621–622

Deutsch S, Krumholz B, Benjamin I 1978 The utility and selection of laboratory tests in the diagnosis of polycystic ovary syndrome. Journal of Reproductive Medicine 20: 275–282

DeVane G W, Czekala N M, Judd H L, Yen S S C 1975 Circulating gonadotropins, estrogens, and androgens in polycystic ovarian disease. American Journal of Obstetrics and Gynecology 121: 496–500

DiZerega G S, Turner C K, Stouffer R L, Anderson L D, Channing C P, Hodgen G D 1981 Suppression of follicle-stimulating hormone-dependent folliculogenesis during the primate ovarian cycle. Journal of Clinical Endocrinology Metabolism 52: 451–456

DiZerega G S, Goebelsmann U, Nakamura M 1982 Identification of protein(s) secreted by the preovulatory ovary which suppresses the follicle response to gonadotropins. Journal of Clinical Endocrinology Metabolism 54: 1091–1096

Dorrington J H, Armstrong D T 1979 Effects of FSH on gonadal functions. Recent Progress in Hormone Reserch 35: 301–342

Dorrington J H, Gore-Langton R E 1982 Antigonadal action of prolactin: further studies on the mechanism of inhibition of follicle-stimulating hormone-induced aromatase activity in rat granulosa cell cultures. Endocrinology 110: 1701–1710

Duignan N M, Shaw R W, Rudd B T, Holder G, Williams J W, Butt W R, Logan-Edwards R, London D R 1975 Sex hormone levels and gonadotrophin release in the polycystic ovary syndrome. Clinical Endocrinology 4: 287–295

Eddy W A 1978 Endometrial carcinoma in Stein-Leventhal syndrome treated with hydroxyprogesterone caprote. American Journal of Obstetrics and Gynecology 131: 581–582

Eddy C A, Asch R H, Balmaceda J P 1980 Pelvic adhesions following microsurgical wedge resection of the ovaries. Fertility Sterility 33: 557–561

Edwards R G 1980 Conception in the Human Female, p 290, Academic Press, London

Erickson G F, Hsueh A J W 1978 Secretion of inhibin by rat granulosa cells in vitro. Endocrinology 103: 190–193

Erickson G F, Hsueh A J W, Quigley M E, Rebar R W, Yen S S C 1979 Functional studies of aromatase activity in human granulosa cells from normal and polycystic ovaries. Journal of Clinical Endocrinology Metabolism 49: 514–519

Falaschi P, Del Pozo E, Rocco A, Toscano V, Petrangeli E, Pompei P, Frajese G 1980 Prolactin release in polycystic ovary. Obstetrics and Gynecology 55: 579–582

Farber M, Millan V G, Turksoy R N, Mitchell G W Jr 1978 Diagnostic evaluation of hirsutism in women by selective bilateral adrenal and ovarian venous catheterization. Fertility and Sterility 30: 283–288

Farber M, Madanes A, O'Briain D S, Millan V G, Turksoy R N, Rule A H 1981 Asymmetric hyperthecosis ovarii. Obstetrics and Gynecology 57: 521–525

Fechner R E, Kaufman R H 1974 Endometrial adenocarcinoma in Stein-Leventhal syndrome. Cancer 34: 444–452

Franchimont P, Channing P 1981 Intragonadal Regulation of Reproduction. Academic Press, New York

Frolich M, Vader H L, Walma S T, de Rooy H A 1980 The influence of long-term treatment with cyproterone acetate or a cyproterone acetate-ethynyl estradiol combination on androgen levels in blood of hirsute women. Journal of Steroid Biochemistry 12: 499–502

Futterweit W, Krieger D T 1979 Pituitary tumors associated with hyperprolactinemia and polycystic ovarian disease. Fertility and Sterility 31: 608–613

Gambrell R D Jr 1976 Regression of polycystic ovaries by estrogen therapy. Obstetrics and Gynecology 47: 569–574

Garm, O 1949 A study on bovine nymphomania; with special reference to etiology and pathogenesis. Acta Endocrinologica (suppl 3): 1–144

Genazzani A R, Pintro C, Corda R 1978 Plasma levels of gonadotropins, prolactin, thyroxine, and adrenal and gonadal steroids in obese prepubertal girls. Journal of Clinical Endocrinology Metabolism 47: 974–979

Gibson M, Lackritz R, Schiff I, Tulchinsky D 1980 Abnormal adrenal responses to adrenocorticotropic hormone in hyperandrogenic women. Fertility and Sterility 33: 43–48

Giorgi E P, Addis M, Colombo G 1969 The fate of free and conjugated oestrogens injected into the Graafian follicle of equines. Journal of Endocrinology 45: 37–50

Givens J R, Wiser W L, Coleman S A, Wilroy R S, Andersen R N, Fish S A 1971 Familial ovarian hyperthecosis: a study of two families. American Journal of Obstetrics and Gynecology 110: 959–972

Givens J R, Anderson R N, Wiser W L, Fish S A 1974 Dynamics of suppression and recovery of plasma FSH, LH, androstenedione and testosterone in polycystic ovarian disease using an oral contraceptive. Journal of Clinical Endocrinology Metabolism 38: 727–735

Givens J R, Andersen R N, Ragland J B, Wiser W L, Umstot E S 1975a Adrenal function in hirsutism I. Diurnal change and response of plasma androstenedione, testosterone, 17-hydroxyprogesterone, cortisol, LH and FSH to dexamethasone and 1/2 unit of ACTH. Journal of Clinical Endocrinology Metabolism 40: 988–1000

Givens J R, Andersen R N, Wiser W L, Donelson A J, Coleman S A 1975b A testosterone-secreting, gonadotropin-responsive pure thecoma and polycystic ovarian disease. Journal of Clinical Endocrinology Metabolism 41: 845–853

Givens J R, Andersen R N, Ragland J B, Umstot E S 1976a Effects of norgestrel and metyrapone on pituitary-adrenal-ovarian function. Obstetrics and Gynecology 48: 392–396

Givens J R, Andersen R N, Umstot E S, Wiser W L 1976b Clinical findings and hormonal responses in patients with polycystic ovarian disease with normal versus elevated LH levels. Obstetrics and Gynecology 47: 388–394

Givens J R, Wiedeman E, Andersen R N, Kitabchi A E 1980 β-endorphin and β-lipotropin plasma levels in hirsute women: correlation with body weight. Journal of Clinical Endocrinology Metabolism 50: 975

Goldenberg R L, Vaitukaitis J L, Ross G T 1972 Estrogen and follicle stimulating hormone interactions on follicle growth in rats. Endocrinology 90: 1492–1498

Goldzieher J W 1968 The interplay of adrenocortical and ovarian function. In: Mack H C (ed) The Ovary, pp 106–129 Charles C. Thomas, Springfield

Goldzieher J W, Green J A 1962 The polycystic ovary. I Clinical and histologic features. Journal of Clinical Endocrinology Metabolism 22: 325–338

Goldzieher J W, Axelrod L R 1963 Clinical and biochemical features of polycystic ovarian disease. Fertility and Sterility 14: 631–653

Goldzieher J W, Axelrod L R 1969 Polycystic ovary. In: Rashad M N, Morton W R M (eds) Selected Topics on Genital Anomalies and Related Subjects, pp 642–683. Charles C Thomas, Springfield

Goldzieher J W, de la Pena A, Chenault C B, Cervantes A 1975 Comparative studies of the ethynyl estrogens used in oral contraceptives III. Effect on plasma gonadotropins. American Journal of Obstetrics and Gynecology 122: 625–636

Goldzieher J W, Dozier T S, Smith K D, Steinberger E 1976 Improving the diagnostic reliability of rapidly fluctuating hormone levels by optimized multiple-sampling techniques. Journal of Clinical Endocrinology Metabolism 43: 824–830

Goldzieher J W, Kleber J W, Moses L E, Rathmacher R P 1970 A cross-sectional study of plasma FSH and LH levels in women using sequential, combination or injectable steroid contraceptives over long periods of time. Contraception 2: 225–248

Govan A D T, Black W P 1981 Some observations on the histology of polycystic ovarian disease. In: Coutts J R T (ed) Functional Morphology of the Human Ovary, pp 157–159 University Park Press, Baltimore

Grattarola R 1969 Misdiagnosis of endometrial adenocarcinoma in young women with polycystic ovarian disease. American Journal of Obstetrics and Gynecology 105: 498–502

Green J A, Goldzieher J W 1965 The polycystic ovary IV. Light and electron microscope studies. American Journal of Obstetrics and Gynecology 91: 173–181

Groffman A, Moult P J A, Gaillard R C, Delitala G, Toff W, Rees L H, Besser G M 1981 Opioid control of LH and FSH release: effects of a met-enkephalin analogue and naloxone. Clinical Endocrinology 14: 41–47

Gual C, Scaglia H E, Midgley R A Jr, Alcocer J, Echeverria-Rivas Y, Lichtenberg R 1975 Regulatory effects of steroids on the pituitary response to LH RH. Journal of Steroid Biochemistry 6: 1067–1074

Guzick D S, Rock J A 1981 Estimation of a model of cumulative pregnancy following infertility therapy. American Journal of Obstetrics and Gynecology 140: 573–578

Gyory G, Kiss C, Feher T, Poteczin E 1975 Concentration of unconjugated adrenogenic hormones and their precursors in normal and polycystic ovaries. Endokrinologie 64: 181–190

Hagino N, Goldzieher J W 1970 Effect of timing and quantity of estrogen on gonadotropin-induced ovulation in immature rats. Endocrinology 86: 29–23

Hagino N, Goldzieher J W 1975 The effect of testosterone and other adrenal steroids on PMS-induced ovulation in the immature rat. Neuroendocrinology 17: 27–39

Harman S M, Louvet J P, Ross G T 1975 Interaction of estrogen and gonadotropins on follicular atresia. Endocrinology 96: 1145–1152

Hillier S G 1981 A consideration of the roles of C 19 steroid aromatase and 5alpha reductase enzymic activities in the local control of follicular development in the human ovary. In: Coutts J R T (ed) Functional Morphology of the Human Ovary pp 94–100 University Park Press, Baltimore

Hillier S G, van de Boogaard A M J, van Hall E V 1979 5 Alpha-reduced androgen metabolites competitively inhibit aromatization of testosterone by isolated granulosa cells in vitro. Endocrine Society, 61st Annual Meeting, Anaheim, California. Program and Abstract #194 p 121

Hillier S G, van den Boogaard A M J, Reichert L E Jr 1980 Intraovarian sex steroid hormone interactions and the regulation of follicular maturation, aromatization of androgens by human granulosa cells in vitro. Journal of Clinical Endocrinology Metabolism 50: 640–647

Hirschowitz J, Soler N G, Wortsman J 1968 Hypersuppression of LH in the management of the polycystic ovary syndrome. Endocrine Society, 60th Annual Meeting, Miami, Florida. Abstract 847 p 50

Horton R, Hawks D, Lobo R 1982 3 alpha, 17 beta androstanediol glucuronide in plasma. A marker of androgen action in idiopathic hirsutism. Journal of Clinical Investigation 69: 1203–1206

Hunzicker-Dunn M, Birnbaumer L 1976 Adenylyl cyclase activities in ovarian tissues III. Regulation of responsiveness to LH, FSH and PGE$_1$ in prepubertal, cycling, pregnant and pseudopregnant rats. Endocrinology 99: 198–210

Jafari K, Javaheri G, Ruiz G 1978 Endometrial adenocarcinoma and the Stein-Leventhal syndrome. Obstetrics and Gynecology 51: 97–100

Jaffee W, Russell V, Longcope C, Vaitukaitis J 1978 Hyperprolactinemia among women with polycystic ovary syndrome, Endocrine Society, 60th Annual Meeting, Miami, Florida, Program and Abstracts (71) p 110

Johansson E D B, Wide L, Gemzell C 1971 Luteinizing hormone (LH) and progesterone in plasma and LH and oestrogens in urine during 42 normal menstrual cycles. Acta Endocrinologica 68: 502–512

Johnson J F Jr 1967 Outcome of pregnancies following clomiphene citrate therapy. In: Westin B, Wiqvist N (eds) Proceedings of the 5th World Congress of Fertility Sterility Amsterdam, Excerpta Medica Findings p 101.

Jones P B C and Hsueh A J W 1982 Regulation of ovarian 3 beta-hydroxysteroid dehydrogenase activity by gonadotropin-releasing hormone and follicle-stimulating hormone in cultured rat granulosa cells. Endocrinology 110: 1663–1671

Judd H L, Rigg L A, Anderson D C, Yen S S C 1976 The effects of ovarian wedge resection on circulating gonadotropin and ovarian steroid levels in patients with polycystic ovary syndrome. Journal of Clinical Endocrinology and Metabolism 43: 347–355

Kahn C R, Flier J S, Bar R S, Archer J A, Gorden P, Martin M M, Roth J 1976 The syndromes of insulin resistance and acanthosis nigricans. Insulin-receptor disorders in man. New England Journal of Medicine 294: 739–745

Kamrava M M, Seibel, M M, Berger M J, Thompson I, Taymor M L 1982 Reversal of persistent anovulation in polycystic ovarian disease by administration of chronic low-dose follicle-stimulating hormone. Fertility and Sterility 37: 520–523

Kandeel F R, Butt W R, London D R, Lynch S S, Logan-Edwards R, Rudd B T 1978 Oestrogen amplification of LH-RH response in the polycystic ovary syndrome and response to clomiphene. Clinical Endocrinology 9: 429–441

Kaplan S A, Nakamura R, Chang J 1982 Insulin resistance in nonobese patients with polycystic ovarian disease. Endocrine Society, 64th Annual Meeting, San Francisco, California, Program and Abstract # 1011 p 332

Katz M, Carr P J 1976 Abnormal luteinizing hormone response patterns to synthetic gonadotrophin releasing hormone in patients with polycystic ovarian syndrome. Journal of Endocrinology 70: 163–171

Katz M, Carr P J, Cohen B M, Millar R P 1978 Hormonal effects of wedge resection of polycystic ovaries. Obstetrics and Gynecology 51: 437–444

Kauppila A, Leinonen P, Vihko R, Ylostalo P 1982 Metoclopramide-induced hyperprolactinemia impairs ovarian follicle maturation and corpus luteum function in women. Journal of Clinical Endocrinology and Metabolism 54: 955–960

Kemeter P, Friedrich F, Breitenecker G 1979 Endocrine profile of preovulatory follicular fluid and blood. Human Ovulation 3: 133–148

Kemmann E, Tavakoli F, Shelden R M, Jones J R 1981 Induction of ovulation with menotropins in women with polycystic ovary syndrome. American Journal of Obstetrics and Gynecology 141: 58–64

Kim M H, Rosenfield R L, Hosseinian A H, Schneir H G 1979 Ovarian hyperandrogenism with normal and abnormal histologic findings of the ovaries. American Journal of Obstetrics and Gynecology 134: 445–452

Kirschner M A, Jacobs J B 1971 Combined ovarian and adrenal vein catheterization to determine the site of androgen overproduction in hirsute women. Journal of Clinical Endocrinology Metabolism 33: 199–209

Koritnik D R, Rotten J, Serron-Ferre M, Laherty R F, Jaffe R B 1980 Does LH stimulate dehydroepiandrosterone sulfate secretion in the neonatal monkey? Endocrine Society, 62nd Annual Meeting, Washington DC, Program and Abstracts 164 p 115

Laatikainen T J, Apter D L, Paavonen J A, Wahlstrom T R 1980 Steroids in ovarian and peripheral venous blood in polycystic ovarian disease. Clinical Endocrinology 13: 125

Lachelin G C L, Barnett M, Hopper B R, Brink G, Yen S S C 1979 Adrenal function in normal women and women with the polycystic ovary syndrome. Journal of Clinical Endocrinology and Metabolism 49: 892–898

Ledwitz-Rigby F, Rigby B W, Gay V L, Stetson M, Young J, Channing C P 1977 Inhibitory action of porcine follicular fluid upon granulosa cell luteinization in vitro: assay and influence of follicular maturation. Journal of Endocrinology 74: 175–184

Legros J J, Coomans C, Lecomte R, Sulon J, Franchimont P 1975 The relation between the release of pituitary LH under the influence of LRH and the level of plasma testosterone in women. Comptes Rendus Societe Biologique 169: 1644–1647

Leung P C K, Armstrong D T 1980 Interactions of steroids and gonadotropins in the control of steroidogenesis in the ovarian follicle. Annual Review of Physiology 42: 71–101

Lisse K, Schurenkamper P, Friedrich W, Rutkowsky J 1980 Diurnal change of serum androstenedione and testosterone and response to hCG and dexamethasone in women with polycystic ovaries, adrenal hyperandrogenism and unexplained hirsutism. Acta Endocrinologica 93: 216–222

Lobo R A, Goebelsmann U 1980 Adult manifestation of congenital adrenal hyperplasia due to incomplete 21-hydroxylase deficiency mimicking polycystic ovarian disease. American Journal of Obstetrics and Gynecology 138: 720–726

Lobo R A, Goebelsmann U 1981 Evidence for reduced 3 beta-ol-hydroxysteroid dehydrogenase activity in some hirsute women thought to have polycystic ovary syndrome. Journal of Clinical Endocrinology and Metabolism 53: 394–400

Lobo R A, Granger L, Goebelsmann U, Mishell D R Jr 1981 Elevations in unbound serum estradiol as a possible mechanism for inappropriate gonadotropin secretion in women with PCO. Journal of Clinical Endocrinology and Metabolism 52: 156–158

Lobo R A, Kletzky O A, DiZerega G S 1982 Elevated serum bioactive LH concentrations in women with PCO. Fertility and Sterility 37: 301–302

Lorber D L, McKenna T J, Rabinowitz D 1978 Plasma pregnenolone and 17-OH-pregnenolone in hirsute amenorrhoeic patients. Acta Endocrinologica 87: 566–576

Louvet J P, Harman S M, Schreiber J R, Ross G T 1975 Evidence for a role of androgens in follicular maturation. Endocrinology 97: 366–372

Louvet J P, Vaitukaitis J L 1976 Induction of follicle-stimulating hormone (FSH) receptors in rat ovaries by estrogen priming. Endocrinology 100: 128–133

Mahesh V B 1980 Current concepts of the pathophysiology of the polycystic ovary syndrome. In: Tozzini R I, Reeves G, Pineda R L (eds) Endocrine Physiopathology of the Ovary pp 275–294 Elsevier/North-Holland Biomedical Press, Amsterdam

Mahesh V B, Toledo S P A, Mattar E 1978 Hormone levels following wedge resection in polycystic ovary syndrome. Obstetrics and Gynecology 51: 64s–69s

Makris A, Ryan K J 1980 The source of follicular androgens in the hamster follicle. Steroids 35: 53–64

March C M, Goebelsmann U, Nakamura R M, Mishell D R Jr 1979 Roles of estradiol and progesterone in eliciting the midcycle luteinizing hormone and follicle-stimulating hormone surges. Journal of Clinical Endocrinology and Metabolism 49: 507–513

Marder M L, Channing C P, Schwartz N B 1977 Suppression of serum follicle stimulating hormone in intact and acutely ovariectomized rats by porcine follicular fluid. Endocrinology 101: 1639–1642

Maschler I, Salzberger M, Finkelstein M 1976 Ovarian enzymatic divergence in patients with polycystic ovary syndrome excreting urinary pregnanetriolone. Acta Endocrinologica 82: 366–379

Mathur R S, Moody L O, Landgrebe S, Williamson H O 1981 Plasma androgens and sex hormone-binding globulin in the evaluation of hirsute females. Fertility and Sterility 35: 29–35

McArthur J W, Ingersoll F M, Worcester J 1958 The urinary excretion of interstitial-cell and follicle-stimulating hormone activity by women with disease of the reproductive system. Journal of Clinical Endocrinology and Metabolism 18: 1202–1215

McDonald T W, Malkasian G D, Gaffey T A 1977 Endometrial cancer associated with feminizing ovarian tumor and polycystic ovarian disease. Obstetrics and Gynecology 49: 654–658

McDonough P G, Mahesh V B, Ellegood J O 1972 Steroid, follicle-stimulating hormone, and luteinizing hormone profiles in identical twins with polycystic ovaries. American Journal of Obstetrics and Gynecology 113: 1072–1078

McGoogan L S 1954 Sterility and ovarian pathology. Obstetrics and Gynecology 3: 254–262

McNatty K P 1979 Relationship between plasma prolactin and the endocrine microenvironment of the developing human antral follicle. Fertility and Sterility 32: 433–438

McNatty K P, Sawers R S 1975 Relationship between the endocrine environment within the Graafian follicle and the subsequent rate of progesterone secretion by human granulosa cells in vitro. Journal of Endocrinology 66: 391–400

McNatty K P, Henderson K M, Sawers R S 1975 Effects of prostaglandin F_2 and E_2 on the production of progesterone by human granulosa cells in tissue culture. Journal of Endocrinology 67: 231–240

McNatty K P, Makris A, DeGrazia C, Osathanondh R, Ryan K J 1979a The production of progesterone, androgens and estrogens by granulosa cells, thecal tissue, and stromal tissue from human ovaries in vitro. Journal of Clinical Endocrinology 49: 687–699

McNatty K P, Makris A, Reinhold V N, DeGrazia C, Osathanondh R, Ryan K J 1979b Metabolism of androstenedione by human ovarian tissues in vitro with particular reference to reductase and aromatase activity. Steroids 34: 429–443

McNatty K P, Mooresmith D, Makris A, Osathanondh R, Ryan K J 1979c The microenvironment of the human antral follicle: interrelationships among the steroid levels in antral fluid, population of granulosa cells, and the status of the oocyte in vivo and in vitro. Journal of Clinical Endocrinology Metabolism 49: 851–860

McNatty K P, Smith D M, Makris A, Osathanondh R, Ryan K J 1979 The microenvironment of the human antral follicle: interrelationships among the steroid levels in antral fluid, the population of granulosa cells, and the status of the oocyte in vivo and in vitro. Journal of Clinical Endocrinology and Metabolism 49: 851–860

McNatty K P, Smith D M, Makris A, De Grazia C, Tulchinsky D, Osathanondh R, Schiff I, Ryan K J 1980 The intraovarian sites of androgen and estrogen formation in women with normal and hyperandrogenic ovaries as judged by in vitro experiments. Journal of Clinical Endocrinology and Metabolism 50: 755–759

Mennin S P, Gorski R A 1975 Effects of ovarian steroids on plasma LH in normal and persistent estrous adult female rats. Endocrinology 96: 486–491

Merrill J A 1963 The morphology of the prepubertal ovary: relationship to the polycystic ovary syndrome. Southern Medical Journal 56: 225–229

Mondschein J S, Schomber D W 1981 Growth factors modulate gonadotropin receptor induction in granulosa cell cultures. Science 211: 1179–1181

Moon Y S, Tsand B K, Simpson C, Armstrong D T 1978 17 beta-estradiol biosynthesis in cultured granulosa and theca cells of human ovarian follicles: stimulation by follicle-stimulating hormone. Journal of Clinical Endocrinology Metabolism 47: 263–267

Morris J M, Scully R E 1958 Endocrine Pathology of the Human Ovary p 42 Mosby, St. Louis

Mortimer R H, Lev-Gur M, Freeman R, Fleischer N 1978 Pituitary response to bolus and continuous intravenous infusion of luteinizing hormone-releasing factor in normal women and women with polycystic ovarian syndrome. American Journal of Obstetrics and Gynecology 130: 630–634

Mossman H W, Koering M J, Ferry D J 1964 Cyclic changes of interstitial gland tissue of the human ovary. American Journal of Anatomy 115: 235–255

Nebel L, Safriel O J, Salzberger M, Finkelstein M 1971 coelomic mesotheliumlike cells in the ovarian stroma of patients with the polycystic ovary syndrome (Stein-Leventhal syndrome). American Journal of Obstetrics and Gynecology 111: 766–772

Netter A, Bloch-Michel H, Salomon Y, Thervet F, Grouchy J de, Lamy M 1961 Study of karyotype in Stein-Leventhal syndrome. Annals of Endocrinology 22: 841–849

Nimrod A, Lindner H R 1976 A synergistic effect of androgen on the stimulation of progesterone secretion by FSH in cultured rat granulosa cells. Molecular Cellular Endocrinology 5: 315–320

Parker L, Odell W 1977 Control of adrenal androgen secretion by a new pituitary factor: cortical androgen stimulating hormone (CASH). Clinical Research 25: 299A

Parker R, Ming P L, Rajan R, Goodner D M, Reme G 1980 Clinical and cytogenetic studies of patients with polycystic ovarian disease. American Journal of Obstetrics and Gynecology 137: 656–660

Patton W C, Berger M J,,Thompson I E, Chong A P, Grimes E M, Taymor M L 1975 Pituitary gonadotropin response to synthetic luteinizing hormone-releasing hormone in patients with typica and atypical polycystic ovary disease. American Journal of Obstetrics and Gynecology 121: 382–386

Quigley M E, Rakoff J S, Yen S S C 1981 Increased luteinizing hormone sensitivity to dopamine inhibition in polycystic ovary syndrome. Journal of Clinical Endocrinology and Metabolism 52: 231–234

Raj S G, Thompson I E, Berger M J, Taymor M L 1977 Clinical aspects of the polycystic ovary syndrome. Obstetrics and Gynecology 49: 552–556

Raj S G, Thompson I E, Berger M J, Talbert L M, Taymor M L 1978 Diagnostic value of androgen measurements in polycystic ovary syndrome. Obstetrics and Gynecology 52: 169–171

Raj S G, Raj H G M, Talbert L M, Sloan C, Hicks B 1981 Normalization of plasma testosterone levels by a low estrogen oral contraceptive in polycystic ovary disease. Endocrine Society, 63rd Annual Meeting, Cincinnati, Ohio, Program and Abstracts 452

Rajaniemi H J, Ronnberg L, Kauppila A, Ylostalo P, Vihko R 1980 Luteinizing hormone receptors in ovarian follicles of patients with polycystic ovarian disease. Journal of Clinical Endocrinology Metabolism 51: 1054–1057

Rao M C, Richards J S, Midgley A R Jr, Reichert L E Jr 1977 Regulation of gonadotropin receptors by LH in granulosa cells. Endocrinology 101: 512–523

Rao M D, Richards J S, Midgley A R Jr 1978 Hormonal regulation of cell proliferation in the ovary. Cell 14: 71–78

Rebar R, Judd H L, Yen S S C, Rakoff J, Vandenberg G, Naftolin F 1976 Characterization of the inappropriate gonadotropin secretion in polycystic ovary syndrome. Journal of Clinical Investigations 57: 1320–1329

Rebar R W, Harman S M, Vaitukaitis J L 1978 Differential responsiveness to LRF after estrogen therapy in women with hypothalamic amenorrhea. Journal of Clinical Endocrinology and Metabolism 46: 48–54

Reichert L E, Abou-Issa H 1977 Studies on a low molecular weight testicular factor which inhibits binding of FSH to receptor. Biology of Reproduction 17: 614–621

Resko J A, Ellinwood W E, Knobil E 1981 Differential effects of progesterone on secretion of gonadotropic hormones in the rhesus monkey. American Journal of Physiology 240: 489E

Richards J S 1975 Content of nuclear estradiol receptor complex in rat granulosa cells during follicular development: modification by estradiol and gonadotropins. Endocrinology 97: 1174–1184

Richards J S 1978 Hormonal control of follicular growth and maturation in mammals. In: Jones R E (ed) The Vertebrate Ovary pp 331–360 Plenum Press, New York

Richards J S, Midgley A R Jr 1976 Protein hormone action: a key to understanding ovarian follicular and luteal cell development. Biology of Reproduction 14: 82–94

Roberts D W T, Haines M 1960 Is there a Stein-Leventhal syndrome? British Medical Journal 2: 1709–1710

Rodriguez-Rigau L J, Smith K D, Tcholakian R K, Steinberger E 1979 Effect of prednisone on plasma testosterone levels and on duration of phases of the menstrual cycle in hyperandrogenic women. Fertility and Sterility 32: 408–413

Ropert J F, Quigley M E, Yen S S C 1981 Endogenous opiates

modulate pulsatile luteinizing hormone release in humans. Journal of Clinical Endocrinology and Metabolism 52: 583–585

Ross G T, Lipsett M B 1978 Hormonal correlates of normal and abnormal follicle growth after puberty in humans and other primates. Clinics in Endocrinology and Metabolism 7: 561–575

Sanyal M K, Berger M J, Thompson I E, Taymor M L, Horne H W Jr 1974 Development of Graafian follicles in adult human ovary. I. Correlation of estrogen and progesterone concentration in antral fluid with growth of follicles. Journal of Clinical Endocrinology Metabolism 38: 828–835

Schneider G, Genel M, Bongiovanni A M, Goldman A S, Rosenfield R L 1975 Persistent testicular delta 5-isomerase-3 beta-hydroxysteroid dehydrogenase (delta 5–3 beta HSD) deficiency in the delta 5–3 beta-HSD form of congenital adrenal hyperplasia. Journal of Clinical Investigation 55: 681–690

Schoemaker J, Wentz A C, Jones G S, Dubin N H 1978 Stimulation of follicular growth with 'pure' FSH in patients with anovulation and elevated LH levels. Obstetrics and Gynecology 51: 270–277

Schreiber J R, Reid R, Ross G T 1976 A receptor-like testosterone-binding protein in ovaries from estrogen-stimulated hypophysectomized immature female rats. Endocrinology 98: 1206–1213

Schwartz N B, Channing C P 1977 Evidence for ovarian inhibin suppression of the secondary rise in serum follicle stimulating hormone levels in procstrus rats by injection of porcine follicular fluid Proceedings of the National Academy of Sciences of the USA 74: 5721–5724

Shapiro A G 1981 Pituitary adenoma, menstrual disturbance, hirsutism and abnormal glucose tolerance. Fertility and Sterility 35: 226–229

Shaw R W, Duignan N M, Butt W R, Logan-Edwards R, London D R 1975 Hypothalamic-pituitary relationships in the polycystic ovary syndrome, serum gonadotrophin levels following injection of oestradiol benzoate. British Journal of Obstetrics and Gynaecology 82: 952–957

Shaw R W, Duignan N M, Butt W R, Logan-Edwards R, London D R 1976 Modification by sex steroids of LH-RH response in the polycystic ovary syndrome. Clinical Endocrinology 5: 495–502

Smith K D, Steinberger E, Perloff W H 1965 Polycystic ovarian disease (PCO). A report of 301 patients. American Journal of Obstetrics and Gynecology 93: 994–1001

Smith K D, Rodriguez-Rigau L J, Tcholakian R K, Steinberger E 1979a The relation between plasma testosterone levels and the lengths of phases of the menstrual cycle. Fertility Sterility 32: 403–407

Smith R G, Besch P K, Dill B, Buttram V C Jr 1979b Saliva as a matrix for measuring free androgens: comparison with serum androgens in polycystic ovarian disease. Fertility and Sterility 31: 513–517

Sommers S C, Wadman P J 1956 Pathogenesis of polycystic ovaries. American Journal of Obstetrics and Gynecology 72: 160–169

Steinberger E, Rodriguez-Rigau L J, Smith K D 1982 The prognostic value of acute adrenal suppression and stimulation tests in hyperandrogenic women. Fertility and Sterility 37: 187–192

Stevens V C, Goldzieher J W 1968 Urinary excretion of gonadotropins in congenital adrenal hyperplasia. Pediatrics 41: 421–427

Symonds D A, Driscoll S G 1973 An adrenal cortical rest within the fetal ovary: report of a case. American Journal of Clinical Pathology 60: 562–564

Tamada T, Matsumoto S 1969 Suppression of ovulation with human chorionic gonadotropin. Fertility and Sterility 20: 840–848

Tanaka T, Fujimoto S, Kutsozawa T 1978 The effect of ovarian wedge resection and incision on circulating gonadotropin in patients with polycystic ovarian disease. International Journal of Fertility 23: 93–99

Taymor M L, Berger M J, Thompson I E, Karam S K 1972 Hormonal factors in human ovulation. American Journal of Obstetrics and Gynecology 114: 445–453

Toaff R, Toaff M E, Peyser M R 1976 Infertility following wedge resection of the ovaries. American Journal of Obstetrics and Gynecology 124: 92–96

Tsafrir A, Channing C P 1975 An inhibitory influence of granulosa cells and follicular fluid upon porcine oocyte meiosis in vitro. Endocrinology 96: 922–927

Valkov I M, Dokumov S I 1977 Effect of ovarian wedge resection for the Stein-Leventhal syndrome on plasma FSH, LH, oestradiol and testosterone levels and on the responses of the pituitary to intravenous LH-RH. British Journal of Obstetrics and Gynaecology 84: 539–542

Valkov I M, Dokumov S I 1977 Plasma follicle-stimulating and luteinizing hormones and the macroscopic characteristics of the ovaries in patients with Stein-Leventhal syndrome. Response to LH-RH in Stein-Leventhal syndrome. Endokrinologie 15: 55–58

Vara P, Niemineva K 1951 Small cystic degeneration of ovaries as incidental finding in gynecological laparotomies. Acta Obstetrics and Gynecologica Scandinavica 31: 94–107

Vasquez S B, Sotos J F, Kim M H 1982 Massive edema of the ovary and virilization. Obstetrics and Gynecology 59: 95S–98S

Vejisted H, Albrechtsen R 1976 Biochemical and clinical effects of ovarian wedge resection in the polycystic ovary syndrome. Obstetrics and Gynecology 47: 575–580

Vierhapper H, Waldhausl W, Nowotny P 1979 Gonadotrophin-release upon intravenous administration of a long-acting analogue of luteinizing hormone-releasing hormone in females with increased plasma-androgens. Acta Endocrinologica 91: 577–590

Vigersky R A, Loriaux D L 1976 An androgen binding protein in the cyst fluid of patients with polycystic ovary syndrome. Journal of Clinical Endocrinology Metabolism 43: 817–823

Vigersky R A, Mehlman I, Glass A R, Smith C E 1980 Treatment of hirsute women with cimetidine. New England Journal of Medicine 303: 1042

Wajchenberg B L, Achando S S, Peixoto S, Cszeresnia C, Okada H, Lima S S 1981 Peripheral, ovarian and adrenal vein androgen dynamics in polycystic ovary syndrome. Endocrine Society, 63rd Annual Meeting, Cincinnati, Ohio, Program and Abstracts #1083

Wang C F, Gemzell C R 1980 The use of human gonadotropins for the induction of ovulation in women with polycystic ovarian disease. Fertility and Sterility 33: 479–486

Welschen R, Hermans W P, Dullaart J, DeJong F H 1977 Effect of an inhibin-like factor present in bovine and porcine follicular fluid on gonadotropin levels in hypophysectomized rats. Journal of Reproduction and Fertility 50: 129–131

Wentz A C, Jones G S, Sapp K 1976 Pulsatile gonadotropin output in menstrual dysfunction. Obstetrics and Gynecology 47: 309–318

Wentz A C, White R I Jr, Migcon C J, Hsu T H, Barnes H V, Jones G S 1976 Differential ovarian and adrenal vein catheterization. American Journal of Obstetrics and Gynecology 125: 1000–1007

Williams R F, Hodgen G D 1980 Disparate effects of human chorionic gonadotropin during the late follicular phase in monkeys: normal ovulation, follicular atresia, ovarian acyclicity, and hypersecretion of follicle-stimulating hormone. Fertility and Sterility 33: 64–68

Wilson E A, Erickson G F, Zarutski P, Finn A E, Tulchinsky D, Ryan K J 1979 Endocrine studies of normal and polycystic ovarian tissues in vitro. American Journal of Obstetrics and Gynecology 134: 56–63

Wortsman J, Hirschowitz J S 1980 Galactorrhea and hyperprolactinemia during treatment of polycystic ovary syndrome. Obstetrics and Gynecology 55: 460–463

Wortsman J, Singh K B, Murphy J 1981 Evidence for the hypothalamic origin of the polycystic ovary syndrome. Obstetrics and Gynecology 58: 137–141

Yen S S C, Chaney C, Judd H L 1976 Functional aberrations of the hypothalamic-pituitary system in polycystic ovary syndrome: a consideration of the pathogenesis. Proceedings of the Serono Symposium 7: 373–385

Ying S Y, Guillemin R 1980 Gonadocrinins: Peptides in ovarian follicular fluid stimulating the secretion of pituitary gonadotropins, of the Endocrine Society, 62nd Annual Meeting, Washington DC, Program and Abstracts #158 p 114

Yuzpe A A, Rioux J E 1975 The value of laparoscopic ovarian biopsy. Journal of Reproductive Medicine 15: 57–59

Zarate A, Canales E S, De la Cruz A, Soria J, Schally A V 1973 Pituitary response to synthetic LH-RH in Stein-Leventhal syndrome and functional amenorrhea. Obstetrics and Gynecology 41: 803–808

Zeleznik A J, Midgley A R Jr, Reichert L E Jr 1974 Granulosa cell maturation in the rat: increasing binding of human chorionic gonadotropin following treatment with FSH in vivo. Endocrinology 95: 818–825

Ian D. Cooke

Hirsutism and virilism

Hirsutism is the occurrence of increased hair growth in women in areas where it does not usually occur. This involves the beard area, the chest, the upper parts of the back, abdomen, the insides of the thighs and the dorsal areas of the toes, but beard hairs are almost always found. There may be just a few terminal hairs or almost a full beard. The hirsutism is a result of increased circulating androgens acting on the hair follicles and may be associated with greater activity of the pilosebaceous unit resulting in addition in seborrhoea and acne vulgaris.

Virilism is a more extreme form of the above where the effects of hyperandrogenaemia result in menstrual disturbance and ultimately increased clitoral growth, deepening of the voice and increased muscularity of the female with an altered body fat deposition pattern leading to a more male phenotype.

PLASMA ANDROGENS

During puberty, the androgens androstenedione and testosterone increase about five-fold to the levels found in the follicular phase of an ovulatory cycle. In the early part of the cycle both steroids are secreted equally from each ovary. During the late follicular phase the ovary containing the dominant follicle secretes much more androstenedione and oestradiol than that of the contralateral side and in the luteal phase again androstenedione is secreted significantly but to a lesser extent than in the pre-ovulatory phase. Androstenedione and testosterone are interconverted in both theca cells, whence it appears in the ovarian vein blood, and in the granulosa cells, whence it diffuses into the follicular fluid and after transport from theca to granulosa cells is aromatised into oestradiol (McNatty et al, 1976). In addition, the stroma produces both androgens into postmenopausal life.

In the male testosterone concentrations are 10–30 times higher than in the female in whom normally about 25 per cent comes from the ovaries, 25 per cent the adrenals and apart from direct secretion about 50 per cent from the

peripheral conversion of androstenedione in liver, skin and lungs. Androstenedione concentrations may normally be twice as high in the female as in the male. Other androgens are of relatively minor importance in the female as only about 0.5 per cent of the daily production of testosterone is derived from dehydroepiandrosterone (DHA) and only about 0.02 per cent from Δ^5 androstenediol (Kirschner et al, 1973).

In idiopathic hirsutism, age (puberty and menopause), race and heredity may play a role in determining the degree of increased hair growth but elevated plasma testosterone and/or androstenedione have always been found. The production rate (metabolic clearance rate × plasma concentration) for testosterone in idiopathic hirsutism is two or three times higher than in a healthy woman. It is now generally assumed that the increased formation of testosterone and its precursor androstenedione arise from the ovary and not the adrenal cortex as well as from increased peripheral conversion (Kirschner et al, 1976) but many American studies still show quite a large proportion of cases of idiopathic hirsutism attributed to excess adrenal production (see later).

Androgens circulate bound to plasma proteins which then have regulatory as well as transport functions. Albumen constitutes 60 per cent of plasma proteins but binds only 20 per cent of testosterone in women. Sex hormone binding globulin (SHBG) binds oestrogens and androgens and in the female binds 78 per cent of testosterone. Hirsute women have reduced SHBG values irrespective of the cause of the increased biologically active testosterone, which only amounts to 1 per cent in the normal state (Wagner, 1978). SHBG is also low in hypothyroidism. Testosterone is activated peripherally by the enzyme 5-α-reductase (3-oxo-5-α steroid Δ^4 hydrogenase) in androgen-dependent tissue to form dihydrotestosterone on the intracellular endoplasmic reticulum (Fig. 21.1). The dihydrotestosterone is then thought to be bound to a unique steroid-binding effector protein termed a receptor and the steroid-receptor complex formed in the cytoplasm migrates into the nucleus where it exerts various influences

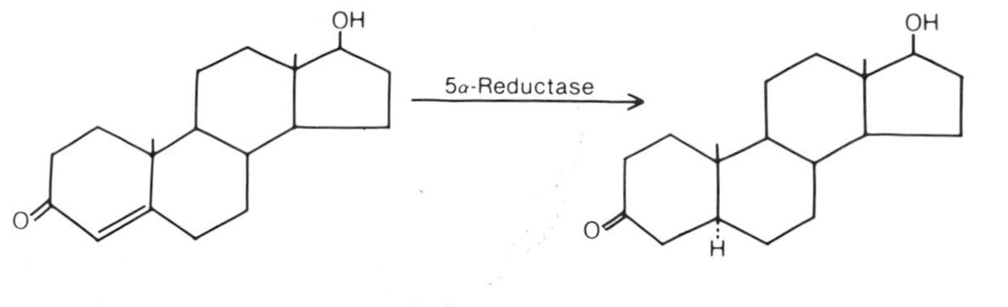

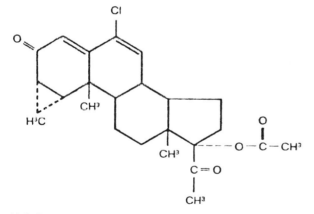

Fig. 21.1 The conversion of testosterone to dihydrotestosterone (DHT) takes place under the influence of the enzyme 5-α reductase

on the properties of DNA including its transcription by RNA polymerase. By inducing protein synthesis, messenger RNA effects the androgenic response. Anti-androgen to be effective must reduce the concentration of effective dihydrotestosterone (DHT) in tissue by 90 per cent. Cyproterone acetate (Fig. 21.2) probably exerts its effect by acting as a competitive inhibitor of the binding of DHT to androgen receptors. Receptor translocation to the nucleus is prevented and the nuclear concentration of free DHT is reduced (Bruchovsky, 1980). Dihydrotestosterone (which also circulates in the plasma at about half the plasma testosterone concentration) binds to SHBG about three times more strongly than testosterone and is not bound to transcortin so it is preferred as the ligand for assay of SHBG. Radiolabelled DHT is equilibrated with the unknown SHBG sample in plasma and the result expressed as nmol DHT bound/litre.

Fig. 21.2 Cyproterone acetate

THE PILOSEBACEOUS UNIT

With respect to endocrine responses of hair follicles, *sexual hair* — such as that occurring in the beard area in the male — is dependent on plasma androgen levels. *Ambisexual hair* — such as that occurring in women in the axilla and in the lower pubic triangle — has its growth stimulated by plasma androgen levels and *non-sexual* hair — e.g. the eyebrows — is independent of the effect of androgens.

Hair growth in follicles is not continuous but is a cyclic process consisting of three different phases. The growth phase, or anagen, is associated with the largest follicle size and a bulbous cleft base to the hair, the root sheaths being quite large. The regression phase, or catagen, features a reduction in the size of the follicle and its sheath and the end embedded in the skin becomes more rounded and club-shaped. The final phase of the cycle is telogen or the resting phase when the whole sheath is very small and just an epithelial sac and the proximal end is also club-shaped, the latter two giving rise to the term 'club' hairs when extracted hairs are inspected.

Paradoxically androgens may not only stimulate hair growth as in hirsutism but can also cause hair loss and baldness in persons with an appropriate genetic disposition. However, in the female alopecia occurs predominantly in the parietal region and male-type baldness in the female requires extremely high plasma testosterone concentrations (Ludwig, 1977).

Hair root steroid metabolism has been examined in anagen and telogen and significantly more DHT is formed in regions with incipient baldness than in other scalp areas and is thought to be aetiologically related. This is due to increased 5-α-reductase activity and may be shown by incubation with androstenedione of hair roots from all areas of the male and female body (Schweikert & Wilson, 1974). Aromatisation to oestrogen is also possible but the role of oestrogens in hair growth is not clear.

Hair follicles may also be divided into three other categories depending on the hair rudiment and the size of the sebaceous glands. Vellus hair, which replaces the embryo's lanugo hair, is fine and non-pigmented and following the rise of plasma androgens at puberty changes to terminal hair which is coarse and pigmented in the areas of sexual hair distribution. At puberty the sebaceous glands develop; they have a relatively small hair rudiment, large lobulated sebaceous gland acini and a wide infundibulum connecting the acini with the exterior, filled with horn cell material. These sebaceous follicles are particularly numerous in the face, in the V-shape on the back, on the upper part of the chest and the first third of the upper arms (Luderschmidt, 1980).

The amount of sebum secreted can be estimated by absorbing it from a carefully defined area on the forehead (10 cm²) on cigarette papers, eluting the lipid with organic solvent and then weighing it (Strauss & Pochi, 1961). As sebaceous glands are androgen-dependent, sebum produced can be shown to be at least doubled to a mean of 2.6 mg.10 cm^{-2}.3 h^{-1} (Ebling et al, 1977) in patients with idiopathic hirsutism.

Acne vulgaris is not an endocrine disease but a hormone-influenced skin disease. All patients with acne vulgaris do not have elevated plasma testosterone activity but probably an increase in follicle 5-α-reductase activity. Certainly testosterone and dihydrotestosterone stimulate increased sebum production but the characteristic lesion of acne is excessive keratinisation of the infra-infundibulum and solid cohesion of the horny cell masses leading to retention hyperkeratosis producing the comedo. Primarily anaerobic *Corynebacteria* settle in the lower levels of the excretory ducts and free fatty acids are split from the triglycerides by their lipases. In the higher levels of the ducts, aerobic coagulase negative *Staphylococci* settle. It takes 2–3 weeks for these changes to occur.

Oestrogens inhibit sebum production and the anti-androgen cyproterone acetate inhibits sebocyte proliferation but not when used topically. It is also presumed to have an effect in reducing the disturbed keratinisation of the infra-infundibulum hence by this combined action reducing sebum production and acne.

ANTI-ANDROGENS

The management of hirsutism has been strikingly influenced by the introduction of anti-androgens. The pharmacology of the most effective, cyproterone acetate, has been reviewed by Neumann et al (1980). A pharmacokinetic study in the human has shown that the 50 mg tablet is absorbed completely when given orally having a second phase half-life of 1.5 h and achieving a maximum plasma

level of 690 nmol/l after 3.4 h. After a 2 mg oral dose a maximum concentration of 17.5 nmol/l was achieved at about 3 h. The radiolabelled metabolites amount to three-fold these values but the curve of each was parallel so the cyproterone acetate radioimmunoassay may be regarded as a valid indication of concentration. Bioavailability studies suggest that cyproterone acetate is not subjected to activation after first pass through the liver. Urinary excretion was 30 per cent and 58 per cent was eliminated at the same rate in the bile but it is considerably slower than other gestagens (the half-life of cyproterone acetate is about 2 days in the bile). There tends to be some accumulation in the plasma but this reaches a maximum after about 5–8 days of treatment at which time the 24 h basal value is about two to three times the concentration following single administration (Hümpel et al, 1980).

Effects of cyproterone acetate are maximised by combination with ethinyl oestradiol in a reversed sequential regime as described by Hammerstein et al (1975). Intermittent anti-androgen administration results in prolonged maintenance of the progestogenic effect on the endometrium because of the protracted excretion pattern. The administration of ethinyl oestradiol throughout the cycle (days 5–25) results in predictable withdrawal bleeding as in the oral contraceptive regimes. The efficacy of this regime on hair growth has been measured by Ebling et al (1977). They showed that by comparing the measured length of 1000 hairs from the thighs there was a reduction after 6 months' therapy of from 8 to 11 mm to a length of from 4 to 6 mm. In the untreated state, more than 1 per cent of hairs had lengths of 18 mm and from the thighs shaven after treatment, more than 1 per cent had a length of 13 mm (Fig. 21.3). There must have been complete replacement of hairs during this course of treatment and the data imply a reduction in the average length of terminal or club hairs induced by this therapy. Fig. 21.4 shows the

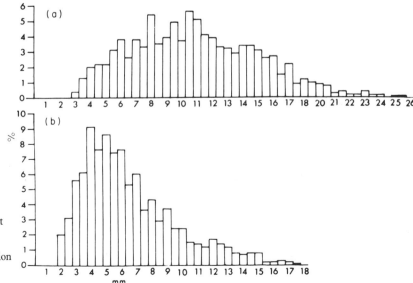

Fig. 21.3 Percentage distribution of lengths of hair shaved from (a) the left thigh of a hirsute patient before treatment (1000 hairs with a total weight of 50.00 mg and (b) the right thigh of the same patient during the seventh cycle of treatment with cyproterone acetate and ethinyl oestradiol (1204 hairs with a total weight of 28.23 mg) (By permission of Ebling et al, 1977, British Journal of Dermatology 97: 371–381)

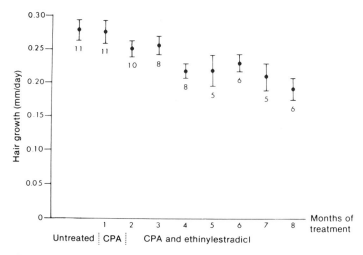

Fig. 21.4 Rate of growth of thigh hair, as measured by the length of hairs cut at skin level 4 weeks after shaving. For each patient the average rate was calculated on the basis of about 50 selected hairs (mean value ± s.d. for the number of patients shown). Each patient received 100 mg cyproterone acetate (CPA)/24 h from the 5th to the 14th day of each cycle and 0.05 mg ethinyl oestradiol/24 h from the 5th to the 25th day of the second and each subsequent cycle (By permission of Ebling et al, 1980, In: Androgenization in Women, 1979, 240–243. Excerpta Medica, Amsterdam)

rate of growth of thigh hair at 4-weekly intervals and there is a reduction to 80 per cent of the initial value after 4 months of treatment. Ebling et al (1980) pointed out that the anti-androgen may also reduce the length of anagen, i.e. the period of follicular activity. Similarly mean hair diameter also decreased progressively reaching a level of about 80 per cent of the initial value after 4 months' therapy (Fig. 21.5).

In addition to the changes in growth rate and diameter, the form of the medulla of the hair also changed. Prior to treatment, each thigh hair had a central portion with an unbroken or spasmodically interrupted medulla. At the distal or more usually the proximal end, the medulla may become fragmented or disappear. However, after six to seven treatment cycles only 10 per cent had a fully medullated segment. This medullary change may or may not occur within a single period of anagen as the hairs are continuously being shed and replaced (Ebling et al, 1980) but clinically there is a lightening of colour during treatment.

Figure 21.6 shows the reduction in the amount of sebum obtained from the forehead of the patients with idiopathic hirsutism under treatment. The cyproterone acetate alone had a significant effect on sebum production even without the additional oestrogen. These data indicate that cyproterone acetate is a potent anti-androgen particularly when supplemented with ethinyl oestradiol, whose principal effect is primarily to increase the sex hormone binding globulin. Most therapy is given using the reversed sequential regime and the cyproterone acetate is usually prescribed at a dose of 100 or 50 mg daily. Twenty-five mg daily has some effect on hair growth rate but the effect of the 10 mg daily dose is difficult to demonstrate, at least in small numbers of subjects. The 2 mg dose given as a combined oral contraceptive formulation is effective against seborrhoea and acne but not against hirsutism itself.

The availability of this anti-androgen has strikingly influenced the approach to management and therefore our investigative and diagnostic approaches. We have had access to this compound for 8 years and have been involved specifically with management of hirsute patients during that time. We report below our experience of 102 patients (Table 21.1) investigated and managed within our 'Hirsute Clinic'. The frequency of disorders diagnosed has presumably been influenced by referral patterns. Our Gynaeco-

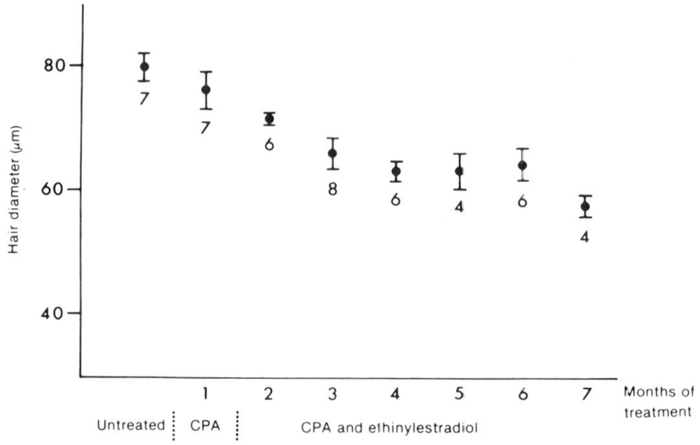

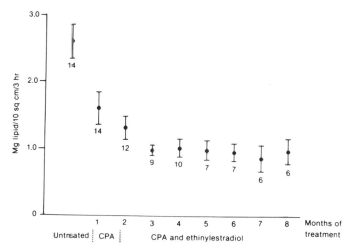

Fig. 21.5 Mean hair diameters in hirsute patients under reverse sequential therapy with cyproterone acetate (CPA) and ethinyl oestradiol (other details as in Fig. 21.4) (By permission of Ebling et al, 1980, In: Androgenization in Women, 1979, 240–243, Excerpta Medica, Amsterdam)

Fig. 21.6 Mean amount of sebum from the forehead of a patient under reverse sequential therapy with cyproterone acetate (CPA) and ethinyl oestradiol (other details as in Fig. 21.4) (By permission of Ebling et al, 1980, In: Androgenization in Women, 1979, 240–243, Excerpta Medica, Amsterdam)

Table 21.1 Diagnosis in patients investigated in hirsute clinic 1976–1983

Adrenal carcinoma	1
21-hydroxylase deficiency	3
Hilus cell tumour of ovary	1
Cushing's syndrome	1
Polycystic ovary syndrome	13
Hyperprolactinaemia	1
Idiopathic hirsutism	82
Total	102

logical Clinic was known to have had endocrine and infertility interests and only latterly specifically included hirsutism. Nevertheless, the experience accumulated has an interesting distribution and is sufficiently large for us to have reconsidered our diagnostic approach which has therefore evolved. Other causes of hirsutism not mentioned are deliberately omitted as it has been felt that if the primary reason for referral is hirsutism, then our experience of these numbers ought to be representative.

CLINICAL ASSESSMENT

History

The presentation may consist of a simple statement that increased hair growth has been noted for a particular time. This may date from puberty, be linked to a specific stressful event or be of greater severity for a shorter period. Aesthetic control measures may no longer be keeping pace with the growth rate or the scarring or expense of the electrolysis therapy may have led to its being abandoned. Anxiety may be focused on facial or periareolar hirsutes, the development of a male escutcheon or concern over generalised increased hair growth. A change in hairstyle may have followed a recognition of temporal thinning. The type and extent of treatments used should be noted: depilatory creams, waxes, shaving as well as electrolysis and their frequency of use. The time of last use will of course influence the scoring (Ferriman & Gallwey, 1961) later and the patient should be asked to return after an interval without treatment to complete an adequate assessment.

Skin greasiness is increased and acne may be a problem extending to chest and back. There is increased hair greasiness with a greater frequency of washing. A family history may be helpful, especially in the Indian ethnic group where constitutional hirsutism is a feature in most female relatives providing a standard against which the patient's degree of affection may be judged.

The menstrual pattern provides useful data. A change — particularly to amenorrhoea — suggests a more serious problem of excess steroid secretion when linked to a change in hair growth status. However, oligomenorrhoea may

always have been a feature of polycystic ovarian disease. Deepening of the voice we have only noted in association with an androgen-secreting tumour and that quite late in its course if benign. Changes in body contour and increase in muscle mass we have only seen in long term uncontrolled adrenal hyperplasia, first manifest at puberty. Any weight change, particularly obesity should be noted.

Physical examination

An immediate appraisal of voice and facial hair growth is possible but a systematic recording of body hair, graded according to site, provides the most comprehensive documentation and there should be available a chart on which are the diagrams of numbered body surfaces as in Fig. 21.7 and the scoring system with its description as in Table 21.2. It is then possible to generate a Ferriman & Gallwey (1961) score providing a careful quantitation. Not only is this useful to evaluate severity (grades 0–4 at each site) but

Table 21.2 Scoring system for hirsute areas

Site	Grade	Definition
Upper lip	1	A few hairs at outer margin
	2	A small moustache at outer margin
	3	A moustache extending halfway from outer margin
	4	A moustache extending to mid-line
Chin	1	A few scattered hairs
	2	Scattered hairs with small concentrations
	3, 4	Complete cover, light and heavy
Chest	1	Circumareolar hairs
	2	With mid-line hair in addition
	3	Fusion of these areas, with three-quarter cover
	4	Complete cover
Upper back	1	A few scattered hairs
	2	Rather more, still scattered
	3, 4	Complete cover, light and heavy
Lower back	1	A sacral tuft of hair
	2	With some lateral extension
	3	Three-quarter cover
	4	Complete cover
Upper abdomen	1	A few mid-line hairs
	2	Rather more, still mid-line
	3, 4	Half and full cover
Lower abdomen	1	A few mid-line hairs
	2	A mid-line streak of hair
	3	A mid-line band of hair
	4	An inverted V-shaped growth
Arm	1	Sparse growth affecting not more than a quarter of the limb surface
	2	More than this cover still incomplete
	3, 4	Complete cover, light and heavy
Thigh	1, 2, 3, 4	As for arm
Forearm	1, 2, 3, 4	Complete cover of dorsal surface; two grades of light and two of heavy growth
Leg	1, 2, 3, 4	As for arm

Grade 0 at all sites indicates absence of terminal hair (after Ferriman & Gallwey, 1961).

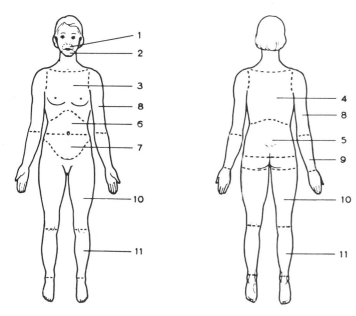

Fig. 21.7 Facsimile of chart used to classify hirsute areas. For legend of numbers and grading see Table 21.2 (By permission of Ferriman & Gallwey, 1961)

loss then quite remarkable improvements may be seen, frequently culminating in conception without further treatment. Adiposity of an unusual distribution and the presence of striae would only be found in well developed Cushing's syndrome. The blood pressure may be elevated in Cushing's syndrome or an 11β-hydroxylase deficiency associated with congenital adrenal hyperplasia.

After general examination, attention is directed to the clitoris but this is unlikely to be enlarged unless there is amenorrhoea. The shaft must be palpated but on retraction of the prepuce the glans may be unusually prominent. A pelvic examination is then performed but as many of these patients are *virgo intacta*, a satisfactory bimanual pelvic examination is not possible in the clinic. A rectal examination is less satisfactory, certainly to the gynaecologist, but may be sufficient to confirm that there is no obvious ovarian enlargement. If there is any enlargement noted in these patients, it is probably best further assessed by ultrasound when consistency may also be evaluated. It would be preferable to have the endocrine evaluation available before proceeding to examination under anaesthesia or a further surgical procedure, as ovarian enlargement may be due to an incidental lesion.

Laboratory investigation

There is a spectrum of assays available for characterising hirsutism, but the hormones measured should provide some diagnostic discrimination and be therapeutically useful. The choice depends on the drugs available. Cyproterone acetate is not generally available in some countries, such as the United States, so low dose glucocorticoids are widely used to treat hirsutism diagnosed as of adrenal or mixed adrenal/ovarian origin. In that situation therefore, discrimination of the source becomes important. However, where cyproterone acetate is available, it is so effective on the pilosebaceous unit in the less severe forms of hirsutism that it only becomes important to distinguish the major categories that require different therapy. Using this rationale, a regime is set out in Table 21.3. Although we prefer to complete it in 36 h as an in-patient, it may be managed as an out-patient. It includes a plasma cortisol diurnal rhythm, overnight dexamethasone suppression and short ACTH stimulation test which is sufficient for routine screening purposes as required in our first 100 cases. Abnormal tests may be repeated selectively or supplemented when the nature of the diagnosis is clearer. Duplicate samples may be deleted for economic reasons but serve as useful confirmation of results to calculate a mean to minimise the impact of episodic fluctuation and as a back-up in case individual samples are lost in some assays. If patients already have clinical stigmata of more severe disease, then specific more extensive endocrine investigation may be instituted. The reasons for using these specific assays are as follows.

in some fair-skinned individuals, where even a small amount of unwanted hair can be unacceptable, it is possible to determine that the scoring is within the normal range. Thus Ferriman & Gallwey (1961) found that 95 per cent of their normal subjects not complaining of hirsutism scored no more than 8 and none more than 13. These values were obtained from the total score which included components for the forearm and lower leg which are not primarily hormone-responsive. Thus the hormonal score, areas 1–9, may add up to 36 and the total score, areas 1–11 to 44. Generalised increased hair growth, or hypertrichosis, may be noted in conditions such as porphyria, following head injury or induced by diphenylhydantoin or corticosteroids. Nerve injury, or local skin irritation may cause increased hair growth on the limbs (Maroulis, 1981).

Head-hair greasiness and seborrhoea are noted with the extent and degree of acne. Body weight appears to be of importance. Weight and height should be measured and a Garrow chart constructed (Garrow, 1979) so that Caucasian women should fall between the values of 19–24 when the relationship is expressed as the Quetelet Index (weight in kg/height^2 in metres). Mathur et al (1982) recently examined the association of plasma sex hormone binding globulin concentration and body weight and concluded that there was a lower SHBG in obese hirsute women than in non-obese hirsute women and that the mechanism probably did not involve androgens. Bates & Whitworth (1982) documented a highly significant reduction in plasma androstenedione and testosterone in obese women losing more than 15 per cent of their body weight. Calculation of ideal body weight, or the 95th centile (24 on the Garrow chart) allows of target setting for the individual. If therapy, especially for infertility is made contingent on the weight

Table 21.3 Hirsutism investigation protocol

Day	Time	Drugs	Venous blood samples
			Investigation
1	21.00		1. Cortisol
2	09.00		1. Cortisol 2. 17-α-hydroxyprogesterone 3. Testosterone 4. Oestradiol, progesterone 5. Androstenedione 6. Sex hormone binding globulin (SHBG) 7. FSH, LH, prolactin 8. Thyroid function tests 9. Full blood count
	21.00		1. Cortisol
	23.00	1.5 mg dexamethasone*	
3	09.00	Repeat all samples (1–7 incl) except thyroid function tests and full blood count from day 2	
		then 0.25 mg Synacthen IM*	
	+ 30 min		1. Cortisol 2. 17-α-hydroxyprogesterone 3. Testosterone†

* Dates and times of drug administration to be recorded in notes for later interpretation of data, especially samples 1, 2 and 3 on days 2 and 3

† Steinberger et al (1982)

(a) *Plasma cortisol.* An elevated plasma cortisol, loss of the diurnal rhythm, an inadequate response to overnight dexamethasone suppression and an exaggerated response to β1–24 tetracosactrin test all point to Cushing's syndrome or disease.

(b) *Plasma 17-α-hydroxyprogesterone.* Adrenal hyperplasia (C_{21} hydroxylase deficiency) may only present post-puberty and the diagnosis is readily made from an elevated plasma 17-α-hydroxyprogesterone concentration. The plasma cortisol may be subnormal or not capable of further stimulation with a short ACTH test. As ACTH is elevated, the other androgens measured, androstenedione and testosterone will also be elevated (See Ch. 18).

(c) *Plasma testosterone.* Plasma testosterone may be at the upper limit of normal or slightly elevated in polycystic ovarian disease (PCO) or idiopathic hirsutism. It tends to be significantly elevated in adrenal hyperplasia and grossly elevated in adrenal carcinoma and ovarian tumours. Steinberger et al (1982) used the suppressibility of plasma testosterone by overnight dexamethasone as an indication of an adrenal source of androgen and therefore as a guide to long-term prednisone therapy for the treatment of hirsutism and infertility (Steinberger et al, 1981).

(d) *Plasma androstenedione.* Plasma androstenedione is more frequently elevated in idiopathic hirsutism than is testosterone and in association with a reduced SHBG provides the most secure diagnosis of androgen abnormality. Because of the doubt about the source of the androgen and the reason for the reduced SHBG, the term 'idiopathic hirsutism' is used when no other endocrine abnormalities have been identified. Androstenedione tends to be elevated as well in PCO, adrenal hyperplasia and in the adrenal and ovarian tumours. In these latter conditions it is only helpful when the concentrations are very high; its greatest value lies in the support for the diagnosis of idiopathic hirsutism when only the SHBG is also abnormal.

(e) *Plasma progesterone and oestradiol.* The female sex steroid results are of more value as aids to management than to diagnosis. Provided the sample is obtained for progesterone in the second half of a regular menstrual cycle, it can provide evidence of ovulation. Otherwise timed in the proliferative phase or in a cycle longer than 35 days it has no value and may be omitted. The chances of obtaining a result suggestive of ovulation (> 18 nmol/l) in an oligomenorrhoeic woman (cycle length 35 days to 6 months) are slim and there is little point in seeking evidence of ovulation in an amenorrhoeic woman. The plasma oestradiol value is used as evidence of oestrogen status in amenorrhoeic women who are infertile as a guide to subsequent induction of ovulation. If it is less than 100 pmol/l then there will be insufficient oestrogen for an anti-oestrogen such as clomiphene to be effective and recourse must be had to human menopausal gonadotrophin (hMG) (Ch. 27), luteinising hormone releasing hormone (LHRH) (Ch. 26) or human follicle stimulating hormone (hFSH) administration. If more than 100 pmol/l, then clomiphene should be used in the first instance. Oestrogen status excluding possible clomiphene therapy may also be determined by urinary total oestrogen excretion (> 45 µmol/24 h) or failure of an attempt to induce progestogen withdrawal bleeding (medroxyprogesterone acetate 5 mg b.d. for 7 days).

(f) *Sex hormone binding globulin.* A reduced plasma sex hormone binding globulin is extremely useful as a feature associated with an increase in circulating biologically active androgens. It is expressed as nmol of dihydrotestosterone bound/l (normal range 34–75). It is most helpful when the only other abnormality is an elevated plasma androstenedione as supporting evidence for a diagnosis of idiopathic hirsutism. Elevated androstenedione or testosterone levels associated with other ovarian or adrenal causes will always be associated with depressed SHBG concentrations which then lose their diagnostic value.

(g) *Gonadotrophin data.* These allow calculation of a luteinising hormone/follicle stimulating hormone (LH/FSH) ratio which Rebar et al (1976) showed was elevated in the proliferative phase of regularly cycling patients with PCO. These data are useful in supporting a diagnosis of PCO in the presence of plasma testosterone and androstenedione values at or above the upper limit of normal. The ratio would need to be within the normal range to support a diagnosis of idiopathic hirsutism.

(*h*) *Plasma prolactin.* Hyperprolactinaemia is rarely associated with hirsutism and a causative relationship must be in doubt. Nevertheless, an appreciation of the normal range will reduce the frequency of the apparent association. Our 95th centile is taken as 880 mU/l (Standard MRC 75/504; Lenton et al, 1979). Isolated elevated values should be checked using an indwelling cannula to obtain repeated basal concentrations before instituting further neuro-radiological investigations.

(*i*) *Serum thyroxine.* Thyroid function assessment is of dubious value. We have found no patients that have presented with hirsutism so far who have alterations in thyroid function. We frequently encounter subclinical hypothyroidism but our centre is located on the edge of a goitre belt. In any case, a confirmed elevation of plasma prolactin should point to the need for further investigation, including thyroid function. Menstrual cycle irregularity or amenorrhoea will also lead to assessment of thyroid function.

Other assays have been used for the assessment of hirsutism and these have been reviewed recently by Maroulis (1981). Serum-free testosterone is technically more difficult to estimate as a separation is required. Although salivary testosterone measures free testosterone, the concentration is much lower than in plasma and hence a much more sensitive assay is required. As large numbers of samples are not required, there seems little advantage in the latter method. Dihydrotestosterone, although the most potent androgen, does not provide more useful information from its plasma concentration than testosterone itself. Plasma DHA is massively elevated in adrenal tumours as is dehydroepiandrosterone sulphate (DHAS) and the latter is probably easier to measure nowadays. Plasma androstenediol has little discriminant value. Group determinations such as plasma 17β-hydroxysteroids and the free 17β-hydroxysteroid index add little and may be normal in hirsute patients. Urinary assays are now rarely used; assay of total 17-oxo (keto) steroids was formerly widely used, hirsute patients had values at or just above the upper limit of normal although those with tumours had grossly elevated levels. As a group determination, the main source is the adrenal cortex in females and includes compounds such as androsterone and aetiocholanolone and their 11β-hydroxy or 11β-oxo derivatives as well as epiandrosterone and dehydroepiandrosterone. Using chromatographic methods these could be fractionated to provide more helpful evidence of selective elevation but the data are still not good enough to provide diagnostic precision. Testosterone glucuronide is usually within the normal range and although androstanediol is usually elevated, its assay is not widely used. Urinary pregnanetriol assay has been almost completely replaced by the assay of plasma 17-α-hydroxy-progesterone, its plasma precursor for diagnosis of adrenal hyperplasia.

Suppression and stimulation procedures

(*a*) *Adrenal suppression.* Dexamethasone suppression of steroid output is used to confirm normal adrenal function or identify an abnormality. A normal adrenal gland may be suppressed by dexamethasone 2 mg four times daily given for 2 days but the time required for this demonstration can be reduced to an overnight examination for most patients when adequate suppression is expected. By giving 1.5 mg dexamethasone (the range used by different workers is 1–2 mg) at 23.00, the same degree of suppression may be obtained on sampling at 09.00 the following morning. In this way, after obtaining samples for the diurnal rhythm of plasma cortisol at 09.00 and 21.00, the normally higher morning plasma cortisol may be suppressed to well below the evening concentration in the normal patient. Failure of suppression occurs in Cushing's syndrome.

As a diagnosis of Cushing's syndrome is unusual in a woman presenting with hirsutism, it is more economical to perform an overnight suppression test and have the patient return for fuller investigation if there is failure of suppression. It may be seen in the lower part of Table 21.4 that subsequent investigation of the patient showed a failure of suppression (although the values are now within the normal range) during a 2-day suppression test, during which 0.5 mg dexamethasone was given every 6 h but that at the higher dose of 2 mg every 6 h effective suppression

Table 21.4 Plasma cortisol data from a patient with Cushing's syndrome presenting with hirsutism

Time and diagnostic test		Plasma cortisol (nmol/l)
Day 1	09.00	798
	21.00	755
Day 2	09.00 after overnight 1.5 mg dexamethasone	726
	09.00 after 0.25 mg i.v. tetracosactrin	1600
Day 3	09.00 after 2 mg/24 h dexamethasone*	586
Day 4	09.00 after 2 mg/24 h	437
Day 5	09.00 after 8 mg/24 h	52
Day 6	09.00 after 8 mg/24 h	40
Day 8	09.00	638

Normal range plasma cortisol 166–660 nmol/l
* see text

occurs, signifying adrenal hyperplasia which was subsequently confirmed as Cushing's syndrome.

Autonomous adrenal tumours, adenoma or carcinoma, do not suppress even on 8 mg dexamethasone per 24 h. Apart from examining plasma cortisol responses to this regime, it may be important to assay androgens which are likely to be relatively more elevated than cortisol as the patient has presented with hirsutism and not overt signs of hypercortisolism. Thus plasma testosterone and androstenedione may be massively elevated and fail to respond to suppression even if it is extended to 5 days at the higher 8 mg/24 h dose level. Other tumour markers may be sought such as DHA and DHAS and a gas chromatographic screen of 24 h urine samples obtained in the suppressed state may identify those steroids at greatest concentration which may be unusual but which may be used as markers to follow any response to therapy.

Suppression of other steroids, such as 17-α-hydroxyprogesterone is also sought to make a diagnosis of adrenal hyperplasia (Table 21.5).

The elevated 17-α-hydroxyprogesterone concentration is well suppressed after the overnight corticosteroid. Although the first plasma cortisol in Table 21.5 is elevated, as was the previous day's (not shown), there is a normal diurnal rhythm and the overnight dexamathasone suppression is effective. These data would confirm the excess circulating 17-α-hydroprogesterone and indicate that there was a partial enzyme block of the C_{21} hydroxylase. Steinberger et al (1982) have included plasma testosterone estimations in the regime as a prognostic device. If any suppression of plasma testosterone occurs after 1 mg overnight dexamethasone then this can be used as an indication of the efficacy of long term prednisone therapy for patients in whom fertility is required; failure of suppression is associated with failure of long-term reduction of plasma testosterone concentration on 7.5 mg prednisone per 24 h.

(b) Adrenal stimulation. A short ACTH test may be carried out using 0.25 mg synthetic β1–24 ACTH (tetracosactrin, Synacthen — Ciba) given either intravenously or intramuscularly, the second sample after the zero control sample being taken exactly 30 min after administration of the ACTH; longer stimulation tests are unnecessary for the differential diagnosis of hirsutism. A normal response, if the investigational sequence follows that of Table 21.3 where it is preceded by the overnight dexamethasone suppression, is to have the plasma cortisol concentration return to the normal range. An example of the excessive response in a patient with Cushing's syndrome is shown in Table 21.4 acting as further supporting evidence to the loss of diurnal rhythm and the failure of overnight suppression.

Similarly, Table 21.5 shows the excessive response of 17-α-hydroxyprogesterone after overnight dexamethasone suppression in a patient with adrenal hyperplasia due to C_{21} hydroxylase deficiency.

In a patient with an autonomous tumour, there is no response to this trophic hormone.

Gibson et al (1980) have attempted to define incomplete forms of enzyme defects in anovulatory or oligoovulatory women who are hyperandrogenic. They gave intravenous ACTH equivalent to 0.25 mg tetracosactrin and measured the ratios of steroid increments above basal values at 30 min to assess individual enzyme competence. By expressing the ratio of a precursor as numerator to product as denominator, a large increase in the ratio would signify precursor build-up. In this way, 17-α-hydroxypregnenolone over 17-α-hydroxyprogesterone or DHA over cortisol would assess 3β hydroxysteroid dehydrogenase Δ^{4-5} isomerase, 11-deoxycortisol over cortisol would examine 11β-hydroxylase and 17-hydroxyprogesterone over 11-deoxycortisol would evaluate 21-hydroxylase. This approach may be of interest if fertility is important and the patient does not ovulate regularly, as it would suggest a role for longer term low dose corticosteroid therapy. However, the authors caution against using it as a diagnostic procedure

Table 21.5 Diagnostic data from a patient with adrenal hyperplasia presenting as hirsutism

Time and diagnostic test		Plasma cortisol (nmol/l)*	Plasma 17-α-hydroxyprogesterone (nmol/l)†	Urinary pregnanetriol (μmol/24 h)°
Day 2	09.00	684	41	11.0
	21.00	303		
Day 3	09.00	488	26	9.0
Day 4	09.00		49	8.6
Day 5	09.00 after overnight 1.5 mg dexamethasone	43	4	
	09.30 30 min after 0.25 mg i.v. tetracosactrin	445	150	

* Plasma cortisol normal range 166–660 nmol/l

† 17-α-hydroxyprogesterone normal range <18 nmol/l

° 24 h collection completed at 09.00 h. Normal range 0.3–5.3 μmol/24 h

and our own use confirms that it is not helpful when there is evidence of regular ovulation as all our results in this situation have fallen within the normal range. This of course, applies to the majority of hirsute women.

It must be said however, that adrenal suppression and stimulation tests are of little help in the vast majority of hirsute women. Although it is generally accepted (Huq et al, 1976) that dexamethasone does not cause ovarian suppression, greater degrees of ovarian suppression can be achieved after periods longer than the overnight or 2-day test periods and 2 weeks is probably required for maximum impact (Abraham et al, 1976). Nevertheless, the diagnostic suppression tests described above are adequate for detecting the uncommon problem presenting as hirsutism. Adrenal stimulation is less certain. Although Givens et al (1975) showed that half their hirsute patients responded to ACTH by increased peripheral plasma androstenedione concentrations, this is not particularly useful diagnostically.

(a) *Ovarian suppression*. Ovarian suppression is not usually attempted. Oestrogen alone is not as effective as a combined oestrogen/progestogen oral contraceptive formulation but the degree of suppression varies according to the dose of oestrogen and type and dose of progestogen (Maroulis, 1981) and it would require 3–4 weeks administration to be effective. Nor is it helpful prognostically as long-term suppression with conventional combined oral contraceptives is not as effective on the pilosebaceous unit as the recently introduced 50 μg ethinyl oestradiol combined with the antiandrogen cyproterone acetate 2 mg as the progestogen (Diane–Schering).

Partial androgen suppression of ovarian and adrenal tumour androgens may be induced by ovarian suppression so it is not useful diagnostically.

(d) *Ovarian stimulation*. Ovarian stimulation using human chorionic gonadotrophin (hCG) produces variable and inconsistent results and Abraham et al (1975) claim that the information gained does not add to that derived from the adrenal suppression test. In addition, hCG may stimulate adrenal tumour androgens (Givens et al, 1974) and ACTH may act similarly on ovarian tumours (Louros et al, 1966).

Sequence of investigations

The fact that the patient is hirsute can be established at the time of the first visit by means of the history and physical examination although if a particular depilatory effort has been made, it may be desirable to wait until such time as the patient believes that another depilation is necessary (and that time interval is useful to note) and then repeat the Ferriman & Gallwey scoring. Short-term admission for endocrine evaluation, including the adrenal suppression and stimulation tests should be arranged at the time of the first visit with a review when the results are available. This will allow the diagnosis of idiopathic hirsutism to be

confirmed by exclusion or attention drawn to a particular diagnostic category requiring more intensive investigation. Thus very high androgen levels suggesting a tumour would require further admission for localisation and a diagnosis of adrenal hyperplasia due to C_{21} hydroxylase deficiency would suggest admission for a 24 h profile of plasma cortisol and 17-α-hydroxyprogesterone after corticoid therapy had been started to gauge the efficacy of control. When the major questions had been resolved, the fertility aspirations of the patient could be considered. If the diagnosis of polycystic ovary syndrome or hyperprolactinaemia has been made and pregnancy is the objective, then drug therapy should be started only after completing infertility investigations. Semen analysis and assessment of tubal patency by laparoscopy would be the first steps.

Diagnosis and differential diagnosis

Case histories will be used to illustrate the diagnostic categories and the rarest and most serious causes will be considered first.

(a) *Androgen-secreting adrenal tumour*. A 49-year-old woman had become hirsute 2 years earlier and had noted virilising changes more recently. Her voice had been deep for 4 months. She had a male pattern hair distribution with temporal recession and shaved daily. She was an intelligent woman but had deferred seeking advice as her husband was dying with a cerebral tumour; she sought help only after he died. On examination she had angular features but denied weight loss. Her blood pressure was 170/100 mmHg. There was obvious hepatomegaly with a right sided mass deeply felt below the liver. The clitoris was enlarged but pelvic examination revealed no other abnormality. Her ESR was 32 mm/h, a chest X-ray showed multiple small lung metastases. An intravenous pyelogram revealed a paucity of gas shadows and a downward displacement of the right kidney by a large suprarenal mass. Ultrasound scan showed a 7 cm diameter right sided adrenal mass with presumed central necrosis and several solid liver lesions were confirmed on a liver scan with ^{99m}Te-labelled albumen. A seleno-cholesterol scan demonstrated a reduced adrenal uptake and none in the liver or lung metastases. The plasma testosterone was 14 nmol/l (normal range 0.5–2.5 nmol/l), plasma androstenedione varied from 28 to 43.5 nmol/l (1.6–5.7 nmol/l). There were very high concentrations of plasma DHA and DHAS and none of these four were suppressible by 2-days dexamethasone at 8 mg per 24 h. The plasma cortisols were within the normal range 169–642 nmol/l (166–660 nmol/l) but there was loss of the diurnal rhythm and a failure of response to tetracosactrin. A urinary screen for steroids using gas chromatography revealed massive concentrations of DHA and 16-α-hydroxy-DHA and there were large amounts of androsterone and aetiocholanolone, androstenediol, tetrahydrocortisone and tetrahydrocortisol.

The patient clearly had disseminated adrenal carcinoma and treatment was started with o,p'-DDD, replacement therapy, antiandrogen and symptomatic support. In spite of improvement in some laboratory parameters, her clinical condition deteriorated and she died 6 months later at home having elected to stop treatment. Histological confirmation was not obtained.

This history shows that a diagnosis of tumour can be suggested by the very high concentration of the androgens routinely assayed in the protocol and the lack of dexamethasone suppressibility. Clinical examination and basic investigation revealed metastatic disease. Precise documentation of the often bizarre steroid secretion pattern, although of interest, does not help management unless a steroid is to be used as a marker for efficacy of treatment when DHA would serve. These points serve to emphasise that the routine examination of a wider range of steroids even including DHA, adds little. If the patient had presented earlier, it is likely that she would still have had very high androgens as hirsutism was her presenting problem. She may not have been virilised as that was a late development. The lack of androgen and secondarily of cortisol suppressibility by high dose dexamethasone, the latter limited to the loss of the diurnal rhythm of plasma cortisol and failure of ACTH response, would have suggested an adrenal site and a tumour not controlled by trophic or feedback influence. Ultrasound and gamma scan of the adrenal were helpful examinations for localisation and recourse was not needed to adrenal vein catheterisation by percutaneous femoral vein puncture. The latter may give erroneous results because of technical difficulty or episodic adrenal steroid output, but may need to be done if the suppression test data are difficult to interpret. Maroulis (1981) claims that suppression tests are unreliable in determining the source of androgens in the presence of a virilising tumour. Finally, computerised tomography using a whole body scanner may also be helpful.

(b) *Cushing's syndrome.* A nulliparous woman had noticed increased hair growth for 4 years from the age of 23. When seen she was having weekly electrolysis of the beard area, upper lip, breasts and lower abdomen but even this could not control the growth rate. She had taken no oral contraception for 6 months. She had noticed headaches for a year but no visual change. There had been no voice change and no loss of libido. She had become amenorrhoeic 6 months earlier. For 6 years she had suffered from scalp psoriasis and had used Betnovate cream. On examination her Ferriman & Gallwey score was 23 and there were obvious electrolysis scars. There was no temporal recession or acne. Her blood pressure was 140/90 mmHg, there was no classical morphology of Cushing's syndrome. There was no clitoral hypertrophy and pelvic examination was normal. No aetiological diagnosis could be made at that stage so routine investigations were begun. Her plasma testosterones were 3.1 and 2.7 nmol/l (normal range

Table 21.6 Adrenal suppression tests in a patient with Cushing's syndrome presenting as hirsutism

Time and diagnostic test	Plasma cortisol (nmol/l)*	Plasma ACTH (ng/l)†	
Day 1	731	330	
Day 2	666	143	
Day 3	469	133	
Day 6	after 2 mg/24 h DXM° for 48 h	437	203
Day 8	after 8 mg/24 h DXM° for 48 h	40	10

* Plasma cortisol: normal range 166–660 nmol/l

† Plasma ACTH: normal range 10–80 ng/l

° DXM: dexamethasone

0.5–2.5 nmol/l). The plasma cortisols were as in Table 21.4 showing elevation, loss of diurnal rhythm, failure of suppression and excessive stimulation. The urinary free cortisol concentration was 1300 nmol/24 h (normal range 97–331 nmol/24 h). The plasma 17-α-hydroxyprogesterone concentration, plasma prolactin, gonadotrophins and thyroid function tests were normal. These data confirmed the hypercortisolism and demanded further investigation.

High levels of plasma ACTH (Table 21.6) excluded an autonomous lesion of the adrenal, adenoma or carcinoma. The elevated plasma cortisols failed to suppress on low dose dexamethasone 2 mg/day for 48 h (compare with a similar failure of overnight suppression seen in Table 21.4) but did so on high dose dexamethasone, 8 mg/day for 48 h. As the plasma ACTH concentrations also fell to below normal on the high dose of dexamethasone, very strong support for a pituitary-driven lesion was provided. A chest X-ray showed no tumour as a possible ectopic source of ACTH. Dynamic anterior pituitary function testing was carried out using an insulin hypoglycaemia (0.3 units/kg) and the plasma cortisol (638 nmol/l) failed to rise in response to adequate hypoglycaemia. Growth hormone and prolactin showed normal increments, TSH responded well to TRH and the gonadotrophins to LHRH.

Skull X-rays and tomography of the pituitary fossa were normal. Computerised axial tomography, with attention to the adrenal and pituitary areas were normal. Metrizamide cisternography confirmed the lack of suprasellar extension and bilateral carotid angiography excluded an aneurysm allowing the conclusion that the lesion was probably a pituitary basophil adenoma. At transnasal trans-sphenoidal exploration of the pituitary gland, a small abnormal area in the midline superiorly was noted and about one quarter of the gland was excised.

Immediately post operatively there were very low plasma cortisols. Subsequently she will need repeat pituitary function testing and stabilisation on any replacement therapy in general which, depending on the pituitary damage, may include cortisol, thyroxine, bromocriptine or desmopressin. When her general condition has been stabilised, her plasma testosterone level may be checked and careful note taken of her hair growth pattern. Her ultimate fertility prospects will depend on her gonadotrophin responses to LHRH which are likely to be markedly impaired. If they are, then she is likely to be amenorrhoeic and fail to respond to clomiphene requiring gonadotrophins for induction of ovulation when conception is required. Otherwise low dose sequential oestrogen/progestogen replacement therapy should be offered.

(c) *Ovarian hilus cell tumour.* A 65-year-old woman presented with a 20-year history of excessive hair growth in the beard area. For 10 years she had had gross male type balding and a deep voice for 4 years. For 2 years she had had hair growth on her abdomen, chest and shoulders. At 40 she had become menopausal. She was obviously virilised with marked balding. On pelvic examination she had moderate clitoral hypertrophy but no ovarian enlargement or palpable irregularity. Chest and skull X-rays were normal as was an intravenous pyelogram. Tomography of the adrenal areas and ultrasonography of the adrenal and ovaries showed no obvious lesions. Plasma cortisols had a normal diurnal rhythm and suppressed readily on low dose dexamethasone. Although urinary 17 oxo-, oxogenic steroids and pregnanetriol were normal, plasma testosterone fluctuated from high to very high. Prior to dexamethasone suppression it was 35 nmol/l (normal range 0.5–2.5 nmol/l), low dose suppression caused it to fall to 6 nmol/l but high dose suppression caused a further reduction only to 4–6 nmol/l, still above the upper limit of normal. Plasma androstenedione fluctuated also but from within the normal range (1.6–5.7 nmol/l) to just above it. Sex hormone binding globulin was reduced to 34 nmol DHT bound/l (normal range 43–74 nmol DHT bound/l). Thyroid function was normal, plasma oestradiol 164 pmol/l and plasma FSH and LH were 24 and 34 iu/l respectively with a normal response to LHRH.

There was no abnormality in cortisol dynamics and the elevated testosterone levels could not be suppressed to below the normal range suggesting that the adrenal gland function was normal and that the source of the testosterone was more likely ovarian although Louros et al (1977) and Tucci et al (1973) describe inappropriate suppression responses in ovarian tumours. The fact that testosterone was the major steroid produced excessively was consistent with its being predominantly produced by an ovarian tumour. Meldrum & Abraham (1979) found it so in 84 per cent of women with masculinising ovarian tumours and in their report the serum testosterone was usually greater than 6.7 nmol/l. Hyperthecosis (Nagamani et al, 1981), hilus cell hyperplasia or diffuse stromal hyperplasia were unlikely even in this postmenopausal woman because of the gross elevation of the plasma testosterone. Although the sex cord tumours (arrhenoblastoma, granulosa, theca and

lipoid cell) are the commonest, they tend to occur in younger women and a 20-year history is more likely to be consistent with a benign than a malignant lesion. This tends to exclude dysgerminoma and gonadoblastoma. The normal size of the ovaries does not help as only about half of the hilus cell or adrenal rest tumours are palpable and they are usually unilateral (Maroulis, 1981). Final localisation of the lesion could be attempted by ovarian vein catheterisation and comparison with peripheral testosterone concentration on one side with the other but ovarian vein steroid levels may be diluted by blood from other sources. In the event it was decided to proceed directly to laparotomy, laparoscopy being ruled out as there was no palpable enlargement and a hilus cell tumour would lie deeply in the ovarian substance and was unlikely to be visible. Bivalving of each ovary would be necessary to exclude a small tumour, at least in the contralateral ovary once one was identified and ovarian vein blood samples for later steroid analysis were also wanted.

At operation a 6 mm diameter nodule was noted on longitudinal opening of the left ovary so after bilateral and peripheral venous sampling, unilateral oophorectomy was performed, the ovarian surface being smooth and normal. Histologically this was a hilus cell ovarian tumour. The operative steroid assay data showed that the peripheral vein plasma testosterone and androstenedione were 9.0 and 6.7 nmol/l respectively, the left ovarian vein values were more than 52 and more than 29 nmol/l respectively and the right ovarian vein 14.0 and 13.5 nmol/l respectively. Postoperatively the plasma testosterone concentrations were normal when checked 1 week later, 1.0 nmol/l but plasma androstenedione levels were still slightly elevated at 7.1 nmol/l.

(d) *Adrenal hyperplasia due to C_{21} hydroxylase deficiency.* At the Family Planning Clinic, a patient on oral contraception was noted to be hypertensive and hirsute attending for electrolysis. Her oral contraceptive was stopped but her blood pressure remained elevated so she was referred. Her increased hair growth had developed shortly after puberty and was most marked on her face (see Fig. 21.8), breasts and lower abdomen apart from the non-hormonal areas of arms and legs. Her voice was normal, she had a regular menstrual cycle of 4/28 days. On examination the Ferriman & Gallwey score was 21, there was a male escutcheon but the clitoris was not enlarged. Pelvic examination was unremarkable. Her blood pressure was 160/95 mmHg but on subsequent admission was 110/80 mmHg. Her weight was 59 kg for 1.55 m giving her a Quetelet Index of 24.6, just above the upper limit of normal (Garrow, 1979). Investigation revealed data as shown in Table 21.5. She had a normal plasma cortisol and diurnal rhythm which suppressed normally on dexamethasone and responded adequately to synthetic ACTH stimulation. However, her basal plasma 17-α-hydroxyprogesterone concentration was elevated although it suppressed readily. There was an

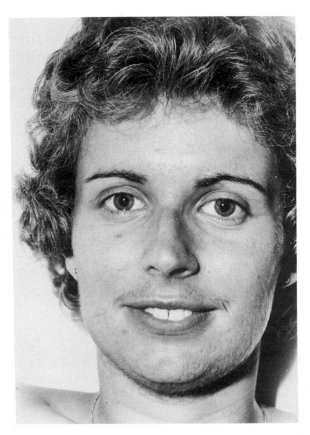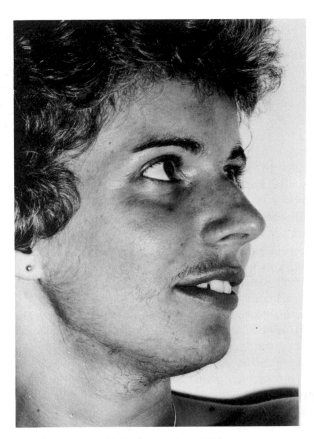

Fig. 21.8a & b Facial hirsutism seen in a patient with adult onset adrenal hyperplasia due to partial C_{21} hydroxylase deficiency

excessive response to ACTH stimulation. Her plasma testosterone values ranged from 3.2 to 4.1 nmol/l (normal range 0.5–2.5 nmol/l).

She was begun on 2.5 mg prednisone b.d. but this was increased to t.d.s. because of mid-afternoon lethargy and the dose on rising increased to 5 mg in the light of a mid-morning 17-α-hydroxyprogesterone of 26.3 nmol/l (normal <18 nmol/l). Subsequently a profile taken throughout a 24 h period during admission showed good suppression of 17-α-hydroxyprogesterone throughout the 24 h although her plasma cortisol in the evening was still subnormal (Table 21.7).

Table 21.7 Twenty-four-hour profile of plasma 17-α-hydroxyprogesterone and cortisol in a patient with adrenal hyperplasia on prednisone*

Time (h)	Plasma 17-α-hydroxyprogesterone (nmol/l)†	Plasma cortisol (nmol/l)°
12.00	3.0	132
16.00	2.5	201
20.00	3.1	58
24.00	2.3	105
08.00	2.8	252

* Patient taking oral prednisone t.d.s. at 5 mg, 2.5 mg and 2.5 mg

† Normal: < 18 nmol/l

° Normal range: 166–660 nmol/l

Thus her regime of 5 mg on rising (08.00), 2.5 mg mid-afternoon (15.00) and 2.5 mg on retiring (23.00) was adequate for excellent suppression. (but see Jones & Klingensmith, Ch. 18). Following this stabilisation she noted an obvious reduction in hair growth rate such that the frequency of the electrolysis was reduced from weekly to monthly. Her skin greasiness was reduced and her hair was much improved (she was a hairdresser). After 12 months she wished to conceive and did so within 2 months. She is currently in late pregnancy which is proceeding satisfactorily.

This patient had adrenal hyperplasia with a partial 21-hydroxylase deficiency accounting for the plasma cortisol levels within the normal range (Table 21.5) and the pubertal onset. The fact that she seemed hypertensive initially suggested the possibility of 11-β-hydroxylase defect although in this rare variant hypertension does not always occur (Cathelineau et al, 1980). However, in this form there is a prepubertal onset of virilism and incomplete fusion of the external genitalia. Elevated levels of urinary 11-desoxycortisol and tetrahydro-11-deoxycortisol have been reported (Glenthøj et al, 1980). Our patient had normal plasma 11-deoxycortisol levels.

Attenuated forms of 21-hydroxylase deficiency have been reported in parents or siblings of patients found to have congenital adrenal hyperplasia and although they have post-pubertal hirsutism with normal external genitalia, they were not described as having presented with hirsutism. Rosenwaks et al (1979) attribute this to the heterozygous state, the homozygous form of the autosomal recessive trait being the so-called adult onset congenital adrenal hyperplasia. The heterozygotes have a normal basal 17-α-hydroxyprogesterone whereas the plasma cortisol is slightly lower than normal. The diagnostic feature is the response to ACTH stimulation (0.25 mg tetracosactrin intramuscularly) when there is a massive increase in 17-α-hydroxyprogesterone and a small increase in plasma cortisol. Bouchard et al (1981) gave 1 mg tetracosactrin intravenously and noted a similarly large response in 17-α-hydroxyprogesterone and progesterone but no response in plasma cortisol. The usual presentation at or soon after puberty may be associated with primary amenorrhoea or with oligomenorrhoea or secondary amenorrhoea respectively and hirsutism progresses to virilism. However, two of our three cases had quite gross hirsutism which had not progressed to virilism over a long time period and was still associated with an irregular menstrual cycle. This emphasises the need to look diligently for this treatable condition using a systematic protocol.

(e) *Hyperprolactinaemia*. Three years after stopping oral contraception, a 26-year-old woman had become hirsute but she retained her regular 2/28-day cycle. On investigation her plasma cortisols and diurnal rhythm were normal but there was an exaggerated response to tetracosactrin from a basal value of 600 to a stimulated 1300 nmol/l. The urinary free cortisol excretion was normal. Her plasma testosterone level was normal but plasma androstenedione was elevated at 10.0 to 15.8 nmol/l (normal range 1.6–5.7 nmol/l) and this was supressible to normal with 48 h of 2 mg/24 h dexamethasone. The sex hormone binding globulin was low varying from 16 to 28 nmol DHT bound/l (normal range 43–74 nmol DHT bound/l). Plasma prolactin was more than 2000 mU/l on four occasions. At this stage the patient moved to another city before the results were available and was started on a reversed sequential regime of ethinyl oestradiol and cyproterone acetate with remarkable resolution of her hirsutism. Subsequently pursuing the earlier results, she was found on lateral tomography of the pituitary fossa to have marked expansion of the right side of the fossa. There was also a left homonymous defect in her visual fields and she was treated with bromocriptine. Unfortunately, because of the sequence of treatments, the question of whether the hyperprolactinaemia was stimulating the adrenal cortex was not resolved as no opportunity was taken to test the response to a dopamine agonist alone.

Hyperprolactinaemia has been reported as being associated with abnormal adrenocortical function (Carter et al, 1977). Normal androstenedione and testosterone levels and elevated DHA and DHAS concentrations are described (Vermeulen & Ando, 1978; Kandeel et al, 1978). Although Belisle & Menard (1980) showed no increase of metabolic clearance rates of DHA and DHAS, and no reduction of circulating levels of these two steroids on bromocriptine, their ten patients studied only had mild hyperprolactinaemia whereas Carter et al (1977) did show a reduction after 6 months bromocriptine therapy in patients with higher prolactin concentrations. Although this case did not unequivocally demonstrate the relationship between hyperprolactinaemia and hyperandrogenaemia leading to hirsutism, the possibility exists so that estimations of plasma prolactin should be retained in the protocol as a screening mechanism.

(f) *Polycystic ovarian disease*. This diagnosis is usually a difficult one to make. Classically obesity, oligomenorrhoea, infertility, hirsutism and bilaterally symmetrically enlarged ovaries comprise the syndrome described in 1935 but this is now regarded as being at one end of the spectrum of conditions that is associated with increased ovarian androgen production although some types originate from increased adrenal androgen production and others produce excess androgens from both sources (see Goldzieher & diZerega, Ch. 20.).

From the management viewpoint, fertility is often not an immediate requirement and from the clinical diagnostic perspective, the patient may not be obese nor may she have detectable ovarian enlargement. In a hirsute clinic, this sign is the reason for presentation. Anovulation is present and frequently oligomenorrhoea or amenorrhoea (more than 6 months). The two major therapies to induce ovulation are clomiphene or corticosteroids and a choice needs to be made between the two, at least initially when pregnancy is the objective, but if not we believe that these two drug treatments should not be offered and the agent of first choice should be cyproterone acetate/ethinyl oestradiol in a reversed sequential regime as it is a more effective treatment for hirsutism. This being so, if fertility is not required, there seems little point in attempting to distinguish ovarian and adrenal sources of the mild degree of hyperandrogenaemia and the prime objective of investigation is to exclude the more serious conditions already described above. If pregnancy is subsequently desired, then if oligomenorrhoea exists, clomiphene may be used but if regular apparently ovulatory cycles occur then it would seem to be not unreasonable to allow regular exposure to pregnancy to occur before attempting further treatments, i.e. corticoids.

A 29-year-old woman presented with hirsutism. She had been investigated and treated extensively elsewhere for 4 years for primary infertility with ovulation induction regimes but without success and had decided that she no longer wished to pursue her infertility and only have her hirsutism controlled. Her menarche was at the age of 11 and hirsutism developed at age 14 and had been stable since 16. It mainly affected her face in the beard area but also her abdomen and legs. This required plucking initially and later shaving until she needed recourse to electrolysis for her face. Her skin and hair were greasy and she had a little acne. Her menstrual pattern was unpredictable ranging from 5/21–56 days. There was no family history of increased hair growth. She had taken no oral contraception. Laparoscopy had revealed no abnormality apart from sclerocystic ovaries.

She was obese but her breasts were normal and the Ferriman & Gallwey score was 29. Her blood pressure was normal, no other abnormality was noted on systemic or pelvic examination.

On investigation she was anovulatory, the plasma progesterone was 3 nmol/l and on day 4 since her last period the plasma LH was 17 and FSH 4.3 iu/l, LH: FSH ratio being 3.95. The plasma testosterone was elevated only once, 3.7 nmol/l in five estimations (normal range 0.5–2.5 nmol/l). Plasma androstenedione was 7.4 nmol/l (normal range 1.6–5.7 nmol/l) and SHBG 10 nmol DHT bound/l (normal range 34–75 nmol DHT bound/l). Plasma cortisols were 145 and 344 nmol/l at 21.00 and 09.00 and were suppressed to 91 nmol/l after overnight 1.5 mg dexamethasone responding adequately to tetracosactrin from a basal of 413 to a +30 min value of 759 nmol/l. The 17-α-hydroxyprogesterone concentration was 5 nmol/l. The urinary 17-oxosteroid values were at the upper limit of normal, 52 μmol/24 h (normal range 18–53 μmol/24 h). Plasma prolactin and thyroid function were normal. Because of her considerable degree of hirsutism and the possibility that she was still young enough to pursue a pregnancy, an attempt was made to assess possible partial enzyme defects, identification of which would provide a rationale for long-term corticoid therapy which would possibly facilitate any subsequent infertilty management after the previous failures. These results are shown in Table 21.8 and proved to be normal. They are based on the steroid pathway sequence of 17-α-hydroxypregnenolone (via 3β-hydroxysteroid dehydrogenase Δ^{4-5} isomerase enzyme) to 17-α-hydroxyprogesterone (via 21-hydroxylase enzyme) to 11-deoxycortisol (via 11β-hydroxylase enzyme) to cortisol. These normal results bear out the ACTH stimulation data of Lachelin et al (1979) which failed to demonstrate an adrenal androgen defect in established PCO and attributed the increased androgens to the ovary and suggest that the adrenal role is different, perhaps related to function at adrenarche but as yet, not adequately defined. Her only identifiable source of additional androgens therefore was the androstenedione although the SHBG seemed to be unusually low for the relatively small increment in androstenedione. This raises the question as to whether the abnormal SHBG concentration arises from a primary defect. The LH/FSH ratio was increased with a higher plasma LH and lower plasma FSH concentration early in the follicular phase as described by Rebar et al (1976); indeed Deutsch et al (1978) found a single plasma LH value to be the most useful diagnostic endocrine parameter.

As the hirsutism was severe, treatment was started with the reversed sequential regime of cyproterone acetate/ethinyl oestradol with considerable improvement in her seborrhoea and hair greasiness and then a reduction in apparent hair growth rate. She was very happy on this regime and has continued now for almost 1 year.

The failure to demonstrate a relative increase of precursor in relation to product (Table 21.8) after stimulation of the steroid pathway excludes an enzyme insufficiency but still does not provide information as to whether the adrenals or the ovaries or both are producing the increased androgen. Although as detailed above, Steinberger et al (1981) have described suppression of testosterone as a rationale for corticosteroid administration, we would not wish to use this modality in the absence of a wish to pursue pregnancy and in the light of the excellent response to the reversed sequential regime. For the same

Table 21.8 Partial enzyme defect assessment in a patient with polycystic ovarian disease

Steroid (nmol/l)	17-α-OH pregn* (A)	17-α-OH prog† (B)	11-Desoxycortisol (C)	Cortisol (D)
Basal°	4.8	1.3	22	260
+ 30 min‡§	26.8	3.1	35	540
Increment	22.0	1.8	13	280

Enzyme	Ratio	Value	Normal range**
3β-OH △ 4–5 isomerase	A/B	22/1.8 = 12.2	2–24
11β-OH dehydrogenase	C/D	13/280 = 0.05	<0.12
21-OH dehydrogenase	B/C	1.8/13 = 0.14	<1.9

* 17-α-hydroxypregnenolone.

† 17-α-hydroxyprogesterone.

° After 1.5 mg oral dexamethasone at 23.00 the previous evening.

‡ Steroid estimation after 0.25 mg intravenous tetracosactrin.

§ Data obtained at +60 min provided no different information.

** From Gibson et al (1980).

reason we did not proceed to adrenal and ovarian vein catheterisation. Ovarian biopsy was not obtained as it would add little. One may find a thickened capsule, even a number of small follicles and no evidence of recent luteinisation but the biopsy is small if obtained laparoscopically and possibly unrepresentative. One may assess the appearance of the ovaries at laparoscopy noting multiple small follicles and a thickened white capsule.

(g) *Idiopathic hirsutism.* This is currently a diagnosis of exclusion, the conditions being excluded are those that have already been described above. The diagnosis does not assume any ratio of adrenal to ovarian source of androgens but rests on a clinical documentation of the hirsutism and a demonstration of elevated plasma androgens (testosterone and/or androstenedione) and a reduced SHBG concentration. We are uncertain whether the apparently ovulatory regularly cycling women are infertile as a result of the endocrine changes leading to their increased hair growth in the absence of adequate documention of the causes of their infertility; bias may be introduced if they present to an infertility clinic.

A 32-year-old unmarried woman first noted excessive hair growth at age 16. There was no family history of hirsutism. She had normal regular menses and was normotensive. Her weight for height was within the normal Garrow range. A Ferriman & Gallwey score was 22, most marked on the upper lip and chin. Seborrhoea was apparent but acne was not a major problem. General and pelvic examinations revealed no abnormality. Laboratory investigation demonstrated that plasma cortisols and the diurnal rhythms and plasma 17-α-hydroxyprogesterone were normal. There was adequate plasma cortisol suppression with dexamethasone although the tetracosactrin stimulation was suboptimal from 286 to 371 nmol/l. The plasma testosterone varied from 1.8 to 2.2 nmol/l (normal 0.5–2.5 nmol/l) suppressible to 1.1 nmol/l and plasma androstenedione was elevated at 12.2 to 13.8 nmol/l but suppressed readily to 5.4 nmol/l (normal range 1.6–5.7 nmol/l). The SHBG was very low at less than 10 nmol DHT bound/l. These date confirm hyperandrogenaemia supported by the low SHBG and exclude any adrenal abnormality, even showing adequate suppression of the elevated androstenedione with dexamethasone. Presumably, therefore, the ovaries are the source of the increased androgen secretion although this makes little difference to our management. The patient was ovulatory and the gonadotrophins and plasma prolactin were normal but the above laboratory data are little different to that of a patient with polycystic ovarian disease considered above except for the lack of an increased LH/FSH ratio. The clinical picture differed in that this patient was not obese and did not have an irregular cycle.

The suboptimal response to adrenal stimulation might suggest a partial enzyme block but this was not pursued further. The patient had had no suggestion of relative adrenal insufficiency associated with intercurrent illness or previous operations and had no plans for childbearing and so the possibility of corticosteroid treatment was not raised. Treatment was primarily with the reversed sequential anti-androgen regime.

Ovarian hyperthecosis has been described again recently in five overweight patients (Nagamani et al, 1981). They had gross hirsutism and were obese. The plasma testosterone was markedly elevated as was 17-α-hydroxyprogesterone and androstenedione less so. Effective reduction in hirsutism only followed bilateral oophorectomy so it seems that cyproterone acetate/ethinyl oestradiol could be the preparation of first choice. The diagnosis may be suggested by the considerably elevated plasma testosterone concentration (in some cases just within the 'tumour range' referred to earlier) but the 17-α-hydroxyprogesterone is also elevated and the plasma progesterone increased over that usually found in the proliferative phase but not reaching levels indicative of ovulation. Abraham et al (1976) suggest that it may be due to a partial defect in the enzyme 17–20 desmolase involved in the $\triangle^4$–3-oxo steroid pathway. This enzyme removes the sidechain from progesterone (via 17-α-hydroxyprogesterone) to produce the C_{17} androgens. The histological diagnosis is unlikely to be sought as it shows increased luteinisation of stromal cells deep in the medulla and does not usually have a polycystic appearance. The LH/FSH ratio is not increased.

Management

After appropriate investigation, the diagnosis will have been suggested or at least major serious abnormality excluded and a diagnosis of idiopathic hirsutism reached.

(a) Specific therapy will of course be indicated similar to that described above for adrenal tumours but if more usually a mass is not palpable then localisation of non-suppressible androgens and corticoids may be supplemented by computerised tomography, adrenal arteriography, retrograde venography or adrenal and ovarian vein catheterisation in addition to the techniques described above. The definition of a smaller adrenal lesion would suggest exploration and excision or adrenalectomy. This would be associated with a plasma testosterone of more than 7 nmol/l and a plasma DHAS concentration that was increased more than 4–5 fold.

(b) Adrenalectomy is also envisaged for Cushing's disease when plasma ACTH is suppressed and there is no pituitary or ectopic lesion.

(c) An ovarian tumour is likely if only testosterone is in the tumour range but an adrenal tumour cannot be ruled out (Givens et al, 1974) so an intravenous pyelogram should be used as a screening procedure. At laparotomy, as the endocrinologically active tumours may more usually be potentially malignant, careful staging and removal of as much of any spread as possible should be attempted. If the tumour is small and well localised without apparent spread, the usual washings from the Pouch of Douglas and para-colic gutters and scrapings from the undersurface of the diaphragm should be taken. Any malignant cells should be pursued vigorously with chemotherapy. At least with the steroid-secreting cells a tumour marker is likely to be available for follow up. Second-look laparotomy should also be used. Aesthetic measures are of course necessary for the redundant hair.

(d) Adrenal hyperplasia requires optimisation of plasma 17-α-hydroxyprogesterone concentrations at perhaps the mid-point of the normal range throughout the day and 24 h profiles should be checked at intervals (cf Jones & Klingensmith, Ch. 18). The patient needs to be issued with a steroid warning card to carry with her with the record of dosage and she and her general practitioner need to be warned of the need for increased dosage in the event of infection, stress or trauma. Adequate control of the adrenal steroidogenesis however, is likely to bestow normal fertility so attention needs to be paid to effective contraception as this may not have been necessary previously. Oral or barrier contraception or an IUD are appropriate. Local attention to the increased hair growth will need to continue but probably at a decreasing rate and electrolysis for example could be suspended. Cycle regularity will return and any attempt at pregnancy should be deferred until there is evidence of regular ovulation achieved on a stable basis. Short-term barrier contraception is useful at this time. Other routine infertility investigations should be deferred for at least 6 months depending on the patient's age and antecedent indications as fertility should now be normal.

(e) For obese patients who are diagnosed as having polycystic ovarian disease, we are now exhorting them to lose weight down to the upper limit of the Garrow range (weight [kg]/height [m]^2 = 24) prior to instituting further therapy and there is a suggestion that regular ovulation may return in quite a number or that responses to ovulation induction are more effective in achieving pregnancy. Clomiphene, beginning at a dose of 25 mg daily for 5 days from day 2, has been the drug of first choice if pregnancy is desired but not otherwise. Ultrasonic monitoring of ovarian responses to stimulation may suggest that lower doses of clomiphene cause less disorganisation of follicle dynamics but more extensive study is required. Clomiphene efficacy of course, depends on there being adequate circulating oestrogen levels, e.g. a plasma oestradiol of more than 100 pmol/1. If clomiphene is unsuccessful even at 50–100 mg dose level, then gonadotrophin therapy could be used for these oligomenorrhoeic women although results are poorer for those patients with adequate peripheral oestrogen levels of more than 100 pmol/1 plasma oestradiol than those with lower levels (less than 100 pmol/1). Pulsatile LHRH may be appropriate but may provoke a high LH output that is inappropriate.

Many of these women do not in fact wish to conceive, at least in the near future, or may not even wish to use contraception. A reversed sequential regime of cyproterone acetate would be appropriate. The usual starting dose is 30 μg ethinyl oestradiol daily from days 5–25 inclusive and cyproterone acetate 50 mg daily from days 5–15. If the hirsutism is gross, 100 mg cyproterone acetate may be used. The choice of 30 μg ethinyl oestradiol is related to the general data on low dose oral contraceptive regimes which associated that dose with minimal vascular complications. For this reason smoking, obesity, hypertension and family histories of myocardial infarction, diabetes and hyperlipidaemia would all be regarded as risk factors. The objective is to maintain therapy for at least 6–9 months and patients should be informed that any acne is likely to show maximal improvement by 4 months and hair growth to be maximally reduced at about 7 months therapy. Improvement is often noted by 2 months but it is important to appreciate the extended time scale.

Prednisone (Rodriguez-Rigau et al, 1979) and dexamethasone (Abraham et al, 1975) have also been used on the basis of increased adrenal androgen activity contributing to the hyperandrogenic state. Most of the patients of Abraham et al (1976) had at least oligomenorrhoea and DHAS suppression was inadequate on short-term dexamethasone. They used long term dexamethasone therapy taking 0.5 mg (more if body weight was more than 70 kg) on retiring to suppress the overnight ACTH surge and claimed considerable improvement in menstrual status, hirsutism and acne on more than 6 months therapy. (It is interesting that they nevertheless used clomiphene as first line treatment for anovulatory infertility.) Dexamethasone is used as it is associated with less weight gain than other corticosteroids. Therapy for 1 year and then stopping is associated with maintained improvement after cessation of treatment one year later (Maroulis et al, 1981) and androgen levels are also said to be frequently normal. This last point appears to be the only one that provides a rational reason for using corticosteroid suppression in preference to cyproterone acetate.

Wedge resection of the ovaries has largely fallen into disuse because of post operative adhesions (Weinstein & Polishuk, 1975) and because improvement tends to be short-lived. Certainly fertility may not be required until some time later yet relief from acne and hirsutism may be required immediately. Sometimes poor responses or inappropriate excessive responses occur after clomiphene. We have found small dermoid cysts in a number of these patients and they may be bilateral (Babaknia et al, 1976). If wedge resection is required, and Jewelewicz (1975) suggested it after 7–8 cycles of unsuccessful treatment, then a microsurgical technique is required. This involves use of a heparinised Ringer's solution for constant lavage and respect for serosal surfaces avoiding glove contact and dry swabs and packs. Non-absorbable sutures 6/0 are used on the ovarian capsule and apposition of cut edges is achieved. Instillation of cortisone acetate 75 mg in 500 ml warmed saline into the peritoneal cavity at the end of the procedure is thought to reduce subsequent adhesion formation but the effect is more likely to be due to the careful handling of tissues and the use of the fine new suture material.

(f) Idiopathic hirsutism is a diagnosis that in our view should be restricted to those women with regular cycles and ideally who have demonstrable evidence of ovulation. Many of these women are unmarried, indeed their social activities have been restricted primarily because of their hirsutism and acne. Fertility is therefore often potential and in the future; exposure to pregnancy is often not a current risk but one that comes from successful treatment and an altered social expression of this. The principal treatment is the reversed sequential regime of cyproterone acetate/ethinyl oestradiol, the former usually starting at the 50 mg dose. The patients are warned about weight gain and lethargy which are the two main side-effects but the weight usually stabilises at an acceptable level.

Initially the current aesthetic measures used to control the excess hair, such as waxing and electrolysis, are continued and the patient reduces the frequency of treatments as the need decreases. She notices a reduction in seborrhoea, acne and head hair greasiness resulting in a major improvement in morale, altered hair styling and greater extroversion. This regime may be continued without a break for a long as the patient wishes. We have now had patients taking it for up to 7 years without problems. Although anxiety was initially generated that adrenal insufficiency was a possibility, as found in the treatment of precocious puberty, we have tested adrenal function in our long-term patients and found no significant impairment apart from a slight increase in serum potassium which remains unexplained. Liver tumours have been found in rats, in which they have also been induced by progesterone and of course, hepatic adenoma is a rare complication of taking oral contraceptives. As the regime suppresses ovulation, there is no need to use supplementary contraception and the patient should be told of this. A 2 mg cyproterone acetate/50 μg ethinyl oestradiol combined oral contraceptive preparation is available (Diane, Schering) and although this is effective against acne, the dose of cyproterone acetate seems to be too low to cause effective suppression of excess hair growth. On cessation of therapy there is usually a slow offset comparable to the slow onset of effect. However, if the patient wishes to attempt conception she should wait at least 1 month using barrier contraception for that time. We have found that plasma cyproterone acetate concentrations fall to unmeasurable levels within 10 days of stopping the 100 mg daily dose regime even after some months' therapy. It is important to ensure that the body fat stores of the 15-β-hydroxy

derivative are excreted, as anti-androgenic effects during the organogenetic period of the fetal male genital tract may lead to anomalies. Administration of a reversed sequential preparation to patients over the age of 35 years presumably carries the general risks of oestrogen/progestogen combinations although the anti-androgen preparations have not been studied epidemiologically after administration to large numbers of patients. Further, the sequential format is different to the sequential oral contraceptive preparations formerly used as the oestrogen dose, in that far from being high, is as low as that directed by the large scale oral contraceptive epidemiological studies. The efficacy of the oestrogen lies in its effect of increasing the SHBG concentration so that the anti-androgen alone would be expected to be less effective. In the absence of better data, and in line with the above background, we prescribe a 30 μg ethinyl oestradiol component of the reversed sequential regime to the small number of patients over the age of 35, provided they do not have identifiable risk factors such as smoking, obesity or a family history of ischaemic heart disease. Fortunately the demand from older patients is quite small. The problem may of course arise with long continued use by patients who began therapy before the age of 35 and that is problem yet to be faced.

Conclusion

It can be seen that cyproterone acetate availability has transformed the approach to investigation and management of hirsutism. It is to be hoped that a wider experience can lead to its taking a major role in treatment of these hyperandrogenic disorders.

Acknowledgements

The hirsute patients have been supervised in turn by Dr A K Thomas, Mr R S Sawers and most recently by Dr S K Smith.

The trichological expertise has been contributed by Professor F J G Ebling and Dr Valerie Dew (née Randall).

The SHBG and androstenedione assays have been performed by Professor S L Jeffcoate, Department of Biochemical Endocrinology, Chelsea Hospital for Women, London.

The assistance with the partial enzyme defect assays has been provided by Dr D Anderson, Department of Medicine, Hope Hospital Salford and Dr J G Ratcliffe, Department of Chemical Pathology, University of Manchester, Hope Hospital, Salford.

Comprehensive secretarial assistance has been provided by Mrs Barbara Laing.

To all of these, my grateful thanks.

REFERENCES

Abraham G E, Chakmakjian L H, Buster, J E, Marshall J R 1975 Ovarian and adrenal contributions to the peripheral androgens in hirsute women. Obstetrics and Gynecology 46: 169–173

Abraham G E, Maroulis G B, Buster J E, Chang R J, Marshall J R 1976 Effect of dexamethasone on serum cortisol and androgen levels in hirsute patients. Obstetrics and Gynecology 47: 395–402

Babaknia A, Calfopoulos P, Jones Jr H W 1976 The Stein-Leventhal syndrome and coincidental ovarian tumours. Obstetrics and Gynecology 47: 223–224

Bates G W, Whitworth N S 1982 Effect of body weight reduction on plasma androgens in obese, infertile women. Fertility and Sterility 38: 406–409

Belisle S, Menard J 1980 Adrenal and androgen production in hyperprolactinaemic states. Fertility and Sterility 33: 396–400

Bouchard P, Kuttenn F, Mowszowicz I, Schaisun G, Raux-Eurin M-C, Mauvais-Jarvis P 1981 Congenital adrenal hyperplasia due to partial 21-hydroxylase deficiency. A study of five cases. Acta Endocrinologica (Kbh) 96: 107–111

Bruchovsky N 1980 Molecular action of androgens and antiandrogens. In: Hammerstein J, Lachnit-Fixson U, Neumann F, Plewig G (eds) Androgenization in Women, p. 7. Excerpta Medica, Amsterdam

Carter J N, Tyson J E, Warne G L, McNeilly A S, Faiman C, Friesen H G 1977 Adrenocortical function in hyperprolactinaemic women. Journal of Clinical Endocrinology and Metabolism 45: 973–980

Cathelineau G, Brerault J-L, Fiet J, Julien R, Dreux C, Canivet J 1980 Adrenocortical 11 β-hydroxylation defect in adult women with post-menarchial onset of symptoms. Journal of Clinical Endocrinology and Metabolism 51: 287–291

Deutsch S, Krumholz B, Benjamin I 1978 The utility and selection of laboratory tests in the diagnosis of polycystic ovary syndrome. Journal of Reproductive Medicine 20: 275–282

Ebling F J, Thomas A K, Cooke I D, Randall V A, Skinner J, Cawood M 1977 Effect of cyproterone acetate on hair growth, sebaceous and endocrine parameters in a hirsute subject. British Journal of Dermatology 97: 371–381

Ebling F J G, Cooke I D, Randall V A, Sawers R S, Thomas A K, Skinner J 1980 The influence of cyproterone acetate on the activity of hair follicles and sebaceous glands in man. In: Hammerstein J, Lachnit-Fixson U, Neumann F, Plewig G (eds) Androgenization in Women p. 239. Excerpta Medica, Amsterdam

Ferriman D, Gallwey J D 1961 Clinical assessment of body hair growth in women. Journal of Clinical Endocrinology and Metabolism 21: 1440–1447

Garrow J S 1979 Weight penalties. British Medical Journal 2: 1171–1172

Gibson M, Lackritz R, Schiff I, Tulchinsky D 1980 Abnormal adrenal responses to adrenocorticotropic hormone in hyperandrogenic women. Fertility and Sterility 33: 43–48

Givens J R, Andersen R N, Wiser W L, Coleman S A, Fish S A 1974 A gonadotropin-responsive adrenocortical adenoma. Journal of Clinical Endocrinology and Metabolism 38: 126–133

Givens J R, Andersen R N, Ragland J B, Wiser W L, Umstot F S 1975 Adrenal function in hirsutism. I. Diurnal change and response of plasma androstenedione, testosterone, 17 hydroxyprogesterone, cortisol, LH and FSH to dexamethasone and 1/2 unit of ACTH. Journal of Clinical Endocrinology and Metabolism 40: 988–1000

Glenthøj A, Damkjaer Nielsen M, Starup J K 1980 Congenital adrenal hyperplasia due to 11β-hydroxylase deficiency: final diagnosis in adult age in three patients. Acta Endocrinologica (Kbh) 93: 94–99

Hammerstein J, Meckies J, Leo-Rossberg I, Matzl L, Zielkse F 1975 Use of cyproterone acetate (CPA) in the treatment of acne, hirsutism and virilism. Journal of Steroid Biochemistry 6: 827–836

Hümpel M, Nieuweboer B, Düsterberg B, Wendt H 1980 Pharmacokinetics of cyproterone acetate in man. In: Hammerstein J, Lachnit-Fixson U, Neumann F, Plewig G (eds) Androgenization in Women, p. 209. Excerpta Medica, Amsterdam

Huq M S, Pfaff M, Jespersen D, Zucker I R, Kirschner M A 1976 Concurrence of aldosterone, androgen and cortisol secretion in adrenal venous effluents. Journal of Clinical Endocrinology and Metabolism 42: 230–238

Jewelewicz R 1975 Management of infertility resulting from anovulation. American Journal of Obstetrics and Gynecology 122: 909–920

Kandeel F R, Ridd B T, Butt W R, Logan Edwards R, London D R 1978 Androgen and cortisol. Responses to ACTH in women with hyperprolactinaemia. Clinical Endocrinology (Oxf) 9: 123–130

Kirschner M A, Sinhamahapatra S, Zucker I R, Loriaux L, Nieschlag E 1973 The production, origin and role of dehydroepiandrosterone and △5-androstenediol as androgen prehormones in hirsute women. Journal of Clinical Endocrinology and Metabolism 37: 183–189

Kirschner M A, Zucker I R, Jesperson D 1976 Idiopathic hirsutism — an ovarian abnormality. New England Journal of Medicine 294: 637–640

Lachelin G C L, Barnett M, Hopper B R, Brink G, Yen S S C 1979 Adrenal function in normal women and women with polycystic ovary syndrome. Journal of Clinical Endocrinology and Metabolism 49: 892–898

Lenton E A, Brook L M, Sobowale O, Cooke I D 1979 Prolactin concentrations in normal menstrual cycles and conception cycles. Clinical Endocrinology (Oxf) 10: 383–391

Louros N C, Batrinos M L, Carcatzoulis S 1966 Individual 17-ketosteroid excretion in a case of arrhenoblastoma and its response to corticotropin and human chorionic gonadotropin stimulation and to dexamethasone inhibition. Journal of Clinical Endocrinology and Metabolism 26: 645–650

Luderschmidt C 1980 Pathogenesis of acne vulgaris. In: Hammerstein J, Lachnit-Fixson U, Neumann F, Plewig G (eds) Androgenization in Women, p 75. Excerpta Medica, Amsterdam

Ludwig E 1977 Classification of the types of androgenetic alopecia (common baldness) occurring in the female sex. British Journal of Dermatology 97: 247–254

McNatty K P, Baird D T, Bolton A, Chambers P, Corker C S, McLean P 1976 Concentration of oestrogens and androgens in human ovarian venous plasma and follicular fluid throughout the menstrual cycle. Journal of Endocrinology 71: 77–85

Maroulis G B 1981 Evaluation of hirsutism and hyperandrogenaemia. Fertility and Sterility 36: 273–305

Mathur R S, Moody L O, Landgrebe S C, Peress M R, Rust P F, Williamson H O 1982 Sex-hormone-binding globulin in clinically hyperandrogenic women: association of plasma concentrations with body weight. Fertility and Sterility 38: 207–211

Meldrum D R, Abraham G E 1979 Peripheral ovarian venous concentrations of various steroid hormones in virilizing ovarian tumours. Obstetrics and Gynecology 53: 36–43

Nagamani M, Lingold J C, Gomez L G, Garza J R 1981 Clinical and hormonal studies in hyperthecosis of the ovaries. Fertility and Sterility 36: 326–332

Neumann F, Schleusener A, Albring M 1980 Pharmacology of anti-androgens. In: Hammerstein J, Lachnit-Fixson U, Neumann F, Plewig G (eds) Androgenization in Women, p 147. Excerpta Medica, Amsterdam

Rebar R, Judd H L, Yen S S C, Rakoff J, Vandenberg G, Naftolin F 1976 Characterization of the inappropriate gonadotropin secretion in polycystic ovary syndrome. Journal of Clinical Investigation 57: 1320–1329

Rodriguez-Rigau L J, Smith K D, Tcholakian R K, Steinberger E 1979 Effect of prednisone on plasma testosterone levels and on duration of phases of the menstrual cycle in hyperandrogenic women. Fertility and Sterility 32: 408–413

Rosenwaks Z, Lee P A, Jones G S, Migeon C J, Wentz A C 1979 An attenuated form of congential virilizing adrenal hyperplasia. Journal of Clinical Endocrinology and Metabolism 49: 335–339

Schweikert H U, Wilson J D 1974 Regulation of human hair growth by steroid hormones. II. Androstenedione metabolism in isolated hairs. Journal of Clinical Endocrinology and Metabolism 39: 1012–1019

Steinberger E, Rodriguez-Rigau L J, Smith K D 1981 The infertile couple: a quantitative approach to the evaluation of each partner. In: Insler V, Bettendorf G (eds) Advances in Diagnosis and Treatment of Infertility, p 179. Elsevier/North Holland, Amsterdam

Steinberger E, Rodriguez-Rigau L J, Smith K D 1982 The prognostic value of acute adrenal suppression and stimulation tests in hyperandrogenic women. Fertility and Sterility 37: 187–192

Strauss J S, Pochi P E 1961 The quantitative gravimetric determination of sebum production. Journal of Investigative Dermatology 36: 293–298

Tucci J R, Zah W, Kalderon A E 1973 Endocrine studies in an arrhenoblastoma responsive to dexamethasone, ACTH and human chorionic gonadotropin. American Journal of Medicine 55: 687–694

Vermeulen A, Ando S 1978 Prolactin and adrenal androgen secretion. Clinical Endocrinology (Oxf) 8: 295–303

Wagner R K 1978 Extracellular and intracellular steroid binding proteins. Properties, discrimination, assay and clinical application. Acta Endocrinologica (Kbh) Supp 1 88: 218

Weinstein D, Polishuk W Z 1975 Role of wedge resection of the ovary as a cause for mechanical sterility. Surgery, Gynecology and Obstetrics 141: 417–418

Endometriosis

INTRODUCTION

Endometriosis is an enigmatic disease affecting women and perhaps females of other species of primates. Men may be susceptible to the disease if their hormonal milieu is disastrously changed as indicated by the documented cases of two men developing endometriosis of the urinary bladder following the prolonged use of oestrogens for the treatment of prostatic carcinoma.

Although the term 'endometriosis' was not coined until 1921 by Sampson, the condition had been recognised as an unnamed entity for many decades prior to that. The first recorded reference to endometriosis is usually credited to Von Rokitansky who described an adenomyoma in 1860, although symptoms characteristic of the disease are recorded in the Papyrus Ebers dating back to 1600 BC. As one traces gynaecological complaints through more modern times of the Greeks, of the Romans, and of the late European cultures, one notes the increasing concern of the practitioners regarding dysmenorrhoea and sterility among the many other complaints in this specialty.

There has always been some confusion as regards definitions of endometriosis and its allied conditions. The terms 'internal endometriosis' and 'external endometriosis' are misleading as to specific locations. It is usual now to term 'internal endometriosis' as adenomyosis and to shorten the term 'external endometriosis' simply to endometriosis. By definition, endometriosis is the presence of functioning endometrial glands and stroma outside their usual location lining the uterine cavity.

Histogenesis of endometriosis

To date there have been at least eleven theories of explanation of the histogenesis of endometriosis. In addition to these published theories many competent observers have formulated their own ideas of explanation. Generally speaking the theories of endometriosis can be categorised as follows:

1. The theory, now proven, suggesting that endometrial tissue is transplanted from the uterus to ectopic locations by regurgitation, by 'benign' metastasis or by direct extension.
2. The theory suggesting that ectopic endometrial tissue developes *in situ* from local tissues.
3. Those suggesting a combination of the transportation and/or the development *in situ* theories.

Implantation theory. Sampson, in his exhaustive studies, surmised that actual transplantation of endometrial cells could occur, although, at first, retrograde menstruation through the Fallopian tubes was doubted or at least thought most uncommon. Gynaecological endoscopy has shown that such is not the case. The viability of these transported cells was also strongly doubted initially. The well-designed animal experimentation of Te Linde & Scott (1950) proved that endometriosis could occur in monkeys following the inversion of the uterus to divert the menstrual flow into the peritoneal cavity; however, six or more menstrual cycles were necessary to produce this. Ridley (1961) subsequently demonstrated the development of endometriosis at the site of implantation of desquamated endometrium in the human. As a result, Sampson's theory became a proven fact, although the theory failed to explain certain observations such as the time taken for the development of endometriosis.

Coelomic metaplasia theory. The easiest explanation of this theory is that certain cells under certain stimuli may change their character and even physiological function. Meyer is stated to be the apparent champion of this theory in the histogenesis of endometriosis. His writings (Meyer, 1919) indicate that he believed that endometriosis occurred as a result of an infective process or through an unknown stimulus, either hormonal, which he did not fully accept, or by some other influence.

Hormonal stimulation theory. The theory of the origin of endometriosis by hormonal stimulation has not been substantiated. It is an accepted fact that implants of endometriosis are directly influenced, and in the same manner influenced as the endometrium itself. This phenomenon is not related to the theory that hormones can initiate the formation of endometrium.

Induction phenomenon theory. The question of the induction of endometriosis is based on the assumption of the presence of specific substances which may be liberated from the endometrium in the uterus, and transported by blood and lymph streams, subsequently leading to activation of an omnipotent blastoma to endometrium formation. Doubt exists that this is true endometriosis because of the absence of stroma.

Mechanical transplantation theory. Endometrial tissue is easily transplanted to other areas of the body and every experienced gynaecologist will have observed instances of such mechanically transplanted endometrium and exercise care to prevent this transplantation of endometrium from actually occurring either within the peritoneal cavity or in operative scars.

Benign metastasis theory. Halban (1924) reported the occurrence of endometriosis along the course of lymphatics draining the pelvic area and reference was also made to the occurrence of the lesion in the inguinal, sacro-iliac and parametrial nodes. Lymphatic interchange between the internal genitalia and the umbilicus occurs and many references have indicated the presence of endometrial cells in the lymphatics and lymph glands. Another suggested route of benign metastasis is the venous channels, similar to that which occurs in the transportation of trophoblast in pregnancy to the lung parenchyma. Sporadic case reports of the occurrence of endometriosis in rare and unusual locations emphasise the possibility of distant metastasis via the lymph or blood stream. Isolated locations of endometriosis within the abdominal cavity as seen on the appendix, omentum, small bowel, without continuity to pelvic endometriosis may be explained by the migration of these benign viable cells which have arisen initially as a result of transtubal regurgitation.

Direct extension theory. The direct extension of endometrial tissue into the myometrium resulting in adenomyosis has been stated to be due to the possible 'destructive action' of the advancing endometrium, or to extension along lymphatic pathways. Similarly the extension may occur along the line of least resistance through a given tissue. This process of direct extension may also occur in tissue of non-Müllerian origin as can be observed in the extension of endometrial growth through the wall and into the lumen of either the rectosigmoid or the bladder. Such benign invasion can destroy planes of cleavage and disrupt anatomy and in some cases can alter the physiological functions of the affected tissue. For these reasons, surgical procedures involved with extensive endometriosis may offer considerable technical difficulties.

Cell rest theories. The activation of cell rests or paramesonephric (Müllerian) or mesonephric (Wolffian) origin to form functioning endometrium has never been widely accepted, as there has been inconsistency of the distribution of the lesion expected from such cell rests.

Composite theories. Javert (1949) proposed a composite theory which created wide interest. This theory included the phenomena of endometrial homeoplasia (ability of tissue to reproduce itself), direct extension, exfoliation and implantation and metastasis by the lymphatic and blood streams.

The uterotubal theory has been proposed to explain the so-called 'salpingitis isthmica nodosa' seen in association with pelvic endometriosis. The tubal lesion is in reality adenomyosis of the tube and most likely demonstrates the direct invasion of Müllerian epithelium through the tubal wall, the viable endometrium being the result of retrograde migration from the uterine cavity.

Aetiology of endometriosis

Many of the so-called aetiological factors although recognised as definite possibilities remain in the realm of theory.

Mechanical factors. Endometrium may be transplanted to ectopic sites accidentally, experimentally and on occasions therapeutically. Animal experiments have proved that tubal insufflation may cause abdominal endometriosis. This can no doubt play a part also in the human when tubal insufflation is performed by either gas or contrast media. For this reason these tests are not carried out immediately after curettage or whilst the patient is menstruating.

Congenital abnormalities of the genital tract. Reports of endometriosis in the young girl shortly after the menarche are almost exclusively confined to those with associated congenital abnormalities, especially in those associated with stenosis or atresia of the lower Müllerian tract. No cases of endometriosis have been reported in proven agenesis of the uterus and tubes, which points strongly to the theory of transtubal regurgitation.

Retroversion of the uterus. Laparotomy performed at the time of menstruation in the woman with a retroverted uterus has been found to be associated with a high incidence of menstrual blood trickling from the tubal fimbriae. Examination of this material which pools in the Pouch of Douglas has shown endometrial cells and is further supportive evidence of Sampson's theory. Frequently the uterus in the pelvis in endometriosis is retroverted with limited mobility but it remains unknown whether this is contributory to the aetiology or a result of endometriotic adhesions.

Hormonal factors. Normal endometrial tissue has an orderly and fairly predictable pattern of behaviour due to the influences of the pituitary-ovarian axis and the hormones of pregnancy. Such is not always true in the case of ectopically situated endometrium where the variations, although similar, are much less predictable. Such a difference may be due to a variable blood supply to the ectopic endometrium because of either the location of the lesion or the amount of associated scar tissue. Other observers have suggested that the variation of response seen in ectopic endometrium may be explained by the varying response of the individual layers of the endometrium, the more superficial layers being more sensitive than the basal layers. These hormonal effects form the basis of the conservative management of endometriosis by nonsurgical means.

Inflammatory factors. The macroscopic presence of serosal adhesions in pelvic endometriosis, together with the microscopic evidence of inflammatory cells in the lesion suggested to Sampson (1927) that the regurgitating menstrual blood or liberated endometriotic cyst contents were irritating to the peritoneal surface and facilitated implantation on the more receptive areas. Secondary invasion of endometriotic areas by pyogenic bacteria may also occur.

Race. It has been noted that endometriosis occurs most frequently in white women between the ages of 30 and 40. With the advent of improved diagnostic procedures, the diagnosis has been made with increasing frequency in black Americans and in Japanese women (Miyazawa, 1976). There is a well-established association between primary infertility and endometriosis. In 23 per cent of patients with infertility endometriosis was diagnosed at laparoscopy by Cohen (1976), and a comparable incidence (25 per cent) was found in 459 consecutive patients with primary infertility investigated at The Johns Hopkins Hospital by Jones & Rock (1977).

Infertility and endometriosis

Rubin reported in 1940 that the expectation of pregnancy with endometriosis was approximately one-half that of the general population. Advances in diagnostic procedures have allowed for the earlier diagnosis and earlier treatment of the disease and the significance of the degree of involvement is now known to influence pregnancy rates, the rate being as high as 66 per cent in patients with minimal endometriosis.

Several theories have been postulated to explain infertility in association with endometriosis. In the presence of peritoneal adhesions and dense scarring around the foci of ectopic endometrium the reason is obviously a mechanical one. The distortion of the normal anatomy may likewise be responsible for the symptoms associated with endometriosis. Cul-de-sac endometriosis involving the utero-sacral ligaments and the posterior aspects of the uterus even in the absence of fixed retroversion of the uterus will result in dyspareunia and reduction in frequency of coitus. Ovarian endometriosis may result in destruction of ovarian cortex with subsequent oligo- or anovulation or perhaps corpus luteum inadequacy.

However, such explanations are not the answer to infertility seen in the presence of minimal or average amounts of endometriosis. These patients may indeed have no symptoms apart from infertility.

One currently accepted suggestion for such is that the ectopic endometrium results in the release of prostaglandins which impairs tubal motility and ovum transport (Meldrum et al, 1977). In their study, prostaglandin E (PGE) and prostaglandin $F_{2\alpha}$ (PGF) were assayed in fluid obtained by aspiration of the cul-de-sac at laparoscopy. In patients in whom minimal endometriosis was noted the concentration of prostaglandins was similar to that obtained in the circulating blood and the PGF:PGE ratio was consistently less than one. In the presence of large amounts of endometriosis there was a ten-fold increase in PGF and the PGF:PGE ratio showed a marked reversal. Fluid obtained from ovarian endometriomas was found to have prostaglandin concentration in excess of 100-fold the blood levels.

An auto-immune basis for the infertility has also been suggested (Weed & Arguembourg, 1980). An auto-immune process can develop in an animal as a result of the release within the animal of an antigen not recognised by its tissues as a normal acceptable substance. In endometriosis the aberrant endometrium responds to stimulation of hormones in a manner comparable to normally situated endometrium. In the endometrioma the numerous endometrial proteins in the menstrual fluid are not removed from the body and must be phagocytised and destroyed by the host. Such proteins may be recognised by the host as foreign and may trigger an auto-immune response.

As there is a varying degree of host reaction there will therefore be a varying degree of auto-immune response. Such would explain the variability of fibrosis seen in endometriosis. Although the exact nature of the antigen has not yet been identified complement has been observed to be deposited around normally sited endometrial glands in curettings of women with endometriosis. Such an immune response may result in infertility by either interfering with sperm passage through the uterus or by causing the rejection of early implantation of the embryo.

Anovulation and corpus luteum inadequacy have also been incriminated as the cause of the associated infertility in pelvic endometriosis. The coexistence of anovulation and endometriosis is well documented although opinion differs as to the incidence. Soules et al (1976) reported an incidence of 17 per cent. Subsequent studies of plasma progesterone levels by Brosens et al (1978) failed to support this incidence which is now considered to be approximately 10 per cent — a figure closely approaching the overall incidence of anovulation among infertile patients. This latter study indicated the major cause of the infertility to be due to a disturbance or failure of ovum release, the luteal phase being found to be somewhat shorter and variable in duration. Luteinisation of the unruptured follicle was also thought to be more common. This latter point has more recently been disproved by Dmowski et al (1979).

Symptomatology

The symptoms of endometriosis bear little relation to the extent of the disease. The extent of the symptoms is dependent partly upon the site of involvement. Dysmenorrhoea which is often said to be the prime symptom of the disease may not be progressive with the disease and the only symptom may in fact be the complaint of infertility. Pelvic discomfort or pain may be present as may deep dyspareunia. The diagnosis should be suspected in patients with nodularity of the utero-sacral ligaments and a retroverted uterus.

In the past decade renewed interest has been shown in the determination of the extent of the disease. Laparoscopy has become the most common method for visualisation of the pelvic organs; endometriosis can be diagnosed, its location and extent evaluated and pelvic inflammatory disease also assessed. The findings may then be utilised to decide on the need for surgical or medical treatment.

Classifications of endometriosis are not new. Riva et al (1961) suggested a classification based on the location and extent of endometriosis recorded at the time of culdoscopy. In 1973, Acosta et al proposed a classification (Table 22.1) which also took into consideration the importance of para-ovarian and peri-tubal adhesions in the assessment of the severity of the disease whilst Kistner et al's classification (1977) (Table 22.2) was based on the natural history of the disease.

Because of the failure of any classification to receive general acceptance it has been extremely difficult to compare treatment results.

In an attempt to resolve this problem and to also allow classification of unilateral disease a further classification has been suggested by the American Fertility Society (1979). This new classification which is based on the natural progression of the disease is hoped to serve as a basis for the evaluation of various therapies and to provide information on pregnancy rates and prognosis in all grades of endometriosis.

Table 22.1 Classification of pelvic endometriosis by Acosta et al (1973) From Acosta et al: A proposed classification of pelvic endometriosis. Reprinted with permission from the American College of Obstetricians and Gynecologists (Obstetrics and Gynecology 42: 19–25, 1973)

Classification	Characteristics
Mild	Scattered, fresh lesions (i.e. implants not associated with scarring or retraction of the peritoneum) in the anterior or posterior cul-de-sac or pelvic peritoneum Rare surface implant on ovary, with no endometrioma, without surface scarring and retraction and without peri-ovarian adhesions No peritubular adhesions
Moderate	Endometriosis involving one or both ovaries, with several surface lesions, with scarring and retraction, or small endometriomas Minimal periovarian adhesions associated with ovarian lesions described Minimal peritubular adhesions associated with ovarian lesions described Superficial implants in anterior and/or posterior cul-de-sac with scarring and retraction; some adhesions, but no sigmoid invasion
Severe	Endometriosis involving one or both ovaries (usually both) with endometrioma > 2 × 2 cm One or both ovaries bound down by adhesions associated with endometriosis, with or without tubal adhesions to ovaries One or both tubes bound down or obstructed by endometriosis; associated adhesions or lesions Obliteration of the cul-de-sac from adhesions or lesions associated with endometriosis Thickening of the uterosacral ligaments and cul-de-sac lesions from invasive endometriosis with obliteration of the cul-de-sac Significant bowel or urinary tract involvement.

Table 22.2 Classification of endometriosis by Kistner et al (1977) From Kistner R W, Siegler A M, Behrman S J: Suggested classification for Endometriosis: Relationship to Infertility. Reproduced with permission of the publisher, the American Fertility and Society (Fertility and Sterility 28: 1008–1009, 1977)

Stage	Characteristics
I	Endometriosis on posterior pelvic peritoneum, uterosacral ligaments, or broad ligament (5 mm diameter) Avascular adhesions may involve tubes Fimbriae uninvolved Ovaries may have avascular adhesions; no fixation Bowel and appendix normal

IIA	Endometriosis on posterior pelvic peritoneum, uterosacral ligaments, and broad ligament (<5 mm diameter)
	Avascular adhesions may involve tubes
	Fimbriae free
	Ovarian involvement:
	    IIA–1) Endometrial cyst or surface area 5 cm
	    IIA–2) Endometrial cyst or surface area 5 > cm
	    IIA–3) Ruptured endometrioma
	Bowel and appendix normal

IIB	Posterior leaf broad ligament covered by adherent ovarian tissue Tubal adhesions endoscopically non removable Fimbriae free Ovaries fixed to broad ligament with areas of endometriosis (>5 mm diameter) Multiple implants in cu-de-sac Bowel non adherent Uterus mobile Bowel and appendix normal
III	Posterior leaf broad ligament may be covered by tube or ovary Fimbriae covered with adhesions Ovaries adherent to broad ligament and tube (endometricsis or endometrioma may not show) Multiple implants in cul-de-sac Bowel non adherent Uterus mobile Bowel and appendix normal Endometriosis involves bladder serosa Uterus fixed retroversion Cul-de-dac covered with adherent bowel or obliterated by fixed uterus Bowel adherrent to cul-de-sac, uterosacral ligaments, or uterus Appendix may be involved

Laparoscopy

The principal role of laparoscopy in the management of endometriosis has been to define more accurately the incidence of the disease. Prior to the advent of endoscopy the condition was frequently diagnosed on clinical impression alone, which resulted in inaccuracies in the analysis of the effectiveness of treatments and of the pregnancy rate following treatments in patients suffering from infertility. It is now generally accepted that, except where major lesions make open surgery obligatory, laparoscopy will accurately define the presence and extent of the endometriosis. During this examination each area of the pelvis should be examined in a set order. One of the advantages of the recent American Fertility Society classification (Fig. 22.1) is that it enables the sites of endometriosis to

Patient's name _____

Total score _____

Stage _____

Stage I (mild)	1–5 points
Stage II (moderate)	6–15 points
Stage III (severe)	16–30 points
Stage IV (extensive)	31–54 points

Associated pathology _____

Means of observation _____

Finding			Size and Characteristics
			PERITONEUM
Endometriosis	<1 cm	1–3 cm	>3 cm
Score	1	2	3
Adhesions	Filmy	Dense with partial cul-de-sac obliteration.	Dense with complete cul-de-sac obliteration.
Score	1	2	3
			OVARY
Endometriosis	<1 cm	1–3	>3 cm or ruptured endometrioma.
Score: R	2	4	6
L	2	4	6
Adhesions	Filmy	Dense with partial ovarian closure.	Dense with complete ovarian closure.
Score: R	2	4	6
L	2	4	6
			TUBE
Endometriosis	<1 cm	>1 cm	Tubal occlusion.
Score: R	2	4	6
L	2	4	6
Adhesions	Filmy	Dense with tubal distortion	Dense with tubal enclosure
Score: R	2	4	6
L	2	4	6

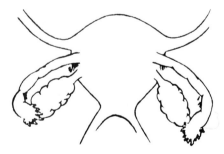

Fig. 22.1 Chart for determining stage of endometriosis according to American Fertility Society classification. Determination of the stage or degree of endometriosis involvement is based on a point system. Although distribution of points has been arbitrarily determined and may require revision or refinement as knowledge of the disease increases, the basis of the classification is the natural progression of the disease with allowances made for unilateral involvement.

To ensure complete evaluation, inspection of the pelvis in a clockwise or counterclockwise fashion is encouraged. Number, size, and location (peritoneum, ovary, or tube) of endometrial implants, plaques, or endometriomas are noted. For example, five separate 0.5 cm endometrial implants of the peritoneum (2.5 cm total) would be assigned 2 points. (The surface of the uterus should be considered peritoneum.) Points assigned may be circled or placed in the left hand column and totaled. Aggregation of points indicates stage of disease (mild, moderate, severe, or extensive).

Presence of endometriosis of the appendix, cervix, skin, etc, should be recorded. Pathology observed should be depicted as specifically as possible on the sketch of pelvic organs, and means of observation should be noted

be charted. Where facilities exist many people also keep a photographic or video tape record. At laparoscopy, the macroscopic identification of most lesions poses no problem but occasionally tiny haemorrhagic areas may make one suspicious of the disease without being diagnostic. The coexistence of well-developed scar tissue around the small endometrioma is generally regarded as being pathognomonic of the lesion, but its absence does not necessarily exclude the possibility. Biopsy may be employed for final confirmation and for this most pathologists require both glandular and stromal elements to be present. Very occasionally a non-encysted area of endometriosis can be found in the pelvis. This is usually seen in the Pouch of Douglas or on the utero-sacral ligaments and appears as a small velvety raised lesion. Histologically, these may be identical to strips of endometrium removed by curettage from within the uterine cavity.

Laparoscopy is also very useful in assessing the response to medical treatment. Small lesions will often have disappeared completely; lesions in which significant fibrosis has occurred will have lost all glandular activity and only scar tissue remains. In such review laparoscopies, the value of earlier charting of lesions becomes obvious as it is sometimes difficult to know whether new lesions have developed or whether old ones have remained active. On occasions it is possible to find new lesions of endometriosis actually developing during a period of definitive medical treatment even when the laparoscopy is carried out during or immediately following that treatment period.

Medical management of endometriosis

As endometriosis is intimately related to ovarian function many efforts have been made to bring the disease under control by changing the hormonal environment. It must be remembered that such action does not often really cure the endometriosis but mostly causes regression for a variable period.

Effect of pregnancy on endometriosis

More than half a century ago Sampson (1924) noted a retrogression of the lesions of endometriosis with pregnancy. The ectopic endometrium undergoes the same changes as uterine endometrium, that is, hypertrophy, increased vascularisation, oedema and decidualisation. The Arias-Stella phenomenon may on occasions be noted in the ectopic endometrial sites, although the visual pattern seen is one of flat glandular epithelium with suppressed activity. With advancing pregnancy atrophic changes have been observed in areas of ectopic endometrium. It is as a result of these changes, specifically due to the increased activity of oestrogens and progesterone in pregnancy, that pregnancy is usually stated to have a beneficial effect on both the symptoms and findings of endometriosis. Such is not always so, and reports have appeared of a worsening of

symptoms and increase in size of endometriomas in association with pregnancy. McArthur & Ulfelder (1965) following an extensive literature review, concluded that symptomatic worsening of the disease and increase in lesion size was more frequently associated with the first trimester of pregnancy. Quiescent disease was more frequently activated at this time. On the other hand, symptomatic improvement and decrease in lesion size was frequently noted in the third trimester, the puerperium and lactational period.

During the 5 years following pregnancy, permanent regression of the disease was encountered much less frequently than was manifest persistent disease. The effect of pregnancy on subsequent fertility appeared also to be negligible: only about 20 per cent of patients who had coincidental pregnancy and endometriosis conceived again regardless of whether or not persistent disease was noted. This apparent progressive compromise of reproductive function in women with endometriosis indicates the need for urgency of treatment in women with endometriosis and known infertility.

Effect of menopause on endometriosis

The symptoms and clinical findings of endometriosis are dependent upon the cyclical stimulation of the lesions by ovarian hormones. With the cyclic fall in circulating levels of hormone at the time of menstruation the ectopic endometrium undergoes congestion and bleeding which results in aggravation of symptoms.

With the cessation of ovarian activity, which may occur either physiologically or surgically, regression of the disease and symptom relief commence.

The physiological menopause results in a gradual decrease of circulating hormone and loss of cyclic production. As oestrogen production may continue well past the menopause active endometriosis may remain. Ranney (1971) in a series of 350 patients with endometriosis reported the incidence of postmenopausal women as 4.8 per cent (17 patients). In seven of these, the endometriosis was an incidental finding, whilst it was responsible for symptoms in ten.

Surgical menopause is associated with the abrupt and complete removal of ovarian hormones which results in a prompt and complete atrophy of both uterine and ectopic endometrium. Coincident with this is the healing of the endometriotic lesions which may be associated with the development of fibrous adhesions and result in further symptomatology.

Reactivation of the disease may occur should exogenous oestrogens be administered to the patient who has had either a surgical or physiological menopause. In the series reported above, exogenous oestrogen administration could have been incriminated in two of the ten postmenopausal patients.

Hormonal approach to the treatment of endometriosis

In consideration of an effective hormonal therapeutic approach to endometriosis many factors must be taken into consideration. The age of the patient, the extent of the disease and the severity of symptoms together with the duration of infertility, if such is a problem, should influence the form of treatment chosen. It should be remembered that hormonal therapy seldom really cures endometriosis and mostly will cause regression only for a given period. Patients with severe disease who are concerned by infertility are not usually ideally suited to hormonal therapy alone. In early endometriosis where the ovaries are not involved and the lesions are confined to the pelvic peritoneum the primary use of hormonal therapy is justified. Where fixation of the ovaries has occurred with resultant tubal distortion reversibility is not possible with hormonal therapy alone. Conservative surgery in such cases would offer the best chance of pregnancy and relief of symptoms. It is in cases such as this that a combination of endocrine and surgical treatment is indicated.

Many efforts have been made to change the hormonal environment and over the years oestrogens, androgens, progestogens and oral contraceptives have been used with varying degrees of success. The efficacy of the individual methods is extremely difficult to determine as few authors relate success of treatment to the stage of the endometriosis.

Oestrogens

Initially, oestrogens were advocated by Karnaky (1948) who considered that in adequate dosage, oestrogenic preparations such as diethyl stilboestrol would not only eliminate cyclic ovarian function but also result in a state of exhaustion atrophy of the ectopic endometrium. The recommended dosage regimen consisted of gradually increasing doses of diethyl stilboestrol up to 100 mg daily which was then maintained for 3 months following which it was gradually reduced. Some symptomatic improvement was noted on this regimen, although the associated risks of the therapy have now seen the cessation of this form of treatment. These risks included the development of cystic glandular hyperplasia and adenomatous hyperplasia of the endometrium and also thrombo-embolic disease. These risks together with the troublesome gastrointestinal side-effects and mastodynia make this form of treatment, in which the reported pregnancy rate was 15 per cent (Haskins & Woolf, 1955) no longer acceptable.

Androgens

The beneficial effects of androgens such as methyl testoterone are also well documented, such effect being thought due to the direct action of the androgen on the endo-metrium, for in the dosage used, there is an inconsistent suppression of ovulation. The commonly employed dose consists of methyl testosterone linguettes given in a dosage of 5 mg daily for approximately 6 months.

Side-effects of therapy include hirsutism, acne, voice changes and clitoral enlargement. The failure of therapy consistently to inhibit ovulation makes this simple regime useful in patients in whom infertility is a problem. Patients must, however, immediately discontinue the drug if menstruation is delayed to avoid possible masculinisation of the female fetus. Symptomatic improvement in the severity of dysmenorrhoea, dyspareunia and pelvic pain has been reported in about 75 per cent of patients with androgens alone (Hammond et al, 1976). However, in most patients, the relief is only partial and of limited duration, the symptoms tending to recur with the efflux of time following cessation of treatment.

Although not widely employed, the average pregnancy rate reported following androgen therapy for the management of endometriosis is 36 per cent (Hirst, 1947; Creadick, 1950; Preston & Campbell, 1953; Katayama et al, 1976).

Progestins

Progestational preparations alone have also been found effective in the management of endometriosis by the production of decidual changes in the ectopic endometrium. The response of the normally situated endometrium to the progestin frequently results in an increased incidence of break-through bleeding. An increase in progestin dosage with each episode of break-through bleeding is usually advocated in an attempt to produce an amenorrhoeic pseudo-pregnancy state for 6–9 months. Such a regimen may lead to atrophy of the normally situated endometrium and necessitate the addition of oestrogen to the therapeutic regimen.

The progestin used may be either a derivative of nor-testosterone (norethisterone acetate, norethynodrel or lynoestrenol) or of progesterone (dydrogesterone or medroxyprogesterone acetate). The results of treatment with progestogens alone are comparable to those obtained with the combined oestrogen-progestogen combinations. The recurrence rate of endometriosis after such treatment relates to the duration of the follow-up. The use of such a regime immediately following conservative surgery has been noted to be associated with a lower pregnancy rate than that expected with the use of a pseudo-pregnancy regime (Jones & Rock, 1980). This, apparently, is considered due to suppression of ovulation at a time when conception is most likely. Because of this finding it has been suggested that any pseudo-pregnancy regime is not indicated immediately following conservative surgery and should preferably be withheld for a period of 12 months.

Delayed resumption of ovulation is frequently seen

following the use of long-acting parenteral progestogens such as depomedroxyprogesterone. For this reason, this form of therapy should not be used in the management of the patient with endometriosis desirous of fertility. However, it is extremely useful in the management of the older patient in whom infertility is not the problem and in whom there is a contraindication to surgery.

Oestrogen-progestin combination

The observation that pregnancy induces both subjective and objective improvement in patients with endometriosis is the basis for the administration of combined oestrogen and progestin in a manner simulating the hormonal profile in pregnancy. Similar to true pregnancy, the pseudo-pregnant state results in the endometrium, both normally situated and aberrant, undergoing decidual transformation, necrosis and resorption.

The exogenous steroids suppress ovulation by their feedback effect on the hypothalamus with resultant suppression of LHRH. The secretion of FSH and LH from the pituitary is therefore suppressed and ovarian inactivity follows. The oestrogen and progestin administered causes initial stimulation of the endometrium which may be reflected in some exacerbation of symptoms. These rapidly settle within 2–3 months.

A common regimen involves the continuous use of the higher dose oral contraceptives commencing with an initial dosage of one tablet daily. After several weeks this is increased to two or three tablets daily, the increase frequently being made at the time of break-through bleeding. Treatment is usually continued for 6–9 months. Kistner, who introduced this form of therapy in 1958, recommends the pseudo-pregnancy regime only for those patients who are infertile and in whom moderate degrees of surface ovarian endometriosis are demonstrated (Kistner, 1975).

Subjective improvement has been reported to be as high as 90 per cent with the pseudo-pregnancy regime. Spontaneous ovulation usually occurs 6–8 weeks following cessation of therapy. Recurrence of symptoms has been found to occur in approximately one-third of patients, commonly within 1 year (Kistner, 1959). Pregnancy rates following treatment vary from 26 to 72 per cent. Interpretation of this is extremely difficult because of the variety of preparations used and lack of standards for therapy and patient selection.

Side-effects of treatment are numerous and include weight gain, depression, breast tenderness, headaches and nausea. The contraindications and potential complications of pseudo-pregnancy are the same as those associated with the use of oral contraceptives. Spontaneous rupture of endometriomas has been reported in some patients with severe disease treated by a pseudo-pregnancy regime (Hammond & Haney, 1978).

Danazol (Danocrine)

Induction of a pseudomenopause in the treatment of endometriosis is a relatively new concept. Danazol, a synthetic steroid derivative is an orally active pituitary gonadotrophin inhibitory agent which has no oestrogenic or progestational activity. Administration of Danazol results in the inhibition of ovulation by the suppression of the cyclic release of pituitary FSH and LH with resultant inhibition of ovarian steroidogenesis. Evidence also suggests that this synthetic (2.3-isoxyl) derivative of 17α-ethinyl testosterone also has direct actions at both gonadal and endometrial levels with probable competitive blocking of oestrogen and progesterone receptors. Following the administration of Danazol peripheral changes similar to those seen with castration or the menopause are seen. Amenorrhoea usually begins with the commencement of treatment, and atrophy of the vaginal mucosa, uterine endometrium and aberrant endometrium occurs. Studies evaluating the effect of Danazol therapy on pituitary, thyroid, and adrenal function have shown a decrease in thyroid-stimulating hormone (TSH), thyroid-binding globulin, T_3, and T_4 with slight increases in free T_4 and free T_3 index (Thorell et al, 1979). Assessment of the adrenal glands response to challenge with metyrapone indicates the maintenance of a normal ability of the pituitary to secrete adrenocorticotrophic hormone (ACTH) and of a normal response by the adrenal gland (Young & Blackmore, 1977). Glucose tolerance and cortisol levels are unaffected by Danazol therapy, as also are serum concentrations of prolactin and testosterone. Likewise, no changes have been demonstrated in coagulation and platelet function (Young & Blackmore, 1977).

Although Danazol is rapidly absorbed, and metabolised, several studies have indicated that the biological effect is by Danazol itself and not by its metabolites (Fraser, 1979). As anticipated from its chemical structure some androgenic and anabolic properties are shown by Danazol. Such side-effects are dose-dependent. Side-effects attributable to suppression of ovarian function include vasomotor instability as evidenced by hot flushes and sweating.

Their incidence has been reported between 1.54 and 4.5 per cent (Dmowski, 1981). Side-effects related to the androgenic activity of Danazol include acne (13.4 per cent), hirsutism (5.8 per cent), oedema (5.8 per cent), voice change (2.8 per cent), weight gain (2.8 per cent) and increased oiliness of skin (1.8 per cent).

The above side-effects were those encountered in patients treated with Danazol in a dosage of 800 mg daily. Studies currently in progress indicate that the incidence of side-effects is lessened with reduction in dosage (Chalmers & Sherington, 1979). Studies still in progress with lower doses (600, 400 and 200 mg daily) suggest that relief of symptoms continues to occur with such dosage reduction (Ward, 1977).

Treatment with Danazol should commence on the first day of the menstrual cycle. Such timing minimises the problems of irregular bleeding which may be encountered should therapy be commenced later in the cycle and also avoids any possibility of the drug being administered during early pregnancy. The length of therapy is dependent upon the extent of the original disease. The average duration of therapy advocated is 6 months although therapy may be adjusted individually in both dose and duration — dependent on the basis of the initial extent of the disease and the clinical response of the individual patient. Subjective symptomatic improvement occurs within a few weeks of commencement of therapy. Amenorrhoea develops promptly and any palpable lesion usually rapidly regresses in size. As therapy progresses some patients may have intermittent vaginal spotting or scanty bleeding from the atrophic endometrium.

Post-treatment laparoscopy is sometimes advocated although this is usually withheld for 6–12 months after the discontinuation of therapy. There is no contraindication to the repeated use of Danazol in the presence of recurring endometriosis.

Within 1–4 months of ceasing therapy regular ovulatory menses usually resume. The efficacy of Danazol in treating infertility associated with endometriosis has been evaluated by post-treatment follow-up. Pregnancy rates have been reported to be 43 per cent at 3 months, 50 per cent at 6 months and 56 per cent at 1 year. Up to 52 months of follow-up care in one study, allowing for correction for other possible responsible factors, gave a pregnancy rate of 72 per cent, the rate being related to the initial severity of the disease (Dmowski & Cohen, 1978).

Luteinising hormone-releasing hormone agonists

A potential new treatment of endometriosis has recently been reported although further evaluation is needed before any conclusions can be reached as to its efficacy. It is well established that repetitive administration of pharmacological doses of luteinizing hormone (LH-RH) or LH-RH agonists have paradoxical anti-fertility effects. Subcutaneous or intranasal administration of LH-RH agonists inhibits ovulation in regularly menstruating women (Berquist et al, 1981), and results in the development of inactive endometrial glands with slightly atrophic stroma with prolonged usage. Lemay & Quesnel (1982) reported the use of therapy with the LH-RH agonist (D-Ser[TBU]^6-des-Gly-NH$_2$^{10}), LH-RH ethylamide, given intranasally for 173 days. Symptomatic relief was obtained and regression of the lesions was noted at subsequent laparoscopy. Resumption of ovulation occurred rapidly following the cessation of the therapy which was relatively free of side-effects.

Surgical management of endometriosis

Surgery has been the traditional time honoured approach to the treatment of endometriosis. Such an approach enables direct visualisation of the lesion and an affirmative diagnosis.

Laparoscopy

Laparoscopically directed diathermy is used as a definitive means of treatment of individual lesions. Provided proper care is taken, this is a simple and quick method of treatment. It has the advantage of not deferring attempts at pregnancy which necessarily attend more extensive surgical intervention or prolonged periods of medical treatment. Recurrence rates and pregnancy rates following such intervention vary enormously. Because it is necessary to use unipolar diathermy exposed dessicated areas are left within the peritoneal cavity. These can and do generate quite extensive adhesion formation. Inadvertent damage to an underlying ureter can be a problem where diathermy has been applied to lesions overlying that organ.

Definitive conservative surgery

Opinions vary widely as to the most appropriate application of this form of treatment. Generally it is now accepted that for very mild endometriosis not involving the ovarian cortex medical treatment is the preferred primary form of treatment. For extensive disease involving the ovarian cortex particularly, there is total agreement that surgery is the primary line of treatment. The area of debate exists where there is very mild endometriosis in association with any cortical ovarian involvement. Lesions measuring 1 cm or more which have infiltrated into the substance of the ovarian cortex respond poorly to any recognised medical treatment. Smaller sized endometriomas may be justifiably treated at least in the first instance with Danazol or some other preferred form of medication and subsequently reviewed laparoscopically.

Conservative surgery in such patients must follow two underlying principles. Firstly, such surgery aims to preserve the reproductive capacity of the patient and, every attempt must be made to minimise surgical trauma. To this end all the techniques that have been learnt from the use of gynaecological microsurgery must be applied:

(a) as glove powder is a powerful irritant and will generate adhesion formation, all powder must be removed from the surgeon's gloves by washing under running water prior to commencement of surgery;

(b) all peritoneal and serosal surfaces must be kept moist throughout the period of the surgery;

(c) bleeding should be minimal throughout the course of the procedure, as any blood that is spilt will quickly clot and the development of fibrin plaques on serosal surfaces virtually guarantees post operative adhesion formation;

(d) minimal tissue trauma is achieved by the use of fine instruments, glass rods and minimal use of diathermy which should be bipolar where possible;

(e) fine non-reactive non-absorbable · suture materials should be used to repair the ovary and peritoneal deficiencies;

(f) all surfaces should be reperitonealised prior to closure.

The second principle must be the maximal eradication of the disease and its attendant scarring.

Possibly the most promising results published to date involve the use of conservative surgery followed by a period of 3 months therapy with Danazol. Malinak and his co-workers at the Baylor Medical Centre in Houston employ all the above techniques surgically and have produced pregnancy rates approaching 80 per cent following such combined therapy and a detailed study of their work is to be commended (Malinak, 1980).

Radical surgery

In those patients in whom there is no desire for further pregnancy and who have severe symptoms, or where conservative surgical or medical treatments have failed repeatedly to arrest the progress of the disease, radical surgery offers the only permanent solution to their problem. It is imperative in this situation to remove all the ovarian substance and while this may appear self-evident it can in practice be extremely difficult.

Such surgery will lead to severe and immediate symptoms of oestrogen deprivation for which oestrogen replacement either in the form of implants or tablets will be required. On rare occasions this may lead to reactivity of minor endometriomas which have been missed at surgery. These can be readily controlled by the associated use of either a progestogen or Danazol over a period of 6–9 months.

If surgery is required in a relatively young patient, assessment and counselling prior to surgery is essential to prevent the occurrence of psychological disturbances post-operatively.

Recurrence of endometriosis post treatment

Regardless of whether treatment has been by conservative surgery or by medical treatment, in many patients recurrence of endometriosis is observed. It has not yet been established whether such a recurrence occurs from the activation of residual endometriotic tissue or from the development of fresh lesions. Variance has been observed in the time interval taken for the recurrence to manifest itself as has also the actual incidence of recurrence.

Following a pseudo-pregnancy regime, Kistner (1962) reported a 16.6 per cent recurrence period after 10.9 months; Riva et al (1961), using similar therapy, reported an incidence of 17.8 per cent over a comparable period. The annual recurrence rate found by Dmowski & Cohen (1978) after pseudomenopause induced with Danazol was found to be 23 per cent during the first year, 5 per cent during the second and 9 per cent during the third year. In the 37 months of observation in that study, 29 per cent of patients had recurrence of symptoms. The time interval between cessation of Danazol and recurrence of the disease was variable. Although no data are available for the annual recurrence rate of endometriosis after conservative surgery, repeated surgical intervention has been required by 40.6 and 46.6 per cent of patients in two individual series (Andrews & Larsen, 1974; Schenken & Malinak, 1978). In those patients in whom conception occurred following the original surgery, it was noted that further surgery was required in only 3.7 per cent.

It is generally felt that the time interval to recurrence is dependent upon the extent of disease noted at time of operation, and that the need for subsequent surgery is directly related to the extent of the disease at the time of initial surgery (Hammond et al, 1976).

The above findings indicate the need for relating potential therapy in endometriosis to the anatomical extent of the disease. In minimal disease, a period of observation may result in pregnancy and remission of the disease. In infertile patients with moderate degrees of surface ovarian endometriosis hormone therapy may be used to induce a pseudo-pregnancy or pseudomenopausal state. Hormonal therapy alone has no place where adhesions are observed in association with infertility. In this group of patients there is a place for conservative surgery. Should conception fail to occur within 6–9 months of such, hormonal therapy may be initiated.

The objectives of conservative treatment for endometriosis include improvement in fertility and preservation of the patients reproductive function. The importance of patient selection cannot be overstressed, the outcome of treatment being directly related to the extent of initial disease. Primary surgery remains the most effective method of treatment for patients with moderate and severe disease.

The role of in vitro fertilisation in endometriosis

Despite all the treatment modalities discussed previously, between 20 and 40 per cent of patients who have received all the appropriate medical and surgical treatment will continue to be infertile. The mechanisms of their continuing infertility is, of course, uncertain as indeed is the mechanism of the infertility associated with all endometriosis. It has now been shown to be possible to produce successful pregnancies in such patients by means of IVF. This is adding a completely new dimension to the overall treatment of these patients.

As most of the ova are obtained by laparoscopy, this must be given consideration in designing the conservative surgical approach and when discussing the possibility of radical surgery in more resistant and severe cases. To this end, the pelvis that has been severely affected by endometriosis and the attendant surgery where there is little chance for a natural pregnancy may best be treated by relocation of the ovaries into the utero-vesical pouch. Although this virtually prohibits naturally occurring pregnancy, it leaves the ovary in the most accessible position for laparoscopic ovum pick-up with or without associated ultrasonic control. It also removes the possibility of ovaries again adhering to the utero-sacral ligaments or to the ovarian fossa thereby allowing the patient's symptom complex to recur. It has been our experience that ovaries so relocated continue to ovulate quite normally and are certainly able to establish and maintain a normally implanted pregnancy achieved by IVF. Should such relocation procedures be used, it is probably preferable to perform bilateral salpingectomy at the time of relocation to prevent the possibility of a tubal pregnancy occurring in association with embryo transfer following IVF.

In The Royal Women's Hospital IVF programme, 15 per cent of the patients are in this category and several of them have apparently normal pregnancies while eight have been delivered of healthy children following long periods of infertility.

It is important to point out that the modern gynaecological surgeon dealing with endometriosis needs to have the skill and the patience of the microsurgeon, as well as the anatomical competence of the cancer surgeon. Anything less is unacceptable.

REFERENCES

Acosta A A, Buttram V C Jr, Besch P K, Malinak L R, Franklin R R, Van Der Heydon J D 1973 A proposed classification of pelvic endometriosis. Obstetrics and Gyecology 42: 19–25

American Fertility Society 1979 Classification of endometriosis. Fertility and Sterility 32: 633–634

Andrews W C, Larsen G D 1974 Endometriosis, treatment with hormonal pseudo-pregnancy +/or operation. American Journal of Obstetrics and Gynecology 118: 643–651

Berquist C, Nillius S J, Wide L, Lindgren A 1981 Endometrial patterns in women on chronic luteinizing hormone-releasing hormone agonist treatment for contraception. Fertility and Sterility 36: 339–421

Brosens I A, Koninckx P R, Corvelleyn P A 1978 A study of plasma progesterone, oestradiol 17B, porlactin, and LH levels, and of the luteal phase appearance of the ovaries in patients with endometriosis and infertility. British Journal of Obstetrics and Gynecology 85: 246–250

Chalmers J A, Shervington P C 1979 Follow-up of patients with endometriosis treated with danazol. Postgraduate Medical Journal 55 (Suppl 5): 44–47

Cohen M R 1976 Endoscopy In: Greenblatt R B. Recent Advances in Endometriosis. Proceedings of a Symposium Augusta, Georgia 1975, pp 18–31. Excerpta Medica, Amsterdam

Creadick R N 1950 The non-surgical treatment of endometriosis. North Carolina Medical Journal 11: 576–577

Dmowski W P 1981 Current concepts in the management of endometriosis. In: Wynn R M (ed) Obstetrics and Gynecology Annual, pp 279–311. Applton-Century-Crofts New York

Dmowski W P, Cohen M R 1978 Antigonadotrophin (Danazol) in the treatment of endometriosis: evaluation of post treatment fertility and three year follow up data. American Journal of Obstetrics and Gynecology 130: 41–48

Dmowski W P, Rao R, Scommegna A 1979 The luteinized unruptured follicle syndrome and endometriosis. Fertility and Sterility 33: 30–34

Fraser I S 1979 Danazol — a steroid with a unique combination of actions. Scottish Medical Journal 24: 147–150

Halban J 1924 Metastatic hysteroadenosis. Wiener Klinische Wochenschrift (Wien) 37: 1205–1222

Hammond C B, Haney A F 1978 Conservative treatment of endometriosis. Fertility and Sterility 30: 497–509

Hammond C B, Rock J A, Parker R T 1976a Conservative treatment of endometriosis: the effects of limited surgery in hormonal pseudo pregnancy. Fertility and Sterility 27: 756–766

Hammond M G, Hammond C B, Parker R T 1976b Conservative treatment of endometriosis externa: the effects of methyl testosterone therapy. Fertility and Sterility 29: 651–654

Haskins A L, Woolf R B 1955 Stilboestrol induced hyperhormonal amenorrhea for the treatment of pelvic endometriosis. Obstetrics and Gynecology 5: 113–122

Hirst J C 1947 Conservative treatment and therapeutic test for endometriosis by androgens. American Journal of Obstetrics and Gynecology 53: 483–487

Javert C T 1949 Pathogenesis of endometriosis based on endometrial homeoplasia, direct extension, exfoliation and implantation, lymphatic and haematogenous metastasis. Cancer 2: 399–410

Jones Jr H W, Rock J A 1977 Regulation of Female Infertility In: Diczfalusy E (ed) Regulation of Human Fertility. WHO Symposium 1976. Scriptor, Moscow

Jones Jr H W, Rock J A 1980 Other factors associated with infertility: Endometriosis externa, fibromyomata uteri. In: Pepperell R J, Hudson B, Wood C (eds) The Infertile Couple, pp 147–163. Churchill Livingstone, Edinburgh

Karnaky K J 1948 The use of stilboestrol for endometriosis: preliminary report. Southern Medical Journal 41: 1109–1111

Katayama P K, Manuel J, Jones Jr H W, Jones G S 1976 Methyl testosterone treatment of infertility associated with pelvic endometriosis. Fertility and Sterility 27: 83–86

Kistner R W 1958 The use of newer progestins in the treatment of endometriosis. American Journal of Obstetrics and Gynecology 75: 264–278

Kistner R W 1959 The treatment of endometriosis by inducing pseudo pregnancy with ovarian hormones. Fertility and Sterility 10: 539–545

Kistner R W 1962 Infertility with endometriosis: a plan of therapy. Fertility and Sterility 13: 237–245

Kistner R W Management of endometriosis in the infertile patient. Fertility and Sterility 26: 1151–1157

Kistner R W, Siegler A M, Berhrman S J 1977 Suggested classification for endometriosis: relationship to infertility. Fertility and Sterility 28: 1008–1009

Lemay A, Quesnel G 1982 Potential new treatment of endometriosis: reversible inhibition of pituitary-ovarian function by chronic intranasal administration of a luteinizing hormone-releasing hormone (LH-RH) agonist. Fertility and Sterility 38: 376–379

McArthur J W Ulfelder H 1965 Th effectof pregnancy on endometriosis. Obstetrical and gynecological Survey 20: 709–733

Malinak L R 1980 Infertility and Endometriosis: Operative technique, clinical staging and prognosis. Clinical Obstetrics and Gynecology 23: 925–935

Meldrum S I, Clark K E, Rubenstein L M, Lebhere T B 1977 The relationship of prostaglandins to infertility associated with endometriosis. Abstract, Pacific Coast Fertility Society

Meyer R 1919 Uber den stande der frage der adenomyosites adenomyoma in allgemeinen und insbesondere uber adenomyonites seroepithelialis und adenomyometitis sarcomatosa. Zentralblatt fur Gynakologie 36: 745–759

Miyazawa K 1976 Incidence of endometriosis among Japanese women. Obstetrics and Gynecology 48: 407–409

Preston S N, Campbell H B 1953 Pelvic endometriosis: treatment with methyl testosterone. Obstetrics and Gynecology 2: 152–157

Ranney B 1971 Endometriosis III Complete operations Reasons Sequelae Treatment. American Journal of Obstetrics and Gynecology 109: 1137–1144

Ridley J H 1961 The validity of Sampson's theory of endometriosis. American Journal of Obstetrics and Gynecology 82: 777–782

Riva H L, Wilson J H, Kawaski D M 1961 Effects of norethynodrel on endometriosis. American Journal of Obstetrics and Gynecology 82: 109–118

Rubin I C 1940 Sterility. In: Lewis D (ed) Practice of Surgery, Vol 10, Ch 9. W F Prior Co

Sampson J A 1921 Perforating haemorrhagic (chocolate) cysts of the ovary. Their importance and especially their relation to pelvic adenomas of endometrial type ('adenomyoma' of the uterus, rectovaginal septum, sigmoid, etc.). Archives of Surgery 3: 245–261

Sampson J A Benign and malignant endometrial implants in the peritoneal cavity, and their relation to certain ovarian tumours. Surgery Gynecology and Obstetrics 38: 287–302

Sampson J A 1927 Peritoneal endometriosis due to menstrual dissemination of endometrial tissue into peritoneal cavity. American Journal of Obstetrics and Gynecology 14: 422–469

Schenken R S, Malinak L R 1978 Reoperation after initial treatment of endometriosis with conservative surgery. American Journal of Obstetrics and Gynecology 131: 416–424

Soules M R, Malinak L R, Bury R, Poindexter A 1976 Endometriosis and anovulation, a coexisting problem in the infertile female. American Journal of Obstetrics and Gynecology 125: 412–417

Te Linde R W, Scott R B 1950 Experimental endometriosis. American Journal of Obstetrics and Gynecology 60: 1147–1173

Thorell J I, Rannevik G, Dymling J F 1979 Effect of Danazol on thyroid function in women. Postgraduate medical Journal 55 (Suppl 5): 33–36

Ward G D 1977 Dosage aspects of danazol therapy in endometriosis. Journal of International Medical Research 5 (Suppl 3): 75–78

Watkins R E 1938 Uterine retrodisplacement, retrograde menstruation and endometriosis. Western Journal of Surgery 46: 480–494

Weed J C, Arquembourg P C 1980 Endometriosis: Can it produce an autoimmune response resulting in infertility. Clinical Obstetrics and Gynecology 23: 885–893

Young M D, Blackmore W P 1977 The use of danazol in the management of endometriosis. Journal of International Medical Research 5 (Suppl 3): 86–91

Neuroradiology in human reproductive biology

INTRODUCTION

The patient suspected of having a pituitary or hypothalamic tumour presents the neuroradiologist with an interesting diagnostic challenge. This is perhaps nowhere more evident than in the case of prolactin-secreting adenomas. Only a decade ago, complete neuroradiological investigation of this problem consisted of plain films, complex-motion tomograms, angiography, and gas encephalography of the sella turcica region. Tumour detection was based upon pathological alterations in normal structures surrounding the pituitary gland, such as sellar erosion or expansion, vascular displacement or staining, and deformities of the gas-filled third ventricle and chiasmatic cistern. Even in the best of hands, accuracy was limited to medium and large-sized lesions and in the case of intracranial air studies, information was gained only at the cost of considerable patient morbidity.

With refinements in prolactin bioassay methods, the endocrinologist could begin to suspect the presence of prolactinomas at a much earlier stage, often before conventional radiological studies revealed any abnormality (Hsu et al, 1976; Malarky & Johnson, 1976; Robertson & Newton, 1978; Cowden et al, 1979). The operating microscope made possible selective trans-sphenoidal adenomectomy, with preservation of normal pituitary tissue (Anonymous, BMJ, 1980; Teasdale et al, 1980). Moreover, the therapeutic success of bromocriptine with some tumours offered an alternative to surgical treatment in many cases, making precise radiological assessment of tumour size and configuration more important than ever to appropriate clinical management (Jacobs, 1976; Geehr et al, 1978; Anonymous, Lancet, 1980; Bonneville et al, 1982).

These developments indicated the need for a non-invasive method of imaging the pituitary gland directly and in sufficient detail to discriminate small sub-total glandular adenomas as well as larger ones. Five years after the introduction of computer-assisted tomography, the first thin section (1.5 mm) high resolution CT images of the sella turcica and its contents were produced. With intravenous iodinated contrast media, axial and coronal scans could now distinguish the enhancing pituitary gland, the infundibular stalk, the hypothalamus and adjacent structures in a degree of detail never attained by earlier CT images. In combination with the intra-thecal water-soluble contrast agent metrizamide, these high-resolution scans yielded excellent CT cisternograms of the supra- and parasellar regions, greatly aiding in the diagnosis of small hypothalamic and pituitary stalk lesions, and complementing information gathered from intravenously enhanced scan studies when suprasellar tumour extension was present.

As a result of these developments, the neuroradiological approach to pituitary and hypothalamic lesions in general, and prolactinomas in particular, has been revised fundamentally (Sakoda et al, 1981). Pneumoencephalography and angiography are now infrequently performed, except in special circumstances which will be mentioned later, thus eliminating most of the risk and morbidity involved in a complete radiological evaluation (Robertson et al, 1981). Instead, high resolution CT scanning with appropriate contrast media, complemented on occasion by sellar polytomography, has become the procedure of choice in the diagnosis of pituitary adenomas. It is sensitive, specific, non-invasive, and provides an excellent means of monitoring the response of known tumours to surgical and medical treatment on progress examinations (Fig. 23.1A–C) (Bonneville et al, 1982).

The following pages will be devoted to acquainting the reader with current attitudes in the neuroradiological assessment of prolactin-secreting pituitary tumours. The roles of plain films, complex motion tomography, angiography, gas encephalography and CT scanning will be discussed, with emphasis on the latter, and examples of normal and pathological pituitary conditions will be illustrated. References to secreting pituitary adenomas of other types, such as hGH and ACTH producing tumours, are made where appropriate.

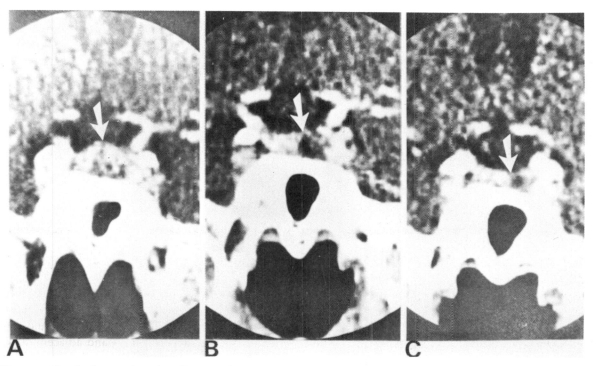

Fig. 23.1 Response of prolactin-secreting microadenoma to bromocriptine. Note progressive reduction in gland volume and tumour size over a 6 month course of therapy

NEURORADIOLOGICAL EVALUATION OF PROLACTIN-SECRETING PITUITARY ADENOMAS

Plain films and complex-motion tomography

Until recently, radiological diagnosis of pituitary adenoma has centered on analysis of the sella turcica, as viewed in plain films and tomograms. Currently accepted criteria for abnormality are (1) thinning of the double layer of cortical bone (lamina dura) forming the sellar floor, (2) focal erosion of the lamina dura, (3) abnormal sellar shape, (4) pathological double contour, and (5) subjective sellar enlargement (McLachlan et al, 1970). Bony changes occur earlier and are more sensitive indicators of pituitary pathology than sellar enlargement. The number, nature, and degree of these abnormal findings in any given patient depend upon a tumour's location within the gland (central or peripheral, midline or lateral) and its size at clinical presentation. The hGH secreting adenomas, which are the largest of the secretory adenomas at diagnosis (Robertson & Newton, 1978), are accompanied by radiographic sellar abnormalities on 90 per cent of plain films and 98.6 per cent of polytomograms (McLachlan et al, 1970). The ACTH and prolactin-secreting tumours, however, are considerably smaller when first diagnosed (Kricheff, 1979). Most are less than 10 mm in diameter, and are designated as microadenomas. In this group, 50–70 per cent of plain films demonstrate no abnormality of sellar size or shape (Robertson & Newton, 1978; Teasdale et al, 1981). Carefully performed complex-motion tomograms at 1 mm intervals reveal alterations in sellar contour, local erosions, or cortical thinning in 96 per cent of prolactinomas and 85 per cent of ACTH-secreting adenomas (Robertson & Newton, 1978; Richmond et al, 1980b).

Thinning of the lamina dura is the earliest sign, followed by focal erosive change (Kricheff, 1979). With the prolactin-secreting adenomas, these erosions are commonest in lateral portions of the anterior quadrants of the sellar floor, where they begin as small pit-like excavations (Richmond et al, 1980a). With larger tumours, the contour of the anterolateral floor of the sella becomes expanded, with forward erosion undercutting the anterior clinoids. If the tumour lies just beneath the surface of the gland, tomographic sellar abnormalities are likely to be detected much earlier than if it lies centrally (Raji et al, 1981). With progressive growth the entire ipsilateral half of the sellar floor is eroded, so that two distinct cortical floor contours may become visible in the lateral plain films. The spectrum of these progressive sellar abnormalities is illustrated in Fig. 23.2A–F. By far the commonest cause of 'double sellar floor' on plain film examination is imperfect radiographical positioning, not tumour (Kricheff, 1979). The appearance may also be produced by a sloping sellar floor, a coronal slope of up to eight degrees being considered within normal sellar variation if corroborating pathological changes are not present (Dubois et al, 1979). The contour of the floor is affected by variations in sphenoid sinus development and septation (Fig. 23.3A–B), as well as by bony grooves produced in the lateral aspects of the sellar floor by the carotid arteries and intercavernous sinus anastomoses (Bruneton et al, 1979; Kishore et al, 1979).

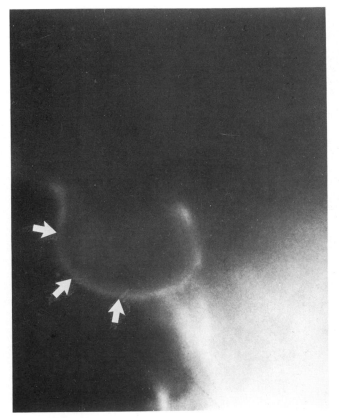

Fig. 23.2A Normal sella turcica. Note smooth, uniform lamina dura (arrows)

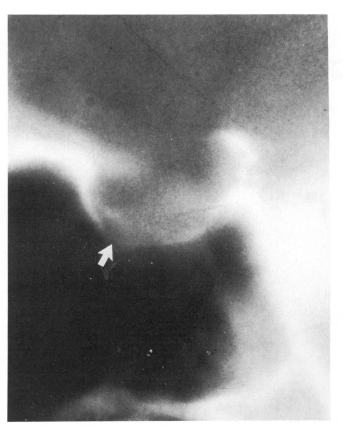

Fig. 23.2C Thinned lamina dura accompanied by pit-like focal erosion (arrow)

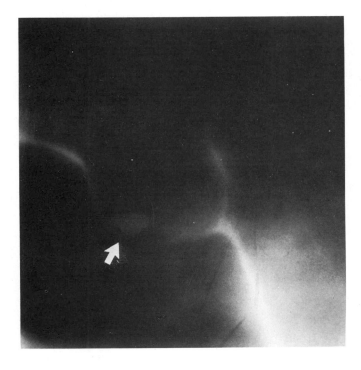

Fig. 23.2B Early abnormal sella. Lamina dura is thinned anteroinferiorly

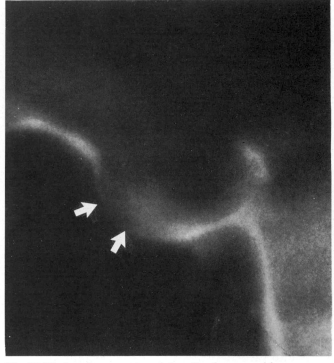

Fig. 23.2D Anterior expansion of the sellar floor caused by more extensive erosion (arrows)

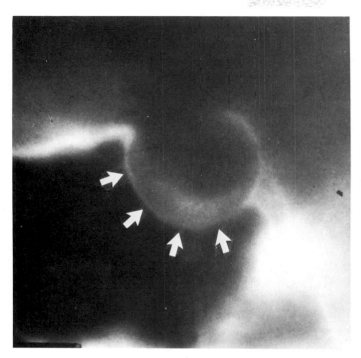

Fig. 23.2E Unilaterally expanded sellar floor resulting in double sellar

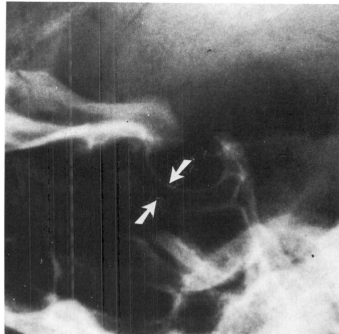

Fig. 23.3A Non-pathological double contour, lateral view, simulating tumour expansion

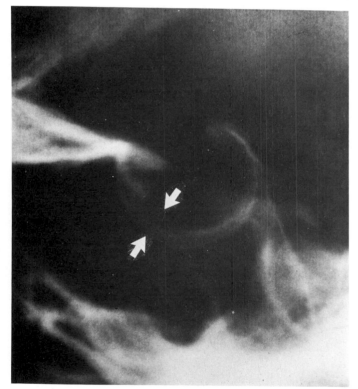

Fig. 23.2F Double sellar contour appearance on plain film examination

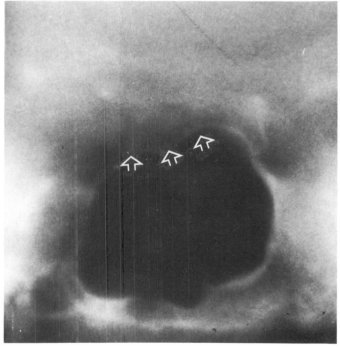

Fig. 23.3B The appearance is due to developmental asymmetry in pneumatisation of the sphenoid sinus

It has been claimed that accurate pre-operative tumour localisation within the gland by tomograms alone is possible in up to 85 per cent of prolactinomas (Teasdale et al, 1981). With the smallest tumours, however, difficulties in interpretation arise regarding the significance of minimal

changes of sellar contour and various configurations of its floor (Turski et al. 1981). Tomographic studies of the sella in large unselected autopsy series indicate that the range of normal sellar contour is broad, the thickness and smoothness of the normal lamina dura are variable, and that plain films reveal little of this variation (Bergland et al, 1968; Banna et al, 1978; Muhr et al, 1981). Moreover, the reported incidence of pituitary microadenomas at autopsy ranges from 2.7 to 27 per cent, of which slightly less than half are prolactinomas (Anonymous, Lancet, 1980; Burrow et al, 1981). Tomographic sellar changes interpreted as abnormal have been described in 20 per cent of subjects having no adenoma (false positive) with a similar frequency of false negative interpretations, giving sellar tomography an overall accuracy of 60 per cent in the general population. Even among true positive cases, sellar abnormalities show valid anatomical correlation with actual tumour site in less than 70 per cent of subjects (Burrow et al, 1981; Raji et al, 1981). Therefore, although carefully performed pluridirectional sellar tomography is more sensitive than the plain film examination in detecting the presence of microadenomas minor bony changes, sloping of the sellar floor, and sharpening of its lateral edges should be interpreted with caution and with a clear understanding of the clinical and hormone assay information available (Kricheff, 1979; Turski et al, 1981). Both anteroposterior and lateral views must be compared section-by-section before a correct radiological assessment of the sella is possible. Even then, sellar pathology may be indistinguishable from normal variation (Banna et al, 1978; Cowden et al, 1979). As a result of earlier clinical and laboratory diagnosis, the neuroradiologist finds himself looking for smaller and smaller tumours. It must be concluded that, in the detection of microadenomas, pluridirectional tomography of the sella turcica is at best a sensitive but non-specific study. Its limitation lies in the fact that it 'sees' a pituitary

microadenoma only in terms of subtle pre-established patterns of sellar asymmetry, the significance of many of which is now in doubt (Bruneton et al, 1979; Muhr et al, 1981; Robertson et al, 1981).

Gas and positive contrast encephalography

Complex motion sellar tomography following intrathecal introduction of air, oxygen, carbon dioxide, or metrizamide has been used to define the presence and extent of extrasellar growth of pituitary adenomas and the relationship of this growth to adjacent structures, such as the carotid siphons, optic system, and hypothalamus. It has also been employed to establish the diagnosis of empty sella, where this has been suspected from plain film examination, with or without coexistent intrasellar adenoma.

When gas is used as the contrast agent, it must be carefully manipulated through the basal CSF pathways into the suprasellar cistern and anterior third ventricle (McLachlan et al, 1971). The superior surface of the normal pituitary gland is usually flat (Fig. 23.4A) or slightly concave (Bergland et al, 1968; Renn & Rhoton, 1975; Syversten et al, 1979; Hall & McAllister, 1980). When the gland is expanded by a small tumour, the superior surface develops a convex upward bulge. In large lesions mushrooming out of the sella, the suprasellar tumour component may fill the cistern, its upper surface capped and demarcated by a thin crescent of gas (Fig. 23.4B). In advanced cases, the cistern may be obliterated, the anterior third ventricle elevated and distorted, and it may be impossible to manipulate the gas between tumour surface and adjacent hypothalamus or

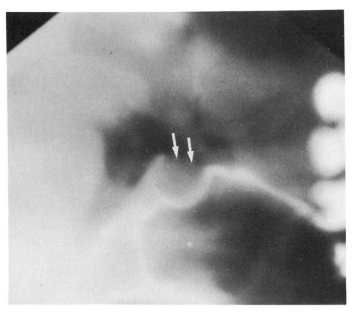

Fig. 23.4A Normal suprasellar air encephalogram. Note the flat superior surface of the pituitary gland (arrows)

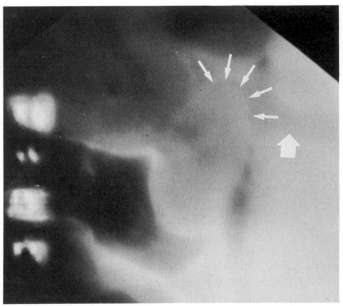

Fig. 23.4B Large prolactinoma with suprasellar extension. Air can be observed outlining and capping the tumour's superior surface (small arrows). The anterior recesses of the third ventricle (large arrow) are deformed

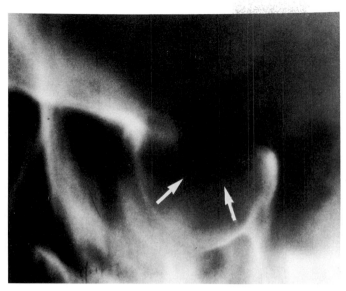

Fig. 23.5 Partially empty sella. Note downward protrusion of the air-filled suprasellar cistern into the upper half of the sella (arrows)

optic chiasm. The empty sella (Fig. 23.5) is readily recognised by the intrasellar entry of cisternal gas from the chiasmatic cistern. Coexistent adenoma is heralded by the detection of bulging or distortion of the gland within the sellar depths, although this is often difficult to distinguish from the effects of non-pathological gland distortion produced by intrasellar herniation of the chiasmatic cistern (Domingue et al, 1978).

Positive contrast polytomocisternography using intrathecal metrizamide provides essentially the same information as gas encephalography, but is easier to perform (Sheldon & Molyneux, 1979; Davis et al, 1980; Kuuliala et al, 1981). The water soluble contrast agent mixes with CSF and flows by gravity, because of its higher density. The surface tension problems of intrathecal air are eliminated, so that the smallest clefts and recesses are filled without difficulty (Gross et al, 1979). Suprasellar extension of small and medium-sized adenomas is accurately delineated, as well as their relationship to the optic chiasm. Large suprasellar masses, however, are not well visualised, particularly if they reach the foramen of Monro and create obstructive hydrocephalus, in which case metrizamide will not reliably pass over the top of the lesion (Hall & McAllister, 1980; Kuuliala et al, 1981).

Gas encephalography, until recently a widely popular pre-operative investigation in the workup of prolactinomas, has in many centres been largely abandoned since the advent of high resolution CT cisternography. It is poorly tolerated by patients, and, if done well, requires special care, skill, complex equipment, and considerable time (Robertson et al, 1981). It is now used mainly in circumstances where a precise pre-operative knowledge of the anatomical relationship of suprasellar tumour to the optic system is necessary, and a high resolution CT scanner is not available (Hall & McAllister, 1980).

While metrizamide polytomocisternography is easier to perform than gas encephalography, high volumes and concentrations of contrast agent are required for cisternal opacification on conventional X-rays. The amounts used are the same as for myelography. The known side-effects of intrathecal metrizamide are dose-related, and include headache (38 per cent), nausea (37 per cent), and vomiting (29 per cent), beginning as early as 3 hours post-procedure, clearing in most cases within 24 hours (Gross et al, 1979). In high concentrations neuronal toxicity manifests itself as transient seizures, vision impairment, diplopia, perceptual alterations and frontal lobe signs. Chronic alcoholism, severe dehydration, previous seizure disorder, or use of neuroleptic drugs and phenothiazines constitute contraindications to the use of intrathecal metrizamide. The information provided by metrizamide polytomocisternography in the evaluation of pituitary tumours can now be duplicated by high resolution CT cisternography using much smaller and more dilute quantities of contrast agent with lower morbidity and better patient tolerance. For this reason, it is infrequently used by most centres in the diagnosis of prolactinomas.

Angiography

Since the development of CT scanning, the indications for cerebral angiography in the diagnosis of pituitary lesions have come under critical re-evaluation (Richmond et al, 1980). In the past, this procedure was considered to be useful in four main respects. (1) It delineated the source of blood supply and the degree of tumour vascularity (Powell et al, 1974). (2) It defined the suprasellar extent of tumour by its capillary blush and parasellar extent by lateral displacement or encasement of the cavernous carotid artery segments (Baker, 1972; Bonneville et al, 1976). (3) It provided pre-operative reassurance that internal carotid anomalies or aneurysms were not the cause of sellar abnormalities seen on plain films and tomograms (Anderson, 1976; Boyce & Huckman, 1976; Richmond et al, 1980a; Robertson et al, 1981). (4) It also excluded other lesions such as suprasellar meningiomas and chiasmal gliomas (Baker, 1972). With large pituitary adenomas, particularly those with extrasellar extension, the contributions of angiography in previous years cannot be disputed. It was the only radiological study of those times which imaged the tissue of the pituitary gland itself, and, because of radiologists' dependence upon it, angiographic interpretation skills became highly refined in spite of equipment limitations.

Today, the role of carotid angiography in diagnosis of prolactin-secreting adenomas is regarded by most neuroradiologists as limited to defining cavernous-carotid anomalies of position (contiguous siphons in an empty sella, intrasellar location) or perisellar aneurysm prior to transsphenoidal surgery or when the cause of sellar asymmetry or the diagnosis of adenoma are in doubt (Drayer et al, 1979; Kishore et al, 1979; Boyce et al, 1981; Daniels et al, 1981). Lateral displacement of the siphons is an unreliable sign of parasellar extension (60 per cent false positive, 15 per cent false negative) (Pripstein et al, 1978; Richmond et al, 1980a). Tumour staining is rarely seen in small lesions, even with the best magnification-subtraction methods. The time-honoured sign of elevation of the proximal anterior cerebral arteries (Fig. 23.6) as an indicator of suprasellar tumour extension has been referred to in many textbooks. It is often absent in obvious suprasellar involvement, however, and has no relevance in cases of pituitary microadenoma.

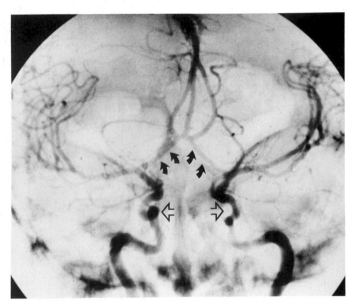

Fig. 23.6 Elevation of the A-1 segments (arrows) of the anterior cerebral arteries caused by suprasellar extension of prolactinoma. This is not a sensitive angiographic sign, and may be absent in the presence of documented suprasellar involvment by pituitary tumour. The internal carotid siphons are indicated by the open arrows

Refined CT scanning techniques can now reliably distinguish pituitary adenomas from other perisellar tumours in the differential diagnosis. Knowledge of tumour vascular supply is less important with small lesions, especially when transsphenoidal selective adenomectomy is now possible (Geehr et al, 1978). Because of these considerations, and because of the risk involved, cerebral angiography is no longer routinely included in the neuroradiological investigation of prolactinomas and other pituitary lesions. Its use is confined to those circumstances described above when the required information cannot be provided by other less invasive studies (MacPherson & Anderson, 1981). Cavernous sinus venography is probably a more sensitive test of lateral and anteroposterior expansion (Theron et al, 1979), but it has not gained acceptance as a routine investigation of tumour suspects (Robertson et al, 1981).

Computerised tomography

Because of its unique ability to image the pituitary gland itself in detail, as well as the sella and surrounding cisterns, high-resolution computerised tomography has surpassed conventional pluridirectional sellar tomography as the procedure of choice in the radiological diagnosis of pituitary adenomas (Bonafé et al, 1981). The best scanning instruments are capable of detecting microadenomas as small as 3–4 mm in diameter, as well as accurately assessing the extrasellar extent of larger tumours (Pripstein et al, 1978). Many neuroradiologists now feel that if high resolution CT is available and is used appropriately, pluridirectional sellar tomography can be eliminated altogether from the work-up of pituitary adenomas without loss of information (Syversten et al, 1979). In those institutions lacking advanced scanners, however, it must continue to complement information provided by standard CT images (Wolpert et al, 1979).

Scanning techniques

Axial scans of the sella and pituitary are performed in planes of section parallel to the canthomeatal line, beginning at the level of the sphenoid sinus, and progressing superiorly through the sella to the suprasellar cistern, hypothalamus, and third ventricle. Slice thicknesses of less than 5 mm are essential in avoiding the effects of volume averaging and image artifact (Earnest et al, 1981). For those scans passing directly through the sella, a thickness of 1.5 mm is optimum, but if this is not attainable, an overlapping technique of 4 mm thick scans taken every 2–3 mm usually images the pituitary gland sufficiently well to demonstrate microadenomas in the 4–6 mm size range (Fig. 23.7A). Contrast-infused scans may be preceded by a non-contrast scan series to detect areas of calcification or haemorrhage.

Although axial scanning methods do provide much useful information, most neuroradiologists agree that the sella and pituitary gland are best evaluated in the coronal plane (Syversten et al, 1979). Small tumours in the sellar depths are more easily imaged (Fig. 23.7B), and the degree of suprasellar tumour extension and its relationship to the hypothalamus and optic system are more precisely defined. Moreover, this method is better suited to the evaluation of empty sella, with or without associated microadenoma. Direct coronal scans are performed preferably perpendicular to the sellar floor, from the anterior clinoid processes to the dorsum sellae, using the same thin-section or overlapping technique as for axial scanning. However, care must be taken in positioning the patient in the scanner, so that image artifacts related to dental work are avoided (see Fig. 23.12). When severely ill patients or those with limited cervical extension are unable to maintain the prone or supine extended position required for direct coronal

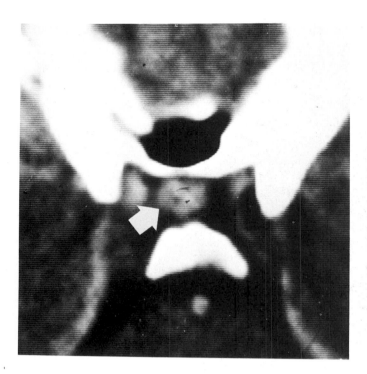

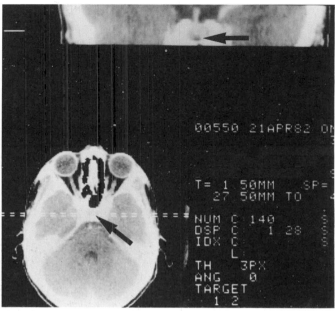

Fig. 23.8 Reformatted coronal CT image generated from axial scan information confirms existence of a small intrasellar prolactinoma (arrow) suspected on the axial study

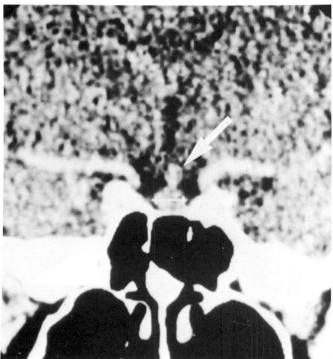

Fig. 23.7A Thin-section high resolution axial CT scan of a 7 mm intrasellar prolactinoma (arrow). B Direct coronal CT scan, 1.5 mm section thickness. Better definition of tumour contour and extent than in A. A small suprasellar tumour component is also present (arrow)

scanning, computerised manipulation of axial scan data can be used to produce reformatted images of the sella and pituitary in coronal, sagittal, or oblique planes (Fig. 23.8) (Earnest et al, 1981). Their resolution characteristics, however, are lower than those of direct coronal scans, and multiple thin axial sections are required for their recon-

struction. Direct coronal scanning is now regarded as the method of choice in the CT evaluation of the sella and pituitary gland (Syversten et al, 1979). Because little additional information is gained by precontrast scanning of uncomplicated or 'routine' suspected adenomas, it is usually sufficient to obtain contrast-infused scans alone in such patients, provided they have had no previous surgery in or around the sella. However, pre-contrast scans are mandatory in any case of suspected pituitary apoplexy. Post-operative follow-up scans should be performed with and without intravenous contrast, to distinguish areas of haemorrhage from residual tumour enhancement.

Coronal CT metrizamide cisternography is employed when questions regarding the degree of suprasellar tumour extension and its relation to the optic chiasm and hypothalamus cannot be answered by standard contrast-infused scans, or when hypothalamic tumour is suspected (Drayer et al, 1977). A conventional lumbar puncture is performed and 3–5 cm³ of concentrated metrizamide solution is injected slowly into the subarachnoid space with the patient in a 15–20 ° Trendelenburg decubitus position. When the contrast has reached the basal cisterns, the patient is rolled 360 ° to distribute it evenly, and thin-section overlapping coronal scans are then obtained at 2–4 mm intervals. There is disagreement about the necessity of CT metrizamide cisternography in the diagnosis of empty sella (Rozario et al, 1977). Difficulty in recognising the empty sella by conventional CT techniques derives from diverse intrasellar cystic structures that are not distinguished from it, unless the pituitary stalk can be positively identified within the sella. This can usually be achieved by 1.5 mm thick intravenously-enhanced high-resolution coronal scans (Fig. 23.9A). However, when the infundibulum is not

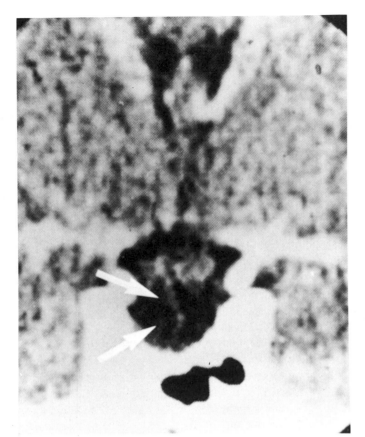

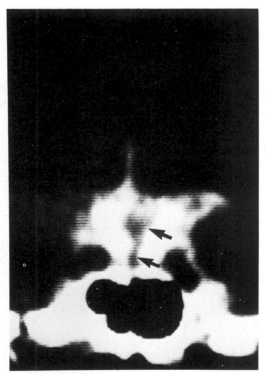

demonstrated by this technique, intrathecal metrizamide is required for the diagnosis of empty sella (Fig. 23.9B) (Haughton et al, 1980).

Normal CT anatomy of the sella turcica and pituitary gland

Viewed in the coronal plane, the pre-contrast appearance of the normal pituitary gland is homogeneous and isodense with brain tissue. Following contrast infusion, it usually enhances uniformly although local areas of low density may be observed due to the presence of pars intermedia cysts, a normal variation observed in up to 20 per cent of autopsy specimens. The upper surface of the gland is flat or concave in 98 per cent of cases, and its height is between 2 and 7 mm, depending on sellar variation and the downward extent of the suprasellar cistern (Syversten et al, 1979). The infundibular stalk can be identified descending to the superior surface of the pituitary from the infundibular recess of the third ventricle. It measures 1–2 mm in diameter and although it is usually in the mid-sagittal plane, it is observed in an off-midline or angled position in some normal glands. The diaphragma sellae is not

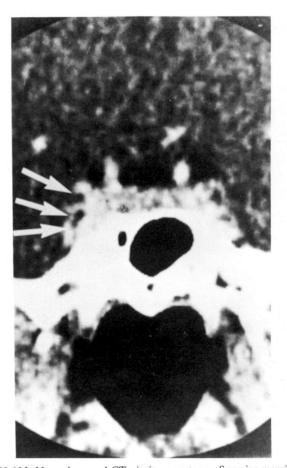

Fig. 23.9A Intravenously enhanced high resolution coronal scan confirms presence of empty sella by demonstrating the infundibulum within its depths, thereby excluding intrasellar cystic or necrotic tumour. B Documentation of empty sella by metrizamide CT cisternography. Pituitary stalk outlined (arrows) within the chiasmatic cistern. Note that here and in A the stalk is angled and off midline, although no adenoma is present

Fig. 23.10A Normal coronal CT pituitary anatomy. Superior margin of the gland is flat. Enhancement is relatively homogeneous. Third, fourth, and sixth cranial nerves (arrows) are visible within the enhancing cavernous sinuses

defined even by high-resolution CT. The superior surface of the pituitary interfaces directly with the suprasellar cisternal space. Before contrast infusion, the cavernous sinuses are only slightly denser than brain tissue. They enhance to the same degree as the cavernous carotid arteries, which cannot be readily differentiated from them. However, the supraclinoid carotid arteries are easily distinguished in the suprasellar cistern with special enhancement techniques (Hayman et al, 1979). Defects in lateral cavernous sinus enhancement can be shown to correspond to the third, fourth, and sixth cranial nerves (Syversten et al, 1979). Within the suprasellar cistern the optic chiasm and nerves can be identified, and above them, the hypothalamus and third ventricle. The bony sellar floor, clinoids and dorsum are easily defined using bone window image settings and size, symmetry and septation of the sphenoid sinus may also be assessed. These CT features of the normal pituitary gland and adjacent anatomy are illustrated in Fig. 23.10A–C.

Viewed in the axial plane (Fig. 23.11A, B), the pituitary gland appears less dense than in the coronal projection and contrast enhancement is more difficult to evaluate due to volume averaging of gland tissue with underlying sellar bone (Earnest et al, 1981). The infundibulum is perceived as a small circular dot within the suprasellar cistern, just anterior to the dorsum sellae, and usually in the midline. Cavernous sinuses are well-defined on enhanced images, but their medial margins are difficult to distinguish from the enhanced gland. The suprasellar cistern is seen as a

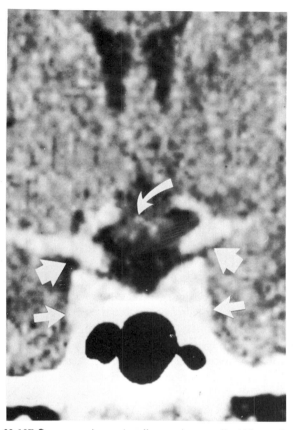

Fig. 23.10B Cavernous sinuses (small arrows), supraclinoid internal carotid arteries (large arrows), and optic chiasm (curved arrow)

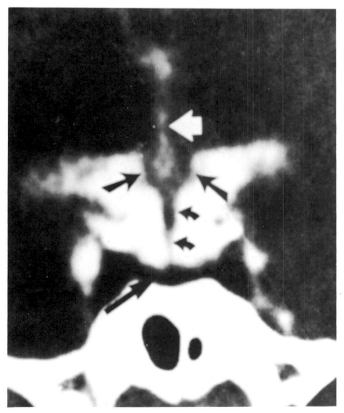

Fig. 23.10C Infundibulum (small arrows), hypothalamus (large arrows), and third ventricle (white arrow) outlined by intrathecal metrizamide

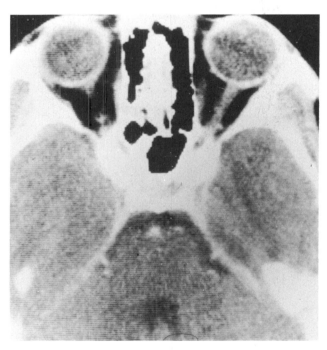

Fig. 23.11A Normal axial CT pituitary anatomy. Gland enhancement is more difficult to evaluate than in coronal sections. Small difference in degree of enhancement between cavernous sinuses and normal pituitary makes their interface indistinct

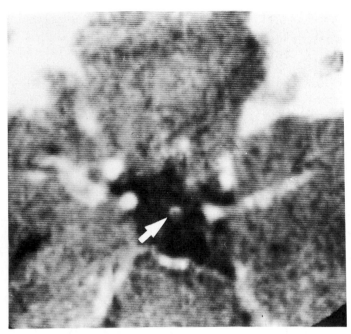

Fig. 23.11B Suprasellar cistern with infundibulum (small arrow) and Circle of Willis (large arrows)

pentagonal low-density space overlying the sella and bounded by the enhancing vessels of the circle of Willis. The optic chiasm is readily discerned within it, anterior to the dorsum sellae. The size and shape of the suprasellar cistern show wide normal variation (Kuuliala, 1980).

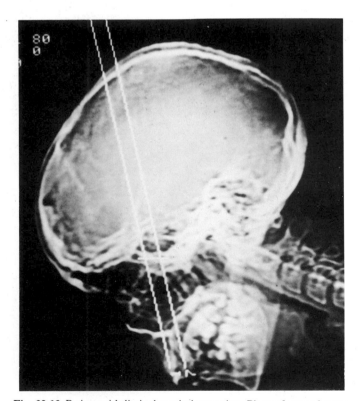

Fig. 23.12 Patient with limited cervical extension. Plane of coronal scans chosen to avoid image artifacts due to dental work

In spite of improved scanning technology and instrumentation, image artifacts continue to be encountered which interfere with the accurate interpretation of sellar and pituitary CT studies. These are commonest in the axial plane, they relate to the bones of the skull base and are identified in up to 60 per cent of high-resolution CT images (Earnest et al, 1981). They can be minimised by using very thin (1.5 mm) scan sections, and employing planes of scan which avoid the petrous bone, the foramen magnum, jugular tubercles, and dental work whenever possible. Direct coronal scanning generates negligible intrasellar artifact and is therefore the preferred method of pituitary CT evaluation (Fig. 23.12).

High resolution CT pathology in prolactin-secreting pituitary adenomas

As mentioned earlier, prolactin and ACTH-secreting pituitary adenomas tend to be smaller than chromophobe and hGH-secreting varieties at the time of radiological diagnosis. Many are less than 1 cm in diameter and are therefore true microadenomas. The value of high-resolution CT scanning in the detection of these lesions is now well established (Smaltino et al, 1980; Robertson et al, 1981; Sakoda et al, 1981). Diagnosis depends upon alterations in the configuration and contrast enhancement of the pituitary gland, both of which are best evaluated on direct coronal scans at right angles to the sellar floor (Syversten et al, 1979).

Abnormalities of pituitary volume and contour

Prolactin-secreting microadenomas usually produce an increase in gland volume. When this expansion is subtotal or focal, a small hump may appear on a portion of the upper margin of the gland (Fig. 23.13A). When the mass effect is more diffuse the entire superior surface of the pituitary develops an upward convex bulge (Fig. 23.13B). A height of more than 7 mm in females and 5 mm in males is probably abnormal, and one which exceeds 9 mm with a convex surface strongly suggests the presence of a microadenoma (Syversten et al, 1979). The infundibular stalk is readily identified in direct coronal scans and in most normal subjects, has a vertical course in or near the mid-line. In the presence of asymmetric gland expansion due to microadenoma, it may be tilted or angled off the saggital plane (Fig. 23.13C, D). As an isolated finding with an unequivocally normovolumic pituitary gland, however, tilting of the infundibulum is probably not of pathological significance. Since the height of the average female pituitary is 5 mm, adenomas as small as 3–4 mm would be expected to produce measurable gland enlargement. This is, in fact, the case with prolactinomas (Fig. 23.13E). ACTH-secreting tumours, however, are very small at presentation, sometimes less than 2 mm in diameter, and

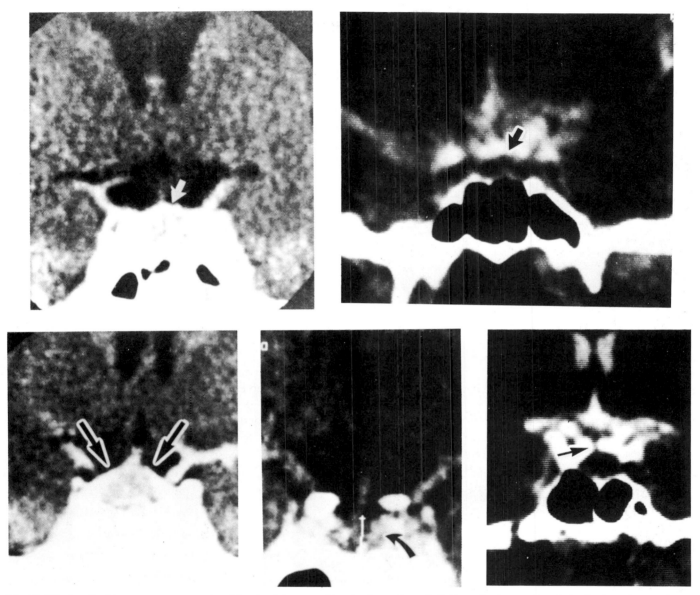

Fig. 23.13A Localised hump on upper margin of the gland due to small prolactinoma (arrow). B Generalised expansion of gland volume from a 10 mm prolactinoma. Convex superior surface, distorted infundibulum. C Tilting of infundibulum associated with prolactin-secreting microadenoma (arrow). D Same changes as in (C) in another patient, demonstrated by metrizamide CT cisternography. E Minimal increase in pituitary gland volume caused by a proven 3 mm prolactinoma at operation

frequently no visible alteration in gland volume or sellar contour is appreciated.

Abnormalities of pituitary enhancement

Alterations in gland enhancement caused by pituitary adenomas are more complex than the changes in volume they produce. Initially, prolactin-secreting adenomas were described as hypodense with respect to the remainder of the contrast-enhanced pituitary gland (Syversten et al, 1979). It is now evident that they can appear either more or less dense than the enhancing gland, with approximately 20 per cent being hypodense and 60 per cent exhibiting some pattern of abnormal enhancement (Wolpert et al, 1979; Gardeur et al, 1981). Areas of relative hypodensity

represent not only microadenomas, but also other diverse changes, including pars intermedia cysts, focal tumour necrosis, cystic degeneration, infarction, haemorrhage, or abscess formation, or even sites of metastasis. Careful correlation with clinical and laboratory information is therefore required to interpret correctly their significance in any given patient (Chambers et al, 1982). ACTH and mixed-cell microadenomas usually demonstrate little or no enhancement (Gardeur et al, 1981). If they are situated centrally in the gland and are smaller than 2 mm in diameter, they are likely to produce no alteration in gland volume or height, and may escape radiological detection. When no volume or enhancement abnormality is present, the location of a microadenoma may sometimes be inferred from a local erosion of the sellar floor. Large intra-supra-

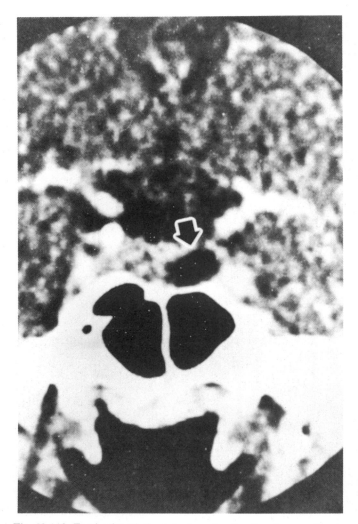

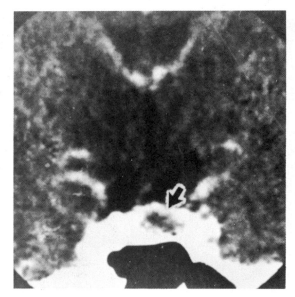

Fig. 23.14B Small prolactinoma showing mixed enhancement features with some hypodensity and a slight increase in gland volume. The tumour has displaced the infundibulum (arrow)

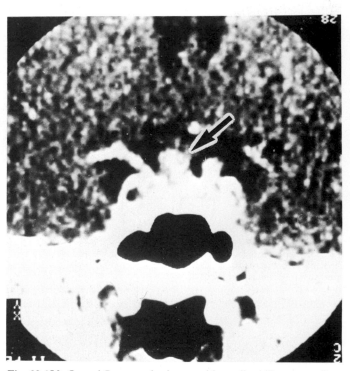

Fig. 23.14A Focal subtotal glandular hypodensity. Significance of such a finding can be diverse, unless clinical and laboratory data are known. In this patient with elevated serum prolactin, the hypodense zone was felt to represent a small partially necrotic or cystic tumour, showing no visible enhancement or volume alteration

Fig. 23.15A Central 7 mm prolactinoma with small midline suprasellar component (arrow). No hypodense regions are visible within the adenoma or the remainder of the pituitary gland

sellar dumbbell macroadenomas, by comparison, also present diverse patterns of abnormal enhancement on contrast-infused scans. Regardless of the pattern, however, their intrasellar components enhance less strongly than their suprasellar portions, and in general, the overall enhancement intensity of macroadenomas is greater than that of microadenomas. Examples of the enhancement spectrum of micro- and macroprolactinomas are illustrated in Figs 23.14 and 23.15.

A partially empty sella does not alter contrast enhancement within the pituitary gland, but appears as a low density region within the sella (Fig. 23.9A). Identification of the infundibular stalk allows this entity to be distinguished from a cystic or necrotic intrasellar tumour. When the stalk cannot be reliably imaged, metrizamide CT cisternography, as described earlier, is required to establish the diagnosis (Haughton et al, 1980). The coexistence of partially empty sella and intrasellar microadenoma is well known and usually poses no diagnostic problems if scan

sections are carefully reviewed for changes in gland contour and enhancement (Domingue et al, 1978; Smaltino et al, 1980).

Metrizamide CT cisternography is occasionally necessary to define the upper surface of a suprasellar tumour extension, when its proximity to the optic chiasm makes differentiation of that structure impossible by intra-

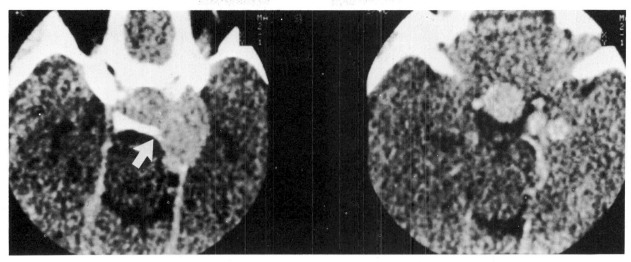

Fig. 23.15B Homogeneously enhancing macroadenoma with suprasellar and right parasellar extension. The lateral aspect of the dorsum has been eroded.

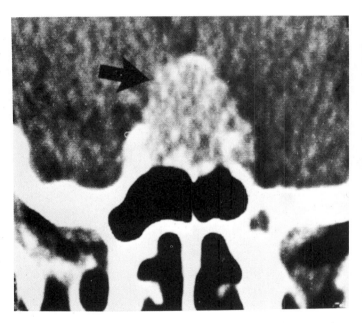

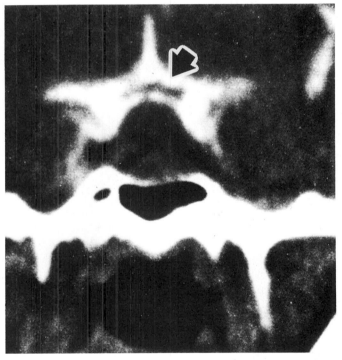

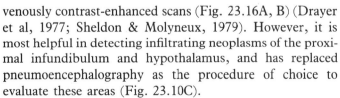

Fig. 23.16A Macroadenoma with suprasellar extension. The tumour's anatomic relationship to the optic system is not apparent. B CT metrizamide cisternogram in another patient enables tumour and optic chiasm (arrow) to be readily distinguished from one another

venously contrast-enhanced scans (Fig. 23.16A, B) (Drayer et al, 1977; Sheldon & Molyneux, 1979). However, it is most helpful in detecting infiltrating neoplasms of the proximal infundibulum and hypothalamus, and has replaced pneumoencephalography as the procedure of choice to evaluate these areas (Fig. 23.10C).

Whether a prolactin-secreting microadenoma enhances or is hypodense, the changes in enhancement it produces are usually seen in lateral portions of the gland, away from the midline, where these tumours originate. With progressive growth, the entire gland becomes involved, and alterations in enhancement are more diffuse. Both homogeneous and heterogeneous patterns are observed, and in

the latter, the exact margins and size of the adenoma may be difficult to recognise if surrounding normal pituitary gland enhancement is not available as a reference (Fig. 23.17). It is sometimes helpful to analyse the bony contours of the sellar floor, using appropriate CT image settings, to determine the probable size and extent of poorly defined intrasellar lesions (Sakoda et al, 1981). Moreover, where transsphenoidal surgery is contemplated, the pattern of sphenoid sinus septation and pneumatisation must be demonstrated to aid in the operative approach.

The postoperative pituitary is more difficult to evaluate. Haemorrhagic and calcific changes should be differentiated from residual or recurrent tumour enhancement by scan-

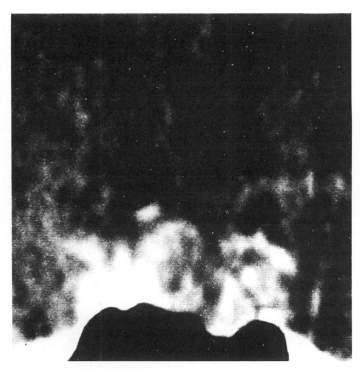

Fig. 23.17 Patchy inhomogeneous enhancement in a prolactin-secreting adenoma. Although the volume of the gland is increased, the actual margins, and therefore the dimension, of the tumour are difficult to define. The hypodense areas are felt to indicate areas of cystic degeneration or necrosis, but zones of infarction or haemorrhage could have an identical appearance

ning before, as well as after, contrast-infusion. Some years ago, it was a common practice for neurosurgeons to place a metallic clip on the diaphragma sellae following tumour removal, so that its position could be monitored postoperatively by plain skull X-rays. A change in the clip alignment or position suggested regrowth of tumour. This practice is now being actively discouraged because the image artifacts it produces make an adequate CT follow-up of known tumour patients virtually impossible.

Although the statements made above pertaining to the CT appearance of the pathological pituitary gland with micro- and macroadenomas represent the general concensus of neuroradiological experience to date, they must be qualified by the fact that no study has yet established standards for the CT appearance of the unequivocally normal pituitary gland. For this purpose it would be necessary to perform complete CT scans of the sella in asymptomatic patients, and later obtain surgical or autopsy confirmation that their pituitary glands were truly normal, free of incidental pathology. Separate standards of normal gland size and appearance should be established for nulliparous, pregnant, and multiparous females, as well as for males, before

pathology and normal gland variation can be reliably distinguished (Gardeur et al, 1981).

SUMMARY

In conclusion, high resolution CT has revolutionised the neuro-radiological evaluation of pituitary disease, particularly where endocrine-secreting microadenomas produce problems of growth and infertility. It has surpassed other more traditional imaging methods whose value and accuracy relied on changes in sellar contour for diagnosis of adenomas. Gland enlargement is more often detected by CT, than true sellar erosion is distinguished on conventional pluridirectional tomography. Furthermore, hyperprolactinaemia secondary to other causes, such as medication or hypothalamic neoplasm can be reliably differentiated from prolactinoma by CT. It is more sensitive and specific than tomography in the diagnosis of microadenoma, even in patients whose symptoms are of short duration. Tomography does, however, remain a primary diagnostic tool where high resolution CT is not available. CT metrizamide cisternography, although infrequently necessary, has replaced gas encephalography in the investigation of suspected empty sella or in delineating suprasellar tumour extent and its relationship to the optic system. Angiography is no longer routinely performed in the work-up of prolactinoma except where the diagnosis is in doubt (e.g. other intra-suprasellar tumours),or where perisellar vascular anomalies or aneurysms are suspected from dynamic CT scans (Hayman et al, 1979; Banna, 1980) and a trans-sphenoidal surgical approach is contemplated.

The patient referred to radiology with elevated or suspicious prolactin levels and amenorrhoea with or without galactorrhoea should first undergo direct coronal thin-section CT scanning of the sella with contrast enhancement. The results obtained should then dictate which, if any, additional procedures must be performed. In most uncomplicated prolactinomas, however, high quality CT studies alone can suffice as a complete neuro-radiological evaluation, reducing not only the financial cost, but also the risks and radiation exposure involved in the investigation of this important clinical problem.

Acknowledgements

I should like to express appreciation to Mr Lee Willis, Dr Jonathan Leicester, and Mrs Frances Stapelfeldt who directly or indirectly helped in the preparation of this chapter and its illustrations.

REFERENCES

Anonymous 1980 Hyperprolactinemia: Pituitary tumour or not? Lancet i: 517–519

Anonymous 1980 Trends in the management of Prolactinomas. British Medical Journal 281: 338–339

Anderson R D 1976 Tortuousity of the cavernous carotid arteries causing sellar expansion simulating pituitary adenoma. American Journal of Roentgenology 126: 1203–1210

Baker H L 1972 The angiographic delineation of sellar and parasellar masses. Radiology 104: 67–8

Banna M 1980 The computed tomographic arteriography of microadenoma. Journal of Computer Assisted Tomography 4: 690–692

Banna M, Nicholas W, McLachlan M 1978 The borderline pituitary fossa in patients with amenorrhea and/or galactorrhea. Neuroradiology 16: 440–442

Bergland R M, Ray B S, Torack R M 1968 Anatomical variations in the pituitary gland and adjacent structures in 225 human autopsy cases. Journal of Neurosurgery 28: 93–99

Bonafé A, Sobel D, Manelfe C 1981 Relative value of computed tomography and hypocycloidal tomography in the diagnosis of pituitary microadenoma – a radio-surgical correlative study. Neuroradiology 22: 133–137

Bonneville J F, Bugault R, Van Effenterre R, Pertuiset B, Metzger J 1976 Delineation of pituitary adenomas by angiotomography. Neuroradiology 11: 49–51

Bonneville J F, Poulignot D, Cattin F, Conturier M, Mollet E, Dietemann J L 1982 Computed tomographic demonstration of the effects of bromocriptine on pituitary microadenoma size. Radiology 143: 451–455

Boyce D W, Huckman M S 1976 Contiguous internal carotid arteries in empty sella syndrome. Radiology 120: 120

Bruneton J N, Drouillard J P, Sabatier J C, Elie G P, Tavernier J F 1979 Normal variants of the sella turcica. Radiology 131: 99–104

Burrow G N, Wortzman G, Rewcastle N B, Holgate R C, Kovacs K 1981 Microadenomas of the pituitary and abnormal sellar tomograms in an unselected autopsy series. New England Journal of Medicine 304: 156–158

Chambers E F, Turski P A, La Masters D, Newton T H 1982 Regions of low density in the contrast enhanced pituitary gland : Normal and pathologic processes. Radiology 144: 109–113

Cowden E A, Thomson J A, Doyle D, Ratcliffe J G, Macpherson P, Teasdale G M 1979 Tests of prolactin secretion in diagnosis of prolactinomas. Lancet i: 1155–1158

Daniels D L, Williams A L, Thornton R S, Meyer G A, Cusick J F, Haughton V M 1981 Differential diagnosis of intrasellar tumours by computed tomography. Radiology 141: 697–701

Davis K R, Zito J L, Hesselink J R, Taveras J M, Kjellberg R N 1980 Metrizamide saggital tomography: Adjunct to CT cisternography of the sellar region. American Journal of Roentgenology 134: 1205–1208

Domingue J N, Wing S D, Wilson C B 1978 Coexisting pituitary adenomas and partially empty sellas. Journal of Neurosurgery 48: 23–28

Drayer B P, Rosenbaum A E, Kennerdell J S, Robinson A G, Bank W O, Deeb Z L 1977 Computed tomographic diagnosis of suprasellar masses by intrathecal enhancement. Radiology 123: 339–344

Drayer B P, Kattah J, Rosenbaum A, Kennerdell, Maroon J 1979 Diagnostic approaches to pituitary adenomas. Neurology 29: 161–169

Dubois P J, Orr D P, Hoy R J, Herbert D L, Heinz E R 1979 Normal sellar variations in frontal tomograms. Radiology 131: 105–110

Earnest F, McCullough E C, Frank D A 1981 Fact or artifact: An analysis of artifact in high-resolution computed tomographic scanning of the sella. Radiology 140: 109–113

Gardeur D, Naidich T P, Metzger J 1981 CT analysis of intrasellar pituitary adenomas with emphasis on patterns of contrast enhancement. Neuroradiology 20: 241–247

Geehr R B, Allen W E, Rothman S L G, Spencer D O 1978 Pluridirectional tomography in the evaluation of pituitary tumours. American Journal of Roentgenology 130: 105–109

Gross C E, Binet E F, Esguerra J V 1979 Metrizamide cisternography in the evaluation of pituitary adenomas and the empty sella syndrome. Journal of Neurosurgery 50: 472–476

Hall K, McAllister V L 1980 Metrizamide cisternography in pituitary and juxtapituitary lesions. Radiology 134: 101–108

Haughton V M, Rosenbaum A E, Williams A L, Drayer B 1980 Recognising the empty sella by CT: the infundibulum sign. American Journal of Neuroradiology 1: 527–529

Hayman L A, Evans R A, Hinck V C 1979 Rapid high dose (R H D) contrast computed tomography of perisellar vessels. Radiology 131: 121–123

Hsu T H, Shapiro J R, Tyson J E, Leddy A L, Paz-Guevara A T 1976 Hyperprolactinemia associated with empty sella syndrome. Journal of the American Medical Association 235: 2002–2004

Jacobs H S 1976 Prolactin and amenorrhea. New England Journal of Medicine 295: 954–956

Kishore P R S, Kaufman A B, Melichar F A 1979 Intrasellar carotid anastomis simulating pituitary microadenoma. Radiology 132: 381–383

Kricheff I I 1979 The radiologic diagnosis of pituitary adenoma. Radiology 131: 263–265

Kuuliala I 1980 The normal suprasellar subarachnoid space in computed tomography. Clinical Radiology 31: 155–159

Kuuliala I, Katevuo K, Ketonen L 1981 Metrizamide with hypocycloid and computed tomography in sellar and suprasellar lesions. Clinical Radiology 32: 403–407

Macpherson P, Anderson D E 1981 Radiological differentiation of intrasellar aneurysms from pituitary tumours. Neuroradiology 21: 177–183

Malarkey W B, Johnson J C 1976 Pituitary tumours and hyperprolactinemia. Archives of Internal Medicine 136: 40–44

McLachlan M S F, Wright A D, Doyle F H 1970 Plain film and tomographic assessment of the pituitary fossa in 140 acromegalic patients. British Journal of Radiology 43: 360–369

McLachlan M S F, Lavender J P, Edwards C R W 1971 Polytome-encephalography in the investigation of pituitary tumours. Clinical Radiology 22: 361–369

Muhr C, Bergstrom K, Grimelius L, Larsson S G 1981 A parallel study of the roentgen anatomy of the sella turcica and the histopathology of the pituitary gland in 205 autopsy specimens. Neuroradiology 21: 55–65

Powell D F, Baker H L, Laws E R 1974 The primary angiographic findings in pituitary adenomas. Radiology 110: 589–595

Pripstein S, Danoff B, Schnapf D, Lee K F, Kramer S 1978 The value of computed tomography in delineating suprasellar extension of pituitary adenomas. Neuroradiology 16: 462–463

Raji M R, Kishore P R S, Becker D P 1981 Pituitary microadenoma: a radiological-surgical correlative study. Radiology 139: 95–99

Renn W H, Rhoton A L 1975 Microsurgical anatomy of the sellar region. Journal of Neurosurgery 43: 288–298

Richmond I L, Newton T H, Wilson C B 1980a Indications for angiography in the preoperative evaluation of patients with prolactin-secreting pituitary adenomas. Journal of Neurosurgery 52: 378–380

Richmond I L, Newton T H, Wilson C B 1980b Prolactin secreting pituitary adenomas: Correlation of radiographic and surgical findings. American Journal of Roentgenology 134: 707–710

Robertson W D, Newton T H 1978 Radiologic assessment of pituitary microadenomas. American Journal of Roentgenology 131: 489–492

Robertson H J, Rose A, Ehmi B, England G, Meriweather R 1981 Trends in the radiological study of pituitary adenoma. Neuroradiology 21: 75–78

Rozario R, Hammerschlag S B, Post K D, Wolpert S M, Jackson I 1977 Diagnosis of empty sella on CT scan. Neuroradiology 13: 85–88

Sakoda K, Mukada K, Yonezawa M, Matsumura S, Yoshimoto H, Mori, Uozumi T 1981 CT scan of pituitary adenomas. Neuroradiology 20: 249–253

Sheldon P, Molyneux A 1979 Metrizamide cisternography and computed tomography for the investigation of pituitary lesions. Neuroradiology 17: 83–87

Smaltino F, Bernini F P, Muras I 1980 Computed tomography for diagnosis of empty sella associated with enhancing pituitary adenoma. Journal of Computer Assisted Tomography 4: 592–599

Swanson H A, du Boulay G 1975 Borderline variants of the normal pituitary fossa. British Journal of Radiology 48: 366–369

Syversten A, Haughton V M, Williams A L, Cusick J F 1979 The computed tomographic appearance of the normal pituitary gland and pituitary microadenomas. Radiology 133: 385–391

Teasdale G M, Ratcliffe J G, Thomson J A, Cowden E A 1980 The prolactinoma problem. Lancet i: 925–926

Teasdale E, Macpherson P, Teasdale G 1981 The reliability of radiology in detecting prolactin-secreting pituitary microadenomas. British Journal of Radiology 54: 566–571

Theron J, Chevalier D, Delvert M, Laffont J 1979 Diagnosis of small and micropituitary adenomas by intercavernous sinus venography. Neuroradiology 18: 23–30

Turski P A, Newton T H, Horten B H 1981 Sellar contour : Anatomic-polytomographic correlation. American Journal of Roentgenology 137: 213–216

Wolpert S M, Post K D, Biller B J, Molitch M E 1979 The value of computed tomography in evaluating patients with prolactinomas. Radiology 131: 117–119

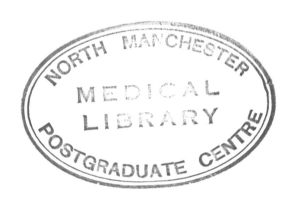

Primary amenorrhoea

INTRODUCTION

The overwhelming majority of girls presenting with primary amenorrhoea have aetiologies with roots in disturbances of the embryogenesis and/or the endocrinology of sexual differentiation and maturation. There is considerable overlap between the problems of intersexuality and primary amenorrohea. It would be nice to believe that any person reading this chapter would aready have read the section dealing with intersexuality (Ch. 17). Working on the principle that nice beliefs are rarely fulfilled, this chapter will begin with a summary of embryogenesis discussed in detail in Chapter 17 and will then deal with the difficult problem of the embryology of the Fallopian tubes, uterus and vagina. This will be followed by a classification of primary amenorrhoea. Finally a clinical approach to the problem, including differential diagnosis and management, will be presented.

EMBRYOGENESIS AND ENDOCRINOLOGY

In summary, the important concepts of sexual differentiation are that:

1. XX is usually needed for normal ovarian development and maintenance. Ovarian development including germ cell migration will occur in the presence of a single X but this is almost invariably followed by rapid disappearance of these follicles, two X chromosomes normally being required for follicular maintenance.

2. The H-Y antigen probably evokes the testis as long as there are specific receptors. However, it will not, by itself, induce germ cell colonisation of the gonads.

3. In the absence of a gonad, female development is the neutral or asexual norm.

4. The Sertoli cells of the testis produce anti-Mullerian factor. A male intersex lacking AMF will have a uterus, tubes and vagina.

5. Fetal testosterone evokes Wolffian structures but has no effect on Müllerian ducts.

6. Fetal testosterone will virilise the cloaca if it is bound to the target cells and can be converted to DHT.

7. A relative deficiency of 5α-reductase will impair the cloacal response to testosterone, but will not effect Wolffian evocation, the latter being dpendent on testosterone without need of conversion.

8. Abnormal or ectopic androgen stimuli, depending on timing and biological potency, may cause variable even almost complete masculinisation of the female cloaca but never effects Müllerian development in chromosomal or gonadal females.

Full amplification of this summary will be found in Chapter 17.

Embryology of the fallopian tubes, uterus and vagina: uterovaginal agenesis

Although there are firm experimental and clinical data related to the control of Müllerian inhibition and Wolffian evocation in a normal male, the same cannot be said about the mechanisms of Müllerian induction in a normal female. Varying degrees of uterovaginal agenesis form one of the single largest groups of patients presenting with primary amenorrhoea (Mashchak et al, 1981; Reindollar et al, 1981; Shearman & Roberts, 1982) and these patients frequently have associated abnormalities of the renal and skeletal systems.

It seems to be almost a truism of clinical medicine that an eponymic cloak masks ignorance of mechanisms; as mechanisms emerge more precise names are given to clinical syndromes. For those who collect eponyms, uterovaginal agenesis is a delight and a full flourish could be given in the title 'Mayer-Rokitansky-Kuster-Hauser syndrome!' The first descriptions of this go back to Mayer (1829; quoted by Griffin et al, 1976) but almost certainly this condition has existed since the heterogametic male human started to produce progeny from a homogametic female. The concurrence of abnormalities of the genital tract, renal tract and vertebral column may fire the imagination but this has not yet produced solid experimental evidence of cause and effect such as relates, for example, to the persistance of the Müllerian duct in one of the rarer forms of XY female (see Ch. 17). The embryology of the problem has been discussed by Griffin et al (1976) and Evans et al (1981).

Although previously called Müllerian agenesis (Shearman 1968, 1981a), uterovaginal agenesis is probably a more acceptable term. But the full spectrum of abnormalities seen in these girls can only, still, be encompassed in the splendid eponym described earlier.

The fact that the fimbrial ends of the Fallopian tubes are often present means that more than the Müllerian ducts (or less) are involved and this is confirmed by the frequent finding of vestigial myometrial tissue, usually uncanalised. The association of renal tract abnormalities indicates that the metanephric duct is involved but common ground must also embrace skeletal deformities — even to the full blown Klippel-Feil syndrome — contained within this group of patients. The skeletal abnormalities of the Klippel-Feil syndrome are well known in their relationship to a malformation of the kidney but not nearly as well documented with Müllerian tract abnormalities (Griffin et al, 1976).

There seems to be general agreement that the cephalic end of the Müllerian duct develops into the Fallopian tubes while the caudal end fuses to form the usually single human uterus. The embryogenesis of the vagina is not so clear. For example, in the syndrome of testicular feminisation, the fact that the lower third of the vagina is usually normal suggests that this comes from the urogenital sinus, everything above this level being inhibited by Müllerian inhibiting factor. However, the girl with uterovaginal agenesis has completely normal external genitals and only a vaginal 'dimple' suggesting that it is not just a simple lack of androgens that allows the lower third of the vagina to

develop. The problem is complicated further by the relatively infrequent problem of 'imperforate hymen' causing amenorrhoea where the suggested embryogenesis is non-canalisation of the vaginal plate (Marshall, 1978). It is likely that the Müllerian ducts are dependent for their normal development on the Wolffian ducts which seem to be parasitised by the Müllerian ducts during their normal evolution.

Knowledge of the control of Müllerian duct development (as distinct from it's inhibition) has not really advanced since the fundamental work of Gruenwald (1959). A general outline is shown in Fig. 24.1. The cephalic portion, derived from coelomic epithelium is joined to the caudal, probably derived from, or in association with the Wolffian duct. Its genesis begins cephalically when there is an evagination of the coelomic epithelium immediately lateral to the mesonephros — what will become the mesonephric kidney. The caudal end of this proximal evagination becomes so closely related to the Wolffian duct that they are not separated even by a basement membrane. This relationship is so intimate that is not clear whether the Müllerian duct then evolves caudally separate from the Wolffian duct or whether the Wolffian duct acts as a template for caudal extension. It does seem that Müllerian duct development in a caudal direction cannot take place in the absence of Wolffian structures. At the most distal end of this caudal extension, the Müllerian duct fuses with the urogenital sinus, an intimate fusion that results in the formation of the originally solid vaginal plate which in turn canalises. It is still uncertain how much of the definitive vagina is of Müllerian and how much of urogenital origin.

The commonest clinical constellation is to find normal ovaries — although these are frequently much higher in the

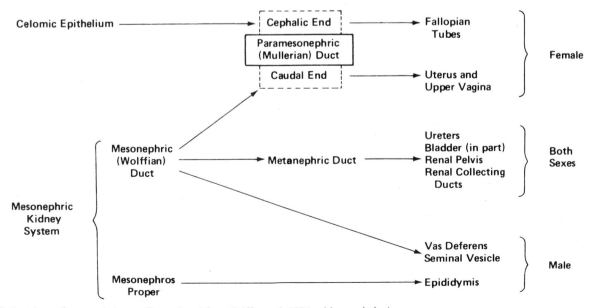

Fig. 24.1 Embryology of uro-genital tract (Reproduced from Griffin et al, 1976, with permission)

pelvis than normal or even in the abdominal cavity — normal tubal fimbriae or even completely normal Fallopian tubes, an absent uterus or occasional islands of non-canalised myometrium and no vagina, even to the lower third. Conflict about the varying embryogenesis of the lower vagina apart, this is the lesion that would be expected if the cephalic end of the Müllerian duct from the coelomic epithelium had developed normally but the caudal end, dependent on the Wolffian duct for its growth and structure was impaired. Recognising that the definitive kidney arises from the metanephric (Wolffian) rather than the mesonephric kidney, difficulty in embryogenesis would also account for the renal abnormalities, most frequently congenital absence of one kidney or a solitary pelvic kidney.

With a small leap of the imagination this would also embrace the skeletal problem. At the 10–11 mm stage when the mischief that affects the Müllerian ducts occurs (and recollecting that the metanephros is derived from mesoderm) there may be concurrent difficulties in the mesoderm that will ultimately form the vertebral column at the same somite levels as the metanephros.

Endocrinology. Brown et al (1959) indicated that ovarian function was normal in three of these patients. A more detailed and longer study by Fraser et al (1973) showed normal hormonal indices of ovulation and corpus luteum function; this has also been the experience in the patients I have studied. The case report of concurrence between a Turner karyotype/phenotype and uterovaginal agenesis (Phansey et al, 1981) is almost certainly coincidental.

Aetiology. There is no known cause of uterovaginal agenesis. Although there are several reports of sisters with the same anomaly, a genetic trait is unlikely as there are data on sets of monozygous twins who did not share this anomaly (Evans et al, 1981). The embryological equivalent of this condition in the male is congenital absence of the vas deferens and seminal vesicles which is well recognised but also of unknown aetiology.

Gonadal failure

It is evident from the discussion on ovarian findings in Turner's syndrome that even though the ovary may start normally in the fetus, it ends up with complete depletion of primordial follicles long before the age of normal puberty. It is also evident that abnormalities of the chromosomes short of full X deletion may relate to the same ovarian problem and for this reason the terminology 'chromosomally incompetent ovarian failure' used by Reindollar et al (1981) has much to recommend it.

Any variant of the 'XY female' (Ch. 17) may present with amenorrhoea. Those with 46,XY gonadal agenesis or 45,X/46,XY gonadal dysgenesis may be due to absence of the H-Y antigen or its receptor. However, this does not explain the relatively common problem of pure gonadal

agenesis in women who have primary amenorrhoea and a normal 46,XX karyotype. Although an autosomal recessive mode of inheritance, intra-uterine viral infection or childhood mumps had been suggested as mechanisms to explain this syndrome (Aleem, 1981) the whole spectrum of XX gonadal agenesis remains an enigma. In our own series of 140 patients with primary amenorrhoea, twenty had 46,XX ovarian agenesis (Shearman & Roberts, 1982 and I have since seen one pair of sisters with the same anomaly.

Any of the recognised causes of premature ovarian failure that may present with secondary amenorrhoea (Ch. 25) may also, if the timing is right, present with primary amenorrhoea. For example, the increased survival of children with various forms of leukaemia and lymphoma who have been treated with combined radiotherapy/chemotherapy will mean that more young girls present with ovarian failure for those reasons. Ovarian failure is more common if comprehensive chemotherapy and whole body irradiation has been given than if either of these therapies had been given alone. Autoimmune causes of ovarian failure before the age of menarche are also recognised. As expected hypothyroidism, hypoparathyroidism and/or autoimmune Addison's disease may be associated. It may surprise some to note that a well documented clinical association with autoimmune prepubertal ovarian failure is the Candida endocrinopathy syndrome (Dempsey et al, 1981).Galactosaemia may result in ovarian failure and primary amenorrhoea (Kaufman et al, 1981, and see also Ch. 25).

It should be clear that all patients in these categories will have high levels of FSH and LH — in other words they have hypergonadotrophic hypogonadism. It might be noted that gonadotrophin producing pituitary adenomata may occur in these patients (Woolf & Schenk, 1974), just as they may in castrates.

The hypothalamus and primary amenorrhoea

This provides the largest single group of patients in our own and other published series. Within this substantial subset, those with an isolated deficiency of gonadotrophin releasing factor (GnRF) form the largest number of patients. The deficiency may be sporadic but is not infrequently familial, when it is associated with anosmia and craniofacial deformities including cleft palate. The latter group may be called Kallman's syndrome (Kallman et al, 1944). These patients present with primary amenorrhoea, sexual infantilism and normal or increased height. A common feature is the inability to release FSH and LH under normal circumstances (Valk et al, 1980). However, LH and FSH release can be normalised by pulsatile infusions of GnRF (Hammond et al, 1979; Valk et al, 1980) indicating that everything 'below' the hypothalamus is potentially normal including the ability to respond to exogenous gonadotrophins (Shearman, 1981b, and see Ch. 26).

1 am not aware of any rational explanation that provides a link between anosmia and hypogonadotrophic hypogonadism. It is of interest that piglets rendered anosmic immediately after delivery have the same sexual destiny as their human counterparts. Perhaps it is the mysterious pheromone!

It is usually assumed that idiopathic delay in the onset of menstruation in a girl with an otherwise normal puberty represents a delay in hypothalamic maturation. Such a diagnosis can only be made in retrospect. The commonest presentation is that of a girl in her mid-teens who has had an otherwise normal puberty but has failed to menstruate. The usual examinations show that she has normal levels of gonadotrophins, a normal vagina and uterus and there is no evidence of virilism. In our own series of patients nine with this diagnosis had all begun to menstruate spontaneously by the age of 21.

Children with growth hormone deficiency will usually cross the clinical horizon long before the age of normal puberty and menarche. These patients will often have a delay in menarche but there is a group of asexual ateliotic dwarfs (Rimion et al, 1968) who in addition to their growth hormone problem also lack the template to make GnRF.

The hypothalamus is also the area under attack in patients with previously undiagnosed or under-treated congenital adrenal hyperplasia (see Ch. 18) and it is usually the hypothalamus at fault as the driving force in the uncommon problem of Cushing's disease in this age group.

Although weight loss has long been recognised for its close relationship with secondary amenorrhoea (Ch. 25) it has more recently become evident that it may be associated with primary amenorrhoea. The full-blown form of anorexia nervosa, although far more common in girls than boys, rarely occurs before the time of puberty but may do so and then relate to primary amenorrhoea. Far more common is a decrease in body fat mass well short of that seen in anorexia nervosa in girls who are in heavy athletic training and/or ballet dancing (Frisch et al, 1981). These patients are usually of normal height and unlike those with hypogonadotrophic hypogonadism will usually have fairly well developed secondary sexual characteristics without having menstruated.

Polycystic ovaries were responsible for primary amenorrhoea in six of our 140 patients (Shearman & Roberts, 1982). Although the most frequent presentation of this multifacetad condition is either oligomenorrhoea or secondary amenorrhoea (Ch. 20) it should be suspected in patients with primary amenorrhoea who have normal secondary sexual characteristics with varying degrees of acne and hirsutism. The fundamental disturbance is in the hypothalamus with an elevated and non-cyclic increase in LH secretion and a high LH:FSH ratio. Maschak et al (1981) found this condition in two of their 62 patients while

17 of the 252 patients studied by Reindollar et al (1981) had polycystic ovaries.

Although hyperprolactinaemia will be found in about 30 per cent of patients with secondary amenorrhoea this remains a relatively uncommon cause of primary amenorrhoea. As in secondary amenorrhoea, hyperprolactinaemic patients may or may not have detectable pituitary tumours. In the series of Maschak et al (1981) five of 62 patients with primary amenorrhoea had hyperprolactinaemia while we have only found one in our total of 140. Reindollar et al (1981) found three hyperprolactinaemic women in their series of 252 with primary amenorrhoea.

Organic intracranial disease

Occasionally hydrocephalus related to events around the time of birth may ultimately lead to primary amenorrhoea and the same may also occur after severe head injury, presumably from damage to the hypothalamus. An intracranial neoplasm should always be suspected until proven otherwise. While those with hyperprolactinaemia may have a pituitary adenoma, more commonly an endocrinologically inert tumour such as a craniopharyngioma or malignant cerebral tumour may be found. The craniopharyngioma operates by interrupting the portal circulation from the hypothalamus to the pituitary gland. These patients will often, therefore, have short stature as well as sexual infantilism and primary amenorrhoea. It is a grave error to assume that every short patient has Turner's syndrome.

Intersexuality and primary amenorrhoea

These relationships are fully discussed in Chapter 17 and some of them have been referred to under the section dealing with gonadal failure. It is apparent that intersexuality will be one of the differential diagnoses in any individual presenting at puberty with primary amenorrhoea and virilism.

The XY female. Although dealt with fully in Chapter 17 these patients are such an important subgroup in any large series with primary amenorrhoea that they must be discussed here briefly. The classification in our own group of patients is shown in Table 24.1. Those with 46,XY true gonadal agenesis will present with primary amenorrhoea, normal or increased stature, sexual infantilism — in other

Table 24.1   XY Female and primary amenorrhoea (15 of 140 patients)

Category	Number of patients
46,XY gonadal agenesis	5
45,X/46,XY gonadal dysgenesis	2
5α-reductase deficiency	3
Testicular feminisation	3
True hermaphrodite	1
Anti-Müllerian factor deficiency	1

From Shearman & Roberts (1982)

words a picture identical to the patient with 46,XX gonadal agenesis. Like them the 46,XY patients will also have high levels of gonadotrophins. Most patients with 45,X/46,XY gonadal dysgenesis are of short stature. Some of these may be known to have partially virilised genitals from birth and others will develop some clitoromegaly at the time of puberty. However, in some the external genitals will be quite normal and the diagnosis will not be considered until the karyotype is available. The clinician must be aware of the high frequency of dysgenetic tumours in this group (Ch. 17).

Patients with 5α-reductase deficiency will be born with equivocal external genitals. Before the nature of this deficiency was recognised, these girls went under a variety of names including 'cryptorchid hypospadiac male intersex' (Shearman, 1968). At birth the statistically more likely diagnosis of congenital adrenal hyperplasia is excluded by finding a male karyotype, normal levels of serum 17-hydroxyprogesterone and complete absence of the uterus and Fallopian tubes. If left untreated, the steroidogenically competent testes will produce normal amounts of testosterone at puberty causing rapid virilism in a child who has probably been brought up as a female until then.

It is very rare for testicular feminism to present before puberty unless a testis is found in the inguinal hernia of a small girl. The diagnosis should be suspected in a patient with amenorrhoea, normal breast development, normal height, scanty or absent pubic and axillary hair and a short blind vagina. Endocrinological confirmation would come from finding a male karyotype, normal or slightly increased levels of FSH and LH and normal male levels of testosterone. Dysgenetic tumours may occur in these undescended testes but are less common than in other XY females. Dewhurst & Spence (1977) put the frequency at no more than 5 per cent, although this incidence will increase substantially by the age of 30 or 40 years.

The majority of true hermaphrodites have an XX karyotype and are reared as apparent males, sometimes presenting with penile bleeding in a cyclic fashion at the time of puberty. However, a substantial minority have XY karyotypes and/or are reared as girls (Shearman et al, 1964). Unlike other forms of the XY female, the nature of the true hermaphrodite will usually not be recognised until each gonad is submitted to open biopsy and frozen section.

Anti-Müllerian deficiency is one of the rarest forms of the XY female and we have only one in our series of patients with primary amenorrhoea. As indicated in Chapter 17 these individuals have a karyotype of 46,XY, testes that are histologically normal for the age of the patient and their intra-abdominal site, normal Fallopian tubes, uterus and upper vagina but varying and sometimes substantial virilism of the external genitals (Shearman, 1968). If left untreated they will virilise at puberty. On technical grounds the appropriate treatment still seems to be bilateral gonadectomy before puberty and reconstruction of the external genitals before the age of 3. If they present after puberty — and with luck those days may now have passed — they will have an inappropriate puberty by virilising with normal male levels of testosterone and gonadotrophins. In other words the laboratory data may be exactly the same as those for the girl with testicular feminising syndrome but nobody could confuse the two clinically.

CLASSIFICATION OF PRIMARY AMENORRHOEA

Since first writing about this problem in 1968 I have been through many classifications, none of which was or is

Table 24.2 Classification of primary amenorrhoea

Hypergonadotrophic hypogonadism
  Chromosomally incompetent ovarian failure includes classic Turner, all other X deletions and 45,X/46,XY
  Chromosomally competent ovarian failure 46,XX
    (i) True agenesis
    (ii) Premature ovarian failure (radiation chemotherapy, autoimmune)
    (iii) Galactosaemia
    46,XY

Hypogonadotrophic hypogonadism
  Reversible
    Physiological delay
    Weight loss/anorexia nervosa/heavy exercise
    Primary hypothyroidism
  Irreversible
  (a) Congenital
    Isolated GnRF deficiency (with or without anosmia)
    Partial or total hypopituitarism
    Congenital CNS defects
  (b) Acquired
    Hyperprolactinaemia (no tumour)
    Pituitary adenoma:
      (i) Prolactinoma
      (ii) Mixed activity (i + acromegaly or Cushing's)
      (iii) producing gonadotrophins
      (iv) Inert
    Empty Sella
    Craniopharyngioma
    Other intracranial tumours
    Trauma (including surgery)

Eugonadal
  Anatomical
    Uterovaginal agenesis
    Imperforate hymen (including transverse septum)
  Polycystic ovaries
  Testicular feminisation
  Noonan's syndrome

Virilising
  Adrenal hyperplasia
  Tumour (adrenal, ovary)
  5α-reductase deficiency
  Partial androgen receptor complex deficiency
  Absent anti-Müllerian factor
  True hermaphrodite

Adapted and expanded from Reindollar et al (1981)

satisfactory. Any classification should satisfy the dictates of good sense, clinical experience, cytogenetics and endocrinology. The classification shown in Table 24.2 is adapted and expanded from Reindollar et al (1981).

THE CLINICAL PROBLEM

Ross (1979) has suggested that primary amenorrhoea should be investigated if sexual infantilism persists until the chronological age of 16 or if, irrespective of the normality of secondary sexual characteristics, menstruation has not occurred by the age of 18. My own view is that if normal menstruation has not begun within 2 years of the onset of an otherwise normal puberty — providing there is no other immediately obvious clinical manifestation beforehand — then congenital absence of the uterus/vagina should be excluded. If puberty is inappropriate (for example virilising) or if abnormal gonadal tissue has been demonstrated prior to puberty then full investigation is mandatory.

Clinically, it is often possible to arrive at a fairly firm provisional diagnosis from the history and results of physical examination. In most of these girls the investigations are straightforward and can be done on an outpatient basis. Only a small minority will require hospitalisation for more complex investigation and very few will even need hospitalisation for treatment.

The patient with sexual infantilism

The most important initial distinction is whether the patient is sexually infantile or whether there is evidence of secondary sexual characteristics. The importance of this distinction should be clear. A girl of 15 or 16 who has no secondary sexual characteristics obviously has not been exposed to any form of stimulation from gonadal hormones. This may be because the gonads have not been stimulated or it may be that she has been born without gonads. The patient's height is important. If she is less than 140 cm tall (4 ft 10 in) statistical probability will be in favour of chromosomally incompetent ovarian failure but other conditions such as intracranial tumour, particularly craniopharyngioma, the various forms of hypopituitarism and Noonan's syndrome (Noonan, 1968) must be considered if only to be excluded.

The classic Turner's syndrome, in addition to short stature and sexual infantilism, will have webbing of the neck, widely spaced nipples, pectus cavum, shortening of the fourth metacarpal and sometimes congenital heart disease, particularly coarctation of the aorta (Fig. 24.2). Clinically, Noonan's syndrome is the most likely to be confused with the Turner phenotype. This syndrome occurs in both phenotypic males and females. Delayed puberty may occur in both sexes but is more common in

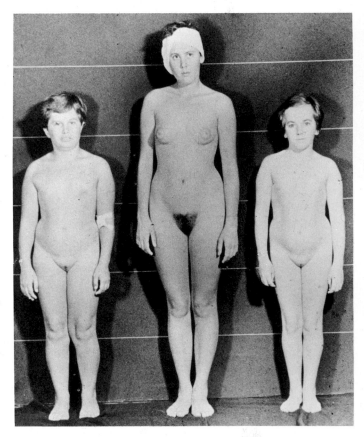

Fig. 24.2 Normal 14-year-old in middle flanked by two patients with Turner's syndrome of the same age (Reproduced from Shearman, 1982, with permission)

the male. However, in the female there may be delayed puberty and then delayed menarche. In addition to short stature they may have webbing of the neck, pectus cavum and congenital heart disease. However, unlike Turner's syndrome, these children are remarkably similar in facial appearance (Fig. 24.3). Any clinician who has seen one of these girls is unlikely to miss the diagnosis.

It is evident then that not every short girl with sexual infantilism and a webbed neck has Turner's syndrome. It is equally clear that not every girl with X chromosome deletion, complete or incomplete, has the full-blown Turner phenotype. A substantial minority will have spontaneous breast development up to Tanner II and further evidence of sexual maturation may be present, even to relatively normal secondary sexual characteristics (Wray et al, 1981). If on examination there is some degree of clitoromegaly and perhaps partial labial fusion then mixed gonadal dysgenesis (45,X/46,XY) must be considered but the same appearance may rarely occur with Turner mosaics (Mead et al, 1981).

Girls with panhypopituitarism will almost always have

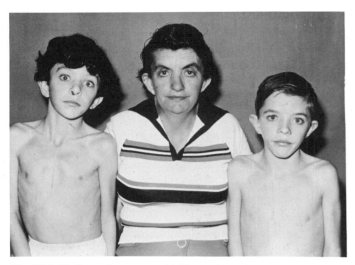

Fig. 24.3 Mother and two sons with Noonan's syndrome (by courtesy of Dr Robert Vines)

entered the clinical arena long before primary amenorrhoea becomes but one further manifestation of their fundamental problem. Similarly those with growth hormone deficiency will, in most developed countries, have been treated with growth hormone well before the age of normal menarche. Delay in puberty and menarche is common in patients with an isolated growth hormone deficiency but in the asexual ateliotic dwarf, sexual infantilism and amenorrhoea is the rule unless specific treatment is introduced. If the short amenorrhoeic patient has headaches this might suggest an intracranial lesion but the absence of headaches does not exclude major intracranial pathology.

The investigations in this group of patients are: chromosomal analysis and karyotype which must include G and C banding. Serum LH and FSH should be measured and X-rays of the skull, pituitary fossa, wrists and metacarpals are needed. The chromosomally incompetent group including 45,X/46,XY patients will be evident by their abnormal karyotype and in these girls FSH and LH will be substantially increased. Patients with Noonan's syndrome, apart from their typical appearance will have a normal female karyotype and low or normal levels of FSH and LH. Growth hormone deficient patients at the age of normal puberty will usually remain sexually infantile. Some of these girls will develop a delayed but otherwise normal puberty. The asexual group will have persistent infantilism unless they receive replacement therapy. The integrated gonadotrophic response to GnRF infusion may help to discriminate between these patients, who on clinical grounds may be indistinguishable (Bourguignon et al, 1982). The commonest organic lesion in this age group will be a craniopharyngioma which typically and fortunately is calcified. These patients in addition to low or normal levels of FSH and LH often have increased levels of prolactin and a diminished ability to release growth hormone. Bone age will be substantially retarded in all of these girls. Laparoscopy is unnecessary but neurosurgery will be appropriate

in some and laparotomy essential in those carrying Y chromosomes.

For the taller patient with sexual infantilism the diagnosis usually lies between true gonadal agenesis and hypogonadotrophic hypogonadism. Some mosaic Turners may be of relatively normal height.

This group of patients should also always be asked about their sense of smell and this can be assessed objectively and rapidly by the 'smell kit' beloved of neurologists. If the tall sexually infantile patient has anosmia she almost certainly has hypogonadotrophic hypogonadism (olfacto-genital dysplasia). There may be a family history of similar problems and in such families there is an increased incidence of cleft palate and harelip. Karyotype in these patients will usually be 46,XX. Clinically in patients of this type with a normal sense of smell I know of no way to distinguish hypogonadotrophic hypogonadism from the less frequent instance of true gonadal agenesis. The distinction will be quite clear after assay of FSH and LH as these will be substantially increased in the girl with gonadal agenesis and low normal or rarely even undetectable in those with hypogonadotrophic hypogonadism. If the karyotype is 46,XY then gonadal agenesis will be certain and levels of FSH and LH will be increased. Laparoscopy is meddlesome and unnecessary in these girls but laparotomy is essential in the 46,XY group.

The patient with primary amenorrhoea and an otherwise normal female puberty

Delay in menstruation in these patients is a different problem. If the patient has some female secondary sexual characteristics, then obviously she has been exposed to some endogenous sex steroid stimulation. This statement is only valid if one can be certain that this sexual maturation has not been induced by prolonged administration of exogenous steroids in unwise attempts to induce vaginal bleeding before a proper diagnosis has been made. Frequently a patient in her late teens or early twenties will present with 'secondary amenorrhoea'. On careful questioning it emerges that all of her periods have been induced by intermittent hormone therapy given over many years. By the time of presentation neither the patient, nor her mother, can recall whether the secondary sexual characteristics preceded or followed this treatment.

If the patient has a normal female habitus then a local abnormality of the genital tract should be excluded forthwith. Uterovaginal agenesis is one of the most frequent causes of primary amenorrhoea in any large series and in our own group of 140 patients there were 24 in this category (Shearman & Roberts, 1982). Inspection of the genitals will show a normal vulva but only a vaginal dimple. On rectal examination the uterus cannot be felt. This examination is better done under anaesthesia in most teenagers. Intravenous pyelography is mandatory as 30 per

Table 24.3 Uterovaginal agenesis (24 of 140 patients with primary amenorrhoea)

Somatic abnormality	Number of patients
Renal tract	8
Scoliosis	2
Klippel-Feil Syndrome	1
Cervical Rib and pectus excavatum	1

From Shearman & Roberts (1982)

cent will have a substantial abnormality of the renal tract, most frequently unilateral absence of one kidney or a solitary pelvic kidney. About 20 per cent of the patients will have abnormalities of the vertebral column. The types of abnormalities are shown in Table 24.3. Laparoscopy is, as a rule, unnecessary and I would only do this if there was a history of cyclic lower abdominal pain. This suggests the presence of uncanalised myometrial tissue which causes the characteristic pain of primary dysmenorrhoea. Very rarely, there may be a non-communicating rudimentary uterus with haematometra and this differentiation can only be made at laparoscopy. However, for the usual patient with uterovaginal agenesis and no pain, laparoscopy should be avoided.

Imperforate hymen is much less frequent than uterovaginal agenesis and would be suspected with a history of progressively severe cyclic lower abdominal pain and sometimes abdominal distension. On examination there is a convex occlusion just within the vulva and characteristic chocolate fluid may be seen behind this on transillumination. The karyotype in both of these types of patient is 46,XX and all hormonal indices show normal pituitary and ovarian function. The findings in testicular feminisation are described earlier.

If after full assessment of patients in this category, a normal uterus, vagina and normal levels of gonadotrophins are found the most likely diagnosis is idiopathic delay of menarche and spontaneous menstruation can be awaited with a degree of confidence. All nine patients in whom this diagnosis was made in our series of 140 girls with primary amenorrhoea began spontaneous menstruation by the age of 21.

Primary amenorrhoea with hirsutism or virilism

Patients who have a predominantly feminine puberty but associated acne/hirsutism and amenorrhoea will usually prove to have either polycystic ovaries of the peripubertal type or late onset adrenal hyperplasia. The former can be determined by finding the typically increased levels of LH and a high LH/FSH ratio. Plasma testosterone is usually at the upper end of the normal range or slightly above and androstenedione may be increased. An increase in dehydro-epiandrosterone sulphate is compatible with this diagnosis as secondary adrenal involvement is well documented

(Shearman & Cox, 1965). Plasma 17-hydroxyprogesterone will be normal. Adrenal hyperplasia would be suggested sometimes by a positive family history and confirmed by finding normal levels of LH and FSH together with a substantial increase in 17-hydroxyprogesterone. Late onset (or late recognised) adrenal hyperplasia is usually due to a mild 21-hydroxylase deficiency.

A fully virilising and, therefore, inappropriate puberty could be due to any of the conditions listed towards the bottom of Table 24.2. Since this chapter is dealing with primary amenorrhoea we are by definition only dealing with individuals brought up as girls. Undiagnosed or under-treated adrenal hyperplasia may be associated with virilism at puberty as may masculinising tumours of the adrenal cortex or ovary. These subjects are discussed in Chapters 18 and 21.

Patients with 5α-reductase deficiency will have been recognised usually before the age of puberty but it is important to recognise that if the testes are left *in situ* gross virilism will occur at the time of puberty — a disaster for an individual brought up until then as a little girl. If confirmation of the diagnosis is needed, stimulation with human chorionic gonadotrophin will cause a normal increase in testosterone but a subnormal increase in dihydrotestosterone.

A similar sexual destiny awaits the girl with absent anti-Müllerian factor but this diagnosis should have been reached long before the age of puberty, as it was in the only patient I have seen.

The clinical constellation covered by the true hermaphrodite is so broad that there is no 'typical' feature that will alert the clinician to this possibility. Finding male levels of testosterone in somebody undergoing a virilising puberty will suggest the presence of a testis. This possibility is unlikely to be neglected if the karyotype is 46,XY. If, however, these levels of testosterone are found in an individual with a karyotype 46,XX the true diagnosis may not be entertained until the time of laparotomy and studies of frozen section.

TREATMENT

Stature

Most girls with growth hormone deficiency will be recognised and treated before the age of normal puberty. In the unlikely event that a growth hormone deficiency is recognised for the first time when a patient presents with primary amenorrhoea, treatment with growth hormone should be introduced to allow linear growth before oestrogen/progestin therapy is introduced. While that approach would defer induction of secondary sexual characteristics this is preferable to precipitate use of gonadal steroids as these will cause rapid epiphyseal fusion.

There are important growth determinants on both the

short and long arms of the X chromosome so that the short stature of girls with chromosomally incompetent ovarian failure is scarcely surprising. It is not clear how this disturbance is mediated. Growth hormone levels in these children are normal. It has been suggested (Simpson & Labo, 1981) that the prolonged cell cycle typical of the X deleted cell might cause the statistically small size at birth seen in Turner's syndrome and their poor post-natal growth. They suggested that anabolic steroids might increase ultimate height in these patients. Rudman et al (1980) have, in fact, shown a significantly synergistic effect on linear growth in these patients treated with human growth hormone and an anabolic steroid — in this instance oxandrolone. However, until quantities of growth hormone are increased by the use of recombinant DNA technology, supplies are both at a premium and extremely expensive. Currently, therefore, attempts to secure increased growth in these girls before introduction of gonadal steroids is probably not justified but it should be born in mind for the future.

Oestrogens and progestins

This treatment should never be introduced until a firm diagnosis has been reached. Once this has been done exogenous steroids will be needed in all patients with sexual infantilism. There is no uniformly accepted therapeutic regime. My own practice is to introduce oestrogens in a low dose, using 10 μg of ethinyl-oestradiol twice daily for 21 days, repeating this after a 1 week gap and continuing for 5 or 6 months. This will usually cause primary breast bud development and the patient will become accustomed to exogenous oestrogens. Withdrawal bleeding rarely occurs with this dose. After about 6 months the dose of oestrogens is increased and a progestin added both because of the positive effect of the progestin on breast tissue and the highly undesirable effect of long-term unopposed oestrogens on the endometrium. The continued use of unopposed oestrogens — still seen most frequently in Turner's syndrome — can and has led to the development of endometrial carcinoma. The cheapest and simplest way to introduce oestrogens and progestins is to use a combined oral contraceptive. Most girls will achieve adequate development with any combination pill containing 50 μg of ethinyloestradiol and an appropriate progestin. Some will need higher doses of oestrogen. The patient should be warned that it will take about 2 or 3 years to achieve full breast development. For reasons that have never been clear to me those with an XY karyotype appear to have less satisfactory breast development even with very high doses of oestrogens and in some of these girls augmentation mammoplasty might be considered.

After this, because there are some concerns about long-term metabolic and cardiovascular effects of combined oral contraceptives (Ch. 33) my own preference is to use oestra-

diol valerate in a dose of 1 or 2 mg daily for 21 days, repeating this after a 7 day gap and to give oral medroxyprogesterone acetate in a dose of 10 mg for the last 10 days of each treatment cycle. This is the same regime that is often used in long-term hormonal replacement therapy of the normal menopausal woman. The reasons for preferring this combination relate mainly to the relatively benign effect on HDL cholesterol.

For those capable of ovulation, such as the patient with hypogonadotrophic hypogonadism it is meddlesome to induce ovulation until the patient wishes to use the ova — that is until she wishes to become pregnant. Induction of ovulation is discussed fully in Chapters 26 & 27.

Corticosteroids. The only role for corticosteroids in this group of patients is in the treatment of adrenal hyperplasia. This is discussed in Chapter 18.

Bromocriptine. Hyperprolactinaemia is rarely associated with primary amenorrhoea. Nevertheless when this is found, treatment with bromocriptine will permit spontaneous and normal ovulatory activity to occur. This treatment is described fully in Chapter 26.

Antiandrogens

These would only be used in patients with substantial hirsutism and most of these will be in the inter-sexuality group. Occasionally the hirsutism in peripubertal polycystic ovaries can be extreme. The role and use of gonadal steroids, cyproterone acetate, spironolactone and other antiandrogens is dealt with fully in Chapter 21.

Embryo transfer

Although not yet achieved, there is no scientific reason why embryo transfer using donated ova should not be practicable in agonadal women (even 46, XY agenesis) within the forseeable future.

Prostaglandin synthetase inhibitors

Some patients with uterovaginal agenesis experience severe 'dysmenorrhoea' from uncanalised vestigial uterine tissue. Although this can be excised surgically, good control can usually be achieved medically by the use of fenamates used in the same dosage as in true primary dysmenorrhoea (Ch. 31).

Surgery

Neurosurgery is unequivocally indicated in patients with craniopharyngioma and pituitary lesions producing Cushing's disease. There is much more controversy about the use of surgery in patients with prolactinomas and to a lesser extent with mixed tumours producing acromegaly and hyperprolactinaemia. Many clinicians, including this

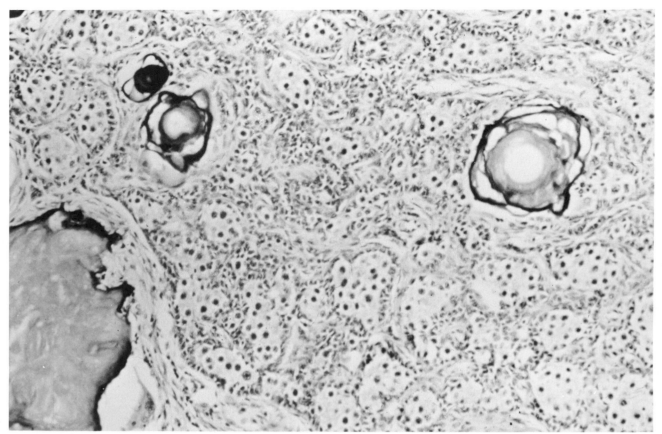

Fig. 24.4 Gonadoblastoma from 45, X/46, XY female

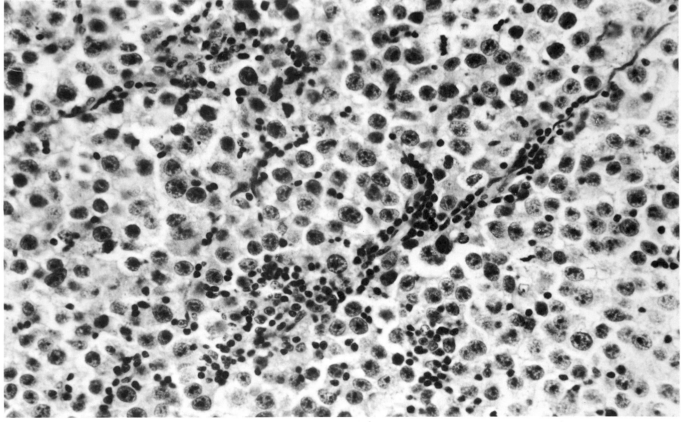

Fig. 24.5 Dysgerminoma from another patient with 45, X/46, XY gonadal dysgenesis (H & E, × 400) (by courtesy of Professor R. Pepperell)

writer, believe that medical treatment is more appropriate for most of these patients and this is discussed fully in Chapter 25.

Surgery will be indicated in all patients with an XY karyotype. In the case of abdominal testes there is an increased risk of dysgerminoma. This is mainly in patients with testicular feminising syndrome where the only justification for surgical removal is to prevent neoplasm. In the intersex primary amenorrhoea group, such as 5α-reductase deficiency and the girl with absent anti-Müllerian factor, gonadectomy is indicated not just to reduce the risk of neoplasm but also to avoid the singularly unpleasant effects of normal adrogen levels at puberty in an individual who regards herself as a girl.

The streak and dysgenetic gonads of other XY females are particularly likely to be the site of dysgenetic tumours. Since this risk is in the vicinity of 25–30 per cent, bilateral excision of the streaks must be undertaken. As most of these girls would like to have menstrual bleeding it is preferable to remove the streak and tube on each side but to leave the uterus *in situ*.

The commonest lesion is a gonadoblastoma (Fig. 24.4) and these are of such low grade malignancy that radiotherapy is not indicated. If, however, there is suggestion of malignancy or frank dysgerminoma (Fig. 24.5) then, ideally, a full staging laparotomy should be performed followed by appropriate adjuvant therapy. Recognising that dysgerminomas are exquisitely sensitive to radiotherapy, this is one of the few ovarian neoplasms where chemotherapy is not, as a rule, indicated. It is obvious that when this type of surgery is done, facilities for frozen section to identify the type of neoplasm should be available. This will avoid the need for early repeat laparotomy.

Formation of the vagina

This is relevant to the large group of patients with uterovaginal agenesis and to the much smaller group of girls with 5α-reductase deficiencies and androgen/receptor defects. Most patients with testicular feminising syndrome develop quite normal vaginal capacity when intercourse commences and do not need surgery. The surgical management of congenital absence of the vagina has a long and chequered career, initially using isolated loops of ileum and moving to the more successful surgical approach of dissecting a passage between the urethra and rectum placing a skin graft *in situ* over a mould (McIndoe & Bannister, 1938). But this operation has a substantial morbidity and even with appropriate use of the mould secondary contracture of the artificial vagina is common. In 1938 Frank described a simple method of developing vaginal depth by repeated pressure against the vaginal dimple with a dilator. Because of the complication rate following operative surgery the Frank approach should always be tried first. In fact, none of my patients in this category have needed surgical procedures during the last 12 years. The simplest device is the graduated glass dilator. The patient will need instruction in the method of use. The procedure should commence with the smallest dilator and consists of firm pressure (firm enough to produce some discomfort) against the vaginal dimple for between 5 and 10 minutes each morning and evening. Within 4 weeks there is usually an appreciable vagina and with increasing size and pressure normal vaginal capacity is usually achieved within 6 months. Most patients adapt remarkably well to this procedure and appear to prefer it to the alternative of complex surgery. Once regular intercourse is initiated, the dilators need not be used any longer. An intriguing modification of this technique using a bicycle seat has been described by Ingram (1981) but it is difficult to believe that patients would prefer this procedure to simple manual pressure with a glass dilator.

The vulval/vaginal abnormalities in most XY females I have seen do not lend themselves so readily to the pressure technique as there is usually no recognisable dimple nor does this area of the perineum in these patients indent readily even with firm pressure. For these few patients a surgical procedure of the McIndoe type is probably the most appropriate. There is not, as a rule, enough 'vulval' skin to use the Williams' operation.

In essence, the treatment of patients with primary amenorrhoea should be directed to initiation of full reproductive potential for those in whom it is possible. For those in whom fertility is impossible, it is very rare that appropriate surgical and medical management will not allow adequate physical development and normal coital relations.

Acknowledgement

Some of this text has been published in Shearman & Roberts (1982).

REFERENCES

Aleem F A 1981 Familial 46,XX gonadal dysgenesis. Fertility and Sterility 35: 317–320

Bourguignon J P, Vanderschueren-Lodeweychx M, Wocter R, Malvaux P, Craen M, Du Caju M V L, Ernold C, Franckimont P 1982 Hypopituitarism and idiopathic delayed puberty: a longitudinal study in an attempt to diagnose gonadotropic deficiency before puberty. Journal of Clinical Endocrinology and Metabolism 54: 733–744

Brown J B, Kellar R, Matthew G D 1959 Preliminary observations on urinary oestrogen excretion in certain gyecological disorders. Journal of Obstetrics and Gynecology of the British Commonwealth 66: 177–211

Dempsey A T, de Swiet M, Dewhurst J 1981 Premature ovarian failure associated with the Candida endocrinopathy syndrome. British Journal of Obstetrics and Gynecology 88: 563–565

Evans T N, Poland M L, Boving R L 1981 Vaginal malformations. American Journal of Obstetrics and Gynecology 141: 910–917

Frank R T 1938 The formation of an artifical vagina without operation. American Journal of Obstetrics and Gynecology 35: 1053–1055

Fraser I S, Baird D T, Hobson B M 1973 Cyclical ovarian function in women with congenital absence of the uterus and vagina. Journal of Clinical Endocrinology and Metabolism 36: 634–637

Frisch R E, Gotz-Welbergen A V, McArthur J W, Albright T. Witschi J, Bullen B, Birholz J, Reed R B, Hermann H 1981 Delayed menarche and amenorrhea of college athletes in relation to age of onset of training. Journal of the American Medical Association 246: 1559–1563

Griffin J E, Edwards C, Madden J D, Harrod M J, Wilson J D 1976 Congenital absence of the vagina. The Mayer-Rokitansky-Kuster-Hauser syndrome. Annals of Internal Medicine 85: 224–236

Gruenwald P 1959 Growth and development of the uterus: the relationship of epithelium to mesenchyme. Annuals of the New York Academy of Sciences 75: 436–440

Hammond C B, Wiebe R H, Haney A F, Yancy J G 1979 Ovulation induction with luteinizing hormone releasing factor in amenorrheic infertile women. American Journal of Obstetrics and Gynecology 135: 924–939

Ingram J M 1981 The bicycle seat stool in the treatment of vaginal agenesis and stenosis: A preliminary report. American Journal of Obstetrics and Gynecology 140: 867–871

Kallman F J, Schonfield W A, Barerra S E 1944 The genetic aspects of primary eunuchoidism. American Journal of Mental Deficiency 48: 203

Kaufman F R, Kogut M D, Donnell G N, Goebelsman U, March C, Koch R 1981 Hypergonadotropic hypogonadism in female patients with galactosemia. New England Journal of Medicine 304: 994–998

McIndoe A H, Banister J B 1938 An operation for the cure of congenital absence of the vagina. Journal of Obstetrics and Gynecology of the British Empire. 45: 490–494

Marshall F F 1978 Vaginal abnormalities. Urologic Clinics of North America 3: 155–159

Mashchak C A, Kletzky O A, Davajan V, Mishell D R 1981 Clinical and laboratory evaluation of patients with primary amenorrhea. Obstetrics and Gynecology 57: 715–721

Meade K W, Wachtel S S, Davis J R, Lighner E S 1981 H-Y antigen in XO/X, iso(X) mosaic Turner syndrome. Obstetrics and Gynecology 57: 594–599

Noonan J A 1968 Hypertelorism with Turner phenotype: A new syndrome with associated congenital heart disease. American Journal of Diseases in Children 116: 373–380

Phansey S A, Tsai C C, Williamson H O 1981 Vaginal agenesis in association with gonadal dysgenesis. Obstetrics and Gynecology 57: 56–57

Reindollar R H, Byrd J R, McDonough R 1981 Delayed sexual development: a study of 252 patients. American Journal of Obstetrics and Gynecology 140: 371–380

Rimion D L, Merimee T S, Rabinowitz D, McKusick V A 1968 Genetic aspects of clinical endocrinology. Recent Progress in Hormone Research 24: 365–437

Ross G T 1979 Diagnosis and management of primary aemorrhea, secondary amenorrhea and dysfunctional uterine bleeding. In: de Groot L J (ed) Endocrinology, pp 1419–1433

Rudman D, Goldsmith M, Kutner M, Blackston D 1980 Effect of growth hormone and oxandrolone singly and together on growth rates in girls with X chromosome abnormalities. Journal of Pediatrics 96: 132–135

Shearman R P 1968 A physiological approach to the differential diagnosis and treatment of primary amenorrhoea. Journal of Obstetrics and Gynecology of the British Commonwealth 74: 1101–1107

Shearman R P 1981a Primary amenorrhoea. In: Dewhurst C J (ed) Integrated obstetrics and gynecology for postgraduates. 3rd edn, ch 5, pp 49–55. Blackwell Scientific Publications, Oxford

Shearman R P 1981b The diagnosis and management of secondary amenorrhoea. In: Dewhurst C J (ed) Integrated obstetrics and gynecology for postgraduates. 3rd edn, ch 6, pp 56–66. Blackwell Scientific Publication, Oxford

Shearman R P, Cox R I 1965 Clinical and chemical correlations in the Stein-Leventhal syndrome. American Journal of Obstetrics and Gynecology 92: 747–754

Shearman R P, Roberts J 1982 The embryology and endocrinology of primary amenorrhoea: a study of one hundred and forty patients. Clinical Reproduction and Fertility 1: 117–130

Simpson J L, Lebeau M M 1981 Gonadal and statural determinants on the X chromosome and their relationship to in vitro studies showing prolonged cell cycles in 45,X; 46,X del(X) (p11); 46,X del(X) (g13); and 46,X del(X) (g22) fibroblasts. American Journal of Obstetrics and Gynecology 141: 930–938

Valk T W, Corley K P, Kelch R P, Marshall J C 1980 Hypogonadotripic hypogonadism: Hormonal response to low dose pulsatile administration of gonadotropin-releasing hormone. Journal of Clinical Endocrinology and Metabolism 51: 730–738

Woolf P D, Schenk E A 1974 An FSH-producing pituitary tumour in a patient with hypogonadism. Journal of Clinical Endocrinology and Metabolism 38: 561–568

Wray H L, Freeman M V R, Ming P-M L 1981 Pregnancy in the Turner syndrome with only 45,X chromosomal constitution. Fertility and Sterility 35: 509–514

Rodney P. Shearman

Secondary amenorrhoea

INTRODUCTION

In this chapter the term secondary amenorrhoea is applied to women of reproductive age who have secondary absence of menstruation for 12 months not due to pregnancy, physiological lactation or, of course, hysterectomy. Premature menopause is defined here as secondary ovarian failure before the age of 35. While being fully aware that many other writers use intervals of amenorrhoea substantially less than 12 months, this duration avoids any potential confusion with the problems of oligomenorrhoea. It is obvious that not all women who menstruate ovulate. The two major causes of anovulatory menstrual bleeding — dysfunctional uterine bleeding and polycystic ovarian disease are covered fully in Chapters 31 and 20.

The fascinating history of secondary amenorrhoea has been reviewed elsewhere (Shearman, 1965). The condition is as old as recorded history and there is not really much that is new under the sun. The flood of publications dealing with inappropriate hyperprolactinaemia and amenorrhoea was very neatly and pithily anticipated by Hippocrates when he wrote from his — or their — retreat on the island of Cos several thousand years ago 'if a woman who is not with child, nor has brought forth, have milk, her menses are obstructed' (Adams, 1939). It is a condition subject to the whims and dictates of fashion. In the century between 1750 and 1850 the most frequently recognised cause of secondary amenorrhoea was chlorosis or 'green sickness or the virgins' disease', a condition that we would probably now call anorexia nervosa (Loudon, 1980). Modern therapeutics has weighed in with it's own contribution, seen in the hyperprolactinaemic amenorrhoea associated with phenothiazine treatment and possibly following oral contraceptives. The urge felt by a large number of the younger generation to express themselves in severe physical exertion has more recently resulted in the recognition of 'joggers amenorrhoea' (see below).

AETIOLOGY

Given a sufficiently obsessional personality it would be possible to cover several pages of closely typed manuscript with individual causes of secondary amenorrhoea. This, however, does not seem to increase comprehension of this subject. For this reason a systems approach will be used, a system in which the uterus, ovary and particularly the cranium dominate causation with a miscellaneous group of lesser clergy such as liver, thyroid disease and renal failure following the major trinity.

Uterus

Many women with secondary amenorrhoea have very low levels of oestrogens and as a result a very small uterus. Older literature often attributed the amenorrhoea to this uterine super-involution but this is a coincidental finding. While it is possible that amenorrhoea could develop in an individual who lacked endometrial receptors for oestradiol, I have never seen such a condition nor have I read of a well documented case. This could be an example of the Eiffel Tower Syndrome. In this syndrome, the writer denies the existence of the Eiffel Tower because he has not been to Paris. The only documented causes of uterine amenorrhoea are Asherman's Syndrome, endometrial tuberculosis and missed abortion.

Asherman's syndrome (amenorrhhoea traumatica). This is due to obliteration of the endometrial cavity following curettage (Asherman, 1950). Almost invariably this curettage is for secondary postpartum bleeding after full-term delivery; much less frequently it follows curettage for induced or incomplete abortion. Very rarely indeed, it may follow diagnostic curettage — an association I have yet to see. The commonest history is of curettage for secondary postpartum bleeding followed by complete amenorrhoea. If histological tissue is available from the curettage, regenerating endometrium and myometrium will both often be present. Incomplete obliteration is more common than complete; although not relevant to this chapter this may cause scanty uterine bleeding, dysmenorrhoea, infertility or alternatively increased risk of spontaneous abortion. Sometimes the adhesions are limited to an area just above the internal os and haematometra is curiously uncommon. The diagnosis should be suspected when the typical history is obtained. Confirmation may be secured by inability to fill the uterine cavity during attempted hysterosalpingography. While hysteroscopy is also diagnostic, this technique should be kept for treatment of those women who want more children. Pituitary and ovarian function are normal.

Endometrial tuberculosis. Genital tract tuberculosis is very rare in most developed countries and is usually diagnosed during investigation of infertility. Endometrial involvement must be extensive and advanced before amenorrhoea will occur. The condition should be kept in mind by those practising in areas where genital tract tuberculosis is common but diagnosis and treatment to restore fertility may be difficult, or in the case of the latter impossible (Schaefer, 1970).

Missed abortion This uncommon but quite definite cause of secondary amenorrhoea is well documented in most old textbooks of obstetrics and gynaecology but receives little or no mention in most of the modern literature. Missed abortion can cause months, years or even decades of secondary amenorrhoea. The longest such association I have seen is 38 months of secondary amenorrhoea. The diagnosis was not suspected until 'ghost' villi were found on histological examination of uterine curettings. Under these circumstances curettage is both diagnostic and therapeutic. Although rare, the diagnosis, like the abortion, will usually be missed unless efforts are made to obtain endometrial tissue for histological examination in women with secondary amenorrhoea.

Ovary

Premature ovarian failure

Premature menopause, the resistant ovary syndrome, autoimmune ovary failure, galactosaemia and ovarian destruction following radiotherapy or chemotherapy, may all cause secondary amenorrhoea. There is a surprising heterogeneity of histology in these women which we have described in a discussion of nineteen open ovarian biopsies (Russell et al, 1982).

True premature menopause. The clinical history is usually of progressive oligomenorrhoea proceeding to complete amenorrhoea. Weight change is uncommon and the presence of typical flushes may provide the only clinical clue to the true diagnosis. These women will have persistent elevation of FSH and LH, normal chromosomes, and usually no detectable autoantibodies. The mechanisms involved remain unclear. Ovarian biopsy may show a picture typical of the type of ovary expected in a woman in her sixties — that is a well defined cortex, corpora albicantia and occasional follicles. However, in an identical clinical circumstance the biopsy may show tissue that is indistinguishable from a 'streak' of the type seen in patients with gonadal agenesis, even though such a patient presenting with secondary amenorrhoea may have proven her fertility by having had children. It is difficult to believe that the mechanisms are the same in these two types of patient.

Chromosomally incomplete ovarian failure. The majority of patients with these problems (the classic Turner's syndrome, Turner mosaics, Xp or Xq deletions) will have primary amenorrhoea and are dealt with fully in Chapter 24. But some of these women will achieve a normal puberty and a few may even have children. While many of these patients will be of short stature, some will have normal height and the diagnosis will not be entertained until the karyotype is available. Chromosome analysis with G and C banding is needed in all patients with hypergonadotrophic amenorrhoea. Gonadotrophins will be persistently elevated. In the presence of documented aneuploidy ovarian biopsy is not necessary. If it is done, then findings typical of a true menopause will be found. Premature ovarian failure is said to be more frequent in the XXX female although I have not personally seen this clinical problem.

The resistant ovary. This condition was first documented by Kinch et al (1965) followed by Jones & de Moraes-Ruehsen (1969). The clinical presentation will be the same as in true premature menopause, gonadotrophins will be persistently increased, but on open ovarian biopsy ovarian tissue with large numbers of primordial follicles will be found. Very few of these will have progressed to the antral stage and while corpora albicantia may indicate previous ovulation there is no histological evidence of current or recent ovulation (Fig. 25.1). The condition may also cause primary amenorrhoea (Dewhurst et al, 1975). Apparent reversal has been noted following hormone replacement therapy with oestrogens and a progestin but spontaneous remission may also occur. Because of this Tulandi & Kinch (1981) have suggested the alternative name of 'the insensitive ovary syndrome'. There is no readily acceptable explanation for the mechanism of ovarian insensitivity in these women. The elevated gonadotrophins are immuno-reactive and bio-active so an attractive but unproven hypothesis would be an ovarian problem with gonadotrophin receptors. Ovarian biopsy through an operating laparoscope may be quite misleading as insufficient tissue will usually be obtained. Definitive diagnosis is reached properly by open ovarian biopsy at formal laparotomy.

Auto-immune ovarian failure. Although this may cause primary amenorrhoea (Ch. 24) it is more frequently recognised as a cause of secondary amenorrhoea. Multiple autoantibodies may be present — for example, to the thyroid, gastric parietal cells, adrenal cortex and parathyroid.

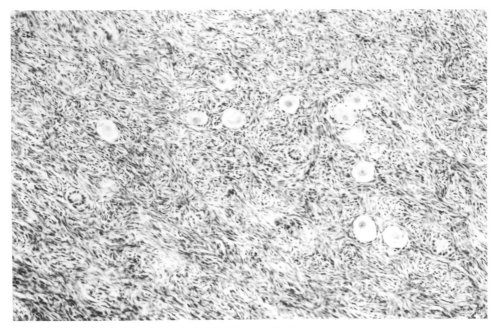

Fig. 25.1 Resistant ovary syndrome. Patient with galactosaemia (H & E, × 125) (From Russell et al, 1982, with permission)

Multiple system disease may be present or may develop in these women. In a review of the subject, Irvine & Barnes (1974) indicate that while lymphocytic infiltration of the follicles is frequently seen, occasionally there may be streak gonads or complete absence of primordial follicles. Immuno-fluorescence will show antibody binding to steroid producing cells in the granulosa and theca. Elder et al (1981) have indicated that gonadal autoimmunity in the absence of adrenocortical autoantibodies is extremely rare but this has not been our experience. In our patients of this type, the woman with the highest level of ovarian auto-antibodies had no other detectable antibodies and on biopsy had typical streak stroma, although there was a clear history of previous ovulation. On the other hand one of our patients with the most typical histological picture of autoimmune ovarian failure (Fig. 25.2) had no detectable autoantibodies.

Gonadotrophin levels will be persistently increased in these patients. Tissue antibody screen should be done in any woman where the diagnosis of premature ovarian failure is being entertained. Although there is no evidence that immuno-suppressive therapy will help these patients to restored fertility (just as there is no evidence it will not), they may be at increased risk of pernicious anaemia,

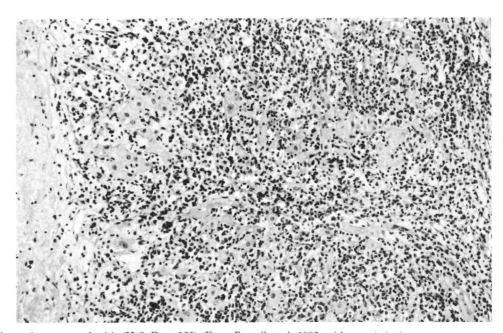

Fig. 25.2 Presumed auto-immune oophoritis (H & E, × 125) (From Russell et al, 1982, with permission)

Addison's disease and hypoparathyroidism. This has clear implications in their follow-up.

Galactosaemia. This disorder is due to a deficiency of the enzyme galactose-1-phosphate uridyl transferase and is an inborn error of galactose metabolism. Hepatic, renal, lenticular and neurological abnormalities are well documented. Early diagnosis and institution of the appropriate diet permit good health and survival in these children.

The relationship to hypogonadism has been documented more recently (Kaufman et al, 1981). Twelve of eighteen female patients had hypergonadotrophic hypogonadism, five with primary amenorrhoea, six with secondary amenorrhoea and one with oligomenorrhoea. There was some evidence that normal reproductive function was more likely if the diagnosis was made at the time of birth. They speculate that the mechanism of ovarian failure is accumulation in the ovary of galacticol and/or galactose-1-phosphate causing damage to oocytes and ovarian stroma culminating in ovarian failure. However, there was no histological diagnosis in their series and the postulated cause of ovarian failure does not match the increase in oestrogens observed when one of two of these patients was treated with human menopausal gonadotrophins. One of our own patients with galactosaemia and secondary amenorrhoea (Russell et al, 1982) had ovaries that were indistinguishable from the resistant ovary syndrome, with a high density of primordial follicles. There was no morphological evidence of oocyte damage and the patient was consistently hypergonadotrophic. We do not yet know whether this patient's gonadotrophins are biologically active but her amenorrhoea is difficult to accept on the basis of ovarian damage. The cause of ovarian failure in galactosaemia remains moot.

Radiotherapy/chemotherapy. As already noted when dealing with primary amenorrhoea (Ch. 24) the increased survival of girls and women with lymphoma and some forms of leukaemia after treatment with combined radiotherapy/chemotherapy will lead to an increased number of women presenting with secondary amenorrhoea and ovarian failure. They are hypergonadotrophic. The risks of ovarian failure are greater if both therapeutic regimes have been used rather than radiotherapy or chemotherapy alone. The normal procedure of repositioning the ovaries behind the uterus at the time of staging laparotomy in Hodgkin's disease seems to offer little protection from irradiation, at least in the patients I have seen. It would be reasonable to assume, however, that those in whom ovarian function continued would not present to a gynaecologist. With radiotherapy alone, there is a relationship between the number of rads used and the risk of long-term amenorrhoea (Jansen & Shearman, 1981).

Functioning ovarian tumours

Although amenorrhoea in women with these tumours is mediated by the effect of this aberrant steroid production on the hypothalamus it seems reasonable to classify these patients under ovarian amenorrhoea because that is the primary site of their disturbance. Feminising neoplasms such as granulosal cell tumours are more likely to produce episodes of dysfunctional uterine bleeding rather than prolonged amenorrhoea, but virilising tumours may cause complete amenorrhoea of abrupt onset associated with hirsutism, male type baldness, acne and voice changes. Arrhenoblastoma remains the classic tumour of this type but it should be recognised that secondary ovarian malignancy, which in its primary site has no hormonal action, may induce excessive androgen production from the ovarian stroma with amenorrhoea and virilism.

The cranium

In any large series of patients studied with secondary amenorrhoea intracranial causes will dominate in more than 90 per cent. While this may be a non-specific effect of increased intracranial pressure from any cause, such as hydrocephalus or cerebral neoplasm, most frequently the changes are in the hypothalamus, pituitary stalk or the pituitary gland itself.

The hypothalamus

Weight change. Although many texts draw attention to the relationship between obesity and amenorrhoea, even in countries cursed with epidemic obesity such as Australia and the United States of America, uncomplicated obesity rarely presents to the clinician with amenorrhoea. Undoubtedly many patients with polycystic ovarian disease are obese (Ch. 20) but the major relationship of weight change to amenorrhoea seen clinically is weight loss. The classic relationship of amenorrhoea to anorexia nervosa is well recognised (Beumont & Russel, 1982). At the nadir of weight loss, LRF stimulation shows that these girls lack the ability to release gonadotrophins, an ability that will be restored as weight approaches ideal weight for height. However, in a gynaecological practice the number of women who, having regained weight, remain amenorrhoeic is impressive. Far more frequently, a gynaecologist is presented with secondary amenorrhoea associated with weight loss that falls short of that required for a diagnosis of anorexia nervosa. The commonest history is that of a mildly overweight teenager who goes onto a 'crash diet'. The onset of amenorrhoea is usually abrupt, as a rule precedes significant weight loss and often persists even when the lost weight is regained. The history is of importance in making this association. These patients look and feel well, are usually of above average intelligence and tend to be the children of professional families who are often over-achievers. In other words the personality profile is very close to that of the classic case of anorexia nervosa.

These girls, however, are usually quite frank about the diets they have been pursuing unlike the more extreme cases of anorexia where there will be denial of dieting — particularly denial of induced vomiting after normal food intake. The patients will show normal levels of gonadotrophins, normal levels of prolactin, radiology will exclude intracranial pathology and there is about a 30 per cent prospect of spontaneous cure, particularly if some weight can be gained.

There is no clear delineation between these non-threatening forms of weight loss and anorexia nervosa. If a history of vomiting can be elicited and/or if there is obvious evidence of emaciation or if electrolytes show evidence of hypokalaemia the gynaecologist or endrocrinologist who is not well versed in handling anorexia nervosa would be well advised to enlist the support of a psyhiatrist or clinical psychologist. Anorexia nervosa is one of the few causes of secondary amenorrhoea where death may be the regrettable and finite end-point.

Much more attention has been paid recently to the association of subtle changes in body mass distribution (between fat and muscle) and amenorrhoea and its relationship to heavy athletic training. The relationship of ballet dancing to secondary amenorrhoea is well documented (Abraham et al, 1982). Wentz (1980) has indicated that a loss of 30 per cent of body fat mass is sufficient to induce menstrual dysfunction. In women in heavy exercise this is often associated with a negligible change in body weight because of the concurrent increase in muscle mass. Amenorrhoea in this type of patient will often remit spontaneously if the amount of exercise is reduced. In a practical sense advice to reduce exercise works as well as telling most fat people that they should lose weight or most underweight people that they should gain it.

The relationship between amenorrhoea and acute or chronic exercise programmes is now well documented (Editorial Comment, 1982). While changes in body fat mass explain much of the problem, exercise induced changes in plasma β-endorphin may be involved (Colt et al, 1981). Increases in β-endorphin will cause transient hyperprolactinaemia and a decrease in LH levels. There seems to be a high degree of probability that a combination of endorphin increase and a reduction in body fat mass induce amenorrhoea in these women. Anecdotally, the β-endorphin increase has been related to the 'high' that comforts the loneliness of the long-distance runner. It is also thought to relate to the difficulties in unhooking these patients from their commitment to an exercise programme that seems irrational to those of us who are more sedentary. The fact that gonadotrophin release is normal after a bolus of LRF given intravenously puts the site of the disturbance firmly in the hypothalamus, whatever the mediating mechanisms may ultimately turn out to be.

In amenorrhoea associated with weight loss there is possibly a preference for hepatic oestradiol metabolism to move away from its predominant normal hydroxylated product oestriol to the catechol-oestrogen, 2-hydroxyoestrone which can inhibit GnRF (Fishman et al, 1975).

Stress. Major environmental stress is often associated with amenorrhoea. It is seen short-term in university students around the time of examinations or in girls who leave a home in the country for life in the city. It was extremely common during the second World War in women entering concentration camps and the amenorrhoea became evident long before there was significant weight loss. In a contemporary sense, amenorrhoea is sometimes seen in girls from Australia who make a ritual tour of the United Kingdom. They have their last period when they board the aircraft to leave the country and menstruate again when they return. The mediating mechanisms in this type of amenorrhoea are not clear but almost certainly the hypothalamus is the centre of mischief.

Polycystic ovarian disease. This is discussed in Chapter 20. It is sufficient to say here that the primary disturbance is within the hypothalamus with a non-cyclic release of LH of the male pattern and a high LH:FSH ratio.

Drugs. Most drugs associated with amenorrhoea produce this effect by increasing prolactin secretion (Table 25.1 and see below).

While opiate addiction may increase prolactin production (Burger & Healey, 1981) in many addicted patients the associated malnutrition and severe weight loss may also be

Table 25.1 Causes of Inappropriate Hyperprolactinaemia

Pharmacological:	Psychotropic drugs
	Phenothiazines
	Butyrophenones
	Imipramine
	Dibenzazephine derivaties
	Anti-hypertensives
	Methyldopa
	Rauwolfia derivatives
	Hormones
	Thyrotrophin-releasing factor
	Oestrogens
	Oral Contraceptives
	Opiates
	Morphine
	Anti-emetics
	Metoclopramide
	Antihistamines
	Meclozine
	Cimetidine
Pathological:	Idiopathic
	Pituitary
	Prolactinoma
	Mixed Tumour — Acromegaly
	Mixed Tumour — Cushing's disease
	Empty Sella
	Lymphocytic adenohypophysitis
	Hypothalamic
	Craniopharyngioma
	Pinealoma
	Hypothyroidism (primary)
	Chronic renal failure
	Prolonged postpartum

operative through hypothalamic mechanisms. The most frequent syndrome seen clinically is the development of amenorrhoea that becomes apparent in time after treatment with oral contraceptives is stopped. This relationship was first described by Shearman (1966) and an association between the use of combined oral contraceptives and subsequent amenorrhoea now appears to be clear (Shearman, 1975; Shearman & Fraser, 1977). What is not so clear is whether this relationship is causal or casual. Many patients with this problem give a history of late menarche, previous menstrual irregularity and quite frequently weight loss or low absolute weight (Wentz, 1980). Although there must be a high index of suspicion that this association is causal, absolute proof that it is so has yet to be obtained (Vessey et al, 1978). About one-third of these patients have hyperprolactinaemia, with or without a detectable adenoma while the remaining two-thirds appear to have hypothalamic secondary amenorrhoea (Shearman & Fraser, 1977; Rowe et al, 1979). A valid relationship between oral contraceptive intake and hyperprolactinaemia is beginning to emerge (Badaway et al, 1981).

Hyperprolactinaemia. Causes of inappropriate hyperprolactinaemia are shown in Table 25.1. Thirty per cent of our own patients with secondary amenorrhoea have hyperprolactinaemia but it is important to recognise that not all patients with hyperprolactinaemia have galactorrhoea and that a small minority of patients with galactorrhoea will have normal prolactin levels (Shearman, 1983). While no cause for the hyperprolactinaemia may be found a careful drug history is mandatory. In clinical practice, in Australia, phenothiazines relate most frequently to hyperprolactinaemia. Prolactin is normally under the control of prolactin inhibitory factor (very probably dopamine). It is not known whether these drugs act by reducing the availability of dopamine or by competing for binding sites with dopamine. It is possible that both mechanisms may be involved with different drugs. It should be evident that compounds such as phenothiazines and rauwolfia relate to concurrent use whereas oral contraceptives, if they are related, may have an ongoing effect for many years after the pill is stopped. The relationships of hypothyroidism and renal failure to hyperprolactinaemia will be discussed separately below.

Amenorrhoea/galactorrhoea may arise spontaneously and this condition used to be called the Argonz del Castello Syndrome. If the same clinical situation was associated with an evident pituitary tumour the name changed to the Forbes-Albright syndrome, whereas inappropriate prolonged galactorrhoea and amenorrhoea after childbirth was called the Chiari-Frommel Syndrome. With the passage of time and the ability to measure prolactin these eponyms have sunk into history, if not into obscurity, and all could be grouped as inappropriate hyperprolactinaemia with amenorrhoea.

In our own hyperprolactinaemic patients 47 per cent had post-pill amenorrhoea, 14 per cent developed amenorrhoea postpartum and 39 per cent noted spontaneous onset of secondary amenorrhoea unrelated to oral contraptives or pregnancy (Rowe et al, 1979). Very similar findings have been noted by Schlechte et al (1980).

Clinically the commonest presentation is secondary amenorrhoea with concurrent infertility or with concern about future fertility. A small minority will volunteer the information that they have noticed a milky secretion from their breasts and a slightly larger number will recollect this on specific questioning. But almost 50 per cent of women with hyperprolactinaemia have no recollection of having experienced galactorrhoea. The majority of these women feel well and look well. Examination is unremarkable except for the presence of galactorrhoea when it is demonstrable, but it must be remembered that a substantial number of patients with unquestionable hyperprolactinaemia have no demonstrable galactorrhoea at any time. Prolactin levels are increased persistently. The ability of stress, including vaginal examination and breast palpation to cause a significant increase in prolactin levels has probably been exaggerated but ideally blood for this estimation should be taken in a relatively quiescent stage sometime during the morning. FSH and LH levels will usually be within the normal range and in the absence of organic disease such as primary hypothyroidism, renal failure or detectable pituitary tumour no other abnormalities will emerge.

Biologically most circulating prolactin is 'little' prolactin with a molecular weight of 22 000 daltons. Occasionally there may be over-production of 'big, big' prolactin with a molecular weight in excess of 100 000. While this may cause galactorrhoea, ovulatory function is usually intact (Whittaker et al, 1981). Although it has been suggested that hyperprolactinaemia mediates secondary amenorrhoea by direct action on the ovary, using ovarian response to exogenous gonadotrophins, we have not been able to confirm this (Fraser et al, 1978). The mechanism is probably and predominantly a feed-back action of high levels of prolactin on GnRF in the hypothalamus.

Pseudo-Cyesis (phantom pregnancy). I have the impression that this condition was more common 20 years ago than it is now. Certainly I have seen it more often in my boxer bitch than in humans! However, no doubt it will recur clinically. The onset of amenorrhoea is usually abrupt, followed by nausea, breast enlargement, abdominal swelling and even simulated labour. These patients often have an excessive wish for or fear of pregnancy, gonadotrophin levels are normal but prolactin levels may be raised. Under anaesthesia the distended abdomen deflates like a pricked balloon but some of these women may require objective evidence of the lack of a fetus by X–ray or ultrasound before they accept the true situation.

Trauma. Any severe head injury may be associated with

amenorrhoea but the clinical situation of such a patient is scarcely conducive to any investigation unnecessary for life support. However, the amenorrhoea may persist when the patient recovers. In women of this type I have seen, investigations have pointed to the hypothalamus by finding normal levels of FSH, LH and prolactin with skull X–rays that, while bearing the evidence of the trauma, show no other evidence of intracranial pathology. Occasionally diabetes insipidus may be associated with this condition and then it is reasonable to believe that the injury must have involved the pituitary stalk. Traumatic amenorrhoea may also result from the deliberate incursions of the neurosurgeon in an attempt to extirpate a substantial intracranial neoplasm particularly those arising in the pituitary and extending beyond it, or surgery for craniopharyngiomata.

Irradiation. Irradiation is still used occasionally in the management of pituitary adenomata and was widely used as an adjunct to surgery in the treatment of prolactinomas. Continuing amenorrhoea secondary to panhypopituitarism may develop in these patients. The first such example I saw followed irradiation using a linear accelerator as source but increasingly in the last 7 years we have seen this following external irradiation with a cobalt source (Shearman, 1981). It is not clear whether this is a continuing effect of irradiation on the pituitary itself or the hypothalamus.

Suprasella tumour

Any intracranial lesion that compresses the hypothalamus may produce amenorrhoea and hypopituitarism. While diabetes insipidus is uncommon, growth hormone production may be severely depressed as may the ability to release TSH. Although prolactin levels may be normal, they may be sufficiently increased to cause galactorrhoea. It is not good medical practice to see a patient with such a lesion — for example a craniopharyngioma — who has been treated by bromocriptine, a drug that cannot be effective in this potentially life threatening condition.

In these women FSH and LH will usually be low or normal, basal levels of TSH and other pituitary hormones will also be normal while prolactin may be normal or increased. The true extent of pituitary compromise will not usually be evident unless a multiple pituitary stimulation is performed (see below). Neoplasms such as gliomas or secondary malignancy may not always be obvious on plain radiology of the skull. Fortunately the commonest of the lesions — the craniopharyngioma — is usually calcified. Visual acuity may be impaired and papilloedema may indicate increased intracranial pressure. Testing of visual fields will often show hemianopia.

Adenohypophysis

Necrosis. The classic cause of this is Sheehan's Syndrome (Sheehan & Davis, 1968). Typically the history is of a substantial postpartum haemorrhage with shock. Again, classically, lactation is impaired, in severe cases there will be diabetes insipidus followed by persistent amenorrhoea and progressive evidence of panhypopituitarism with hypothyroidism (not myxoedema) atrophy of the vulva and genital tract and loss of axillary and pubic hair. In clinical practice in developed countries this condition is now very rare, presumably because of better obstetric care and, more importantly, greater availability of blood for immediate transfusion. I have not seen a case of Sheehan's Syndrome since I was a medical student in the late 1940s. With the typical history it does not require a great leap of the intellect to suspect the diagnosis which could be confirmed by identifying low or low–normal levels of FSH, LH and prolactin and low levels of TSH. Because full multiple pituitary stimulation involves the administration of insulin this should never be done if a diagnosis of panhypopituitarism is suspected but GnRF and TRF stimulation will show the typical flat response of hypopituitarism. In these patients human pancreatic tumour GH-releasing factor may be a safe alternative to insulin (Evans et al, 1983). Although uncommon, pituitary apoplexy due to haemorrhage into a pituitary adenoma during pregnancy is a more frequent cause of pituitary necrosis these days than Sheehan's Syndrome. I have also seen this problem arise as a complication of pneumoencephalography when attempting to delineate the extent of a pituitary tumour.

Pituitary tumour. Pituitary tumour must be a constant phantom in the mind of any clinician who is investigating a patient with secondary amenorrhoea, either to prove its existance or to indicate it absence. While most gynaecologists are now quite familiar with the need to exclude a prolactinoma in patients with secondary amenorrhoea there is still insufficient recognition of the possible concurrence of mixed tumours producing hyperprolactinaemia and acromegaly or hyperprolactinaemia and Cushing's Syndrome. Nor is there sufficient awareness of the problem of multiple endocrine neoplasia which may include carcinoid of the gut and phaechromocytoma. This concurrence is most frequently recognised in acromegaly and Cushing's Syndrome (Anderson et al, 1981; Leveston et al, 1981) but an association between phaeochromocytoma and prolactinoma has been described (Meyers, 1982), facts of relevance in patients with both hypertension and secondary amenorrhoea.

Prolactinoma. Despite some claims to the contrary, it is almost certain that the apparent epidemic of prolactinomas identified in the last 10 years is not due to an increase in prevalence but rather an increased ability to make the diagnosis. It should be recognised that pituitary adenomata are a common finding in autopsies in patients who had no symptoms referable to the adenoma. Burrow et al (1981) found an incidence of 27 per cent. Almost half of these adenomata contained prolactin secreting cell — in other words more than 10 per cent of the population have asymptomatic prolactinomas during their lives. It is also apparent that an adenoma may not be found in a patient with hyperprolactinaemic amenorrhoea and radiological evidence of such a tumour (Nachtigall et al, 1980). Identifiable pituitary tumours may be found in approximately one-third of patients with hyperprolactinaemia (Rowe et al, 1979). It is of paramount importance to exclude the presence of tumour in any patient with hyperprolactinaemia whether this becomes evident as prolonged amenorrhoea after delivery, as amenorrhoea after oral contraceptives or arises spontaneously without any such clinical association. The majority of these lesions will be microadenomata confined to the pituitary fossa but a substantial minority will be macroadenomata extending beyond the fossa, above into the third ventricle with consequent risk of optic nerve compression, laterally or inferiorly into the cavernous sinus.

There is a substantial overlap in the prolactin levels between patients with and those without detectable tumours (Rowe et al, 1979). Methods of radiological assessment are described in Chapter 23. Visual field impairment may rarely be present in the absence of radiologically detectable tumour so that this is an integral part of investigation. Patients with uncomplicated prolactinomas have a normal capacity to release other pituitary hormones including gonadotrophins. The older thought that the amenorrhoea was due to compression of normal pituitary tissue is no longer tenable. In this group of patients all other pituitary hormones will be within the normal range in the basal state.

The natural history of a prolactinoma is not clear. Long-term follow-up remains incompletely documented but in the series of March et al (1981) and our own group of 117 patients (Rowe et al, 1979) large tumours were usually evident at the time of presentation while significant growth of a microadenoma is really very uncommon. In fact, in our own series there was only one such patient, a woman who had previously undergone bilateral adrenalectomy for Cushing's Syndrome and who subsequently developed Nelson's Syndrome with hypersecretion of prolactin as well as ACTH. Haemorrhage into these tumours is uncommon and when it does occur, is more likely during pregnancy.

Pituitary tumour and hypothyroidism. The relationship of thyroid disease to secondary amenorrhoea will be discussed in more detail later but in the meantime it should be noted that in long-standing primary hypothryroidism a pituitary tumour may be recognised. While this may be a true adenoma, such an enlarged fossa may also be due to hyperplasia of the pituitary prolactin secreting cells (Stoffer et al, 1981).

Acromegaly and hyperprolactinaemia. About one-third of all patients with acromegaly have hyperprolactinaemia and this is seen even more frequently in women (De Pablo et al, 1981; Kanie et al 1983). The mechanism of hyperprolactin-

aemia is not clear in all of these patients but mixed secretory activity may occur. With large growth hormone producing tumours there may be compression of the stalk. Two distinct tumours may be present (Tolis et al, 1978). Finding hyperprolactinaemia may be of some interest to the general endocrinologist who has already made the diagnosis of acromegaly. If, however, the patient presents to a gynaecologist, having found hyperprolactinaemia he may miss the diagnosis of acromegaly unless he is aware of this association and carries out the appropriate investigations (see below). If the treatment of the two conditions was always similar such a clinical oversight may not be important; but only a minority of acromegalics will have growth hormone suppression if they are treated with bromocriptine (see below).

The patient may present with gross acromegaly — facial coarsening, palpable peripheral nerves — but the patients that I have seen, presenting with predominant concerns of amenorrhoea and infertility have had minimal clinical evidence of acromegaly but undoubted endocrinological confirmation.

Cushing's syndrome with hyperprolactinaemia. Turney et sl (1981) have indicated that the association between Cushing's Syndrome and amenorrhoea/hyperprolactinaemia is uncommon. In reviewing the literature and reporting two cases of their own it is clear that this clinical complex is thought to be sufficiently rare for isolated case reports to continue. I have seen several cases. In one of these the Cushingoid element dominated the clinical picture with a round plethoric face, striae, easy bruising, hypertension and glycosuria. But in two others, the clinical evidence of Cushing's Syndrome was not nearly as strong and became evident after these patients were referred from other gynaecologists when their hyperprolactinaemic amenorrhoea had not responded to bromocriptine (Shearman, 1983, and see below). While a pituitary tumour will be evident in most of these women, sometimes no organic lesion in the pituitary or hypothalamus can be demonstrated (Berlinger et al, 1977).

Other pituitary tumours. Endocrinologically inert adenomas may be associated with secondary amenorrhoea and varying degrees of panhypopituitarism (Bauserman et al, 1978). Hypogonadism in the presence of pituitary tumours secreting FSH (Woolf & Schenk, 1974) LH and FSH (Snyder & Sterling, 1976) or FSH and TSH (Koide et al, 1982) has been recognised more frequently in men than in women. Nevertheless, this possibility should always be entertained in women with secondary amenorrhoea with obvious relevance to those with apparent premature ovarian failure.

Lymphocytic adenohypophysitis. This unusual condition is usually associated with hypopituitarism and there may be evidence of enlargement of the pituitary fossa (Mayfield et al, 1980). However, galactorrhoea and presumably hyperprolactinaemia, may occur (Cebelin et al, 1981). In all published cases they have declared themselves either by symptoms of hypopituitarism or actual death within 14 months postpartum. The most likely mechanism is autoimmune. There is not, at this stage, any known method of antemortem diagnosis.

Empty sella syndrome. The pathophysiology of this condition is not clear. Normally the dura mater forms a watertight seal around the pituitary stalk excluding the subarachnoid space from the pituitary fossa. Occasionally the arachnoid and subarachnoid space can herniate into the fossa and the resulting pressure from cerebrospinal fluid will compress and flatten the pituitary gland. While endocrine function of the pituitary may be normal, hypopituitarism may be evident (Farber et al, 1975). Occasionally, a coexisting microadenoma may be present deep in the fossa (Domingue et al, 1978) and then be associated with hyperprolactinaemia or hypersecretion of other pituitary tumours (Jansen, 1981). On routine radiology, the pituitary fossa may appear to be enlarged and the true diagnosis will not be entertained until pneumoencephalography, CT scanning or other contrast scanning is carried out (Ch. 23). In those patients with a coexisting hypersecretion of pituitary hormones, it is tempting to believe that the empty sella arises from pituitary apoplexy, but it is very difficult to prove this.

Liver disease

Severe liver disease may be associated with secondary amenorrhoea. The commonest type that I have seen, possibly because it is more common in younger women, is active chronic hepatitis (Bearn et al, 1956). In none of these women has the secondary amenorrhoea been a predominant or even substantial symptom as the liver disease, including portal hypertension, dominates management. The mechanism of secondary amenorrhoea in these patients is not clear.

Thyroid disease

Hyperthyroidism may be associated with normal menstrual function, scanty menstrual bleeding or amenorrhoea. It is very uncommon for amenorrhoea to be the presenting symptoms; most frequently these women present with symptoms dominated by the hyperthyroidism and the amenorrhoea is a subsidiary issue.

In hypothyroidism menstrual function is often normal but dysfunctional uterine bleeding or amenorrhoea may occur. For women with florid hypothyroidism menstrual dysfunction is usually of secondary importance. However, 4 per cent of the patients I see with hyperprolactinaemia and secondary amenorrhoea have primary hypothyroidism and in most of these women at the time of presentation the hypothyroidism is compensated. In other words, measurements of thyroxin or tri-iodothyronine are normal and the only clue is an increased level of TSH. Early compensated

hypothyroidism with amenorrhoea is more likely to present to the gynaecologist, at least in Australia, whereas those with clinically evident hypothyroidism are more likely to be referred to a general endocrinologist. FSH and LH levels are usually within the normal range while in those presenting gynaecologically prolactin will be increased and, of course, high TSH levels will be found. Hyperprolactinaemia occurs because thyrotrophin releasing factor, in addition to stimulating release of thyroid stimulating hormone, will also cause release of prolactin.

Chronic renal failure

Any clinician who sees women with chronic renal failure advanced to the state where chronic dialysis is necessary will be aware that amenorrhoea is the rule. The probable mechanism is a reduction in the metabolic clearance rate of LH but not of FSH while prolactin levels are increased in about 70 per cent of these patients (Sieverston, 1980). In my own experience it is very uncommon for secondary amenorrhoea to be the presenting symptom of any patient with renal failure, the reproductive disturbance being of secondary importance. However, it is reasonable — and not expensive — to check renal function by measurement of creatinine and blood urea in patients with secondary amenorrhoea. Our own experience, which is by no means unique, is that successful renal transplantation is followed by restoration of ovulatory function and many of these women have now had successful pregnancies.

Adreno-cortical neoplasm

Any adrenal tumour whether benign or malignant and whether causing Cushing's disease or hirsutism/virilism may be associated with secondary amenorrhoea. The clinical presentation tends to be dominated by overproduction of androgens, as discussed fully in Chapter 21.

THE CLINICAL PROBLEM

As in any other branch of medicine an adequate history is essential. The spontaneous history given by the patient is valuable but specific questioning will usually be necessary to elicit relevant information in the very large group of women who feel and look perfectly well and whose only concern is the secondary amenorrhoea with actual infertility or concern about potential fertility. Recollecting the multitudinous causes of secondary amenorrhoea already discussed it is obvious that some patients will have presenting symptoms such as hirsutism, virilism, those related to hyperthyroidism or florid hypothyroidism when the amenorrhoea is relatively unimportant. Here, the clues to subsequent investigations will become manifest during the history and physical examination. However, the apparently well woman with secondary amenorrhoea may be harbouring quite nasty pathology such as mild Cushing's Syndrome, acromegaly, craniopharyngioma, compensated hypothyroidism or chronic renal failure, diagnoses that may be missed unless the possibility of co-existance is borne in mind constantly.

Events relating to the onset of amenorrhoea are important. A history of curettage for secondary postpartum bleeding or repeat curettage after spontaneous or induced abortion suggests the diagnosis of Asherman's Syndrome. Substantial postpartum haemorrhage with a history of failed lactation raises the probability of Sheehan's Syndrome. Patients should be asked specifically about weight change and it must be recognised that the weight change relates to the time of the onset of amenorrhoea rather than what has happened since the amenorrhoea developed. Continued amenorrhoea after completion of physiological lactation should suggest hyperprolactinaemia.

A careful drug history is mandatory. Current intake of psychotrophic drugs, particularly phenothiazines, or hypotensive drugs such as methyldopa is relevant while in the case of oral contraceptives, if these are related to amenorrhoea, the effect may continue for years after cessation of treatment.

The only clinical clues to premature ovarian failure may be the presence of hot flushes and the patient should be asked specifically about these. Any change in hair growth should be noted and the patient should be asked about acne and how often she washes her hair. These problems may relate to polycystic ovarian disease, mild adrenal disturbances or be secondary to the slight overproduction of adrenal androgens seen in some patients with hyperprolactinaemia.

The patient should be asked about the presence of inappropriate galactorrhoea. Many will recollect this when asked specifically even though they have not volunteered the information but the absence of this history does not exclude the presence of galactorrhoea nor, must it be said again, does the absence of galactorrhoea exclude hyperprolactinaemia.

Significant headache is really quite uncommon in these women. When headaches relate to pituitary pathology they are usually temporal. Visual field defects will as a rule only become obvious during the appropriate examination and I have only ever seen one patient who volunteered the information that her ability to see objects laterally had become reduced.

Physical examination

This should be meticulous and include assessment of blood pressure, thyroid status, the presence of otherwise of acne and/or abnormal hair growth pattern and, of course, the presence or absence of galactorrhoea. About 10 per cent of patients with otherwise uncomplicated hyperprolacti-

naemia have greasy hair and skin with some acne and minor hirsutism. If the patient has a florid round face, some hirsutism and hypertension then it would be appropriate to think of Cushing's disease. Classical and advanced acromegaly might be suggested by coarse features, palpable peripheral nerves and the other manifestations of the older textbook pictures. In practice, early but unequivocal acromegaly may be found on laboratory criteria only.

Vaginal examination is important. I am still surprised at the reluctance with which general endocrinologists perform this examination, but functioning ovarian tumours related to amenorrhoea are usually big enough to be felt, polycystic ovaries may be palpably and symmetrically enlarged and uterine size needs to be assessed. Uterine size relates far more to endogenous oestrogen levels than it does to the primary cause of secondary amenorrhoea.

Further investigation

If there is any suspicion of organic disease, it is mandatory to undertaken the fullest investigation necessary to reach a precise diagnosis. Those steps will be evident from a perusal of aetiological factors.

The remainder of this section will deal with the very common problem of the patient with no abnormal physical finding or at most marginal evidence of underlying organic disease. In the clinically well woman who is concerned only with the reason for the amenorrhoea but not with her future fertility, investigations need be directed only to the exclusion of otherwise asymptomatic organic disease. Almost without exception the only problems here are an otherwise asymptomatic pituitary tumour, hypothyroidism or renal failure.

Mandatory investigations in this group are X–ray of the skull and pituitary fossa, assay of prolactin and thyroid stimulating hormones. Since prolactin levels are susceptible to stress blood for this examination should, ideally, be taken at a time well removed from physical examination — particularly efforts to express milk and vaginal examination.

If prolactin levels, X–ray of the skull and pituitary fossa and TSH are normal, then no further investigation is warranted in this otherwise well woman.

If the patient is concerned by actual or potential infertility then obviously further investigations are needed. FSH and LH should be assayed. High levels of both suggest premature ovarian failure. These findings, however, do not permit a differentiation between a true early menopause, the resistant ovary syndrome, autoimmune ovarian failure of other causes of hypergonadotrophic secondary amenorrhoea discussed above. In this group, galactosaemia will be excluded on the history, induced ovarian failure will be evident by a history of previous radiotherapy and/or chemotherapy, autoimmune failure may be suggested by evidence of antibodies against the ovary and the concurrent presence of other antibodies such as gastric parietal cells, the parathyroid, adrenal cortex or thyroid microsomes. Karyotype will be necessary to exclude early ovarian failure due to chromosomal incompetence and the only method of differentiating the resistent ovary syndrome from a true premature menopause is open ovarian biopsy.

Although not all women with a provisional diagnosis of ovarian failure will wish to have this final proof, the clinician should be cautious in giving a prognosis without such evidence. Spontaneous ovulation may recur in these women and the practitioner may face an embarrassing situation by being presented with one of these patients obviously pregnant having been told that this could not possibly occur. O'Herlihy et al (1980) have discussed these difficulties. There is not yet enough knowledge of the natural history of this condition to know whether such an occurence represents long-term remission or whether it is the last ecstatic ovulatory fling of an ovary doomed to fail in the near future. This is seen not uncommonly in women around the age of a normal menopause who produce the dreaded 'change of life baby'.

X-rays of the pituitary fossa should be viewed with a great deal of care. Relevant neuroradiology is discussed in Chapter 23 but in summary in addition to plain radiology, polytomography, pneumoencephalography, carotid arteriography, and CT scanning may be indicated.

Very few machines for CT scanning have the resolution to detect suprasellar extension without concurrent enhancing techniques. There is no endocrinological method of being certain whether a tumour is present or not. The empty sella syndrome may be suspected on CT scanning but confirmation will require the introduction of some contrast material into the subarachnoid space. With high resolution CT scanning the latter may not be necessary.

Multiple pituitary stimulation (MPS) can be extremely valuable (Mortimer et al, 1973). This is a complex investigation that generates a large number of radioimmunoassays and substantial cost. Basal levels of growth hormone,

cortisol, TSH and prolactin, LH and FSH are assessed and then measured further after a bolus injection of insulin (0.1 μ/kg body weight) gonadotrophin releasing factor (GnRF 100 μg) and TRF (200 μg). It is indicated in patients who are candidates for surgery and/or radiotherapy and it is extremely helpful if there is a clinical or other reason for some unease about the diagnosis of a pure prolactinoma. This unease may be based on clinical intuition, something that should never be dismissed, or it may be that C.T. scanning has shown a central pituitary lesion. Recollecting that the prolactin secreting cells and, therefore, prolactinomas are almost always lateral (hence 'doubling' of the floor of the fossa in cone views) a central lesion should always raise the possibility of a mixed acromegalic or Cushingoid nature. A craniopharyngioma is usually calcified and an MPS can clearly show the related hypopituitarism. However, it should be noted that some prolactinomas may also be calcified (Phansey et al, 1981). Assay of somatomedin C will be invaluable if acromegaly is suspected (Phillips & Vassilopoulou-Sellin, 1980) either on clinical grounds or because of the central nature of pituitary neoplasm. If the patient is hypertensive appropriate steps should be made to exclude a phaeochromocytoma (Shearman, 1982) while if Cushing's disease is considered, assay of urinary free cortisol and morning and evening ACTH will be helpful.

It would not be possible to discuss all of these potential permutations without devoting a full text to the problem. However, some specific examples might be of assistance. Table 25.2 shows a typical MPS in a patient with an uncomplicated prolactinoma. Table 25.3 shows the findings of a patient with Cushing's Syndrome. This patient was referred with a diagnosis of hyperprolatinaemic amenorrhoea. There was clinical evidence of Cushing's Syndrome with a plethoric face, mild hirsutism, striae and hypertension and she had a central pituitary tumour. It should be noted that the MPS shows only mild hyperprolactinaemia, a substantial increase in plasma cortisol and blunting of all other pituitary parameters. Urinary free cortisol is substantially increased.

Table 25.2 Multiple pituitary stimulation in uncomplicated prolactinoma

Time	Insulin hypoglycaemia			TRF stimulation		GnRF stimulation	
	Glucose (mmol/l)	Plasma Cortisol (nmol/l)	hGH (ng/ml)	TSH (uμ/ml)	Prolactin (ng/ml)	LH (iu/l)	FSH (iu/l)
0	4.9	250	1	2	245*	13	10
10	2.3		2				
20	0.9		10				
30		430		25	250*	86	25
45	1.9		13				
60	2.8	520	13	12	235*	61	25
90	3.8	350	4	7		51	22
120	4.7		1	4		45	10
150	4.3		1		240*		
180	4.4		1				

* Normal range 3–13

Table 25.3   Multiple pituitary stimulation with Cushing's Syndrome and hyperprolactinaemia

Time	Insulin hypoglycaemia			TRF stimulation		GnRF stimulation	
	Plasma Cortisol (nmol/l)	hGH (ng/ml)	TSH Prolactin (uμ/ml)	(ng/ml)		LH (iu/l)	FSH (iu/l)
0	710*	1	3	34*		4	2
10		2					
20		2					
30	725*	2		90*		10	4
45		2	4				
60	690*	1	4	54*		11	5
90	665*	1	4			10	6
120		1	4	45*		11	6

* Result above normal range. Subnormal release of hGH, TSH, FSH, LH. Urinary free cortisol 1366 nmol/ 24 h (normal <250)

Table 25.4   Multiple pituitary stimulation with acromegaly and hyperprolactinaemia

Time	Insulin hyperglycaemia			TRF stimulation		GnRF stimulation	
	Plasma Cortisol (nmol/l)	hGH (ng/ml)	TSH Prolactin (uμ/ml)	(ng/ml)		LH (iu/l)	FSH (iu/l)
0	689*	5	2.3	52*		2.8	2.3
10		47*					
20		49*					
30	533	43*	14.4	102*		61.9	14.4
45		40*					
60	371	30*	14.4	84*			14.1
90	273	19*	12.3	51*		12.3	4.7

* Result above normal range. Somatomedin C 3.57 u/ml (0.6–1.5)

Table 25.5   Multiple pituitary stimulation with craniopharyngioma

Time	Insulin hypoglycaemia			TRF stimulation		GnRF stimulation	
	Glucose (mmol/l)	Plasma Cortisol (nmol/l)	hGH (ng/ml)	TSH (uμ/ml)	Prolactin (ng/ml)	LH (iu/l)	FSH (iu/l)
0	5.8	135	<1.6	2.8	19	1.9	2.6
10	4.6		<1.6				
20	2.3		<1.6				
30	3.0	237	1.8	3.1	33	5.2	4.5
45	4.1		<1.6				
60	4.1	292	<1.6	2.9	27	5.0	4.6
90	5.3	262	<1.6	3.2		5.4	5.1
120	5.6		1.8	3.1	21	3.1	5.5
150	5.8		<1.6				
180	5.9		<1.6				

Mild hyperprolactinaemia. Inadequate release of all other pituitary hormones. Inverted LH:FSH ratio.

Table 25.4 shows the findings in a patient with acromegaly. Neither at the time nor in retrospect was there any clinical evidence of acromegaly. However, she did have a central tumour and only a modest increase in basal prolactin. It should be noted that although her basal levels of growth hormone were normal she had a gross over-response to induced hypoglycaemia and the diagnosis was confirmed by finding increased levels of somatomedin C.

Table 25.5 shows the findings in a patient with craniopharyngioma. There was no clinical evidence of panhypopituitarism and the patient's only symptoms were of post-pill amenorrhoea and galactorrhoea. She had no headaches and physical examination was completely normal. Radiology had, however, shown a calcified suprasellar lesion and MPS showed low levels of all pituitary hormones except prolactin and all, except prolactin had a very blunted response.

Visual fields should be checked. It is unlikely that this would be neglected in a patient with evidence of a pituitary tumour on radiology but I have seen several women with completely normal radiology who had hemianopia due to suprasellar extension without any enlargement of the bony fossa. This assessment should be done formally, with both a red and white spot.

TREATMENT

Surgery

Neurosurgery. It may appear presumptuous for a gynae-cologist to become involved in an argument about the place of neurosurgery. However, neither the neurosurgeons themselves nor their cohort of internists are certain about the place of surgery.

There is general agreement that intracranial surgery is indicated in women with craniopharyngioma or Cushing's Syndrome. Medical treatment has no place in the primary management of these women. The use of surgery in acro-megaly remains unresolved; just as with tumours causing pure hyperprolactinaemia, surgery is usually incomplete. Bromocriptine is sometimes successful in lowering growth hormone levels to normal and in causing tumour shrinkage but external therapeutic radiation probably remains the primary treatment for most acromegalic women. Until relatively recently there seemed to be general agreement that a prolactinoma with extension outside the pituitary fossa should be treated surgically. While this surgery was very rarely curative (in the sense that menstrual function was restored and prolactin levels return to normal) there was a very real fear that if pregnancy occurred in these women, rapid enlargement due to the high oestrogen levels of pregnancy might lead to abrupt enlargement of the tumour or even pituitary apoplexy. More recently it has become evident that even very large tumours will show a rapid reduction in size during treatment with bromocrip-tine and even if tumour growth should progress in preg-nancy bromocriptine is usually able to control it. Medical management is discussed fully in Chapter 26.

The position is not much clearer for the patient with a microadenoma. Although high cure rates may be obtained after transphenoidal excision of these tumours (Turksoy et al, 1980; Woosley et al, 1982) not all neurosurgical units can achieve these results. In addition, there is now very good evidence that with appropriate supervision, clinically significant pituitary enlargement of a microadenoma is uncommon during pregnancy (Divers & Yen 1983). If this should occur bromocriptine may still be used (Ch. 26). It is probably fair to say that at the time of writing this manu-script, the neurosurgeons are losing the race.

Bilateral ovarian wedge resection. This operation still has a place in the management of polycystic ovaries. The treatment of choice for those who are hirsute is medical and the treatment of first choice for those who want children is clomiphene (Chs 21 and 26). But some patients with this condition who do not ovulate in response to clomiphene will find bilateral ovarian wedge resection a very attractive alternative to the hazards of treatment with human gona-dotrophins (Ch. 27). If this operation is to be performed it must be done meticulously with obsessive attention to haemostasis. It is a disaster to find infertility due to surgically induced peritubal adhesions in a patient whose

anovulation has been cured by this operation.

Uterine surgery. This is indicated in those patients with secondary amenorrhoea due to intra-uterine synechiae who wish to have more children. Earlier treatment was to break down intra-uterine adhesions blindly with a uterine sound followed by the insertion of an intra-uterine device such as a Lippes loop to keep the uterine walls apart while the basal endometrium regenerated. While this may be successful in re-establishing menstrual bleeding and preg-nancy will frequently follow, there is a very high incidence of morbid pregnancy mainly related to pathological adher-ence of the placenta (Jewelewicz et al, 1975). Division of these adhesions under direct vision using an operating hysteroscope, followed by oral oestrogens and progestins appears to have a better reproductive outcome (March et al, 1978; Siegler & Kontopoulos, 1981). After division of the adhesions and insertion of a Lippes loop size B or C a reasonable hormonal regime is to give ethinyloestradiol in a dose of 0.1 mg daily for 21 days together with oral Provera 10 mg for the last 10 days of each treatment cycle, repeating this after a 7 day gap. After 3 months of this treatment the Lippes loop should be removed and normality of the uterine cavity confirmed by either hyster-osalpingography or repeat hysteroscopy.

Surgery for functioning tumours of the ovary or adrenal. Virilising ovarian tumours associated with secondary amenorrhoea are usually detectable clinically and need to be removed surgically. Virilising tumours of the adrenal cortex may be more difficult to detect but whole body CT or gallium scanning may locate the tumour. Treatment is again surgical.

Medical treatment

Induction of ovulation with clomiphene, gonadotrophins, GnRF, bromocriptine and other dopamine agonists is discussed in Chapters 26 & 27. Corticosteroids to treat adrenal hyperplasia are discussed in Chapter 18.

Thyroxine. Hyperprolactinaemic patients who have compensated or uncompensated primary hypothyroidism should be treated with thyroxine. This will resolve both the hypothyroidism and the hyperprolactinaemia. Thyroxine has no place otherwise in the management of secondary amenorrhoea.

Osteoporosis. Because of the low oestrogenic environment in many women with secondary amenorrhoea, osteoporosis will develop and this is best documented in those with hyperprolactinaemia (Schlechte et al, 1983). The preven-tion of this problem is still controversial. Patients with hyperprolactinaemia can expect to have a further increase in prolactin levels if oestrogens are used. Very long-term treatment with bromocriptine in those who do not need it either for infertility or to reduce tumour size remains controversial. In other women with, for example, hypo-thalamic amenorrhoea, induction of ovulation followed by pregnancy will usually be the first priority and will resolve the problem of bone demineralisation. However, in patients with prolonged secondary amenorrhoea who do not wish to have children, hormone replacement therapy such as described in Chapter 7 for the post-menopausal woman should be considered very seriously.

Management of weight loss

Patients with weight loss short of anorexia nervosa or amenorrhoea related to heavy exercise can usually be managed on the basis of ordinary common sense. However, many obsessive exercisers are reluctant to change their lifestyle. For the patient with anorexia nervosa, particularly those with electrolyte disturbances, many clinicians including this writer feel inadequate to manage the problem and would refer them for appropriate psychiatric care (Beumont, 1982).

LONG-TERM FOLLOW-UP

Follow-up appropriate to the various clinical conditions described above should be an integral part of management. The natural history of patients with hyperprolactinaemic amenorrhoea remains unknown. Spontaneous cure is singularly uncommon. Development of a large pituitary tumour is rare, in our experience, in those patients presenting either with no detectable lesion or a microadenoma but this might occur (Rowe et al, 1974). After full initial assessment, in my own practice, I have relied on measurement of prolactin alone. I have yet to see a large tumour develop without a substantial increase in the patient's initial prolactin level. More detailed follow-up will be needed for patients who have had radiotherapy. Repeated polytomography should be avoided as there is a substantial risk of inducing lenticular opacities from the radiation. Many years will elapse before the true natural history of this condition is well documented. A national register along the lines described by Pepperell (1981) is a logical way to determine this.

REFERENCES

Abraham S F, Beumont P J V, Fraser I S, Llewellyn-Jones D 1982 Body weight, exercise and menstrual status among ballet dancers. British Journal of Obstetrics and Gynaecology 89: In press

Adams F 1939 The Genuine Works of Hippocrates, Aphorism 39, p 310

Anderson R J, Lufkin E G, Sizemore G W, Carney J A, Sheps S G, Silliman Y E 1981 Acromegaly and pituitary adenoma with phaeochromocytoma: a variant of multiple endocrine neoplasia. Clinical Endocrinology 14: 605–612

Asherman J G 1950 Traumatic intra-uterine adhesions. Journal of Obstetrics and Gynaecology of the British Empire 57: 892–896

Badaway S Z A, Rebscher F, Kohy L, Wolfe H, Oates R P, Moses A 1981 The relation between oral contraceptive use and subsequent hyperprolactinaemia. Fertility and Sterility 36: 464–467

Bauserman S C, Hardman J M, Schochet S S, Earle K M 1978 Pituitary oncocytoma. Archives of Pathology and Laboratory Medicine 102: 456–459

Bearn A G, Kunkel H G, Slater R J 1956 The problem of chronic liver disease in young women. American Journal of Medicine 21: 3–15

Berlinger F G, Ruder H J, Wilber J F 1977 Cushing's syndrome associated with galactorrhea, amenorrhea and hypothyroidism: a primary hypothalamic disorder. Journal of Clinical Endocrinology and Metabolism 45: 1205–1210

Beumont P J V, Russel J 1982 Anorexia nervosa In: Beumont P J V, Burrows G D (eds) Handbook of Psychiatry and Endocrinology, Ch 3, p 63–96. Elsevier Biomedical, Amsterdam

Burger H G, Healy D L 1981 Disorders of prolactin secretion: diagnosis and therapy. Australian Prescriber 5: 8–10

Burrow G N, Wortzman G, Rewcastle N B, Holgate R C, Kovacs K 1981 Microadenomas of the pituitary and abnormal sellar tomograms in an unselected autopsy series. New England Journal of Medicine 304: 156

Cebelin M S, Velasco M E, De Las Mulas J M, Druet R L 1981 Galactorrhoea associated with lymphocytic adenohypophysitis. British Journal of Obstetrics and Gynaecology 88: 675–680

Colt E W, Wardlaw S L, Frantz A G 1981 The effect of running on plasma β-endotrophin. Life Science 28: 1637–1640

Dewhurst C J, De Koos E B, Ferreira H P 1975 The resistant ovary syndrome. British Journal of Obstetrics and Gynaecology 82: 341–345

Divers W A, Yen S C C 1983 Prolactin-Producing Microadenomas in Pregnancy. Obstetrics and Gynecology 61: 425–429

Domingue J N, Wing S D, Wilson C B 1978 Co-existing pituitary adenomas and partial empty sellas. Journal of Neurosurgery 48: 23–28

Editorial Comment 1982 Menstrual cycle and its disorders. Obstetrical and Gynecology Survey 37: 193–195

Elder M, Maclaren N, Riley W 1981 Gonadal autoantibodies in patients with hypogonadism and/or Addison's disease. Journal of Clinical Endocrinology and Metabolism 52: 1137–1142

Evans W S, Borges J L C, Kaiser D L, Vance M L, Sellers R P, MacLoed R M, Vale W, Rivier J, Thorner M O 1983 Intranasal administration of Human Pancreatic Tumour GH-Releasing Factor-40 stimulates GH release in normal men. Journal of Clinical Endocrinology and Metabolism 57: 1081–1083

Farber M, Turksoy R N, Rogers J 1975 The primary empty sella syndrome. Obstetrics and Gynecology 49 (Suppl): 2–5

Fishman J, Boyar R M, Hellman L 1975 Influence of body weight on estradiol metabolism in young women. Journal of Clinical Endocrinology and Metabolism 41: 989–991

Foix A, Bruno R O, Davison T, Lema B 1966 The pathology of post-curettage intrauterine adhesions. American Journal of Obstetrics and Gynecology 96: 1027–1033

Fraser I S, Markham R, Shearman R P 1978 Plasma prolactin levels and ovarian responsiveness to exogenous gonadotropins. Obstetrics and Gynecology 51: 548–551

Irvine W J, Barnes E W 1974 Addison's disease and autoimmune ovarian failure. Journal of Reproduction and Fertility (Suppl) 21: 1–3

Jansen R P S 1981 Amenorrhea In: Pauerstein C J (ed) Gynecological Disorders, Differential Diagnosis and Treatment, Ch 2, pp 11–50. Grune & Stratton, New York

Jansen R P S, Shearman R P 1981 Oncological Endocrinology In: Coppleson M (ed) Gynecologic Oncology, Ch 8, p 96. Churchill Livingstone, Edinburgh

Jewelewicz R, Khalof S, Neuwirth R S, Vande Wiele R L 1976 Obstetric complications after treatment of intrauterine synechiae (Asherman's syndrome). Obstetrics and Gynecology 47: 701–705

Jones G S, De Moraes-Ruehsen M 1969 A new syndrome of amenorrhea in association with hypergonadotropism and apparently normal ovarian follicular apparatus. American Journal of Obstetrics and Gynecology 104: 597–600

Kanie N, Kageyama N, Kuwayama A, Nakane T, Watanabe M, Kawaoi A 1983 Pituitary Adenomas in Acromegalic patients. Journal of Clinical Endocrinology and Metabolism 57: 1093–1101

Kaufman F R, Kogut M D, Donnell G M, Goebelsman U, March C, Koch R 1981 Hypergonadotrophic hypergonadism in female patients with galactosemia. New England Journal of Medicine 304: 994–998

Kinch R A H, Plunkett E R, Smout M S, Carr D H 1965 Primary ovarian failure. American Journal of Obstetrics and Gynecology 91: 630–644

Koide Y, Kugai N, Kimura S, Fujita T, Kameya T, Azokizawa M, Ogata E, Tomono Y, Yamashita K 1982 A case of pituitary adenoma with possible stimultaneous secretion of thyrotropin and follicle stimulating hormone. Journal of Clinical Endocrinology and Metabolism 54: 397–403

Leveston S A, McKeel D W, Buckley P J, Deschryver K, Greider M H, Jaffe B M, Daughaday W H 1981 Acromegaly and Cushing's syndrome associated with a foregut carcinoid tumour. Journal of Clinical Endocrinology and Metabolism 53: 682–689

Loudon I S L 1980 Chlorosis, anaemia and anorexia nervosa. British Medical Journal 281: 1669–1675

March C M, Israel R, Marchad 1978 Hysteroscopic management of intra-uterine adhesions. American Journal of Obstetrics and Gynecology 130: 653–657

March C M, Kletzky O A, Davajan V, Teal J, Weiss M, Apuzzo M J L, Marrs R P, Mishell D R 1981 Longitudinal evaluation of patients with untreated prolactin-secreting adenomas. American Journal of Obstetrics and Gynecology 139: 835–844

Mayfield R K, Levine J H, Gordon L, Powers J, Galbraith R M, Rawe S E 1980 Lymphoid adenohypophysitis (LAH) presenting as a pituitary tumour. Annals of Internal Medicine 69: 619–623

Meyers D H 1982 Association of phaeochromocytoma and prolactinoma. Medical Journal of Australia 1: 13–14

Mortimer C H, Besser G M, McNeilly A S, Turnbridge W M G, Gomez-Pan A, Hall R 1973 Interaction between secretion of gonadotrophins, prolactin, growth hormone, thyrotrophin and corticosteroid in man. The effects of LSH/FSH-RH, TRH and hypoglycaemia alone and in combination. Clinical Endocrinology 2: 317–326

Nachtigall R D, Monroe S E, Wilson C B, Jaffe R B 1981 Prolactin-secreting adenomas in women. American Journal of Obstetrics and Gynecology 140: 303–308

O'Herlihy C, Pepperell R J, Evans J H 1980 The significance of FSH elevation in young women with disorders of ovulation. British Medical Journal 281: 1447–1450

De Pablo F, Eastman C, Roth J, Gordon P 1981 Plasma prolactin in acromegaly before and after treatment. Journal of Clinical Endocrinology and Metabolism 53: 344–352

Pepperell R J 1981 Prolactin and reproduction. Fertility and Sterility 35: 267–274

Phansey S, Powers J M, Sagel J, Hungerford G D, Rawe S E, Williamson H O 1981 Calcified pituitary prolactinoma. Obstetrics and Gynecology 57: 62–66

Phillips L S, Vassilopoulou-Selin R 1980 Somatomedins. New England Journal of Medicine 302: 371–446

Rowe T C, Shearman R P, Fraser I S 1979 Antecedent factors and outcome of amenorrhea-galactorrhea. Obstetrics and Gynecology 54: 535–543

Russell P, Bannantyne P, Shearman R P, Fraser I, Corbett P 1982 Premature hypergonadotrophic ovarian failure: clinicopathological study of nineteen cases. International Journal of Gynecological Pathology In press

Schaefer G 1970 Tuberculosis of the female genital tract. Clinical Obstetrics and Gynecology 13: 965–998

Schlechte J, Sherman B, Halmi N, Van Gilder J, Chapler F, Dolan K, Granner D, Duello T, Harris C 1980 Prolactin-secreting pituitary tumours in amenorrheic women: a comprehensive study. Endocrine Reviews 1: 295–308

Schlechte J A, Sherman B, Martin R 1983 Bone Density in Amenorrheic Women with and without Hyperprolactinaemia.

Shearman R P 1965 Induction of Ovulation. Thomas, Springfield

Shearman R P 1966 Amenorrhoea after treatment with oral contraceptives Lancet ii: 1110–111

Shearman R P 1975 Secondary amenorrhea after oral contraceptives — treatment and follow-up Contraception 11: 123–132

Shearman R P 1981 Secondary amenorrhoea. In: Dewhurst C J (ed) Integrated Obstetrics and Gynaecology for Postgraduates 3rd edn, Ch 6, pp 56–66.

Shearman R P 1982 Prolactin-secreting pituitary adenoma. Medical Journal of Australia 2: 314

Shearman R P 1983 Inappropriate hyperprolactinaemia and secondary amenorrhoea. In: Studd J (ed) Progress in Obstetrics and Gynaecology, Vol 3, pp 257–266. Churchill Livingstone, Edinburgh

Shearman R P, Fraser I S 1977 Impact of new diagnostic methods on the differential diagnosis and treatment of secondary amenorrhoea. Lancet i: 1195–1197

Sheehan H L, Davis J C 1968 Pituitary necrosis. British Medical Bulletin 24: 59–70

Siegler A M, Kontopoblos V G 1981 Lysis of intrauterine adhesions under hysteroscopic control. Journal of Reproductive Medicine 26: 372–374

Sieverston G D, Lim V S, Nakawatase C, Frohman L A 1980 Metabolic clearance and secretion rates of human prolactin in normal subjects and in patients with chronic renal failure. Journal of Clinical Endocrinology and Metabolism 50: 846–852

Snyder P J, Sterling F H 1976 Hypersecretion of LH and FSH by a pituitary adenoma. Journal of Clinical Endocrinology and Metabolism 42: 544–550

Stoffer S S, McKeel D W, Randall R V, Laws E R 1981 Pituitary prolactin cell hyperplasia with autonomous prolactin secretion and primary hypothyroidism. Fertility and Sterility 36: 682–685

Tolis G, Bertrand G, Carpenter S, McKenzie J M 1978 Acromegaly and galactorrhea-amenorrhea with two pituitary adenomas secreting growth hormone or prolactin. Annals of Internal Medicine 89: 345–348

Tulandi T, Kinch R A H 1981 Premature ovarian failure. Obstetrical and Gynecological Survey (Suppl) 36: 521–527

Turksoy R N, Farber M, Mitchell G W 1980 Diagnostic and therapeutic modalities in women with galactorrhea. Obstetrics and Gynecology 56: 323–329

Turney T H, Ruyter H, Vigersky R A 1981 Cushing's disease presenting as amenorrhoea with hyperprolactinaemia: Report of two cases. Clinical Endocrinology 14: 539–545

Vessey M P, Wright N H, McPherson K, Wiggins P 1978 Fertility after stopping different methods of contraception. British Medical Journal 1, 265–267

Wentz A C 1980 Body weight and amenorrhea. Obstetrics and Gynecology 56: 482–487

Whittaker P G, Wilcox T, Lind T 1981 Maintained fertility in a patient with hyperprolactinaemia due to big, big prolactin. Journal of Clinical Endocrinology and Metabolism 53: 863–866

Woolf P D, Schenk E A 1974 An FSH producing pituitary tumour in a patient with hypogonadism. Journal of Clinical Endocrinology and Metabolism 38: 561–568

Woosley R E, King J S, Talbert L 1982 Prolactin secreting pituitary adenomas: neurosurgical management of 37 patients. Fertility and Sterility 37: 54–60

Induction of ovulation with clomiphene, bromocriptine and gonadotrophin-releasing hormone (GnRH)

INTRODUCTION

Clomiphene, bromocriptine and gonadotrophin-releasing hormone (GnRH) are effective ovulatory stimulants for patients with disorders of ovulation providing the serum FSH level is not elevated. The decision as to which of these agents should be prescribed usually depends on the serum PRL level; clomiphene is usually tried initially if the PRL level is normal whereas bromocriptine is employed when the PRL level is elevated. In the past when treatment with either or both of these two agents did not result in ovulation, gonadotrophin therapy was usually employed. The recent successful use of pulsatile injections of GnRH in such patients may well mean that fewer patients will be treated with gonadotrophin in the future as GnRH would appear to be much less likely to result in ovarian hyperstimulaton.

Each of these ovulatory stimulants acts at the level of the hypothalamus and/or pituitary gland and an understanding of the physiology of the hypothalamo-pituitary axis in normal and anovulatory subjects is essential if a rational approach to therapy is to be achieved.

GONADOTROPHIN-RELEASING HORMONE (GnRH)

History and physiological considerations

The identification of the intimate role of the hypothalamus in the secretory control of gonadotrophin release from the anterior pituitary via a closed portal circulation (Green & Harris, 1947) initiated a quest both for the humoral neuroendocrine factor responsible and for the location of the steroidal feedback centres. These investigations culminated over a decade ago in the isolation and synthesis of a single decapeptide gonadotrophin-releasing hormone (GnRH) with a specific amino acid sequence (Amoss et al, 1971; Arimura et al, 1972) (Fig. 26.1). Since then further intensive research in both primate and human subjects has provided further understanding of the role of this hormone

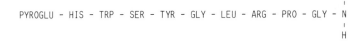

Fig. 26.1 The structural amino-acid sequence of human gonadotrophin-releasing hormone

in the physiology and pathology of the endocrine regulation of the menstrual cycle.

The central nervous system is now recognised as the primary site of functional disturbances which lead to disordered ovulation. These influences are mediated through the hypothalamus, that part of the diencephalon situated in the floor of the third ventricle, which acts as the final pathway for functional co-ordination of higher centres and the reproductive endocrine system. It derives this potential from its peptidergic neural cells, which share characteristics of both neurones and endocrine glandular tissue, being capable of responding to both nervous and chemically transmitted stimuli (McCann, 1980). These cells lying in the arcuate nucleus of the medial basal hypothalamus (Plant et al, 1978) synthesise GnRH in cytoplasmic ribosomes whence it is actively transported by axonal flow to the nerve terminal for secretion into the pituitary portal system. The arcuate nucleus thus acts as a neuroendocrine interface by translating the frequency of neuronal signals into alterations in circulating hormone levels.

Indirect evidence from observation of the pulsatile pattern of luteinising hormone (LH) release in the human female (Yen et al, 1972) together with direct experimental evidence following pituitary stalk transection in the rhesus monkey (Nakai et al, 1978) indicate that GnRH control of gonadotrophin secretion is obligatorily intermittent. Continuous pituitary exposure to GnRH leads to the desensitisation phenomenon of 'down regulation', whereby prolonged GnRH levels flood the gonadotroph receptors preventing their regeneration. This phenomenon has also been demonstrated with other agonal hormones such as growth hormone and LH (Roth et al, 1975; Hsueh et al, 1977).

On the other hand pituitary exposure to intermittent GnRH pulses with a frequency of one every 60–120 min is followed by physiological secretion of both FSH and LH in arcuate lesioned monkeys (Knobil, 1980). Further treatment using identical GnRH stimuli during the peri-ovulatory, as well as the early stages of the cycle, leads to the typical mid-cycle LH surge, indicating that no essential change is necessary in GnRH pulsatility to achieve ovulation. However in the intact reproductive system several other influences, including progesterone and endogenous opiates (Quigley & Yen, 1980), may modulate the basic frequency of the arcuate nucleus oscillator. Pulse frequencies shorter than 30 min are associated with a progressive decline in pituitary response to each releasing hormone stimulus and conversely, prolongation of the interval beyond 120 min upsets the normal circulating FSH:LH ratio due to increased FSH release with each pulse possibly combined with differences in the metabolic clearance rates of the two gonadotrophins. Changes in GnRH pulse amplitude appear to hold less potential for physiological control than frequency alterations since the effective dosage range is relatively narrow (Wildt et al, 1979) in both primate and human subjects.

In the presence of adequate GnRH stimulation the pituitary secretes gonadotrophins in a pattern characterised by an early cycle FSH peak and mid-cycle peaks of both LH and, to a lesser extent, FSH. At an ovarian level the developing cohort of follicles develop first FSH and then oestradiol receptors which in turn induce development of LH receptors in the dominant pre-ovulatory follicle. Oestradiol from this dominant follicle feeds back to exert a major degree of control over its own maturation process. In a further series of primate ablational experiments Knobil et al (1980) have demonstrated that the site of this oestrogen feedback centre lies in the pituitary and not at a hypothalamic level and that the characterstic pre-ovulatory positive feedback of oestradiol on LH can occur even in the temporary absence of GnRH. The function of the hypothalamus has, therefore, been shown to be merely permissive, rather than it acting as the regulator of ovarian function as was formerly believed. This concept, together with the elucidation of intricate intra-ovarian controls of follicular selection and differentiation (McNatty et al, 1979), has gone some way to establishing the ovary, through the dominant follicle, as the controlling centre of the ovulatory cycle and the determinant of this cyclicity. The sites at which progesterone exerts its feedback effect are less well defined but these probably exist at both hypothalamic and pituitary levels.

While feeding back on the anterior pituitary during the pre-ovulatory phase, oestradiol inhibits both synthesis and storage of FSH, while inhibiting only secretion of LH, leading to the formation of a large, readily releasable LH pool (Wang et al, 1976). This balance between LH storage and release is disrupted when the rapidly rising oestradiol concentrations 2 days before ovulation attain a critical threshold (Knobil, 1974). A massive LH discharge is thus induced by this positive feedback mechanism and ovulation ensues without any further GnRH stimulation being necessary.

The majority of cases of disordered ovulation, in the absence of permanent ovarian failure or hyperprolactinaemia, stem from a hypothalamic aetiology, which may in turn be triggered by higher neural influences, such as psychological stress. Whatever the primary cause, this hypothalamic anovulation is characterised initially by a reduction and later possibly by a disappearance of the pulsatile fluctuations in LH concentrations in the circulation. Progressive observation of such women may identify a spectrum of transition from luteal phase insufficiency, through anovulatory cycles culminating in amenorrhoea and it is likely that this disorder is the result of gradually reducing pulsatile GnRH release (Leyendecker, 1979).

Diagnostic usefulness of GnRH measurements and GnRH tests
Tests

GnRH pulses once released into the pituitary portal circulation have a half-life lasting only a few minutes (Gallo, 1980), just long enough to exert its local effects. Very minute amounts find their way into the general circulation and it has thus proved an extremely difficult task to assay peripheral GnRH levels satisfactorily (Jonas et al, 1975; Mortimer et al, 1976). The methodological problems involved have cast doubt on the results obtained which even then have proved of little diagnostic value. Using a specific radioimmunoassay Aksel (1979) has documented peripheral GnRH concentrations throughout the cycle and has found them to be relatively constant with no quantitative relationship to plasma FSH and LH and no fluctuations corresponding with ovulation or the mid-cycle LH surge. Because of its confined mode of action it appears unlikely that peripheral GnRH measurement has any potential value in diagnosis or treatment.

On the other hand, dynamic testing of the pituitary–ovarian axis using aliquots of the synthetic decapeptide has been widely employed in the investigation of ovulatory disorders in addition to its administration at different phases of the normal cycle (Yen et al, 1972). A normal response to a standard 100 μg intravenous bolus given during the early follicular phase consists of a rapid, four-fold rise in basal LH concentration, reaching a peak within 30 min and followed by a gradual decline (Fig. 26.2); the observed rise in FSH is less dramatic (Nillius & Wide, 1972). Such a response in an amenorrhoeic subject indicates an intact pituitary gonadotrophin reserve, whereas the response will be deficient in primary hypopituitarism or in conditions associated with deficient

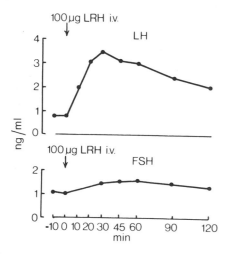

Fig. 26.2 The effect of GnRH (100 μg bolus) on serum LH and FSH levels when given during the early follicular phase of the cycle

hypothalamic GnRH production, such as anorexia nervosa.

The observation that oestrogen administration augments the pituitary response to GnRH in normal women (Shaw et al, 1975) has been employed in an attempt to predict the therapeutic response of anovulatory patients to conventional induction agents, such as clomiphene citrate. It has been suggested that only those demonstrating this positive oestrogen amplification following a single dose of GnRH will subsequently ovulate on clomiphene citrate therapy (Shaw, 1978); however, in many patients with negative responses the addition of mid-cycle hCG as an LH substitute is all that is necessary to achieve ovulation. The oestrogen amplified response also appears unreliable when assessing patients treated with more than standard clomiphene dosage (O'Herlihy et al, 1981). For standard clinical practice dynamic pre-treatment testing with GnRH is not essential and probably adds little information to what can be discerned from the initial therapeutic effects of clomiphene itself.

Therapeutic use of GnRH

When synthetic GnRH was first introduced for clinical trials in the early 1970s, reports appeared of successful ovulation induction in small numbers of amenorrhoeic women (Kastin et al, 1971; Nillius & Wide, 1975). This initial clinical experience raised great expectations of its potential value as a replacement for established drugs, including exogenous human gonadotrophins of menopausal urinary (hMG) or pituitary (hPG) origin. GnRH has considerable theoretical advantages over gonadotrophin therapy, particularly in terms of its cost and availability. In addition, the elaborate daily monitoring of ovarian response essential during gonadotrophin administration would be rendered unnecessary with GnRH through preservation of the intrinsic physiological feedback control mechanisms between the pituitary and ovary, making

hyperstimulation and multiple conception probably no more likely than during spontaneous ovulatory cycles.

Despite its anticipated therapeutic superiority, clinical experience with GnRH was disappointing for several years. In general it was administered subcutaneously thrice daily in doses varying between 100 and 500 μg (Nillius et al, 1975). While it effected follicular maturation in some subjects, as evidence by increased oestrogen concentrations, with a small number of pregnancies resulting, the patient response to this regimen was unpredictable (Zarate et al, 1976); overall ovulation rates rarely exceeded those reported following placebo treatment (Evans et al, 1967). Selection of the minority likely to respond to this intermittent GnRH regimen proved difficult and FSH values tended to decline with continued treatment. Pre-ovulatory hCG was usually necessary even when follicular growth had been induced and GnRH was an inadequate substitute in these circumstances. Nasally administered releasing hormone was more effective than that given by injection (Potashink et al, 1978) but this route is much less dose-efficient and more costly. Superactive analogues such as D-Ser(TBU)[6]-desGly[10]-GnRH (Hoechst 766) were introduced to counter the very short half-life of the naturally occurring hormone but these have proved even less effective and may in fact be more useful as anovulant contraceptive agents (Nillius et al, 1978) or in the suppression of inappropriate gonadotrophin release such as during precocious puberty.

The gradual evolution of our understanding of the physiology of pituitary exposure to GnRH throughout the ovulatory cycle, as summarised above, has now satisfactorily explained the relative lack of success of intermittent thrice daily GnRH therapy. Most of the phenomena observed have been manifestations of 'down regulation' of the pituitary gonadotroph receptors caused by excessively large and too widely-spaced GnRH pulses. The introduction of continuous 60–120 min pulsatile parenteral GnRH therapy has renewed enthusiasm for its use in the successful treatment of several forms of anovulatory infertility.

During the past 3 years several groups have reported on the therapeutic efficacy of pulsatile GnRH (Crowley & McArthur, 1980; Leyendecker et al, 1980; Reid et al, 1981; Schoemaker et al, 1981; Hurley et al, 1982). The pulse frequency used has been 90 min and ovulation and pregnancy have been achieved within the first four treatment cycles. The aetiology of anovulation among the patients treated has included congenital hypogonadotrophic hypogonadism (Kallmann's Syndrome), anorexia nervosa and functional hypothalamic amenorrhoea suggesting that this treatment is suitable for all forms of hypothalamic dysfunction in which pulsatile GnRH production is absent or severely diminished.

The mode and pattern of GnRH administration has varied but the maintenance of regular 90 min pulses for 2 weeks or more has been followed by an endocrinologically normal follicular phase culminating in ovulation. It appears possible to abandon treatment after ovulation provided the luteal phase is supported with supplementary injections of hCG (1500 U) every 3 days until menstruation or pregnancy ensues (Reid et al, 1981). Elaborate pre-ovulatory monitoring can also be dispensed with, since ovarian hyperstimulation is unusual and adequate information on pre-ovulatory follicular growth can be obtained using intermittent ultrasound examination of the ovaries (O'Herlihy et al, 1980). Schoemaker et al (1981) have induced ovulation with patient-administered intravenous 2-hourly pulses for 16 hours per day but with the current commercial availability of small automated portable infusion pumps it seems likely that these will be most widely used to administer the GnRH. The optimal dosage of the hormone appears to vary between 10–25 μg per pulse with little difference in effectiveness noted between intravenous or subcutaneous routes; the latter would therefore seem preferable in terms of patient convenience and safety with change of the infusion site (usually abdominal wall) every 4–5 days. When pulses smaller than 10 μg are used only the intravenous route is reliable (Reid et al, 1981) while doses larger than 25 μg are likely to induce receptor desensitisation.

It now seems likely that in a large proportion of patients with hypothalamic amenorrhoea, the application of physiological principles to GnRH therapy has revolutionised its usefulness. Mild forms of disordered ovulation may still best be treated with established agents such as clomiphene citrate which can be taken orally over a short period. However, since pulsatile GnRH appears equally, if not more, effective in profound forms of hypothalamic depression it is likely to replace exogenous gonadotrophin therapy in the majority of resistant anovulatory patients with consequent distinct advantages in terms of cost, patient convenience and a lowering of multiple pregnancy rates following ovulation induction therapy. Hurley et al (1982) recently reported the successful treatment of three women who had previously had high multiple pregnancies (triplets or worse) following treatment with hPG. Each conceived

within two cycles of treatment with GnRH and singleton pregnancies resulted.

GnRH has yet to be shown to be effective in disorders of ovulation due to PCO, in which pituitary sensitivity to GnRH is over- rather than under-stimulated. In this condition standard or incremental clomiphene therapy is more likely to induce ovulation successfully, until some method of abolishing the intrinsic hypothalamic pulsatility is devised.

CLOMIPHENE CITRATE

History and physiological considerations

Clomiphene citrate, with the formula 2[P-(2-chloro-1, 2 diphenylvinyl) phenoxy] triethylamine dihydrogen citrate, (Fig. 26.3), has become established during the past two decades of widespread clinical use as the most effective simple agent in the treatment of anovulation due to mild to moderate hypothalamic disorders, including polycystic ovarian disease (PCO). It is an orally active non-steroidal compound related in structure to the synthetic oestrogen diethylstilboestrol. This structural similarity to an oestrogenic substance in fact endows it with oestrogenic properties in some mammals (Wood et al, 1968) and because of this it was initially considered as a potential oral contraceptive (Holtkamp et al, 1960). In prepubertal children or in adults with very low circulating oestrogen levels its oestrogen-like effects can predominate, resulting in induction of breast development. However, early trials in adults demonstrated clomiphene's effectiveness as an ovulation promoting agent consistent with predominant anti-oestrogenic properties (Kistner & Smith, 1960; Greenblatt et al, 1961). This action has been found to be mediated through a transient increase in pituitary secretion of gonadotrophins, which in turn triggers and promotes pre-ovulatory follicular maturation.

Other drugs with anti-oestrogenic potential, such as tamoxifen, have subsequently been used successfully to induce ovulation (Williamson & Ellis, 1973) but clomi-

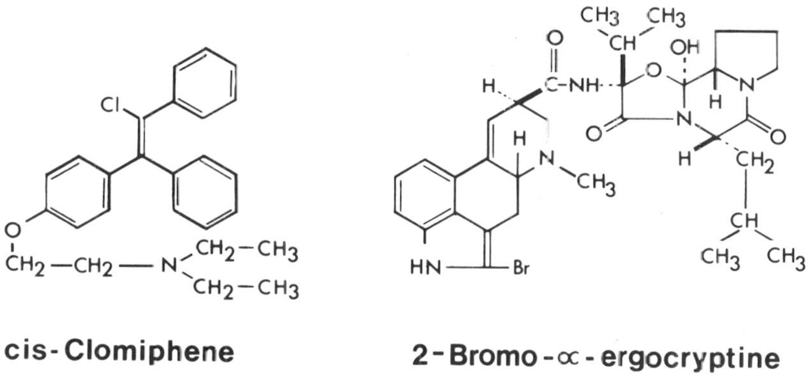

cis-Clomiphene   **2-Bromo-α-ergocryptine**

Fig. 26.3 Structure formula of cis-clomiphene and bromocriptine

phene remains the most effective in this category. It is marketed ('Clomid', Merrell) as a racemose mixture of its two stereo-isomers, cis-and trans-clomiphene, the former being five times more potent as an anti-oestrogen (Korenman, 1966) while the latter is ten times more effective in inducing vaginal cornification (Ross et al, 1973); hence its potential in non-oestrogenised subjects to depress rather than stimulate gonadotrophin release.

At a cellular level oestrogens, in common with other steroids, exert their effect on target cells by specifically binding to cytoplasmic receptor sites prior to translocation of this oestrogen-receptor complex into the nucleus. Clomiphene also has the ability to bind to these cytoplasmic oestrogen receptors and be transferred to the nucleus (Clark et al, 1973). There the clomiphene-receptor complex may have some weak oestrogenic actions, such as increasing pituitary gonadotroph responsiveness to GnRH stimulation (Hsueh et al, 1978) but it fails to stimulate the replenishment of the cytoplasmic receptor, possibly due to a failure to dissociate from nuclear chromatin (Chan & O'Malley, 1976). This leaves the target tissues unresponsive to subsequent oestrogen stimulation (Clark & Peck, 1974) so that a reduction in preferential oestrogen binding is detectable in the pituitary, hypothalamus and uterus (Roy et al, 1963). The resultant disturbance in the oestrogen–gonadotrophin feedback relationship at a pituitary level leads to increased FSH and LH secretion during clomiphene exposure (Wu, 1977). This transient gonadotrophin surge is more important in respect to FSH, which can initiate growth in a cohort of primary ovarian follicles which may culminate in ovulation some days later.

Although the effects of clomiphene on gonadotrophin secretion are the most important in terms of ovulation induction, it has also been found to act on other tissues in the female reproductive system. It binds to the ovary where it increases conversion of androgens to oestrogens (Smith, 1966), an action which may be potentiated by reducing agents such as ascorbic acid (Igarashi, 1977). Clomiphene's anti-oestrogenic effects have also been documented on the endometrium (Lamb et al, 1972) while its depressant action on mid-cycle cervical mucus production has long been recognised and recently quantified (O'Herlihy et al, 1982). It has long been held that clomiphene exerted its stimulatory effect on gonadotrophin secretion at the level of the hypothalamus (Van Look, 1978). But the elegant primate studies which have localised both the positive and negative oestrogen–gonadotrophin feedback centres to the pituitary rather than the hypothalamus (Nakai et al, 1978) suggest that clomiphene's principal site of action also lies there. It will evoke a prepubertal, or oestrogenic, response when GnRH pulsatility is absent since some priming of the pituitary gonadotrophs by GnRH is necessary to enable it to interfere with oestrogen feedback. However, in less profound forms of hypothalamic depression three forms of pituitary–ovarian response may be obtained (Table 26.1).

Table 26.1 Responses to clomiphene therapy based on mid-luteal urinary oestrogen and pregnanediol excretion values, in relation to subsequent recommended treatment

Response	Mid-luteal hormone excretion Oestrogen (μg/24 h)	Pregnanediol (mg/24 h)	Further therapy
No response	< 20	< 1.0	Increase dosage
Follicular response without ovulation	50–150	< 1.0	Add mid-cycle hCG
Follicular maturation with luteal deficiency or late ovulation	20–100	1.0–1.9	Repeat treatment with same dose. Then increase dose if repeat treatment unsuccessful
Satisfactory ovulation	> 20	> 2.0	Repeat treatment with same dose

Minor fluctuations in FSH secretion will be followed by minimal ovarian follicular stimulation. This results in a transient rise in oestrogen production but arrested follicular development before the Graafian stage. Greater gonadotrophin increments during clomiphene therapy will lead to a rise in circulating oestrogen into the pre-ovulatory range. Suboptimal follicular growth in these circumstances may still be followed by a failure of positive oestrogen-LH feedback with consequent late follicular atresia rather than ovulation. This fault usually responds to a single mid-cycle injection of hCG (Kistner, 1966) in a subsequent treatment cycle, although dosage should be minimised to 3000–5000 iu to reduce the possibility of multiple ovulation (Healy & Burger, 1978). The third consequence of a 5-day course of clomiphene is the successful induction of ovulation, where follicular growth is brisk enough to stimulate a pre-ovulatory LH surge. Each of these therapeutic responses can be clearly differentiated by means of mid-luteal sampling of oestrogen and progesterone production in blood or urine (Pepperell et al, 1975) in time to plan the next course of treatment.

As with synthetic GnRH, clomiphene has been proposed as a potentially useful tool in the pre-treatment assessment of likely patient response. Given in a dosage varying between 50 and 200 mg daily for 5 days, a two-fold increment in basal FSH and LH during the 5 days of treatment is indicative of an intact negative feedback mechanism (Newton & Dixon, 1971). Similarly, intact positive feedback release of LH can be demonstrated following a small dose of exogenous oestrogen, since an LH surge will follow within 48–96 h (Shaw, 1976). However, the most widely used predictive pre-treatment test is that of progesterone withdrawal (Leyendecker, 1979). Progesterone or, more usually, a synthetic progestogen such as norethisterone or medroxyprogesterone, if given for 5 days will elicit shedding of an oestrogen-stimulated endometrium within a few days of its cessation. Failure of this withdrawal bleeding identifies patients with low endogenous oestrogen production who are unlikely to respond to standard clomiphene treatment. However, since some hypo-oestrogenic subjects may unexpectedly ovulate when treated, a short trial of clomiphene is usually recommended in all suitably selected anovulatory patients. An additional advantage of an induced withdrawal bleed is that it ensures that clomiphene is not given during a period of unsuspected spontaneous ovarian activity when an excessive cumulative response to treatment might otherwise be more likely.

Standard treatment regimen

Because of its simple mode of administration clomiphene is established as the first choice treatment for patients with hypothalamic amenorrhoea and normal serum prolactin levels. While ovulation induction with clomiphene is possible in the presence of hyperprolactinaemia, positive oestrogen feedback is almost always absent and much more impressive therapeutic results can now be obtained with dopamine-agonist drugs, such as bromocriptine. Clomiphene has also proved particularly effective in cases of polycystic ovarian disease (PCO), a syndrome first identified by Stein & Leventhal (1935) (Ch. 20).

Clomiphene is usually prescribed for a 5-day period, generally days 5–9 or 2–6, after a spontaneous or progestogen-induced menstrual bleed. The standard starting dose is 50 mg/day but this should be reduced to 25 mg/day in patients with clinical features of PCO, who may be particularly sensitive to the drug and may develop ovarian cysts on higher doses. The monitoring of therapeutic response is most often based on observation of a rise in basal body temperature of about 0.5°C between 5 and 12 days after completion of treatment; such a biphasic temperature record is supportive evidence of ovulation mediated through the thermogenic effects of progesterone secretion from the corpus luteum. But many temperature records are not clearly interpretable, even when ovulation has been confirmed biochemically (Lenton et al, 1977b) and this is thus a crude index of ovulation. More informative are mid-luteal phase measurements of progesterone in blood or pregnanediol in urine. A single luteal serum progesterone value exceeding 3 μg/ml (Israel et al, 1972) or a urinary pregnanediol value of 2 mg/24 h or more (Pepperell et al, 1975) can be considered as diagnostic of an ovulatory response.

The value of a coincident oestrogen measurement in the interpretation of anovulatory treatment cycles has been well documented. A rise in oestrogen without ovulation may, in the next cycle, be corrected by increasing the amount of clomiphene given or by adding mid-cycle hCG; however, when the levels of both steroids remain low a larger dose will always be required. Dosage increments of 50 mg/day up to a maximum of 200–250 mg/day are used if no response is obtained. Large amounts of clomiphene frequently induce its commonest side-effect — hot flushes

— which may restrict the ultimate dosage used. These flushes are similar to those occurring at the climacteric but their mechanism has not been established, although they may represent a direct hypothalamic effect; flushes appear to occur more commonly when an ovarian response has been induced (O'Herlihy et al, 1981).

Other unwanted effects of treatment include minor gastrointestinal symptoms, such as nausea and vomiting and abdomino-pelvic tenderness which may represent mild ovarian hyperstimulation. In the absence of endocrine monitoring, ovarian palpation is recommended at the beginning of each treatment cycle to avoid cumulative ovarian enlargement. Severe forms of hyperstimulation with cyst formation and ascites are unusual when adequate clinical supervision is maintained. Visual symptoms, such as blurring or scotomata rarely occur but are considered contraindications to further treatment, although permanent eye damage has not been reported. Multiple pregnancies, usually twins, are achieved in about 10 per cent of induced conceptions; high multiples, such as may occur with exogenous gonadotrophin therapy, are very rare.

The incidences of abortion and congenital malformation in pregnancies induced with clomiphene are overall slightly higher than those documented following spontaneous conceptions. These complications are however no commoner than among other relatively infertile patients (Ahlgren et al, 1976; Harlap, 1976). Isolated cases of fetal malformation, including neural tube defects, have been described among infants conceived during clomiphene-stimulated cycles (Berman, 1975; O'Herlihy et al, 1982) and the drug is known to persist in the mother during the early weeks of pregnancy, because of its predominant enterohepatic route of excretion. Based on the structural similarity between clomiphene and diethylstilboestrol (DES), an oestrogenic effect on the developing genital tract of the rat fetus has been postulated following antenatal clomiphene exposure (Clark & McCormack, 1980) but there is to date no evidence of any DES-like stigmata in human offspring when ovulation has been induced with this drug.

Although pre-ovulatory positive oestrogen-LH feedback is usually preserved in clomiphene-treated patients with PCO, many women with hypothalamic amenorrhoea will manifest a significant rise in oestrogen production without ovulation and will require adjuvant hCG therapy. The timing of this single mid-cycle injection has until recently been determined empirically, usually 5–7 days after completion of clomiphene, to coincide with peak preovulatory follicular maturation (Kistner, 1966). However, conception rates with such a regimen have proved disappointing (Swyer et al, 1975). Once a mature follicle has developed, hCG 3000 iu induces ovulation within 34–40 hs of administration (Edwards & Steptoe, 1975) but if it is given other than at the peak of follicular maturity, by which time adequate LH receptors have developed, hCG

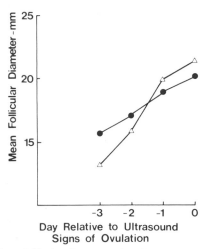

Fig. 26.4 Mean follicular diameter values in 28 clomiphene stimulated cycles (filled circles) and spontaneous ovulatory cycles (open triangles) illustrating more rapid follicular growth with clomiphene. Reprinted with permission from The American College of Obstetricians and Gynecologist (Obstetrics and Gynecology, 1982, 59: 40–45)

can cause follicular atresia and thus actively inhibit ovulation (Williams & Hodgen, 1980).

The pattern of follicular growth in ovulatory clomiphene-stimulated cycles has recently been studied using serial ovarian ultrasound examinations (O'Herlihy et al, 1982). It has been shown that while clomiphene induces more rapid pre-ovulatory growth than that observed during spontaneous cycles, the ranges of mean follicular diameter are similar (18–25 mm), and the mean diameter approximately 36 h before ovulation is 18 mm (Fig. 26.4). Using this information it has proved possible to time, precisely and optimally, hCG in a group of patients with deficient positive feedback by deferring its administration until at least one follicle of 18 mm or more has developed. No patient required hCG before day 14 while the median day of administration was day 15; in some cycles hCG was not given until day 19. Timing of treatment in this way was almost invariably (92 per cent) associated with ovulation and a pregnancy rate of 70 per cent was achieved. The use of ultrasound would now seem to be a desirable prerequisite to treatment with adjuvant hCG.

Results of treatment. Provided patients with ovarian failure and hyperprolactinaemia are excluded, clomiphene will succeed in inducing ovulation in between about 50 and 80 per cent of women with hypothalamic causes of anovulation (MacGregor et al, 1968; Kistner, 1975; Pepperell, 1978). The most successful treatment subgroup is that which includes patients with relatively high basal oestrogen production, in particular those with PCO. However, despite satisfactory rates of ovulation, conception rates in several series have been disappointingly low. This discrepancy between ovulation and conception rates has been ascribed to several factors, including the anti-oestrogenic effects of clomiphene on cervical mucus and on the endometrium (Lamb & Guderian, 1966; Lamb et al, 1972), ovum entrapment (Whitelaw et al, 1970) and follicular

luteinisation without ovulation (Kase et al, 1967). In practice, many anovulatory women are treated with clomiphene prior to the assessment of other potential causes of infertility, such as seminal or tubal abnormalities. Furthermore, the diagnosis of ovulation is often based on relatively unreliable criteria such as basal temperature recordings (Hancock & Oakey, 1973), so that reported ovulation rates may not be a true representation of the facts.

The more accurate timing of ovulation using ultrasound and hCG (O'Herlihy et al, 1982) and the use of life table analysis suggests that clomiphene pregnancy rates in otherwise healthy couples are comparable with the normal spontaneous rates (Gorlitsky et al, 1978; Hull et al, 1979), though they do not approach the results achieved with exogenous gonadotrophin therapy (Brown et al, 1969). A failure to achieve pregnancy within at most six ovulatory treatment cycles therefore strongly suggests that another significant anti-fertility factor coexists. In unsuccessfully treated patients the role of adjuvant therapy, other than preovulatory hCG, has not been established. While a definite antagonistic effect of clomiphene on mid-cycle cervical mucus production has been repeatedly demonstrated, this effect is of doubtful therapeutic significance once ovulation has been satisfactorily induced. Indeed attempts to improve the mucus quality or quantity with the administration of supplemental oestrogen (Taubert & Dericks-Tan, 1976) appears to be more likely to interfere with ovulation (O'Herlihy et al, 1982).

Other forms of clomiphene therapy

The administration of clomiphene during the early cycle phase in regularly ovulating women induces increased gonadotrophin output from the pituitary (Vandenberg & Yen, 1973) which also appears to enhance pre-ovulatory follicular growth. This effect has been employed in two evolving forms of infertility practice. It has proved useful for regulating or synchronising ovulation in women undergoing artificial insemination (Klay, 1976) and it has more recently been introduced into the rapidly developing technique of *in vitro* fertilisation and embryo transfer (IVF and ET). Laparoscopic oocyte collection for this procedure has been attempted during both spontaneous ovulatory cycles and also after stimulation with exogenous gonadotrophins with limited success. Considerably more promising results have been obtained, in terms of oocytes harvested and fertilisation rates, using clomiphene 100 mg/day in early cycle (days 5–9) followed by hCG given when at least one mature follicle is identified by ultrasound scanning (Hoult et al, 1981). This regimen is currently the most suitable for permitting the more widespread introduction of IVF.

Luteal phase insufficiency, a syndrome characterised by suboptimal progesterone production in association with normal menstrual rhythm, has received considerable attention as a cause of infertility. Several treatments have been recommended including bromocriptine, hCG and progesterone supplements. However, despite its name, the fundamental abnormality probably results from deficient early cycle FSH secretion (Sherman & Korenman, 1974) which can be corrected with clomiphene therapy, although not always with satisfactory results (MacNaughton et al, 1978).

Before the criteria for its optimum dosage and duration of treatment had been established, clomiphene was given in early clinical studies in relatively large amounts for protracted periods. This frequently resulted in ovarian hyperstimulation due to excessive endogenous gonadotrophin secretion in responsive subjects (Southam & Janovski, 1962; Roy et al, 1963). By the mid-1960s it was realised that a safe and adequate ovarian response could be obtained by restricting treatment to 5 days and limiting total dosage to a maximum of 1000–1500 mg/cycle (Kistner, 1975). As many as one-third of patients with hypothalamic amenorrhoea fail to show any increase in ovarian oestrogen production with this protocol, even when the maximum dose of 250 mg/day is given for 5 days. This group includes many women with profound and persistent weight loss or with severe forms of PCO who have subsequently been successfully treated with exogenous human gonadotrophins of either pituitary (hPG) or menopausal urinary origin (hMG).

Studies of ovarian function under stimulation with hPG have led Brown (1978) to propose that the follicular requirement for FSH operates within a very narrow range, involving changes in concentration of only 10–30 per cent between the threshold and maximum stimulation required for follicular development. This threshold hypothesis has recently been introduced to clomiphene therapy in patients unresponsive to the standard dosage (O'Herlihy et al, 1981). It has proved possible to titre clomiphene dosage, by means of incremental increases of 50 mg/day every 5 days, against ovarian responsiveness. This has involved total doses of the drug of up to 3750 mg/cycle (Fig. 26.5) given continuously over 25 days; with this treatment over two-thirds of previously unresponsive patients ovulated successfully and a minority conceived. Twice weekly oestrogen assessment was adequate during this incremental regimen to prevent ovarian hyperstimulation since clomiphene administration was stopped when oestrogen values rose significantly above baseline. Serial ultrasound examinations were then used to assess late follicular growth and to time the pre-ovulatory hCG injection.

In responsive patients incremental therapy was associated with increases in FSH and LH while clomiphene was given but positive LH feedback was almost invariably absent; hCG given when a mature follicle was identified on ultrasound examination overcame this problem. Ovulation was frequently induced with dosages less than the 1000 mg which had earlier failed during standard 5 day therapy in

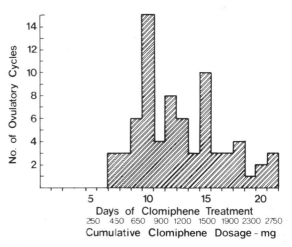

Fig. 26.5 The cumulative clomiphene dosage and duration of therapy necessary to induce ovulation during incremental clomiphene treatment. Reprinted with permission from The American College of Obstetricians and Gynecologists (Obstetrics and Gynecology, 1981, 58: 535–545)

the same patients, suggesting that duration of exposure is as important as the amount of clomiphene given in eliciting a response. With the monitoring protocol used, unwanted effects did not present problems. In the majority of cycles two follicles of ovulatory size were visible with ultrasound, usually in the same ovary, at the time of ovulation but in only a small minority were three or more present. Multiple ovulation does not seem invariably to follow, even in the presence of multiple large follicles. This suggests that, contrary to the experience in hPG-stimulated cycles, multiple follicular growth stimulated by clomiphene occurs in series rather than in parallel, significantly reducing the risk of multiple conception.

Although it is considerably more costly than standard modes of clomiphene treatment, incremental administration remains more cost-effective and less complicated and potentially dangerous than exogenous gonadotrophins, hitherto the only alternative in unresponsive patients; hPG or hMG may still be used should incremental therapy fail. Pulsatile GnRH treatment is probably still cheaper than either of these methods and requires even less monitoring during its administration. It is particularly suited to anovulatory states where intrinsic GnRH pulsatility has disappeared.

BROMOCRIPTINE

The virtual simulataneous discovery of a method to measure serum PRL levels and a drug to reduce elevated serum PRL levels (bromocriptine — Parlodel, Sandoz) revolutionised the evaluation and management of patients with disorders of ovulation. Although an association between galactorrhoea and amenorrhoea had been described by Hippocrates, it was not until the mid 1970s that it was realised that 20 per cent of patients with secondary amenorrhoea and 7.5 per cent of those with oligomenorrhoea had elevated PRL levels (Pepperell, 1978; Flückiger et al, 1982), approximately 30–40 per cent of patients with elevated PRL levels had pituitary tumours (Jacobs, 1980) and that bromocriptine therapy resulted in ovulation and pregnancy in at least 80 per cent of subjects with elevated PRL levels (Pepperell et al, 1977a).

Physiology of prolactin secretion

The secretion of prolactin by the anterior pituitary gland has been shown to be under the tonic inhibitory control of the hypothalamus. It is now widely accepted that this inhibition is mediated by dopamine (MacLeod & Fontham, 1970) which is secreted from tubero infundibular neurones into the portal venous system leading to the pituitary gland (Ben-Jonathan et al, 1977; Gibbs & Neill, 1978). Although other catecholamines such as noradrenaline and adrenaline also inhibit prolactin secretion they are much less potent than dopamine.

In addition to inhibiting release of prolactin, dopamine also inhibits prolactin synthesis, thus resulting in a dual mechanism of reducing prolactin levels (MacLeod et al, 1980). Presumably these two actions are mediated by dopamine acting at separate sites on the pituitary lacto-troph cells as different dopamine agonist drugs vary in their degree of inhibition of these two separate processes.

Although various hormones have been proposed as stimulators of prolactin secretion, thyrotrophin releasing hormone (TRH) is best known for this effect. Other-stimulatory hormones discovered so far include vasoactive intestinal peptide, metenkephalin, β-endorphin, and sero-tonin (5-HT). The physiological relevance of these hormones to the stimulation of prolactin secretion in both the normal and hyperprolactinaemic subjects is still unclear however.

The functional role of prolactin during the normal menstrual cycle has not been established clearly although the effect of elevated prolactin levels on reproductive function has been studied extensively. Hyperprolactinaemia has been described in association with primary and secondary amenorrhoea, oligomenorrhoea, ovulation associated with deficient corpus luteum function and the premenstrual syndrome. Although the exact mode of action of the hyper-prolactinaemia in these conditions has not been fully elucidated, the major effect would appear to be at the level of the hypothalamus. High PRL levels have been shown to stimulate hypothalamic dopamine turnover in rats (Höhn & Wuttke, 1978) and probably inhibit GnRH release from the hypothalamus. These effects presumably result in the decreased LH secretion observed in many hyperprolactinaemic subjects. In addition to its effect at the level of the hypothalamus, PRL has also been shown to reduce progesterone production by human ovarian granu-losa cells in tissue culture (McNatty et al, 1974) and elevated PRL levels have been associated with a reduction

in progesterone secretion by the corpus luteum of preg-nancy (Pepperell et al, 1977b).

Physiology and pharmacology of bromocriptine

Bromocriptine — a dopamine agonist derived from the ergot alkaloid group of drugs (Fig. 26.3) — inhibits PRL secretion of all species of fishes and mammals tested so far (Flückiger, 1976) under basal conditions or under conditions in which PRL output is stimulated by physio-logical, pharmacological or surgical means.

Bromocriptine achieves its PRL suppression by acting at both hypothalamic and pituitary levels. Its direct effect on the pituitary is clearly evident when it is added to pitui-taries in vitro or to pituitary cell cultures, and it also blocks TRH stimulation of prolactin secretion in vivo. Although its effect on the hypothalamus is not as well documented it does slow dopamine turnover which, in turn, lowers pituitary prolactin levels.

Bromocriptine, like dopamine, inhibits not only the release but also the synthesis of PRL and thus probably acts at the two separate sites postulated on the lactotroph cell. Lisuride, an ergoline with dopamine agonist proper-ties, only inhibits PRL release yet serum PRL levels are still suppressed (MacLeod et al, 1980).

Apart from reducing PRL secretion and release, brom-ocriptine also diminishes DNA synthesis and reduces mitotic activity in the pituitary (Lloyd et al, 1975, 1978). Similar effects are observed on prolactinoma cells and there have now been several reports of a reduction in tumour size during treatment with bromocriptine, as determined by improvement in visual field defects or by radiological means (Corenblum, 1978; McGregor et al, 1979; Wass et al, 1979).

The peak blood level of bromocriptine occurs 3 h after ingestion however PRL suppression is maintained for the subsequent 8 h despite falling plasma levels of the drug (Thorner et al, 1980b). Its long duration of action means that twice or thrice daily doses are sufficient to keep PRL levels suppressed throughout the day.

Following withdrawal of bromocriptine therapy, circu-lating PRL levels usually return to their pretreatment values. However Eversmann et al (1979) have reported lower post-treatment PRL levels in patients with macro-prolactinomas. Surprisingly, in patients with microprolac-tinomas, significant long-lasting suppression of PRL secretion was not observed.

Clinical use of bromocriptine in anovulatory subjects

In ovulation induction, bromocriptine is a specific treat-ment for a specific defect, namely anovulation due to raised prolactin production. The drug is administered orally and the dose increased at intervals until a satisfactory ovulation occurs. Apart from mild nausea and postural hypotension, the treatment is virtually free of side-effects. The incidence of multiple pregnancy is not increased and, although the drug is commonly stopped as soon as pregnancy is confirmed, no teratogenic effects have been described.

Bromocriptine is commenced in the low dose of 1.25 mg (half a tablet) twice daily for 1 week. This is taken with meals to reduce the gastrointestinal side-effects and the low dose allows the patient to become accustomed to the drug and able to tolerate higher doses. After a week, the dose is increased to 2.5 mg twice daily and maintained at this level.

Approximately 21 days after commencing therapy, the response is assessed by determining the urinary oestrogen and pregnanediol excretion (or plasma oestradiol and progesterone levels) and the serum prolactin level, and by examining for the persistence of galactorrhoea if this was present initially (60 per cent of hyperprolactinaemic patients have this symptom). In the absence of a response, as judged by lack of change in the hormone levels or in galactorrhoea, the dose of bromocriptine is doubled to 5 mg twice daily. The assessment is repeated monthly and, in the absence of a response, the dose is then doubled. It is unusual to exceed a maximum dose of 20 mg twice daily (40 mg/day).

Alternatively, but not ideally, in the absence of laboratory facilities, the dosage can be increased empirically until a response, as indicated by bleeding or pregnancy, is obtained. If conception does not occur within 3 to 4 months on this empirical regime, it is necessary to reassess the situation by measurement of the serum PRL values to determine whether suppression of the hyperprolactinaemia has been adequate. Most patients respond to treatment with bromocriptine at a daily dose of 5–10 mg and the great majority who conceive do so within six ovulatory cycles, the mean number of ovulatory cyles per conception being 1.9.

Once ovulation occurs during treatment with bromocriptine, regular ovulation usually continues for as long as the drug is administered or until conception results. It has been usual to stop bromocriptine as soon as a positive pregnancy test is obtained. Following cessation of this agent, serum PRL levels rise rapidly to values similar to those which were present prior to treatment and which are significantly higher than those seen at the same time in normal pregnancy (Pepperell et al, 1977b). Although this elevation in prolactin levels is accompanied by a significant fall in urinary pregnanediol excretion between 11 and 14 weeks of gestation, all pregnancies where a fetus is present continue normally without supplemental progesterone therapy and the overall abortion rate following this treatment is not increased above normal.

The hormonal responses to therapy are illustrated in Fig. 26.6. The elevated PRL levels are rapidly suppressed to normal, and galactorrhoea, if present initially, subsides. However, ovarian activity often does not commence until

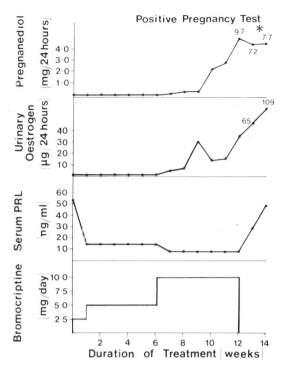

Fig. 26.6 Weekly serum PRL and urinary oestrogen and pregnanediol values during treatment with bromocriptine in a patient who conceived following the first induction of ovulation

the serum PRL level is suppressed below 10 ng/ml. In at least half of the patients treated the initial ovarian response is not that of normal ovulation as follicular development without ovulation, or ovulation with deficient corpus luteum function is observed. These partial responses often evolve into full ovulatory responses in subsequent cycles even without an increase in the dose of bromocriptine administered (Pepperell et al, 1977a).

Concurrent use of other agents. Most hyperprolactinaemic patients respond as illustrated above however, in about 5 per cent of subjects, adequate PRL suppression is not associated with a return of ovarian function. Administration of clomiphene citrate, in addition to the continuing treatment with bromocriptine, commonly restores ovulation under these circumstances and it has been assumed that a dual hypothalamic–pituitary cause has been the cause of the ovulatory disorder.

In a further 5 per cent of hyperprolactinaemic subjects, the serum PRL level cannot be suppressed to normal despite the administration of exceedingly large doses of bromocriptine (up to 80 mg/day). Some of these subjects have obvious suprasellar or pituitary tumours, others have small adenomas only evident with sophisticated computerised axial tomography (CAT) scanning techniques but in many the reason for the failure of PRL suppression remains obscure. In some of these subjects the PRL level prior to treatment is only two to three times the upper limit of normal and the failed response comes as a complete surprise. Because of the high cost of bromocriptine and the fact that the administration of 80 mg/day is rarely much more effective than 20 mg/day in lowering PRL levels in such patients, it has been usual to reduce the maintenance dose to 20 mg/day and administer thyroxine as well, even though thyroid function has previously been shown to be normal. Theoretically, the administration of thyroxine should reduce PRL levels by reducing the serum TSH levels, however little change usually occurs in serum PRL levels during this therapy. Where a return of ovarian function still does not occur, clomiphene citrate is then given, usually in a dose of 100–150 mg/day for 5 days, in addition to bromocriptine and thyroxine and in six of the eight subjects so treated ovulation has occurred. This ovulatory response has been observed even though the serum PRL level is still mildly elevated. However it has not been observed where the serum PRL was still greater than twice the upper limit of normal.

Use of bromocriptine in patients with pituitary tumours

Although Hardy et al (1978) achieved normalisation of PRL secretion in 91 per cent of a group of patients with microadenomas and in 78 per cent of those with intrasellar macroadenomas when treated surgically, these results have not been reproduced by other workers. The vast majority of patients have thus been left with elevated PRL levels following surgery.

External irradiation of the pituitary (usually 4500–5000 rads given over 20–25 days), although effective in reducing PRL levels in many patients, rarely leads to complete normalisation of PRL levels. Any decrease in PRL levels occurs slowly, taking at least 6–12 months to occur (Gomez et al, 1977). Even where a slow return to normality of PRL levels does occur it is common for other trophic hormone production by the pituitary to be compromised (Franks et al, 1977).

Because of the damage to pituitary hormone secretion which often follows surgical attack on the pituitary or irradiation of that region, it is often necessary to administer gonadotrophin therapy to such patients when they wish to conceive. Administration of bromocriptine to lower their prolactin level is often not associated with a resumption of cyclical menstrual activity and the addition of clomiphene citrate is rarely effective in restoring ovulation.

The failure of surgical and/or radiotherapeutic treatment to effect a cure has led to the use of prolactin antagonists, particularly bromocriptine, in patients with both microadenomas and macroadenomas of the pituitary. This therapy not only reduces elevated PRL (and growth hormone) levels but also markedly reduces the likelihood of further tumour growth and, in many instances, has resulted in a significant reduction of tumour size (Corenblum, 1978; McGregor et al, 1979; Wass et al, 1979).

Most patients, even those with markedly elevated PRL levels, have their PRL level suppressed to normal while taking bromocriptine in a dosage of 5–10 mg per day,

Table 26.2 Radiological classification of sella turcica

Grade 0	Normal sella
Grade I	The sella is within normal limits in size. Its floor is intact but shows discrete modifications such as localised blistering, thinning, bulging or double contour
Grade II	The sella is asymmetrically or globally enlarged. It exceeds standard measurements but tomography shows integrity of its bony walls
Grade III	The sella may or may not increased in size. Its floor is locally eroded or destroyed, suggesting tumour tissue has transgressed its boundaries and herniates into the sphenoid sinus or basisphenoid.
Grade IV	The bony walls of the sella are definitely destroyed. In most of these cases, the tumour fills entirely the sphenoid sinus and may invade the clivus or the cavernous sinuses

Each of these grades has subgroups ∅, A, B and C.

∅ — no suprasellar extension.
A — extension to the anterior recesses.
B — extension to the floor of the third ventricle.
C — huge expansion to the foramen of Munro.

however some patients will not achieve this effect even when given 80 mg of bromocriptine per day. Because of the varying dose requirement, the dose of bromocriptine should be increased in a step-wise fashion every 3–4 weeks if the PRL level remains elevated. As many patients with large tumours will still not establish menstrual cycles even though the PRL has been suppressed to normal — presumably due to damage to the FSH and LH producing mechanisms — the measurement of serum PRL levels is essential if adequate control is to be achieved.

It has now been almost universally accepted that bromocriptine is the treatment of choice for patients with prolactin producing pituitary micro- or macroadenomas, especially where suprasellar extension of tumour is not present and the tumour is of grade I or grade II in type (Table 26.2). Where suprasellar extension of tumour is present, or where the tumour is grade III or IV in type, there is considerable controversy as to the most appropriate treatment. Surgical removal of the tumour, usually with post-operative radiotherapy, should protect against optic chiasmal compression. However, this treatment rarely results in normal PRL secretion and treatment with bromocriptine is therefore still required. Primary treatment with bromocriptine, withholding surgery and radiotherapy initially, is now being used in many centres. Because of the reduction in tumour size which accompanies therapy it is hoped that this will transform a macroprolactinoma into a surgically resectable tumour (if surgery is required at all) as operative procedures in such patients without prior treatment with bromocriptine are rarely curative (Thorner et al, 1980a).

How long bromocriptine therapy should be continued and what happens to PRL secretion and tumour growth when treatment is ceased is not yet known. In some patients, particularly those with macroadenomas, significant long-lasting suppression of PRL levels after ceasing bromocriptine has been observed (Eversmann et al, 1979).

Where the patient is asymptomatic, not desirous of pregnancy and has a grade I or grade II tumour with no evidence of suprasellar extension, there is debate as to whether bromocriptine therapy should be given. Until recently there have been no long-term follow-up studies of patients with prolactin producing pituitary tumours, although it was known that most tumours increased in size slowly, if at all. A recent report (March et al, 1981) indicating that progression of tumour growth was seen in only 4.3 per cent of such patients followed for a period of 3–20 years, raises the possibility that bromocriptine therapy could be withheld until progressive tumour growth was evident except in patients with troublesome galactorrhoea or those desirous of pregnancy.

Pregnancy following treatment with bromocriptine

It is well established that the normal pituitary enlarges during pregnancy (Erdheim & Stumme, 1909; Goluboff & Ezrin, 1969; Pasteels, 1972), this enlargement being due to lactotroph cell growth consequent upon stimulation by increased oestrogen levels. In addition to normal pituitary tissue, adenomatous tissue growth is also stimulated by oestrogen (Peillon et al, 1970) and enlargement of pituitary tumours during pregnancy, leading to optic chiasmal compression is well documented (Child et al, 1975; Gemzell & Wang, 1979).

The likelihood of tumour complications during pregnancy in women with previously untreated prolactinomas has been widely debated but the consensus of opinion currently is that the risk is low. Nillius et al (1980), reviewing reports from 11 separate groups, found a 5.6 per cent tumour complication rate in 146 such patients (162 pregnancies). This low complication rate suggests there is no need for potentially harmful therapy such as pituitary surgery or radiotherapy to minimise the risk of tumour growth during pregnancy, except in patients with large adenomas in whom a 35 per cent incidence of clinically significant pituitary enlargement during pregnancy can be reduced to 7 per cent by such therapy (Gemzell & Wang, 1979).

The current practice in Melbourne is to cease treatment with bromocriptine as soon as the pregnancy test is positive, except in patients with grade III or IV tumours, and those with grade II tumours with suprasellar extension who have not been treated surgically, where therapy is continued throughout pregnancy in the same dose used to induce ovulation. Irrespective of whether bromocriptine therapy is ceased or continued, visual field examination should be performed at least every third month during the pregnancy in order that tumour growth can be recognised early and treated appropriately. This assessment should be performed even when there has been no evidence of a pituitary adenoma prior to pregnancy, as a small tumour, too small to be recognised by the less sophisticated radiological techniques commonly used, can grow quickly and cause marked chiasmal compression.

During the last 5 years it has only been necessary to recommence treatment with bromocriptine in three of 150 bromocriptine induced pregnancies at the Royal Women's Hospital in Melbourne. In two instances severe headache was the reason for recommencing treatment; in the other patient development of a visual field defect necessitated reinstitution of therapy.

No increase in congenital abnormalities has been identified in patients taking bromocriptine at the time of conception whether the drug was ceased as soon as a positive pregnancy test was obtained or continued throughout pregnancy (Griffith et al, 1978; Flückiger et al, 1982).

Use of bromocriptine in other infertile subjects

Although bromocriptine was initially thought to be effective in inducing ovulation in anovulatory patients with normal PRL levels, further experience in treating such patients has been most disappointing. Ovulation and pregnancy rates of about 15 per cent have been observed, these values being virtually identical to those following placebo therapy (Evans et al, 1967).

Bromocriptine has also been employed in the treatment of patients with unexplained infertility as the mean serum PRL level in such patients has been shown to be higher than that of control subjects (Lenton et al, 1977a). Although these workers reported an increased pregnancy rate following treatment with bromocriptine, their results have not been confirmed in two double-blind placebo controlled trials (Wright et al, 1979; McBain & Pepperell, 1982).

REFERENCES

Ahlgren M, Källen B, Rannevik G 1976 Outcome of pregnancy after clomiphene therapy. Acta Obstetrica et Gynecologica Scandinavica 55: 371–375

Aksel S 1979 Luteinizing hormone-releasing hormone and the human menstrual cycle. American Journal of Obstetrics and Gynecology 135: 96–101

Amoss M, Burgus R. Blackwell R, Vale W, Fellows R, Guillemin R 1971 Purification, amino acid composition and N-terminus of the hypothalamic luteinizing hormone releasing factor (LRF) of ovine origin. Biochemical Biophysical Research Communications 44: 205–210

Arimura A, Matsuo H, Baba Y, Debeljuk L, Sandow J, Schally A V

520 CLINICAL REPRODUCTIVE ENDOCRINOLOGY

1972 Stimulation of release of LH by synthetic LH-RF in vivo. I. A comparative study of natural and synthetic hormones. Endocrinology 90: 163–168

Ben-Jonathan N, Oliver C, Weiner H J, Mical R S, Porter J C 1977 Dopamine in hypophysial portal plasma of the rat during the estrous cycle and throughout pregnancy. Endocrinology 100: 452–458

Berman P 1975 Congenital malformations associated with maternal clomiphene ingestion. Lancet ii: 878–881

Brown J B 1978 Pituitary control of ovarian function — Concepts derived from gonadotrophin therapy. Australian and New Zealand Journal of Obstetrics and Gynaecology 18: 47–54

Brown J B, Evans J H, Adey F D, Taft H P, Townsend L 1969 Factors involved in the induction of fertile ovulations with human gonadotrophins. Journal of Obstetrics and Gynaecology of the British Commonwealth 76: 289–307

Child D F, Gordon H ,Mashiter K,Joplin G F 1975 Pregnancy, prolactin and pituitary tumours. British Medical Journal 4: 87–89

Chan L, O'Malley B W 1976 Mechanism of action of the sex steroid hormones. New England Journal of Medicine 294: 1322–1328

Clark J H, McCormack S A 1980 The effect of clomid and other triphenylethylene derivatives during pregnancy and the neonatal period. Journal of Steroid Biochemistry 12: 47–53

Clark J H, Peck E J Jr 1974 Oestrogen receptors and antagonism of steroid hormone action. Nature 251: 446–448

Clark J H, Anderson J N, Peck E J Jr 1973 Estrogen receptor-anti-estrogen complex: atypical binding by uterine nuclei and effects on uterine growth. Steroids 22: 707–718

Corenblum B 1978 Bromocriptine in pituitary tumours. Lancet ii: 786

Crowley W F Jr, McArthur J W 1980 Stimulation of the normal menstrual cycle in Kallman's syndrome by pulsatile administration of luteinizing hormone-releasing hormone (LHRH). Journal of Clinical Endocrinology and Metabolism 51: 173–175

Edwards R G, Steptoe P C 1975 Induction of follicular growth, ovulation and luteinisation in the human ovary. Journal of Reproduction and Fertility (Suppl) 22: 121–163

Erdheim J, Stumme E 1909 Über die Schwangerschaftsveränderung in der Hypophyse. Beiträge zur Pathologischen Anatomie und zur Allgemeinen Pathologie 46: 1–132

Evans J H, Taft H P, Brown J B, Adey F D, Johnstone J W 1967 Induction of ovulation by cyclical hormone therapy. Journal of Obstetrics and Gynaecology of the British Commonwealth 74: 367–370

Eversmann T, Fahlbusch R, Rjosk H K, von Werder K 1979 Persisting suppression of prolactin secretion after long-term treatment with bromocriptine in patients with prolactinomas. Acta Endocrinologica 92: 413–427

Flückiger E 1976 The pharmacology of bromocriptine. In: Bayliss RIS, Turner P, Maclay WTP (eds) Pharmacological and Clinical Aspects of Bromocriptine (Parlodel), pp 12–26. MCS Consultants, Tunbridge Wells

Flückiger E, del Pozo E, von Werder K 1982 Incidence of hyperprolactinemia. In: Flückiger E, del Pozo E, von Werder K (eds) Prolactin: Physiology. Pharmacology and Clinical Findings. Springer Verlag, New York

Franks S, Jacobs H S, Hull M G R, Steele S J, Nabarro J D N 1977 Management of hyperprolactinaemic amenorrhoea. British Journal of Obstetrics and Gynaecology 84: 241–253

Gallo R V 1980 Neuroendocrine regulation of pulsatile luteinising hormone release in the rat. Neuroendocrinology 30: 122–131

Gemzell C and Wang C F 1979 Outcome of pregnancy in women with pituitary adenoma. Fertility and Sterility 31: 363–372

Gibbs D M, Neill J D 1978 Dopamine levels in hypophysial stalk blood in the rat are sufficient to inhibit prolactin secretion in vivo. Endocrinology 102: 1895–1900

Goluboff L G, Ezrin C 1969 Effect of pregnancy on the somatotroph and the prolactin cell of the human adenohypophysis. Journal of Clinical Endocrinology and Metabolism 29: 1533–1538

Gomez F ,Reyes F I, Faiman C 1977 Nonpuerperal galactorrhea and hyperprolactinemia. American Journal of Medicine 62: 648–660

Gorlitsky G A, Kase N G ,Speroff L 1978 Ovulation and pregnancy rates with clomiphene citrate. Obstetrics and Gynecology 51: 265–269

Green J D, Harris G W 1947 The neurovascular link between the neurohypophysis and adenohypophysis. Journal of Endocrinology 5: 136–146

Greenblatt R, Barfield W E, Jungck E C, Roy A W 1961 Induction of ovulation with MRL-41. Journal of the American Medical Association 178: 101–108

Griffith R W,Turkalj I, Braun P 1978 Outcome of pregnancy in mothers given bromocriptine. British Journal of Clinical Pharmacology 5: 227–231

Hancock K W, Oakey R E 1973 The low incidence of pregnancy following clomiphene therapy. International Journal of Fertility 18: 49–56

Hardy J ,Beauregard H, Robert F 1978 Prolactin secreting pituitary adenomas: transphenoidal microsurgical treatment. In: Robyn C, Harter M (eds) Progress in Prolactin Physiology and Pathology, pp 361–70. Elsevier/North-Holland Biochemical Press, Amsterdam

Harlap S 1976 Ovulation induction and congenital malformations. Lancet ii: 961

Healy D L, Burger H G 1978 An hypothesis for high multiple pregnancies after clomiphene. Australian and New Zealand Journal of Obstetrics and Gynaecology 18: 242–246

Höhn K G, Wuttke W O 1978 Changes in catecholamine turnover in the anterior part of the mediobasal hypothalamus and the medial preoptic area in response to hyperprolactinemia in ovariectomized rats. Brain Research 156: 241–252

Holtkamp D E, Greslin J G, Root C A, Lerner L J 1960 Gonadotrophin inhibiting and anti-fecundity effects of clomiphene. Proceedings of the Society of Experimental Biology and Medicine 105: 197–210

Hoult I J, de Crespigny L Ch, O'Herlihy C, Speirs A L, Lopata A, Kellow G, Johnston I, Robinson H P 1981 Ultrasound control of clomiphene/human chorionic gonadotropin stimulated cycles for oocyte recovery and in vitro fertilization. Fertility and Sterility 36: 316–319

Hsueh A J W, Dufau M L, Catt K J 1977 Gonadotropin-induced regulation of luteinizing hormone receptors and desensitization of testicular 3':5'-cyclic AMP and testosterone responses. Proceedings of the National Academy of Sciences 74: 592–595

Hsueh A J W, Erickson G F, Yen S S C 1978 Sensitisation of pituitary cells in luteinising hormone releasing hormone by clomiphene citrate in vitro. Nature 273: 57–59

Hull M G, Savage P E, Jacobs H S 1979 Investigation and treatment of amenorrhoea resulting in normal fertility. British Medical Journal 1: 1257–1259

Hurley D, Brian R, Outch K, Stockdale J, Burger H G 1982 Pituitary and ovarian responses to pulsatile subcutaneous gonadotrophin-releasing hormone in hypothalamic amenorrhoea: reliable ovulation and pregnancy. Proceedings of the Endocrine Society of Australia, 25th Annual Meeting, Sydney. Abstract 40

Igarashi M 1977 Augmentative effect of ascorbic acid upon induction of human ovulation in clomiphene-ineffective anovulatory women. International Journal of Fertility 22: 168–173

Israel R, Mishell D R, Stone S C, Thorneycroft I H, Moyer D L 1972 Single luteal phase serum progesterone assay as an indicator of ovulation. American Journal of Obstetrics and Gynecology 112: 1043–1046

Jacobs H S 1980 Management of prolactin secreting pituitary tumours. In: Studd J W W (ed) Progress in Obstetrics and Gynaecology, Vol I, pp 263–276. Churchill Livingstone, Edinburgh

Jonas H A, Burger H G, Cumming I A, Findlay J K, de Kretser D M 1975 Radioimmunoassay for luteinizing hormone-releasing hormone (LHRH): its application to the measurement of LHRH in ovine and human plasma. Endocrinology 96: 384–393

Kase N, Mroueh A, Olson L E 1967 Clomid therapy for anovulatory infertility. American Journal of Obstetrics and Gynecology 98: 1037–1047

Kastin A J, Zarate A, Midgley A R, Canales E S, Schally A V 1971 Ovulation confirmed by pregnancy after infusion of porcine LH-RH. Journal of Clinical Endocrinology and Metabolism 33: 980–982

Kistner R W 1966 Use of clomiphene citrate, human chorionic gonadotropin, and human menopausal gonadotropin for induction of ovulation in the human female. Fertility and Sterility 17: 569–583

Kistner R W 1975 Induction of ovulation with clomiphene citrate. In:

Behrman S J, Kistner R W (eds) Progress in Infertility, 2nd ed, pp 509–536. Little, Brown and Company,Boston

Kistner R W, Smith O W 1960 Observations on use of non-steroidal estrogen antagonist: MER-25. Surgical Forum 10: 725–729

Klay L J 1976 Clomiphene-regulated ovulation for donor artificial insemination. Fertility and Sterility 27: 383–388

Knobil E 1974 On the control of gonadotropin secretion in the rhesus monkey. Recent Progress in Hormone Research 30: 1–46

Knobil E 1980 The neuroendocrine control of the menstrual cycle. Recent Progress in Hormone Research 36: 53–88

Korenman S G 1969 A mechanism of action of estrogen inhibitors. Clinical Research 17: 144

Lamb E J, Guderian A M 1966 Clinical effects of clomiphene in anovulation. Obstetrics and Gynecology 28: 505–512

Lamb E J, Colliflower W W, Williams J W 1972 Endometrial histology and conception rates after clomiphene citrate. Obstetrics and Gynecology 39: 389–396

Lenton E A, Sobowale O S, Cooke I D 1977a Prolactin concentrations in ovulatory but infertile women: treatment with bromocriptine. British Medical Journal 2: 1179–1181

Lenton E A, Weston G A, Cooke I D 1977b Problems in using basal body temperature recordings in an infertility clinic. British Medical Journal 1: 803–805

Leyendecker G 1979 The pathophysiology of hypothalamic ovarian failure: Diagnostic and therapeutical considerations. European Journal of Obstetrics, Gynecology and Reproductive Biology 9: 175–186

Leyendecker G, Wildt L, Hansmann M 1980 Pregnancies following chronic intermittent (pulsatile) administration of Gn-RH by means of a portable pump ("Zyklomat") — A new approach to the treatment of infertility in hypothalamic amenorrhea. Journal of Clinical Endocrinology and Metabolism 51: 1214–1216

Lloyd H M, Meares J D, Jacobi J 1975 Effects of oestrogen and bromocriptine on in vivo secretion and mitosis in prolactin cells. Nature 255: 497–498

Lloyd H M, Jacobi J M, Meares J D 1978 DNA synthesis and depletion of prolactin in the pituitary gland of the male rat. Journal of Endocrinology 77: 129–136

MacLeod R M, Fontham E H 1970 Influence of ionic environment on the in vitro synthesis and release of pituitary hormones. Endocrinology 86: 863–869

MacLeod R M, Nagy I, Login I S, Kimura H, Valdenegro C A, Thorner M O 1980 The roles of dopamine, cAMP and calcium in prolactin secretion. In: MacLeod R M, Scapagnini U (eds) Central and Peripheral Regulation of Prolactin Function, pp 27–42. Raven Press, New York

March C M, Kletzky O A, Davajan V, Teal J, Weiss M, Apuzzo M L J, Marrs R P, Mishell D R 1981 Longitudinal evaluation of patients with untreated prolactin-secreting pituitary adenomas. American Journal of Obstetrics and Gynecology 139: 835–841

McBain J C, Pepperell R J 1982 Use of bromocriptine in unexplained infertility. Clinical Reproduction and Fertility 1: 145–150

McCann S M 1980 Control of anterior pituitary hormone release by brain peptides. In: Cumming I A, Funder J W, Mendelsohn F A (eds) Endocrinology 1980, pp 25–34. Elsevier/North Holland, Amsterdam

MacGregor A H ,Johnson J E,Bunde C A 1968 Further clinical experience with clomiphene citrate. Fertility and Sterility 19: 616–622

McGregor A M, Scanlon M F, Hall R, Hall K 1979 Effects of bromocriptine on pituitary tumour size. British Medical Journal 2: 700–703

McNatty K P, Sawers R S, McNeilly A S 1974 A possible role for prolactin in control of steroid secretion by the human graafian follicle. Nature 250: 654–655

McNatty K P, Smith D M, Makris A, Osathanondh R, Ryan K J 1979 The micro-environment of the human antral follicle: Interrelationships among the steroid levels in antral fluid, the population of granulosa cells, and the status of the oocyte in vivo and in vitro. Journal of Clinical Endocrinology and Metabolism 49: 851–860

Macnaughton M C, Fleming R, Carswell W, Black W P, England P, Craig A, Coutts J R T 1978 Treatment of the defective luteal phase.

In: Jacobs H S (ed) Advances in Gynaecological Endocrinology, pp 92–101. RCOG, London

Mortimer C H, McNeilly A S, Ress L H, Lowry P J, Gilmore D, Dobbie H G 1976 Radioimmunoassay and chromatographic similarity of circulating endogenous gonadotropin releasing hormone and hypothalamic extracts in man. Journal of Clinical Endocrinology and Metabolism 43: 882–888

Nakai Y, Plant T M, Hess D L, Keogh E J, Knobil E 1978 On the sites of the negative and positive feedback actions of estradiol in the control of gonadotropin secretion in the rhesus monkey. Endocrinology 102: 1008–1014

Newton J, Dixon P 1971 Site of action of clomiphene and its use as a test of pituitary function. Journal of Obstetrics and Gynaecology of the British Commonwealth 78: 812–821

Nillius S J, Wide L 1972 The LH-releasing hormone test in 31 women with secondary amenorrhoea. Journal of Obstetrics and Gynaecology of the British Commonwealth 79: 874–882

Nillius S J, Wide L 1975 Gonadotrophin-releasing hormone treatment for induction of follicular maturation and ovulation in amenorrhoeic women with anorexia nervosa. British Medical Journal 3: 405–408

Nillius S J, Fries H, Wide L 1975 Successful induction of follicular maturation and ovulation by prolonged treatment with LH-releasing hormone in women with anorexia nervosa. American Journal of Obstetrics and Gynecology 122: 921–928

Nillius S J, Bergquist C, Wide L 1978 Inhibition of ovulation in women by chronic treatment with a stimulatory LRH analogue — a new approach to birth control? Contraception 17: 537–545

Nillius S V, Bergh T, Larsson S G 1980 Pituitary tumours and pregnancy. In: Derome P J, Jedynak C P, Peillon F (eds) Pituitary Adenomas: Biology, Physiopathology and Treatment, pp 103–111. Asclepios Publishers, France

O'Herlihy C, de Crespigny L J Ch, Robinson H P 1980 Monitoring ovarian follicular development with real-time ultrasound. British Journal of Obstetrics and Gynaecology 87: 613–616

O'Herlihy C, Pepperell R J, Brown J B, Smith M A, Sandri L, McBain J C 1981 Incremental clomiphene therapy: a new method for treating persistent anovulation. Obstetrics and Gynecology 58: 535–542

O'Herlihy C, Pepperell R J, Robinson H P 1982 Ultrasound timing of human chorionic gonadotropin administration in clomiphene-stimulated cycles. Obstetrics and Gynecology 59: 40–45

Pasteels J L 1972 Morphology of prolactin secretion. In: Wolstenholme GE W, Knight J (eds) Lactogenic Hormones, pp 241–255. Churchill, Livingstone, Edinburgh

Peillon F, Vila-Porcile E, Olivier L, Racadot J 1970 L'action des oestrogens sur les adénomes hypophysaires chez l'homme. Annals of Endocrinology (Paris) 31: 259–270

Pepperell R J 1978 Clinical investigation and assessment of amenorrhoea. Proceedings of the 6th Asia and Oceania Congress of Endocrinology, Singapore, pp 389–392. Endocrine and Metabolic Society of Singapore

Pepperell R J, Brown J B, Evans J H, Rennie G C, Burger H G 1975 The investigation of ovarian function by measurement of urinary oestrogen and pregnanediol excretion. British Journal of Obstetrics and Gynaecology 82: 321–332

Pepperell R J, McBain J C, Healy D L 1977a Ovulation induction with bromocriptine (CB154) in patients with hyperprolactinaemia. Australian and New Zealand Journal of Obstetrics and Gynaecology 17: 181–191

Pepperell R J, McBain J C, Winstone S M, Smith M A, Brown J B 1977b Corpus luteum function in early pregnancy following ovulation induction with bromocriptine. British Journal of Obstetrics and Gynaecology 84: 898–903

Plant T M, Krey L C, Moossy J, McCormack J T, Hess D L, Knobil E 1978 The arcuate nucleus and the control of gonadotropin and prolactin secretion in the female rhesus monkey (Macaca mulatta). Endocrinology 102: 52–62

Potashnik G, Homburg R, Eshkol A, Insler V, Lunenfeld B 1978 Hormonal and clinical responses in amenorrheic patients treated with gonadotropins and a nasal form of synthetic gonadotropin-releasing hormone. Fertility and Sterility 29: 148–152

Quigley M E, Yen S S C 1980 The role of endogenous opiates on LH secretion during the menstrual cycle. Journal of Clinical Endocrinology and Metabolism 51: 179–181

Reid R L, Leopold G R, Yen S S C 1981 Induction of ovulation and pregnancy with pulsatile luteinizing hormone releasing factor: Dosage and mode of delivery. Fertility and Sterility 36: 553–559

Ross J W, Paup D C, Brant-Zawadzki M, Marshall J R, Gorski R A 1973 Effects of cis- and trans-clomiphene in the induction of sexual behavior. Endocrinology 93: 681–685

Roth J, Kahn C R, Lesniak M A, Gorden P, De Meyts P, Mesyesi K et al 1975 Receptors for insulin, NSILA-s, and growth hormone: Applications to disease states in man. Recent Progress in Hormone Research 31: 95–135

Roy S, Greenblatt R B, Mahesh V B, Jungck E C 1963 Clomiphene citrate: Further observations on its use in induction of ovulation in the human and on its mode of action. Fertility and Sterility 14: 575–580

Schoemaker J, Simons A H M, van Osnabrugge G J C, Lugtenburg C, van Kessel H 1981 Pregnancy after prolonged pulsatile administration of luteinzing hormone-releasing hormone in a patient with clomiphene-resistant secondary amenorrhoea. Journal of Clinical Endocrinology and Metabolism 52: 882–885

Shaw R W 1976 Tests of the hypothalamic pituitary ovarian axis. Clinical Obstetrics and Gynecology 3: 485–503

Shaw R W 1978 Diagnostic tests. In: Jacobs H S (ed) Advances in Gynaecological Endocrinology, pp 35–45. RCOG, London

Shaw R W, Butt W R, London D R 1975 The effect of oestrogen pretreatment on subsequent response to luteinizing hormone releasing hormone in normal women. Clinical Endocrinology 4: 297–304

Sherman B M, Korenman S G 1974 Measurement of plasma LH, FSH, estradiol and progesterone in disorders of the human menstrual cycle: The short luteal phase. Journal of Clinical Endocrinology and Metabolism 38: 89–98

Smith O W 1966 The effect of clomid on estrogen secretion and metabolism. American Journal of Obstetrics and Gynecology 94: 440–446

Southam A L, Janovski N A 1962 Massive ovarian hyperstimulation with clomiphene citrate. Journal of the American Medical Association 181: 443–446

Stein I F, Leventhal M L 1935 Amenorrhea associated with bilateral polycystic ovaries. American Journal of Obstetrics and Gynecology 29: 181–191

Swyer G I M, Raowanska E, McGarrigle H H G 1975 Plasma oestradiol and progesterone estimation for the monitoring of induction of ovulation with clomiphene and chorionic gonadotrophin. British Journal of Obstetrics and Gynaecology 82: 794–804

Taubert H D, Dericks-Tan J S E 1976 High doses of estrogens do not interfere with the ovulation-inducing effect of clomiphene citrate. Fertility and Sterility 27: 375–382

Thorner M O, Evans W S, MacLeod R M, Hunley W C Jr, Rogol A D, Morris J C, Besser G M 1980a Hyperprolactinemia: current concepts of management including medical therapy with bromocriptine. In: Thorner M O, Calne D B, Lieverman A, Goldstein G (eds) Ergot Compounds and Brain Function — Neuroendocrine and Neuropsychiatric Aspects, pp 165–189. Raven Press, New York

Thorner M O, Schran H F, Evans W S, Rogol A D, Morris J L, MacLeod R M 1980b A broad spectrum of prolactin suppression by bromocriptine in hyperprolactinemic women: A study of serum prolactin and bromocriptine levels after acute and chronic administration of bromocriptine. Journal of Clinical Endocrinology and Metabolism 50: 1026–1033

Vandenberg G, Yen S S C 1973 Effect of anti-estrogenic action of clomiphene during the menstrual cycle: evidence for a change in the feedback sensitivity. Journal of Clinical Endocrinology and Metabolism 37: 356–365

Van Look P 1978 Diagnostic and therapeutic use of clomiphene. In: Jacobs H S (ed) Advances in Gynaecological Endocrinology, pp 170–190. RCOG, London

Wang C F, Lasley B C, Lein A, Yen S S 1976 The functional changes of the pituitary gonadotropins during the menstrual cycle. Journal of Clinical Endocrinology and Metabolism 42: 718–722

Wass J A H, Thorner M O, Charlesworth M, Moult P J A, Dacie J E, Jones A E, Besser G M 1979 Reduction of pituitary tumour size in patients with prolactinomas and acromegaly treated with bromocriptine with or without radiotherapy. Lancet ii: 66–69

Whitelaw M J, Foster T N, Graham W H 1970 Hysterosalpingography and tubal insufflation. Journal of Reproductive Medicine 4: 56–63

Wildt L, Marshall G, Hausler A, Plant T M, Belchetz P E, Knobil E 1979 Amplitude of pulsatile GnRH input and pituitary gonadotropin secretion. Federation Proceedings (Federation of American Societies for Experimental Biology) 38: 978

Williams R F, Hodgen G D 1980 Disparate effects of human chorionic gonadotropin during the late follicular phase in monkeys: Normal ovulation, follicular atresia, ovarian acyclicity and hypersecretion of follicle-stimulating hormone. Fertility and Sterility 33: 64–68

Williamson J G, Ellis J D 1975 Factors influencing the pregnancy and complication rates with human menopausal gonadotrophin therapy. British Journal of Obstetrics and Gynaecology 82: 52–57

Wood J R, Wrenn T R, Bitman J 1968 Estrogenic and antiestrogenic effects of clomiphene MER-25 and CN55, 945–27 on the rat uterus and vagina. Endocrinology 82: 62–74

Wu C H 1977 Plasma hoemones in clomiphene citrate therapy. Obstetrics and Gynecology 49: 443–448

Yen S S 1980 The polycystic ovary syndrome. Clinical Endocrinology 12: 177–207

Yen S S C, Tsai C C, Naftolin F, Vandenberg G, Ajabor L 1972 Pulsatile patterns of gonadotropin release in subjects with and without ovarian function. Journal of Clinical Endocrinology and Metabolism 34: 671–675

Zarate A, Canales E S, Soria J, Forsbach G, Kastin A J, Schally A V 1976 Therapeutic use of gonadoliberin (follicle-stimulating hormone/luteinizing hormone-releasing hormone) in women. Fertility and Sterility 27: 1233–1239

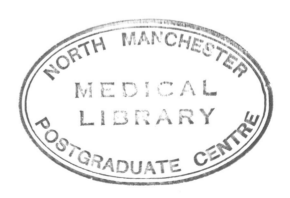

Induction of ovulation with gonadotrophins

INTRODUCTION

Probably the most far-reaching discovery ever made in reproductive biology was the relevation in the mid-1920s that the male and female reproductive systems are under the functional control of the anterior hypophysis. The first firm evidence (Zondek 1926a, b, Zondek & Ascheim, 1927) was obtained by demonstrating that implantation of anterior pituitary glands evoked a rapid development of sexual puberty in immature animals. At the same time, another group led by Smith (1926; Smith & Engle, 1927) was able to show that hypo physectomised immature male or female animals failed to mature sexually. They also noted in the adult hypophysectomised animal a rapid regression of sexual characteristics. Shortly afterwards, three gonadotrophic factors were discovered: (1) follicle-stimulating hormone (FSH), which as its name indicates is primarily responsible for follicular growth and ripening; (2) luteinising hormone (LH), responsible for the final maturation of the FSH stimulated follicles, ovulation, and the transformation of the follicular remnants into functional corpora lutea; and (3) human chorionic gonadotrophin (hCG), the hormone secreted by the trophoblastic cells, which has biological actions similar to LH.

CHEMISTRY AND BIOSYNTHESIS

During the last 20 years, the major elements of the mechanism of action, control and regulation of secretion of gonadotrophins were elucidated and more recently their structure was determined. They were found to be glycoproteins with molecular weights around 30 000 daltons and containing about 20 per cent carbohydrate. The carbohydrate moieties in their molecules are fucose, manose, acetylglucosamine and N-acetylneuroaminic acid (Butt & Kennedy, 1971). They consist of two noncovalently associated α and β subunits that can be dissociated into the individual subunits by denaturing agents (De la Liosa & Jutisz, 1969). All the gonadotrophins as well as thyroid-

stimulating hormone (TSH) share a common α subunit of 92 amino acid residues in the same sequence with five disulphide bonds. The β subunits (of FSH, LH and hCG) are unique to each hormone and confer their biological specifity; they have amino acid chains of variable lengths (116–147 amino acid residues) and contain six disulphide bonds. Methodologies which have allowed the analysis of genes and gene products have shown that the two subunits of the gonadotrophic hormones are translated from separate messenger RNAs (Fiddes & Goodman, 1979). The nascent polypeptide α and β subunits are then glycosylated by enbloc attachment of high complex type oligosacharide to two aspargine residues of each subunit. Excess mannose and glucose residues are trimmed from the intermediates.

Thereafter peripheral monosacharides N-acetylglucosamine, galactose, and N-acetylneuroaminic acid are attached sequentially to complete the oligosacharide structures. The α and β subunits then combine noncovalently in a two step reaction to form the biological, active glycoproteins (Hussa, 1980).

PRINCIPLES OF GONADOTROPHIC THERAPY

To stimulate follicular maturation both FSH and LH are required; biologically pure FSH is unable to do so. For this reason, all gonadotrophic preparations used for therapeutic purposes contain both FSH and LH in various proportions. While the FSH content of the preparation is essential for follicular development, final maturation of the follicles and subsequent ovulation are brought about by a surge of LH secretion. Thus two different gonadotrophic preparations are required for induction of ovulation: one providing the required amount of FSH + LH and another providing LH or LH-like material (hCG) of sufficient quantity to provoke ovulation and corpus luteum formation. During the last 45 years, gonadotrophic hormones have been extracted from various sources: mammalian pituitary glands, serum of pregnant mares, urine of pregnant women, and more recently, from postmortem human hypophyses and human postmenopausal urine. All these extracts have been shown to be potent gonadal stimulants in laboratory mammals. Numerous researchers have applied these hormones in clinical trials to stimulate the ovaries to induce ovulation and corpus luteum formation, which could then be followed by pregnancy (see extensive reviews Zondek & Shulman, 1945; Loraine, 1956, Albert, 1956, Kotz & Herrmann, 1961; Netter & Belaisch, 1962). Gonadotrophins of animal origin gave inconsistent results due to the formation of neutralising antibodies to heterologous gonadotrophins following repeated or prolonged administration. Usually an initial ovarian stimulation can be evoked. The extent of such stimulation depends on the time of appearance and the quantity of circulating neutralising antibodies. Continuous administration of pregnant mares serum gonadotrophin (PMSG) has stimulated antigonadotrophin in the blood of treated patients. To avoid therapeutic failure as a result of neutralising antibodies, only gonadotrophins from human sources are now used for clinical treatment

Gonadotrophins of human origin were obtained from postmortem pituitary glands or human postmenopausal urine. Both are used in conjunction with hCG. In 1958, Gemzell et al reported on a procedure for the extraction of a FSH-like substance from human postmortem pituitary glands. This preparation (HPFSH), in conjunction with hCG, produced polycystic enlargement of the ovaries, ovulation in four out of five patients, and secretory transformation of the endometrium in three out of these five patients. Ovulation was followed by a marked increase of both urinary oestrogens and pregnanediol. In 1967, Gemzell summarised his results in induction of ovulation in 100 amenorrhoeic infertile women. Ninety per cent of them ovulated, and 50 per cent became pregnant following the treatment.

Other authors using the same, similar, or different extraction procedures, obtained potent gonadotrophic extracts from human postmortem pituitary glands and reported on successful induction of ovulation (Buxton &

Herrmann, 1961; Crooke et al, 1962, 1963; Rosemberg et al, 1963, Brown, 1969, Shearman, 1966). Of particular significance is the report of Bettendorf (1966) who induced ovulation followed by pregnancy with human pituitary gonadotrophins in hypophysectomised patients. This finding clearly indicates that purified gonadotrophic extracts may successfully substitute the endogenous gonadotrophins in patients lacking these hormones.

Data from the Australian Department of Health (ADH), Canberra indicate that by the end of 1981, 1056 patients were treated with HPFSH through 4008 cycles, and 552 pregnancies occurred.

The scarcity of human postmortem pituitary glands required for the production of HPFSH, greatly restricted its widespread use in all other countries. Thus attention was directed towards the extraction of gonadotrophins from human postmenopausal urine.

The initial urinary extract was prepared by the kaolin-acetone method purified first by ammonium acetate ethanol and then by DEAE-cellulose. The resulting material was further purified by permutit. Borth et al (1954, 1957) showed that human menopausal gonadotrophins (HMG) were effective gonadal stimulators in hypophysectomised laboratory mammals. Borth et al reported in 1961 that this preparation was a potent ovarian stimulator in the human. Lunenfeld et al (1962) were able to enlarge these studies and report in detail on 16 courses of treatment in ten women, with three resulting pregnancies.

Reports indicate that gonadotrophic therapy with extracts prepared from pituitary glands (HPFSH) or from postmenopausal urine (HMG) have an identical effect on the ovary and give similar results (Lunenfeld & Insler, 1978; Bettendorf, 1966). Thus they will be considered together in this chapter.

A survey of several large series of gonadotrophin therapy, published during the last several years, indicates that this therapy has become universally accepted. This survey includes 15 740 treatments given to 5747 patients which resulted in 2525 pregnancies (Table 27.1).

Table 27.1 Induction of ovulation with human gonadotrophins: a literature survey of results obtained

Author		Patients	Cycles	Pregnancies	Pregnancy Rate (%)
Bettendorf et al	(1981)	756	1585	224	33.0
ADH	(1981)	1056	4008	552	52.3
Butler et al	(1970)	134	438	31	23.1
Caspi et al	(1976)	101	343	62	61.4
Ellis & Williamson	(1975)	77	322	43	55.8
Gemzell	(1970)	228	463	101	44.3
Spadoni et al	(1974)	62	225	26	41.9
Thompson & Hansen	(1970)	1190	2798	334	28.1
Lunenfeld et al	(1982)	1107	3646	424	38.3
Goldfarb	(1982)	442	1098	118	26.7
Tsapoulis et al	(1978)	320	?	163	50.9
Schwartz et al	(1980)	232	655	136	58.6
Healy et al	(1980)	40	159	33	82.5
Total		5747	15740	2525	43.9

The overall results of this large survey are not very precise since statistical methods used in the analysis of data have not kept pace with diagnostic and therapeutic advances in the field of reproduction. The infertility specialist might find it difficult to state, with any precision, what defines a couple with a fertility problem and what prognosis can be given to them. Thus a detailed analysis of results was carried out on our own material, which is large enough to provide a valid assessment and has the singular advantage of being uniform so far as the classification of patients, gonadotrophic preparation, treatment schedules, type of monitoring, and follow-up of patients are concerned. Only a few such studies exist (ADH, 1981; Bettendorf et al 1981; Lunenfeld et al, 1982). This report is based on computer tabulations of pooled data from 1107 patients to whom 3646 treatment cycles with HMG were administered during the past 20 years.

Selection of patients

The suitability of patients for gonadotrophic treatment is essentially determined by the very nature of this therapy. Being a replacement therapy (Lunenfeld & Insler, 1978) it may be effective in patients lacking endogenous gonadotrophins but having ovaries capable of responding normally to gonadotrophic stimuli. The presence of normal, sensitive ovaries is *sine qua non* for effective HMG-hCG therapy. For clinical purposes and for the comparison of results obtained by HMG-hCG therapy we used a simple classification (Insler et al, 1968) with patients separated into two main groups:

Hypothalamic-pituitary failure (group I), included women with primary or secondary amenorrhoea, low levels of endogenous gonadotrophins, and lack of endogenous oestrogen activity. The treatment of choice for this group of patients is gonadotrophic therapy. Hypothalamic-pituitary dysfunction (group II), included patients with anovulation associated with a variety of menstrual disorders (including amenorrhoea) whose urinary or serum gonadotrophin levels were within the normal range and who had evidence of endogenous oestrogen activity.

The treatment of choice for patients belonging to group II is a chlorotrianisene analogue, such as clomiphene citrate alone or in conjunction with oestrogen and/or hCG. About one-third of such patients will become pregnant with this treatment regimen. Patients who fail to ovulate or conceive within a reasonable time are considered 'Clomiphene failures' and if after reassessment of the couple no mechanical, cervical, or male factors are detected, they can be considered for HMG therapy.

Before initiation of HMG treatment one has to rule out general systemic diseases or endocrinopathies that may be the cause of the infertility. Pituitary tumours should be sought, particularly in amenorrhoeic patients, and more so among those exhibiting high prolactin levels. Lateral skull radiography and tomography of sella turcica, visual fields, and periodic prolactin determinations are mandatory in these cases. Ovarian, tubal, cervical, and male factors should be meticulously checked. If any abnormality is discovered, the patients should be excluded from gonadotrophic treatment, at least until the abnormality has been corrected.

Monitoring of therapy

Menotrophins (HMG) are given daily by intramuscular injections in order to stimulate follicular development; ovulation is actually induced by hCG. The daily dose of HMG given in a particular cycle depends upon the ovarian response of the patient in that particular cycle. The response is reflected by an anatomical growth of follicles accompanied by biochemical changes mainly with respect to increased synthesis and secretion of steroidal hormones. The follicular enlargement can be visualised by ultrasonographic measurement, while oestrogen secretion values can be estimated directly by urine or blood measurement or evaluated by their effect on secondary targets such as the cervical glands.

The monitoring of treatment serves to assess the dose that is effective in evoking an ovarian response and the length of time required for follicular maturation and the appropriate time for induction of ovulation with hCG. Furthermore, it should aim to prevent hyperstimulation or at least to detect it as early as possible. For these purposes, a combination of ultrasonography and oestrogen determination ideally should be used, since exogenous gonadotrophic stimulation usually induces the development and growth of several follicles. The levels of oestrogens reflect the total oestrogen secretion of all growing follicles.

It was observed that in gonadotrophin treated-women, the mean level of E_2, in cycles with one maturing follicle 1 day prior to ovulation, was 320.4 pg/ml. In cycles with several growing follicles, the mean E_2 concentration was 972.9 pg/ml. The mean follicular diameters in these two groups of the largest follicle were almost indentical, 22.0 and 22.2 mm respectively (Nitschke-Dabelstein et al, 1981).

Sonographic visualisation may thus discriminate between single and multiple follicular growth, and their measurement may aid in the interpretation of the meaning of the oestrogen levels. Evidence is accumulating that only follicles of diameters between 19 and 22 mm will ovulate. Thus, sonography can be a more precise indicator for the determination of the time for ovulation induction.

Endogenous oestrogen production affects several cervical parameters. These parameters were assessed by a points scoring system — the cervical score. This score is a semiquantitative index of the response of the cervix to oestrogens. It is scaled from 0 to 12 by giving points (0 to 3) for each of: amount of mucus, degree of ferning of mucus, degree of spinbarkeit of mucus, and opening of the cervical ostium. The score shows a reasonably good correlation with oestrogen levels and is a particularly useful guide in establishing the effective daily dose and the time when oestrogen determination should be initiated. Treatment can be thus monitored sequentially — first by the cervical score which indicates oestrogenic secretion by growing follicles and, when the score is about 8 or more, by actual oestrogen determinations. When urinary oestrogens reach 80 μg/24h or serum estradiol 250 pg/ml, ultrasonographic visualisation of the ovaries should be performed as an additional aid in timing hCG administration.

In practice, the individualy adjusted treatment schemes is monitored as shown in Fig. 27.1. The treatment is started on the fifth day of spontaneous or induced bleeding. The initial HMG dose is usually one to two ampoules per day. If the patient received gonadotrophic therapy within the last 3 months, treatment is usually started at the highest effective dose of the previous course. Patients are instructed to keep daily morning BBT records and are examined at frequent intervals, about every 1 or 3 days, as required. The examination includes palpation of the ovaries, estimation of the cervical score, postcoital tests when indicated, and a short interview with the patient as to her general wellbeing. It is also important to be aware of the presence of abdominal pain or discomfort, nausea, diarrhoea, or any other symptoms possibly related to treatment.

If the cervical score does not change, or if oestrogen levels do not rise, and there are no alarming clinical signs, the initial dose of HMG is continued for 5–7 days, and then increased by one ampoule. Monitoring by oestrogen levels can be postponed until the cervical score reaches 8 and more, provided that a cervical factor has been excluded previously. Treatment is continued until the effective daily dose — the dose of HMG which causes a significant and

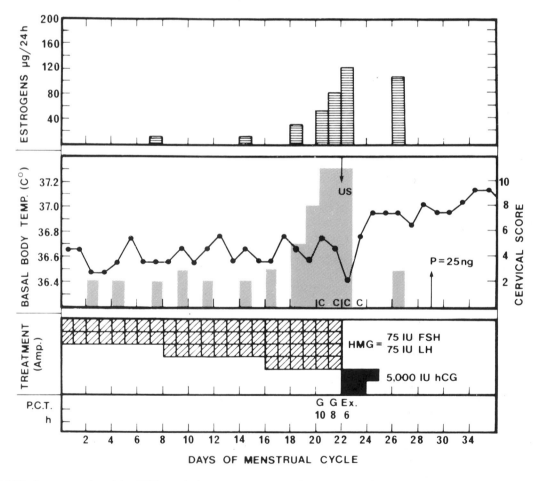

Fig. 27.1 HMG/hCG therapy monitored by BBT, cervical score, oestrogens and progesterone (P), and ultrasound (US). Therapy was started with two ampoules per day. Since the cervical score was persistently low, the dose of HMG was increased on the 9th and 17th day to three and four ampoules respectively. On the 19th day of treatment, the cervical score reached 5 and increased thereafter steadily, reaching 11 points on the 21st day. Daily urinary oestrogen measurements increased steadily from the time of maximal cervical score to reach 120 μg/24 h on day 23 (i.e. 5 days after the cervical score became positive). Ultrasonic examination showed one follicle of 20 mm in the right side and two follicles of 10 $\pm$ 13 mm on the left side. hCG was administered on 3 consecutive days; the patient conceived, and delivered a single child. Note that a post-coital test (PCT) was performed 10, 8, and 6 h after coitus (C) and was good (G) and excellent (Ex.) between day 20 and day 22

steady oestrogen rise — is achieved. From this day on, the patient is examined daily or on alternate days. If urinary oestrogens or plasma oestradiol levels increase too rapidly and the day difference exceed the geometric rise, the HMG dose is reduced by 30–50 per cent and treatment is continued at this reduced dosage. If the oestrogen rise is steady and not excessive, the same dose is continued until urinary oestrogens reach the level of 80 μg/24h (250 pcg/ml). At this stage an ultrasonic visualisation of follicular development is advisable.

If ultrasonic examination reveals only one single follicle, the HMG dose is continued until this follicle reaches the size of 20–22 mm. In that case, the oestrogen level on the day of induction with hCG will not likely exceed 150 μg/24h urine, (320 pcg/ml plasma).

In case of multifollicular development, one will obtain much higher levels of oestrogens when one or more of the follicles will reach a diameter of 20 mm. In this case the decision to inject hCG should be carefully weighed against the risk of hyperstimulation or multiple pregnancies. In cases of multifollicular development and urinary oestrogens levels above 250 μg/24h or plasma oestrogens above 1500 pg/ml, hCG should definitely be withheld since, in our experience, hyperstimulation is likely to complicate the treatment.

On the day a satisfactory follicular diameter is reached and oestrogen levels are in acceptable range, a thorough clinical examination is carried out and if the ovaries are not excessively enlarged and the patient is not reporting any ususual symptoms, the first ovulatory dose of 10 000 iu hCG is given. The same dose is administered on the next day, and 5000 iu are administered on the third day. Some centers have used less than 3000 iu hCG to induce ovulation, and some of these supported luteal phase with hCG injection. However, the higher dose obviates the need for further hCG doses during the luteal phase, and does not increase the hyperstimulation or multiple pregnancy rate (tabulated computerised information obtained from Australian Department of Health (ADP) (1981) and our own data). The patient is instructed to have intercourse daily on these 3 days.

After induction of ovulation, the patient is examined on days 3–5 and 7–9 following the first hCG injection. Special care is taken not to overlook possible ovarian enlargement, abdominal pains, or tenderness. Again, blood (for plasma progesterone) or urine (for pregnanediol) analyses should be performed. The patient is then instructed to report back if abdominal pain, nausea, vomiting, or diarrhoea appear concomitant with bleeding or, 3 weeks following the ovulatory dose of hCG, if neither hyperstimulation nor menstruation occured. If a sustained high phase of BBT lasting for about 15 days is noted, a serum sample should be analysed the next day for a specific hCG determination.

Results

The pregnancy rate in patients with hypothalamic pituitary failure (group I) following gonadotrophic therapy is high; of 279 patients in our series, 82 per cent conceived. Similarly, out of 139 such patients treated with HPG-hCG, 60 per cent conceived (Australian Department of Health (ADP), 1981).

Pregnancy rate however, does not give the true estimate of treatment efficacy, since it does not take into consideration the number of treatments each patient received at any given time; furthermore drop out of patients after short treatment periods will falsify the true expected pregnancy rate. To overcome this bias, cumulative pregnancy rate using the life table analysis has been designed (Lamb & Cruz, 1972).

The cummulative pregnancy rate for patients of group I was 91.2 per cent after six cycles of treatment. This is approximately 30 per cent higher than the cummulative pregnancy rate in the normal nulliparous population (17 patients of group I who conceived following HMG/hCG therapy returned for further treatment). The cummulative pregnancy rate for the second conception was 87.9 per cent after six cycles and 93.6 per cent after eight cycles of treatment.

In 117 patients with hypothalamic pituitary dysfunction (group II), who failed to conceive following clomid therapy, the pregnancy rate following HMG/hCG was only 21.4 per cent. ADP reported in 1981 on 110 patients suffering from oligomenorrhoea or regular menses (similar to our group II). They obtain a pregnancy rate of 35.4 per cent following HPG/hCG.

The difference in pregnancy rates between group I and II may be explained by the fact that patients belonging to group II are negatively selected, i.e. many of these patients failed to conceive following clomiphene therapy, although many of them did ovulate. It is possible that additional factors may contribute to the low success rate.

Age affected the cumulative pregnancy rate significantly (Dor et al, 1980). In both groups the cumulative pregnancy rates were higher in the younger women (Fig. 27.2 and 27.3). The cumulative pregnancy rate in group I patients under 35 years was 95.1 per cent after six cycles and in patients above 35 years it was only 60.1 per cent. In group II, of 14 patients who commenced treatment after the age of 40 years, only one conceived.

The success rates (the percentage of women who took home at least one living child) were 60.6 per cent in group I and 11.5 per cent in group II. Altogether, 424 children were born to women who conceived following treatment with HMG; 60 women are still pregnant. The mean number of treatment cycles per patient were 3.15 in group I and 3.17 in group II. Among the women of group I who conceived, 90 per cent did so within four treatment cycles,

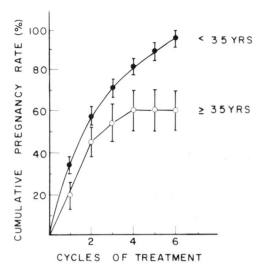

Fig. 27.2 Cumulative pregnancy rates after gonadotrophin therapy in group I patients less than 35 years and 35 years or more. The vertical bars represent the 67 per cent confidence limits

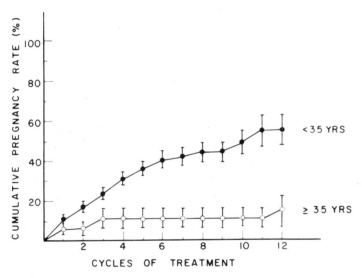

Fig. 27.3 Cumulative pregnancy rate after gonadotrophin therapy in group II patients less than 35 years and 35 years or more. The vertical bars represent the 67 per cent confidence limits

and of the group II patients, 86 per cent did so within four treatment cycles, and 94 per cent within five treatment cycles (Table 27.2). The results together with the pattern of the cumulative pregnancy rates calculated from the life table analysis method indicate that patients who have not become pregnant after five treatment cycles will only rarely achieve pregnancy thereafter.

The considerable individual variations in treatment response preclude exact prediction of an individual dose requirement of HMG for any given patients. Thus, standardised dosage schemes are less effective and dangerous in some cases. However, some basic difference of response to gonadotrophic stimulation in various groups of patients have been observed. Such data, although rough and

Table 27.2 Cumulative pregnancy rate as a function of the number of treatment cycles with HMG/hCG

Treatment cycle	Group I (%)	Group II (%)	Total
1	47	39	45
2	71	57	66
3	84	75	81
4	90	86	89
5	94	93	95
6		97	97
7			98

approximate, may assist in the planning and monitoring of therapy and in estimating its cost. The mean number of ampoules of HMG* per treatment cycle was 40.2 in group I patients as compared to 18.2 ampoules in patients of group II.

Assessment of complications

All complications of gonadotrophin therapy are essentially due to ovarian stimulation and induction of ovulation. To the best of our knowledge, direct side-effects of the drug itself have not been reported. The main complications of gonadotrophic treatment are hyperstimulation syndrome, high incidence of multiple pregnancy, and pregnancy wastage by abortion.

The most serious complication of treatment results from ovarian overstimulation, 'the hyperstimulation syndrome' (Paseto & Montanino, 1964; Neuwirth et al, 1965; Vande Wiele, & Turksoy, 1965; Mozes et al 1965).

The reaction occurs when ovaries respond with the formation of too many follicles and, after administration of hCG, develop ovarian follicular and corpus luteum cysts. Lunenfeld et al (1969) presented a comprehensive classification of the hyperstimulation syndrome into six grades. This was later modified into three grades (WHO, 1976) (Table 27.3).

Grade I includes patients with variable ovarian enlargement and sometimes small cysts. Laboratory findings include urinary oestrogen levels over 150 μg/24h and pregnanediol excretion of over 10 mg/24h. Treatment is not necessary. It is important, however, that patients report back immediately if additional symptoms appear, since severe complications may develop from initially innocent looking disturbances.

Grade II (mild hyperstimulation) comprises patients with distinct ovarian cysts, accompanied by various additional symptoms, such as abdominal distention, nausea, vomiting, and diarrhea. Women with grade II hyperstimulation should be hospitalised and watched carefully. Usually, only symptomatic treatment is required, and the patient may be discharged after several days.

---

* The preparation used was Pergonal.

Table 27.3 Hyperstimulation classification

Laboratory and clinical findings	Adverse reaction					
	Mild				Severe	
	I		II		III	
	I	II	III	IV	V	VI
Excessive steroid production	+	+	+	+	+	+
Ovarian enlargement		+	+	+	+	+
Abdominal discomfort		+	+	+	+	+
Ovarian palpable cysts		?	+	+	+	+
Abdominal distension			+	+	+	+
Nausea			+	+	+	+
Vomiting				+	+	+
Diarrhea				?	+	+
Ascites					+	+
Hydrothorax						+
Severe haemoconcentration					+	
Thromboembolic phenomena						?

* WHO, (1976)
† Lunenfeld et al (1969)

Grade III (severe hyperstimulation) includes patients with large ovarian cysts, ascites and sometimes hydrothorax. The pathogenesis of ovarian hyperstimulation is not entirely clear; part of the syndrome is certainly due to acute hyperoestrogenism and some symptoms are probably a secondary result of abdominal distention and peritoneal irritation. Several facts we have learned empirically may help to explain the syndrome better. Ovarian hyperstimulation is the result of massive luteinisation of the follicles. Clinical symptoms usually appear 5 to 10 days following the first dose of hCG. To provoke hyperstimulation, both HMG and hCG have to be administered; hCG alone, even in large doses, does not lead to severe side-effects. On the other hand, if sufficient endogenous luteinising hormone (LH) is available, HMG not followed by hCG may result in ovarian enlargement, sometimes with cyst formation and ovulation. Hyperstimulation in such cases, however, is extremely rare, because the endogenous feedback mechanism is usually able to prevent massive luteinisation.

Abnormally high levels of ovarian steroids (e.g. oestradiol, oestriol, progesterone, 17 hydroxy progesterone, pregnanediol, pregnanetriol, testosterone, and $\triangle^5$ steroids) have been found. The abnormal hormonal secretion apparently leads to capillary damage and permeability, with loss of fluid from the intravascular compartment, hypovolaemia, haemoconcentration and decreased renal perfusion, together with increased blood viscosity and coagulation abnormalities. Aldosterone production also increases sodium retention.

If not promptly recognised, and treated, the syndrome may be complicated by the occurrence of dangerous thromboembolic phenomena. Ovarian hyperstimulation could be prevented by indomethacin, a blocker of prostaglandins. Thus, Shenker postulated that increased capillary permeability might be due to an excess of prostaglandins secreted by the ovary after gonadotrophin stimulation (Shenker, 1978).

The treatment of severe hyperstimulation syndrome is directed primarily to correction of the disturbed fluid and electrolyte balance. A careful intake/output record should be kept and 5 per cent glucose in water may be administered initially. Diuretic agents should be used with caution, if at all, since the artificially induced diuresis may diminish further the intravascular volume but be unable to cause reduction of the ascites or hydrothorax. Plasma expanders seem to be a much more logical treatment and should be used early. Abdominal pulmonary symptoms may be alleviated or, at least, diminished by puncture and drainage of fluid from the abdominal and/or pleural cavities. Anticoagulant therapy is usually not necessary if the aforementioned steps are employed promptly. Except for torsion or rupture of cysts and internal haemorrhage there is no reason for contemplating laparotomy. The cysts are so large and so extremely brittle that surgery attempted as a palliative procedure will almost certainly end with oophorectomy. In our 20 years experience with gonadotrophin therapy, we have encountered only eight patients with severe hyperstimulation.

The close observation of clinical conditions is useful in preventing, or at least reducing, the incidence of clinical hyperstimulation. The most important hint is the slope of ascent and level of urinary or blood oestrogens. A steep increase of oestrogen, i.e. when for 2 or 3 consecutive days the level of blood oestrogen is more than doubling itself, should be regarded as a serious warning sign, and the decision whether, when, and what dosage hCG should be administered should be carefully evaluated. It has been recommended that whenever urinary oestrogen levels exceed 200 μg/24h or plasma oestrogens are above 1500 pg/ml, the administration of hCG to induce ovulation should be withheld in that treatment cycle (WHO, 1976). We generally adhere to this rule; however, since strict adherence may be overconservative and cause a fall in pregnancy rate, in special cases we have given hCG when oestrogen levels have been up to, but not exceeding 250 μg/24h. Under well-controlled conditions, but prior to the introduction of ultrasonography, the incidence of severe hyperstimulation was less than 2 per cent (Table 27.4).

Ultrasonographic visualisation of follicles may help in deciding whether the oestrogen secretion reflects one or more growing follicles and serve therefore as an additional tool in the monitoring of the therapy. The uniformity of results reported in Table 27.4 may be due to careful selection of patients, based on similar diagnostic criteria and meticulous monitoring of treatment. It is true that only some of the patients who received hCG, despite inappropriate ascent or excessive levels of oestrogen, developed ovarian hyperstimulation. It is however, certain that all

Table 27.4 The incidence of hyperstimulation following gonadotrophin therapy

Authors		No. of treatment cycles	Mild hyperstimulation (%)	Severe hyperstimulation (%)
ADH	(1981)	4008	3.7	0.9
Caspi et al	(1976)	343	6.0	1.2
Ellis & Williamson	(1979)	322	5.0	0.6
Spadoni et al	(1974)	225	4.4	1.8
Thompson & Hansen	(1970)	2798	?	1.3
Lunenfeld et al	(1982)	3646	3.1	0.25
Total		11343	3.4	0.84

women who did develop the syndrome had abnormally high pre-ovulatory oestrogen levels. Only future statistical analyses will demonstrate if the additional use of sonography enables a further reduction in the rate of hyperstimulation or multiple birth.

Pregnancy wastage

A review of the fate of 1048 terminated pregnancies (Table 27.5) showed abortion rates between 12 and 31 per cent. The overall abortion rate in our own material was 25.2 per cent for all pregnancies.

There was no significant difference between patients belonging to group I or II. However, a significant difference in the abortion rate between the first and second pregnancy following HMG/hCG treatment was observed. Whereas it was 28 per cent in the first pregnancy, the abortion rate for the second pregnancy was only 8 per cent. After the first pregnancy following HMG/hCG therapy, 23 patients conceived a second time without any therapy, and of these 13 per cent aborted. A spontaneous abortion rate of 14 per cent in normal pregnancies without ovulation induction has been reported.

Although the factors leading to the relatively high abortion rate following induction of ovulation with HMG/hCG have not been fully elucidated, severe hyperstimulation seems to be at least one factor, since 50 per cent of patients with severe hyperstimulation aborted.

Multiple gestation

The incidence of multiple birth after gonadotrophin therapy is excessive and ranges from 11 to 44 per cent

(Hack et al, 1970; Thomson & Hansen, 1970; Gemzell, 1975). The composition of the diagnostic sample could explain this rather wide range of results, since in our series multiple pregnancy rate in group I was 34 per cent and in group II only 14.3 per cent. In our own series the overall multiple pregnancy rate was 26.6 per cent. Of the 378 terminated pregnancies 13 (3.7 per cent) resulted in triplets, four (1 per cent) in quadruplets, and one quintuplet.

Of terminated pregnancies reported by Bettendorf et al (1981) 113 (69.8 per cent) were single 41 (25.3 per cent) twins, five were triplets (3.1 per cent) and three were quadruplets (1.8 per cent).

Despite the widespread publicity given to this high incidence of multiple deliveries, the multiple births should theoretically be considered as treatment failures rather than as successes, since possible complications may arise. However, a couple treated for several years for primary infertility usually welcome the possibility of twins rather than fear it as a complication. The chance of producing a multiple pregnancy appears to be smaller if urinary oestrogen levels do not exceed 100 μg/24 hrs the day preceding hCG administration (Serr et al, 1975).

The course of pregnancy, mode of delivery, and postnatal development of children born following induction of ovulation with HMG/hCG is being recorded continuously. Apart from the incidence of abortion discussed before, and some obstetric complications due to multiple pregnancy, the course of gestation appeared to be normal. Analysis of the mode of delivery showed a high incidence of interventions, breech extraction, vacuum extraction, forceps delivery and Caesarean sections. The high incidence of obstetric interventions may be explained by the high multiple preg-

Table 27.5 Abortion rate in pregnancies following induction of ovulation with HMG/hCG

Authors		No. of patients	No. of pregnancies	Abortion rate (%)
Bettendorf et al	(1981)	756	239 (9)	21.7
ADH	(1981)	1065	552	14.6
Caspi et al	(1976)	101	62	28
Ellis & Williamson	(1975)	77	43	12
Spadoni et al	(1974)	62	26	31
Lunenfeld et al	(1982)	1107	424 (52)	25.2

nancy rate and primiparity ratios and also in terms of the possible psychological influences involved in delivering a 'premium child' in patients of longstanding infertility.

Sex ratio

The sex ratio (M/F) of the single births was 1.06 (54 per cent boys) and of the twins 0.72 (42 per cent boys). The numbers of triplets were too small to analyse. Caspi et al (1976) reported 32 males and 50 females in the single births (39 per cent boys) with a twin M/F ratio of 0.78.

In the series reported by Bettendorf et al (1981), the incidence of male children in single pregnancies was 51.8 per cent. However, in the above author's series the incidence of male children in twins and triplets was 53.8 per cent and 66.7 per cent respectively.

The normal sex ratio at 28 weeks is considered to be 106 boys to 100 girls (1.06) (Tricomi et al, 1960; Serr & Ismajovich, 1963). This excess birth of boys reflects the interplay between the primary sex ratio and sex differences in early pre-natal mortality. It is known that the number of boys decreased with an increasing number of children at birth. This is regarded as being due to the better survival of the female and an absolute and relative loss of males (Benirshke & Kim, 1973; Nichols, 1952). The sex ratio (M/F) for twins was found by Nicols (1952) to be 1.043 for triplets 1.007 and for quadruplets 0.940. The high incidence of girls in our own twin series and the high incidence of male children in twins and triplets in the series of Bettendorf et al (1981), are probably due to rather small series. However, by combining all the three series, one approaches the expected sex ratios. This indicates clearly the importance of sufficient large numbers in order to estimate sex ratio.

Congenital malformations

During the period until 1970, Hack et al (1970) reported major malformations in four out of 122 infants born. Between 1970 and 1972 (Hack & Lunenfeld, 1979), no major malformations occurred among the 87 infants examined during the neonatal period. Minor malformations included one infant with a malformed kidney and normal intravenous pyelogram, two infants with pre-auricular polyps and one with a functional murmur.

Caspi et al (1976) reported on 157 infants born after gonadotrophin therapy. Four infants were classified as having major malformations: one with a sacrococcygeal teratoma and three infants with a ventricular septal defect, but in two of these infants the diagnosis was clinical only. Eleven children had various minor malformations.

Harlap (1976) presented preliminary data on 66 infants born as a result of HMG/hCG treatment after 28 weeks gestation. One infant had a major malformation and five had minor malformations (ratios of 15.21/1000 and 75.8/1000, respectively). This frequency did not differ significantly from the 10.3/1000 minor and 72.4/1000 major malformations frequencies reported for the population as a whole. The incidence of congenital malformations in normal population has been reported to be 12.7/1000 after 28 weeks gestation, with a range of 3.1–22.5 (Stevenson et al, 1966). There is further rise to 23.1/1000 up to the age of 5 years (McKeown, 1960). Hendricks (1966) reported a rate of 3 per cent in the neonatal period, with twice as many malformations in twin birth, mostly monozygotic twins. The clinical evidence presented here does not indicate that babies born after HMG/hCG ovulation induction are at any greater risk of malformations that the population as a whole.

Post-natal development

It appears that post-natal development of children born after induction of ovulation does not differ from those observed in the control population. Of the girls born, 28 are to date above the age of 10 years. Although this number is too small to reach final conclusions, it seems that their growth rate and pubertal development were similar to that of the control population. Menarche occurred at a mean age of 12, with a range of 10.5–14 years.

Finally, one additional remark should be made in respect to the complications of gonadotrophin therapy. The possibility that the induction of ovulation, and particularly pregnancy, may cause enlargement of previously existing but not diagnosed pituitary tumour should be kept in mind. It has been shown that during pregnancy the pituitary gland undergoes a 'physiological' hypertrophy and increase in size. In a woman with a normal hypophysis, this transient hypertrophy is of no consequence, but in patients harbouring an undiagnosed pituitary tumour, pregnancy may turn the previously silent and innocent lesion into a major catastrophe. Amenorrhoea and the resulting anovulation and infertility may thus be regarded not only as symptoms of a disease but also as signs of adaptation of the organism to reach a certain homeostasis. Gonadotrophic therapy inducing ovarian activity, ovulation and pregnancy can be an effective therapeutic measure but it may also disturb the homeostasis of the hypothalamic-pituitary-ovarian axis, and, for that matter, of the whole body.

This review, which includes the results of our own studies initiated 20 years ago, may serve to delineate criteria for selection of patients, monitoring treatment and assessing the effectiveness of HMG/hCG therapy by considering not only the benefits but also the risks involved.

Acknowledgement

Our deep thanks are due to residents and colleagues, past and present, whose constant help and efforts enabled the 20 years follow-up of gonadotrophic therapy.

This investigation received financial support from the Special Programme of Research, Development and Research Training in Human Reproduction of the World Health Organization.

REFERENCES

Australian Department of Health (ADH) Canberra, Australia 1981 Computer print out, provided by the courtesy of Professor R. Shearman. The Human Pituitary Advisory Committee

Albert A 1956 Human urinary gonadotropin. Recent Progress in Hormone Research, Academic Press, Vol 12, p 227. New York

Benirshke K, Kim C K 1973 Multiple pregnancy. New England Journal of Medicine 288: 1276

Bettendorf G 1966 Ovarian stimulation in hypophysectomized patients by human gonadotropins. Proceedings of the Vth World Congress on Fertility and Sterility. Excerpta Medica International Congress 133: 46

Bettendorf G, Braendle W, Sprotte Ch, Weise Ch, Zimmermann R 1981 Overall results of gonadotropin therapy. In: Insler V, Bettendorf G (eds) Advances in Diagnosis and Treatment of Infertility, p 21. Elsevier/North Holland, Amsterdam

Borth R, Lunenfeld B, de Watteville H 1954 Activite gonadotrope d'un extrait d'urines de femmes en menopause. Experientia 10: 266

Borth R, Lunenfeld B, Riotton G, de Watteville H 1957 Activite gonadotrope d'un extrait des femmes en menopause (2e communication). Experientia 13: 115

Borth R, Lunenfeld B, Menzi A 1961 Pharmacologic and clinical effects of a gonadotropin preparation from human postmenopausal urine. In: Albert A, Thomas M C (eds) Human Pituitary Gonadotropins. p 255. Charles Thomas, Illinois

Butler J K 1970 Oestrone response patterns and clinical results following various pergonal dosage schedules. In: Butler J K, (ed) Development in the Pharmacology and Clinical Uses of Human Gonadotropins, p 42. G D Searle & Co. Ltd, High Wycombe

Butt W R, Kennedy J F 1971 Structure-activity relationships of protein and polypeptide hormones. In: Margoulis M, Greenwood F C (eds) Protein and Polypeptide Hormones, p 115. Excerpta Medica, Amsterdam

Buxton C L, Herrmann W 1961 Induction of ovulation in the human with human gonadotropins (preliminary report). American Journal of Obstetrics and Gynecology 81: 585

Caspi E, Ronen J, Schreyer P, Goldberg M D 1976 Pregnancy and infant outcome after gonadotropin therapy. British Journal of Obstetrics and Gynaecology 83: 967

Crooke A C, Butt W R, Morris R, Palmer R 1962 Pregnancy following treatment with human pituitary follicle stimulating hormone and chorionic gonadotropin. Acta Endocrinologica 67: 132

Crooke A C, Butt W R, Palmer R F, Morris R, Logan R, Anson C J 1963 Clinical trial of human gonadotrophins. I. The effect of pituitary and urinary follicle stimulating hormone and chorionic gonadotropin on patients with idiopathic secondary amenorrhea. Journal of Obstetrics and Gynecology of the British Commonwealth 70: 604

Dor J, Itzkowic D J, Mashiach S, Lunenfeld B, Serr D M 1980 Cumulative conception rates following gonadotropin therapy. American Journal of Obstetric and Gynecology 136: 102

Ellis J D, Williamson J G 1975 Factors influencing the pregnancy and complication rates with human menopausal gonadotrophin therapy. British Journal of Obstetrics and Gynaecology 82: 52

Fiddes J C, Goodman H M 1979 Isolation, Cloning and sequence analysis of the cDNA for the α-subunit of human chorionic gonadotrophin. Nature 281: 351

Gemzell C A 1967 Treatment of sterility with human gonadotropins. In: Marcus S Z, Marcus C C (eds) Advances in Obstetrics and Gynecology. Williams and Wilkins Co. Baltimore, Md. p 386

Gemzell C A, 1975 Induction of ovulation. Acta Obstetrica et Gynecologica Scandinavica (Suppl) 44: 21

Gemzell C A, Diczfalusy E, Tillinger K G 1958 Clinical effect of human pituitary follicle stimulating hormone (FSH). Journal of Clinical Endocrinology and Metabolism 18: 1333

Hack M, Lunenfeld B 1979 The influence of hormone induction of ovulation on the fetus and newborn. Pediatric and Adolescent Endocrinology 5: 191

Hack M, Brish B, Serr D M, Insler V, Lunenfeld B 1970 Outcome of pregnancy after induced ovulation. Follow-up of pregnancies children born after gonadotropin therapy. Journal of American Medical Association 211: 791

Harlap S 1976 Ovulation induction and congenital malformations. Lancet i: 961

Healy D L, Kovacs G T, Pepperell R J, Burger H G 1980 A normal cumulative conception rate after human pituitary gonadotropin. Fertility and Sterility 34: 341

Hendricks C H 1966 Twinning in relation to birthweight. Mortality and congenital malformations. Obstetrics and Gynecology 27: 47

Hussa R O 190 Biosynthesis of human chorionic gonadotropin. Endocrine Reviews 1: 268

Insler V, Melmed H, Mashiach S, Monseliese, Lunenfeld B, Rabau E 1968 A functional classification of patients selected for gonadotropic therapy. Obstetrics and Gynecology 32: 620

Kotz H L, Herrmann W 1961 A review of the endocrine induction of human ovulation. Fertility and Sterility 12: 375

Lamb E J, Cruz A L 1972 Data collection and analysis in an infertility practice. Fertility and Sterility 23: 310

De la Llosa P, Jutisz M 1969 Protein and polypeptide hormones. In: Margoulis M (ed) p 229. Excerpta Medica, Amsterdam

Loraine J A 1956 Bioassay of pituitary and placental gonadotropins in relation to clinical problems in man. Vitamins and Hormones, Academic Press New York 14: 305

Lunenfeld, Insler V 1978 Infertility, Diagnosis and Treatment of Functional Infertility. Grosse Verlag, Berlin

Lunenfeld B, Sulimovici S, Rabau E et al 1962 L'Induction de l'ovulation dans les amenorhees hypophysaires par un traitment combine de gonadotrophines urinaires menopausiques et de gonadotrophines chorioniques. Comptes rendus de la societe Francais de Gynecologie 5: 287

Lunenfeld B, Insler V, Rabau E 1969 Induction de L'ovulation par ler gonadotrophines. In: Moricard R, Ferin J (eds) L'ovulation, Masson & Cie Paris p 291

Lunenfeld B, Insler V, Eshkol A, Birenboim N 1974 Pituitary responsiveness to gonadotrophin releasing hormone. Hormone and Metabolic Research, (Suppl) 5: 184

Lunenfeld B, Eshkol A, Tikotzky D, Serr D M, Mashich S, Oelsner G et al 1982 HMG/hCG therapy of anovulation. In: Van der Molen H, Klopper A, Lunenfeld B, Neves e Castro M, Sciarra F, Vermeulen A (eds) Hormonal Factors in Fertility, Infertility and Contraception p 259. Excerpta Medica

McKeown T 1960 Malformations in a population observed for 5 years. Ciba Foundation Symposium on Congenital Malformations, p 2. J & A Churchill, London

Mozes M, Bogokowsky H, Antebi E, Lunenfeld B, Rabau E, Serr D M et al 1965 Thromboembolic phenomena after ovarian stimulation with human gonadotrophins. Lancet ii: 1213

Netter A, Bellaisch J 1962 In: Beclere C (ed) Les Gonadotropines en Gynecologie p 197. Masson et Cie, Paris

Neuwirth R S, Turksoy R N, Vande & Viele R L 1965 Acute Meigs' Syndrome secondary to ovarian stimulation with menopausal gonadotropins. American Journal of Obstetrics and Gynecology 91: 977

Nichols J B 1952 Statistics of births in the USA, 1915–1948. American Journal of Obstetrics and Gynecology 64: 376

Nitschke-Dabelstein S, Hackeloer B J, Sturm G 1981 Die bedeutung endokrinologischer und klinischer parameter fuer die beurteilung der follikelreifung, ovulation und corpus luteum Gildung inter beruecksichtigung de im ultra-schall darstellbaren strukturveraenderungen des follikel-tragenden ovaras (thesis). Phillips University of Marburg, Department of Obstetrics and Gynecology

Pasetto N, Montanino G 1964 Human urinary gonadotropins (HMG and HCG) in the therapy of amenorrhea. Minerva Gynecology 16: 377

Rosemberg E, Coleman J, Damany M, Garcia C R 1963 Clinical effect of human urinary postmenopausal gonadotropin. Journal of Clinical Endocrinology and Metabolism 23: 181

Schwartz M, Jewelewicz R, Dyrenfurth I, Tropper P, Vande Wiele R L 1980 The use of human menopausal and chorionic gonadotropins for induction of ovulation. Sixteen years' experience at the Sloane Hospital for Women. American Journal of Obstetrics and Gynecology 138: 801

Serr D M, Ismajovich B 1963 Determination of the primary sex ratio for human abortions. American Journal of Obstetrics and Gynecology 87: 63

Serr D M, Homburg R, Blankstein J, Lunenfeld B, Snyder W, Insler V 1975 Multiple pregnancy following gonadotropin therapy. 'Abstract' European Society for the Study of Sterility, Madrid.

Shearman R P 1966 Induction of ovulation. Australasian Annals of Medicine 15: 266

Shenker J Y 1978 Ovarian hyperstimulation syndrome. In: Hafes E S E (ed) Human Ovulation: Mechanisms, Prediction, Detection and Induction, p 32. North-Holland, Amsterdam

Spadoni L R, Cox D W, Smith D C 1974 Use of human menopausal gonadotropin for the induction of ovulation. American Journal of Obstetrics and Gynecology 120: 988

Smith P E 1926 Hastening development of female genital system by daily hemoplastic pituitary transplants. Proceedings of the Society for Experimental Biology and Medicine 24: 131

Smith P E, Engle E T 1927 Experimental evidence regarding role of anterior pituitary in development and regulation of genital system. American Journal of Anatomy 40: 159

Stevenson A C 1966 Congenital malformations: a report of a study of a series of consecutive births in 24 centres. Bulletin of the World Health Organization 334: 14

Thompson L R, Hansen L M 1970 Pergonal (menotropins): a summary of clinical experience in the induction of ovulation and pregnancy. Fertility and Sterility 21: 844

Tricomi V, Serr D M, Solish G 1960 The ratio of male and female embryo as determined by the sex chromatin. American Journal of Obstetrics and Gynecology 79: 504

Tsapoulis A D, Zourlaz P A, Comninos A C 1978 Observations on 320 infertile patients treated with human gonadotropins (human menopausal gonadotropin/human chorionic gonadotropin). Fertility and Sterility 29: 492

Vande Wiele R L, Turksoy R N 1965 The use of human menopausal and chorionic gonadotropins in patients with infertility due to ovulatory failure. American Journal of Obstetrics and Gynecology 93: 632

WHO Scientific Group Report 1976 Agent stimulating gonadal function in the human. World Health Organization, Technical Report Series Number 514

Zondek B 1926a Ueber die funktion des ovariums. Deutsche Medizinische Wochenschrift, 18: 343

Zondek B 1926b Ueber die funktion des ovariums. Zeitschreft fur Geburtschilde und Gynaekologie 90: 372

Zondek B, Aschheim S 1927 Das hormon des hypophysenvoderlappens; testobject zum nachweis des hormons. Klinische Wochenschrift 6: 248

Zondek B, Sulman F 1945 Mechanism of action and metabolism of gonadotropic hormones in organism. Vitamins and Hormones 3: 297

In vitro fertilisation and embryo transfer

INTRODUCTION

The birth of a baby after the laparoscopic aspiration of an oocyte, *in vitro* fertilisation (IVF), and the subsequent transfer of the embryo (ET) (Steptoe & Edwards, 1978), was an event of both great sensational interest and scientific importance, as it showed that the treatment of infertility by this technique could become a reality.

The first documented pregnancy after IVF was a tubal ectopic pregnancy reported by Steptoe & Edwards (1976). This had confirmed that human embryos fertilized and cultured *in vitro* were capable of implantation. At this time it was not known whether viable offspring could be produced by IVF and ET and it took a further 2 years to demonstrate this. The very rapid advance of the technique and application to treatment of infertility in the last few years has been reviewed by Trounson & Conti (1982).

MAJOR DEVELOPMENTS IN IVF TECHNOLOGY

The methodology of recovery of human oocytes, their *in vitro* fertilisation and culture had been under close investigation since the late 1960s.

Initially the ovary was exposed at laparotomy and the oocytes identified by examination of follicular aspirates (Edwards, 1965; Morgenstern & Soupart, 1972; Lopata et al, 1974). Other methods used for obtaining oocytes included mincing the excised ovary (Jacobsen et al, 1970), dissecting the intact follicle prior to puncture, excising the ovary or an ovarian wedge, and dissecting follicles under the microscope.

These procedures required major surgery, caused extensive damage to the ovary and their application was therefore rather limited. The development of gynaecological laparoscopy was a major advance in oocyte recovery and it became possible to aspirate ovarian follicles with minimal invasive surgery and relative safety. It also enabled repeated attempts at oocyte collection in the same patient.

Steptoe & Edwards (1970) reported their experience of laparoscopy in 49 patients resulting in 118 oocytes. They also introduced the classification of pre-ovulatory, non-ovulatory and atretic oocytes based on microscopic evaluation.

The basic technical procedures for the fertilisation and culture of human embryos were described by the British researchers (Steptoe & Edwards, 1970; Edwards, 1973; Edwards & Steptoe, 1975). The utilisation of these experimental techniques resulted in a transient pregnancy in Melbourne in 1973 (de Kretser et al, 1973) and a tubal pregnancy by Steptoe & Edwards (1976). Studies on the fertilisation of human oocytes were also being carried out by groups in North America (Morgenstern & Soupart, 1972; Soupart & Strong, 1974).

Collection of oocytes in monovular species is normally carried out after superovulation with gonadotrophins. Similarly, most of the early work in the human was performed after superovulation with clomiphene citrate or gonadotrophins (Steptoe & Edwards, 1970; Talbot et al, 1976; Lopata et al, 1978). In 1977 Steptoe & Edwards began the recovery of a single mature oocyte developing during the natural ovulatory cycle. Using the unstimulated cycle and relying on the spontaneous surge of luteinising hormone (LH), four intra-uterine pregnancies were established (Steptoe et al, 1980). This success was reproduced by the Australian group using spontaneous ovulation in the natural cycle (Lopata et al, 1980). It was felt that the stimulated ovulatory cycle with controlled ovulation may provide too many difficulties to establish the correct endocrine situation and to sustain a normal pregnancy. However, hormonally controlled cycles have clinical and physiological advantages over the spontaneous ovulatory cycle and as shown by Trounson et al (1981a, b), pregnancies may be achieved by IVF in cycles controlled with clomiphene citrate and hCG. This report demonstrated unequivocally that it was feasible to use hormones to stimulate follicular development and to control the time of ovulation. This procedure with minor modifications has been adopted almost universally for IVF.

SELECTION OF PATIENTS

The criteria for selection of patients for IVF have been comprehensively reviewed by Trounson & Wood (1981) and Wood & Trounson (1982). Prior to the establishment of IVF as a clinical procedure, treatment of damaged or non-functional Fallopian tubes was limited to surgical repair. However, success rates of surgery in terms of live births have been low (Siegler, 1960; Winston, 1981) and even with the use of microsurgical techniques, the treatment of fimbrial occlusion, which is the most common and most intractable tubal problem, has a pregnancy rate of less than 25 per cent. In a review evaluating the place of tubal surgery and IVF, Camus & Trounson (1982) concluded that IVF was likely to replace surgery as the treatment for tubal infertility except for cases of sterilisation reversal.

Other approaches to the cure of tubal infertility include ovarian implantation, either as a pedicle or a free graft into or continuous with the cavity of the uterus (Estes & Heitmeyer, 1934), tubal transplantation (Wood et al, 1976) and the replacement of tubes by an artificial graft (Wood et al, 1971). However only the first of these approaches has resulted in term pregnancies, and then only infrequently (Adams, 1979).

IVF may also be appropriate for patients with unexplained (idiopathic) infertility. This group may account for up to 15 per cent of couples attending an infertility clinic (Kovacs, 1979). Possible explanations for this syndrome would include fertilisation failure, early embryonic death, or the failure of implantation through genetic or physiological mechanisms. IVF and embryo culture was thought to be a useful method for diagnosing problems of fertilisation and early embryonic development (Wood & Trounson, 1982). An initial study comparing results for patients with unexplained infertility with tubal infertility, suggested that failure of or abnormal fertilisation may have contributed to infertility (Trounson et al, 1980a). However, further investigation of couples with idiopathic infertility suggested that IVF and ET is also a useful therapeutic method as well as a diagnostic test. Pregnancy rate following IVF in patients with idiopathic infertility is similar to that for patients with tubal infertility (Trounson et al, 1981b; Camus & Trounson, 1982). Recent results comparing the two groups are shown in Fig. 28.1. Idiopathic infertility is now an accepted condition for inclusion into IVF programmes and these patients are now treated in many other clinics besides our own.

The lower limit for sperm concentration in semen usually accepted for normal fertility is about 15 to 20 million per ml (Hudson et al, 1980), and the chance of a man with a sperm concentration of less than 5 million per ml producing pregnancy is 10 per cent per annum (Baker, 1982, unpublished data). For IVF as little as 10 000 to 50 000 motile spermatozoa per ml are required, although there must be a high proportion of morphologically normal

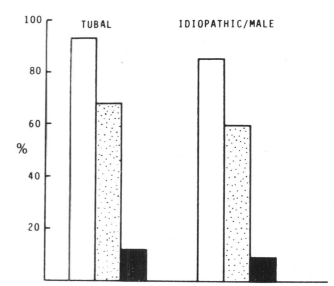

Fig. 28.1 Comparison of outcome between tubal and idiopathic infertility patients. Oocytes recovered (open columns); embryos developed (stippled columns); pregnancies <9 weeks (solid columns)

spermatozoa with forward progressive motility. It is possible that in cases of severe oligospermia there may be sufficient motile spermatozoa for IVF, although the chance of producing pregnancy in vivo is minimal. In our experience the use of oligospermic semen reduces fertilisation rate although fertilisation and early embryonic development may be achieved with very low semen concentration (<2 million per ml). Further research is necessary to determine the extent to which IVF may be used to treat various forms of male infertility.

Another area of infertility where current diagnosis and therapy are disappointing is the hostile cervical factor (Kovacs & Burger, 1982). IVF and ET could be used to bypass the potential problem if cervical hostility is suspected.

Potential therapeutic roles of IVF in the future may include the treatment of infertility due to non-functional or inaccessible ovaries and infertility due to an absent or non-functional uterus (Trounson, 1982b). In the former an oocyte could be donated by a donor which could be inseminated by the husband's spermatozoa in vitro and the developing embryo transferred to the infertile recipient. In the case of absent or non-functional ovaries, exogenous steroid replacement would be necessary. In the case of an absent uterus, oocytes recovered from the patient could be fertilised in vitro and the embryos transferred to a surrogate mother for the period of pregnancy.

ASSESSMENT OF PATIENTS

Before couples can be included in the IVF programme they have to fulfil a number of criteria. The female partner must be physically fit to carry a resultant pregnancy and have no medical contraindications to the surgical procedures involved. At present laparoscopy under general anaesthesia is normal for oocyte collection although oocyte recovery may be performed under local or regional anaesthesia. Follicles may also be aspirated under ultrasonic guidance rather than under laparoscopic vision (Lenz et al, 1981). Obesity and previous abdominal operations make oocyte collection more difficult and more hazardous.

It has previously been considered that the woman must be ovulating spontaneously, but with the routine use of clomiphene and hMG for IVF in the stimulated cycle, this is no longer essential. It suffices that the patient should be able to respond to ovulation induction.

To recover oocytes by laparoscopy for IVF the woman's ovaries need to be accessible. Before including women in the programme it is important to ensure that this is the case, especially if they have had previous pelvic surgery. If the ovaries are obscured by adhesions, preliminary laparotomy and ovariolysis may need to be performed. Impeccable operative techniques especially with regards to haemostasis and tissue handling should be observed to minimise the chance of recurrence of adhesions. Ovariopexy, with fixing of the ovary to the uterine cornu or round ligament is often undertaken, but it is important not to restrict ovarian mobility as this will make manipulation at oocyte collection more difficult. In difficult cases, relaparoscopy may be indicated prior to inclusion in the programme. With the numerous difficulties involved with each stage of the programme, and the high chance of failure, prospective couples need to be well informed before deciding to enter the programme.

Finally, the woman must have a uterus capable of accepting and harbouring a pregnancy to term. It is also important that the cervix can be negotiated by the transfer catheter, which is routinely performed without anaesthesia. If difficulty is experienced in negotiating the cervical canal regional anaesthesia may be used. However pregnancies are usually associated with easy passage of the transfer catheter (Wood et al, 1981a; Leeton et al, 1982). An alternate route for embryo transfer is through the fundus. At present this has only been performed under direct laparoscopic vision requiring repeated anaesthesia, but other simple modifications are under investigation.

TREATMENT OF PATIENTS FOR IVF

While patients are on the waiting list their rubella status is ascertained and if necessary, they are immunised. They also record the commencement of each of their menstrual cycles for at least 6 months to enable the 95 per cent confidence interval to be calculated for the day of the spontaneous LH surge (McIntosh et al, 1980). This interval is used to assist the decisions for admitting the patient to hospital, urine sampling for the LH surge and administration of hCG to control the final stages of follicular and

oocyte maturation (Trounson et al, 1983; Trounson, 1982b).

Methods for patient treatment

Basically three types of treatment may be offered to patients for IVF (Table 28.1). In the natural cycle no ovarian stimulation is given and the spontaneous LH surge is detected by urine or plasma sampling at 3–6 hourly intervals. For the stimulated cycle, clomiphene and/or human menopausal gonadotrophin (hMG) is given to stimulate multiple follicular development but the spontaneous LH surge is detected in plasma or urine. If hMG is used alone it may be necessary to administer hCG because the spontaneous LH surge may be inhibited. In this circumstance, follicular oestrogen secretion falls and follicular atresia is initiated. This may also occur in some patients treated with clomiphene. The controlled cycle requires administration of human chorionic gonadotrophin (hCG) at the optimum stage of follicular maturation as judged by follicular growth monitors (Table 28.1). The advantages

Table 28.1 Methods for the treatment of patients for IVF

	Natural	Stimulated	Controlled
Ovarian stimulation	Not applicable	Clomiphene Human menopausal gonadotrophin (hMG) Clomiphene with hMG	Administration of hCG (3000–5000 iu) Laparoscopy 32–36 h after hCG injection
Follicular growth monitors	Day of menstrual cycle (95% confidence limits for LH release) Urinary or plasma oestrogen levels (daily) Ultrasonic assessment of follicular size (2–3 days apart) Cervical mucus score Plasma progesterone (to confirm suspected ovulation)		
Decision for oocyte recovery	Spontaenous LH surge (3 hourly urine or plasma samples) Laparoscopy 21–28 h after start of LH surge		

Table 28.2   Advantages of the stimulated cycle

Several follicles available for aspiration
A larger number of mature oocytes obtained
Increased number of embryos available for transfer
Might be higher success rate per cycle of treatment (Trounson et al, 1981b)
Increased rate of pregnancy if two or more embryos transferred
If one follicle has ovulated others are still available for aspiration
High levels of oestrogen — easier to detect and interpret (Trounson, 1982a)
Multiple births — family can be completed with one successful treatment
If both ovaries are not totally accessible, there is still a chance of collecting oocytes
Possibility of cryopreservation of excess embryos to implant in subsequent cycles without need for further laparoscopy

---

Table 28.3   Disadvantages of stimulated cycle

Hormone levels are more difficult to interpret as they vary with the number of follicles maturing
Ultrasonic scaning to assess the number of developing follicles is usually mandatory
Hormonal environment is abnormal
Defective luteal phase more common (Edwards et al, 1980a)
Conception rate in cycles which are clomiphene induced are lower than in spontaneous cycles (Edwards, 1981)
Variable rate of growth and development of multiple follicles, but all have to be aspirated simultaneously
Some patients fail to respond to clomiphene
It has been postulated that more abnormal oocytes may be collected
Multiple pregnancy may result with increased risk of abnormality, premature labour and complication of pregnancy
Risk of hyperstimulation

Table 28.4   Advantages and disadvantages of the spontaneous cycle

---

Advantages
Responsible for early term pregnancies (Steptoe & Edwards, 1978; Lopata et al, 1980)
Provides natural hormonal environment for embryo transfer

Disadvantages
Only one follicle available for aspiration therefore there is an absolute necessity to recover the only oocyte
Lower chance of success at every step of the process
Both ovaries must be totally accessible so that follicle is not hidden

---

Table 28.5   Advantages and disadvantages of controlled ovulation

---

Advantages
Laparoscopy can be programmed at a time convenient to the IVF team
Better utilisation of resources by appropriate timing and reduction of night work
Reduces patient anxiety as operation can be planned for in advance
Shorter hospital stay
Fewer hormone assays
Injection to laparoscopy time very precise
36 Hours notice for laparoscopy

Disadvantages
Difficulty of predicting the optimum time for hCG administration
The time of hCG administration may not be appropriate for all the pre-ovulatory follicles

---

Table 28.6   Advantages and disadvantages of spontaneous ovulation

---

Advantages
Natural hormonal environment
Better maturity, the LH rise is in response to maturation of the oocyte

Disadvantages
Oocyte pickup depends on determining the LH rise appropriately
Multiple sampling and assays required 24 h a day
Difficulty of defining the commencement of the LH rise
Laparoscopy needs to be performed at fairly short notice, sometimes as little as 8 h

---

and disadvantages of the three methods of treatment for IVF are shown in Tables 28.2, 28.3, 28.4, 28.5 & 28.6.

Initial studies suggest that the stimulated or controlled cycles have a higher success rate, whether expressed as oocytes collected, embryos transferred or pregnancies obtained (Trounson et al, 1981a; Johnston et al, 1981).

As stimulated and controlled cycles are easier to manage and they appear to be at least as effective as natural cycles, our unit has used them exclusively since 1981. It is also our aim to administer hCG so that laparoscopy can be timed electively, 26–37 hours after the injection. About 20 per cent of patients normally have a spontaneous LH rise before the hCG is administered. For this reason checking of urinary LH excretion is performed in all patients admitted to hospital. Should there be a natural LH rise, laparoscopy is timed 21 to 28 hours after the onset of the rise.

Ovarian stimulation

Having decided that the stimulated cycle is the treatment of choice, the dose of clomiphene used was investigated. After examination of a number of dose levels and regimes, 150 mg given daily from the fifth to the ninth day of the cycle was found to be most suitable (Trounson, 1983). The use of lower doses of 50 mg or 100 mg per day, or administration for 5 days earlier in the cycle produced no better results. Some patients do not respond to the routine 5-day course of clomiphene and it has been suggested that prolonged administration for as long as 10 days might be helpful. However, this will also prolong the anti-oestrogenic effects of clomiphene, which may decrease uterine receptivity for embryo implantation. This unfavourable effect on the uterine endometrium was reported by Garcia et al (1977) in 50 per cent of women treated with clomiphene and was associated with an increased spontaneous abortion rate.

In contrast this increased rate of abortion has not been observed with gonadotrophin-induced pregnancies. The rate of conception is higher in women stimulated with gonadatrophin (one in three ovulatory cycles: Kovacs et al, 1982) than in clomiphene induced ovulation (one in eight cycles: Edwards, 1981).

A trial of hMG for follicular stimulation has been

undertaken and pregnancies have been obtained by this method. One disadvantage of hMG is the increased cost and thus a combination of clomiphene and hMG has also been investigated again resulting in pregnancies (Trounson, 1982c).

However, there are dangers of hyperstimulation when regularly cycling women are given hMG. There is the risk that the resultant endocrinological environment may not support a pregnancy, and there is the risk of hyperstimulation syndrome. It is our experience that when excessive hyperstimulation results in a large number of follicles, pregnancy is not initiated. There is also danger to the patient with hyperstimulation syndrome resulting in abdominal discomfort, ascites, pleural effusion, and thromboembolic phenomena (Mozes et al, 1965). These iatrogenic complications have resulted in several deaths (Schenker & Polishuk, 1975). One of our patients needed hospitalisation with 'Meigs-like Syndrome' following stimulation with 225–300 in hMG daily, but recovered spontaneously after several days. In Australia, the use of gonadotrophins for ovulation has been strictly controlled by the Human Pituitary Advisory Committee (Cox, 1976). This has resulted in very high standards, and minimisation of complications. It would be a pity if such standards of excellence were discarded because of indiscriminate use of gonadotrophins for IVF.

Monitoring ovarian stimulation

As parameters of follicular development can vary from patient to patient and cycle to cycle, the system for monitoring approaching ovulation should use several indicators. These may include: statistical prediction of the day of the LH surge, determined on the basis of previous menstrual cycle lengths (McIntosh et al, 1980); the temperature chart; changes in the cervical mucus score; plasma or urinary oestrogen levels; ultrasonic determination of follicular size; detection of the LH surge and plasma progesterone determinations.

Although statistical prediction of the day of expected LH rise is a useful adjunct to the detection of ovulation in the spontaneous cycle (McIntosh et al, 1980), its accuracy of prediction in the stimulated ovulatory cycle is yet to be fully evaluated.

The usefulness of the temperature chart is rather limited, although the pre-ovulatory nadir or post-ovulatory rise in temperature can act as a warning to check hormone results.

Changes in cervical mucus (Kovacs & Burger, 1982) are an indicator of follicular development, and its usefulness for timing ovulation has been clearly demonstrated in the practise of artificial donor insemination (Kovacs & Lording, 1980). Cervical mucus score usually begins to increase about 5 days before the LH surge, is maximal the day before, and falls sharply on the day of the LH surge

(Trounson, 1983). The test is quick, cheap and non-invasive and may be used to assist in decision making in both stimulated and natural cycles.

The precise timing of the LH surge or hCG injection may be more easily determined by examining sequential plasma or urinary oestrogen levels (Trounson et al, 1982a, Trounson, 1983). Estimation of oestrogen secretion has always been an important parameter for assessing follicular maturation (de Kretser et al, 1973; Lopata et al, 1978; Steptoe et al, 1980, Trounson, 1982b). Oestrogen levels may be determined in 24 hr urine collections by the established method of Brown et al (1968) or modifications of this procedure. More rapid determination of oestrogen levels which may be more appropriate for prospective treatments such as those involved in IVF include the radioimmunoassay for urinary oestrone-3 — glucuronide, which is very satisfactory for clinical practice (Kovacs et al, 1982), and the rapid radioimmunoassay for plasma oestradiol-17β(E_2) (Trounson 1983; Trounson et al, 1982a). Although IVF pregnancies have been obtained by the use of simple monitors such as cervical mucus changes and the assessment of follicular size by ultrasound (Trounson et al, 1981a), the success rate of IVF is improved dramatically if oestrogen assays are also incorporated into the protocol. (Trounson, 1983; Trounson et al, 1982a).

Follicular oestrogen is intimately involved with priming the hypothalamo-pituitary axis for the LH surge, with maturation of the oocyte, and for granulosa cell integrity and function. It is essential that oestrogen secretion continuously increases over the 5–7 days prior to the LH surge (Fig. 28.2). The critical nature of high levels of E_2 for the success of IVF has been clearly demonstrated in the studies of Carson et al (1982). Analysis of follicular fluid collected at the time of oocyte recovery showed that oocytes from the follicle with the highest oestrogen concentration are most likely to develop to normal fetuses after IVF and ET. In fact this appears to be the most significant single factor associated with successful IVF that has been identified to date (Trounson, 1982d). According to Carson et al (1982) 90 per cent of oocytes which fertilise and develop to fetuses have concentrations of E_2 7nmol/ml or more, compared with only 30 per cent of oocytes which fail to continue development after ET. These data show it is essential that follicles receive the LH or hCG stimulus for the final phase of maturation when oestrogen secretion is maximal. Treatment of patients for IVF must allow for the continued growth and development of follicles, particularly the capacity for continued oestrogen secretion. Loss of this functional capacity could indicate the onset of follicular atresia and a consequent reduction of oocyte viability. Abnormalities of oestrogen secretion, such as the absence of a steady rise, or a fall in oestrogen without any obvious LH surge, are indicative of an abnormal follicular condition and IVF should not be contemplated under such circumstances. Some patients may not respond to clomi-

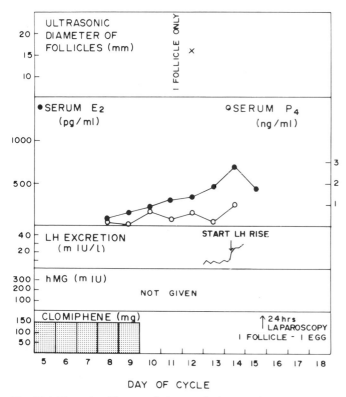

Fig. 28.2 Example of hormonal changes during a typical treatment cycle

phene and it may be more appropriate to use hMG in such cases.

Unfortunately, even in unstimulated cycles the absolute level of oestrogen secretion shows such variation that it cannot be used to predict the day of ovulation. Edwards et al (1980b) reported on 35 patients undergoing IVF in the natural cycle and found total urinary oestrogen levels varying between 18 and 70 μg/day on the day prior to and 27 and 112 μg/day on the day of the LH rise. Following ovarian stimulation with clomiphene or hMG a number of developing follicles will make varying contribution to the circulating oestrogen pool. Unless the number of follicles can be determined by ultrasound, it is extremely difficult to predict the exact level to which plasma or urinary oestrogen levels will rise.

The normal procedure used for management of ovarian stimulation in our own IVF programme has been described in detail previously (Trounson et al, 1982a; Trounson, 1982a, b).

Blood sampling for plasma E_2 usually commences on the eighth day of the menstrual cycle and an initial ultrasound examination is performed when plasma E_2 concentrations begin increasing to about 500 pg/ml. If the average diameter of the largest follicle is less than 1.4 cm a second ultrasound is done 2 or 3 days later. If E_2 levels increase above 1 ng/ml or the largest follicle exceeds 1.7 cm (Fig. 28.2), three hourly urine specimens are collected to detect a spontaneous LH surge (Trounson et al, 1980b; Trounson, 1983).

The use of diagnostic ovarian ultrasound to measure the number of follicles present and their size has been valuable in the diagnosis of ovulation (Renaud et al, 1980) and for ovulation induction with gonadotrophins (Kovacs et al, 1982). However, the accuracy of assessment of the number and size of the follicles is limited by pelvic adhesions, endometriosis, distortion of ovarian position and shape, the presence of hydrosalpinges, obesity, position of the bowel, the quality of equipment and the experience of the operator. The ultrasonic examination can be enhanced by distension of the bladder.

Follicular diameter may not be indicative of follicular function because the largest follicles following ovarian stimulation may not be the most oestrogenic and may even be atretic. For this reason it is not possible to use ultrasound alone to determine the time of hCG administration.

There is also theoretical concern of possible harmful effects of the energy transmitted to the genetic material in the oocyte at the time of examination. However the Bio Effects Committee of the American Institute of Ultrasonic Medicine advised that machines currently used in clinical practice would emit such a low dose of energy, that deleterious effects on the genetic constitution of the oocyte would be most unlikely.

Even with these reservations in mind the use of ovarian ultrasound is important in the stimulated cycle, as only by determining the number of preovulatory follicles can hormone levels be adequately interpreted. The ultrasound information on the size and position of follicles is of value at the time of laparoscopy for oocyte collection, particularly when ovaries are partially obscured.

The spontaneous LH surge

All successful IVF programmes have centered their attention on the detection of the LH peak (Edwards et al, 1980a; Trounson et al, 1981a), for the accurate prediction of the time of ovulation. If laparoscopy is performed after ovulation has taken place, there is little chance of recovering the oocyte. If the collection of the oocyte preceeds ovulation by more than 6 hours, it is unlikely that normal fertilisation will result, although recent experience with maturing oocytes in vitro prior to insemination may make timing of oocyte recovery less critical (Trounson et al, 1982b).

LH can be assayed in urine either by haemagglutination assay (Higonavis, Mochila Pharmaceuticals, Tokyo, Japan), or by rapid radioimmunoassay (Trounson et al, 1980b). Whichever assay is used, it must be sensitive, accurate, rapid and reliable.

Although either blood (Testart et al, 1981) or urine samples can be used for the detection of the LH surge, as frequent repeated sampling (3–6 hourly) is required, most patients prefer urine samples. For the urinary assay to be interpreted accurately, urinary excretion should be limited to 100–200 ml per 3 hours by the control of fluid intake.

In our experience twice daily assay of 3-hourly urine samples for LH can predict the time of ovulation accurately and enable laparoscopic recovery of mature preovulatory oocytes for IVF. Sampling of urine over longer periods of time may result in mis-timing of ovulation, with an increased rate of ovulation before laparoscopy, or the aspiration of immature oocytes which reduce rates of fertilisation or increase abnormalities of fertilisation and early embryonic development.

Plasma progesterone concentrations begin to rise at the same time as the spontaneous LH surge in naturally cycling women (Trounson et al, 1980b; Trounson, 1983) and may begin to increase 24 hours prior to the LH surge in stimulated cycles (Trounson, 1982c). Elevation of plasma progesterone usually indicates that a spontaneous LH surge will occur within the next 24 hours (Fig. 28.2). There is often a failure of plasma progesterone levels to rise or for the rise to be maintained in patients where oocytes fail to fertilise or develop abnormally (Trounson, 1983).

Plasma progesterone determinations may also be used to confirm suspected ovulation or spontaneous luteinisation of follicles (Trounson, 1982c).

Now that hCG is used to control the time of ovulation, the main role for LH determination is to ensure that a spontaneous rise has not commenced before the decision to administer hCG has been made. In about 20 per cent of our patients the rise in LH will preceed the hCG injection (Wood & Kovacs, 1983). If an LH rise is detected, laparoscopy is timed 21–28 hours after the mid-point of the first urine sample which showed elevated levels of LH (Trounson & Wood, 1981; Trounson, 1983). It is sometimes difficult to determine the exact sample with the first elevated LH level. This decision is made statistically by calculating the mean of all previous baseline levels, then adding two standard deviations. The LH surge is confirmed by three consecutive samples above the mean plus two standard deviations (Trounson & Wood, 1981).

Administration of hCG

In the majority of patients (>80 per cent) ovulation can be controlled by the administration of hCG (4000 iu Pregnyl, Organon). The decision to administer hCG is made on the basis of the day of the menstrual cycle, absolute levels and changes in the levels of oestrodial 17β, follicular size and number from ultrasonic examinations and cervical mucus score (Trounson, 1983; Trounson & Conti, 1982).

E_2 levels often plateau as the follicle approaches maturity. If only a single follicle is present this plateau is usually in the range of 500–800 pg E_2 per ml plasma. If multiple follicles are present, it is appropriate to consider that follicular maturation may be complete when plasma E_2 levels approach about 500 pg/ml for each large follicle present.

The cervical mucus score should be in agreement with the rising oestrogen levels and the score of 10–12 out of 12 is expected at the time when hCG is administered (Trounson, 1983).

The ultrasonic scan should confirm that there are one or more follicles of at least 1.9 cm in diameter. If the follicles are smaller than this, hCG is delayed until the follicles are estimated to be pre-ovulatory in size (> or = 19 mm diameter). In our experience, follicles grow at the rate of 1.4–1.6 mm per 24 hours during the 3–6 days before the spontaneous LH surge.

It is also important that urinary LH levels have not risen from the baseline at the time that hCG is administered. If an LH rise has taken place, hCG is withheld and laparoscopy is timed as discussed previously. In patients with no indication of a spontaneous LH surge, laparoscopy is timed for 28–36 hours after the hCG injection.

OOCYTE RECOVERY

The aspiration apparatus and techniques used for oocyte collection in our own group have been reported previously (Renou et al, 1981; Wood et al, 1981b).

The apparatus

Since Steptoe & Edwards (1970) first described their oocyte recovery equipment the principles have not changed. A needle is inserted into the follicle and the follicular contents aspirated under negative pressure. The vacuum can be supplied manually such as described by Morgenstern & Soupart (1972) or by controlled suction (Lopata et al, 1974). Using these techniques of collection, oocyte recovery rates were consistently below 50 per cent. Steptoe & Edwards (1970) reported that 33 per cent of oocytes were recovered and rates up to 46 per cent were reported by Lopata et al (1974). Although our group obtained a recovery rate of 81 per cent with the original apparatus (Trounson et al, 1980a), in a programme to maximise the yield at each stage of the IVF procedure, an improved system was designed (Renou et al, 1981).

The aspiration apparatus was designed specifically taking into consideration the following factors:–
1. Size of oocyte and cumulus mass.
2. A minimum of fluid dead space.
3. Maximum velocity of fluid flow.
4. Minimum of friction.
5. Non-turbulent continuous flow with the elimination of joins where oocytes should become trapped.

These aims were achieved by using a stainless steel needle 23 cm in length with an external diameter of 2.1 mm and an internal diameter 1.6 mm. The needle is lined by Teflon tubing resulting in an internal diameter of 1.0 mm. The length of the tubing is 52 cm and it is continuous from the sharp bevel, along the needle and through a silicone rubber bung into a 5 ml or 10 ml tissue culture tube. The total fluid dead space within the needle and its tubing is only 1.2 ml. An 18 gauge needle also perforates the rubber bung and is connected to a suction pump operated by a foot pump. The oocyte recovery rate using the modified collecting system is consistently in excess of 85 per cent.

Laparoscopy technique

Laparoscopies are normally all performed under general anaesthesia, although the possibility of regional or local anaesthesia is being explored. The surgical technique is the same as diagnostic laparoscopy except that a third puncture is performed with a trocar and cannula under laparoscopic vision, aiming for the follicles that are to be aspirated. Special care also has to be taken to avoid the bowel as many of these patients have undergone previous surgery. As carbon dioxide is potentially less dangerous to the patient should an embolism occur, this is used in preference to a nitrogen mixture (nitrogen 90 per cent, oxygen 5 per cent, carbon dioxide 5 per cent; Edwards et al, 1980a; Lopata et al, 1980). Other workers advocate the use of the nitrogen mixture because this is more physiological and is the gas used for embryo culture. In our experience with careful surgical technique in obtaining an airtight fit within the follicle, carbon dioxide can be used without any deleterious effect on oocytes (Trounson, 1982b). Pregnancies have been obtained after prolonged exposure of the ovaries to carbon dioxide after recovery of oocytes from ovulated follicles and in free fluid within the Pouch of Douglas (Wood et al, 1981a; Trounson, 1982b). Because of its increased safety we advocate the use of carbon dioxide as the gas of choice for insufflation of the peritoneal cavity.

Further difficulties are sometimes experienced due to the presence of omentum or adhesions overlying the ovary. These can often be dealt with by diathermy or laparoscopic scissors. Ovarian manipulation is carried out by grasping the ovarian ligament, and gently elevating it so that its total surface can be inspected. Extra difficulty may be experienced if the patient is obese or if there has been previous surgery distorting the anatomy, or if there are adhesions. Uterine manipulation is strongly discouraged and no instrument should be placed inside the uterine cavity as this may disturb the endometrial lining for subsequent implantation. Gentle manipulation of the uterus was undertaken in the early days, but with more experience with surgical technique, this is rarely necessary. Before aspiration is attempted, the suction apparatus is tested with culture medium. It is imperative that the suction apparatus should be working when the follicle is entered, otherwise spillage of fluid and loss of the oocyte may result. The principle of needling the follicle aims for minimal disturbance of the theca and granulosa and a tight fit between the needle and follicle wall. This prevents loss of follicular

fluid or entry of carbon dioxide into the follicle. The site of entry should be at the bulging topmost part of the follicle. The follicle should be entered gently so it is not torn, because this will destroy a good fit between the needle and follicular wall. The suction provided by the vacuum pump should be of the order of 80–100 mm of mercury.

Technique of aspiration

The initial procedure is to aspirate totally the follicular fluid. The volume of fluid within a mature ovulatory follicle is usually from 4 ml to 12 ml, with a mean of 8 ml. Follicular fluid should be straw coloured, but it may become contaminated with blood. As soon as blood appears in the tubing leading from the needle to the tissue culture tube heparinised culture medium should be added to the aspirate. If a blood clot forms within the aspirate the ovum may be hard to identify, and may also be entrapped within a fibrin mass, making it difficult to isolate and less likely to be fertilized. Usually it is possible to see the walls of the follicle collapsing as the fluid is aspirated. At this stage the aspirates should be sent to the laboratory. If the oocyte is identified further aspiration is not necessary. However, if the oocyte is not present in the initial aspirate, repeated flushing of the follicle with heparinised culture medium is performed. Enough culture medium is injected via the needle to distend the follicle under laparoscopic vision, and the injected fluid is then reaspirated. This may be repeated as often as is necessary until the oocyte is recovered. On the completion of the aspiration of each follicle the needle is washed with fresh culture medium. Ova that fertilise are rarely recovered from follicles smaller than 1.5 cm (Trounson, 1983). However, it is sometimes difficult to estimate the size of the follicle accurately at laparoscopy because some follicles are situated beneath the ovarian surface and most of their volume is within the ovarian tissue.

If the follicle has ruptured it is worthwhile to try and flush the follicular cavity because oocytes are sometimes recovered from ovulated follicles. Aspiration of any fluid in the Pouch of Douglas is also worthwhile as a pregnancy has resulted from an ovulated oocyte recovered under this circumstance (Trounson, 1982b).

IN VITRO FERTILISATION AND EMBRYO CULTURE

Oocyte recovery and treatment

Follicular fluid and aspirates are examined under the microscope and the mucinous cumulus mass containing the oocyte identified. Identification of the oocyte is made more difficult if there is no cumulus mass (naked oocytes), or if it is entrapped in a fibrin clot. The oocyte should be handled and manipulated gently at all times.

Careful interpretation of follicular monitors and precision in timing the interval between LH surge or hCG injection and laparoscopy is required to obtain fully mature oocytes. Trounson et al (1982b) showed that the rate of fertilisation and subsequent embryo development could be improved significantly by a short period of culture in vitro of oocytes after collection and before insemination.

Electron-microscopic studies of oocytes confirm that cortical granule maturation takes place during this preincubation (Sathanantham & Trounson, 1982). Insemination of oocytes that are immature may result in polyspermy or failure of fertilisation. It is now known that pregnancy may result from insemination immediately after oocyte recovery to 14 hours after oocyte recovery, so that there is probably a very large variation in the maturational state of oocytes recovered from the follicle. In our own studies we incubate oocytes for 5–10 hours after oocyte recovery depending on the estimated maturity of follicles and oocytes.

The culture media

Although modified Ham's F10 medium was used initially for fertilisation and embryo culture (Steptoe & Edwards, 1976; Lopata et al, 1980; Trounson et al, 1980a) other more simple media have been examined. As a result of these experiments, successful in vitro fertilisation has also been obtained with Earl's solution, modified Whitten's culture medium, and Whittinghams T6 (Trounson 1983, 1982d). A controlled trial is presently being conducted with these four media to compare the relative fertilisation, embryo development and pregnancy rates.

Whatever medium is being used it is essential that quality control is carried out regularly (Wood & Trounson, 1982). As our culture media are prepared weekly, each batch is tested for its suitability by culturing mouse embryos from the 2 cell to blastocyst stage. This ensures that embryo-toxic chemicals and instruments are not being introduced. The development of fertilisation and embryo culture in test tubes (Trounson et al, 1980a), and the use of the same medium for both fertilisation and embryo culture has simplified the fertilisation and culture techniques.

Preparation of semen

The procedures for preparing spermatozoa for insemination have been described in detail (Trounson et al, 1982b), and are essentially similar to those performed by all the groups working with IVF. A specimen is collected on site by masturbation, 60–90 min before insemination. After liquefaction, the semen is centrifuged and the resultant sperm pellet is then resuspended in culture medium. After recentrifugation the washed spermatozoa are incubated in culture medium at 37 °C for 30–60 min and a sample is taken from the surface layer containing the most active spermatozoa for insemination. A total of 10 000–50 000 motile spermatozoa are added in 10–20 μl to the 1 ml of culture medium containing the oocyte.

Mammalian embryos are more sensitive than any other cell line when cultured in vitro, and meticulous care is required to ensure success at this stage of the procedure. This has been described in detail by Edwards et al (1980a) and by Trounson et al (1982b). After insemination the oocyte is left for 12–23 hours, before being inspected. Examination of the oocyte is performed in a Petri dish containing culture medium and the cumulus removed with a micro-pipette. The oocyte is examined for the presence of two pronuclei and two polar bodies. Any abnormality such as the presence of multiple pronuclei, granulation or vesciculation of the cytoplasm or any abnormal shape of the oocyte, is also noted. The first cleavage division should take place within 24–30 hours of insemination, and each subsequent division should occur within 10–12 hours (Trounson et al, 1982b). The rate of cleavage of embryos which have subsequently produced developing fetuses is important. If cleavage does not occur within 24 hours, or if further development is arrested for 24 hours or more, this would indicate that the oocyte or embryo was abnormal. Oocytes which fail to fertilise and embryos which are abnormal are not transferred but are examined by light and electron microscopy.

Apart from the assessment of the rate of development of embryos, and their morphological appearance, there is no really effective way of assessing the viability of embryos prior to transfer by non-invasive tests (Mohr et al, 1982). To prevent the transfer of non-viable embryos, or to select the best embryos for transfer, a rapid non-invasive test is required. The fluorescein diacetate test (Mohr & Trounson, 1980) appeared promising, but has doubtful value in the human, because of its close correlation with the morphological appearance of oocytes and embryos.

It has been suggested that one of the cells of a multicellular embryo could be removed and be examined by electron microscopy. Apart from the practical difficulty of this manoeuvre, the cell obtained may not be representative of the whole embryo as normal and degenerating cells may be present in the one embryo. Furthermore, even with the appearance of apparently normal ultrastructure, normal biological function is not assured.

TIME OF EMBRYO TRANSFER

The best time to transfer embryos to the uterus has not yet been determined. Pregnancies have resulted from the transfer of 1–8 cell (Trounson et al, 1981a; Trounson, 1982b) 8 cell (Lopata et al, 1980) and 8 and 16 cell (Edwards et al, 1980a) embryos, but the transfer of more advanced embryos has not been successful (Edwards et al, 1980a).

Prolonged culture of embryos *in vitro* may reduce their viability and thereby reduce pregnancy rate. However, early stage embryos may not survive well within the uterus. Normally the embryo is retained in the Fallopian tube until the 8 to 16 cell stage. There is not yet sufficient information to decide the best time for transfer of the embryo, but preliminary data suggested that the 2 to 4 cell stage may give the best results (Trounson, 1982d).

It has been shown conclusively that the chance of subsequent pregnancy increases with the number of embryos transferred. However, this has to be considered carefully in view of the increased obstetric risks associated with multiple pregnancy. In our programme the number of embryos transferred in each case is decided upon after joint consultation between the doctor and patient, taking such factors into consideration.

Technique of embryo transfer

All pregnancies reported to date have resulted from embryo transfer through the cervical canal (Leeton et al, 1982). All embryo transfers in our programme are performed in the operating theatre where it is easy to position the patient, there is good lighting, aseptic surroundings and quiet conditions are ensured. The husband is encouraged to be present at the time of transfer and/or a sympathetic companion for the woman has been found to be helpful. Premedication is with 10 mg diazepam (Valium), given orally to the patient.

No anaesthesia or analgesia is needed as a rule, although occasional regional epidural analgesia has been used if the cervical canal cannot be negotiated. A sterile bivalve vaginal speculum is gently inserted to visualise the cervix. The external os and exocervix is then gently cleansed with a sterile swab soaked with culture medium. The length of the uterine cavity is measured during the preliminary ultrasonic examination. The principles of embryo transfer are not to cause bleeding, to minimise the introduction of mucus into the uterine cavity that may entrap the embryo, and to stimulate the minimum amount of uterine activity. Premedication with anti-prostaglandins (mefenamic acid) to reduce uterine contractility has been tried but was not beneficial.

The patient is placed in the knee-chest or lithotomy position with enough head-down tilt to ensure the fundus is lower than the cervical canal. The uterus is manipulated gently to align the cervical canal and uterine cavity. When the cervix is exposed and ready for transfer, the embryo is drawn into a Teflon catheter in 10 μl of tissue culture medium. Teflon is used because of its low adhesiveness which reduces the chance of carrying cervical secretions into the uterine cavity. The catheter has an external diameter of 1.27 mm and an internal diameter of 1 mm. The Teflon catheter is then passed down an outer Teflon sheath which protects the inner catheter from vaginal contamination. The outer cannula can also be used to gently dilate and negotiate the cervical canal if there is any difficulty in passing the fine cannula. The metal introducer tried previously (Lopata et al, 1980) has been abandoned as it is considered to be too traumatic. The catheter is inserted into the uterine cavity just short of the fundus using the information on the distance from the fundus to external cervical os, provided by ultrasound. The embryo is gently injected in 15–20 l of culture medium and catheter and cannula are slowly withdrawn. The catheter is then checked under the microscope to ensure that the embryo has been expelled.

The transfer technique has been improved with the development of a special catheter (Leeton et al, 1982). The majority of transfers are performed by the one experienced clinician. In the initial study of this technique 26 per cent of 56 transfers resulted in pregnancy (Leeton et al, 1982).

If difficulty is experienced with transfer an alternative bullet ended cannula may be used with a side-opening exit hole (Leeton et al, 1982). The uterine position can sometimes be altered by gentle manipulation and counter pressure may be applied to straighten the cervical canal by grasping the anterior lip of the cervix with a volsellum forcep. In our experience the chance of pregnancy is much higher if the transfer is easy and non-traumatic (Wood et al, 1981a; Leeton et al, 1982). Incorrect placement of the catheter, or the use of excessive quantity of fluid for transfer may lead to the expulsion of the embryo from the uterine lumen or possible tubal pregnancy. This complication has been reported by a number of groups (Steptoe & Edwards 1976; Tucker et al, 1981), and recently our own group has seen a tubal pregnancy.

After transfer the patients are advised to rest in bed for 2–3 hours and to abstain from intercourse for at least a week. Currently no post-transfer hormonal support is given. A randomised trial of Proluton Depot (Schering AG) showed no beneficial effect. Other hormones that have been suggested include hCG, bromocriptine, clomiphene or hydroxyprogesterone hexanoate but none of these individually or in combination have improved pregnancy rate (Trounson, 1983).

Although an initial report (Kerin et al, 1980) suggested a reduction in serum 17β E$_2$ levels in the mid luteal phase after oocyte aspiration, this difference was not statistically significant. It appears from our own experience that there is no inadequacy of luteal progesterone or oestrogen levels after oocyte collection (Trounson, 1982b). Further evidence for a satisfactory hormonal environment is the increasing chance of pregnancy with the transfer of multiple embryos. This suggests that the major reason for failure of implantation is due to abnormal embryos or to faulty transfer technique, rather than to defective hormone levels in the recipient.

PREGNANCY CARE

The clinical features of our first eight pregnancies have been reported (Wood et al, 1982). Serum hCG, progesterone, and E_2 levels are assayed weekly until 12 weeks of gestation to assess feto-placental and corpus luteum function. Progesterone is then measured monthly, and oestriol (E_3) fortnightly from 26 weeks of gestation until delivery, to ensure that feto-placental function is adequate. Antenatal tococardiography is also performed fortnightly from 30 weeks of gestation.

Amniocentesis is offered at 14–16 weeks to ensure chromosomal normality, but with the miscarriage of an IVF pregnancy after amniocentesis (Lopata et al, 1981) most of our patients so far have refused this investigation.

Obstetric ultrasound is performed at 7–8 weeks to confirm the presence of an intra-uterine pregnancy and to determine the number of fetuses. This is repeated at 12–13 weeks to confirm feto-placental viability and at 16–17 weeks to detect any malformation. Another scan is undertaken at 30 weeks of gestation to determine fetal growth.

The initial miscarriage rate in our programme was nearly 50 per cent with 20 of our first 42 pregnancies miscarrying (Wood et al, 1981c). However, the abortion rate has now decreased. In judging this high rate of miscarriage, it has to be kept in mind that many natural pregnancies miscarry subclinically, and are thus not recorded (Craft, 1982).

The mode of delivery must be determined after considering all the obstetric factors. Because these patients as a group are older, and they have often had utero-tubal surgery, the rate of Caesarian section is high.

At the present time in our group all IVF pregnancies are routinely monitored in labour by toco-cardiography. Although our Caesarian section rate is high, indications have included breech presentation with a contracted pelvis, obstructed labour, foetal distress during labour, premature labour at 29 weeks of gestation, and spontaneous term labour with failure to progress.

At present it is not possible to be certain whether IVF will result in any increased or decreased rate of congenital abnormality. Our group has only experienced one congenital abnormality (Wood et al, 1982), which was probably unrelated to IVF. However, other groups have reported triploidy in aborted material (Steptoe et al, 1980), and trisomy.

REFERENCES

Adams C E 1979 Consequence of accelerated ovum transport, including a re-evaluation of Estes' operation. Journal of Reproduction and Fertility 55: 239–246

Brown J B, MacLeod S O, MacNoughton C, Smith B, Smith M A 1968 A rapid method for measuring oestrogens in human urine using a semi-automatic extractor. Journal of Endocrinology 42: 5–15

Carson R S, Trouson A O, Findlay J K 1982 Succesful fertilization of human oocytes in vitro: concentration of estradiol-17β, progesterone and androstenedione in the antral fluid of donor follicles. Journal of Clinical Endocrinology and Metabolism 55: 798–800

Camus M, Trounson A O 1982 The place of microsurgery and in vitro fertilization. Patient Management. Birkenhead, N.Z. ADIS Press 11: 39–45

Cox L W Human Pituitary Advisory Committee 1976. Ovulation induction by human FSH — the results of the Australian Programme. Australian and New Zealand Journal of Obstetrics and Gynaecology 16: 106–110

Craft I 1982 In virto fertilization — a fast changing technique: a discussion. Journal of the Royal Society of Medicine 75: 253–257

Edwards R G 1965 Maturation in vitro of human ovarian oocytes. Lancet ii: 926

Edwards R G 1973 Physiological aspects of human ovulation, fertilization and cleavage. Journal of Reproduction and Fertility 34 (Suppl 18): 87–101

Edwards R G 1981 Test-tube babies 1981. Nature 293: 253–256

Edwards R G, Steptoe P C 1975 Induction of llicular growth, ovulation and luteinization in the human ovary. Journal of Reproduction and Fertility 22: 121–56

Edwards R G, Steptoe P C, Purdy J M 1970 Fertilization and cleavage in vitro of preovulatory human oocytes. Nature 227: 1307–1309

Edwards R G, Steptoe P C, Purdy J M 1980a Establishing full-term human pregnancies using cleaving embryos grown in vitro. British Journal of Obstetrics and Gynaecology 87: 737–756

Edwards R G, Steptoe P C, Fowler R E, Baillie J 1980b Observations on preovulatory human ovarian follicles and their aspirates. British Journal of Obstetrics and Gynaecology 87: 769–779

Estes W L, Heitmeyer P L 1934 Pregnancy following ovarian implantation. American Journal of Surgery 24: 563–581

Garcia J, Jones G S, Wentz A C 1977 The use of clomiphene citrate. Fertility and Sterility 28: 707–717

Hudson B, Baker H W G, de Kretser D M 1980 The abnormal semen sample. In: Pepperell R J, Hudson B, Wood C (eds) The infertile couple, p 84. Churchill Livingstone, Edinburgh

Jacobson C B, Sites J G, Arias-Bernal L F 1970 In vitro maturation and fertilization of human follicular oocytes. International Journal of Fertility 15: 103–114

Johnston I, Lopata A, Speirs A, Hoult I, Kellow G, Du Plessiss Y 1981 In vitro fertilization: the challenge of the eighties. Fertility and Sterility 36: 699–706

Kerin J F, Edmonds D K, Warnes G M, Ralph M M, Broom T, Seamark R F, Cox L W 1980 Human luteal phase function following follicular fluid aspiration of the immediate preovular Graafian follicle (abstract) In: Proceedings of the 22nd British Congress of Obstetrics and Gynaecology, p 7

Kovacs G T 1979 Infertility — a flow chart approach. The Australian and New Zealand Journal of Obstetrics and Gynaecology 19: 220–224

Kovacs G T, Lording D W 1980 Artificial insemination with donor semen — a review of 252 patients. Medical Journal of Australia 2: 609–612

Kovacs G T, Burger H G 1982 Cervical mucus assessment. In: Donald R A (ed) A Guide to the Diagnosis of Endocrine Disorders. Marcel Dekker, New York

Kovacs G, Brian R, Burger H, Dennis P, Outch K 1982 Induction of ovulation with human pituitary gonadotrophins. 1982 Proceedings of the Fertility Society of Australia, p 70

de Kretser D, Dennis P, Hudson B, Leeton J, Lopata A, Outch K, Talbot J, Wood C 1973 Transfer of a human zygote. Lancet ii: 728–729

Leeton J F, Trounson A O, Jessup D, Wood C 1982 The technique for human embryo transfer. Fertility and Sterility 35: 156–161

Lenz S, Lauritsen J G, Kjellow M 1981 Collection of human oocytes for in vitro fertilization by ultrasonically guided follicular puncture. In: Follicular Maturation and Ovulation, IVth Reiner de Graaf Symposium, pp 338–341. Excerpta Medica, Amsterdam

Lopata A, Johnston I W H, Leeton J F, Muchnicki D, Talbot J M,

Wood C 1974 Collection of human oocytes at laparoscopy and laparotomy. Fertility and Sterility 25: 1030–1038

Lopata A, Brown J B, Leeton J F, Talbot J Mc, Wood C 1978 In vitro fertilization of pre-ovulatory oocytes and embryo transfer in infertile patients treated with clomiphene and human chrionic gonadotrophin. Fertility and Sterility 30: 27–35

Lopata A, Johnston I W H, Hoult I J, Speirs A I 1980 Pregnancy following intrauterine implantation of an embryo obtained by in vitro fertilization of a preovulatory egg. Fertility and Sterility 33: 117–120

Lopata A, Kellow, G N, Johnston I W H, Speirs A L, Hoult I J, Pepperell R J, du Plessis Y P 1981 Human embryo transfer in the treatment of infertility. Australian and New Zealand Journal of Obstetrics and Gynaecology 21: 156–158

McIntosh J E A, Matthews C O, Crocker J M, Brown T J, Cox L W 1980 Predicting the Luteinizing Hormone Surge: Relationship between the duration of the follicular and luteal phases and the length of the human menstrual cycle. Fertility and Sterility 34: 125–130

Mohr L R, Trounson A O 1980 The use of fluorescein diacetate to assess embryo viability. Journal of Reproduction and Fertility 58: 189–196

Mohr L R, Trounson A O, Leeton J F, Wood C 1982 Evaluation of normal and abnormal human embryo development during procedures in vitro. In: Beier H M, Lindner H R (eds) Fertilization of the Human Egg In Vitro: Biological Basis and Clinical Applications pp 209–219. Springer-Verlag, Berlin

Morgenstern L L, Soupart P 1972 Oocyte recovery from the human ovary. Fertility and Sterility 23: 751–758

Mozes M, Bogokowski H, Antebi E, Lunenfeld B, Rabau E, Serr D M, David A, Salomy M 1965 Thromboembolic phenomena after ovarian stimulation with human gonadotrophins. Lancet ii: 1213–1215

Renaud P L, Macler J, Dervain I, Ehret M C, Aron C, Plas-Roser S, Spira A, Pdlack H 1980 Echographic study of follicular maturation and ovulation during the normal menstrual cycle. Fertility and Sterility 33: 272–276

Renou P, Trounson A O, Wood C, Leeton J F 1981 The collection of human oocytes for in vitro fertilization. 1. An instrument for maximizing oocyte recovery rate. Fertility and sterility 35: 409–412

Sathananthan H, Trounson A O 1982 Ultrastructural observations on cortisol granules in human follicular oocytes cultural in vitro. Gamete Research 5: 191–198

Schenker J G, Polishuk W Z 1975 Ovarian Hyperstimulation Syndrome. Obstetrics and Gynecology 46: 23–28

Siegler A M 1960 Tubal plastic surgery, the past, the present and the future. Obstetrical and Gynecological Survey 15: 680–701

Soupart P, Strong P A 1974 Ultrastructural observations on human oocytes fertilized in vitro. Fertility and Sterility 25: 11–44

Steptoe P C, Edwards R 1970 Laparoscopic recovery of pre-ovulatory human oocytes after priming of ovaries with gonadotrophins. Lancet i: 683–689

Steptoe P C, Edwards R G 1976 Reimplantation of a human embryo with subsequent tubal pregnancy. Lancet i: 880–882

Steptoe P C, Edwards R G 1978 Birth after the re-implantation of a human embryo. Lancet ii: 366

Steptoe P C, Edwards R G, Purdy J M 1980 Clinical aspects of pregnancies established with cleaving embryos grown in vitro. British Journal of Obstetrics and Gynaecology 87: 757–768

Talbot J M, Dooley M, Leeton J, Lopata A, McMaster R, Wood C 1976 Gonadotrophin stimulation for oocyte recovery and in vitro fertilization in infertile women. Australian and New Zealand Journal of Obstetrics and Gynaecology 16: 111–118

Testart J, Frydman R, Feinstein M C, Thebault A, Roger M, Scholler R 1981 Interpretation of plasma luteinizing hormone assay for the collection of mature oocytes from women: definition of a luteinizing hormone surge-initiating rise. Fertility and Sterility 36: 50–54

Trounson A 1982b Current perspectives of in vitro fertilization and embryo transfer. Clinical Reproduction and Fertility 1: 55–56

Trounson A O 1982c Manipulation of endocrine requirements for in vitro fertilization. Proceedings of the Endocrine Society of Australia, Vol 25, Suppl 1, pp 1–6

Trounson A O 1982d Factors controlling normal embryo development and implantation of human oocytes fertilized in vitro. In: Beier H M, Lindner H R (eds) Fertilization of the human egg in vitro: biological basis and clinical applications. Springer-Verlag, Berlin

Trounson A O 1983 In vitro fertilization. In: Martini L, James V (eds) Current Topics in Experimental Endocrinology 5: 44–73. Academic Press, New York

Trounson A O, Wood C 1981 Extracorporeal fertilization and embryo transfer. Clinics in Obstetrics and Gynecology 8: 681–713

Trounson A O, Conti A 1982 Research in human in vitro fertilization and embryo transfer. British Medical Journal 285: 244–248

Trounson A O, Leeton J F, Wood C, Webb J, Kovacs G 1980a The investigation of idiopathic infertility by in vitro fertilization. Fertility and Sterility 34: 431–438

Trounson A O, Herreros M, Burger H, Clarke I 1980b The precise detection of ovulation using a rapid radio-immunoassay of urinary LH. Proceeding of the Endocrine Society of Australia 23: 73

Trounson A O, Leeton J F, Wood C, Webb J, Wood J 1981a Pregnancies in humans by fertilization in vitro and embryo transfer in the controlled ovulatory cycle. Science 212: 681–682

Trounson A O, Leeton J F, Wood C, Buttery B, Webb J, Wood J, Jessup D, Talbot J M, Kovacs G 1981b A programme of successful in vitro fertilization and embryo transfer in the controlled ovulatory cycle. In: Semm K, Mettler L (eds) Human Reproduction (Proceedings of 111 World Congress), pp 173–180. Excerpta Medica, Amsterdam

Trounson A O, Leeton J F, Wood C 1982a In vitro fertilization and embryo transfer in the human. In: Rolland R, van Hall E V, Hillier S G, McNatty K P, Schoemaker J (eds) Follicular Maturation and Ovulation pp 313–322 (International Congress Series No 560). Excerpta Medica, Amsterdam

Trounson A O, Mohr L R, Wood C, Leeton J F 1982b Effect of delayed insemination on in vitro fertilization, culture and transfer of human embryos. Journal of Reproduction and Fertility 64: 285–294

Tucker M, Smith D H, Pike I, Kemp J F, Picker R H, Saunders D M 1981 Ectopic pregnancy following in vitro fertilization and embryo transfer. Lancet ii: 1278

Winston R M L 1981 Is microsurgery necessary for salpingostomy? The evaluation of results. Australian and New Zealand Journal of Obstetrics and Gynaecology 21: 143–152

Wood C, Trounson A O 1982 In vitro fertilization and embryo transfer. In: Bonnar J (ed) Recent Advances in Obstetrics and Gynaecology, pp 259–282. Churchill Livingstone, Edinburgh

Wood C, Kovacs G T 1983 Extracorporeal fertilization. In: Studd J (ed) Progress in Obstetrics and Gynaecology, Vol 3, pp . Churchill Livingstone, Edinburgh

Wood C, Leeton J, Taylor R 1971 A preliminary design and trial of an artificial human tube. Fertility and Sterility 22: 446–450

Wood C, Downing B, McKenzie I, O'Brien B McC, Paterson P 1978 Microvascular transplantation of the human fallopian tube. Fertility and Sterility 29: 607–613

Wood C, Trounson A, Leeton J, Talbot J M, Buttery B, Webb J, Wood J, Jessup D 1981a A clinical assessment of nine pregnancies obtained by in vitro fertilization and embryo transfer. Fertility and Sterility 35: 502–508

Wood C, Leeton J, Talbot J Mc, Trounson A O 1981b Technique for collecting mature human oocytes for in vitro fertilization. British Journal of Obstetrics and Gynaecology 88: 756–760

Wood C, Renou P, Leeton J, Trounson A, Kovacs G 1981c u Pickup (abstract) In: Walters W A W, Wood C (eds) The Scientific Proceedings of the V111 Asian and Oceanic Congress of Obstetrics and Gynaecology, pp 24–25

Wood C, Trounson A, Leeton J F, Renou P M, Walters W A W, Buttery B W, Grimwade J C, Spensely J, Yu V Y H 1982 Clinical features of eight pregnancies resulting from IVF and ET. Fertility and Sterility 38: 22–29

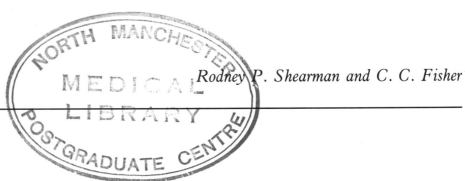

Threatened abortion

DEFINITION

Any definition should be finite. There are immediate difficulties in defining threatened abortion, as the definition of abortion varies between countries. In many countries, a birth is defined as the expulsion of a fetus of more than 400 g and/or more than 20 weeks menstrual age; an abortion is the expulsion of products of conception that does not meet the definition of birth. Partly because of these difficulties, there are widely conflicting data on subjects of fundamental importance such as incidence and outcome. The definition used here is the same as that used by Johannsen (1970): 'Threatened abortion is defined as haemorrhage from the uterus in association with an intra-uterine pregnancy prior to 20 weeks gestation, with the cervix incompletely effaced and the os closed, and irrespective of whether or not uterine contractions are occuring.'

In a book dealing with reproductive endocrinology this definition has the advantage that it excludes the predominantly mechanical problem of threatened abortion and the incompetent cervix.

INCIDENCE

Of those pregnancies that reach the level of clinical consciousness, the quoted incidence of *threatened* abortion varies between 2.4 per cent and 20 per cent (Editorial Comment, 1980). The figure of 16 per cent quoted by Hertig & Livingstone (1944) is still widely used in the literature, perhaps because age has given it a patina of acceptability and authenticity. None of these figures match very well with the usually quoted *spontaneous* abortion incidence of 15 per cent (Shearman, 1980), figures based on clinical data and a total implantation loss of 43 per cent based on endocrinological data (Grudzinskas et al, 1981). The manifest difficulties of arriving at a true estimate of the frequency of spontaneous abortion, let alone threatened abortion, are discussed thoughtfully by Jansen (1982). It

should be recognised that no uniformly accepted figures of the incidence of threatened abortion exist. There are, however, good figures on the numbers of women delivering a viable fetus who had a threatened abortion during that pregnancy. In a carefully documented group of nearly 8000 private patients, Correy (1980) found an incidence of 6.6 per cent of threatened abortion before the sixteenth week of pregnancy dated on menstrual age, but there are no figures in this study to indicate those women who had a threatened abortion and then proceeded to abort.

NATURAL HISTORY

Almost all women who suffer from bleeding in the first half of pregnancy will have several concerns. 'Will I miscarry?', 'Will the baby be premature?', 'If I do not miscarry will the baby be abnormal?'. There is almost no good evidence that therapeutic intervention has any effect on the ultimate outcome. Because of this one might expect that the natural history of this common problem would be well documented but is is not. Almost all the available data come from those women admitted to hospital; in Britain admission to hospital for threatened abortion is confined to 'women with heavy or prolonged bleeding' (Editorial Comment, 1980). The same criteria for hospital admission apply in most other countries. Data based on hospital studies will be heavily biased towards those most likely to abort since there is a relationship between the amount of bleeding and ultimate outcome (Mantoni & Pedersen 1981).

Progression to spontaneous abortion

In a study of 266 patients admitted to hospital with threatened abortion, Johannsen (1970) found that 50.8 per cent proceeded to spontaneous abortion. Abortion occurred within one week in 43.7 per cent and within 1 month in 80 cent of the total aborting. Eriksen & Philipsen (1980) found 35 per cent of patients admitted to hospital with threatened abortion proceeded to abort. Spontaneous abortion in 80 per cent of patients admitted to hospital with threatened abortion has been reported by Evans & Beischer (1970) while in another Australian study, 35 per cent aborted (Ho & Jones, 1980). Joupilla et al (1979) found that 50 per cent of admitted patients aborted. In a small study, Mantoni & Pedersen (1981) found a relationship between the amount of bleeding, assessed by ultrasonic measurement of uterine haematoma size and outcome. Haematomas of less than 35 ml had, in general, a good prognosis, while those larger than 50 ml had a very poor prognosis. The quoted incidence of progression to abortion ranges between 35 and 80 per cent of hospital population studies suggesting that variation relates to the original criteria for admission rather than to differences in the behaviour of the total population.

On purely clinical grounds only two factors of prognostic significance emerge — abortion is more likely when the bleeding occurs early in pregnancy and abortion is more common when the bleeding is heavy. Empiricism also suggests that women with a threatened abortion who have severe nausea are less likely to abort than those who are not nauseated, unless they happen to harbour an hydatidiform mole. It is unfortunate that there are no data on risk in all women with threatened abortion. There is no information on the natural history of this condition that includes women with threatened abortion who were not admitted to hospital.

Subsequent prematurity

In Correy's study of almost 8000 patients, 487 of 524 women with threatened abortion delivered after the thirty-eighth week, an incidence of prematurity that is, in fact, less than the Australian national incidence of prematurity. It is probably significant that all of his subjects were private patients. Social class has a major impact on the incidence of premature labour and the same increased risk is seen in relation to social class in women with threatened abortion (Johannsen, 1970). Correy's study apart, there is a near concensus that threatened abortion is followed by a significant increase in premature delivery and/or birth of small for dates infants. Nineteen per cent of Johannsen's patients delivered prematurely. The largest study relevant to this problem is that of Funderburk et al (1980). The total population consisted of 25 387 consecutive deliveries. Prematurity occurred in 12.7 per cent of women with a history of threatened abortion (5.4 per cent in controls), low birthweight, defined as less than 2500 g in 17.4 per cent (6.9 per cent) and very low birthweight, defined as less than 1501 g in 8.9 per cent (1.3 per cent). These are not trivial figures. In this study, the main clinical clue to an increased risk was a history of heavy bleeding.

Fetal abnormality

Although some studies have shown an increase in the incidence of congenital abnormality, more recent and substantial data have, fortunately, not confirmed this. While an abortion is disappointing for a couple who want a baby and a premature baby a cause of substantial concern the birth of a baby with a major malformation is a tremendous blow. Correy (1980) found 1.9 per cent of major malformations in patients with a history of threatened abortion and a figure of 0.9 per cent in controls, significant at only the 5 per cent level. Funderburk et al (1980) found 2.7 per cent of subsequent births to be associated with fetal abnormality compared with 1.6 per cent in controls and this difference was not significant.

Any clinician faced — as he often is — with a discussion about the risk of congenital malformation is in a 'no win' situation. No pregnancy carries with it a guarantee of fetal normality. The patient who has had a threatened abortion cannot be told there is no risk of fetal abnormality, but she may be told with reasonable confidence that her risk is no greater than if she had not suffered this episode of bleeding.

In summary, about 50 per cent of women admitted to hospital with threatened abortion will ultimately abort. Of those who do not, there is a substantially greater risk of delivering an immature or small for dates baby but no greater risk of delivering an abnormal fetus. Suggestions (Editorial Comment, 1980) that the live born and surviving infant from a pregnancy complicated by threatened abortion faces a greater risk of psychomotor retardation or psychological abnormality remain to be confirmed. Given the great difficulties in studies of this type, no clinician should hold his breath awaiting the outcome.

AETIOLOGY

There are no data on the confused, confusing and controversial problems of the aetiology of threatened abortion that satisfy Kock's postulate! In a volume dealing with endocrinology, it would be nice to produce evidence that endocrine deficiency or imbalance caused abortion. The quickest and simplest way to dispose of this suggestion would be to say that no such evidence exists and, in fact, very little does. This will be discussed further below and in Chapter 30. If one excludes such causes of bleeding as cervical carcinoma or trauma there seems to be general agreement that threatened abortion is due to bleeding from early separation of a normal or abnormal trophoblast. But what causes the bleeding?

Maternal factors

General

A poor socio-economic environment provides an equally poor background for reproductive efficiency and this is seen just as much in threatened abortion (Johannsen, 1970) as it is in a high perinatal mortality, increased risk of prematurity and greater risk of congenital malformation in socially disadvantaged women. Cigarette smoking and alcohol intake increase the risk, but knowledge of the relationship, if any, to other commonly used drugs is meagre or non-existent.

Any maternal infection that causes a high fever, whether this be influenza, pneumonia or typhoid fever increases the risk of both threatened and incomplete abortion. Concurrent fetal infection — rubella, cytomegalo-virus, toxoplasmosis — further and substantially increases the risk. The possible role of chorioamnionitis due to *mycoplasma hominis* or *lysteria monocytogens* is no less obscure now than it was a decade ago.

Maternal occupation

With one exception, there is no good evidence that maternal occupation is causally related to the risk of spontaneous abortion. The exception is exposure to an environment of anaesthetic gases, best documented in female anaesthetists, dentists and nursing staff in the same environment. This anxiety first surfaced in a study from Russia (Vaisman, 1967, quoted by Vessey & Nunn, 1980) where more than 50 per cent of all pregnancies in female anaesthetists were reported to end in abortion. Vessey & Nunn (1980) have summarised and analysed critically all data up to 1980. Despite valid criticism of the methods of data collection (largely questionnaires) and the inadequacy of control, Vessey & Nunn conclude that there is an additional risk of about 40 per cent of abortion and, given the earlier data in this chapter, an even greater excess of threatened abortion. The material analysed came from Russia, the United Kingdom and the United States of America. The most likely cause seems to be too high concentrations of nitrous oxide and possibly, also halothane. Accepting that most operating theatres and dental surgeries do not have adequate scavenging systems and also accepting that there are no hard data that such systems are protective, Vessey & Nunn (1980) conclude: 'On present evidence, a theatre nurse or female anaesthetist becoming pregnant or wishing to become pregnant should be advised to avoid working in an environment contaminated with anaesthetic gases'.

Chromosomal Aneuploidy

There is no longer any doubt that aneuploidy of the conceptus is one of the major causes of early spontaneous abortion and, therefore, of the preceding threatened abortion (Carr, 1971). Earlier studies indicated that between 25 and 50 per cent of all first trimester abortions are associated with aneuploidy of the conceptus, particularly trisomy of the D group and X monosomy. For every live infant born

with Turner's syndrome, ten will abort and in this particular group there is a relationship to young maternal age, while trisomy and triploidy increase with advancing maternal age. The introduction of banding techniques has further increased this association to about 60 per cent of early abortions and 55 per cent overall (*Lauritson*, 1976). For most women this is an isolated 'act of God', a non-dysjunctional problem of that particular ovum or that particular sperm. However, in couples with recurrent abortion there is a balanced translocation in 3.25 per cent which increases the risk of recurrence very substantially (Tsenghi et al, 1976; and see ch. 30).

Endocrine relationships

The history of hormonal inter-relationships in threatened and recurrent abortion is long and complex. It would be nice to say that it has been rewarding, but unfortunately it has not. Far too often investigators have found a pattern of low or falling hormone levels in patients who subsequently aborted and made the grave error that the first caused the second, rather than being both simply related to the fundamental cause of ultimate abortion. These findings became embedded in the folklore of abortion. For historical reasons and particularly because many physicians still believe, emotionally rather than intellectually, that there is such a causal relationship, the evidence in this area warrants careful examination.

(a) *Progesterone and its metabolites.* The majority of spontaneous abortions occur between 9 and 12 weeks of pregnancy. Since the human corpus luteum goes into decline — but not complete retirement — during the eighth week of pregnancy and following Corner's classical purification of progesterone from the corpus luteum, the events were seen to be causally related by many people. This unleashed a mass of uncritical thinking and writing unmatched in almost any other area of medicine.

The first objective evidence of a relationship between threatened and subsequent abortion and low levels of pregnanediol, using a method of assay that fulfilled all reliability criteria, was published by Shearman (1959) (Fig. 29.1). These five women were part of a group being followed serially throughout pregnancy to delineate normal levels of pregnanediol excretion. Assays on each of these five, who ultimately aborted, began before there was any bleeding or other objective evidence of disturbance in the pregnancy. Discussing these results, the senior author of this chapter wrote:

'Since there appears to be a correlation between placental progesterone content and urinary pregnanediol, it is reasonable to say that in some cases of abortion there is an associated fall in progesterone production preceding, in some cases by weeks, the onset of bleeding. However, it is impossible to say yet whether these patients abort because progesterone secretion falls

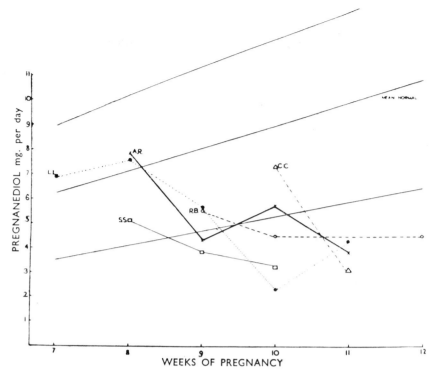

Fig. 29.1 Urinary pregnanediol excretion in five patients with spontaneous abortion. The mean normal and range is shown by parallel lines (from Shearman, 1959.)

or whether the factor responsible for the abortion also causes the fall in progesterone secretion.'

Further work showed that while abortion rarely occurred with normal levels of pregnanediol, in 80 per cent of patients with low or falling levels of pregnanediol there was spontaneous restoration of levels to normality with continuation of pregnancy (Shearman &Garrett, 1963).

Accepting, as we must, that pregnanediol excretion in urine is a very imprecise reflection of progesterone production it should, nevertheless, be noted that there is some relationship between low progesterone levels and subsequent abortion (Eriksen & Philipsen, 1980; Jouppila et al, 1979. This however, does not help to throw further light on aetiology.

(b) Corpus luteum deficiency. Elsewhere in this book, McDonough & Tho define abortion due to corpus luteum deficiency as 'inadequate ovarian production of progesterone' and this problem is fully discussed in Ch. 30. While there is some evidence that a poor corpus luteum built on the shaky foundation of a poor follicle may relate to both infertility and an increased risk of abortion, well-controlled trials indicating that treatment materially affects the outcome are almost non-existent. One such study that could be illuminating (Svigos, 1982) showed a significantly improved salvage rate in women having low serum progesterone levels who were given hCG, compared with those who did not receive treatment. The numbers in this study are small and since treatment started after pregnancy was diagnosed, the results are difficult to reconcile with the poor graafian follicle theory.

(c) Oestrogens. Earlier studies of the urinary excretion of either total oestrogens or oestriol (Klopper & Macnaughton, 1965; Brown et al, 1970) showed the same pattern as that seen with urinary pregnanediol — low or falling levels before abortion. We are not aware of any data to indicate that oestrogen therapy improves the prognosis of threatened abortion.

(d) Human chorionic gonadotrophin (hCG). Low levels of the whole molecule of hCG (Brody & Carlstrom, 1962; Mishell & Davajan 1966, Nygren et al 1973) and of the βsub-unit (Batzer, 1980; Mellows et al, 1980) are found in the majority, but not all, women who are threatening to abort. With the exception of the small study by Svigos (1982), mentioned earlier in this chapter, there is no well-controlled evidence to show that these low levels of chorionic gonadotrophin are causally related to the threatened abortion or to subsequent abortion when it occurs.

(e) Human placental lactogen (hPL). Biswas et al (1980) have found low levels of hPL in those women with threatened abortion who ultimately abort. Like almost all other data in this vexed area, this does not prove causality.

(f) Pregnancy-specific β₁-glycoprotein (SP-1). Like a bitch whelping at every bound, the human placenta continues to be the source of 'new' peptides. Obviously they are not new–only newly discovered–and whether or not they will ultimately fulfill the definitional criteria of a hormone remains to be seen. There are conflicting data on SP-1 levels in patients with threatened abortion probably related to the heterogeneity of this molecule. Ho & Jones (1980) found a positive correlation between low levels of

SP–1 in women threatening to abort and subsequent missed or actual abortion.

What then do all of these endocrinological associations mean? In terms of aetiology almost nothing. In essence, most but not all women with threatened abortion who proceed to abort will have low and/or falling levels of any feto-placental hormone you may care to measure. This is a reflection of the tortured trophoblast and has nothing to do with the aetiology of ultimate abortion. The suggestive data relating corpus luteum inadequacy to a *primary* cause of threatened abortion must, for want of control data, remain in the category of 'not proven'.

Other maternal conditions. While most of these relate to recurrent abortion, each in turn will cause threatened abortion in an index pregnancy. A full review will be found in Shearman (1980) and in Ch. 30.

Of uterine abnormalities, cervical incompetence is not, by definition, relevant to this chapter. However, two uterine abnormalities — one congenital, the other acquired — are relevant. Varying degrees of Müllerian malfusion may be present in any woman threatening to abort. Intra-uterine synechiae may cause complete secondary amenorrhoea (Ch. 24) or increased risk of abortion (Ch. 30, Shearman, 1980).

Immunological causes of abortion may need to be considered particularly in patients with a history of recurrence. Jones (1976) has found a high incidence of abortion, as well as relative infertility, in women with sperm immobilising antibodies. The relationship of lupus erythematosis to recurrent abortion is discussed in Ch. 30. In our own experience it is the group who demonstrate a lupus Type III coagulation inhibitor who are at particular risk of abortion.

CLINICAL FEATURES

The clinical diagnosis of threatened abortion will be entertained in a woman, presumed to be less than 20 weeks pregnant who presents with vaginal bleeding with or without crampy pains and in whom the cervix is closed and uneffaced. The bleeding may be little more than a brown 'show', like that of a normal period, or less frequently, heavier and associated with the passage of clots. Heavy bleeding carries a poor prognosis. A further clinical sign that is helpful is the presence or severity of nausea. Clinically there is a good correlation between morning sickness and continuation of pregnancy. This almost certainly relates to the endocrine associations that precede abortion, discussed earlier in this chapter.

Clinical evidence of severe blood loss should suggest another diagnosis such as incomplete abortion or ruptured tubal pregnancy. Cardiovascular decompensation is exceptionally rare in threatened abortion, although tachycardia

may be present due to understandable and related maternal anxiety.

Threatened abortion is not associated with abdominal tenderness unless there is significant retro-placental bleeding in a pregnancy between 14 and 20 weeks. If such tenderness is present the prognosis for an intra-uterine pregnancy is poor. If abdominal tenderness is present, particularly with rebound and the uterus is not palpable abdominally then ruptured ectopic pregnancy, a twisted or ruptured ovarian cyst or criminal interference should be considered. In those countries where legal abortion is available, illegal interference has, thankfully, almost disappeared. In countries where abortion is illegal, attempted induced abortion should always be kept in mind, particularly if the patient has a fever. An increased temperature almost never occurs in a patient with a simple uncomplicated threatened abortion. There are, however, special problems in the patient with a threatened abortion and an intra-uterine device *in situ*. This is discussed later.

On vaginal examination the cervix will be closed. The uterine size should be evaluated. If it is of the expected size the prognosis is improved. If it is bigger, trophoblastic disease should be considered (and twins and wrong dates). If it is smaller the patient may have a missed abortion or may prove to have an episode of dysfunctional uterine bleeding (or wrong dates). A small uterus with bleeding and tenderness on cervical movement may be associated with ectopic pregnancy. In frank cases of ectopic pregnancy the diagnosis is rarely in doubt, but a chronic ectopic can fool the most experienced clinician.

Vaginal examination must include inspection with a speculum and a good light. Cervical carcinoma may present as a threatened abortion; coital trauma causing injury to the vaginal vault or bleeding from a vascular area of erythroplakia will not be noted unless looked for. Exceptionally rarely, a cervical pregnancy may be seen. In about 50 per cent of patients, threatened abortion will become inevitable and then incomplete. Apart from the clinical clues already described, endocrine and biophysical methods to be discussed below may sometimes be helpful in diagnosis and prognosis.

Differential diagnosis

As well as threatened abortion, bleeding during the first 20 weeks of apparent pregnancy may be due to: dysfunctional bleeding; inevitable or incomplete abortion; hydatidiform mole; ectopic pregnancy; local causes, including carcinoma of the cervix; missed abortion.

Dysfunctional bleeding. Any experienced clinician will be aware how often an episode of dysfunctional bleeding is confused with threatened or incomplete abortion. Many patients who present with a history of 'recurrent abortion' are found to have had recurrent episodes of dysfunctional bleeding if enough trouble is taken to verify histopathology from previous curettages. Clinically most women with dysfunctional bleeding will have a long history of irregular and often heavy menstruation. In the adolescent girl, at least in Australia, a history of 3–4 months amenorrhoea followed by prolonged vaginal bleeding is far more frequently due to juvenile metropathia than it is to one or other of the varieties of abortion. On clinical examination the cervix will be closed, the uterus will be small while endocrine and ultrasonic investigation will exclude pregnancy; the diagnosis is confirmed by diagnostic curettage if this is thought necessary — a rare event in the adolescent girl.

Inevitable or incomplete abortion. Apart from the severity of bleeding, inevitable abortion will always be associated with cervical dilatation. Products of conception may be felt in the cervical canal in either inevitable or incomplete abortion. In a patient with an old incomplete or missed abortion, however, the cervix may be closed, but the uterus will be small.

Hydatidiform mole. These women often have very severe morning sickness and the uterus is frequently larger than it should be on dates; but sometimes and just to make life more difficult, the uterus will be smaller. The presence of bilateral ovarian cysts would strengthen the clinical suspicion of this diagnosis, although these are rarely noted until after the uterus is empty. Ultrasound is of paramount assistance in making or excluding this diagnosis (see below).

Ectopic pregnancy. This remains the great imposter. Every clinician has made a mistaken diagnosis in the short run and most clinicians have made the same mistake in the medium haul as well. The classical ruptured ectopic with gross intraperitoneal bleeding is not the problem; the leaking ectopic is. Shoulder pain, faintness, peritonism and pain on moving the cervix raise the likelihood of ectopic pregnancy. A mass in the fornix increases the probability. Then again, every clinician will sooner or later make this diagnosis and find that he is dealing with a 'leaking' corpus luteum of pregnancy and a threatened abortion. In some cases of ectopic pregnancy the diagnosis may not be suspected until a revealing ultrasound is obtained and in many other patients, final differentiation will only be made after laparoscopy. A ruptured bleeding corpus luteum cyst is more likely to be confused with an ectopic than with threatened abortion.

Most clinicians will go through their lives without seeing a cervical pregnancy. The clinical presentation may be identical to an 'ordinary' threatened abortion, but once seen on inspection of the cervix, neither the appearance nor the frightening clinical course will ever be forgotten (Shearman & Parkin, 1977).

Local causes, including carcinoma of the cervix. Unless adequate inspection through a speculum is a routine part of clinical assessment, this cause of vaginal bleeding will be missed. Vary rarely, bleeding from a ruptured vaginal vault will be so massive that transfusion and suture under anaesthesia are required.

Vascular area of erythroplakia may be differentiated from carcinoma by colposcopy. Cervical carcinoma (the age specific incidence of which continues to drop in most developed countries) will be confirmed by biopsy where there is clinical suspicion. Here, generally, management of the malignancy will take priority over the pregnancy.

Missed abortion. Classically, most of these women suspected clinically will have a long history of bleeding, often slight and a uterus that is either absolutely smaller than it should be or is observed over a week or more to diminish in size. Other evidence of pregnancy such as breast tenderness and enlargement and nausea will have regressed. More recently it has become evident that many women with a short history of bleeding and some with no bleeding at all have a dead, or non-viable embryo, or an anembryonic sac. While clinical evidence may be sufficiently firm to make a diagnosis, most physicians now prefer additional endocrine or more particularly ultrasonic evidence of embryonic death before emptying the uterus.

Other aids to diagnosis

Biophysical methods.

The development and refinement of ultrasonics has made a substantial impact in many areas of obstetrics and gynaecology. During the early 1960s, the most reliable form of ultrasound to find wide acceptance during early pregnancy was the use of Doppler sensors to demonstrate embryonic heart movement (Johnson et al, 1965). In 1972, Robinson described a more sophisticated method by which heart movement could be detected abdominally from 48 days amenorrhoea. He located the embryo using B mode apparatus and then defined heart movement using a time position (M) mode. Heart activity can be identified by this method with 100 per cent accuracy from 7 weeks amenorrhoea. Jouppila & Piiroinen (1975) concluded that in early pregnancy the prognosis was favourable in over 90 per cent of cases in which the viability of the pregnancy was confirmed by ultrasound. Eriksen & Philipsen (1980) and Jouppila et al (1980) subsequently confirmed this. The former authors described a false positive rate of 8 per cent occurring in patients examined at the end of the first trimester, in whom abortion occurred in the presence of fetal heart activity. These women had histories suggestive of cervical incompetence and were similar to a group previously classified by Robinson (1975) as 'late live abortions'. Jouppila et al (1980) concluded that if embryonic heart activity could not be detected after 9 weeks amenorrhoea, the outcome was unsuccessful in 100 per cent of cases. This is the most reliable predictive ultrasonic finding in the investigation of threatened abortion.

Normal pregnancy. The normal ultrasonic findings in

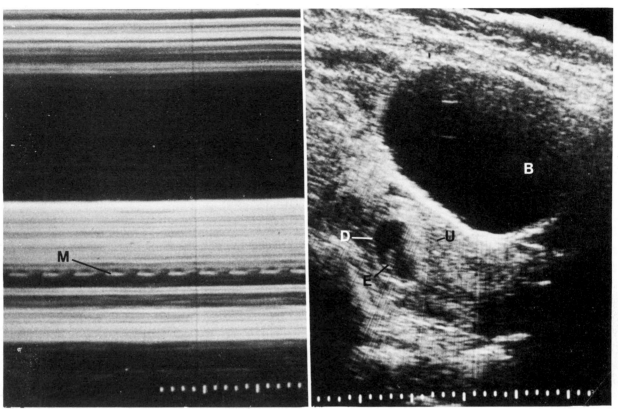

Fig. 29.2 A normal pregnancy at 7 weeks amenorrhoea. The maternal bladder (B) is superior to the uterus (U). The decidual ring (D) is complete and slightly thickened anteriorly, marking the site of future placental development. The embryo (E) lies posteriorly. Cardiac action is demonstrated by M-mode (M)

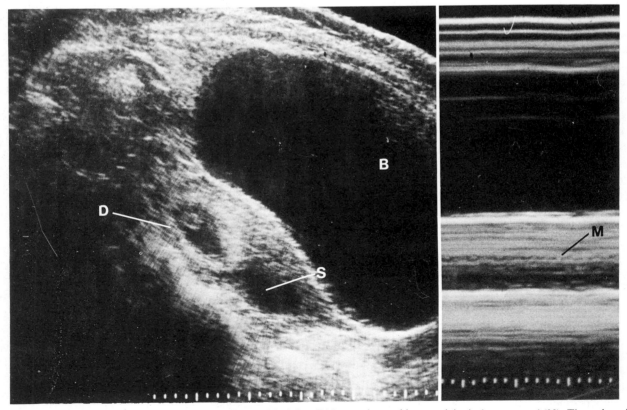

Fig. 29.3 Threatened abortion at 8 weeks amenorrhoea. The decidual ring (D) is complete and heart activity is demonstrated (M). The embryo is seen at the top of the sac. Blood (S) is seen in the uterine cavity below the sac

early pregnancy have been fully documented (Fisher et al, 1976; Fisher, 1982). Normal findings are shown in Fig. 29.2. Initially there is no obvious gestation sac but by 5 weeks the uterus should be obviously enlarged and contain a sac. This is usually spherical, but may be slightly irregular, secondary to uterine contractions or compression from a distended bladder. Surrounding the sac is a complete ring of echogenic decidua which is normally greater than 5 mm thick. An embryo should be demonstrated after 6–7 weeks amenorrhoea and embryonic heart movements should be either seen or recorded (Jouppila & Piiroinen, 1975; Eriksen & Philipsen, 1980).

Based on the data of Jouppila et al (1980) the following ultrasonic diagnoses will be made in a group of women with threatened abortion. Successful outcome will occur in 50 per cent, a blighted ovum diagnosed in 26 per cent, incomplete abortion in 8 per cent, missed abortion in 6 per cent, later spontaneous abortion where embryonic heart activity is recorded in 5 per cent, ectopic pregnancy in 4 per cent and hydatidiform mole in 1 per cent. Even if there is separation of the placenta or membranes, the outcome of the pregnancy will be successful in at least 90 per cent of instances where fetal heart activity is recorded (Fig. 29.3).

Varma (1981) found that where the placenta completely covered or encroached upon the internal cervical os in early pregnancy, the incidence of bleeding and abortion was greater than if the placenta was situated higher in the uterus. While some authors state that finding a sac low in the uterine cavity is a poor prognostic sign, there is no uniformity of opinion about this point.

Anembryonic sac. The term blighted ovum has become synonymous with an anembryonic sac. Donald et al (1972) defined the condition as 'an impregnated ovum whose development has become arrested at an early stage of pregnancy before the completion of the first trimester'. The term anembryonic sac is descriptive and should be used in preference to 'blighted ovum'. The typical appearance is seen in Fig. 29.4. Robinson (1975) stressed the importance of repeat examinations where the gestation sac appears empty in early pregnancy. If the sac volume is less than 2.5 ml and no embryo is seen, the examination should be repeated in 1 week. Pregnancy failure can then be demonstrated if the sac volume is not increased by 75 per cent during that time.

Incomplete abortion. The ultrasonic findings are shown in Fig. 29.5. The uterus is obviously bulky, mainly due to myometrial thickening and disorganised echoes are seen representing debris. A variable amount of fluid is seen in the uterine cavity. Where there is little remaining debris, it may be difficult to distinguish intra-uterine ultrasonic findings from those associated with ectopic pregnancy or normal menstruation.

Missed abortion. Ultrasonically this condition is diagnosed by observing an embryo with no detectable heart

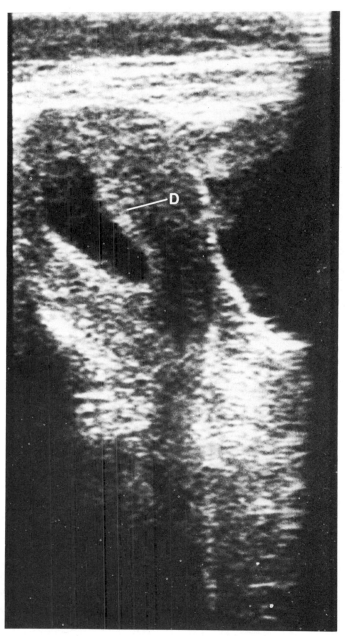

Fig. 29.4 An anembryonic sac. No evidence of an embryo is seen. The echogenic density of the decidua (D) is variable and appears to be broken superiorly

movement (Jouppila & Piiroinen, 1975; Eriksen & Philipsen, 1980). Frequently the sac volume is smaller than expected for the period of amenorrhoea (Robinson, 1975) and may be irregular in shape or poorly defined (Eriksen & Philipsen, 1980). The decidual ring is often noted to be broken, but the reliability of this sign has been disputed.

Ectopic pregnancy. As already discussed, the diagnosis of ectopic pregnancy can be very difficult, particularly the 'chronic' ectopic. In these women the use of serum βhCG (see below) and ultrasound in combination have been helpful in deciding which patients need surgical intervention. Ultrasound when used alone may not be helpful (Kelly et al, 1973). The most reliable finding is that of an

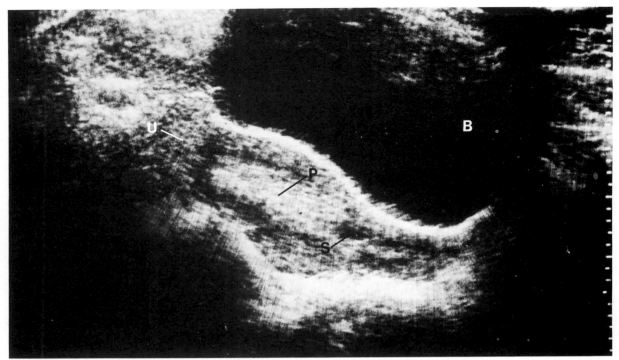

Fig. 29.5 Incomplete abortion at 8 weeks amenorrhoea. The uterus (U) is bulky. No gestation sac is seen. Placental debris (P) is seen on the anterior uterine wall and a small amount of blood (S) is seen low in the uterine cavity

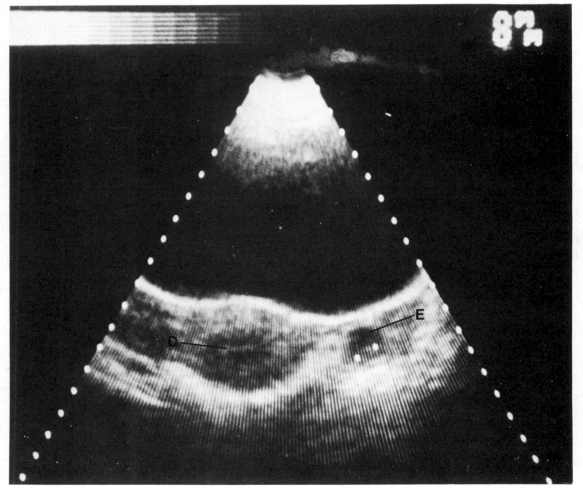

Fig. 29.6 A left tubal pregnancy (E) is shown. The sac contains an 8 mm embryo. A decidual reaction (D) is seen in the uterine cavity

intra-uterine pregnancy in a patient with a positive βhCG which virtually rules out a coexistent ectopic pregnancy.

Confusion may arise because both echogenic decidua and echo free fluid may be seen in the uterus and lead to the mistaken diagnosis of a 'pseudo-sac' for an intrauterine pregnancy (O'Neil et al, 1982). It is of paramount importance to find a fetal pole in the sac before a diagnosis of intra-uterine pregnancy is made and preferably fetal heart activity should be demonstrated (Kadar & Romero, 1982). The combination of an empty uterus and positive pregnancy test is very suggestive of ectopic pregnancy and has been associated with this diagnosis in up to 73 per cent of cases (Brown et al, 1978).

In the presence of any empty uterus, diagnosis can be difficult (Fig. 29.6). An extra-uterine sac may be confused with bowel loops, ovarian swellings, tubo-ovarian inflammatory disease and, of course, the reverse. Administration of a water enema can be a useful adjunct in the examination of these patients. Another finding which may be helpful is demonstration of free fluid in the Pouch of Douglas. However, all clinicians are aware that free fluid in the Pouch of Douglas other than blood is really very common.

Hydatidiform mole. Leopold & Asher (1975) state in reference to hydatidiform mole that 'using ultrasonic techniques, diagnosis can usually be made with a high degree of reliability by the tenth week of amenorrhoea'. However, this optimism is not shared (Wittman et al, 1981). Wittman et al (1981) have shown by repeated ultrasonic scanning that an apparent anembryonic sac may progress to the typical 'snow-storm' appearance of an hydatidiform mole and these changes are shown in Figs 29.7 and 29.8.

Woodward et al (1980) stress the importance of histological examination of all evacuated material in order to avoid missing the diagnosis of hydatidiform mole in what otherwise may be considered an anembryonic sac. Confusion may arise because of hydatidiform degeneration of the placenta in association with missed abortion, but the difference can only be judged microscopically, not ultrasonicly.

Hormonal indices

Although low or falling levels of urinary pregnanediol (Shearman, 1959) or progesterone (Jouppila et al, 1979; Eriksen & Philipsen, 1980) are associated with an

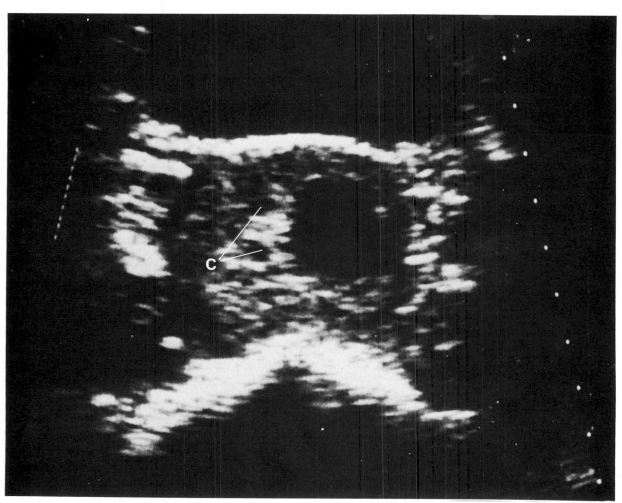

Fig. 29.7 An early hydatidiform mole at 8 weeks amenorrhoea. Cystic spaces (C) are seen in the 'placental' tissue. This condition is indistinguishable ultrasonically from an anembryonic sac

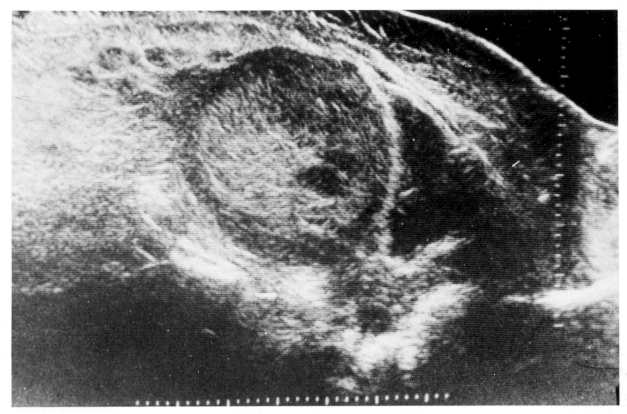

Fig. 29.8 A classical 'snowstorm' appearance of an hydatidiform mole at 13 weeks amenorrhoea

increased risk of abortion, only a minority of such patients abort and in a few women abortion can proceed with normal plasma levels of progesterone. Similarly, a poor index of discrimination is found in women with threatened abortion when plasma oestradiol is assayed (Jouppila et al, 1979). Mellows et al (1980) concluded that 'because of the overlap of hCG ranges in pregnancies that aborted compared with pregnancies that proceeded to term this precludes the use of hCG estimation prognosticly in the management of threatened abortion'. Although Batzer (1980) did not find single assays of hPL useful Biswas et al (1980) found that they were helpful in giving a prognosis, concluding that 'abnormal hPL levels during a bleeding episode are an accurate means of predicting outcome of pregnancy'. There is similar conflict about the prognostic significance of serum levels of pregnancy specific β_1-glycoprotein (SP–1), Jandial et al (1978) finding them of little assistance while Ho & Jones (1980) found them more helpful. However, the latter workers also found normal levels in 35 per cent of pregnancies which subsequently terminated in spontaneous abortion.

In essence, the correlation between clinical outcome and single assays of any of these hormones is too poor to use in clinical management, but serial assays, in association with clinical features and ultrasound are of use in some women.

MANAGEMENT

Prevention

Where known causes are few, prophylaxis is difficult. Women planning pregnancy should be advised not to smoke or to drink alcohol. Female anaesthetists, theatre nurses, dentists and dental assistants exposed to nitrous oxide (and/or halothane) should be advised to change their environment before attempting conception. Advice about smoking and alcohol may, for behavioural reasons, fall on stony ground. Environmental changes for those exposed to anaesthetic gases may be impossible for economic reasons. It is not yet known whether improved scavenging techniques to reduce ambient levels of volatile anaesthetics will alter the outlook but as a general principle, this makes a lot more sense than asking a theatre nurse or female anaesthetist or dentist to give up work.

Treatment

If knowledge of prophylaxis is meagre, knowledge related to effective treatment is almost non-existent although there are some small indicators of help from hormonal treatment in a minority of women with habitual abortion rather than actual threatened abortion (Ch. 30). The saga begins when the pregnant woman, up to that time normal, begins bleeding. Should she stop work? Should she be put to bed? If so should this be at home or in hospital? To stop work may be a financial disaster for the single parent or for the family dependent on two incomes and no-one could say with any honesty that it affects the ultimate outcome. Bedrest at home does not cost anything, but may be socially disruptive if there is no-one else to care for children. Admission to hospital is always expensive, either directly to the patient or to the wider community, depending on the system of health care. Given the frequency of threatened abortion, the total costs of management of the problem are enormous which would be easier to justify if medical intervention made any difference to the outcome. Unlike Dr Pangloss, we live in a real world where physicians look after the total patient. It is unwise to ignore the affective component of threatened abortion. The woman who really wants a child, bleeds and aborts at home, will inevitably think that the outcome may have been different if she had gone to bed or been admitted to hospital. For the same woman admitted to hospital who ultimately aborts, the costs of the hospital bed and investigations may be rationalised along the lines that 'everything possible was done'. This may not be good news for the mandarins who control a nation's health services but is not necessarily bad medicine. It will be a sad day for society if science ultimately replaces completely old fashioned tender loving care. Fortunately in many, if not all societies, there is still room for both.

Lacking any real guidelines, the clinician must make his initial decisions on impressionistic grounds. If there is no pain and if the amount of bleeding is slight then bedrest at home may be advised. If there is any pain or bleeding is heavier than that of a normal menstrual loss, or if there is maternal anxiety for any reason, the patient may be better in hospital. Physical examination should be complete and must include adequate speculum examination. Full differential diagnosis is mandatory. In most cases of threatened abortion there is no clinical doubt of the diagnosis and the physician should not be afraid of relying on his clinical skills alone. Where real doubt exists other investigations described from hormone assays, ultrasound to laparoscopy may be needed to resolve the doubt. However, let us assume that a firm diagnosis of threatened abortion has been reached. First the patient must be reassured. She should be told that there is about a 50 per cent chance that the bleeding will settle and the pregnancy proceed. She can be reassured that there is no increased risk of fetal abnormality if the pregnancy continues, but should be told that there is a slightly increased risk of prematurity and/or retarded intra-uterine growth. She needs to know this because of the implications for management of the rest of the pregnancy.

If the patient is still anxious and concerned an anxiolytic drug such as diazepam may be used for 1 or 2 days; but many women prefer to avoid medication if possible, even if there is no evidence that the drug is teratogenic.

It should be evident that we are therapeutic nihilists as far as hormone therapy for threatened abortion is concerned. We showed (Shearman & Garrett, 1963) in a double blind study that progestins made no difference to the outcome of pregnancy in patients with a history of habitual abortion and similar findings with different progestins were subsequently published by Goldzieher (1964) and Klopper & Macnaughton (1965). Fuchs (1963; quoted in Johannsen, 1970) in a survey of the literature reached the same conclusions regarding progestins and threatened abortion. The abuse of drugs in this area is long and often sad, some of the compounds being actively harmful. Stilboestrol was widely used for threatened abortion in the 1940s and 1950s with no good effect. All it left was a legacy of young women with adenosis and a poor reproductive potential and some young men with oligospermia because of their intra-uterine exposure to this stilbene derivative. The 19 nor-steroids caused a mini epidemic of non-progressive virilism of the female fetus in the 1950s, while medroxyprogesterone acetate (Depo-Provera) was first used as a systemic contraceptive when it became evident that women given the drug for 'pregnancy support' usually had months of anovulatory amenorrhoea either postpartum or after abortion.

The place of corpus luteum inadequacy remains undetermined. Current thinking suggests that if this is to be treated, this needs to be during the phase of the developing follicle rather than after ovulation and certainly well before pregnancy is diagnosed. The only exception to this belief is the unconfirmed work of Svigos (1982) using hCG early in pregnancy.

In most patients, further investigations will not be needed. The threatened abortion will progress to inevitable and incomplete abortion or will resolve and the pregnancy continue. If the bleeding persists for more than a couple of days or if there is doubt about viability of the pregnancy then further investigations are very helpful but not essential. Pregnancy, whether it ends in the delivery of an infant or abortion is finite with the very rare exception of a missed abortion that may stay *in utero*, if untreated, for months or even years. But for the patient, waiting can be both nerve racking and expensive. Of all investigations, ultrasound is the most helpful. Demonstrations of an empty or collapsed sac or a dead fetus on real time is definitive and can be followed by suction curettage without unnecessary delay. In very early pregnancy — before 6 or 7 weeks — even ultrasound in other than the very best units may be misleading or inconclusive. If this circumstance prevails, then serial measurements of β-hCG, hPL or progesterone probably offer the best endocrinological discriminants, but a single assay should never form the sole basis for a clinical decision.

THREATENED ABORTION AND THE INTRA-UTERINE DEVICE (IUD)

The woman who conceives with an intra-uterine device *in situ* is in a class of her own. By definition the pregnancy is unplanned, but is is a mistake to assume that all unplanned pregnancies are unwanted. An intra-uterine pregnancy with a coexisting IUD carries about a 60 per cent chance of abortion. If the tail of the device is visible it should be removed and the risk of abortion will then be reduced to about 30 per cent.

If the tail of the IUD cannot be seen there is a major problem; not just of increased risk of abortion but of septic threatened and incomplete abortion. This illness is explo-sive in onset, rapid in its evolution and carries a high mortality from septicaemia. if the tail of the device cannot be seen the patient and her consort should be advised of the risks. If they so wish and there is no legal impediment, termination of pregnancy should be considered.

Acknowledgements

Some of this text has been published previously (Shearman, 1982).

Mrs Jane Fonda supplied the echograms shown in Figs 2, 3 and 5. Dr Ian McKinnon supplied Fig. 7. Other echograms are from the Department of Diagnostic Ultrasound, Royal Hospital for Women, Paddington.

REFERENCES

Batzer F R, 1980 Hormonal evaluation of early pregnancy. Fertility and Sterility 34: 1–13

Biswas S, Murrey M, Buffoe G, Graves L, Jelowitz J, Dewhurst J 1980 Placental lactogen as a reliable index of fetal outcome in threatened abortion during early pregnancy. Journal of Obstetrics and Gynaecology 1: 75–77

Brown T W, Filly R A, Laing F C, Barlow J 1978 Analysis of ultrasonographic criteria in the evaluation of ectopic pregnancy. American Journal of Roentgenoy 131: 967–971

Brown J B, Evans J H, Beischer N A, Campbell D G, Fortune D W 1970 Hormone levels in threatened abortion. Journal of Obstetrics and Gynaecology of the British Commonwealth 77: 690–700

Carr D H 1971 Advances in Human Genetics. Plenum Press, New York

Correy J F 1980 The outcome of continuing pregnancies complicated by threatened abortion. Asia-Oceania Journal of Obstetrics and Gynaecology 6: 49–52

Editorial Comment 1980 British Medical Journal 281: 470

Ericksen P S, Philipsen T 1980 Prognosis in threatened abortion evaluated by hormone assays and ultrasound scanning. Obstetrics and Gynecology 55: 435–438

Evans J H, Beischer N A 1970 The prognosis of threatened abortion. Medical Journal of Australia 2: 165–168

Fisher C C 1982 Ultrasonic placental ageing. In: Contributions to Gynaecology lbstetrics. Karger, Basel

Fisher C C, Garrett W J, Kossoff G 1976 Placental ageing monitored by grey scale echography. American Journal of Obstetrics and Gynecology 124: 483–488

Funderburk S J, Guthrie D, Meldrom D 1980 Outcome of ancies complicated by early vaginal bleeding. British Journal of Obstetrics and Gynaecology 87: 100–105

Goldzieher J W 1964 Double-blind trial of a progestin in habitual abortion. Journal of the American Medical Association 188: 651–654

Grudzinskas J G, Gordon Y B, Miller J F, Williamson E 1981 Pregnancy wastage following implantation. Australian and New Zealand Journal of Obstetrics and Gynaecology 21: 56

Hertig A-T, Livingstone R G 1944 Spontaneous, threatened and habitual abortion: their pathogenesis and treatment. New England Journal of Medicine 230: 797–806

Ho P C, Jones W R 1980 Pregnancy-specific β_1 -glycoprotein as a prognostic indicator in complications of early pregnancy. American Journal of Obstetrics and Gynecology 138: 253–256

Jandial V, Towler C M, Horne C W H, Abramovich D R 1978 Plasma pregnancy-specific β_1 -glycoprotein in complications of early pregnancy. British Journal of Obstetrics and Gynaecology 85: 832–836

Jansen R P S 1982 Spontaneous abortion incidence in the treatment of infertility. American Journal of Obstetrics and Gynecology 143: 451–473

Johannsen A 1970 The prognosis of threatened abortion. Acta Obstetrica et Gynecologica Scandinavica 49: 89–93

Johnson W L, Stegall H F, Lein J M, Rushmer R F 1965 Detection of fetal life in early pregnancy with an ultrasonic doppler flow. Obstetrics and Gynecology 26: 305–307

Jones W R 1976 In: J J Scott, W R Jones (eds) Iummunology of man Reproduction, p 396. Academic Press, London

Jouppila P, Huhtaniemi I, Tapanainen J 1980 Early pregnancy failure: study by ultrasonic and hormonal methods. Obstetrics and Gynecology 55: 42–47

Jouppila P, Piiroinen O 1975 Ultrasonic diagnosis of fetal life in early pregnancy. Obstetrics and Gynecology 46: 616–620

Kadar N, Romero R 1982 The timing of repeat ultrasound examination in the evaluation of ectopic pregnancy. Journal of Clinical Ultrasound 10: 211–214

Kelly M T, Santos-Ramos R, Duenhoelter J H 1973 The value of omography in suspected ectopic pregnancy. Obstetrics and Gynecology 53: 703–708

Klopper A I, MacNaughton M 1965 Hormones in recurrent abortion. Journal of Obstetrics and Gynaecology British Commonwealth 72: 1022–1028

Lauritsen J G 1976 Aetiology of spontaneous abortion. Acta Obstetrica et Scandinavica (Suppl) 52: 1–29

Leopold G R, Asher W M 1975 Fundamentals of Abdominal and Pelvic Ultrasonography, p 174. W B Saunders, Philadelphia

Mantoni M, Pederson J F 1981 Intrauterine haematoma: an ultrasonic study of threatened bortion British Journal of Obstetrics and Gynaecology 88: 47–51

Mellows H J, Bennett M J, Brackpool P, Gordon Y B, Dewhurst J 1980 Human chorionic gonadotrophin in normal and abnormal pregnancy. Journal of Obstetrics and Gynaecology 1: 7–11

Mishell D R, Davajan V 1966 Quantitative immunologic assay of human chorionic gonadotropin in normal and abnormal pregnancies. American Journal of Obstetrics and Gynecology 96: 231–239

Nygren K G, Johansson E D, Wide L 1973 Evaluation of the pregnosis of threatened abortion from the peripheral plasma levels of progesterone, estradiol and human chorionic gonadotrophin. American Journal of Obstetrics and Gynecology 116: 916–922

O'Neil A G B, Hammond I G, S E 1982 Problems in the diagnosis of ectopic pregnancy: pseudo gestational sac. 22: 94–95

Robinson H P 1972 Detection of fetal heart movement in the first trimester of pregnancy using pulsed ultrasound. British Medical Journal 4: 466–468

Robinson H P 1975 The diagnosis of early pregnancy failure by sonar. British Journal of Obstetrics and Gynaecology 82: 849–857

Shearman R P 1959 Some aspets of the urinary excretion of pregnanediol in pregnancy. Journal of Obstetrics and Gynaecology of the British Empire 66: 1–11

Shearman R P 1980 In: J J Gold (ed) Gynecoogic Endocrinology, 3rd edn, pp 752–759. Harper and Row, Maryland

Shearman R P 1982 Threatened abortion in current topics in experimental endocrinology. In: Martini M (ed) The Endocrinology of Pregnancy and Parturition

Shearman R P, Garrett W J 1963 Double-blind study of the effect of 17-hydroxyprogesterone caproate on abortion rate. British Medical Journal 1: 292–295

Shearman R P, Parkin G M 1977 Cervical pregnancy — case report. Australian and New Zealand Journal of Obstetrics and Gynaecology 17: 105–107

Svigos J 1982 Preliminary experience with the use of human chorionic gonadotrophin therapy in women with repeated abortions. Clinical Reproduction and Fertility 1: 131–135

Tsenghi C, Metaxotou-Stavridaki C, Strataki-Benetou M, Kalpini-

Mavrov A, Matsaniotis N 1976 Obstetrics and Gynaecology 47: 463–68

Varma T R 1981 The implications of a low implantation of the placenta. Acta Obstetrica et Gynecologica Scandinavica 60: 265–268

Vessey M P, Nunn J F 1980 Occupational hazards of anaesthesia. British Medical Journal 281: 696–698

Wittman B K, Fulton L, Cooperberg P L, Lyons E A, Miller C, Shaw D 1981 Molar pregnancy: early diagnosis by ultrasound. Journal of Clinical Ultrasound 9: 153–156

Woodward R M, Filly R A, Callen P W 1980 First trimester molar pregnancy: non specific ultrasonographic appearance. Obstetrics and Gynecology (Supplt) 55: 315–335

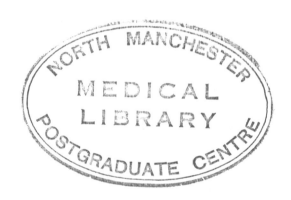

Aetiology and evaluation of repetitive reproductive wastage

Pre-natal loss covers a wide range of abortive processes from fertilisation of the ovum until viability, through pre-implantation, early post-implantation, embryonic and fetal life. An adverse genetic or environmental influence may affect the gametes as well as the conceptus. These influences may alter the blastocyst and prevent implantation. They may disrupt the developmental programme in early organogenesis leading to severe congenital malformations and fetal death or they may damage a single organ system at a later time in gestation. Early pregnancy wastage is known to be extensive. It has been estimated that only 30 per cent of all conceptions survive to birth, 15 per cent end in recognisable miscarriage and the remaining 55 per cent represent undetectable losses at pre-implantation and early post-implantation stages prior to the onset of the first missed menses (Hertig et al, 1959; Lindley, 1979). Preclinical post-implantation wastage can be diagnosed by early serial β-hCG determinations (Miller, 1980; Craft et al, 1982). Release of a specific early pregnancy factor (EPF) by the zygote soon after fertilisation and its rapid disappearance after embryonic death have recently provided an important tool for distinguishing between failure of fertilisation and preimplantation embryonic loss (Rolfe, 1982). With advances in knowledge and techniques, many cases of unexplained infertility might indeed be recurrent subclinical early pregnancy wastage. Clinically recognised abortion represents an event in a spectrum of reproductive failure. An aetiological factor may be operative in such a way that abortions are interspersed with infertility, normal pregnancy, stillbirth, neonatal death, or defective live births. Sporadic fetal abortion is a frequent phenomenon representing 15 per cent of all recognisable pregnancies. The vast majority of single sporadic abortions are caused by non-repetitive errors in gametogenesis or fertilisation. Less frequently they are the result of accidental adverse maternal factors or external teratogenic influences. Recurrent abortion is a problem in approximately one in 200 couples. Clinically, a recurrent factor may be genetic, anatomical, endocrine, or immunological. In a number of couples, these recurrent causes of reproductive failure can

be uncovered by a systematic evaluation accessible to most clinical settings. The same basic clinical workup may identify another large group of couples with recurrent abortions and no recognisable aetiology. Recent heteromorphic banding techniques on the aborted material indicate that recurrent gamete non-disjunction and dispermy play an important role in this group of recurrent abortion couples with an otherwise negative evaluation. The purpose of this review is to place into perspective the relative role of the known and unknown aetiological factors and to draw general guidelines for a practical approach to this complex and enigmatic problem. A rational therapeutic management will be based upon the aetiological factors.

AETIOLOGY

Recognisable genetic factors

Known genetic factors are prevalent in pregnancy wastage. These factors were reported to occur in 25 per cent of the Medical College of Georgia's recurrent abortion population (Fig. 30.1A) (Tho et al, 1979; McDonough & Tho, 1981). A parental chromosomal rearrangement was found in 50 per cent of this known genetic group and multifactorial disorders were uncovered in the remaining half.

Since the 1966 Geneva conference (Geneva Conference, 1966), numerous reports of independent series have shown that balanced chromosomal rearrangements in a parent may predispose to recurrent fetal wastage (De La Chapelle et al, 1973; Papp et al, 1974; Khudr, 1975; Byrd et al, 1977; Tho et al, 1979; Husslein et al, 1982). These studies have indicated that a parent may be a carrier of a cytogenetic abnormality in approximately 4–14 per cent of recurrent abortion couples with or without fetal malformations. A balanced chromosomal translocation in a parent may produce — as a result of a normal meiotic segregation — unbalanced gametes leading to abortions or defective live-born children. It may also give rise to a balanced gamete resulting in a balanced carrier or it may produce a cytogenetically normal gamete. Figure 30.2 illustrates the

100 Patients

15%
Mullerian

23%
Endocrine

37%
Unknown

Known Genetic
12%
Gross parental
cytogenetic abnormalities

13%
Multifactoral

A

110 Patients

12%
Parental chromosomal
variants

5.4%
Gross parental
cytogenetic abnormalities

B

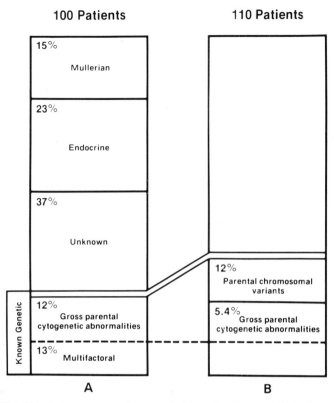

Fig. 30.1 A demonstrates the recognisable and unknown aethiologic categories in 100 couples studied for reproductive failure at the Medical College of Georgia (reproduced with permission from Tho et al, 1979). B illustrates the addition of parental chromosomal variants (12 per cent) in the subgroup of gross parental abnormalities (5.4 per cent) in the most recent series of 110 couples studied for reproductive failure at the Medical College of Georgia. Note the extension of the known genetic group toward the unknown aetiology group (Tho et al, 1983)

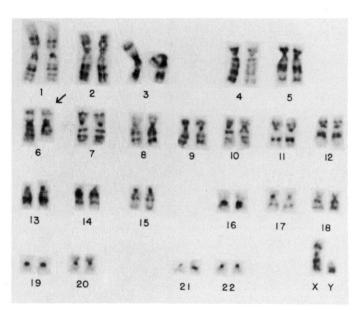

Fig. 30.2 Unbalanced karyotype of male abortus 46,XY, del (6) (pter–q2) with deletion of the long arm of the chromosome 6 (arrow) (reproduced with permission from McDonough & Tho, 1981)

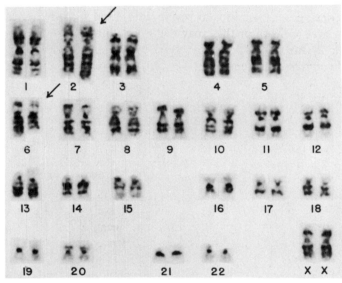

Fig. 30.3 Balanced karyotype of the mother 46,XX,t(2;6) (q3; q2) who produced the abortus in Fig. 30.2. Deleted portion of chromosome 6 has been translocated to chromosome 2. (reproduced with permission from McDonough $ Tho, 1981)

unbalanced karyotype of a male abortus [46,XY, del (6) (pter–q2)]. Figure 30.3 demonstrates the karyotype of the mother who is carrier of the balanced translocation 2/6 [46,XX,t(2;6)(q3;q2)]. In rare instances, the balanced rearrangement may induce non-disjunction of other chromosomes during meiosis, leading to aneuploidic gametes. The Medical College of Georgia series distinguished couples with a pure history of abortions from couples having abortions intermixed with the delivery of liveborn malformed infants. While parental chromosomal rearrangements were found in 12 per cent of the total series, the incidence of parental chromosomal rearrangements in pedigrees with pure abortion history was 9.6 per cent. In couples with a combined history of abortions and fetal malformations, the percentage of cytogenetically rearranged parents within the group increased to 23 per cent (Tho et al, 1979; McDonough & Tho, 1981). Furthermore, among couples with abortion histories, there was a 3:1 predominance of female carriers, and among couples with mixed histories, all carriers were female. Conversely, the risks of a balanced translocation carrier having a liveborn malformed child was higher if an unbalanced translocation was carried by a liveborn offspring rather than by just abortuses. This risk was also higher if a balanced translocation was carried by

a female rather than a male parent. In agreement with the natural history of meiotic chromosomal segregation in these balanced carriers, our observations indicate that these couples produce mixtures of abortions and malformed liveborns or stillborns or mixtures of abortions and normal children rather than consecutive series of abortions.

Recently developed banding techniques make it possible to detect even small structural rearrangements that are not apparent on routine karyotyping. Figure 30.4 illustrates the cytogenetic non-banding study performed on a male parent with three consecutive early abortions. Routine karyotyping was interpreted as normal. However, banding

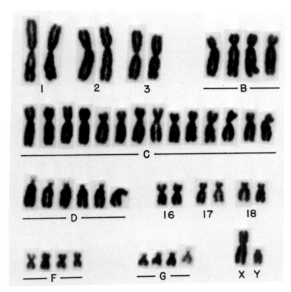

Fig. 30.4 The 'normal' non-banding karyotype of a male parent with three consecutive early abortions (reproduced with permission from McDonough P G et al, 1979 Overall evaluation of recurrent abortion In: Givens J R (ed), The Infertile Female, Year Book Medical Publishers, Chicago, pp 385–404)

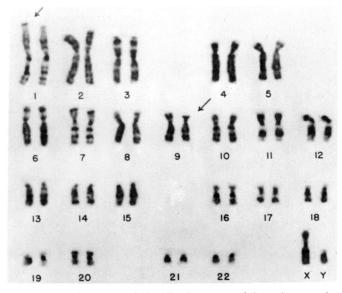

Fig. 30.5 The Giemsa-trypsin banding karyotype of the male parent in Fig. 30.4 which now demonstrates a balanced 1/9 translocation [46,XY, t(1;9) (p3; p2)] (reproduced with permission from McDonough P G et al, 1979 Overall evaluation of recurrent abortion. In: Givens J R (ed), The Infertile Female, Year Book Medical Publishers, Chicago, pp 383–404)

techniques identified the translocation of a small fragment of chromosome 9 to chromosome 1 (Fig. 30.5).

Current banding techniques also permit a better detection of a pericentric inversion. This results from an intrachromosomal breakage on both sides of the centromere followed by a 180° rotation and healing to produce an inverted genetic sequence. Large pericentric inversions have been shown to predispose to aneuploidy in progeny. Homologous chromosomal pairing during meiosis is poss-

ible only with the formation of inversion loops. Chromosomal duplication or deficiency has occasionally resulted from crossing over and subsequent chromosomal breakage of these large inversion loops during meiotic segregation, leading to abortion or malformations (Taysi et al, 1973; Fujimoto et al, 1978).

A small pericentric inversion such as inversion (9)(plql) involves mostly the inactive heterochromatin. Crossing over is absent in these heterochromatic segments. These small pericentric inversions are therefore considered as a chromosome variant or a type of chromosome polymorphism. Other chromosome variants include an enlargement of the heterochromatin such as 9qh+ (Nielson et al, 1974) and a large Y chromosome (Genest, 1979). Chromosome anomalies in the gametes of carriers of small pericentric inversions or chromosome variants may be explained by interchromosomal effects due to the activity of the abnormal heterochromatin during meiosis. Normal segregation of other chromosomes may be prevented (Gagné et al, 1973; Boué et al, 1975c; Stahl et al, 1975). The association of parental chromosome variants and either recurrent abortion or fetal malformation has been a controversial subject (De La Chapelle et al, 1974; Baccichetti et al, 1980). In the most recent Medical College of Georgia series, only 5.4 per cent of the 110 couples studied for reproductive failure were carriers of a gross chromosomal rearrangement. However it demonstrated chromosome variants in 12 per cent of the study population (Fig. 30.1B) (Tho et al, 1982). This incidence represents more than four times that of the general population (2–3 per cent) (Court-Brown, 1967). The reproductive performance of the carriers of pericentric inversion (9) (plql) in this series is extremely poor, with only a 17 per cent success rate. In contrast, it was very good with the recurrent abortion subgroup harbouring other types of chromosome variants (85 per cent success rate). The apparently ominous nature of the pericentric inversion (9) (plql) in our report is concerning. It is, however, in agreement with the findings of Boué et al (1975c) in their ten reported families. More advanced techniques for meiotic studies in the human are necessary to clarify the role of a given chromosomal inversion or variant in recurrent reproductive failure.

Finally, *X chromosome mosaicism* in females has been repeatedly reported in association with recurrent abortion histories. Some of these women have also produced liveborn children with Down's syndrome and X chromosome aneuploidy or mosaicism (Shapiro, 1969; Predescu et al, 1969; Hsu et al, 1972; Singh et al, 1980.) One patient in the Medical College of Georgia series of recurrent pregnancy wastage has 45,X (94 per cent)/46,XX (6 per cent) mosaicism. At the age of 35, she still has functioning ovaries but had a previous history of three early spontaneous abortions followed by protracted infertility. X chromosome aneuploidy in the progeny of these mothers may be explained either by fertilisation of ova with a nullisomy X complement, or by the effect of genes for non-disjunction or anaphase lag.

It may be concluded that a chromosome analysis utilising newer banding techniques and an adequate chromosome count should be performed on couples having a history of recurrent abortion or having a pedigree with one abortion plus one malformed fetus. Parental balanced translocation, pericentric inversion, chromosome variants or X chromosome mosaicism may be uncovered. This detection is important for appropriate counselling and prenatal cytogenetic monitoring.

Some multifactorial conditions that cause early childhood or neonatal death may also cause early fetal loss and spontaneous abortion. This possibility was suggested by the Medical College of Georgia series of eight couples with a combined history of pregnancies ending in abortion and delivery of children having neural tube defects. Two other couples had mixed histories of abortions and fetuses with Potter's syndrome. Anencephaly was the predominant type of neural tube defect and was found in the offspring of five among the 13 couples with multifactorial reproductive loss. Except for one anencephalic whose sex was not mentioned, all anencephalics were female in our study. Figure 30.6 represents the pedigree of a couple who had two female anencephalic newborns at 28 weeks and five early abortions prior to the delivery of two normal male children. Some of the other neural tube abnormalities noted among pedigrees with multifactorial disorders may represent variants of the Meckel's syndrome (Hsia et al, 1971). This is a special type of neural tube defect with an autosomal recessive mode of inheritance. Abnormalities associated with this syndrome also include cleft palate, polycystic kidneys and abnormal genitalia. Careful examination of external and internal structural abnormalities and tissue karyotyping of defective fetuses are essential for a correct diagnosis and proper counselling.

A subsequent term normal child was born to only 32 per cent of the patients in the known genetic group of the Medical College of Georgia series (Fig. 30.7). The poor

PEDIGREE
M.J.B.

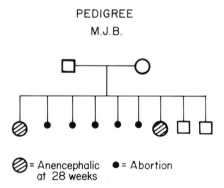

⊘ = Anencephalic   ● = Abortion
at 28 weeks

Fig. 30.6 Pedigree of a couple with two female anencephalic newborns and five early abortions prior to delivery of two normal male children (reproduced with permission from McDonough et al, 1979 Overall evaluation of recurrent abortion In: Givens J R (ed), The Infertile Female, Year Book Medical Publishers, Chicago, pp 385–404)

ETIOLOGY—INCIDENCE	PROGNOSIS FOR NORMAL CHILD AND THERAPY
KNOWN GENETIC FACTORS 25% Chromosomal Multifactorial	NORMAL CHILD 32% Prenatal diagnosis
ANATOMIC FACTORS 15% Uterus Subseptus (thick septum) DES uterus Incompetent cervix Uterine fibroids (severe distortion) Asherman's syndrome	NORMAL CHILD 60%-70% Metroplasty, monitor cervix Progesterone blockade, monitor cervix Cerclage Myomectomy Hysteroscopic lysis of synechiae
ENDOCRINE FACTORS 23% Corpus luteum defect	NORMAL CHILD 90% Prenidation progesterone vaginal suppositories, repeat biopsy Parlodel if prolactin elevated Clomid if follicular dysgenesis suspected
UNKNOWN ETIOLOGY 37% Recurrent aneuploidy: Gamete aging Delayed ovulation Maternal age Delayed fertilization Recurrent euploidic abortion: Corpus luteum defect of early pregnancy Immunologic Infectious Smoking—alcohol consumption	NORMAL CHILD 62% Avoid gamete aging Ovulation control Synchronization of gametes Rarely: Donor male Prenatal diagnosis Serial endocrine studies, empirical vaginal progesterone supplementation Immunologic studies Empirical antimicrobial therapy Counseling

Fig. 30.7 The aethiological categories, their incidence, therapy, and prognosis in the series of 100 couples studied for reproductive failure at the Medical College of Georgia [reproduced with permission from Tho et al (1983), Recurrent Abortion In: Wynn R (ed), Obstetrics and Gynecology Annual, 12th edn]

reproductive outcome in this group may be improved if more couples were to attempt further pregnancies, taking advantage of prenatal monitoring.

Anatomical aetiology

Anatomical causes of recurrent abortion include uterus subseptus, DES* uterus, incompetent cervix, uterine fibroids and Asherman's Syndrome. They usually induce early second trimester abortions and are responsible for 10–15 per cent of recurrent pregnancy wastage.

Absent or incomplete embryonic resorption of the septum which has been produced by midline fusion of the Müllerian ducts gives rise to the *uterus septus* or *subseptus*. This variety of Müllerian anomaly has been recognised as the most common anatomical cause of recurrent abortion (Shearman, 1975; McDonough & Tho, 1981; Jones, 1981). A hysterogram should be part of the basic evaluation of the parents suffering from recurrent pregnancy loss and facilities should be available for an additional pelvic pneumoperitoneum in the same setting. By performing this gynaecogram, both internal and external uterine contours are simultaneously outlined. This additional pelvic pneumoperitoneum technique is not necessary if laparoscopy was previously performed for another indication and a normal external uterine contour was documented. Volu-

---

* DES = Diethylstilboestrol.

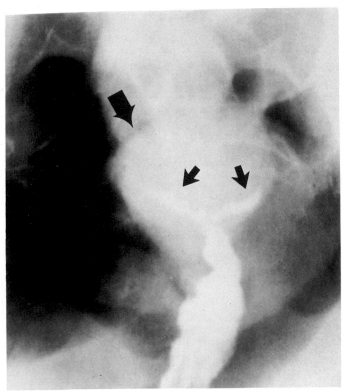

Fig. 30.8 The gynaecogram on a female with three consecutive early abortions, illustrating a thick septum and the slit-like duplicated cavities. The small arrows indicate these very small uterine cavities. The large arrow demonstrates the external uterus [reproduced with permission from Tho et al (1983), Recurrent Abortion In: Wynn R (ed), Obstetrics and Gynecology Annual, 12th edn

metric compromise of the uterine cavity and implantation on the fibrous, poorly vascularised septum are possible explanations for repetitive abortions and premature labour. Figure 30.8 demonstrates a gynaecogram performed on a woman with three early spontaneous abortions. It illustrates an extremely thick septum and the slit-like duplicated cavities. The rate of subsequent pregnancy salvage is good in these patients with surgical unification. Cervical incompetence is not uncommonly seen in asociation with a subseptate uterus. It may also be caused by the removal of the entire septum in the septate uterus. An interesting syndrome, the 'hand-foot-uterus syndrome,' consists of a Müllerian anomaly and malformations of the hands and feet. It was seen in one couple of the Medical College of Georgia series. Renal anomalies should be investigated in all women found to have Müllerian anomalies.

More than two-thirds of the *DES exposed women* have hysterographic Müllerian anomalies such as the T-shaped uterus, the hypoplastic uterus and the uterine constriction band. Intra-uterine polypoid defects and synechiae also occur (Kaufman et al, 1977). DES exposed women with structural abnormalities of the cervix or vaginal epithelial changes have a five times higher chance of having uterine abnormalities that appear on radiological visualisation than those without cervical or vaginal changes. Several recent reports suggest that DES exposure by itself in the absence

of abnormal hysterographic and structural cervical changes do not significantly alter the pregnancy outcome. In contradistinction, DES exposure associated with abnormal radiological and structural anomalies of the upper uterus and cervix is related to a poorer pregnancy outcome (Pillsbury, 1980). Pregnancy complications such as ectopic pregnancy, early abortion, premature labour are more frequent and may result from abnormalities of implantation, uterine fundal dysfunction and cervical incompetency (Berger & Goldstein 1980; Schmidt et al, 1980; Verdiano et al, 1980; Sandberg et al, 1981). Women with recurrent reproductive failure and a positive history of DES exposure should have an adequate evaluation of the upper genital tract and close surveillance of their pregnancy.

The precise role of the *incompetent cervix* in fetal wastage is difficult to delineate because of the multiple variables involved in premature labour and the subjectivity involved in the diagnosis of the incompetent cervix. Women with a history of 'painless labour' during the second trimester and those with repetitive unexplained immaturity or prematurity should be highly suspect for this clinical entity. Although the aetiology of cervical incompetence is often obscure, it is frequently associated with uterine malformations, a DES uterus, a previous history of cervical dilation and manipulation, cervical conisation and obstetric cervical lacerations. The diagnosis is most easily made during pregnancy by observing the cervix for premature effacement and dilatation. In the non-pregnant woman it can be suspected by the ease with which a Foley catheter is passed through the internal os. Radiological confirmation of the diagnosis is controversial. Fetal salvage rate after a simple cerclage approximates 90 per cent.

Uterine fibroids may rarely cause repetitive abortions either by severe cavitary distortion or their submucous location.

Endometrial sclerosis or *Asherman's syndrome* may be a cause of recurrent early abortion if infertility is not a problem. It may be a complication of previous recurrent abortions and curettages rather than a precipitating factor.

Müllerian anomalies and balanced chromosomal rearrangement in the parents are the two well defined and accepted causes of repetitive fetal wastage. Their incidence in the Medical College of Georgia series was 15 per cent and 12 per cent, respectively (Fig. 30.1A). A patient with both aetiologies, uterus subseptus and a balanced translocation state, was found in our series of recurrent abortion. This exemplifies the need for a complete evaluation in all couples.

Endocrine aetiology

Corpus luteum deficiency is responsible for 23 per cent of the recurrent abortion couples in the Medical College of Georgia series (Tho et al, 1979; McDonough & Tho, 1981), and for 35 per cent in other series (Jones, 1975). It is defined as an inadequate ovarian production of progesterone. Progesterone secreted by the corpus luteum prior and subsequent to conception supports the endometrium until the trophoblast assumes sufficient function for maintenance of pregnancy. The actual lifespan of the corpus luteum is extended beyond its usual duration by hCG. The function of the corpus luteum of pregnancy declines after the fourth week of gestation in spite of rising levels of hCG. The placenta subsequently becomes the primary source of progesterone synthesis and secretion. The time of luteoplacental shift is variable but occurs at about the seventh week of gestation. Progesterone plays a crucial role in the successful course of the human pregnancy. It converts the oestrogen primed endometrium of the proliferative phase to a secretory pattern which is receptive for implantation. It induces the decidual change in the stromal tissue of the endometrium so that the fetus is protected from the immunological responses of the mother and the mother is protected from uninhibited invasion by the fetus. This endometrial receptivity for nidation and maintenance of early pregnancy depends upon an appropriate dose and sequential orchestration of the steroidal milieu throughout the menstrual cycle. Current evidence indicates that oestrogen and progesterone binding regulates endometrial functions through nuclear translocation of these hormones. It has been uniformly accepted that patterns of oestradiol and progesterone receptor concentrations in the endometrium are directly influenced by the secretions of the maturing dominant follicle and the functional corpus luteum (Bayard et al, 1978; Kreitmann-Gimbal et al, 1980). With progressive increase of oestrogens during the proliferative phase and more specifically during the pre-ovulatory period, the continuous synthesis of oestrogen receptor in the cytoplasm and the parallel transfer of hormone-receptor complexes into the nuclei result in a steady level in the cytoplasm and an increased concentration in the nucleus. After ovulation, early in the secretory phase the reduction of cytoplasmic oestrogen receptor sites has been attributed to a progesterone effect. The subsequent decrease of nuclear oestrogen receptor sites probably reflects the sustained low levels of cytosol oestrogen receptors. During the follicular phase, progesterone receptor concentrations rise under the influence of increasing oestradiol levels and are primarily in the cytoplasm. After ovulation, the secretion of progesterone by the corpus luteum is accompanied by a rapid nuclear translocation and concomitant decrease in cytoplasmic progesterone receptor. Thereafter, progesterone receptors decline in both nuclei and cytosol. This is attributed to the negative effect of progesterone on its own receptors and also to the decrease of oestradiol effect due to the low levels of oestradiol receptors at this time period. In conclusion, oestrogen binding and nuclear translocation stimulate endometrial growth and proliferation and also enhance endometrial sensitivity to progesterone by increasing the number of cytoplasmic

progesterone receptors (Hsueh et al, 1976). Thus the oestrogen output in the follicular phase is the major determinant for the subsequent progesterone action in the luteal phase. Measurements of total oestradiol and progesterone receptor sites in the endometrium at different locations indicate their highest concentrations in the fundus and their progressive fall to negligible concentrations in the isthmus (Bayard et al, 1978). Often patients with luteal phase defects have below normal levels of circulating oestrogens and progesterone during the follicular and luteal phases of the menstrual cycle, respectively. In rare instances, the endometrial stromal development remains persistently suboptimal in spite of normal serial gonadotrophin and steroid patterns throughout the cycle, and in spite of luteal progesterone supplementation. Binding studies will clarify the absence or reduction of progesterone receptor site or their inability to respond (Keller et al, 1979).

Although it is well known that steroid receptor concentrations and histological changes in the endometrium depend upon the levels of circulating oestradiol and progesterone, the precise pattern of intracellular receptors preparing the endometrium for implantation is incompletely characterised. Recent binding studies on the endometrium at pre-implantation time in monkeys in the conception and non-conception cycles demonstrate a change in oestrogen receptors in nuclei of endometrial cells. The ratio of nuclear oestrone receptor concentration (NE_1R) to nuclear oestradiol receptor concentration (NE_2R) remains below 1 throughout the menstrual cycle. This ratio rises to 2.5 at pre-implantation in the conception cycle. This change was demonstrated to be induced by the abrupt increase of progesterone level during the late luteal phase of the conception cycle. This finding may have future implications in the understanding of reproductive failure related to corpus luteum defects (Kreitmann-Gimbal et al, 1981).

Besides its function on endometrial receptivity for ovo-implantation, progesterone also maintains the early pregnancy following implantation by keeping the uterine myometrial activity fully suppressed. Removal of the corpus luteum within 21 days after the missed menses is promptly followed by a continuous fall in plasma progesterone and a progressive increase of intra-uterine pressure and oxytocin response leading to abortion in most women. There is a possibility that by blocking the increase of oestrogen receptor level in the myometrium, progesterone inhibits the excitatory effect of oestradiol. Abortion can be prevented by exogenous progesterone supplementation in these luteectomised women (Csapo et al, 1973).

It is becoming increasingly evident that adequate follicular maturation in the pre-ovulatory phase is an important determinant of the corpus luteum function. Follicular growth is initiated in the late luteal phase of the previous cycle by an increase of FSH which stimulates the development of a number of primary follicles. Follicular growth is associated with enlargement of the oocyte and with an increase in follicular size due to proliferation of the granulosa cells. During this early follicular phase — known as follicular recruitment phase — FSH stimulates its own receptors and activates the aromatase system which converts the androgens formed in the theca cells into oestradiol. The so-formed oestradiol enhances follicular sensitivity to FSH by increasing FSH receptors on granulosa cells. Most importantly, FSH stimulates the formation of LH receptors on granulosa cells (Lee et al, 1973). FSH is concentrated in the follicular fluid of growing follicles and may exert local effects on follicular growth. Oestrogens accumulate in very high concentration in antral fluid and locally enhance follicular maturation. Oestrogens in large antral follicles inhibit the production of androgens and progesterone by a local intra-ovarian effect. Full follicular development is therefore dependent on the interactions between the gonadotrophins and various steroids. This gonadotrophin-steroid harmonious interplay is operative since early follicular phase resulting in the appearance of a large number of LH responsive granulosa cells. The follicle destined to ovulate has already been selected by this time and oestradiol plays a key role in the selection of the dominant follicle. The oestradiol surge induces a LH surge through positive feedback signals acting on the cyclic centre of the hypothalamus. With the rise of LH, luteinisation of the follicle is induced, associated with cessation of granulosa cell proliferation. As luteinisation proceeds, progesterone levels rise. Oestrogens, LH, and FSH, after achieving their peaks, subsequently regress. The physical rupture of the mature follicle occurs 7–24 hours after LH surge and the newly ruptured follicle differentiates into a corpus luteum. The final determinant for adequate corpus luteum function is the presence of sufficient LH to stimulate the granulosa luteal cells of the corpus luteum to secrete steroids, essentially progesterone. Progesterone rises within one day after ovulation to reach a peak on day 8 when the corpus luteum reaches its maximum stage of development during the menstrual cycle. Then it declines unless pregnancy has begun. Human chorionic gonadotrophin appears in the circulation in detectable amounts by the ninth post-ovulatory day. It rescues the corpus luteum function and enhances progesterone production (Halme et al, 1978). The most important characteristic of luteal phase defective cycles is the inability of the corpus luteum to respond to hCG due to insufficient LH/hCG receptors on the granulosa luteal cells. Since FSH augmented by oestrogen induces the expression of LH receptors during folliculogenesis, FSH availability during the follicular phase is the mainstay for subsequent corpus luteum function. Clinically, luteal phase defects include a spectrum of presentations which are characterised by various deficiencies of progesterone production leading to inappropriate endometrial development and impaired implantation. The

two most accepted features of this disorder were described initially by Moszkowski et al (1962) and later by Sherman & Korenman (1974a, b) as the short luteal phase and the inadequate luteal phase. The short luteal phase is defined as a luteal phase of 8 days or less. In the inadequate luteal phase, progesterone output is lower than expected but the interval from ovulation to menses is normal.

Recently, direct evidence that a FSH deficiency during follicular growth results in defective corpus luteum function has been shown in both the monkey and the human model. Porcine follicular fluid extract (pFF) injected to monkeys in the early follicular phase, selectively suppresses serum FSH levels, without changing serum LH. These treated monkeys experienced either normally timed ovulation followed by luteal dysfunction, or a delay in follicular maturation and ovulation, depending on the dose and duration of pFF therapy. When pFF was injected later in the follicular phase from day 9 to day 11 of the cycle, it induced cessation or delay of final development of the dominant follicle and subsequent luteal phase dysfunction. In these pFF induced luteal phase defects (Stouffer & Hodgen, 1980; diZerega et al, 1981a, b; diZerega & Hodgen, 1981), serum progesterone patterns were similar to those characteristic of spontaneous luteal phase defects in women and monkeys (Wilks et al, 1976). The sequence of events leading to corpus luteum dysfunction seemed to be similar in both early and late FSH suppression. The transient FSH depression was followed by decreased aromatase activity as evidenced by lowered oestradiol production. The final result is the impaired development of LH/hCG receptors on the granulosa luteal cells which become unable to produce sufficient amounts of progesterone.

In the human model, corpus luteum function was induced by subcutaneous injection of a LRF* agonist to five volunteers for 3 consecutive days after the onset of menses (Sheehan et al, 1982). After a transient rise in serum FSH, LH and oestradiol, LH remained unchanged. However, FSH was subsequently depressed to lower levels than in the control cycle and oestradiol started to decrease during the last 4 days of the follicular phase. These hormonal changes induced by LRF agonist were associated with a 9-day delay in the onset of mid-cycle gonadotrophin surge. The LH, FSH and oestradiol peak levels were significantly lower in the treated cycles than in the control cycles. These follicular aberrations were extended into the luteal phase. There was early luteal regression in four subjects as evidenced by the fall in oestradiol and progesterone on the eighth and ninth days following the gonadotrophin surge (Fig. 30.9, left). In the remaining individual, the luteal phase was of normal length, but was characterised by reduced progesterone output (Fig. 30.9, right). In the human model, the same cascade of hormonal

---

* LRF = Luteinising hormone releasing factor.

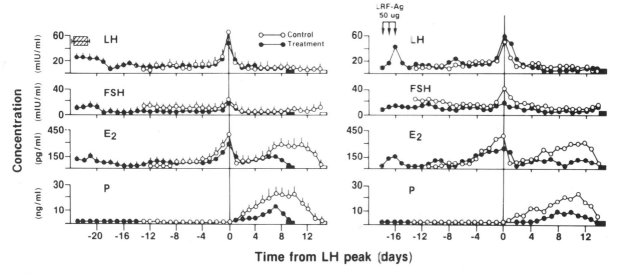

Fig. 30.9 Left = Time course and pattern of circulating LH, FSH, oestradiol (E₂) and progesterone (P) concentrations during the control and LRF agonist (hatched box, top left) treated cycles in four among the five normal volunteers. Ovulation was 9 days delayed, occurring on day 23 of the treated cycle instead of day 14 as in the control cycle. Onset of menses occurred on day 9 in the treated cycles (solid boxes) and day 14 after the midcycle surge in the control cycles (open boxes). Right = Time course and pattern of circulating LH, FSH, oestradiol (E₂) and progesterone (P) concentrations during the control and LRF agonist treated cycles in the remaining subject. Ovulation was 5 days delayed, occurring on day 19 of the treated cycle as compared to day 14 in the control cycles. She also exhibited reduced FSH during the follicular phase, reduced FSH and oestradiol (E₂) during the mid-cycle surge, normal luteal phase length, but reduced oestradiol (E₂) and progesterone (P) during the entire luteal phase. Solid boxes indicate the period of menstruation (reproduced with permission from Sheehan et al, 1982)

defects was observed following the induced FSH depression as in the monkey model.

Finally, decreased luteal LH or hCG could also be the culprit in functional inadequacy of the corpus luteum of the menstrual cycle or the corpus 'luteum rescue' of early pregnancy. Thau et al (1979) have used anti-LH serum in the monkey model. They have induced infertility in these animals as a result of corpus luteum dysfunction. This was demonstrated by reduced peripheral concentrations and production rate of progesterone and shortened luteal phase length in the immunised animals. They have also found significantly suppressed progesterone production rates in early pregnancy in treated animals. The fertility rates were restored with medroxyprogesterone acetate administration during the critical period following fertilisation (Thau & Sundaram, 1980). Human models with induction of corpus luteum dysfunction by suppressing follicular FSH or by depressing luteal LH/hCG and with attempt to restore FSH by clomiphene or by FSH rich HMG preparations or luteal supplementation with natural progesterone in respective situations would be very helpful for a better insight in the current clinical management of corpus luteum dysfunction. Factors that interfere with adequate release of FSH such as hyperprolactinaemia (Del Pozo et al, 1979), and androgen excess (Sarris et al, 1978) will prevent adequate follicular development. Possible consequences include an inadequate ovulatory LH surge and premature corpus luteum regression. A high abortion rate occurring in cycles treated with clomiphene citrate or exogenous gonadotrophins may be related to disorders of

luteal function secondary to abnormal stimulated or exogenous gonadotrophins (Jones et al, 1970; Ross et al, 1970). Physiological ovulation, fertilisation, implantation of the conceptus and development of the placenta as an organ of steroidogenesis are complex endocrine processes of early pregnancy. In the course of these events, potential endocrine mishaps may lead to early abortion. In addition, the completion of meiosis I and II and the fertilisation that follows are critical genetic events that are, in part, hormonally modulated. The only segment of this process that is at least partially susceptible to clinical evaluation is the corpus luteum function.

Corpus luteum deficiency is suggested when a history of recurrent abortion is associated with a short menstrual interval of 21–23 days, interval infertility, ovulation delay, a short luteal temperature rise. It is confirmed by a poor glandular development or a lack of pseudodecidual change or both on a late luteal endometrial biopsy. Parental balanced chromosomal rearrangements may also be discovered in couples with infertility followed by abortion with the suggestion of corpus luteum inadequacy (Sarto & Therman, 1976). Ovulation delay resulting in gamete ageing is a concern in pedigrees of recurrent abortion. When ovulation is late, meiosis I may be delayed and predispose to non-disjunction and pathological gametes.

Prior to pregnancy, corpus luteum function is best evaluated by a late luteal phase endometrial biopsy. Endometrial development at that time is the best bioassay for the total effect of oestrogen and progesterone production on the implantation site. There is no practical and reliable

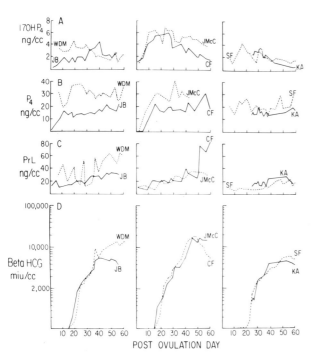

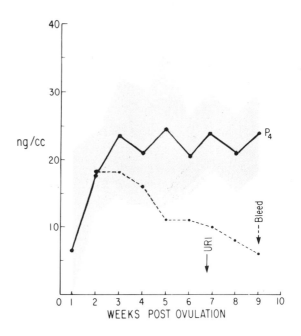

a

Fig. 30.10 The sequential pattern of 17 α-hydroxyprogesterone (170HP₄), progesterone (P), prolactin (Prl), and βhCG values in six normal women in early pregnancy (reproduced with permission from Manganiello et al, 1981)

method to assess the function of the corpus luteum of early pregnancy. Figure 30.10 illustrates the hCG pattern and the steroidogenic activity of the corpus luteum of pregnancy, evaluated by sequential serum assays of progesterone and 17 α-hydroxyprogesterone in six normal pregnant women (Manganiello et al, 1981). Figure 30.11A demonstrates the early and profound decline of the progesterone concentrations below the 95 per cent confidence levels in a patient who aborted a grossly abnormal fetus at 9 weeks post-conception. The levels of 17 α-hydroxyprogesterone also declined, but they were always within the 95 per cent confidence range (Fig. 30.11B). The values of hCG did not fall beneath the 95 per cent confidence range until the eighth week after conception (Fig. 30.11C). It appears from this study that sequential progesterone determinations may have a prognostic value in early pregnancy. Distinguishing between primary failure of the corpus luteum and its failure secondary to a chromosomally defective conceptus which does not secrete sufficient hCG presents a dilemma. Serial β-hCG, oestradiol and progesterone levels may clarify this situation. Low oestradiol and

b

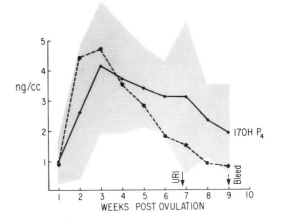

Fig. 30.11A Early and profound decline of progesterone values in a patient who aborted an apparently normal fetus 9 weeks after conception. URI = onset of upper respiratory infection (reproduced with permission from Manganiello et al, 1981). B. A later and less important drop of 17 α-hydroxyprogesterone (170HP₄) values in the same aborting woman. URI = onset of upper respiratory infection (reproduced with permission from Manganiello et al, 1981). C. The much later fall of β-hCG in the same abortion patient. URI = onset of upper respiratory infection (reproduced with permission from Manganiello et al, 1981)

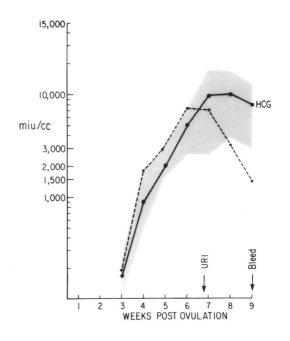

hCG levels may be suggestive of retarded fetal development in defective embryos (Schweditsch et al, 1979).

In recent years, measurements of immunoreactive relaxin in early pregnancy have given more insight into the function of the corpus luteum of pregnancy (Sherwood et al, 1975). Relaxin is a peptide hormone produced only by the corpus luteum of pregnancy. It is undetectable in non-pregnant women. It appears in significant amounts between 14 and 21 days after conception. It may therefore serve as a potential marker for the corpus luteum of pregnancy, since unlike progesterone and oestradiol, it is solely a luteal product. It has been shown that steroid-free extracts of human corpus luteum of pregnancy contain relaxin which inhibits the amplitude of spontaneous human myometrial contractions *in vitro* (Quagliarello et al, 1979). The appearance of relaxin in early pregnancy suggests its important role, together with progesterone, in early pregnancy maintenance. Quagliarello et al (1981) reported simultaneous determinations of serum relaxin and hCG in 18 aborting first trimester pregnancies and also their levels in seven asymptomatic pregnant patients who subsequently aborted within 2 to 6 weeks after sampling. In the aborting group, nine of 18 had normal relaxin levels, five had subnormal values and in four, relaxin was undetectable. hCG values were subnormal in 14 of 18 aborting patients. In the asymptomatic group, four of the seven had subnormal hCG levels at a time when relaxin levels were normal. It was found that low hCG levels were associated with low or normal relaxin levels and that no patients with a high hCG level had a low relaxin level. The data on this small group of patients seems to suggest that there is no primary failure of the corpus luteum of pregnancy and that luteal defect is secondary to trophoblastic failure. However, further prospective investigations with serial determinations of β-hCG, relaxin and progesterone levels on larger series of recurrent loss of karyotypically normal and abnormal conceptuses are necessary for a better delineation of this entity of primary defect of the corpus luteum of pregnancy.

Hyperthyroidism and hypothyroidism are rare causes of recurrent abortion. Patients with Hashimoto's thyroiditis may develop hypothyroidism insidiously. Subtle stress hypothyroid conditions which develop during pregnancy have been identified by noting the absence of the normal pregnancy induced increase in T_4 associated with a decrease in the T_3 resin uptake.

Rare known causes

A small percentage of midtrimester abortions are associated with *abnormalities of placentation*. Circumvallate placenta, and less commonly marginata placenta, are examples of these abnormalities resulting from superficial implantation of a normal ovum. Normally, the placenta tapers at its edge and is continuous with the chorionic membranes. The large thick margin of the marginata, and especially that of the circumvallate placenta, may extend beyond the membranes that gave rise to the original placenta, and invade the decidua vera. The gestational sac tends to herniate into the uterine cavity because of the small size of the chorion. With continued growth, the chorion laeve folds back upon the thick marginal portion of the underlying placenta. Disruption of the adjacent decidua by the radial growth of the placenta may cause persistent bleeding and initiate abortion (Torpin, 1969).

Immunological aetiologies may also complicate gestation by causing abortion. Pregnancy that occurs in the SLE* patient before the disease process is clinically apparent is associated with a higher abortion rate than that of the general population (Estes & Larson, 1965; Fraga et al, 1974). When SLE becomes symptomatic, the abortion rate is high regardless of its clinical manifestation (Fraga et al, 1974; Zurier et al, 1977; Bulmash, 1978). However, it has been agreed that lupus nephritis is associated with the worst maternal and fetal outcome. The reason for spontaneous abortion in patients with SLE is unclear. Recent evidence seems to indicate that fetal wastage is mediated by immunological factors. Bresnihan et al (1977) have demonstrated lymphocytotoxic antibodies which cross-react with trophoblast membrane antigens. This antibody antigen cross-reaction was more frequent in patients with SLE who subsequently aborted than in those with live births. A lupus cell preparation and serum antinuclear antibody assay (ANA) should therefore be included in the basic evaluation of couples suffering from recurrent pregnancy wastage. When SLE is diagnosed, a thorough search for evidence of renal or cardiac disease is mandatory. Frequent serological and clinical testing during pregnancy is necessary to monitor SLE activity and adjust therapy.

Maternal systemic diseases such as severe chronic hypertension, congenital heart diseases, chronic glomerular nephritis, and chronic pyelonephritis may be associated with recurrent pregnancy loss. These processes may cause a marked reduction of uterine blood flow. Women with advanced diabetes are also prone to recurrent fetal wastage. These systemic diseases may be insidious and habitual abortion may be the major manifestation.

Unrecognisable aetiologies

Recurrent aneuploidy constitutes the most important cause of recurrent abortions in couples with chromosomally normal karyotypes and a negative history of malformations in the previous reproductive history. It has been uniformly shown in several large series of sporadic abortions that at least 50 per cent of early pregnancy losses are caused by chromosomal aberrations (Creasy et al, 1976; Hassold et al, 1978; Warburton et al, 1980). Cumulative cytogenetic data

---

* SLE = Systemic lupus erythematosus.

of successive abortions from the same couples further indicate a concordance for the normal or abnormal nature of the chromosomal complements. Karyotypes of successive abortuses to the same parents were most likely either both normal or both abnormal. If the karyotype of the first abortus was normal, about 84 per cent of the second abortuses were also normal. If the karyotype of the first abortus was abnormal, about 66 per cent of the second abortuses were also abnormal, but usually of a different type. When the first abortus was monosomic, 25 per cent of the second abortuses were trisomic and when the first abortus was trisomic, 67 per cent of the second abortuses were also trisomic. Furthermore, these studies demonstrated that triploidic first abortuses were followed by trisomic and triploidic abortuses, 25 and 17 per cent of the time, respectively (Boué & Boué, 1973; Alberman et al, 1975; Kajii & Ferrier, 1978). These data suggest that some couples have a predisposition to non-disjunction.

It is important to know the possible mechanism of origin as well as the parental source of these chromosomal aberrations for appropriate counselling and management. Fortunately, over the last decade, more refined banding techniques have provided for the determination of the mechanism of origin of chromosomal abnormalities in spontaneous abortion. Normal variations of the fluorescent banding patterns of the human chromosomes have been detected. These variations are also referred to as chromosomal heteromorphism or polymorphism. Chromosomal polymorphism is secondary to the variation in size, position or staining properties of the heterochromatic segments. Heterochromatin consists of repetitive DNA sequences and is felt not to contain genetic information. It is most often located near the centromere, is unaffected by crossing over and constitutes an ideal marker for tracing the parental origin and precise mechanism of chromosomal errors in the abortus (Jacobs & Hassold, 1980). Chromosomal abnormalities in the abortuses may arise from an error of gametogenesis in the female or male, from an error of fertilisation or from an error of early cleavage in the zygote.

Gametogenesis in the female occurs in three stages. The oogonia undergo mitotic division from the eighth week to the fifth month of fetal life. Meiosis I is initiated at the fifth month of gestation, is arrested before birth at the dictyotene stage and completed only at ovulation. Meiosis II occurs in the oviduct and is completed after fertilisation. Any factor affecting the first meiotic division might have 20–40 years to exert its action while any factor affecting meiosis II would have to exert its effect in the brief period between ovulation and fertilisation. Non-disjunction in the first or second meiotic division can produce gametes with one or more missing or additional chromosome, leading to an aneuploid conceptus. Trisomy appears to occur more frequently than autosomal monosomy. However, monosomy may be more lethal and abortion may occur before pregnancy is suspected. In trisomic abortions, the

additional chromosome is almost always maternal in origin, irrespective of maternal age (Mattei et al, 1979; Jacobs & Hassold, 1980). It uniformly results from an error in meiosis I of maternal germ cells.

Oocyte ageing caused by increased maternal age or secondary to delayed ovulation has been related to fertilisation errors and the production of abnormal zygotes. Hertig et al, (1959) performed morphological studies on 34 fertilised human ova in timed conceptions. They demonstrated that the proportion of abnormal zygotes to normal ones was 1 to 12 in the eggs ovulated on or before cycle day 14. This proportion of abnormal to normal zygotes becomes 12 to 9 in those eggs ovulated after the fifteenth day of the cycle. Hertig concluded that oocytes remaining longer than day 14 in the follicle had an increased chance of becoming a 'bad egg' when fertilised. Witschi & Laguens (1963) found a high incidence of chromosomal abnormalities in amphibian embryos when release of the ova was experimentally delayed. These aberrations included monosomy, trisomy, polyploidy and mosaicism. Errors in the first or second meiotic division that involve an entire haploid genome can give rise to a diploid oocyte. Fertilisation of a diploid oocyte is called digyny and results in a triploidic zygote. Heteromorphic banding techniques have demonstrated that most of the triploidic conceptuses result from causes other than digyny (Jacobs et al, 1978).

The *male germ cells* undergo a period of mitotic activity during fetal life, then become dormant until puberty. From puberty throughout life, they continue to undergo mitosis to become primary spermatocytes. Meiosis I transforms the primary spermatocytes into secondary spermacytes. Meiosis II transforms the secondary spermatocytes into spermatids. Aetiologic factors affecting mitotic divisions may exert this effect on the male germ cells *in utero* or at anytime after puberty. Factors affecting either the first or the second meiotic division can give rise to gametes with a missing or additional chromosome, leading to aneuploidic fetuses. They can also involve an entire haploid set of chromosomes and produce diploid spermatozoa. Fertilisation of an oocyte by a diploid sperm is called diandry and results in a triploid conceptus. Boué et al (1975a) observed that meiotic chromosomal accidents in the male may result from environmental influences such as radiation. The incidence of diploid spermatozoa is approximately 0.5 per cent (Carrothers & Beatty, 1975). Heteromorphic banding techniques indicate that one-third of the human triploidic conceptuses arise from diploid sperm (Carrothers & Beatty, 1975; Jacobs et al, 1978).

The most important event in the *fertilisation* process is the prevention of polyspermy. Soon after the fertilising spermatozoa has bound to the plasma membrane of the oocyte, cortical granules are discharged. This blocks fertilisation by any other spermatozoa (Wolf & Hamada, 1979). In all species, eggs that are not fertilised for a given period of time after ovulation may lose the mechanism that prevents polyspermy and results in polyploidy (Adams & Change, 1962; Szolollosi, 1975). Recent heteromorphic banding techniques on both parents and their triploid offspring suggest that two-thirds of triploidic human conceptuses are formed by fertilisation with two spermatozoa (dispermy) (Couillin et al, 1978). Ill-timed fertilisation demonstrated by the analysis of basal body temperature curves with known dates of intercourse has been associated with an increased frequency of triploidies (Boué et al, 1975a). Guerrero & Rojas (1975) reviewed 1000 menstrual cycles monitored by basal body temperature charts. They demonstrated that spontaneous abortion was most frequent when patients had intercourse 3 or more days prior to ovulation or 2 or more days after ovulation.

Misdivision of one or more chromosomes by anaphase lag or non-disjunction in the zygote will give rise to a mosaic conceptus. Rarely a failure in cell division with absence of cytokinesis of an early cleavage division will result in a tetraploid fetus. Tetraploidy is not compatible with life and is associated more often with sporadic than with recurrent abortion.

Couples with *recurrent euploidic abortion* of unknown aetiology may have undetected corpus luteum failure of early gestation. Other causes implicated include disorders of the maternal immune system responsible for the tissue acceptance of a foreign fetus and environmental factors such as infectious processes, cigarette smoking and alcohol consumption.

There are no practical means to detect a deficiency of the *corpus luteum* of early pregnancy in a recurrent aborter who had a normal late luteal endometrial biopsy. Sequential determinations of serum progesterone may be of diagnostic value if obtained from implantation until the time of maximum placenta steroidogenesis. Concomitant serial assays of hCG, relaxin and progesterone and sonographic monitoring of fetal growth would aid in the distinction between primary failure of the corpus luteum of pregnancy and its failure secondary to a genetically defective conceptus (Jouppila, 1980).

Recent interest has been focused on the possible *immunological* aetiology of recurrent euploidic abortions of unidentifiable causes. Maternal serum was shown to exert a relatively specific blocking action on sensitised lymphocytes taken from pregnant women (Jenkins & Hancock, 1975). It is known that when circulating lymphocytes are sensitised against a specific antigen, they produce a migration inhibition factor (MIF) that prevents the migration of macrophages. This factor is produced by lymphocytes during a normal pregnancy (Pence et al, 1975). Blocking antibodies, produced during maternal immunisation with paternal antigens, prevent the release of MIF by sensitised lymphocytes. The blocking factor appears to be an IgG and persists for several years after pregnancy (Taylor & Hancock, 1975). A number of women suffering from recurrent abortion fail to produce this blocking factor, and their

lymphocytes may incite direct or indirect damage on the fetoplacental unit. Beer et al (1981) reported their immunological studies on a series of 26 couples with histories of multiple consecutive spontaneous abortions. The 16 couples with a recognisable aetiology served as the control group while the remaining ten couples with negative evaluation served as the experimental group. He observed that the women with recurrent abortions of unknown aetiology had a significantly increased frequency of sharing HLA antigens at the A, B, and D/DR loci with their husbands as compared to those with recurrent abortions of known aetiology. This major histocompatibility complex (MHC) homozygosity was also found in association with hyporeactivity of the maternal lymphocytes when they were stimulated by the husband's lymphocytes in the mixed lymphocyte culture (MLC) reactions. However, these maternal lymphocytes showed good responses to third party HLA incompatible donors. This seems to suggest that the MHC homozygous fetus is less capable of stimulating the mother's immune system along the lines of protective antibody response. However, the protective blocking antibodies have not been fully defined to date, neither their functioning during a successful pregnancy. It is still unclear at this time whether MHC homozygosity between spouses accounts for the female leucocyte hyporeactivity in the MLC *in vitro* assays. Furthermore, Beer's HLA homozygosity hypothesis is controversial until a prospective study is done on a number of couples with good reproductive performance who also share HLA antigens. Since the parents share MHC determinants, the offspring may be homozygous for developmental genes linked to the MHC genes, specifically the analogues of the T locus. Homozygosity of T locus mutants in mice is associated with developmental abnormalities and embryonic death. Schacter et al (1979) observed a high frequency of MHC compatibility in couples suffering from recurrent fetal wastage and neural tube defects. This seems to suggest that the human equivalent of the murine T locus is a lethal neural tube defect gene which is linked or associated with the HLA loci. Three couples in Beer's study who demonstrated significant sharing of antigens between spouses at the HLA-A, B, and D/DR loci and female hyporesponsiveness to spouse antigens were enrolled in the white blood cell immunisation protocol. They were immunised by intradermal injections with viable mononuclear cells prepared from peripheral blood leucocytes of the husband. Pregnancies have been reported in two of the couples. Further investigations are necessary for future diagnostic and therapeutic applications for the immunological group of reproductive failure.

Abortion may be the sequelae of an acute *infectious* process. Syphilis, toxoplasmosis, cytomegalic inclusion diseases, listeriosis, herpes, T-mycoplasma (ureaplasma urealyticum), and chlamydia have all been implicated. There is little sound evidence relating *chronic infection* to recurrent abortion. Stray-Pederson et al (1978) reported that colonisation of T-mycoplasma in the endometrium was significantly more frequent among recurrent abortion and infertility patients than among control subjects. Treatment with doxycycline eradicated that infectious agent from the endometrium leading to an improvement in the outcome of post-treatment pregnancies. Infection as an aetiology of recurrent abortion is included in the unknown group because it is difficult to identify.

Cigarette smoking and alcohol consumption have been implicated as causes of recurrent abortion by some investigators. Butler et al (1972) found that the late fetal death rate was significantly increased in heavy smokers. Boué, in a series of 1500 karyotyped human abortions, found a significant increase in chromosomally normal abortuses among women who inhaled cigarette smoke. This rate was 50 per cent as compared to the non-inhaling mothers who had a rate of 38 per cent (Boué et al, 1975b). Kline et al (1980) studied 657 aborters and their matched controls who delivered after 28 weeks gestation. They correlated exposure to alcohol and tobacco with the abortion rate and with chromosomal and morphological characteristics of the abortion material. Alcohol and/or tobacco exposure were associated with spontaneous abortion of chromosomally normal conceptuses.

EVALUATION OF THE COUPLE WITH REPETITIVE REPRODUCTIVE FAILURE

The following six key points are important in assimilating the historical information:
1. Documentation of previous abortion with histological findings.
2. Detection of a history of malformed children plus abortion.
3. Detection of a neural tube abnormality, especially anencephaly plus abortion.
4. Detection of a history of interval infertility plus abortion.
5. Detection of clues for recurrent aneuploidy.
6. Detection of a history of male abortuses.

Documentation of recurrent abortion. It is not uncommon for patients who have never conceived to be seen for recurrent abortion. Their previous curettings, when reviewed, repeatedly lack histological evidence of products of conception and often demonstrate unopposed oestrogen stimulated endometrium. Couples may actually have infertility rather than recurrent abortion and require evaluation of male, cervical, tubal and ovulatory factors as well (Shearman, 1975; McDonough & Tho, 1981). Review of the microscopic material provides not only for documentation of recurrent abortion but also for clues to a chronic infectious process. The identification of intranuclear inclusion bodies is suggestive of viral infection.

Concurrent history of malformed children. The couple which has a malformed or stillborn child plus abortion or normal children plus abortions is at higher risk than is the couple who has a pure history of recurrent abortion. A parent with a balanced translocation or a pericentric inversion has the potential to produce balanced and unbalanced gametes. Subsequent conception may result in abortion or produce abnormal children, balanced carriers or cytogenetically normal individuals. A careful pedigree analysis is important. In the couple with a mixed history of malformation plus abortion, there is a 23 per cent chance of one of these individuals being a balanced translocation carrier. Couples with a pure history of abortion have a 9.6 per cent chance of this carrier state being present. The chance for identification of a carrier state decreases further as the number of pure abortions in a family increases. Attention should also be brought to the history of recurrent abortion and/or malformation occurring in any generation other than the couple under investigation.

Neural tube abnormalities. Eight per cent of the Medical College of Georgia's recurrent abortion population had neural tube defects plus abortion. Neural tube abnormalities are usually isolated multifactorial disorders and are associated with a 2 per cent risk of recurrence. Mixed reproductive histories that include neural tube defects and abortions might be related to an autosomal recessive gene (e.g. Meckel Syndrome). If the anencephalic or hydrocephalic is male, then an X-linked disorder may be present and the recurrence risk of an early abortion or viable male fetus with a neural tube defect may be 50 per cent.

Interval infertility plus abortion. Unexplained infertility followed by conception with abortion may be related to an ovulation disturbance, resulting in inadequate progesterone production, a suboptimally developed implantation site and an inadequately developed placenta as an organ for steroidogenesis. Short menstrual cycles in the range of 21–23 days or a prolonged proliferative phase with ovulation delayed to cycle day 25 are both suggestive of ovulation disturbances and consequent gonadotrophin-dependent corpus luteum deficiency. A marked asynchrony of endometrial gland and stromal development can be found in the late luteal endometrial biopsy of a regularly menstruating female who has unexplained infertility plus early abortion. The ovulation defects need to be corrected with clomiphene citrate or rarely human menopausal gonadotrophins. Protracted infertility and abortion can also be seen when one of the parents is the carrier of a balanced chromosomal rearrangement or of a pericentric inversion. The gametes of such an individual are frequently abnormal, resulting either in infertility or fertilisation with early spontaneous abortion.

Clues for recurrent aneuploidy. As previously discussed, there is concordance between the normal and abnormal karyotype of two abortuses in the same couple. A cytogenetically normal couple with a history of abortion plus a previous child or a previous fetus with autosomal trisomy would be suspect for recurrent aneuploidy. A careful search should be made for factors that theoretically might predispose to non-disjunction. Pre-ovulatory follicular ageing in cycles with late ovulation and increased maternal age are possibilities. Recurrent extensive molar degeneration in recurrent abortion material suggests triploidic abortuses.

History of male abortuses. Occasionally one sees a woman with recurrent abortion in whom all the abortuses are male. Figure 30.12 is the pedigree of a woman who had eight immature male fetuses by two different husbands. Whether the aetiology is genetic or immunological is not known. The prognosis is poor unless the conceptus is female.

PEDIGREE
M.W.

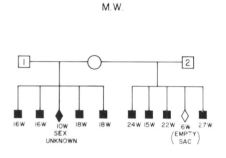

■ = Male Abortuses

Fig. 30.12 Pedigree of a female who had eight immature male fetuses by two different husbands. W = week (reproduced with permission from McDonough et al, 1979 Overall evaluation of recurrent abortion In: Givens J R (ed), The Infertile Female, Year Book Medical Publishers, Chicago, pp 385–404)

Physical examination may disclose medical problems or pelvic pathology that might be associated with the reproductive difficulty. The male's semen should be examined. Rarely hyperzoospermia or a markedly elevated number of abnormal forms are identified in the spermogram of these couples with recurrent abortion.

Appropriate laboratory tests for the female might include a complete blood count, a 2-hour postprandial blood glucose test, renal and hepatic function chemistry, antinuclear antibodies, blood type, indirect Coombs test, serology and urinalysis. Thyroid function studies, including T_4, T_3 resin uptake and TSH are obtained on all patients. Hypothyroidism is rarely a cause of recurrent abortion. Occasionally, the physiological evaluation of T_4 and the concomitant drop of T_3 resin uptake do not occur during early pregnancy. In this situation, it is difficult to differentiate true maternal hypothyroidism from the suboptimal production of oestrogen and its subsequent failure to increment thyroxin binding globulin. The failure to augment T_4 in pregnancy accompanied by a normal decrease in T_3 resin uptake is suggestive of a subtle stress hypothyroid condition of pregnancy. Both partners should have blood leucocyte karyotyping with G and Q banding

to identify small rearrangements or chromosome polymorphism. Meiotic studies on testicular tissues that demonstrate abnormal pairing of chromosomes might confirm the pessimistic prognosis for reproduction and expedite the decision for artificial insemination donor in males with homologous chromosome rearrangement and poor reproductive performance.

The luteal phase is evaluated by recording the basal body temperature and performing a fundal endometrial biopsy between days 11 and 13 of the temperature elevation. In the late luteal phase, glandular and stromal development is at a maximum if the endometrium has been adequately prepared by a normal corpus luteum. Luteal phase defect is defined as an endometrium which is 3 or more days behind dates as determined by the onset of the subsequent menses. It is not uncommon among patients with infertility and recurrent abortion to find evidence of immature glandular development in the endometrium. This histological feature suggests suboptimal glandular oestrogen priming prior to ovulation. It might be appropriately treated by improving the quality and function of the pre-ovulatory follicle using clomiphene or human menopausal gonadotrophins. The endometrial biopsy as a bioassay endpoint is the only reliable clinical parameter to document an adequate endometrial development for implantation. A local defect in endometrial response to a normal progesterone production may result in a non-receptive endometrium for implantation.

In early gestation, serum progesterone and relaxin levels determined in conjunction with β-hCG levels may be of value. Absence of an increase in progesterone and relaxin levels in association with normal increments of β-hCG would indicate primary corpus luteum dysfunction and the need for post-conception progesterone supplementation. In the future, concomitant determinations of sequential serum progesterone, relaxin and β-hCG levels in high risk pregnancies of known and unknown aetiology may be helpful in delineating the primary defect of corpus luteum of pregnancy from the endocrine deficiency in a genetically defective fetus. Ultrasound examination may aid in diagnosing viability and prognosticating outcome, but provides no information on the functional status of the trophoblast.

Hysterography is performed on all patients. It will help identify uterine anomalies and intra-uterine pathology including intra-uterine synechiae. One must distinguish the bicornuate uterus from the subseptate uterus. While the bicornuate uterus causes only minimal problems with reproduction, the subseptate uterus is frequently involved with reproductive failure. The radiological pictures of the uterine cavity may be the same for these two types of uteri. Laparoscopy may be necessary to visualise the normal external contour of the septate uterus. A gynaecogram which provides a simultaneous outline of internal and external uterine contours can also aid in the differential diagnosis of these two varieties of uterine anomalies.

Subclinical fetal wastage which represents the largest portion of reproductive failure should be the most urgent subject for future investigation. Approximately 15 per cent of all recognisable pregnancies result in spontaneous abortion between 4 and 22 weeks after the last menstrual period. Prior to 4 weeks, the rate of pregnancy wastage is unknown because most women are not aware that they are pregnant and that a delayed heavy menstruation is in reality a subclinical abortion. With the advent of the β-hCG radioimmunoassay it is possible to detect with precision and specificity a pregnancy as early as 6–9 days after conception (Vaitukaitus et al, 1972; Braunstein et al, 1977). Serial β-hCG determinations late in the luteal phase would allow the diagnosis of recurrent subclinical abortions in patients who would otherwise be considered as suffering from unexplained infertility. Miller et al (1980), by serially measuring β-hCG from the 21st day until the menstrual onset or until routine pregnancy confirmation diagnosed 152 conceptions in the 623 studied cycles. They found that 43 per cent of these pregnancies were lost before 20 weeks of gestation. Figure 30.13 illustrates serial hCG in three of the 31 patients receiving oocyte and sperm transfer. While in patient A, the hCG excretion pattern is suggestive of a continuing pregnancy, in patient B it is consistent with a conception which aborts at the time of expected menses and in patient C implantation and subsequent trophoblastic activity are not certain (Craft et al, 1982). However, β-hCG determinations detect only the pregnancies in the late post-implantation stage.

One pregnancy specific protein known as early pregnancy factor (EPF) appears in the serum within 48 hours of fertilisation and disappears promptly following embryonic death. EPF is thus a sensitive indicator of embryonic

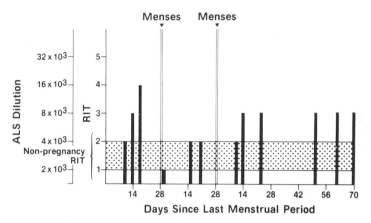

Fig. 30.14 Rosette inhibition titre (RIT) with the serum from one subject sampled at various times for three cycles. RIT with non-pregnancy serum fell between 1 and 2. An RIT of 3 or higher indicates the presence of early pregnancy factor (EPF). In each cycle, intercourse took place at day 13 to day 15 of the cycle. Luteal progesterone levels higher than 10 nmol/l confirmed that ovulation had occurred. In this subject, EPF levels remained elevated throughout the study period. Pregnancy was confirmed by β-hCG assays 12 and 36 days after fertilisation and the pregnancy continued to term

viability during the pre-implantation and early post-implantation periods. Morton et al (1979) reported that EPF augments the immunosuppressive potential of anti-lymphocyte serum as determined by its ability to decrease the number of rosettes formed between lymphocytes and heterologous red blood cells. In this rosette inhibition test, the rosette inhibition titre (RIT) is the highest antileucocyte serum (ALS) in which the number of rosettes formed is less than 75 per cent of the number formed in the tubes containing no ALS. An RIT of 3 or higher indicates the presence of EPF. Figure 30.14 exemplifies the early detection of EPF which remained elevated (RIT = 3) in the third study cycle and the increased RIT was well maintained throughout the study period. Pregnancy was confirmed by β-hCG assays 12 and 36 days after fertilisation and the pregnancy continued to term (Rolfe, 1982). However, rosette inhibition is still a lengthy test requiring strict adhesion to experimental parameters for a predictable reproducibility (Smart et al, 1982).

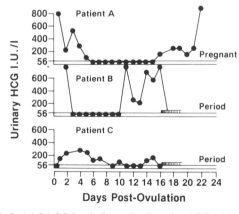

Fig. 30.13 Serial β-hCG levels from the day after hCG administration until and including the expected date of the next menses in three of the 31 women with infertility due to tubal obstructive disease who underwent 'oocyte and sperm transfer to the uterus.' Values in excess of 56 iu/l 6 or more days after hCG administration are indicative of trophoblastic activity. Patient C had positive values for a few days without rise and started menses at the expected time. Patient B, whose urinary hCG excretion was consistent with a continuing pregnancy, also started her menses on time. Patient A is one of the two patients with continuing pregnancy (reproduced with permission from Craft et al, 1982)

TREATMENT OF RECURRENT ABORTION

Therapy should be tailored for each couple, depending upon identified aetiologies as outlined in Fig. 30.7.

Couples identified in the known genetic group with either chromosomal or multifactorial aetiologies should be appropriately counselled. Couples who are carriers of a heterologous balanced translocation or a large pericentric inversion should be encouraged to attempt further pregnancies and to have pre-natal cytogenetic monitoring. Individuals whose karyotypes demonstrate chromosome variants or polymorphism should probably be managed in the same way. All couples should be provided with a sterile physiological solution (i.e. Hank's solution) to preserve the abortus for chromosome study, if that unfortunate event should occur prior to amniocentesis. Couples who are carriers of a translocation of two homologous chromosomes should be discouraged against further pregnancies because a living normal child is not possible. Sterilisation is recommended for a female carrier and artificial insemination by a donor can be an option for the male carrier. Couples who have delivered a previous fetus or newborn with a neural tube defect may attempt to have further pregnancies with α-fetoprotein and serial sonographic monitoring. Should abortion occur, a diligent phenotypic examination of the fetus is in order. The chance for subsequent delivery of a full term normal child approximates 30 per cent in this known genetic group of the Medical College of Georgia series. This figure takes into consideration those couples who elect not to attempt pregnancy.

Surgical treatment of anatomical uterine abnormalities is considered only in selected cases and after exclusion or treatment of other aetiologic factors. One must remember that multiple causes may be operative in some couples and an anatomical abnormality may be merely a coincidental finding with little significance as regards recurrent abortion. Tompkin's metroplasty for a subseptate uterus with marked volume compromise, myomectomy for a fibroid uterus with severe cavitary distortion, hysteroscopic lysis of intra-uterine synechiae followed by re-epithelisation in Asherman's Syndrome, and a McDonald cerclage for an incompetent cervix may be the techniques of choice for these individuals. Certain patients identified with Müllerian abnormalities or distortion of the uterine cavity by fibroids may benefit from bed rest and progesterone myometrial blockade using 17 α-hydroxyprogesterone caproate 250 mg intramuscularly every week from 14 weeks until fetal viability. β-Mimetic agents such as Ritodrine (Yutopar), 10 mg four times a day or Terbutaline (Brethin), 5 mg three times a day could be added to this regimen. Successful reproduction in patients with an anatomical uterine abnormality approximates 70 per cent, depending upon the specific defect and other associated aetiologies.

Ninety per cent of couples diagnosed with corpus luteum defects will have a successful reproductive outcome with appropriate therapy. Corpus luteum deficiency associated with a relatively normal menstrual interval and a physiological ovulation time is best treated with prenidation progesterone supplementation. This therapy utilises natural progesterone in the form of 25 mg vaginal suppositories given twice daily. It is best initiated 3 or 4 days after the temperature shift to improve pre-implantation endometrial development. It should be continued until 60 to 70 days after conception to bridge the gap between the declining function of the corpus luteum and the gradual rise in progesterone production by the placenta. The transfer of progesterone production from the corpus luteum of pregnancy to the placenta occurs during the seventh week of gestation.

Corpus luteum deficiency associated with wide ranging menstrual intervals, a delay in ovulation time and an inordinate lag in endometrial development may be the result of follicular dysgenesis. This aberration of ovulation is best treated with clomiphene therapy. Dosage should be progressively increased until the basal body temperature graph and the endometrial histology are considered normal. The additional use of prenidation progesterone may be beneficial if the endometrial stroma remains immature in spite of satisfactory glandular development. Occasionally a mild hyperprolactinaemia is discovered in the evaluation of the corpus luteum defect. Bromocriptine (Parlodel), 2.5 mg twice a day should be the primary treatment. Clomiphene or progesterone is only added if the basal body temperature curve and the endometrial development are not adequately corrected with bromocriptine therapy alone.

The most difficult couples to manage are those in the unknown aetiologic group. Routine genetic, anatomical and endocrine evaluation is unrevealing for these individuals. Basal body temperatures should be recorded for several months to ascertain the normal timing of ovulation and to plan for a future pregnancy. Delayed ovulation should be treated with clomiphene to avoid intrafollicular ovum overripeness. Empiric antibiotic treatment of both partners can be instituted with doxycycline (Vibramycin), 100 mg twice daily for the first 10 days of the initial cycle in which pregnancy is attempted. Sperm deposition should be synchronised with ovulation to avoid gamete ageing or overripeness. One must caution against long abstinence of ejaculation prior to ovulation for this also may be associated with sperm ageing and subsequent fetal aneuploidy.

The biochemical diagnosis of pregnancy should be established early, utilising a specific radioimmunoassay for β-hCG. Follow-up confirmation of a viable pregnancy is best obtained with real-time ultrasonography after 6 weeks of gestation and is helpful in prognosticating the pregnancy outcome. Patients should be followed with thyroid function studies at 2-week intervals during the first trimester to identify stress hypothyroidism of pregnancy. Synthroid, 0.1 mg daily is instituted for individuals in whom a physiological drop of the T_3 resin uptake assay is not accompanied by an increase in serum T_4 measured by RIA. In selected cases, the sequential measurements of β-hCG and serum progesterone levels are performed to identify postnidation corpus luteum deficiency and allow for progesterone supplementation of early pregnancy. The empirical use of progesterone supplementation might be considered when such frequent endocrine studies are not easily obtained or readily available. Such therapy should be instituted as soon as the diagnosis of pregnancy is established. Couples with second trimester losses might also benefit with the use of condoms to avoid exposure to seminal prostaglandins. Occasionally, it is best to avoid orgasm during this critical period of gestation. If the couple is unfortunate and a planned pregnancy terminates again in abortion, the products of conception should be carefully examined and placed in Hank's solution for cytogenetic studies. This will aid in prognosticating future pregnancy outcome. Amniocentesis with fetal fibroblast karyotyping should be offered for individuals with cytogenetic or phenotypic abortal abnormalities as well as abnormalities of their own karyotypes. Artificial insemination is an option for couples highly suspect for a male aetiology in recurrent fetal aneuploidy. A well-planned pregnancy and appropriate follow-up through early gestation will result in a successful outcome 62 per cent of the time for couples in this unknown group (Fig. 30.7)

SUMMARY

The aetiologies of recurrent reproductive failure are diverse. Many of them are not evident through routine clinical practice and some are still unknown to sophisticated researchers in the field of reproduction. A rational clinical evaluation of the couple will identify the known causes and suggest the unknown aetiologies.

More recently the unknown causes have been further classified because of advances in cytogenetic techniques. Abortion material can now be divided into aneuploidic and euploidic conditions. Heteromorphic banding techniques are useful in exploring both the parental source and the mechanism responsible for recurrent aneuploidy. Ovulation and fertilisation delays may be closely linked to these cytogenetic errors. Identification of euploidic abortuses in the unknown group will allow for diagnosis of endocrine, immunological and teratological aetiologies yet to be discovered. With identification of known aetiologies, the treatment is clear cut. All other couples are at the present time dependent upon the availability of techniques to identify unknown causes. Treatment must centre around normalisation of ovulation, synchronisation of sperm deposition and ovulation, and optimisation of the maternal environment in which fertilisation will occur for these couples of unknown aetiology. Recent advances in techniques will also allow us to recognise pregnancies and their potential loss during the pre-implantation and post-implantation periods, prior to the expected menses. The extended spectrum of recognisable embryonic wastage will bring more insight in the understanding of the various aetiologic categories of recurrent fetal wastage.

REFERENCES

Adams C E, Change M C 1962 The effect of delayed mating on fertilization in the rabbit. Journal of Experimental Zoology 151: 155–158

Alberman E, Elliott M, Creasy M, Dhadial R 1975 Previous reproductive history in mothers presenting with spontaneous abortions. British Journal of Obstetrics and Gynaecology 82: 366–373

Baccichetti C, Lenzina E, Peserico A, Tenconi R 1980 Study on segretation and risk for abnormal offspring in carriers of pericentric inversion of the (p11q13) segment of chromosome 2. Clinical Genetics 18: 402–407

Bayard F, Damilario S, Robel P, Baulieu E E 1978 Cytoplasmic and nuclear estradiol and progesterone receptors in human endometrium. Journal of Clinical Endocrinology and Metabolism 46: 635–648

Beer A E, Quebbeman J F, Ayers J W, Haines R F 1981 Major histocompatibility, complex antigens, maternal and paternal immune responses, and chronic habitual abortions in humans. American Journal of Obstetrics and Gynecology 141: 987–1000

Berger M H, Goldstein D P 1980 Impaired reproductive performance in DES exposed women. Obstetrics and Gynecology 55: 25–27

Boué J, Boué A 1973 Chromosomal analysis of two consecutive abortions in each of 43 women. Human Genetics 19: 275–280

Boué J, Boué A, Lazar P 1975a The epidemiology of human spontaneous abortions with chromosomal anomalies. In: Blandau R J (ed) Aging Gametes, Their Biology and Pathology. International Symposium on Aging Gametes. Seattle, Washington, 1973, pp 330–348. Karger, Basel

Boué J, Boué A, Lazar P 1975b Retrospective and prospective epidemiologic studies of 1500 karyotyped spontaneous human abortions. Teratology 12: 11–26

Boué J, Taillemite J L, Hazael-Massiena L C, Boué A 1975c Association of pericentric inversion of chromosome 9 and reproductive failure in ten unrelated families. Human Genetics 30: 217–224

Braunstein G D, Karow W G, Gentry W D, Wade M E 1977 Subclinical spontaneous abortion. Obstetrics and Gynecology (Suppl) 50: 41s–43s

Bresnihan B, Grigor R R, Oliver M, Lewkomia R M, Hughes G R V, Lovins R E, Faulk W P 1977 Immunological mechanism for spontaneous abortion in systemic lupus erythematosus. Lancet ii: 1205–1207

Bulmash J M 1978 Systemic lupus erythematosus and pregnancy. Obstetrics and Gynecology Annual 7: 153–194

Butler N R, Goldstein H, Ross E M 1972 Cigarette smoking in pregnancy: Its influence on birth weight and perinatal mortality. British Medical Journal 2: 127–180

Byrd J R, Askew D E, McDonough P G 1977 Cytogenetic findings in fifty-five couples with recurrent fetal wastage. Fertility and Sterility 28: 246–250

Carrothers A D, Beatty R A 1975 The recognition and incidence of haploid and polypoid spermatozoa in man, rabbit and mouse. Journal of Reproduction and Fertility 44: 487–500

De La Chapelle A, Schroder J, Kokkonen J 1973 Cytogenetics of recurrent abortion or unsuccessful pregnancy. International Journal of Fertility 19: 215–219

De La Chapelle A, Schroder J, Steustrana K, Fellman J, Herba R, Saarni M, Anttolainen I, Tallila I, Tervila L, Husa L, Tallqvist G, Robson E B, Cook P G L, Sanger R 1974 Pericentric inversions of human chromosomes 9 and 10. American Journal of Human Genetics 26: 746–766

Couillin P, Hors J, Boué J, Boué A 1978 Identification of the origin of triploidy by HLA markers. Human Genetics 41: 35–44

Court-Brown W M 1967 Chromosome studies on the general population. In: Human Population Cytogenetics, Ch 1, p 1. North Holland Publishing Co, Amsterdam

Craft I, Djahanbakhch O, McLeod F, Bernard A, Green S, Twigg H 1982 Human pregnancy following oocyte and sperm transfer to the uterus. Lancet i: 1031–1033

Creasy M R, Crolla J A, Alberman E 1976 A cytogenetic study of human spontaneous abortion using banding techniques. Human Genetics 31: 177–196

Csapo A T, Pulkkinen M O, Wiest W G 1973 Effects of luteectomy and progesterone replacement therapy in early pregnancy patients. American Journal of Obstetrics and Gynecology 115: 759–765

DiZerega G S, Hodgen G D 1981 Luteal phase dysfunction in fertility: a sequel to aberrant folliculogenesis. Fertility and Sterility 35: 489–499

DiZerega G S, Stouffer R L, Hodgen D G 1981a FSH regulation of intrafollicular events in the primate ovarian cycle. In: Channing N P, Franchimont P (eds) Intragonadal Regulation of Reproduction, Ch. II, p 10. Academic Press, New York

DiZerega G S, Turner C K, Stouffer R L, Anderson L D, Channing C P, Hodgen G D 1981b Suppression of FSH dependent folliculogenesis during the primate ovarian cycle. Journal of Clinical Endocrinology and Metabolism 52: 451–456

Estes D, Larson D L 1965 Systemic lupus erythematosus and pregnancy. Clinical Obstetrics and Gynecology 8: 307–321

Fraga A, Mintz G, Orozco J, Ozozco J H 1974 Sterility and fertility rates, fetal wastage and maternal morbidity in systemic lupus erythematosus. Journal of Rheumatology 1: 293–298

Fujimoto A, Towner J W, Turkel S B, Wilson M G 1978 A fetus with recombinant of chromosome 8 inherited from her carrier father. Human Genetics 40: 241–248

Gagné R, Laberge C, Tanguay R 1973 Aspect cytologigue et localisation intranucleaire de l'heterochromatine constitutive des chromosomes C9 chez l'homme. Chromosoma 41: 159–166

Genest P 1979 Chromosome variants and abnormalities detected in 51 married couples with repeated spontaneous abortions. Clinical Genetics 16: 387–389

Geneva Conference 1966 Standardization of procedures for chromosome studies in abortion. Cytogenetics 5: 361–393

Guerrero R, Rojas O 1975 Spontaneous abortion and aging of human ova and spermatozoa. New England Journal of Medicine 293: 573–575

Halme J, Ikonen M, Rutanen E M, Seppala M 1978 Gonadotropin receptors of human corpus luteum during menstrual cycle and pregnancy. American Journal of Obstetrics and Gynecology 131: 728–734

Hassold T J, Matusyama A, Newlands T M, Matusra J S, Jacobs P A, Maueul B, Tsuei J 1978 A cytogenetic study of spontaneous abortions in Hawaii. Annals of Human Genetics 41: 443–454

Hertig A T, Rock J, Adams E C, Menkin M C 1959 Thirty-four fertilized human ova, good, bad and indifferent recovered from two hundred and ten women of known fertility: a study of the biological waste in early human pregnancy. Pediatrics 23: 202–211

Hsia Y E, Bratu M, Herbordt H 1971 Genetics of the Meckel syndrome. Pediatrics 48: 237–246

Hsu L Y F, Carcia F E P, Grossman D, Kutinsky E, Hirshorn K 1972 Fetal wastage and maternal mosaicism. Obstetrics and Gynecology 40: 98–103

Hsueh A J W, Peck Jr, E J, Clark J H 1976 Control of uterine estrogen receptor levels by progesterone. Endocrinology 98: 438–444

Husslein P, Huber J, Wagenbichler P, Schnedl W 1982 Chromosome abnormalities in 150 couples with multiple spontaneous abortions. Fertility and Sterility 37: 379–383

Jacobs P A, Angell R R, Buchanan I M, Hassold T J, Jatusyama A M, Manuel B 1978 The origin of human triploids. Annals of Human Genetics 42: 49–57

Jacobs P A, Hassold T J 1980 The origin of chromosome abnormalities in spontaneous abortion. In: Porter I H, Hook E B (eds) Human Embryonic and Fetal Death, pp 289–298. Academic Press, New York

Jenkins D M, Hancock K W 1972 Maternal unresponsiveness to paternal histocompatibility antigens in human pregnancy. Transplantation 13: 618–619

Jones G S 1975 Luteal phase defects. In: Behrman S J, Kistner R W (eds) Progress in Infertility, Ch. 14, p. 299. Little, Brown and Co, Boston

Jones H W 1981 Reporudctive impairment of the malformed uterus. Fertility and Sterility 36: 137–148

Jones, G S, Maffezzoli R D, Strott C A, Ross G T, Kaplan G 1970 Pathophysiology of reproductive failure after clomiphene induced ovulation. American Journal of Obstetrics and Gynecology 108: 847–867

Jouppila P 1980 Clinical and ultrasonic aspects in the diagnosis and followup of patients with early pregnancy failure. Acta Obstetrica et Gynecologica Scandinavica 59: 405–409

Kajii T, Ferrier A 1978 Cytogenetics of aborters and abortuses. American Journal of Obstetrics and Gynecology 131: 33–38

Kaufman R H, Binder G L, Adam E 1977 Upper genital tract changes associated with exposure in utero to diethylstilbestrol. American Journal of Obstetrics and Gynecology 128: 51–59

Kaufman R H, Adam E, Binder G, Gerthoffer E 1980 Upper genital tract changes and pregnancy outcome in offspring exposed in utero to diethylstilbestrol. American Journal of Obstetrics and Gynecology 137: 299–308

Keller D W, Wiest W G, ASkin F B, Johnson L W, Strickler R C 1979 Pseudocorpus luteum insufficiency: a local defect of progesterone action on endometrial stroma. Journal of Clinical Endocrinology and Metabolism 48: 127–132

Khudr G 1974 Cytogenetics of habitual abortion. Obstetrics and Gynecology Survey 299–310

Kline J. Stein Z, Susser M, Warburton D 1980 Environmental influences on early reproductive loss in a current New York City study. In: Porter I H, Hook E B (eds) Embryonic and Fetal Death, pp 225–240. Academic Press, New York

Kreitmann-Gimbal B, Bayard F, Hodgen D G 1981 Changing ratios of nuclear estrone to estradiol binding in endometrium at implantation: Regulation by chorionic gonadotropin and progesterone during rescue of the primate corpus luteum. Journal of Clinical Endocrinology and Metabolism 52: 133–137

Kreitmann-Gimbal B, Bayard F, Nixon W E, Hodgen D G 1980 Patterns of estrogen and progesterone receptors in monkey endometrium during the normal menstrual cycle. Steroids 35: 471–479

Lauritsen J G 1976 Etiology of spontaneous abortion. Acta Obstetrica et Gynecologica Scandinavica (Suppl) 52: 1–29

Lee C Y, Coulam C B, Jiang N S, Ryan R G 1973 Receptors for human luteinizing hormone in human corpora lutea tissue. Journal of Clinical Endocrinology and Metabolism 36: 148–152

Lindley M 1979 Life and death before birth. Nature 280: 635–646

McDonough P G, Tho P T 1981 Etiology of recurrent abortion. In: Sciarra J J (ed) Gynecology and Obstetrics, Ch 92, p 1. Harper and Row, Hagerstown

Manganiello P D, Nazian S H, Ellegood J O, McDonough P G, Mahesh V B 1981 Serum progesterone, 17 α-hydroxyprogesterone, human chorionic gonadotropin and prolactin in early pregnancy and a case of spontaneous abortion. Fertility and Sterility 36: 55–60

Mattei J F, Mattei M G, Ayme S, Girand F 1979 Origin of the extra chromosome in trisomy 21. Human Genetics 46: 107–110

Miller J F, Williamson E, Glue J, Gordon Y B, Grudzinskas J G, Sikes A 1980 Fetal loss after implantation: a prospective study. Lancet ii: 554–556

Morton H, Nancarrow C D, Scaramuzzi R J, Evison B M, Clunic G J A 1979 Detection of early pregnancy in sheep by the rosette inhibition test. Journal of Reproduction and Fertility 56: 75–80

Moszkowski E, Woodruff J D, Jones G S 1962 The inadequate luteal phase. American Journal of Obstetrics and Gynecology 83: 363–372

Nielson J, Friedrick U, Hreidarsson A B, Zeuthen E 1974 Frequency of 9qh + and risk of chromosome aberrations in the progeny of individuals with 9qh +. Human Genetics 21: 211–216

Papp Z, Gardo S, Dolhay B 1974 Chromosome study of couples with repeated spontaneous abortion. Fertility and Sterility 25: 713–717

Pence H, Petty W M, Rocklin R E 1975 Suppression of maternal responsiveness to paternal antigens by maternal plasma. Journal of Immunology 114: 525–528

Pillsbury S G 1980 Reproductive significance of changes in the endometrial cavity associated with exposure in utero to diethylstilbestrol. American Journal of Obstetrics and Gynecology 137: 178–182

Del Pozo E, Wyss H, Tolis G, Alcaniz J, Campana A, Naftolin F, 1979 Prolactin and deficient luteal function. Obstetrics and Gynecology 53: 282–286

Predescu V, Christodorescu D, Tautu C, Ciovirnache M,

Constantinescu E 1969 Repeated abortions in a woman with XO/XX mosaicism. Lancet ii: 217

Quagliarello J, Steinetz B F, Weiss G 1979 Relaxin secretion in early pregnancy. Obstetrics and Gynecology 53: 62–63

Quagliarello J, Szlachter N, Nisselbaum J S, Schwarta M K, Steinetz B, Weiss G 1981 Serum relaxin and human chorionic gonadotropin concentrations in spontaneous abortions. Fertility and Sterility 36: 399–401

Rocklin R E, Kitzmiller J L, Carpenter C I, Gavovoy M R, David J R 1976 Absence of an immunologic blocking factor from the serum of women with chronic abortions. New England Journal of Medicine 295: 1209–1213

Rolfe B E 1982 Detection of fetal wastage. Fertility and Sterility 37: 655–660

Ross G T, Cargille C M, Lipsett M B, Rayford P L, Marshall Jr, Strott C A, Rodbard D 1970 Pituitary and gonadal induced ovulatory cycles. Recent Program of Hormone Research 26: 1–62

Sandberg E C, Riffle N L, Hidgon J V, Getman C E 1981 Pregnancy outcome in women exposed to diethylstilbestrol in utero. American Journal of Obstetrics and Gynecology 140: 194–205

Sarris S, Swyer G I M, Ward R H T, Lawrence D M, McGarrigle H H, Little V 1978 The treatment of mild adrenal hyperplasia and associated infertility with prednisone. British Journal of Obstetrics and Gynaecology 85: 251–253

Sarto G E, Therman E 1976 Large translocation t(3q; 4p+) as possible cause of semisterility. Fertility and Sterility 27: 784–788

Schacter B, Muir A, Gyves M, Tasin M 1979 HLA-A, B compatibility in parents of offspring with neural tube defects or couples experiencing involuntary fetal wastage. Lancet i: 796–799

Schindler A M, Mikama K 1970 Triploidy in man. Report of a case and discussion on etiology. Cytogenetics 9: 116–130

Schmidt G, Fowler W C, Talbert L M, Edelman D A 1980 Reproductive history of women exposed to diethylstilbestrol in utero. Fertility and Sterility 33: 21–24

Schweditsch M O, Dubin N H, Jones G S, Wentz A C 1979 Hormonal considerations in early normal pregnancy and blighted ovum syndrome. Fertility and Sterility 31: 252–257

Shapiro L R 1969 Repeated abortions in XO/XX mosaicism. Lancet ii: 217

Shearman R P 1975 Habitual abortion. In: Gold J J (ed) Gynecologic Endocrinology, Ch 30, p 534. Harper and Row, Hagerstown

Sheehan K L, Casper R F, Yen S S C 1982 Luteal phase defects induced by an agonist of luteinizing hormone-releasing factor: a model for fertility control. Science 215: 170–172

Sherman B M, Korenman S G 1974a Measurements of serum LH, FSH, estradiol and progesterone disorders of the human menstrual cycle: the short luteal phase. Journal of Clinical Endocrinology and Metabolism 38: 89–93

Sherman B M, Korenman S G 1974b Measurements of LH, FSH, estradiol and progesterone in disorders of the human menstrual cycle: the inadequate luteal phase. Journal of Clinical Endocrinology and Metabolism 39: 145–149

Sherwood O D, Rosentreter K R, Birkhime M L 1975 Development of a radioimmunoassay for porcine relaxin using ^{125}I labeled polytyrosyl-relaxin. Endocrinology 96: 1106–1113

Singh D N, Hara S, Foster H W, Grimes E M 1980 Reproductive performance in women with chromosome mosaicism. Obstetrics and Gynecology 55: 608–611

Smart Y C, Roberts T K, Fraser T S, Cripps A W, Clancy R L 1982 Validation of the rosette inhibition test for the detection of early pregnancy in women. Fertility and Sterility 37: 779–785

Stahl A, Luciani J M, Devictor M, Capoderno A M, Gagné R 1975 Constitutive heterochromatin and micronucleoli in the human oocyte at the diplotene stage. Humangenetik 26: 315–327

Stouffer R L, Hodgen D G 1980 Induction of luteal phase defects in rhesus monkeys by follicular fluid administration at the onset of the menstrual cycle. Journal of Clinical Endocrinology and Metabolism 51: 669–671

Stray-Pederson B, Eng J, Reikvarm T M 1978 Uterine T-mycoplasma colonization in reproductive failure. American Journal of Obstetrics and Gynecology 130: 307–311

Szolollosi D 1975 Mammalian eggs aging in the fallopian tubes. In: Blandau R J (ed) Aging Gametes, Their Biology and Pathology. International Symposium on Aging Gametes, Seattle, Washington, 1973, pp 98–121. Karger, Basel

Taylor P V, Hancock K W 1975 Antigenicity of trophoblast and possible antigen masking effects during pregnancy. Immunology 28: 973–982

Taysi K, Bobrow M, Balci S, Madan K, Atasu M, Say B 1973 Duplication/deficiency product of a pericentric inversion in man: a cause of D, trisomy syndrome. Journal of Pediatrics 82: 263–268

Thau R B, Sundaram K 1980 The mechanism of action of an antifertility vaccine in the rhesus monkey: reversal of the effects of antisera to the β-subunit of ovine luteinizing hormone by medroxyprogesterone acetate. Fertility and Sterility 33: 317–320

Thau R B, Sundaram K, Thornton Y S, Seidman L S 1979 Effects of immunization with the β-subunit of ovine luteinizing hormone on corpus luteum function in the rhesus monkey. Fertility and Sterility 31: 200–204

Tho S P T, Byrd J R, McDonough P G 1979 Etiologies and subsequent reproductive performance of 100 couples with recurrent abortion. Fertility and Sterility 32: 389–395

Tho S P T, Byrd J R, McDonough P G (1982) Chromosome polymorphism in 110 couples with reproductive failure and subsequent pregnancy outcome. Fertility and Sterility 38: 688–694

Torpin R (ed) 1969 Placenta marginata, placenta circumvallata. Two primary developmental varieties of placenta circumvallata. Evolution on placenta circumvallata based upon the Leipman (1906) four month pregnant uterus. In: The Human Placenta, Ch 8, p 43; Ch 9, p 48; Ch 10, p 71. Charles Thomas, Springfield

Vaitukaitus J L, Braunstein G D, Ross G T 1972 A radioimmunoassay which specifically measures human chorionic gonadotropin in the presence of human luteinizing hormone. American Journal of Obstetrics and Gynecology 113: 751–758

Verdiano N P, Dekle I, Rogers J, Tancer M L 1980 Reproductive performance of DES exposed female progeny. Obstetrics and Gynecology 58: 58–61

Warburton D, Stein Z, Kline J, Sussez M 1980 Chromosome abnormalities in spontaneous abortion: Data from the New York City study. In: Porter I H, Hook E B (eds) Human Embryonic and Fetal Death, pp 261–287. Academic Press, New York

Wilks J W, Hodgen G D, Ross G T 1976 Luteal phase defect in the rhesus monkey: the significance in serum FSH:LH ratios. Journal of Clinical Endocrinology and Metabolism 43: 1261–1267

Witschi E, Laguens R 1963 Chromosomal aberrations in embryos from overripe eggs. Developmental Biology 7: 605–616

Wolf D P, Hamada M 1979 Sperm binding to the mosue egg plasmalemma. Biology and Reproduction 21: 205–211

Zurier R B, Argyros M D, Urman J D, Warren J, Rothfield N F 1977 Systemic lupus erythematosus management during pregnancy. Obstetrics and Gynecology 51: 178–180

The 'dysfunctional' uterus: dysmenorrhoea and dysfunctional uterine bleeding

INTRODUCTION

In most present day cultures women are conditioned to expect a state of regular menstrual bleeding at approximately monthly intervals throughout the major part of their reproductive lives, although *Homo sapiens* has until very recently existed in a state where late menarche, early first pregnancy, prolonged lactation and early menopause ensured that regular menstrual cycles were few and far between (Short, 1976). Nowadays, any spontaneous or contraceptive-induced deviation from the regular pattern may be interpreted as undesirable although individual women will often tolerate major changes without undue alarm. It follows that complaints of abnormal menstruation or menstrually-related symptoms are highly subjective and greatly influenced by the local social and cultural environment. Dysmenorrhoea and dysfunctional uterine bleeding (DUB) are examples of conditions which are subject to substantial psychological influences although there is no doubt that both have clear biochemical or endocrine bases in most cases. These menstrual symptoms are mediated through dysfunction of one or more structures within the uterus itself.

As an intellectual diversion it is intriguing to consider why women menstruate at all. The usually quoted reason is that the old uterine lining must be shed to allow regeneration of a new lining which will be more suitable for the next potential implantation. However, the same end is achieved in animals like sheep by remodelling of the endometrium without actual bleeding. Many consider that the human system has been badly designed.

Somewhat surprisingly we still have a relatively poor understanding of the sequence of events which occur during normal menstruation and a discussion of present knowledge of this complex process is fundamental to a rational consideration of dysmenorrhoea and dysfunctional uterine bleeding.

NORMAL MENSTRUATION AND THE NORMAL CYCLE

In women normal menstruation consists of the loss of blood, endometrial tissue and tissue fluid through the cervix and vagina following the withdrawal of trophic hormone support from the corpus luteum. The volume of blood lost per cycle appears to vary in different countries from a median of 20 ml in Egypt through 30–40 ml in Northern Europe to 50 ml in China (Hallberg et al, 1966; Cole et al, 1971; Hefnawi et al, 1980; Gao et al, 1981). In most cases this probably accounts for about 50 per cent of the total volume of the menstrual discharge.

Most authors seem to be in agreement that an arbitrary upper limit for normal menstrual blood loss can be set at about 80 ml, since iron deficiency anaemia appears to become much more common in European women with repeated blood loss in this range (Hallberg et al, 1966). Blood loss may sometimes vary considerably from cycle to cycle in individuals but in some cases the variation is small (Hallberg & Nilsson, 1964b). The amount of endometrial tissue shedding at menstruation has been a subject of much controversy over the years (Bohnen, 1927; McLennan & Rydell, 1965; Flowers & Willborn, 1978), and it seems likely that there is wide individual variation. In some women there is relatively little tissue loss but a major restructuring of the tissue architecture, whereas in others there may be a loss of most of the superficial layers of the endometrium.

Our understanding of the morphological events in the endometrium during menstruation is still based to a great extent on the very elegant and meticulously described observations of Markee (1940) of intra-ocular endometrial transplants in rhesus monkeys. These are now being increasingly supplemented by corroborative morphological data and new biochemical and endocrine data in women.

Spiral arterioles seem to be essential for the process of menstruation, and excessive growth and coiling of these vessels occurs during the secretory phase. The coiling is greatly accentuated during a period of endometrial regression which occurs immediately prior to endometrial break-down (Markee, 1950). The regression merges into a period of intense arteriolar constriction which is most obvious at the myometrial–endometrial junction and in the inner myometrium. This usually precedes bleeding by a few hours. It persists throughout menstruation but intermittent relaxation of individual vessels occurs with consequent bleeding.

The exact causes of the endometrial regression, intense vasoconstriction and vascular breakdown are unknown. In recent years evidence has accumulated to implicate the prostaglandins, especially PGE_2 and $PGF_{2\alpha}$, in the vaso-constriction and regulation of the volume of blood that is lost (Abel, 1979). It is possible that these agents may also cause direct damage to the structure of the vessel walls and help to initiate bleeding. Since prostaglandins and related 'prostanoids' (cyclic endoperoxides, prostacyclin-PGI_2 and thromboxane A_2–TXA_2) have varying actions on blood vessels and platelets (see Ch. 11) it seems likely that a balance between different prostaglandins is important. Interesting new information is compatible with the hypothesis that PGI_2 synthesised in the myometrium from endo-metrial precursors may have a role in the control of endometrial blood flow (Kelly, 1981). It is possible that ischaemia increases free arachidonic acid concentration and that stasis prevents transfer of intermediates to the myometrium. This would lead to a marked increase in endometrial $PGF_{2\alpha}$ concentration and vasoconstriction limiting blood loss.

The sequence of events which links luteolysis and falling levels of oestradiol and progesterone with actual tissue breakdown is also far from clear. There is strongly sugges-tive evidence to implicate lysosomes in the initiation of tissue breakdown (Henzl et al, 1972) but the role could be limited to remodelling of the tissue during and after break-down (Wilson, 1980). The elegant ultrastructural and histochemical study of Henzl et al (1972) demonstrated that acid phosphatase is released from lysosomes into the cyto-plasm and intercellular spaces immediately prior to tissue breakdown. This release appears to be consequent upon a fall in plasma levels of oestradiol and progesterone. In most tissues, lysosome membrane stability is influenced by ambient steroid levels, but at the present time little infor-mation is available on the behaviour of lysosomes of endometrial origin. Additionally, very little is known about the different hydrolase enzymes which could be present in endometrial lysosomes. Of particular interest is the obser-vation that the arachidonic acid mobilising enzyme, phos-pholipase A_2, is sometimes present in lysosomes. This could provide the link between lysosome activity and pros-taglandin release at the onset of menstruation.

Haemostatic mechanisms play a central role in control of the volume of blood lost (Paton et al, 1980; Sixma et al, 1980) and this role is complementary to arteriolar constric-tion. The haemostatic response in the endometrium is highly defective compared with other tissues such as skin. This defective response is almost certainly due partly to the highly active fibrinolytic system within the endometrium (Rybo, 1966) and possibly also to increased release of pros-tacyclin and heparin (Paton et al, 1980). Morphological studies indicate that bleeding begins when gaps appear in the blood vessel walls. Intravascular haemostatic plugs containing platelets and later some fibrin slowly lead to partial or complete occlusion of vessels, but these platelet and fibrin plugs are not seen around the outside of vessels as in other tissues. The haemostatic response is so defective that in the premenstrual phase gaps in vessel walls with exposed collagen may appear without any evidence of platelet plug formation. Platelet plugs only form in the vessel lumina during the first 12–24 hours of menstruation and fibrin is only detectable in small amounts during the first 48 hours. The haemostatic plugs are shed with the superficial tissue layers into the menstrual fluid. Uterine contractility increases markedly at the onset of menstru-ation and encourages rapid drainage of the uterus. All these features seem to be aimed at preventing the deposition of significant amounts of fibrin and true blood clot within the cavity. This aim is obviously highly desirable since organ-isation of a true clot could result in the formation of intra-uterine adhesions with serious consequences for future reproduction.

Since haemostatic plugs and fibrin are only present in the endometrium during the early stages of menstruation, the mechanism of haemostasis during the remainder of menstruation remains unexplained. It is possible that blood loss after the first 12 hours is limited mainly by vasocon-striction and after 48 hours by surface regeneration of the epithelium. The major quantity of blood loss occurs during the first 2 days and usually then tails off rapidly within the next 2–3 days.

The most 'normal' menstrual patterns appear to occur following oestrogen priming of the endometrium for 1–2 weeks followed by oestrogen and progesterone together for a further 2 weeks. Predictable menstruation then occurs following simultaneous withdrawal of oestrogen and progesterone. Any departure from this pattern may be accompanied by abnormalities of menstruation, as is well illustrated by the endocrine patterns with the progestogen-only minipill (Landgren & Diczfalusy, 1980). Conversely, it should be recognised that disturbances of menstruation may sometimes occur when circulating hormone patterns are indistinguishable from normal.

The average menstrual period lasts 5 days with 90 per cent having a duration between 2 and 8 days. Cycle length is also very variable with the mean around 29.4 days (Gray, 1980) and only 80 per cent of women in the mid-reproductive years exhibiting cycles between 25 and 35 days. There is a skewed distribution towards longer cycles and irregular cycles are much more common in adolescence and the perimenopause.

DYSMENORRHOEA

Strictly translated from Greek dysmenorrhoea means 'difficult monthly flow', but it has now come to mean pain with menstruation. Pain is the major feature of the symptom-complex which may also include headache, faintness, dizzyness, nausea, vomiting, diarrhoea, abdominal bloating, backache and leg pains.

Traditionally, dysmenorrhoea is classified into two categories:

Primary dysmenorrhoea. This occurs in the absence of recognisable pelvic disease. Typically it begins in adolescence a few months after the menarche when ovulatory cycles first occur. The pain usually begins at or immediately before the onset of menstruation and persists through the first 12–48 hours of the flow. Pain can sometimes be so severe that the patient is confined to bed for several hours or days. It is usually described as spasmodic and cramping.

Secondary dysmenorrhoea. This is related to pelvic pathology such as endometriosis, adenomyosis or pelvic inflammatory disease. It usually first appears later in reproductive life, e.g. mid-twenties or thirties, and frequently has a different symptom pattern with abdominal bloating, pelvic heaviness and dragging pain being prominent. Pain may begin well before the onset of bleeding and often rises to a peak during early menstruation before declining towards the end of menstruation.

It is not always possible to distinguish these two categories on symptoms and signs alone.

Incidence and associations

The incidence of dysmenorrhoea is not accurately known for any population. However, information is available on the numbers who consult the medical profession or who admit to symptoms of dysmenorrhoea in population surveys.

In the United Kingdom the annual consultation rate per 1000 of the female population for dysmenorrhoea is 12.0 (Office of Population Censuses and Surveys, 1974). Of those women consulting their general practitioners with dysmenorrhoea 9.7 per cent were referred to consultants and 0.7 per cent required in-patient care. Several other studies have indicated that approximately 10–15 per cent of the female population aged between 14 and 50 years will complain of dysmenorrhoea (Kessel & Coppen, 1973; Richards, 1979; Widholm, 1979). However if population surveys are carried out it appears that over half of all menstruating women claim to experience dysmenorrhoea and at least 10 per cent will lose significant time from school or work because of their discomfort (Wood et al, 1979a).

Age is a very important factor. The incidence is low within the first few months of the menarche and then rises rapidly to a peak at the age of 16–18. It has been calculated that 82 per cent of girls will experience dysmenorrhoea between the ages of 15 and 19. The incidence then steadily decreases to around 40 per cent in the mid-reproductive years and may remain as high as 20 per cent at the age of 50 (Wood et al, 1979b; Widholm, 1979). It is said that the onset of sexual activity decreases the incidence but the evidence is not clear. It seems reasonably definite that childbirth is important and a decrease of 11 per cent has been recorded after the birth of one child and a further 19 per cent after the birth of a second child (Wood et al, 1979b). It is of interest that women who experience spontaneous premature labour are twice as likely to have a history of moderate or severe dysmenorrhoea than women who do not have premature labour (Ylikorkala & Kujansuu, 1981).

Most population surveys have some biases but there do seem to be a number of factors which are commoner in women who complain of dysmenorrhoea. These include a strong association with smoking cigarettes and an increased association of taking multiple alcoholic drinks at a time (Wood et al, 1979b). There is a strong correlation with mothers and daughters both experiencing dysmenorrhoea (Widholm, 1979) but level of education and type of employment do not appear to have any effect. Even the degree of physical activity at work does not appear to have any influence. The occurrence of sexual problems may contribute and there is little doubt that personality and psychological factors are important.

There are major socio-economic implications of this disorder in all western societies. The incidence and importance in developing countries is uncertain although preliminary data suggest that the disorder occurs with fairly similar frequency in most societies. In Norway it has been recorded that 1 in 3 factory workers stay in bed for at least 1 day per month because of dysmenorrhoea (Bergsjo, 1979) and this accounts for 3.7 per cent of total female sick leave. It seems likely that many of those who do not take time off work have a reduced working capacity at the time of menstrual pain.

Psychological associations and grading of pain

Pain is clearly a multidimensional experience (Melzack & Torgerson, 1971) and assessment can be a very difficult clinical problem. The sensory input is influenced by many factors, of which psychological processes are among the most important. Numerous psychological studies of dysmenorrhoea have been carried out and have used a variety of menstrual and pain questionnaires (Moos, 1968; Melzack, 1975; Bloom et al, 1978). Melzack has grouped the pain adjectives of the questionnaire into three dimensions reflecting his three factor theory of pain: sensory-discriminative, affective, and evaluative. Others have found this simplistic and grouped the responses into four, five or even seven categories (Reading, 1979). These clearly indicate that dysmenorrhoea has a major emotional significance which may reflect the negative attitude which many women have towards menstruation. A comparative study of intra-uterine device users who exhibit menstrual pain and non-IUCD dysmenorrhoea patients indicated that the dysmenorrhoea patients were more likely to regard their symptoms in affective or emotional terms while the IUCD users were more likely to use sensory terms. It was suggested that the IUCD users may be less distressed by their pain as it can be attributed to a clear physical cause which they have voluntarily accepted and which has positive contraceptive aspects against which the pain can be offset (Reading & Newton, 1977).

Homo sapiens is not the only species to suffer from dysmenorrhoea since several cases have been reported in chimpanzees (Solleveld & Van Zwieten, 1978). It seems unlikely that these were entirely psychosomatic!

It is not surprising that the woman who experiences cyclical severe pain comes to regard this in negative terms and may even become quite psychologically disturbed at the continuing prospect. It is still stated that this syndrome seems particularly common in introverted intellectualised neurotic women of obsessive personality (Carney, 1981), and it may well be that these women are more likely to complain about their symptom than others. However, the converse that all or even most women with dysmenorrhoea have these personality traits is certainly not true. Personality measures indicate that dysmenorrhoea sufferers are not maladjusted but are more likely to have neurotic traits or to be depressed, anxious or introverted (Bloom et al, 1978).

The attitude of male doctors throughout history has tended to emphasise the very negative aspects of menstruation. The classic quotation from Pliny (Pickles, 1979) epitomises a cultural view which engenders negative associations at all levels of the community: 'But nothing could easily be found that is more remarkable than the monthly flux of women. Contact with it turns new wine sour, crops touched by it become barren, grafts die, seeds in gardens are dried up, the fruit of trees falls off, the bright surface of mirrors in which it is merely reflected is dimmed, the edge of steel and the gleam of ivory are dulled, hives of bees die, even bronze and iron are at once seized by rust, and a horrible smell fills the air; to taste it drives dogs mad and infects their bites with an incurable poison'. Although most of this may be fanciful, it comes as a surprise to many that there is reasonable scientific evidence of the existence of a 'menotoxin' which has profound toxic effects on certain plants (Pickles, 1979). However, the relevance of this to human symptomatology is entirely speculative.

Grading of pain is clearly highly subjective and is best achieved using a standardised pain questionnaire. During experimental therapy it is essential to assess responses in an unbiased manner using a double-blind format and in most cases a placebo control. An objective corroboration of symptomatology has been provided by intra-uterine pressure measurements using accurate and error-free transducers and recording instruments (Akerlund et al, 1976; Smith & Powell, 1980), but this approach is impractical except in specialised research studies.

Aetiology

Primary dysmenorrhoea

It is now clear that the pain of primary dysmenorrhoea is associated with increased uterine muscular activity resulting in increased uterine tone and excessive spasmodic contractions (Akerlund, 1979; Smith & Powell, 1980). Baseline intra-uterine pressure may easily reach 50 mmHg and pressures up to 100 mmHg have been recorded; superimposed upon this may be spasmodic pressure rises up to 200–400 mmHg during contractions. This combination of high resting tone and excessive contractions is clearly capable of causing uterine ischaemia. Objective recordings of intra-uterine pressure and endometrial blood flow show that flow decreases during contractions and pain is at a maximum when flow is at a minimum (Akerlund et al, 1976; Fig. 31.1). It is probable that the pain results from ischaemia by a mechanism analagous to that seen in the heart with myocardial ischaemia and cardiac angina.

There is also now irrefutable evidence that prostaglandins are intimately involved in the pathogenesis of primary dysmenorrhoea. Excessively high concentrations of $PGF_{2\alpha}$ (and a high $PGF_{2\alpha}/PGE_2$ ratio) have been recorded in menstrual blood, uterine cavity washings, endometrium and peripheral blood from many but not all of these women (Pickles et al, 1965; Lundström & Green, 1978; Rosenwaks et al, 1981). The normal endometrium appears to develop

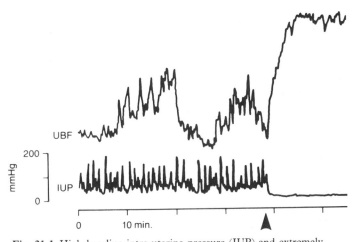

Fig. 31.1 High baseline intra-uterine pressure (IUP) and extremely high pressure contractions in a patient with dysmenorrhoea on day 1 of her menstrual period. Endometrial blood flow (UBF) was initially low and fluctuating but rose markedly after an injection of terbutaline (at arrow). This also abolished contractions and greatly reduced baseline tone (Akerlund et al 1976, with permission)

an increased capacity to synthesise $PGF_{2\alpha}$ even before the onset of menstruation (Downie et al. 1974) and this is exaggerated in dysmenorrhoea. Infusion experiments (intravenous and intra-uterine) have demonstrated that $PGF_{2\alpha}$ can mimic the symptoms of primary dysmenorrhoea, including the often associated systemic symptoms like nausea, vomiting, diarrhoea and headaches (Lundström, 1977). There is clear *in vitro* evidence that $PGF_{2\alpha}$, thromboxane A_2 and the cyclic endoperoxides can all cause excessive contraction of uterine muscle (Bygdeman et al, 1979; see Ch. 11) and therefore have the capability of fulfilling the causative role for primary dysmenorrhoea. On the other hand PGE_2 appears to relax myometrium at menstruation. Gap junctions between adjacent muscle cells facilitate transmission of contractile impulses, and appear with greater frequency in myometrium at the time of menstruation. They appear to be more frequent than usual in women with dysmenorrhoea (Garfield & Hayashi, 1980). It is known that gap junctions can be induced by $PGF_{2\alpha}$ and this is probably the mechanism by which it causes excessive contractions. Perhaps the most persuasive evidence for the involvement of prostaglandins is the dramatic therapeutic benefit obtained with many prostaglandin inhibitors.

What is much less clear is the underlying cause for excessive $PGF_{2\alpha}$ production. Several investigators have demonstrated that prostaglandin secretion from human endometrium and myometrium *in vivo* and *in vitro* is greatly influenced by the stage of the menstrual cycle and by the ambient levels of oestradiol and progesterone. High levels of oestradiol appear particularly important. Therefore, abnormalities in plasma steroid levels could account for the disturbance. In fact, a recent detailed study of daily plasma levels of LH, FSH, prolactin, oestradiol and progesterone has demonstrated a significantly elevated plasma oestradiol level in the late luteal phase (163 pg/ml compared with 93 pg/ml) in women with dysmenorrhoea compared with controls (Ylikorkala et al, 1979). They also found decreased plasma levels of prolactin — a finding of uncertain biological significance. Plasma levels of LH, FSH and progesterone were completely normal. An earlier study of daily urinary excretion of oestrogens and pregnanediol suggested that oestrogen excretion was significantly lower in dysmenorrhoeic than in normal women (Bell & Loraine, 1966), but this has not been confirmed by others and would be difficult to explain with our present knowledge of the effect of oestrogens on prostaglandin synthesis.

Recent *in vitro* experiments have demonstrated that the catechol oestrogens (2-hydroxylated and 4-hydroxylated oestrogens) are even more potent stimulants for prostaglandin synthesis than oestradiol-17β (Kelly, 1981) and the possibility exists that they may have a role in directing synthetic pathways for prostaglandins in menstrual disorders.

It has been known for several years that plasma levels of vasopressin (but not oxytocin) are elevated at the time of menstruation and are higher (by up to 4-fold) in women with dysmenorrhoea but this was generally considered to be a phenomenon secondary to menstrual pain. An interesting therapeutic experiment now indicates that plasma vasopressin levels remain excessively high in women whose dysmenorrhoea is successfully controlled with prostaglandin inhibitors (Strömberg et al, 1981). This suggests that vasopressin could have an aetiological role mediated through uterine prostaglandin synthesis.

Another intriguing clinical experiment involved the removal of venous plasma at the time of severe dysmenorrhoea followed by transfusion back into the same women some weeks later (Irwin et al, 1981). This produced typical abdominal pain and sometimes associated symptoms in eight out of 12 women. Plasma withdrawn at symptom-free periods did not cause pain when retransfused. A fascinating feature is that the pain could be reproduced in some women at a later stage after hysterectomy which suggests that in some women pain may be mediated by other means than uterine hypertonicity. This circulating factor and its effects are speculative.

The extent of involvement of catecholamines and the autonomic nervous system in the mechanism of dysmenorrhoea is unknown. Clearly, dysmenorrhoea can be abolished by presacral neurectomy, but it is also suggested that the decrease in dysmenorrhoea following pregnancy may be related to a marked decrease in autonomic nerve fibres in the uterus at that time (Sjoberg, 1979).

A popular explanation for dysmenorrhoea has been spasm of the nulliparous cervix resulting in high intra-uterine pressure and retrograde menstruation into the peritoneal cavity. It was thought that this excited free pain nerve fibres on the peritoneum in some way. Nowadays it is thought that this is unlikely since retrograde menstruation is probably very common. For example it has been recorded regularly in nine out of 11 women undergoing chronic peritoneal dialysis (Blumenkrantz et al, 1981) even in the absence of dysmenorrhoea.

Secondary dysmenorrhoea

This symptom is most commonly associated with the presence of endometriosis, adenomyosis or pelvic inflammatory disease. It is uncertain how often it occurs with endometrial polyps, mobile uterine retroversion or cervical stenosis, and is probably uncommon with fibroids. Many doubt the existence of that nebulous condition — the pelvic congestion syndrome. Rarely, severe dysmenorrhoea may occur with congenital anomalies of the reproductive tract, such as a rudimentary non-communicating uterine horn (McRae & Kim, 1979). Several studies have suggested that surgical sterilisation is followed by an increase in dysmenorrhoea, although it now seems that this does not occur or is only transient (Lieberman et al, 1978; Goh et al, 1981). Insertion of an intra-uterine device may certainly be followed by an increase in menstrual pain in many women. This is probably a prostaglandin related phenomenon similar to primary dysmenorrhoea. The mechanism of causation of pain in other types of secondary dysmenorrhoea is generally unexplained, but may be through an inflammatory process.

Management

Investigation

The management of primary dysmenorrhoea has been altered dramatically since recognition of the aetiological role of prostaglandins. Before this discovery most doctors believed that psychosomatic factors played a major part in the clinical presentation of this condition, and that management should be planned accordingly. Although nowadays the emphasis has greatly changed, an essential part of the initial approach to treatment continues to be through counselling and explanation.

An important prerequisite to treatment will always be an attempt at diagnosis, although this is not as crucial as in many conditions. The main aim of diagnosis is to distinguish those conditions which cause secondary dysmenorrhoea, especially endometriosis and chronic pelvic inflammatory disease, and treat them appropriately. Since none of these are life threatening a delay in diagnosis is unlikely to be serious. However, it must be recognised that some of these conditions can closely mimic primary dysmenorrhoea and may occur at a young age — even in teenagers. In this situation the laparoscope may prove invaluable, although an initial therapeutic trial of one or more of the medications discussed below may be quite justified.

If the history and clinical findings are unremarkable further investigations are generally not indicated in the teenager with typical symptoms. In fact even a vaginal examination can be deferred if the teenager is still a virgin. If symptoms persist in spite of adequate therapy or abnormal pelvic findings are present laparoscopy with endometrial curettage will probably be necessary to clearly identify or exclude pelvic pathology. Other investigations are generally unhelpful. If pelvic inflammatory disease is suspected endocervical swabs for culture for gonorrhoea, chlamydia and mycoplasma may be helpful, but even when collected under strictly correct conditions will often not identify a causative organism. The place of serology in pelvic inflammatory disease is uncertain, but may be helpful with chlamydial infections.

Treatment

A vast range of medications and procedures have at some time been applied to the management of dysmenorrhoea. Some of these (past, present and proposed) are been listed in Table 31.1. Those which are most relevant to the modern management are in italics.

Clearly severity of the pain and individual tolerance influence the approach to management. It should also be remembered that severe recurrent pain may induce an unpleasant anticipation of menstruation which may initially require stronger medication than later maintenance. Many women experiencing dysmenorrhoea are also susceptible to the temporary power of suggestion known as the placebo effect. In most cases this effect wears off over several cycles of placebo treatment. However it means that assessment of the efficacy of any new method of treatment requires comparison either against placebo or some standard mode of therapy, preferably on a double-blind and cross-over basis. Any trial should preferably also include at least three cycles of treatment on each medication.

An essential part of the management is an explanation

Table 31.1 Treatment for dysmenorrhoea — past, present and proposed

General measures	Pharmacological relief of pain	Hormones	Surgical	Other approaches
Explanation of physiology	*Analgesics*	*Oestrogen-progestogen 'pill'*	Cervical dilatation	*Relaxation therapy*
Counselling	*Prostaglandin synthetase inhibitors*	Oestrogen alone	D & C	Manipulation
Over the counter analgesics	*β-sympathomimetic agonists*	Progestogen alone (oral or injected)	Menstrual extraction	Behaviour modification
Bed rest	Calcium antagonists	Androgen	Ventrosuspension	Biofeedback techniques
Heat	Other 'spasmolytics'	Danazol	Presacral neurectomy	Psychotherapy
Short-wave diathermy	Sedatives	Gonadotrophin releasing-hormone analogues	Hysterectomy	Hypnosis
Alcohol	Amphetamines			Acupuncture
Special diets	Antihistamines			
	Local anaesthetic compresses			

Those approaches in italics are most widely regarded as having some value in modern therapy of straightforward cases of dysmenorrhoea.

of basic reproductive physiology and a reassurance about normality of function, including ovulation and fertility. For an adolescent patient the explanation and reassurance should usually be given in the presence of the mother. The topic of sexual activity should be broached with most adolescents in confidence, and advice given about contraception even if this is not immediately required. In mild to moderate cases supportive measures such as mild analgesia and encouraging normal activity may be helpful. However, there is little good evidence that agents such as aspirin and paracetamol are superior to placebo (Janbu et al, 1979; Rosenwaks et al, 1981). Drugs like propoxyphene hydrochloride may be somewhat superior to placebo (Morrison et al, 1980). Those women who need bed rest and abdominal heat such as a hot water bottle, should usually be given more active pharmacological agents.

It should not be forgotten that pharmacists and other paramedical personnel are likely to be approached before the medical profession and therefore play a very important role in counselling.

More intensive supportive measures appear to be of value although it should be emphasised that no comparative trials against medication of proven value have been reported. These measures do not take away the cause of the symptom but do improve the ability of the individual to cope with her problem. Techniques which have been used in dysmenorrhoea include relaxation therapy, behavioural modification therapy, hypnosis, manipulation, psychotherapy, acupuncture and biofeedback techniques (Chesney & Tasto, 1975; Cox & Meyer, 1978; Silver & Blanchard, 1978; Ben-Menachem, 1980; Denny & Gerrard, 1981).

Medication is usually required for all cases of moderate or severe dysmenorrhoea. Many of these agents will probably work for both primary and secondary dysmenorrhoea although the primary type usually responds very much better. Most of the discussion in this section relates to primary dysmenorrhoea.

The first major decision depends on the requirement for contraception. If contraception is required the obvious choice is a combined oestrogen-progestogen oral contraceptive. Numerous studies have confirmed the value of these agents in primary dysmenorrhoea. It appears that up to 50 per cent of women will experience complete relief of menstrual pain and approximately 90 per cent will experience marked relief (Nakano & Takemwura, 1971; Kremser & Mitchell, 1971). Progestogens alone such as norethisterone 5 mg daily or medroxyprogesterone acetate 5–10 mg daily, given for 3 weeks out of 4 will provide adequate contraception and will usually also produce substantial improvement in dysmenorrhoea. However the combined pill is probably a more satisfactory approach. The use of progestogens during the luteal phase only has been suggested by some but the value of this regimen is doubtful. Dydrogesterone has been used by some with benefit but this will not provide reliable contraception (Gould, 1979). A novel approach is the use of a progesterone releasing intra-uterine device and this has been used with some success (Trobough et al, 1978). Another agent which has been suggested for severe dysmenorrhoea but which is excessively expensive is danazol.

For those who do not wish oral contraceptive cover the medication of choice nowadays is probably the use of a prostaglandin inhibitor administered only for the duration of symptoms. These are recently become extremely popular because of their relatively high degree of efficacy, the simplicity of administration and the relatively low incidence of side-effects. Most studies have reported major benefit in 60–90 per cent of subjects and several different agents have proven very significantly superior to placebo. The clinical value of a prostaglandin inhibitor in women with severe dysmenorrhoea was first convincingly demonstrated by Schwartz et al (1974) using flufenamic acid. The fenamates appear to be particularly valuable agents and the benefits of mefenamic acid have been convincingly demonstrated with excellent relief in up to 89 per cent of women when less than 15 per cent responded to placebo (Anderson et al, 1978; Kintis & Contifaris, 1980). Another drug which has been extensively tested and provides excellent benefit is naproxen and its sodium salt (Henzl et al, 1980; Hamann, 1980). Other agents which may have a similar level of efficacy include ibuprofen, ketoprofen, tolfenamic acid and indomethacin. All of these agents are cyclo-oxygenase inhibitors which therefore switch off the synthesis of all the major classes of prostanoids. In addition, some of these agents have a weak end organ effect which prevents the action of the small amount of prostaglandin which is synthesised. The individual biological half-lives of these drugs are different and therefore recommended dosage schedules vary. Some of these drugs require a loading dose and thereafter individual response usually dictates the frequency of subsequent administration.

Many studies have shown the benefits of prostaglandin inhibitors in terms of reduction in pain, reduction in the use of supplemental analgesia, reduction in hours spent in bed and time off work. There is usually also a substantial reduction in associated symptoms such as nausea, vomiting, headache and diarrhoea. The therapeutic failures are often difficult to explain and do not appear to be due to nausea and vomiting affecting absorption (Ylikorkala et al, 1980). A number of side-effects have been recorded with prostaglandin inhibitors but these are generally uncommon. The gastrointestinal and central nervous effects are most conspicuous. These include dyspepsia, nausea, heart burn, diarrhoea, headache, dizzyness, irritability and drowsiness. More serious effects such as skin reactions, bronchospasm, transient renal failure and blood dyscrasias are fortunately very rare and the newer agents given in short intermittent dosage have a good risk benefit ratio.

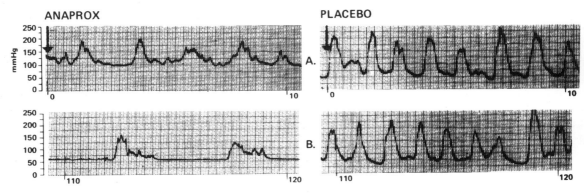

Fig. 31.2 Intra-uterine pressure tracings in two patients with dysmenorrhoea. One patient received oral naproxen sodium (Anaprox) with rapid marked reduction in uterine contractions and baseline tone. The other subject showed no reduction in intrauterine pressure following placebo (Henzl et al 1979, with permission)

Several studies have demonstrated a clear reduction in prostaglandin secretion during therapy with prostaglandin inhibitors. This includes a marked reduction in the $PGF_{2\alpha}$ content of menstrual blood following ibuprofen (Pulkkinen & Csapo, 1979) and a substantial reduction in the circulating levels of the main metabolite of $PGF_{2\alpha}$ with naproxen (Lundstrom & Green, 1978; Rosenwaks et al, 1981). The clear end result of this reduction in prostaglandin secretion is a marked reduction in the intra-uterine tone and contractions (Henzl et al, 1979; Smith & Powell, 1980, 1982; Fig. 31.2).

Another class of drugs which may be extremely beneficial are the betasympathomimetic agonists such as terbutaline and ritodrine (Akerlund et al, 1976; Andersen, 1977). Extensive evidence from Scandinavia has demonstrated their efficacy but the incidence of side-effects may be somewhat higher than with the antiprostaglandin agents. Calcium antagonists such as nifedipine (Sandahl et al, 1979) are also effective but can cause troublesome headaches. Sandahl et al (1980) have also reported the use of ketocaine local analgesic compresses applied locally over the main site of referred pain and giving major relief in 19 out of 23 subjects with a mean of 3 hours of benefit per treatment.

Failure of response to the above agents is rare provided that causative pelvic disease has been excluded. However these rare patients gain dramatic and long lasting benefit from the operation of presacral neurectomy. Since this operation is not entirely without complications it is usually only recommended as a last resort. An alternative surgical approach has been the use of repeated dilatation and curettage but nowadays most authorities agree that this should never be used as a therapeutic procedure in primary dysmenorrhoea. If dilatation and curettage is necessary for diagnostic purposes dilatation should never exceed 7–8 mm.

The treatment of secondary dysmenorrhoea usually requires specific management of the underlying cause. However, many cases will also respond to the approaches discussed above and there is good evidence that some cases of dysmenorrhoea due to endometriosis will respond well to tolfenamic acid (Kauppila et al, 1979). It should not be forgotten that women with dysmenorrhoea which is secondary to an intra-uterine device will usually respond well to antiprostaglandin agents (Buttram et al, 1979).

DYSFUNCTIONAL UTERINE BLEEDING

Dysfunctional uterine bleeding is one of the most poorly understood of common gynaecological conditions. This is partly due to great confusion over definitions and terminology, and few authorities can agree on consistent criteria to delineate the condition. The definition which this author prefers is 'excessively heavy, prolonged or frequent bleeding of uterine origin which is not due to recognisable pelvic or generalised medical disease, or to pregnancy'. Therefore this is a diagnosis of exclusion — a useful 'working diagnosis'. The commonest complaint is of excessively heavy bleeding (menorrhagia) and it is this symptom which is mainly considered in the following review.

There is little doubt that whatever definition is used the aetiology is multifactorial and only a few categories can be defined clearly. Perception of symptoms by the patient can be quite misleading but clearly forms a crucial part of the initial presentation and the clinical assessment. It is convenient to group the women into those with acute or chronic symptoms and ideally also into those who are predominantly ovulatory or predominantly anovulatory.

Incidence

DUB is a common diagnosis, being made in up to 10 per cent of cases attending an out-patient clinic (Taylor, 1965). It may occur at any time between menarche and menopause, but is particularly common in the 10 years leading up to the menopause. It is said that a small peak also occurs in adolescence but this is difficult to demonstrate because most cases are treated without any contact with hospital clinics. This is illustrated by a very large pathological study of DUB where only 4 per cent of patients undergoing curettage were under 20 years (Sutherland, 1949). By contrast 40 per cent were over 40 years and 50 per cent in the 20–40 year age group. Anovulatory DUB is certainly commoner in adolescence and perimenopause, whereas 80 per cent of cases in the mid-reproductive years are ovulatory. For example, cystic glandular hyperplasia (CGH) of the endometrium is mainly seen in the 40–50 year age group although a very small peak occurs in adolescence (Schröder, 1954; Fraser & Baird, 1972). It used to be taught that almost all cases of DUB in young girls were associated with endometrial hyperplasia but this is clearly erroneous and is probably between 5 and 15 per cent (Sutherland, 1949; Fraser & Baird, 1972). The population incidence of adolescent CGH is probably about 5 new cases per million per year.

Population studies of menstrual blood loss indicate that menorrhagia with measured loss over 80 ml per cycle is relatively infrequent (Hallberg et al, 1966; Cole et al, 1971). These studies are subject to many biases but give an indication that perhaps 5–10 per cent of women in a general population will exhibit objective menorrhagia at any one time. This is very different from the subjective complaint of 'menorrhagia' as made by the patient, which is probably much commoner. It is calculated that 5–25 per cent of women will complain of menorrhagia at some time (Richards, 1979; Wood et al, 1979a; National Opinion Poll Research Survey, 1980).

Differential diagnosis

Since dysfunctional uterine bleeding is a diagnosis of exclusion, recognition of other potential causes of excessive uterine bleeding is of central importance.

Pelvic disease causing excessive bleeding

Leiomyomata (fibroids). These are a common cause of menorrhagia (Buttram & Reiter, 1981). Submucous and intramural lesions seem much more likely to cause menorrhagia than subserous ones, although no objective measurements of blood loss have been reported. The mechanism appears to be gross distortion of the vascular architecture around the fibroid (Beilby et al, 1970).

Endometriosis. This has a common clinical association with menorrhagia although again no objective measurements of blood loss have been reported (Sensky & Liu, 1980). The mechanism is unknown but thought to be due to a disturbance of prostaglandin secretion.

Adenomyosis. This is another relatively common association with menorrhagia, although the diagnosis is usually not made until the time of hysterectomy (Vora et al, 1981). Again prostaglandins are thought to be involved in the mechanism of disturbed bleeding.

Chronic pelvic inflammatory disease. This may cause heavy or irregular bleeding, presumably through uterine vascular congestion and dilatation.

Endometrial polyps. These are somewhat mysterious lesions of uncertain aetiology, which are found more frequently in women with anovulation. Use of the hysteroscope suggests that they are probably much commoner than is generally appreciated from routine curettage, and they are undoubtedly associated with a proportion of cases of clinically diagnosed DUB.

Endometrial adenocarcinoma. This usually presents with postmenopausal bleeding but 30–40 per cent present before the menopause with irregular, intermenstrual, postcoital or excessive bleeding. Many of these cases give a preceding history of anovulatory DUB (Chamlian & Taylor, 1970). This is undoubtedly the most serious of all the differential diagnoses of DUB.

Polycystic ovarian disease. This is often associated with infrequent episodes of menorrhagia due to anovulation with elevated circulating oestrogen levels.

Pelvic congestion syndrome. This is a rather nebulous concept which may or may not exist as a distinct entity capable of causing menorrhagia.

Bicornuate uterus. This is said to be associated with menorrhagia due to the increased endometrial surface area, but objective evidence is not available.

Rarities. Those which may be associated with menorrhagia include functional ovarian tumours, endometrial haemangiomata, uterine lymphangiomata, pelvic arteriovenous malformations.

Surface lesions of the genital tract. These may cause irregular or intermenstrual bleeding at any age, although in these cases regular menstruation usually continues normally.

Complications of pregnancy. These must necessarily be excluded in all cases of acute or subacute 'menorrhagia'.

Medical diseases causing excessive bleeding

Disorders of haemostasis. These present as rare causes of menorrhagia (Quick, 1966) but may occur in as many as 20 per cent of adolescents with menorrhagia in whom pelvic pathology has been excluded (Claessens & Cowell, 1981). Any type of haemostatic disorder may cause excessive bleeding in some individuals, but in many, especially those on anticoagulants, menstruation may be completely normal. The disorders most commonly associated with menorrhagia are disturbances of platelet function including thrombocytopoenia, various thrombocytopathies, leukaemia, Von Willebrand's disease and possibly chronic excessive aspirin ingestion.

Hypothyroidism. Classically said to cause anovulation and menorrhagia, although a few will develop amenorrhoea or oligomenorrhoea instead (Scott & Mussey, 1964).

Systemic lupus erythematosus. This may cause menorrhagia either by damage to vascular function or through the action of a circulating coagulation-inhibiting antibody.

Other medical causes. These include congestive cardiac failure, chronic hepatic disease and chronic renal failure following adequate dialysis.

Aetiology and mechanisms

It is convenient to divide these patients into those who are anovulatory and those who are ovulatory although it should be remembered that women with a history suggestive of anovulation will not infrequently have some ovulatory cycles (Fraser & Baird, 1974).

Anovulatory cycles

The classical studies of Brown et al (1959) have thoroughly documented the urinary oestrogen excretion in women with anovulatory cycles. They have shown that oestrogen levels usually fluctuate substantially but may occasionally be relatively constant for some weeks. In their studies heavy menstrual bleeding usually occurred when oestrogen levels were falling but occasionally would occur when levels were steady or even when they were rising. These authors investigated the oestrogen levels in terms of the degree of endometrial proliferation and clearly demonstrated that cystic glandular hyperplasia of the endometrium was associated with high fluctuating levels of oestrogen or with moderate and prolonged unopposed levels of oestrogen (Brown & Matthew, 1962). It is now clear that the condition of 'metropathia haemorrhagica' with multicystic ovaries, cystic glandular hyperplasia of the endometrium and erratic menorrhagia is merely the severe end of the spectrum of anovulatory dysfunctional uterine bleeding (Schröder, 1954; Brown et al, 1959).

It appears that ovarian synthesis and subsequent metabolism of oestrogens is within normal limits in perimenopausal women with anovulatory DUB but the dynamics of oestrogen secretion are disturbed (Fraser & Baird, 1974). In anovulatory women in the late reproductive years significant amounts of oestradiol may be secreted by both ovaries. These may come from large and sometimes multiple follicles suggesting a disturbance of intra-ovarian follicular control mechanisms or abnormalities in gonadotrophin release. A detailed study of perimenopausal women with anovulatory DUB reported results consistent with a variety of defects both in hypothalamic–pituitary and intra-ovarian mechanisms (Van Look et al, 1977). The perimenopausal findings are in striking contrast to the mechanism of anovulatory DUB in adolescents. Detailed investigation has clearly demonstrated that the majority of adolescents with anovulation have a defect in the positive feedback response to oestrogen (Fig. 31.3) (Fraser et al, 1973; Van Look et al, 1978). It is suggested that these girls may be experiencing a delay in the maturation of hypothalamic control.

Hyperprolactinaemia is occasionally recorded in women with anovulatory DUB. Since treatment with bromocriptine rarely cures the condition, it may just be a chance association or more likely may be a consequence of the elevated oestrogen levels.

The erratic, prolonged and excessively heavy bleeding which is typical of anovulatory DUB is clearly associated with the prolonged unopposed stimulation of the endometrium by fluctuating and sometimes excessively high levels of oestradiol. However, the exact mechanism of the abnormal breakdown of the endometrium has not been elucidated. The endometrium is rarely found to be atrophic and generally varies from different degrees of proliferation to cystic glandular hyperplasia or more exaggerated forms such as adenomatous hyperplasia. These atypical forms of hyperplasia do seem to be associated with an increased risk of endometrial malignancy later. Endometrial polyps are sometimes found. The histological findings have been well described by Sutherland (1949). Orderly development of the endometrial vasculature does not occur and there is usually poor spiral arteriole development with exaggerated venous vascularity and the development of venous sinusoids (Beilby et al, 1971).

It is usually stated that bleeding follows a fall in oestrogen levels but this is not necessarily so and the relative importance of different biochemical mechanisms has not been demonstrated. There is increasing evidence to implicate the prostaglandins and two groups of investigators have demonstrated an increased endometrial concentration or synthetic capacity for prostaglandin E_2 in anovulatory DUB (Willman et al, 1976; Smith et al, 1982). There may also be abnormal intra-uterine haemostasis due to excessive fibrinolysis (Rybo, 1966) or to excessive heparin production by endometrial mast cells (Paton et al, 1980). It is not known whether there is any abnormality of endometrial lysosome function although it could be expected that lysosome membrane stability would be reduced in the presence of unopposed oestrogen. Unopposed oestrogen may also lead to an excessive rate of endometrial blood flow at the time of endometrial breakdown. This could be expected to be translated into an excessive blood loss.

Ovulatory cycles

The great majority of women with DUB in the mid reproductive years will experience regular ovulatory cycles. Daily plasma measurements of LH, FSH, oestradiol and progesterone have indicated that these cycles are indistinguishable from normal women (Haynes et al, 1980). This suggests that the disorder is due to a local functional abnormality within the uterus itself or to some unidentified circulating substance.

Most of these women have secretory endometrium which is indistinguishable from normal (Taw, 1975;

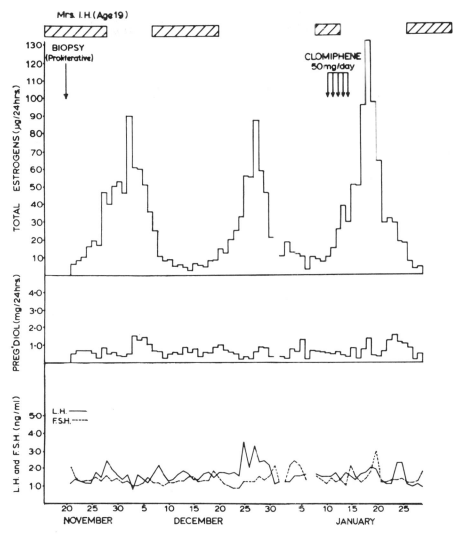

Fig. 31.3 Excretion of total oestrogen and pregnanediol and plasma concentrations of FSH and LH in a 19-year-old patient with anovulatory dysfunctional uterine bleeding. There is no evidence of a midcycle LH surge or ovulation, although excessively high peaks of oestrogen excretion have occurred on three occasions. ▨ represents uterine bleeding (Fraser et al 1973, with permission)

Nedoss, 1971). The literature is replete with descriptions of irregular ripening, irregular shedding and secretory hyperplasia of the endometrium. These appearances are presumably due to an abnormal stromal and/or glandular response to progesterone and perhaps oestrogen. The underlying causes and relative importance of these appearances are unknown. It has also been suggested that increased uterine weight and increased uterine surface area may be important although a recent careful study has not confirmed this (Chimbira et al, 1980).

Increasing evidence again implicates abnormalities of prostaglandin metabolism in the mechanism of bleeding. There is reasonable evidence to implicate a decreased production of prostaglandin $F_{2\alpha}$ (Smith et al, 1982). There is also evidence to indicate that endometria from these patients have an increased capacity to synthesise prostacyclin (Smith et al, 1982). Prostacyclin is a potent vasodilator and inhibitor of platelet aggregation and hence could substantially influence the degree and duration of menstrual bleeding. The factors responsible for the shift in the endometrial conversion of prostaglandin endoperoxides from $PGF_{2\alpha}$ to PGE_2 and PGI_2 are unknown. It will be of interest to look for an abnormality of catechol oestrogen metabolism in these patients (Kelly, 1981). It must be remembered that the endometrium is a highly active tissue biochemically and there may well be abnormalities of fibrinolysis, heparin secretion, lysosome activity, prolactin secretion (Maslar & Riddick, 1979) or even relaxin or the renin angiotensin system.

One study has suggested that iron deficiency and anaemia are causative factors or exacerbate DUB (Taymor et al, 1964), whereas it seems much more probable that the majority of patients who develop iron deficiency anaemia trigger a compensatory mechanism which tends to reduce the menstrual blood loss. Jacobs & Butler (1965) studied 15 women with iron deficiency anaemia and found that in the great majority the blood loss per menstrual period almost doubled following correction of the anaemia. The increase in blood loss was greatest in those women whose initial blood loss was about average. This indicates that the presence of anaemia and iron deficiency may not correlate well with menstrual blood loss. The development of anaemia depends upon a number of factors including the iron intake, the efficiency of iron transport and storage, and the efficiency of the erythropoietic system as well as upon the amount of menstrual blood loss. This is clearly seen in women blood donors who can maintain a normal haemoglobin and therefore compensate for a blood loss at the rate of 300 ml/month (Fowler & Barer, 1942).

For some years it has been alleged that surgical tubal sterilisation may cause menorrhagia and the question is still unresolved. Some have even suggested that sterilisation may ultimately lead to a high incidence of hysterectomy (Muldoon, 1972). Most of the investigations indicating a relationship between tubal interruption and subsequent menorrhagia have been retrospective and based entirely on the woman's perception. However, some of these studies have been adequately controlled and are apparently convincing (Neil et al, 1975; Lawson et al, 1979). On the other hand there are now numerous studies in the literature which have found no evidence of an adverse relationship (Edgerton, 1977; Lieberman et al, 1978; Sapire & Davey, 1980).

The only study which has attempted an objective and prospective evaluation of menstrual blood loss in sterilised women found no increase in measured menstrual loss up to 1 year following operation (Kasonde & Bonnar, 1976). These investigators measured menstrual loss objectively over two to three cycles before sterilisation and at intervals of up to 12 months in 25 women.

It has been suggested that ceasing oral contraceptive use at the time of sterilisation may be responsible for the real increase in perceived menstrual bleeding in many of these women. Clearly this effect may be particularly disturbing for some women who have not experienced normal menstruation for many years because of pregnancies, lactation and prolonged pill use. However, this does not account for all cases and it seems likely that in the majority the problem is one of decreased tolerance of menstruation. For these women recurring menstruation is no longer a reminder of continuing fertility and in addition it may be associated with undesirable features such as pain and premenstrual tension. Nevertheless some women do develop genuine menorrhagia some years following sterilisation and it is impossible to say that this association is not causal in some cases.

If there is a genuine causal association between surgical sterilisation and menorrhagia in a small number of women the mechanism is unknown. Decreased corpus luteum secretion of progesterone has been reported in several studies (Donney et al, 1981) but this type of endocrine disturbance is not noted as a cause of menorrhagia in other situations. The most likely explanation would be interrup-

tion of vascular transport of some unknown factor from the ovary along the utero-tubal arcade. However, further speculation awaits a convincing prospective demonstration that the post-tubal ligation menorrhagia syndrome really exists. In the meantime it is reasonable to manage them as cases of ovulatory dysfunctional uterine bleeding, from which they are indistinguishable in other ways at the present time.

It is important to recognise that many cases diagnosed on clinical grounds as DUB will ultimately be found to have pelvic or systemic pathology of sufficient degree to cause the symptoms. This is shown in a retrospective study from the Chelsea Hospital for Women London, where 40 per cent (105 out of 287) of women undergoing hysterectomy for 'dysfunctional uterine haemorrhage' were found to have substantial pelvic pathology (Beazley, 1970; Table 31.2). There is even the suggestion that some of these cases may be associated with minor degrees or even microscopic deposits of endometriosis.

Table 31.2 Pathology of specimens removed at hysterectomy for 'dysfunctional uterine bleeding' (Beazley, 1970)

Pathology report		Number of specimens	Percentage
No abnormality	} 'true' DUB	114	40
Functional abnormality		56	20
Functional and organic abnormality		26	9
Organic abnormality		89	31
Lost reports		2	—
Total		287	100

Psychological aspects

These are of the utmost importance in the assessment of DUB, since the diagnosis is based almost entirely on the history presented by the patient.

Perception of menstrual bleeding is inaccurate and retrospective recall is unreliable (Gray, 1980). Many women have little idea how their menstrual loss compares with the norm and their recorded perception may bear little relation to measured loss (Hallberg et al, 1966; Chimbira et al, 1980). Hallberg et al (1966) found that 40 per cent of women with menstrual loss exceeding 80 ml considered their periods only moderate or scanty, while 14 per cent of those with a loss of less than 20 ml judged their periods to be heavy. In a recent study of 69 women presenting with good clinical histories of menorrhagia (Fraser et al, 1981) it was found that only 31 per cent had a measured menstrual loss of greater than 80 ml and 22 per cent actually had a loss of less than 35 ml — the mean for the normal population (Fig. 31.4). A more detailed assessment demonstrated that some of these women had difficulty in perceiving major changes in volume from cycle to cycle and even from 1 day to the next (Fraser et al, 1984).

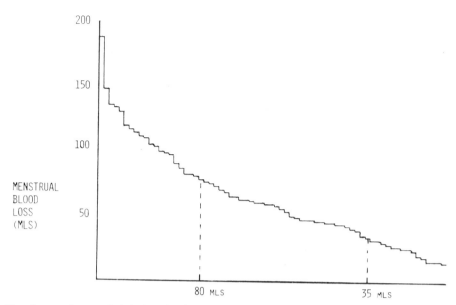

Fig. 31.4 Menstrual blood loss (mean of two cycles) during placebo treatment in 69 individual women presenting with a good clinical history of menorrhagia. 80 ml marks the upper limit of the normal range, and 35 ml marks the mean of most studies of normal populations in developed countries

It seems likely that women under different types of emotional strain may have decreased tolerance of disturbances of menstruation and this may be particularly so in women who have been surgically sterilised. However, objective data are not available.

From time to time anecdotal reports are mentioned of women who have experienced sudden unheralded bleeding in the face of unexpected emotional trauma. The extent of this phenomenon and the possible mechanisms are unclear.

Prognosis

Very little accurate information is available about this aspect of DUB. None of this is based on objective measurements of blood loss.

Single episodes of DUB in adolescence probably have a good prognosis, whereas the adolescent with several episodes of DUB has a poor prognosis in terms of persistent menstrual disturbances (30–80 per cent), repeated need for curettage (40–55 per cent), anaemia (30 per cent), repeated hormone therapy (40 per cent), infertility (45–55 per cent), laparotomy for ovarian cysts (10–30 per cent) and even endometrial carcinoma if inadequately treated (1–2 per cent) (Southam, 1959; Southam & Richart, 1966). This prognosis is particularly bad when CGH is diagnosed (Fraser & Baird, 1972), and is a good reason for curettage in the adolescent with repeated episodes of DUB.

It is said that the prognosis in ovulatory DUB in the mid-reproductive years is good, but convincing evidence is not available. In some communities many of these women undergo hysterectomy and an accurate assessment of prognosis is no longer possible. From published data it appears that the long-term prognosis for anovulatory DUB

in the later reproductive years is poor and recurrence is the rule.

It is often said that curettage leads to long-term reduction in menstrual blood loss in many patients. However, the published data do not confirm this. Objective measurements indicate a reduction in loss in the first cycle following curettage but a return to pre-treatment levels thereafter (Nilsson & Rybo, 1971; Haynes et al, 1977). The persisting subjective benefit which many women experience is presumably related to reassurance about the absence of pathology and a change in tolerance of symptoms.

Assessment of menstrual blood loss

There is only one reliable means of assessing the volume of menstrual loss and that is by direct measurement. This has been recommended by several investigators, but there is a resistance by many doctors to asking patients to collect their sanitary towels for laboratory assessment. This is most unfortunate in view of the major errors which many women make in perception of their menstrual loss. In fact, excessively heavy blood loss (menorrhagia) must be the only common subjective medical complaint upon which treatment decisions of far reaching import are made without any attempt at objective measurement.

Many clinical means have been recommended for quantitating menstrual loss, but none of these is generally helpful. Even the recognition of blood clots in the flow does not correlate well with volume. 'Flooding' is probably the most reliable single symptom followed closely by use of two sanitary towels at a time. Tiredness and lassitude are unhelpful, whereas a previous history of objectively confirmed anaemia is strong supportive evidence. Some doctors still rely on a sanitary towel count to give a measure

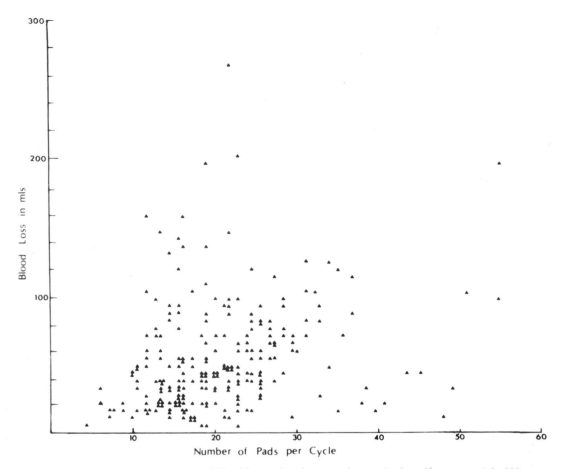

Fig. 31.5 Lack of correlation between measured menstrual blood loss and sanitary towel usage (pads and/or tampons) in 228 menstrual periods

of volume, although several authors have indicated that this is unreliable (Chimbira et al, 1980; Fraser et al, 1981). A recent study of 276 menstrual periods in women complaining of menorrhagia (Fraser et al, 1981) found no significant correlation between objectively measured menstrual loss and the number of pads or tampons used (Fig. 31.5).

Several methods have been proposed for measurement of menstrual blood loss (Cohen & Gibor, 1980) but the one which has gained most popularity because of relative simplicity and reproducibility is that of Hallberg & Nilsson (1964a). This method relies on careful collection of all menstrual pads, tampons and clots followed by extraction of the haemoglobin and conversion to alkaline haematin with 5 per cent sodium hydroxide. The practical application of the method has been greatly increased by the use of a semi-automatic extractor (Newton et al, 1977). More widespread clinical use of objective methods of assessment such as this must occur if progress is to be made in the management of menorrhagia.

Investigations

A presumptive diagnosis of DUB is usually made on the basis of history plus clinical examination and few investigations are usually necessary.

1. Full blood count including haemoglobin, haematocrit, mean corpuscular volume, mean corpuscular haemoglobin concentration, white cell count and platelet count should always be performed. Serum ferritin may be useful for the assessment of early iron deficiency.

2. Diagnostic dilatation and curettage is mandatory in all women with recurrent episodes of DUB except perhaps some young adolescents. The primary reason is to exclude early endometrial adenocarcinoma, but useful diagnostic information about ovulation may be obtained if the procedure is timed to precede the next menstrual period. The presence of submucous fibroids or endometrial polyps may also be detected.

3. Assessment of menstrual blood loss (see above)

4. Other investigations only if indicated.

4.1 Coagulation screen should be seriously considered if the woman has a history of easy bruising or heavy bleeding at minor operations.

4.2 Endocrine studies may include plasma thyroid stimulating hormone and thyroid function tests to exclude hypothyroidism. Plasma prolactin may reveal hyperprolactinaemia and a raised plasma LH/FSH ratio may suggest polycystic ovarian disease.

4.3 Diagnostic laparoscopy may be valuable to confirm or exclude endometriosis, PID, fibroids or other pelvic pathology.

4.4 Diagnostic hysteroscopy (Sugimoto, 1978) may provide confirmation of submucous fibroids, endometrial polyps or other intra-uterine lesions when these have been missed or cannot be confirmed in any other simple manner.

4.5 Hysterosalpingogram has also been used to detect intra-uterine lesions with some success in skilled hands.

4.6 Blood biochemistry including electrolytes, liver function tests and renal function tests may rarely reveal unexpected abnormalities of hepatic or renal function.

4.7 Plasma salicylate levels may occasionally identify chronic aspirin takers who have not given a positive history.

Management of DUB

Acute

Rarely, DUB may be so heavy that urgent therapy is required. Traditionally, most of these patients have been treated by thorough endometrial curettage for both diagnostic and therapeutic reasons. This will stop the bleeding in most cases, but rarely extreme measures, including ligation of the anterior division of the internal iliac arteries or even hysterectomy, may be required.

An alternative approach in the patient who has had a previous diagnostic curettage is the use of intravenous Premarin (Ayerst Labs). This mixture of conjugated equine oestrogens has produced impressive results in anecdotal cases reported over many years but only very recently has good scientific evidence been presented testifying to its efficacy (De Vore et al, 1982). In a double-blind placebo-controlled study of 34 women presenting as emergencies with excessive or prolonged DUB, haemorrhage ceased in 72 per cent after one or two intravenous injections of Premarin 25 mg. However, bleeding also stopped within the same time in 38 per cent who received placebo injections ($P = 0.021$). Premarin is thought to act rapidly on capillary bleeding by multiple effects on blood levels of fibrinogen, factors V and IX, platelet aggregation, tissue reactions to bradykinin, mucopolysaccharides in intercellular tissue and capillary permeability (De Vore et al, 1982). In the long term it will have a beneficial effect by increasing endometrial proliferation and must always be followed by an oral progestogen to produce predictable withdrawal bleeding.

In acute episodes of lesser severity oral progestogens (e.g. norethisterone/norethindrone 5 mg three or four times a day; medroxyprogesterone acetate 10 mg three times a day) may slow the bleeding within 8–12 hours and stop it within 24–48 hours. This will work more effectively in women with anovulation and should be continued for a minimum of 10 days to permit conversion of the proliferative or hyperplastic endometrium into a normal secretory pattern. The subsequent withdrawal bleed should not be excessively heavy and should be of limited duration.

Chronic

There are several possible approaches to the management of recurrent episodes of DUB.

1. *Full explanation and reassurance* about the absence of pathology is essential following diagnostic curettage. If measured menstrual blood loss or haemoglobin and serum ferritin levels are normal it may also be possible to provide strong reassurance that subjective 'menorrhagia' is not a health hazard. This reassurance may be sufficient to allow many women to accept and cope with their perceived symptom without further therapy. Temporary use of a menstrual calender may be a helpful adjunct to this advice by emphasising the doctor's interest in her problem and illustrating the regularity of her cycles. Changing the patient's attitude and increasing tolerance is an integral part of this approach.

2. *Drug therapy* will be required in many cases and before starting treatment it is helpful to know if the patient is predominantly anovulatory or ovulatory. Those women who have iron-deficiency anaemia should obviously receive iron supplements in addition to their other therapy.

2.1 *Hormonal preparations* may be of great value, but must be used in appropriate regimens for each individual.

For the anovulatory woman progestogens alone should usually be the first choice. They should usually be given orally for 7–10 days from day 15–18 of the cycle, e.g. NET 5 mg twice or three times a day or MPA 10 mg twice or three times a day. This will usually permit good secretory change in the endometrium and a predictable withdrawal bleed. However, some women with excessive oestrogen secretion from early in the cycle may need a longer duration of progestogen exposure, for example from day 5 to 25. This regimen has the further advantage that it is contraceptive, and after two to three courses the dosage can often be reduced as low as 5 mg NET or 10 mg MPA daily.

Injectable progestogens (e.g. depot medroxyprogesterone acetate, DMPA) have been used to produce amenorrhoea, but unfortunately the response is unpredictable with many women experiencing irregular scanty bleeding and around 10 per cent having episodes of prolonged or rarely heavy bleeding (see Ch. 34). A novel approach is the use of a progesterone-releasing intra-uterine device which has proved valuable in a small number of women with menorrhagia following haemodialysis for chronic renal failure (Newton et al, 1976). Although these patients obtain a substantial reduction in total volume of blood loss this is often at the expense of an increase in scanty intermenstrual bleeding.

Many women with ovulatory or anovulatory DUB will benefit from a combined oestrogen-progestogen oral

Table 31.3 Incidence of complaints of menstrual disturbance in users and non-users of oral contraceptives in a large prospective cohort study (Royal College of General Practitioners, 1974)

| | Rate per 1000 women years | | Relative risk |
	O.C. users	Controls	
Menorrhagia	12.48	23.82	0.52*
Irregular bleeding	5.19	13.08	0.65*
Intermenstrual bleeding	3.04	5.26	0.72*
Dysmenorrhoea	3.87	10.43	0.37*

* $P < 0.01$.

contraceptive and theoretically this should have a relatively high progestogenic balance. Women using oral contraceptives are much less likely to complain of menorrhagia, irregular bleeding or intermenstrual bleeding (Royal College of General Practitioners, 1974; Table 31.3). Combined oral contraceptives can also be shown to reduce measured menstrual blood loss in women complaining of menorrhagia (Nilsson & Rybo, 1971). However, it appears that at least 20 per cent of patients will not respond.

It must also be accepted that many women have risk factors which make them unsuitable for long-term hormonal therapy. These factors are well known and include smoking, age over 40 years, strong family history of cardiovascular disease, diabetes mellitus, hyperlipidaemia and many others (see Chs 33 and 35).

2.2 Antiprostaglandin agents include several groups of drugs which act mainly by inhibiting the cyclo-oxygenase enzyme system which converts arachidonic acid into cyclic endoperoxides. It has recently been shown that some of these agents may induce a dramatic reduction in menstrual blood loss in some women with menorrhagia. The most extensively investigated preparation is mefenamic acid used in the same manner as for dysmenorrhoea (Anderson et al, 1976; Fraser et al, 1981). This results in a mean reduction in blood loss of 28 per cent, but is usually proportionately greater in those with more excessive loss. The benefit is usually maintained with repeated treatment over long periods (Fraser et al, 1983), and may also be seen in women with menorrhagia due to an IUCD, fibroids, or even Von Willebrand's disease (Guillebaud et al, 1978; Fraser et al, 1981). Very limited published information suggests that flufenamic acid, indomethacin and naproxen may have similar beneficial effects (Anderson et al, 1976; Damarawy & Toppozada, 1976; Davies et al, 1981).

Since the antiprostaglandin agents inhibit synthesis of PGE_2, $PGF_{2\alpha}$, PGI_2 and TXA_2 it has been suggested that their beneficial effect on menorrhagia may be mediated by a relative increase in synthesis of a vasoconstrictive leukotriene. However, not all women will experience a reduction in blood loss with PG inhibitors, and therefore these drugs may act merely by altering the balance of prostanoid synthesis within the uterus. The fenamates also have a weak end-organ action inhibiting prostaglandins that have already been synthesised (Collier & Sweatman, 1968).

2.3 Fibrinolytic inhibitors such as epsilon amino caproic acid (EACA) and tranexamic acid (AMCA) have been used by several investigators with striking benefit in some women with menorrhagia and intermenstrual bleeding (Weström & Bengtsson, 1970; Kasonde & Bonnar, 1975a). Unfortunately, the widespread use of these drugs has been limited by side-effects and concerns about long-term safety. Intra-uterine application may avoid these risks and appears to produce benefit for several cycles following one treatment (Tauber et al, 1977). Several diamidines and guanidines which are potent inhibitors of fibrinolysis are under investigation as potentially valuable therapeutic or preventive agents for IUD-related bleeding problems (World Health Organisation, 1979).

2.4 Ethamsylate is a rather mysterious drug which is said to reduce menstrual blood loss by a reduction in capillary fragility (Harrison & Campbell, 1976) acting perhaps as an anti-hyaluronidase and an anti-prostaglandin agent. A 50 per cent reduction in blood loss in women with spontaneous menorrhagia and a 19 per cent reduction in IUD users has been reported by one group (Harrison & Campbell, 1976) and confirmed by another (Kovacs & Annus, 1978). However, this benefit could not be demonstrated by Kasonde & Bonnar (1975b).

2.5 Other agents include long-acting vasopressin analogues, such as triglycyl lysine vasopressin (Pavlin et al, 1978), anti-heparin agents, including the rather non-specific toluidine blue and protamine sulphate (Rumbolz et al, 1952) and antagonists of histamine, kinins and complement (World Health Organisation, 1979). Distant possibilities include the use of specific thromboxane analogues or prostacyclin inhibitors delivered locally into the uterus. It has been suggested that microcapsules placed in the vagina might migrate through the cervix into the uterus and this might provide a convenient route for the delivery of intra-uterine medication.

2.6 Induction of ovulation may be indicated in women with anovulatory DUB who wish to become pregnant. The usual drug of first choice is clomiphene, but bromocriptine may be appropriate in the occasional patient with mild to moderate hyperprolactinaemia. If these do not work the second line of treatment involves injections of pituitary FSH and LH with midcycle HCG. In general pregnancy rates with all these treatments are lower in women with anovulatory DUB than in similarly treated patients who have amenorrhoea.

3. Surgery is frequently necessary in the therapy of menorrhagia, whether it be due to pelvic disease, medical disorders or DUB. Conservative surgery may include myomectomy for fibroids and bilateral ovarian wedge resection for polycystic ovarian disease. However, the choices with DUB are virtually limited to therapeutic curettage and hysterectomy, although endometrial cryosurgery and laser ablation have been reported.

3.1 Therapeutic curettage has often been advocated for

DUB but the evidence for its efficacy is uncertain. Many women will experience a decrease in measured menstrual loss in the cycle following curettage (Haynes et al, 1977) but this is not usually maintained. However, the subjective benefit may persist and is probably related to reassurance and increased tolerance.

3.2 *Hysterectomy* is probably the most widely used treatment for DUB and is undoubtedly curative. Unfortunately, it involves major abdominal or vaginal surgery and may occasionally be associated with a wide range of short- and long-term complications. It is a highly satisfactory method of treatment for severe or refractory DUB but is increasingly used for less severe cases. A recent survey of health insurance figures concluded that approximately 40 per cent of Australian women will undergo hysterectomy at some time in their lives (Selwood & Wood, 1978). Although some of these cases would be for cancer or uterine prolapse it is obvious that many must have been for menstrual disturbances and particularly 'menorrhagia'. In which case it is highly probable that many women with menstrual blood loss in the normal range have undergone hysterectomy for a symptom which is perceived rather than real. It seems likely that the same situation pertains in many centres in North America and perhaps also in Europe.

One of the major concerns about hysterectomy is the occurrence of post-operative psychological disturbances (Menzer et al, 1957). However, there is increasing evidence that full counselling and ample thinking time prior to finalising the decision for hysterectomy almost eliminate significant adverse reactions. Use of medical agents for control of abnormal bleeding may be a valuable adjunct during this decision making period.

REFERENCES

Abel M 1979 Production of prostaglandins by the human uterus: are they involved in menstruation? Research and Clinical Forums 1: 33–37

Akerlund M 1979 Pathophysiology of dysmenorrhoea. Acta Obstetrica et Gynecologica Scandinavica (Suppl) 87: 27–32

Akerlund M, Anderssen K-E, Ingermarsson I 1976 Effects of terbutaline on myometrial activity, uterine blood flow and lower abdominal pain in women with primary dysmenorrhoea. British Journal of Obstetrics and Gynaecology 83: 673–681

Anderson A B M, Haynes P J, Guillebaud J, Turnbull A C 1976 Reduction of menstrual blood loss by prostaglandin synthetase inhibitors. Lancet i: 774–776

Anderson A B M, Fraser I S, Haynes P J, Turnbull A C 1978 Trial of prostaglandin synthetase inhibitors in primary dysmenorrhoea. Lancet i: 345–348

Andersen A N 1977 Severe primary dysmenorrhoea treated with the selective beta-adrenergic stimulating agent ritodrine chloride. Ugeskr Laeger 139: 1366–1368

Beazley J M 1972 Dysfunctional uterine haemorrhage. British Journal of Hospital Medicine 7: 573–578

Beilby J O W, Farrer-Brown G, Tarbit M H 1971 The microvasculature of common uterine abnormalities excluding fibroids. Journal of Obstetrics and Gynaecology of the British Commonwealth 78: 361–368

Bell E T, Loraine J A 1966 Hormone excretion patterns in patients with dysmenorrhoea. Lancet ii: 519–521

Ben-Menachem M 1980 Treatment of dysmenorrhoea: a relaxation therapy program. International Journal of Gynecology and Obstetrics 17: 340–342

Bergsjo P 1979 Socioeconomic implications of dysmenorrhoea. Acta Obstetrica et Gynecologica Scandinavica (Suppl) 87: 67–68

Bloom L H, Shelton J L, Michael A C 1978 Dysmenorrhoea and personality. Journal of Personal Assessment 42: 272–276

Blumenkrantz M J, Gallagher N, Bashore R A, Tenckhoff H 1981 Retrograde menstruation in women undergoing chronic peritoneal dialysis. Obstetrics and Gynecology 57: 667–670

Bohnen P 1927 Wie weit wird das endometrium bei der menstruation abgestossen? Archiv fur Gynakologie 129: 459–471

Brown J B, Matthew G D 1962 The application of urinary estrogen measurements to problems in gynecology. Recent Progress in Hormone Research 18: 337–373

Brown J B, Kellar R, Matthew G D 1959 Preliminary observations on urinary oestrogen excretion in certain gynaecological disorders. Journal of Obstetrics and Gynaecology of the British Empire 66: 177–211

Buttram V S, Reiter R C 1981 Uterine leiomyomata: etiology, symptomatology and management. Fertility and Sterility 36: 433–445

Buttram V, Izu A, Henzl M R 1979 Naproxen sodium in uterine pain following intrauterine contraceptive device insertion. American Journal of Obstetrics and Gynecology 134: 575–580

Bygdeman M, Bremme K, Gillespie A, Lundstrom V 1979 Effects of the prostaglandins on the uterus: prostaglandins and uterine contractility. Acta Obstetrica et Gynecologica Scandinavica (Suppl) 87: 33–38

Carney M W 1981 Menstrual disturbance: a psychogenic disorder? Clinics in Obstetrics and Gynecology 8: 103–109

Chamlian D L, Taylor H B 1970 Endometrial hyperplasia in young women. Obstetrics and Gynecology 36: 659–665

Chesney M A, Tasto D L 1975 The development of the menstrual symptom questionnaire. Behaviour, Research and Therapy 13: 237–246

Chimbira T, Anderson A B M, Turnbull A C 1980 Relation between measured menstrual blood loss and patients subjective assessment of loss, duration of bleeding, number of sanitary towels used, uterine weight and endometrial surface area. British Journal of Obstetrics and Gynaecology 87: 603–609

Claessens E A, Cowell C A 1981 Acute adolescent menorrhagia. American Journal of Obstetrics and Gynecology 139: 277–280

Cohen B J B, Gibor Y 1980 Anaemia and menstrual blood loss. Obstetrical and Gynecologic Survey 35: 597–618

Cole S K, Billewicz W Z, Thomson A M 1971 Sources of variation in menstrual blood loss. Journal of Obstetrics and Gynaecology of the British Commonwealth 78: 933–939

Collier H O J, Sweatman W J F 1968 Antagonism by fenamates of prostaglandin F_{2c} and of slow reacting substance on human bronchial muscle. Nature 219: 864–866

Cox D J, Meyer R G 1978 Behavioural treatment parameters with primary dysmenorrhea. Journal of Behavioural Medicine 1: 297–310

Damarawy H, Toppozada M 1976 Control of bleeding due to IUDs by a prostaglandin biosynthesis inhibitor. I.R.C.S. Medical Science, Reproduction, Obstetrics and Gynaecology 4: 5–7

Davies A J, Anderson A B M, Turnbull A C 1981 Reduction by Naproxen of excessive menstrual bleeding in women using intrauterine devices. Obstetrics and Gynecology 57: 74–78

Denney D R, Gerrard M 1981 Behavioural treatments of primary dysmenorrhoea — a review. Behaviour Research and Therapy 19: 303–312

De Vore G R, Owens O, Kase N 1982 Use of intravenous Premarin in the treatment of dysfunctional uterine bleeding — a double blind randomised control study. Obstetrics and Gynecology 59: 285–291

Donney J, Nanters M, Thomas K 1981 Luteal function after tubal sterilisation. Obstetrics and Gynecology 57: 65–69

Downie J, Poyser N L, Wunderlich M 1974 Levels of prostaglandins in human endometrium during the normal menstrual cycle. Journal of Physiology 236: 465–469

Edgerton W D 1977 Late complications of laparoscopic sterilisation. Journal of Reproductive Medicine 18: 275–277

Farrer-Brown G, Beilby J O W, Tarbit M H 1970 The vascular patterns in myomatous uteri. Journal of Obstetrics and Gynaecology of the British Commonwealth 77: 967–971

Flowers C E, Willborn W H 1978 New observations on the physiology of menstruation. Obstetrics and Gynecology 51: 16–24

Fowler W M, Barer P A 1942 Rate of hemoglobin regeneration in blood donors. Journal of the American Medical Association 118: 421–423

Fraser I S, Baird D T 1972 Endometrial cystic glandular hyperplasia in adolescent girls. Journal of Obstetrics and Gynaecology of the British Commonwealth 79: 1009–1015

Fraser I S, Baird D T 1974 Blood production and ovarian secretion rates of estradiol 17β and estrone in women with dysfunctional uterine bleeding. Journal of Clinical Endocrinology and Metabolism 39: 564–570

Fraser I S, Michie E A, Wide L, Baird D T 1973 Pituitary gonadotrophins and ovarian function in adolescent dysfunctional uterine bleeding. Journal of Clinical Endocrinology 37: 407–414

Fraser I S Pearse C, Shearman R P, Elliott P M, McIlveen J, Markham R 1981 Efficacy of mefenamic acid in patients with a complaint of menorrhagia. Obstetrics and Gynecology 58: 543–551

Fraser I S, McCarron G, Markham R, Robinson M, Smyth E 1983 Long term treatment of menorrhagia with mefenamic acid. Obstetrics and Gynecology 61: 109–112

Fraser I S, McCarron G, Markham R 1984 A preliminary study of factors influencing perception of menstrual blood loss volume American Journal of Obstetrics and Gynecology (in press)

Gao J, Ma L-Y, Zeng S, Fan H-M, Han L-H 1981 Menstrual blood loss in healthy Chinese women. Contraception 23: 591–601

Garfield R E, Hayashi R H 1980 Presence of gap junctions in the myometrium of women during various stages of menstruation. American Journal of Obstetrics and Gynecology 138: 569–574

Goh T H, Puvan I S, Wong W P, Sivanesaratuam V, Sinnathuray T A 1981 A study of menstrual patterns following laparoscopic sterilisation with silastic rings. International Journal of Fertility 26: 116–119

Gould C H 1979 Dydrogesterone in teenage dysmenorrhoea. A multicentre trial in general practice. Practitioner 222: 718–723

Gray R H 1980 Patterns of Bleeding associated with the use of steroidal contraceptives. In: Diczfalusy E et al (ed) Endometrial Bleeding and Steroidal Contraception, pp 14–49. Pitman Press, Bath

Guillebaud J, Anderson A B M, Turnbull A C 1978 Reduction by mefenamic acid of increased menstrual blood loss associated with intra-uterine contraception. British Journal of Obstetrics and Gynaecology 85: 53–62

Hallberg L, Nilsson L 1964a Determination of menstrual blood loss. Scandinavian Journal of Clinical Laboratory Investigation 16: 244–248

Hallberg L, Nilsson L 1964b Constancy of individual menstrual blood loss. Acta Obstetrica et Gynecologica Scandinavica 43: 352–361

Hallberg L, Hogdahl A M, Nilsson L, Rybo G 1966 Menstrual blood loss — a population study. Acta Obstetrica et Gynecologica Scandinavica 45: 320–351

Hamann G D 1980 Severe, primary dysmenorrhoea treated with naproxen. A prospective, double-blind cross-over investigation. Prostaglandins 19: 651–657

Harrison R F, Campbell S 1976 Double-blind trial of ethamsylate in the treatment of primary and intrauterine device menorrhagia. Lancet ii: 283–285

Haynes P J, Hodgson H, Anderson A B M, Turnbull A C 1977 Measurement of menstrual blood loss in patients complaining of menorrhagia. British Journal of Obstetrics and Gynaecology 84: 763–768

Haynes P J, Anderson A B M, Turnbull A C 1980 Endocrine studies in unexplained menorrhagia. Proceedings of 22nd British Congress of Obstetrics and Gynaecology. Royal College of Obstetricians and Gynaecologists, London

Hefnawi F, El-Zayat A F, Yacout M M 1980 Physiologic studies of menstrual blood loss. International Journal of Gynaecology and Obstetrics 17: 343–352

Henzl M R, Smith R C, Boost G, Tyler E T 1972 Lysosomal concepts of menstrual bleeding in humans. Journal of Clinical Endocrinology 34: 860–875

Henzl M R, Ortega-Herrera E, Rodriguez C, Izu A 1979 Anaprox in dysmenorrhea: reduction of pain and intrauterine pressure. American Journal of Obstetrics and Gynecology 135: 455–460

Henzl M R, Masrey S, Hanson F W, Buttram V C, Rosenwaks Z, Pauls F D 1980 Primary dysmenorrhea: the therapeutic challenge. Journal of Reproductive Medicine 25 (Suppl) 4: 226–235

Irwin J, Morse E, Riddick D 1981 Dysmenorrhea induced by autologous transfusion. Obstetrics and Gynecology 58: 286

Jacobs A, Butler E B 1965 Menstrual blood loss in iron-deficiency anaemia. Lancet ii: 407–409

Janbu T, Lokken P, Nesheim B-I 1979 Effect of acetysalicylic acid, paracetamol and placebo on pain and blood loss in dysmenorrhoeic women. Acta Obstetrica et Gynecologica Scandinavica (Suppl) 87: 81–86

Kasonde J, Bonnar J 1975a Aminocaproic acid and menstrual blood loss in women using intrauterine devices. British Medical Journal 4: 17–19

Kasonde J, Bonnar J 1975b Effect of ethamsylate and aminocaproic acid on menstrual blood loss in women using intrauterine devices. British Medical Journal 4: 21–22

Kasonde J, Bonnar J 1976 The effect of sterilisation on menstrual blood loss. British Journal of Obstetrics and Gynaecology 83: 572–580

Kauppila A, Puolakka J, Ylikorkala O 1979 Prostaglandin biosynthesis inhibitors and endometriosis. Prostaglandins 18: 655–661

Kelly R W 1981 Prostaglandin synthesis in the male and female reproductive tract. Journal of Reproduction and Fertility 62: 293–304

Kessel N, Coppen P 1973 The prevalence of common menstrual symptoms. Lancet ii: 61–64

Kintis G A, Contifaris B 1980 Treatment of primary dysmenorrhea with mefenamic acid. International Journal of Gynecology and Obstetrics 18: 172–175

Kovacs L, Annus J 1978 Effectiveness of ethamysylate in intrauterine device menorrhagia. Gynecological Investigation 9: 161–165

Kremser E, Mitchell G M 1971 Treatment of primary dysmenorrhoea with a combined-type oral contraceptive. A double blind study. Journal of American College Health Associations 19: 195–199

Landgren B M, Diczfalusy E 1980 Hormonal effects of the 300 μg Norethisterone minipill. Contraception 21: 87–99

Lawson S, Cole R A, Templeton A A 1979 The effect of laparoscopic sterilisation by diathermy or silastic bands on post-operative pain, menstrual symptoms and sexuality. British Journal of Obstetrics and Gynaecology 86: 659–663

Lieberman B A, Belsey E, Gordon A G, Wright C S W, Letchworth A T, Noble A D, Niven P A R 1978 Menstrual patterns after laparoscopic sterilisation using a spring-loaded clip. British Journal of Obstetrics and Gynaecology 85: 376–380

Lundstrom V 1977 The myometrial response to intra uterine administration of $PGF_{2\alpha}$ and PGE_2 in dysmenorrhoeic women. Acta Obstetrica et Gynecologica Scandinavica 56: 167–173

Lundstrom V, Green K 1978 Endogenous levels of $PGF_{2\alpha}$ and its main metabolites in plasma and endometrium of normal and dysmenorrhoeic women. American Journal of Obstetrics and Gynecology 130: 640–649

McLennan C E, Rydell A H 1965 Extent of endometrial shedding during normal menstruation. Obstetrics and Gynecology 26: 605–621

McRae M A, Kim M H 1979 Dysmenorrhea in uterus unicornis with rudimentrary uterine cavity. Obstetrics and Gynecology 53: 134–137

Markee J E 1940 Menstruation in intraocular endometrial transplants in the rhesus monkey. Contributions to Embryology (Carnegie Institution of Washington) 28: 219–308

Markee J E 1950 The relation of blood flow to endometrial growth and the inception of menstruation. In: Engle E T (ed) Menstruation and its Disorders, pp 165–185 C C Thomas, Illinois

Maslar I A, Riddick D H 1979 Prolactin production by human endometrium during the normal menstrual cycle. American Journal of Obstetrics and Gynaecology 135: 751–754

Melzack R 1975 The McGill Pain Questionnaire: major properties and scoring methods. Pain 1: 277–299

Melzack R, Torgerson W S 1971 On the language of pain. Anaesthesia 34: 50–59

Menzer D, Morris T, Gates P, Sabbath J, Robey H, Plant T, Sturgis S H 1957 Patterns of emotional recovery from hysterectomy. Psychosomatic Medicine 19: 379–388

Moos R H 1968 The development of a menstrual distress questionnaire. Psychosomatic Medicine 30: 853–867

Morrison J C, Ling F W, Forman E E K, Bates G W, Blake P G Vecchio T J 1980 Analgesic efficacy of ibuprofen for treatment of primary dysmenorrhea. Southern Medical Journal 73: 999–1002

Muldoon M J 1972 Gynaecological illness after sterilisation. British Medical Journal 1: 84–88

Nakano R, Takemura H 1971 Treatment of functional dysmenorrhoea, a double-blind study. Acta Obstetrica Gynecologica Japonica 18: 41–46

National Opinion Poll Research Survey 1980 Menstrual Symptoms in the Community. Commissioned by Parke-Davis Company, United Kingdom

Nedoss B R 1971 Dysfunctional uterine bleeding: relation of endometrial histology to outcome. American Journal of Obstetrics and Gynecology 109: 103–107

Neil J R, Hammond G T, Noble A D, Rushton L, Letchworth A T 1975 Late complications of sterilisation by laparoscopy and tubal ligation. Lancet ii: 699–700

Newton J R, Snowden S A, Parsons V 1976 Control of menstrual bleeding during haemodialysis. British Medical Journal 1: 1016–1017

Newton J, Barnard G, Collins W 1977 A rapid method for measuring menstrual loss using automatic extraction. Contraception 16: 269–282

Nilsson L, Rybo G 1971 Treatment of menorrhagia. American Journal of Obstetrics and Gynecology. 110: 713–720

Office of Population Censuses and Surveys 1974 Second National Study for General Practice, Morbidity Statistics

Paton R C, Tindall H, Zuzel M, McNicol G P 1980 Haemostatic mechanisms in the normal endometrium and endometrium exposed to contraceptive steroids. In: Diczfalusy E, Fraser I S, Webb F T G (eds) Endometrial Bleeding and Steroidal Contraception, pp 325–341. Pitman Press, Bath

Pavlin V, Flynn M J, Mulder J L, Cort J H 1978 The treatment of uterine bleeding with vasopressin hormonogen (Glypressin) — a pilot study. British Journal of Obstetrics and Gynaecology 85: 801–805

Pickles V R 1979 Prostaglandins and dysmenorrhoea: A historical survey. Acta Obstetrica et Gynecologica Scandinavica (Suppl) 87: 7–12

Pickles V R, Hall W J, Best F A, Smith G N 1965 Prostaglandins in endometrium and menstrual fluid from normal and dysmenorrhoeic subjects. Journal of Obstetrics and Gynaecology of the British Commonwealth 72: 185–192

Pulkkinen M O, Csapo A I, 1979 Effect of Ibuprofen on menstrual blood prostaglandin levels in dysmenorrheic women. Prostaglandins 18: 137–142

Quick A J 1966 Menstruation in hereditary bleeding disorders. Obstetrics and Gynecology 28: 37–40

Reading A E 1979 The internal structure of the McGill pain questionnaire in dysmenorrhoea patients. Pain 7: 353–358

Reading A E, Newton J R 1977 A comparison of primary dysmenorrhoea and intrauterine device related pain. Pain 3: 265–276

Richards D H 1979 A general practice view of functional disorders associated with menstruation. Research and Clinical Forums 1: 39–45

Rosenwaks Z, Jones G S, Henzl M R, Dubin N H, Ghodgoankar R B, Hoffman S 1981 Naproxen sodium, aspirin and placebo in primary dysmenorrhea. American Journal of Obstetrics and Gynecology 140: 592–599

Royal College of General Practitioners 1974 Oral contraception and health: an interim report from the Oral Contraceptive Study of the Royal College of General Practitioners. Pitman Medical, New York

Rumbolz W L, Moon C F, Norelli J C 1952 Use of protamine sulphate and toluidine blue for abnormal uterine bleeding. American Journal of Obstetrics and Gynecolcgy 63: 1029–1036

Rybo G 1966 Plasminogen activator in the endometrium. Acta Obstetrica et Gynecologica Scandinavica 45: 411–450

Sandahl B, Ulmsten U, Anderssen K E 1979 Trial of the calcium antagonist nifedipine in the treatment of primary dysmenorrhea. Archiv fur Gynakologie 227: 147–151

Sandahl B, Ulsten U, Anderssen K E 1980 Local application of Ketocaine for treatment of referred pain in primary dysmenorrhea. Acta Obstetrica et Gynecologica Scandinavica 59: 259–260

Sapire K E, Davey D A 1980 The effect of sterilisation by bipolar cautery and Falope ring on menstrual bleeding patterns. South African Medical Journal 58: 275–277

Schröder R 1954 Endometrial hyperplasia in relation to genital function. American Journal of Obstetrics and Gynecology 68: 294–309

Schwarz A, Zor U, Lindner H R, Naor S 1974 Primary dysmenorrhoea: alleviation by an inhibitor of prostaglandin synthesis and action. Obstetrics and Gynecology 44: 709–714

Scott J C, Massey E 1964 Menstrual patterns in myxoedema. American Journal of Obstetrics and Gynecology 90: 161–164

Sensky T E, Liu D T 1980 Endometriosis: associations with menorrhagia, infertility and oral contraceptives. International Journal of Gynaecology and Obstetrics 17: 573–576

Selwood T, Wood C 1978 Incidence of hysterectomy in Australia. Medical Journal of Australia 2: 201–203

Short R V 1976 The evolution of human reproduction. Proceedings of the Royal Society of London B 195: 3–24

Silver B V, Blanchard E B 1978 Biofeedback and relaxation training in the treatment of psychophysiological disorders: or are the machines really necessary? Journal of Behavioural Medicine 1: 217–239

Sixma J J, Christiaens G C M L, Haspels A A 1980 The sequence of haemostatic events in the endometrium during normal menstruation. In: Diczfalusy E et al (ed) Endometrial Bleeding and Steroid Contraception, pp 86–96. Pitman Press, Bath

Sjoberg N-O 1979 Dysmenorrhoea and uterine neurotransmitters. Acta Obstetrica et Gynecologica Scandinavica (Suppl) 87: 57–60

Smith R P, Powell J R 1980 The objective evaluation of dysmenorrhoea therapy. American Journal of Obstetrics and Gynaecology 137: 314–319

Smith R P, Powell J R 1982 Intrauterine pressure changes during dysmenorrhoea therapy. American Journal of Obstetrics and Gynecology 143: 286–289

Smith S K, Abel M H, Kelly R W, Baird D T 1982 Prostaglandins and dysfunctional uterine bleeding. Research and Clinical Forums 4: 39–45

Solleveld H A, Van Zwieten M J 1978 Membranous dysmenorrhoea in the chimpanzee (Pan troglodytes). Journal of Medical Primatology 7: 19–25

Southam A L 1959 The natural history of menstrual disorders. Annals of the New York Academy of Science 75: 840–854

Southam A L, Richart R M 1966 The prognosis for adolescents with menstrual abnormalities. American Journal of Obstetrics and Gynecology 94: 637–643

Strömberg P, Forsling M L, Akerlund M 1981 Effects of prostaglandin inhibition on vasopressin levels in women with primary dysmenorrhoea. Obstetrics and Gynecology 58: 206–208

Sugimoto O 1978 Diagnostic and Therapeutic Hysteroscopy. Igaku-Shoin, Tokyo

Sutherland A M 1949 The histology of the endometrium in functional uterine haemorrhage. Glasgow Medical Journal 30: 1–28

Tauber P F, Wolf A S, Herting W, Zaneveld J J 1977 Hemorrhage induced by intrauterine devices: control by local proteinase inhibition. Fertility and Sterility 28: 1375–1377

Taw R L 1975 Review of menstrual disorders in which a secretory endometrium was found. American Journal of Obstetrics and Gynecology 122: 490–496

Taylor E S 1965 Essentials of Gynecology, 3rd edn, p 429. Lea and Ferbiger, Philadelphia

Taymor M L, Strugis S H, Vonica C 1964 The etiological role of chronic iron deficiency in the production of menorrhagia. Journal of the American Medical Association 187: 323–325

Trobough G, Guderian A M, Erickson R R, Tillson S A, Leong P, Swisher D A, Pharriss P B 1978 The effect of exogenous intrauterine progesterone on the amount of PGF$_{2\alpha}$ content of menstrual blood in dysmenorrheic women. Journal of Reproductive Medicine 21: 153–158

Van Look P F A, Lothian H, Hunter W M, Michie E A, Baird D T 1977 Hypothalamic-pituitary-ovarian function in perimenopausal women. Clinical Endocrinology 7: 13–22

Van Look P F A, Hunter W M, Fraser I S, Baird D T 1978 Impaired estrogen-induced luteinizing hormone release in young women with anovulatory dysfunctional uterine bleeding. Journal of Clinical Endocrinology and Metabolism 46: 816–823

Vora I M, Raizada R M, Rawall M Y, Chadda J S 1981 Adenomyosis. Journal of Postgraduate Medicine 27: 7–11

Weström L, Bengtsson L P 1970 Effect of tranexamic acid (AMCA) in menorrhagia with intrauterine contraceptive devices. A double-blind study. Journal of Reproductive Medicine 5: 41–48

Widholm O 1979 Dysmenorrhoea during adolescence. Acta Obstetrica et Gynecologica Scandinavica (Suppl) 87: 61–66

Willman E A, Collins W P, Clayton S G 1976 Studies in the involvement of prostaglandins in uterine symptomatology and pathology. British Journal of Obstetrics and Gynaecology 83: 337–345

Wilson E W 1980 Lysosome function in normal endometrium and endometrium exposed to contraceptive steroids. In: Diczfalusy E et al (eds) Endometrial Bleeding and Steroidal Contraception, pp 201–218. Pitman Press, Bath

Wood C, Larsen L, Williams R 1979a Menstrual characteristics of 2,343 women attending the Shepherd Foundation. Australian and New Zealand Journal of Obstetrics and Gynaecology 19: 107–110

Wood C, Larsen L, Williams R 1979b Social and psychological factors in relation to premenstrual tension and menstrual pain. Australian and New Zealand Journal of Obstetrics and Gynaecology 19: 111–115

World Health Organisation, Special Programme of Research, Development and Research Training in Human Reproduction 1979 Eighth Annual Report, Geneva

Ylikorkala O, Kijansuu E 1981 Increased rate of primary dysmenorrhea in women with spontaneous premature labour. Prostaglandins in Medicine 6: 213–216

Ylikorkala O, Puolakka J, Kauppila A 1979 Serum gonadrotrophins, prolactin and ovarian steroids in primary dysmenorrhoea. British Journal of Obstetrics and Gynaecology 86: 648–653

Ylikorkala O, Puolakka J, Kauppila A 1980 Comparison between naproxen tablets and suppositories in primary dysmenorrhea. Prostaglandins 20: 463–468

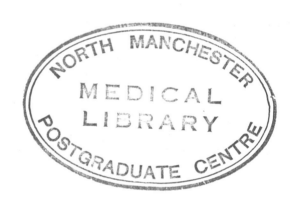

The premenstrual syndrome

INTRODUCTION

Almost every aspect of the premenstrual syndrome (PMS) remains in dispute although a vast amount of research has been performed. Failure to understand the syndrome may be partly explained by the everchanging physiological processes of the menstrual cycle superimposed on which are not only profound somatic disturbances, but a multitude of psychological changes. This, however, is only part of the explanation and the main problems have been due to the imprecise basis on which all our knowledge of the syndrome is based. Fundamentals such as definition, incidence and, most important, measurement techniques are not yet established. Diagnosis, aetiology and treatment are accordingly still poorly understood. The literature on PMS has been plagued by anecdotes, ill-founded dogma, uncontrolled therapeutic studies and scientifically naive measurement techniques. Inconsistencies in the definition of the syndrome and our inability to conclusively diagnose it have led some authors to even question the disease status of the syndrome (Leader, 1981).

Definition

Although the syndrome had not been defined by the beginning of the century, not surprisingly, factors associated with menstruation have been the subject of both medical and mythological interest for many years. Hippocrates probably made the first reference to premenstrual disturbance in his aphorism, 'the blood of females is subject to intermittent 'agitations', and as a result the 'agitated' blood finds its way from the head to the uterus whence it is expelled'. Premenstrual tension was first described by Frank in 1931. He described tension in both its physical and psychological sense in several women and attributed it to oestrogen excess which was the consequence of diminished urinary oestrogen excretion which occurs during the premenstrual phase. He treated these patients with irradiation of the ovaries and reported successful treatment. In 1964 Dalton derived the term 'premenstrual syndrome' to encompass all the possible changes associated with significant disturbances in the premenstrual phase. Sutherland & Stewart suggested that 'any combination of emotional or physical features which occur cyclically in a female before menstruation and which regress or disappear during menstruation' constitute the premenstrual syndrome (Sutherland & Stewart, 1965). The nature of the symptoms need not be specific and a symptom peculiar to a particular patient may be regarded as part of the premenstrual syndrome. (A syndrome is normally regarded as a collection of specific signs and symptoms, and therefore, pedantically speaking, we are not talking about a true syndrome.) More recently, the term 'the premenstrual syndromes' has been used. This may help to subdivide the various symptoms groups, but the term is not yet widely accepted.

For practical purposes a woman may be said to be suffering from premenstrual syndrome (PMS) if she complains of regularly occurring psychological or somatic symptoms (or both) which occur specifically during the luteal phase of the cycle. The symptoms should be relieved with the onset of or during menstruation, but there should be a symptom-free interval of at least a week following menstruation. Often symptoms are seen immediately prior to menstruation, but in many patients they may begin early in the luteal phase, and may continue throughout.

THE SYMPTOMS

The definition above allows a very wide range of symptom types to be included in the syndrome. They can be placed in two groups — psychological and somatic. There are typical or 'key' symptoms. The most commonly reported and typical psychological symptom is the irritability/aggression type of symptom, whilst the most common somatic symptom is that of bloatedness. One or other of these (and quite frequently both) symptoms are invariably present.

Psychological symptoms

Table 32.1 lists the majority of the important psychological symptoms that have been described; the more common of these should be considered.

Depression is commonly reported and may present in several ways from premenstrual crying bouts to sadness and deep depression, parasuicide and actual suicide. Some convincing data is that by MacKinnon & MacKinnon (1956) who studied postmortem uterine specimens in women who had successfully committed suicide. They showed that in the majority of women the histology of the endometrium was in the secretory phase of the cycle.

Tension and anxiety are also commonly reported. There may be changes in appetite and sleep pattern, particularly insomnia, libido changes, though this may be in either direction — some women have more sexual drive and in others it is diminished. A particular problem is that of clumsiness, inability to concentrate and inability to perform tasks as well, which may lead to poorer performance at work or when driving. However, the evidence to support this is largely anecdotal.

We have previously said that the most commonly reported group of symptoms is the irritability and aggression type of symptom. This may range from the snappy, intolerant attitude towards children and the woman's husband. It may be worse, and manifest itself as violent attack. It has been claimed that this may be so severe as to cause intra-familial discord, child battering and violent crime. The evidence on which these assumptions are made is not wholly convincing, but even so, British law has recently recognised premenstrual syndrome as mitigation in several crimes, even though we have no exact means of

Table 32.1 Symptoms of premenstrual syndrome

Psychological symptoms
  Irritability
  Aggression
  Tension
  Anxiety
  Depression
  Lethargy
  Insomnia
  Change in appetite
  Crying
  Change in libido
  Thirst
  Loss of concentration
  Poor coordination/clumsiness/accidents

Somatic symptoms
  Feeling 'bloated'
  Feeling of weight increase
  Breast pain/tenderness
  Swelling of ankles
  Skin disorders
  Hot flushes
  Headache
  Pelvic pain
  Change in bowel habit

diagnosing the syndrome (Brahams, 1981). Patients accused of murder and arson have recently had their sentences drastically reduced on the basis of their temporary inability to control themselves, due to the supposed lack of progesterone during the premenstrum. In the most recent case on these lines the defending counsel attempted to align the case with a woman suffering from hypoglycaemia due to excessive insulin administration (which had previously been proven in 1973). This appeal failed. The Judge concluded that it was the duty of the court to protect the public and that it would be most undesirable for a woman suffering from PMS and prone to violence to be able to go out and commit a series of offences without restraint. This lady had had 45 previous convictions, apparently many of which had occurred in the premenstrual phase.

Premenstrual syndrome has also been related to an increased number of psychiatric admissions; these have usually been exacerbations of previous psychiatric problems (Janowsky et al, 1969). Alcohol abuse has also been shown to increase in the premenstrual phase (Belfer et al, 1971). There are many other supposed consequences of the syndrome; the majority are based on inadequate evidence.

Effect on work and performance

There is some evidence to suggest that concentration, dexterity, and thus performance in school, work and sports are impaired premenstrually. Dalton reports deterioration of schoolgirls' weekly grades and examination results in the paramenstruum (Dalton, 1977).

There also appears to be a decline in industrial and sporting performance (Humke, 1968; Redgrove, 1971) and the effect on industry is further aggravated by the greater incidence of absenteeism premenstrually (Dalton, 1977).

Road accidents appear to be more frequent premenstrually (Landauer, 1974; Dalton, 1977) and two investigators have concluded that women pilots should not be permitted to fly before or during menstruation (Humke, 1968; Landauer, 1974).

Somatic symptoms

Apart from the well-known mood and behavioural changes described above, there are also many physical and somatic symptoms associated with the syndrome (Table 32.1). Typically, women complain of a feeling of bloatedness, weight increase (or a feeling of weight increase), peripheral swelling, water retention symptoms, breast swelling and pain and also headache and premenstrual pelvic pain. There may also occasionally be skin symptoms such as exacerbation of eczema and in many women acne occurs premenstrually. Urinary retention (and occasionally frequency) and constipation are occasionally reported and one or two women complain of hot flushes. Since bloatedness is the most commonly reported symptom (O'Brien, 1979) it would be interesting to look at this in more detail. Of symptomatic women, over 90 per cent reported a feeling of bloatedness as a significantly distressing symptom. Over 40 per cent complained of a feeling of weight increase and only 4 per cent reported ankle oedema. It has long been assumed that water retention is an integral part of the syndrome (Sweeney, 1934), and many have suggested that sodium and water retention is the underlying basis of the syndrome (Janowsky et al, 1973). There have been several studies where fluid and electrolytes have been looked at in relation to weight and mood disturbance, but none of these have really been conclusive. Indeed, there has not even been shown a consistent pattern of weight increase in these patients. The study of Janowsky showed a direct correlation between sodium/potassium ratio and mood change (Janowsky et al, 1973) and Backstrom has shown a direct correlation between weight and mood change (Backstrom & Carstensen, 1974). There have been many other studies looking at weight, electrolytes and mood and these are considered in detail later. A recent study at the University of Nottingham has looked specifically at the relationship between weight and bloatedness and the patient's perceived body image (O'Brien et al, 1982). In this study, measurements were made of actual abdominal size, perceived body image, weight and bloatedness and mood change as assessed by a visual analogue scale. The measurements were made in three groups of women: (1) asymptomatic control; (2) symptomatic women complaining predominantly of bloatedness; (3) symptomatic women whose predominant symptoms were of the psychological type.

There were no consistent increases in weight in any of the three groups, even though there was an increase of feeling of bloatedness to some extent in the 'psychological' group and to a marked extent in the 'bloated' group. Moreover, there was no measurable increase in abdominal dimensions in any of the groups. There was, however, a quite distinct increase in perceived body image in the 'bloated' group during the premenstrual phase of the cycle. In fact, the 'bloated' group over-estimated their abdominal diameters by about 8 cm (mean) when their perceptions were compared with actual measurements.

It seems unlikely that bloatedness can be attributed to water retention if there is no consistent weight increase.

Pelvic pain

Premenstrual pelvic pain has been attributed to a variety of phenomena including prostaglandin secretion, pelvic venous congestion and distension due to fluid. The only supportive evidence for any of these is that of Edlundh & Jansson (1966) who showed by angiographical techniques an increase in pelvic varicosities in the premenstrual phase. However, although these studies were performed in women with premenstrual discomfort, they were not compared with controls.

Pelvic pain is, in fact, quite a common symptom. It must, of course, be distinguished from other causes of pelvic pain such as pelvic inflammatory disease, endometriosis and dysmenorrhoea. These are often confused and hinder diagnosis and treatment.

Breast symptoms

Breast pain and swelling are important symptoms and can be severe to the extent that some women have even requested bilateral mastectomy. Breast pain can be due to numerous causes and Preece et al (1976) made the first serious attempt to classify the different types of breast pain. They studied 232 patients and were able to categorise them into six types (Table 32.2). Of these, however, 19 patients had pain which could not be characterised and were labelled idiopathic, the assumption being that the pain arose from sites other than the breast. One further patient had a fibroadenoma which was excised and another patient realised that she was pregnant shortly after attending the breast clinic. Of their six categories, breast cancer is the most important, though they only actually saw one case within their series. (They did conclude from other data, however, that 10 per cent of breast cancer cases presented with breast pain.) Other categories were sclerosing adenosis and Tietze Syndrome which both presented with mastalgia. Nineteen patients out of the total group presented with pain due to trauma. Sixty-two patients were categorised as ductectasia/periductal mastitis with obvious mammographic appearances. The largest group, however, was of 93 patients which they termed cyclical pronounced mastalgia. This appears to be the sub-group most commonly associated with the premenstrual phase of the cycle. The pain was bilateral in at least 50 per cent of the cases and the breasts were diffusely affected. The usual mammographic finding was fibroadenosis with or without cysts. The terms fibrocystic disease of the breast and/or benign breast disease are probably synonymous with cycli-

Table 32.2 Classification and frequency of mastalgia

Type	No.
Cancer	1
Sclerosing adenosis	11
Trauma	19
Tietze syndrome	25
Ductectasia/periductal mastalgia	62
Cyclical pronounced	93
Not classified	
Miscellaneous	2
Not breast related	2
Idiopathic	17
Total	232

cal pronounced mastalgia and the underlying cause of this has been assumed (though not proven) to be due to hormonal changes. Investigations and treatment have centred around oestrogen, progesterone and prolactin.

INCIDENCE OF PREMENSTRUAL SYNDROME

Since there have been no rigid definitions of the syndrome, it is difficult to give true incidence rates. It is probably for this reason that there is a very wide reported prevalence. An early study (Rees, 1953a) using strict criteria, reported that 5 per cent of women complained of the syndrome. At the other extreme, where the definition of any symptom, but occurring specifically in the premenstrual phase was used, 97 per cent of women were reported to complain of symptoms of PMS (Sutherland & Stewart, 1965). It is well-known that a large percentage of normally healthy women will complain to some degree of one or more premenstrual symptoms. It is probably important to distinguish between these and women complaining of significantly distressing symptoms. Even then, as many as 50 per cent of women would be included as PMS sufferers. These figures will obviously vary with the characteristics of the study population. For example, studies of the general population will probably give lower figures than studies of specific populations such as in psychologists, hospital workers and similar study groups who will obviously be aware of the syndrome.

STUDIES OF THE PREMENSTRUAL SYNDROME AND MEASUREMENT TECHNIQUES

Although we have seen that difficulties in the definition of PMS give rise to inconsistencies in the reporting of incidence, it is even more important when we are considering setting up, analysing and interpreting studies related to the aetiology and the treatment of the syndrome. For this, we need an accurate method of quantifying all aspects of the syndrome including physiological and psychological or an endocrine marker which distinguishes the symptomatic from the control group. In general, we have been dependent on the patient's self-reporting of symptoms. Ideally, an objective numerical measurement of changes would seem the obvious approach and lend credibility to any work produced. Several approaches have already been tried.

Weight

If all PMS patients consistently gained weight this would be a useful parameter to assess the syndrome. Some women do put weight on during the luteal phase of the cycle. However, this is not shown in the majority of women, is inconsistent, and does not occur in a sufficient number of patients to be useful. Moreover, asymptomatic patients may increase their weight premenstrually. There is one study where the measurement of weight only has been used in the assessment. This was in the study by Hoffman (1979) who evaluated the use of a combination of caffeine and the mild diuretic ammonium chloride. Not surprisingly, all patients lost weight on the diuretic; he interpreted that treatment was 100 per cent effective, exemplifying the limitations of weight to measure therapy in this context.

Oedema

Again, the number of patients complaining of frank oedema is insufficient to justify its use in measuring this syndrome. Moreover, methods for measuring oedema are generally cumbersome and inaccurate.

Breast and abdominal measurements

The measurement of breast circumference and abdominal transverse and AP diameters shows no consistent increase premenstrually, and is therefore of no value in evaluating premenstrual syndrome (O'Brien et al, 1982). Measurement of perceived body image showed an increase premenstrually; this was only in the 'bloated' group and would be of no value in the 'psychological' group. Again, we are dependent on the patient's own evaluation.

Psychological performance tests

Although many performance tests have been used in the evaluation of drugs and hormones in the male, these have largely been avoided in the female due to a supposed menstrual fluctuation. Landauer (1974) assessed choice reaction time during the menstrual cycle. Fifty-seven women were assessed; the decision time was found to be prolonged in the immediate premenstrual phase. There was no reference to PMS. In a pilot study by Taylor (1982, unpublished data) there appeared to be no clear change in choice-reaction time of symptomatic or non-symptomatic women. Other studies have shown that performance tests have limited value (Slade & Jenner, 1980) though this type of approach warrants further investigation.

Objective assessment

Objective assessment of mood and behaviour is a familiar tool to clinical psychologists. Measures of galvanic skin potential, flush threshold time and arm steadiness have been used as objective measures of patients' symptoms. However, the results obtained are not directly related to the intensity of symptoms and are probably inadequate for the measurement of PMS (Sampson & Prescott, 1981) though they have not been evaluated in this context. In addition, the well-established techniques of measuring depression and other psychological symptoms in an objective manner have not been evaluated in premenstrual syndrome.

All of these techniques are, in any case, impractical, since evaluation would need to be done on a daily basis. They require formal interviews lasting up to 45 min and would thus be too prolonged and time-consuming for any large study of the syndrome.

Blood measurements

One would hope to find a chemical, enzyme or hormone which would be obviously elevated or diminished in patients with PMS. One might expect there to be a measurable difference in ovarian or pituitary hormone. Various studies have, however, been conflicting and the overlap between study groups is such as to make this method impractical. A single blood sample, for example, taken premenstrually for oestradiol, progesterone, oestrogen/progesterone ratio is of no value in distinguishing between symptomatic and asymptomatic women (O'Brien, 1982). The measurement of sex hormone binding globulin (SHBG) binding capacity has been measured in 50 women with severe premenstrual syndrome and compared with 50 age-matched controls (Dalton, 1981). The binding capacity was significantly lower in the affected group and shw suggests that this may be useful in diagnosis of the syndrome, and also suggests that it may help to explain the aetiology. This, however, has yet to be substantiated.

Psychometric methods

Since attempts to find an objective measure of somatic changes have been unsuccessful we are left solely with evaluation of psychological changes and these methods are dependent on patient self-assessment. These range from a simple menstrual chart to a visual linear analogue scale. Menstrual charts (Fig. 32.1) are well established and have been used for some time in clinical practice. These allow the patient to include any symptoms she chooses. They tell us the timing of menstruation and the timing of the symptoms, which we have already seen is probably the most important factor for diagnosis. However, they give no indication of the severity of the symptoms and are thus of limited value. A three-point severity scale is often used, but these are of limited discriminatory value, though easy to analyse.

There are two adequate methods of measuring psychological symptoms:

(a) The Moos' Menstrual Distress Questionnaire (MDQ) which measures symptoms related to premenstrual syndrome and to menstruation; it is not entirely specific to PMS (Moos, 1977). This mood chart includes 47 symptoms which are rated on a 6-point scale (Fig. 32.2). These symptoms can be factor analysed into seven symptom clusters. These are: (i) a negative affect scale (including the main psychological symptoms of the syndrome); (ii) a pain scale; (iii) an arousal scale; (iv) water retention symptoms; (v) behavioural change; (vi) autonomic reaction; and (vii) concentration. There is also a group of control symptoms (viii) which assess the patient's general tendency to complain. In a study of 19 women complaining of premenstrual syndrome, Sampson & Jenner have used this scale by computing the statistical significance of the ability to fit a sine wave as the means of quantitating symptoms. They concluded that it was a useful method of assessing premenstrual symptoms (Sampson & Jenner, 1977). She has since used the method to evaluate the efficacy of progesterone therapy (Sampson, 1979).

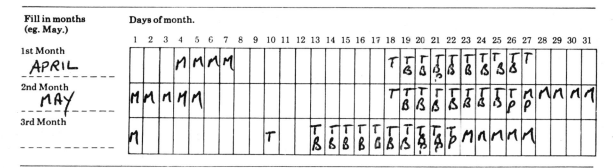

Menstrual Chart

Indicate on the chart the days on which symptoms trouble you using the appropriate letter or letters from the key below.

Key to symptoms:
D depression. P pain – backache or headache. T tension or irritability. F fatigue. B bloated feeling. M menstruation.

Fig. 32.1 Menstrual chart (Duphar Laboratories)

Name   Date

Please complete this form every evening to describe your symptoms in the previous 24 hours
On the page below is a list of symptoms which women sometimes experience. For each symptom choose the descriptive category listed below which best describes your experience of that symptom today. Circle the number of the category which best describes your experience of the symptom today. Even if none of the categories is exactly correct, choose the one that best describes your experience. Please be sure to circle one number for each symptom. Please also remember to put your name and the date in the blank spaces at the top of this page.

Descriptive   1. No reaction at all.   2. Barely noticeable.
Categories   3. Present, mild.   4. Present, moderate.
               5. Present, strong   6. Acute, or partially disabling.

1. Weight gain	1	2	3	4	5	6
2. Insomnia	1	2	3	4	5	6
3. Crying	1	2	3	4	5	6
4. Lowered school or work performance	1	2	3	4	5	6
5. Muscle stiffness	1	2	3	4	5	6
6. Forgetfulness	1	2	3	4	5	6
7. Confusion	1	2	3	4	5	6
8. Take naps of stay in bed	1	2	3	4	5	6
9. Headache	1	2	3	4	5	6
10. Skin disorders	1	2	3	4	5	6
11. Loneliness	1	2	3	4	5	6
12. Feelings of suffocation	1	2	3	4	5	6
13. Affectionate	1	2	3	4	5	6
14. Orderliness	1	2	3	4	5	6
15. Stay at home from work or school	1	2	3	4	5	6
16. Cramps (uterine or pelvic)	1	2	3	4	5	6
17. Dizziness or faintness	1	2	3	4	5	6
18. Excitement	1	2	3	4	5	6
19. Chest pains	1	2	3	4	5	6
20. Avoid social activities	1	2	3	4	5	6
21. Anxiety	1	2	3	4	5	6
22. Backache	1	2	3	4	5	6
23. Cold sweats	1	2	3	4	5	6
24. Lowered judgment	1	2	3	4	5	6
25. Fatigue	1	2	3	4	5	6
26. Nausea or vomiting	1	2	3	4	5	6
27. Restlessness	1	2	3	4	5	6
28. Hot flushes	1	2	3	4	5	6
29. Difficulty in concentration	1	2	3	4	5	6
30. Painful or tender breasts	1	2	3	4	5	6
31. Feeling of well-being	1	2	3	4	5	6
32. Buzzing or ringing in ears	1	2	3	4	5	6
33. Distractable	1	2	3	4	5	6
34. Swelling (e.g. abdomen, breasts, ankle)	1	2	3	4	5	6
35. Accidents (e.g. cut finger, break dish)	1	2	3	4	5	6
36. Irritability	1	2	3	4	5	6
37. General aches and pains	1	2	3	4	5	6
38. Mood swings	1	2	3	4	5	6
39. Heart pounding	1	2	3	4	5	6
40. Depression (feeling sad or blue)	1	2	3	4	5	6
41. Decreased efficiency	1	2	3	4	5	6
42. Lowered motor coordination	1	2	3	4	5	6
43. Numbness or tingling in hands or feet	1	2	3	4	5	6
44. Change in eating habits	1	2	3	4	5	6
45. Tension	1	2	3	4	5	6
46. Blind spots or fuzzy vision	1	2	3	4	5	6
47. Bursts of energy or activity	1	2	3	4	5	6

Fig. 32.2 Moos' Menstrual Distress Questionnaire

(b) The alternative to this method is the use of visual linear analogue scales (Aitkin, 1969). The basis of this method is to use a 10 cm line with opposing adjectives for a particular symptom placed at either end. The patient marks a vertical line at the point on the linear analogue scale appropriate to her symptom at that time (Fig. 32.3). The assessment must be made at the same time each day and should not be compared with previous days. The mood score is determined by measuring the distance of the mark in millimetres from the reference symptom. Various combinations of visual analogue scales have been used and they can be adapted for each particular study (Fig. 32.3) (Herbert et al, 1976; O'Brien et al, 1979, 1982). The symptoms were factor analysed into four groups which were affective score, bloated score, non-alertness and irritability. The method was studied over 148 cycles in 52 women and proved extremely good in discriminating between symptomatic and non-symptomatic subjects. Fig. 32.4 shows the results of three cycles in a symptomatic patient.

To measure premenstrual symptomatology, we have only methods which use self-reporting techniques such as Moos' Menstrual Distress Questionnaire or the combined visual analogue scales. We should, however, continue to seek an objective method of evaluation which would give a more scientific approach to the subject and lend credibility to endocrine studies, studies of aetiology and the evaluation of treatment.

AETIOLOGY

Rosseinsky & Hall (1974) considered PMS to be intrinsic and ineradicable, and, from the evolutionary point of view, beneficial. They suggest that the combination of a week's menstruation at the beginning of the cycle, coupled with the female hostility during the luteal phase of the cycle encourages intercourse to take place around the time of ovulation. They imply that the premenstrual syndrome is the normal state and is advantageous to the species.

Results from a study by Ruble (1977) questioned the existence of the syndrome and validity of self-reporting techniques as a means of symptom evaluation. Women were led to believe that the stage of their cycle, according to their EEG, was different from the actual day. The subjects then reported a higher incidence of premenstrual-like symptoms during this artificial premenstrual phase.

Several workers have considered the syndrome to be purely of psychosomatic origin. This is not an uncommon view, particularly amongst psychiatrists whose referral pattern would obviously tend to favour patients with underlying psychological or psychiatric disorders. It has been reported that women with PMS have higher

Patient Daily Self Assessment Form

Name: _____ Cycle No: _____

Date: _____ Day No: _____

Please rate the way you feel in terms of the dimension below.
Regard the lines as representing the full range of each dimension.
Rate your feelings as they are at the moment.
Mark clearly and perpendicularly across each line.
Please complete at the same time each day.

Measurement
(MM)

Alert	Drowsy
Calm	Excited
Strong	Feeble
Muzzy	Clear-headed
Well Co-ordinated	Clumsy
Lethargic	Energetic
Contented	Discontended
Troubled	Tranquil
Mentally slow	Quick witted
Tense	Relaxed
Attentive	Dreamy
Incompetent	Proficient
Happy	Sad
Antagonistic	Friendly
Interested	Bored
Withdrawn	Sociable
Depressed	Elated
Self-centred	Outward going
Bloated	Thin
Irritable	Calm

Fig. 32.3 Visual analogue scales for assessment of PMS

anxiety levels and tend to complain of similar symptoms at any time of the cycle (Coppen & Kessel, 1963; Moos, 1969).

The number of aetiological theories in this syndrome is enormous (Fig. 32.5). It appears that each new chemical, hormone, vitamin or neurotransmitter discovered is thought to be causative.

Central nervous theories

Recently, several neurotransmitters and their co-enzymes have been implicated. Of particular interest are the endorphins (Reid & Yen, 1981; Halbreich, 1981) and the coenzyme of dopamine and 5-hydroxytryptamine metabolism, vitamin B_6 (pyridoxine) (Brush, 1977). Endorphins are neuropeptides thought to have particular roles in mood control and in the physiology of pain. Cyclical change during the menstrual cycle would implicate them as a possible factor in at least the psychological symptoms of PMS and, indeed, a lengthy review on this subject by Reid & Yen (1981) concluded that the syndrome was a multifactorial psychoneuroendocrine disorder involving the endorphins. They neither produced nor cited data to show that the endorphins fluctuated with the phases of the menstrual cycle, nor reported any studies of endorphins or other neurotransmitters in subjects with PMS. It does remain an interesting hypothesis, and no doubt data will soon be available.

There has been similar enthusiasm and lack of data for the role of vitamin B_6 (pyridoxine) in PMS. Adams

suggested that oral contraception was responsible for the depletion of central nervous pyridoxine with resulting pill-associated depression and has shown effective replacement therapy in a double-blind trial (Adams et al, 1973). This hypothesis was extrapolated to premenstrual syndrome suggesting that the hormonal changes of the menstrual cycle brought about alteration of pyridoxine stores or distribution. The resulting defect in dopamine and seratonin metabolism could be responsible at least for psychological symptoms of PMS and perhaps through complex inter-relationships with prolactin and other hormones of the pituitary–ovarian axis for the somatic symptoms (Brush, 1977). These theories tend to be rather nebulous and again there are no data showing any alteration of pyridoxine level through the menstrual cycle or in patients with PMS. Treatment with pyridoxine replacement gives no further supportive evidence.

Vitamin deficiency

Other vitamin deficiencies have at one time or another been implicated in this syndrome. There have been no assays of vitamin blood levels but 'successful' treatment with various supplements has been cited as evidence for a deficiency state. Unfortunately, none of these early trials were placebo controlled (the placebo effect of this syndrome (40–50 per cent) making this apparent evidence meaningless. Vitamin B (Biskind, 1943) and vitamin A (Argonz & Abinzano, 1950; Block, 1960) have both been looked at.

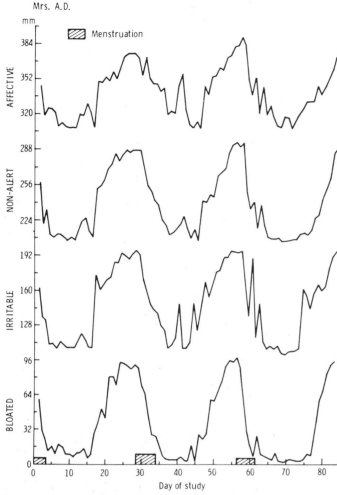

Fig. 32.4 Factor-analysis of visual analogue scales in a premenstrual syndrome patient

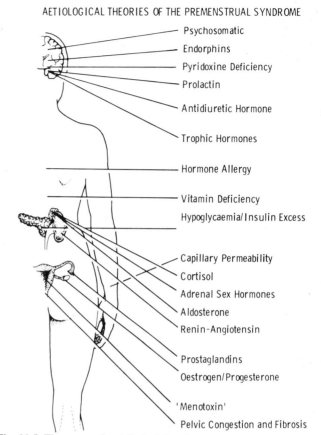

Fig. 32.5 The range of aetiological theories

Sodium and water metabolism

Fluid retention has long been assumed to be an important associated factor in PMS and some authors have suggested that it is the underlying cause of the syndrome (Janowsky et al, 1973). Unfortunately, there is a lot of conflicting evidence and even the changes within the normal menstrual cycle are poorly understood.

Sodium and water metabolism in the normal menstrual cycle and premenstrual syndrome

The variations that occur in the levels of salt-retaining and salt-losing hormones during the menstrual cycle and their potential effect on sodium and water metabolism have been the subject of numerous studies over the last 50 years — mainly because of the belief that disturbances of this balance may provide the mechanism for the premenstrual syndrome. These changes are of particular interest in relation to weight gain during the premenstrual phase of the cycle.

Weight gain — the normal menstrual cycle. In 1933, Okey & Stewart reported daily weight findings on 20 college women and showed that only five of them demonstrated significant weight gain in the premenstrual phase of their cycle. Subsequently, a study on 42 nurses showed that 30 per cent gained 3 pounds or more in weight in the premenstrual phase (Sweeney, 1934); this was substantiated by several further studies. Thorn et al (1938) suggested that premenstrual weight gain was due to salt and water retention, but it was clear that only half of the 50 women in their study gained weight premenstrually, whereas three-quarters did so at mid-cycle.

Chesley & Hellman (1957) failed to show any consistent change in body weight during the menstrual cycle in subjects on controlled sodium and water intake. Reeves et al (1971) demonstrated a significant weight gain in ten asymptomatic women during the five premenstrual days. Janowsky et al (1973) studied 11 female volunteers under controlled conditions and showed a significant luteal phase increase in weight which began 11 days before the onset of menses and decreased at the time of onset of the menses. The weight increase also peaked 1 day and 4 days before the onset of the period. Thus, the data are contradictory in normal women, although the general trend in studies performed in metabolic units suggest that weight gain does occur in the premenstrual phase of some women.

Weight gain — premenstrual tension. Some forms of idiopathic oedema occur on a cyclical basis, but this syndrome bears little or no relationship to the changes seen in the premenstrual tension syndrome. Bruce & Russell (1962) studied 24 women on unrestricted diets and ten women on controlled diets in a metabolic unit with premenstrual symptoms of irritability, depression, bloatedness and breast tenderness. In the group on unrestricted diets, there was no constant weight gain and in the 10 women on a fixed food intake, a small weight gain occurred in the second half of the cycle in five women, but there was no evidence of any association with the severity of symptoms.

Reeves et al (1971) compared premenstrual weight gain in ten asymptomatic women and ten with symptoms associated with premenstrual tension and failed to show any difference between the two groups. Furthermore, no correlation could be established between the severity of symptoms and weight gain in symptomatic women. O'Brien compared weight gain in a group of asymptomatic and 20 symptomatic women (O'Brien, 1979). Both groups demonstrated a small, but not significant weight gain in the premenstrual phase. There was no significant difference between the two groups.

Thus, despite the general belief that premenstrual tension and feelings of bloatedness are related to salt and water retention, there is little experimental evidence to support this hypothesis as far as weight gain is concerned.

If there is no true phase of water retention, it is possible that redistribution of fluid occurs in various compartments, thus giving rise to distension in various tissues. Jones et al (1966) have produced evidence to suggest that there is leakage of albumen and water into tissue spaces during the premenstrual phase of the cycle and Wong et al (1972) have shown changes in the capillary filtration coefficient of cutaneous vessels in women with premenstrual tension. These findings would support a newer hypothesis of oedema due to re-distribution rather than retention of fluid. No consistent differences have been shown between total exchangeable sodium (Klein & Carey, 1957) or total body water (Andersch et al, 1978) when follicular and luteal phases are compared.

Changes in the renin-angiotensin and aldosterone systems in the menstrual cycle and in premenstrual tension

Plasma renin activity is a measure of the rate of generation of angiotensin I in the presence of an angiotensinase inhibitor. Renin activity represents the interaction of both enzyme and substrate and is therefore dependent on the concentration of both factors. Plasma renin concentration is a measurement of the rate of generation of angiotensin I in the presence of standardised substrate concentration and therefore represents enzyme concentration alone. Renin substrate is measured by action of excess renin in plasma and the total generation of angiotensin I when the reaction is carried to exhaustion.

Renin-angiotensin system in the normal menstrual cycle.

Brown et al (1964) first showed that plasma renin concentration was significantly higher in the luteal phase of the cycle and, since then, several investigators have shown that both plasma renin and plasma renin activity are increased in the luteal phase of the cycle (Skinner et al, 1969; Robertson et al, 1971; Sundsfjord & Aakvaag, 1972; Katz & Romph, 1972; Michelakis et al, 1975). The evidence suggests that renin substrate remains constant and therefore the changes are enzyme dependent. There has been considerable speculation as to why the levels of plasma renin concentration increase and it seems likely that the increase results from the natriuretic effects of progesterone in the second half of the menstrual cycle (Landau & Lugibihl, 1961). Both angiotensin II and aldosterone levels also increase in the second half of the menstrual cycle (Reich, 1962; Sundsfjord & Aakvaag, 1970).

Renin-angiotensin system in the premenstrual syndrome. In the premenstrual syndrome, there has been some evidence to suggest that there is a correlation between mood and aldosterone levels (Janner et al, 1967). Perrini & Pilego (1959) demonstrated high levels of urinary aldosterone in patients with premenstrual tension. O'Brien et al (1979) studied plasma aldosterone levels in women with premenstrual syndrome and in an asymptomatic control group and showed that aldosterone levels were higher in both groups of women in the second half of the cycle. They were, however, slightly higher in the controls. Despite these findings, the use of an aldosterone antagonist (Aldactone) in the second half of the menstrual cycle resulted in a significant improvement in symptoms in women with significant premenstrual syndrome. In this same study, levels of both plasma renin activity and renin concentration were higher at all phases of the menstrual cycle in symptomatic women, although these changes did not achieve statistical significance.

Other hormones affecting salt and water metabolism

There are several other hormones which have an effect on fluid and electrolyte balance, which may be relevant to PMS. Prolactin, oestradiol, antidiuretic hormone and cortisol, promote retention of fluid, whereas progesterone and the prostaglandins have a natriuretic and diuretic effect. How relevant these factors are in the light of the unproven relationship between PMS and water retention, remains to be seen.

Ovarian hormones

Although a direct relationship between hormones and water retention has not been shown it would be surprising if the underlying cause of the syndrome was not related to the hormonal fluctuation of the menstrual cycle. This was first suggested by Frank (1931) who thought that diminished excretion of oestrogen gave rise to higher plasma levels which in turn gave rise to physical and psychological tension. Israel (1938) suggested that this was not solely the effect of oestrogen but a breakdown in the oestrogen/progesterone balance. More recently attention has been focused on actual progesterone levels and it has been suggested that the PMS is a progesterone deficiency state (Dalton, 1964).

It appears that the timing of PMS symptoms follows that of progesterone secretion and to postulate a hypothesis of progesterone deficiency seems appropriate for two reasons: (1) progesterone has a direct natriuretic effect on the distal renal tubules by competitively inhibiting aldosterone (Landau & Lugibihl, 1961). A progesterone deficiency state would presumably allow excessive sodium and water retention, though we have seen this phenomenon is still in doubt. (2) progesterone has a central nervous sedative effect (Herrmann & Beach, 1978) so deficiency of progesterone would be expected to allow increased central nervous excitability perhaps accounting for symptoms such as irritability, tension, anxiety and maybe many of the others. Some workers have postulated that the effective treatment of PMS by progesterone replacement and progestagen therapy provides evidence for a deficiency state (Dalton, 1977). Unfortunately, this means of therapy remains unproven. Secondly, it must be remembered that effective treatment with an agent does not prove that there is a deficiency of that agent: 'Headache is not due to aspirin deficiency'. The most serious argument against this theory is the well-established knowledge that progesterone is actually lowest in the first half of the cycle. It is, therefore, impossible to explain the syndrome as simplistically as being due to progesterone deficiency. Oestrogen/progesterone ratio is also greatest in the first half of the cycle and therefore the imbalance of these two hormones is also an insufficient explanation of PMS.

Progesterone levels have been measured in various studies. In the studies by Bäckström and his associates at the University of Umea, Sweden, they concentrated on looking at the oestrogen and progesterone levels in the late luteal phase. In the first study (Bäckström & Carstensen, 1974) he concluded that women with PMS had lower progesterone and higher oestrogen levels than normal women. In the second study, Backstrom & Mattsson (1975) concluded that anxiety and irritability were closely correlated with the oestrogen/progesterone ratio, but not to progesterone levels. He, in fact, concluded that the symptoms were more related to the oestrogen level than the actual progesterone level. Smith (1975) reported significant but very small differences in some patients with PMS during the 7 days preceding the menses. There was no difference in the oestrogen/progesterone ratio and there was considerable overlap with the control group. Studies at Nottingham University, England, have shown significantly higher progesterone levels in symptomatic women immediately following ovulation (O'Brien et al, 1979).

Andersch and his co-workers found no difference in progesterone levels between the two groups (Andersch et al, 1979). There have been two studies by Munday. In her first study (Munday, 1977) she showed that one-third of PMS patients have low progesterone levels compared with their normal laboratory range. A better-controlled study (Munday et al, 1981) showed lower progesterone levels 8 to 9 days before menstruation in symptomatic women.

It is interesting to note that, prior to these more sophisticated endocrine studies, Morton (1950) gave oestrogen to women following oophorectomy and produced bloatedness and irritability. In 1942, Gillman was able to reproduce PMS-like symptoms following the injection of progesterone. Nobody has to date shown that the ovaries actually play a role in genesis of premenstrual symptoms. Bäckström et al (1981) reported to continuance of symptoms following hysterectomy, but no one has systematically evaluated the symptoms following oophorectomy; this would seem to be a fundamental study in the investigation of this syndrome albeit logistically difficult to perform.

It is difficult to explain the various differences in the hormonal findings and the relationship with the symptoms. Differences in definition, patient selection and measurement of symptoms obviously play a part. It may be that the actual dynamic changes of the hormones or the abrupt fall of the hormones at the end of the cycle may be more relevant than the absolute levels. This has also been postulated as a mechanism in postpartum depression where steroid levels, particularly progesterone, fall profoundly. An alternative explanation that total hormone levels are less relevant than the unbound fraction of the hormone has been suggested by Dalton (1977) and studied by Dalton (1981). In this study, a relatively large group of patients with severe premenstrual syndrome and collected from various parts of the country were compared with 50 matched controls. The symptomatic group did contain a rather large number of non-typical patients including those with psychopathic tendencies, other criminal tendencies and baby-batterers. There was also one patient with premenstrual epilepsy. However, measurements of sex hormone binding globulin (SHBG) binding capacity showed significantly lower levels in this symptomatic group. As well as these differences, no overlap in the actual values was shown. Unfortunately, total oestrogen levels were not measured at the same time. Bäckström et al (1976) has previously measured sex steroid binding globulin and found no differences; he concluded that higher differences in oestrogen levels were more important. Even so, the findings of Dalton are interesting and probably warrant further investigation.

Gonadotrophins

Intimately related to the ovarian hormone changes are the changes in gonadotrophin and prolactin excretion.

Andersch et al (1979) looked at gonadotrophin levels. He showed no difference in follicle-stimulating hormone (FSH) or luteinising hormone (LH) in the two groups at any stage of the cycle. Bäckström et al (1976), however, showed slightly elevated levels of FSH in the follicular phase of the cycle which probably parallels his oestrogen findings. O'Brien (1979) showed no difference between FSH or LH measurements between the two groups, nor was there any statistical correlation between the premenstrual mood score and gonadotrophin levels.

Prolactin

There are several reasons why prolactin may be thought to give rise to PMS. First, prolactin causes retention of sodium, water and potassium. Secondly, it has a direct effect on the breasts and may be responsible for at least the breast symptoms. Thirdly, it is well-established that prolactin is secreted in response to stress, and lastly it has an inter-relationship with dopamine metabolism. Horrobin (1973) suggested that the hormone may play a crucial aetiological role, though he did not measure the hormone in either the menstrual cycle or in women complaining of PMS. Many other workers have assessed the significance of prolactin levels during the menstrual cycle. Halbreich and co-workers showed higher levels of prolactin throughout the course of the menstrual cycle in the symptomatic group; there was also a rise in the prolactin levels during the premenstrual phase, but this was found in symptomatic and control subjects. The absolute rise was approximately the same in both groups (Halbreich et al, 1976). Two other studies have shown elevated prolactin levels in the premenstrual phase (Friesen et al, 1972; Vekemans et al, 1977). The remaining studies have not shown such a clearcut picture. In symptomatic subjects, Andersch and colleagues showed lower levels of prolactin in the follicular phase, compared with controls. The luteal phase levels, however, were no different from those of the control group (Andersch et al, 1979). The majority of studies show no difference between control and symptomatic patients (McNeilly & Chard, 1974; Harrison & Letchworth, 1976; Andersen et al, 1977; O'Brien & Symonds, 1982). Because prolactin is released in a pulsatile manner, there are often dramatic fluctuations even throughout the course of a day. The most convincing studies are those in which at least daily samples are taken. In a study by Epstein et al (1975) daily samples were taken and although he confirmed the considerable day-to-day fluctuations, there were no consistent alterations during the course of the menstrual cycle itself. No mention was made in this study of the occurrence of PMS symptoms, but a study by Backstrom & Aakvaag (1981) reported daily values and showed no difference between the symptomatic and asymptomatic subjects.

Anti-diuretic hormone

Although anti-diuretic hormone (ADH) has been measured in PMS, there are no conclusive studies. A preliminary report has shown cyclical ADH variation but these findings have not been confirmed (Charvat & Holececk, 1966).

Testosterone

Testosterone has been measured daily. Epstein et al (1975) showed raised levels of testosterone around the time of ovulation, but no alteration premenstrually. Backstrom & Aakvaag (1981) showed no difference at any stage of the menstrual cycle, nor was there any difference between the symptomatic and control groups.

Adrenal hormones

In addition to the pituitary and ovarian hormones, other endocrine changes have been considered in the aetiology of the syndrome. Adrenal hormones, catecholamines, pancreatic hormones and prostaglandins have all been the subject of hypotheses if not actually studied. There are virtually no good investigative studies of adrenal functions in this syndrome with the exception of aldosterone and testosterone which have previously been discussed. Adrenal sex steroids could theoretically account for the persistence of the syndrome after oophorectomy and after the menopause — a suggestion put forward by Dalton (1964). The amount of adrenal sex steroid produced is much less than that produced by the ovary during reproductive life and a cyclical pattern has not yet been shown. There is as yet no research to confirm these assumptions.

Cortisol is another 'stress' hormone and it also has some mineralo-corticoid activity. Cyclical variation does occur; however this is only slight and is characterised by a slight increase in the premenstrual phase (Silbergeld et al, 1971). Differences between symptomatic and non-symptomatic women have not been demonstrated.

Catecholamines from adrenal or other sympathetic ganglia, may well cause or contribute to the syndrome. Catecholamines exert their effect throughout the body particularly on the cardiovascular system and on the juxta-glomerular apparatus, therefore indirectly affecting sodium handling. However, the role of the sympathetic nervous system remains unknown in PMS.

Pancreatic hormones

There appear to be alterations in glucose tolerance in the menstrual cycle and thus the roles of glucagon, insulin and carbohydrate have been considered. Flattening of the glucose tolerance test occurs premenstrually (Billig & Spaulding, 1974; Morton et al, 1950). This phase of the cycle is sometimes associated with hunger, sweating, nervousness and craving for sweets and it may be that there is some hyper-insulinism at this phase of the cycle. It has been thought that the symptoms of anxiety, irritability and aggression may be related to this in the same way that hypoglycaemia causes similar symptoms in pancreatic tumours. Systematic studies have not been performed to evaluate this although women occasionally attempt to relieve symptoms by increasing carbohydrate intake premenstrually.

Prostaglandins

The ubiquitous nature of the prostaglandins (PG) would make them admirable agents to account for the diverse symptoms of the syndrome. Of particular interest is the relationship between the E and A series prostaglandins which have a direct effect on renal handling of sodium and water (McGiff et al, 1974). Studies on the normal menstrual cycle have shown no significant variation premenstrually of either E or F prostaglandin (Kindahl et al, 1976; Jordan & Pokoly, 1977). There are as yet no data available for the premenstrual syndrome. In any case it is likely that peripheral blood levels will not reflect tissue activity of these hormones. However, the interaction between E series prostaglandins and angiotensin II is now well established (O'Brien et al, 1977; Broughton Pipkin et al, 1981). The prostaglandins suppress the vascular response to angiotensin II in pregnancy. Thus it may be that a breakdown in this balance could be responsible for any renal and cerebral vascular changes associated with PMS. This interaction is currently being studied in the normal menstrual cycle and in PMS.

Despite this lack of information, two studies related to prostaglandins in PMS have been undertaken, looking at both inhibition and supplementing PG production. These are considered under 'Treatment'.

Hypersensitivity

The possibility of hypersensitivity to endogenous hormone has been considered by Zondek & Bromberg, (1945). No studies have shown antibodies to progesterone and there have been no successful studies using desensitisation in the treatment of PMS.

Menotoxin

Finally, Macht (1943) proposed a role for 'menotoxin' produced by the endometrium, found in blood, saliva, tears, sweat, milk and urine. This toxin was apparently able to stop the root growth of plants, stultify the motor performance of rats, emanate rays which could kill yeast spores and could be absorbed with dire consequences through the male genitalia. No further information is available on this 'menotoxin' but the persistence of cyclical symptoms after removal of the endometrium and uterus dispels a 'menotoxin' theory (Bäckström et al, 1981).

TREATMENT

The investigation of treatment in premenstrual syndrome has been affected by many of the same problems as encountered in the studies attempting to determine aetiology. But in addition to the problems of definition and measurement, failure to take account of the markedly significant placebo effect of any therapy has led to a vast number of almost worthless studies. In general, it appears that the results of open studies report a 70–100 per cent improvement rate, whereas controlled studies give a range of 65–80 per cent. Thus, it may be that the use of controlled trials may mask the efficacy of certain drug regimes, though this seems unlikely.

Placebo effect

Placebo effect in this syndrome must be amongst the highest documented. Until recently, this was not really appreciated and has probably accounted for the wide range of regimes which, presumably in good faith, have been reported as highly efficacious. There are, however, several recent studies where placebo has been included. Sampson (1979) conducted a study to compare the effect of progesterone with placebo. This drug regime is well established in the literature as a treatment for PMS. In this study, she found that the response to placebo was 40 per cent which was slightly greater than the effect of the active drug. Day (1979a) reported a 43 per cent placebo effect, whilst other studies have shown even greater levels, for example, the 53 per cent response rate shown in the study by Haspels (1980) when he compared the effect of placebo against dydrogesterone. Part of this placebo response is presumably due to the placebo drug, though a large part of it is due to the psychotherapeutic effect of patient consultation. It has been suggested that the response afforded by placebo therapy is transient, i.e. lasting for only two or three cycles. A problem of inclusion of placebo in therapeutic trials of the mentrual cycle is the carry-over effect from the treatment cycle into the placebo cycle. This is a particular problem when one is testing a deficiency state, for example, vitamin or hormone deficiency. The only way to avoid this is to have long treatment periods and long placebo periods. Unfortunately, long placebo periods are often associated with a high drop-out rate during the placebo phase of the study. There is no other way to avoid this carry-over effect; it is important to appreciate this for statistical analysis and interpretation of the studies.

The range of treatment in PMS

When one considers the large number of aetiological

theories, it is not surprising that there is an equally large range of methods of treatment available. Enthusiastic claims have been made for many of these drugs and, again, this is not surprising in view of the high placebo effect. There have been several approaches to management; one is to assume that one drug may cure all symptoms and that drug is prescribed for every patient; the second is to prescribe any drug in an empirical manner until the correct one is found; the third, and probably most effective method, is to analyse each patient's symptoms in detail and prescribe the drug appropriate to those symptoms. Even this method, however, is not as successful as one would hope and often one has to resort to the random approach. Unfortunately, the treatment of premenstrual syndrome has largely been based on anecdotes or the result of poorly controlled therapeutic trials. Consequently, there has been little to guide the clinician through the maze of the available regimes.

In a syndrome where the placebo effect has been reported as high as 50 per cent and where the prevalence of the condition is as high as 50–90 per cent of all women of reproductive age, it is not surprising that many doctors and drug companies wish to produce the effective drug.

The many reported regimes fall into three main categories. These are (a) without drugs; (b) using non-hormonal drugs; and (c) hormonal therapy. We will look at the whole range of regimes and then pick out the drugs which appear useful.

Non-drug treatment

Formal psychotherapy has been an important tool of the clinical psychologist and psychiatrist for many years for the treatment of other psychological disorders. In 1953 Rees assessed the value of psychotherapy in the treatment of PMS and concluded that it was of value, but only in conjunction with other therapy (Rees, 1953b). A second study (Fortin et al, 1958) showed that 50 per cent of patients were improved by psychotherapy alone (CF placebo effect drugs). Overall, it appears that premenstrual syndrome of any severity will require further treatment in addition to the psychotherapy.

Many of the other non-drug treatments tend to follow current fashion. Diverse approaches such as acupuncture, yoga, transcendental meditation, masturbation, intravaginal electrical stimulation, homeopathy and music have all been suggested, but not adequately tested. We should keep an open mind about these approaches, but remembering that premenstrual syndrome does lend itself to treatment methods which are not readily assessable.

Non-hormonal drug treatment

Psychoactive drugs

Many of the approaches to the treatment of PMS have been particularly aimed at the psychological symptoms. Some psychoactive drugs have profound effects, many with serious side-effects. They should probably be reserved for severe cases and then probably only administered by psychiatrists conversant with the drugs. Their most important role would be where premenstrual syndrome is superimposed on an underlying psychiatric disturbance.

Anti-depressants. There is as yet no anti-depressant which acts immediately or quickly enough to be used intermittently as would be necessary for the treatment of PMS symptoms, and although depression is a frequent symptom of premenstrual syndrome, these drugs have not yet been tested.

Minor tranquillisers. Diazepam must be one of the most frequently prescribed drugs in general practice for 'the neurotic women' which PMS patients have so frequently been labelled. They almost certainly have some benefit as an anxiolytic for patients with irritability and anxiety. However, they may worsen symptoms such as depression and lethargy. Phenobarbitone has been used in conjunction with ergotamine tartrate for both menopausal symptoms and PMS. There has been one double-blind study in which one tablet was prescribed three times daily in the premenstrual phase (Robinson et al, 1977). This showed an improvement in most symptoms compared with placebo. It is, however, becoming increasingly apparent that barbiturate therapy is inadvisable in view of potential dependency. Mephenisin (Swyer, 1955) and meprobamate (Pennington, 1957; Appleby, 1960) have both been claimed to be effective in PMS, but in uncontrolled studies.

Meprobamate has been used in conjunction with bendrofluozide and has for some time been recommended for PMS. It has only recently been evaluated in a placebo-controlled study (Carstairs & Talbot, 1982). The overall improvement rate in this study was a little over 60 per cent. Meprobamate does also have potential dependency problems.

Good results have been claimed for lithium on the basis that the drug alters water and electrolyte balance and because it had been used previously in manic-depressive psychosis, the parallel between them being the periodicity of the two conditions. Good results have been claimed in uncontrolled trials (Altmann et al, 1941; Sletten & Gershon, 1966) though these were not confirmed when tested in a double-blind controlled trial (Singer et al, 1974).

Diuretic therapy

Although it has generally been accepted that water retention is a constant feature of the premenstrual syndrome, we have already seen that the evidence of many good scientific studies has failed to support this. We have also seen that many women complain of a feeling of bloatedness and a feeling that their weight has increased, whilst there has been no measurable increase in weight (O'Brien, 1979). There are many studies of the various diuretics. Simple diuretics such as ammonium chloride have been given in the luteal phase of the cycle with claims of about 90 per cent improvement (Stieglitz & Kimble, 1949; Rees, 1953b). Placebo was not used in these studies. Ammonium chloride, in combination with caffeine, has been used in an over-the-counter preparation. In 22 patients two tablets or placebo were given daily from day 18 to 24 of the menstrual cycle (Hoffman, 1979). The success rate in this study was reported as 100 per cent. This was presumably because they looked only at weight as their means of assessing treatment. Many other diuretics have been used in uncontrolled studies. These include chlorothiazide (Jungck et al, 1959; Appleby, 1960), chlorthalidone (Kramer, 1962), and quinethazone (Baden & Lizcano, 1963). In the double-blind studies that have been performed, chlorthalidone (Mattson & Van Schoultz, 1974) and potassium chloride (Reeves et al, 1971) appeared no better than placebo. Coppen et al (1969) conducted a study using a combination of triamterine and benzthiazide and found it to be more effective than placebo or norethisterone in the treatment of depression and irritability. Surprisingly, norethisterone was superior in the treatment of bloatedness.

Metolazone given from 7 days before and during menstruation up to 5 mg a day was studied in 46 women (Werch & Kane, 1976). Thirty-three patients completed the study. Premenstrual symptom scores were lower in the treatment group compared with the placebo, though lethargy and weakness was a frequent problem, especially at the higher doses. These patients were selected for trial only if they had a weight gain of 3 lb or more in the premenstrual week. A double-blind placebo-controlled study of spironolactone has been carried out (O'Brien et al, 1979). Twenty-five mg spironolactone were given 4 times a day from day 18 to day 26 of the menstrual cycle in 18 patients. There was a significant improvement in premenstrual mood assessment together with a reduction in weight.

Diuretics have been used for some time in clinical practice and this is often the first line therapy of the general practitioner. It is important to note that these drugs have a potential hazard in that they may produce secondary aldosteronism and this may lead to the more severe idiopathic oedema. Often a history of 'diuretic abuse' is found in this type of patient (McGregor et al, 1979). This inappropriate diuretic therapy is often self-prescribed in patients who are either treating themselves for premenstrual syndrome or for weight reduction as an adjunct to dieting. The aldosterone antagonists are therefore preferable whenever diuretic therapy is indicated. Spironolactone or spironolactone combined with thiazide is therefore recommended.

Vitamins

We have previously seen that vitamin deficiency has been postulated as a cause of the syndrome, although levels have never been measured. In therapeutic trials vitamin A (Argonz & Abinzano, 1950; Block, 1960) and vitamin B (Biskind, 1943) have been used with claimed success. These studies were not compared with placebo. The results are therefore difficult to interpret. Much more recently, the use of vitamin B_6 has been popularised. Stokes & Mendels (1972) have previously used the drug in uncontrolled trials. When they studied it in an adequately controlled trial, their results were disappointing. In a more recent study by Kerr et al (1980) 70 patients showed a 50 per cent improvement, particularly for depression, irritability, bloatedness, oedema and headache. This study was uncontrolled. In a later study by Day (1979a) 57 patients received pyridoxine 100 mg daily or placebo in a single blind manner. Forty patients completed the study. He reported an overall improvement rate of 63 per cent and there were no reported side-effects. It is generally thought that vitamin B_6 is a useful drug where psychological symptoms predominate. It is difficult to assess how much of this is placebo effect and how much of this is pharmacological activity.

Hormone treatment of premenstrual syndrome

Although an endocrine cause for PMS still remains unproven, it seems highly likely that in a syndrome where events escalate following ovulation, an endocrine basis probably exists. Accordingly, alteration or correction of the hormonal status would appear an obvious approach to therapy. Hormone treatment has been along one of three approaches: (1) correction of a deficiency or hormonal imbalance; (2) inhibition of the menstrual cycle and ovulation; (3) inhibition of specific hormones. There is occasionally some overlap.

Progesterone

Enthusiastic claims have been made for the use of pure progesterone (Dalton, 1977). It has been accepted for some time that progesterone is inactive when given by mouth, though more recent studies have shown that plasma progesterone levels do rise following oral administration. Treatment has, therefore, rarely been given orally. Dalton has administered progesterone by several routes over the past 20 years. These include daily intramuscular injections, suppositories, pessaries and slow-release implants. If progesterone deficiency is the underlying cause of this syndrome, then one would expect this to be the perfect agent. Timing of therapy is all-important and inaccurate timing of administration is said to be one of the underlying reasons for treatment failure (Dalton, 1977). If premenstrual syndrome is caused by some factor other than progesterone deficiency, progesterone would still be expected to be useful. Firstly, it has a central nervous depressant action and causes sedation (Herrman & Beach, 1978) and, secondly, it has a natriuretic and diuretic action through its competive inhibition of aldosterone at the distal renal tubules. It would, however, be expected to produce a secondary rise in aldosterone and therefore rebound water retention after discontinuing therapy. There are several disadvantages of this therapy. The menstrual pattern may be disrupted in some patients. Regular progesterone injections given intramuscularly are painful, whilst pessaries and suppositories are not always acceptable to the patient. The literature supporting this mode of therapy fails to cite any controlled trials to support the claim.

Two studies have been performed on progesterone treatment. Smith (1975) compared progesterone with spironolactone, progesterone plus spironolactone and placebo. The progesterone dose was 50 mg intramuscularly from day 19 of the menstrual cycle. These were given in a double-blind manner and the authors concluded that there was no improvement in progesterone cycles except in three patients. Moreover, there was no correlation between the degree of effect and the plasma progesterone levels. The second study was performed by Sampson (1979). She administered progesterone either rectally or vaginally at two different dose levels. She concluded that, if anything, the placebo was slightly more effective than progesterone though this was not supported statistically. Dalton has since argued that this failure of therapy was due to misdiagnosis of patients and that the patients were actually complaining of menstrual distress. (She defines menstrual distress as the presence of symptoms throughout the menstrual cycle with an increase in severity during the premenstrual phase and menstruation.)

Gillman was able actually to produce PMS symptoms using injections of pure progesterone (Gillman, 1942). Despite any clear proof of the efficacy of this drug, it remains a popular form of therapy and its popularity is actually increasing. It is interesting to note that improvement of symptoms following treatment has been the main basis on which two charges of murder have been repealed in English law; it is not suggested that this lends any scientific credence to the issue.

Progestogens

A wide range of progestogens has been used over the past 25 years. Some of these have been evaluated adequately, the majority have not. Ethisterone, norethisterone, dimethisterone, medroxy-progesterone and more recently dydrogesterone have all been used (Fig. 32.6). Dydrogesterone is the progestogen which most closely resembles natural progesterone. It is the optical isomer. Whilst it is assumed that the progestogens correct supposed progesterone defi-

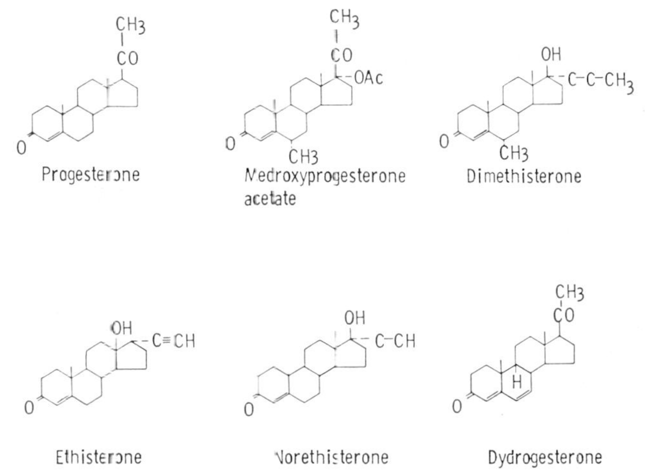

Fig. 32.6 Progesterone and progestagens used in the treatment of premenstrual syndrome

ciency, it is also possible that the synthetic agents are capable of suppressing endogenous progesterone levels. Johansson (1971) has shown that the administration of norethisterone reduces plasma progesterone levels.

The number of progestogen studies without placebo far outweigh those with adequate control. Coppen assessed the efficacy of norethisterone. He compared it with diuretic and placebo and found that norethisterone gave slight improvement in water retention symptoms but no significant difference between placebo or diuretics (Coppen et al, 1969). In a study of medroxyprogesterone acetate and diuretic, Jordheim (1972) showed little difference between progestogen, placebo or progestogen/diuretic combinations. Swyer (1955) compared ethisterone with mephenesin (a minor tranquilliser) and showed neither to be superior to placebo. Apart from dydrogesterone there have been few adequate studies of progestogens. Norethisterone, dimethisterone and ethisterone have been studied on several occasions (Green & Dalton, 1953; Swyer, 1955; Dalton, 1959; Appleby, 1960). Typically, these studies show an improvement in symptoms; unfortunately, one cannot draw adequate conclusions from such uncontrolled studies.

Dydrogesterone. Dydrogesterone is a drug which has become available more recently and has been used to treat various gynaecological disorders including dysmenorrhoea, endometriosis, threatened abortion, infertility, menstrual irregularity and heavy periods. It has been strongly promoted for the treatment of premenstrual syndrome and this is based on the findings of several uncontrolled studies in which improvement rates ranging from 50 to 82 per cent have been shown (Taylor, 1977; Taylor & James, 1979; Piton, 1979; Romanini et al, 1979; Strecker, 1980). Single-blind controlled studies have shown improvement rates of about 70 per cent (Day, 1979a; Kerr et al, 1980). One double-blind study that has been performed is a large multi-centre study including several European countries. Haspels (1981) has reported 123 patients which constitute the Dutch part of the study. Women were considered to

Table 32.3 Percentage of patients showing improvement on dydrogesterone and placebo

Symptoms	Dydrogesterone (N = 70) (%)	Placebo (N = 53) (%)	P (χ²)
50–100% improvement	54	32	0.02
10–49% improvement	19	21	n.s.
Unchanged	24	45	0.2
Worse	3	2	n.s.

have PMS if they had three of the characteristic symptoms occurring in the second half of the cycle only. They were all studied over four cycles. No treatment was given in the first cycle. During the subsequent three cycles the patients were prescribed dydrogesterone or identical placebo. This was given in a double-blind manner from day 12 to the onset of menstruation. The active dose was 10 mg twice daily. Common symptoms were recorded on a 0–3 rating scale. Of a total of 150 patients, 123 completed the study; of these, 70 had taken active drug whilst 53 had placebo. Dydrogesterone gave a greater than 50 per cent improvement in 54 per cent of patients. Nineteen per cent of patients showed improvement rates between 10 and 49 per cent; 24 per cent were unchanged and only 3 per cent made worse. This compared favourably with placebo (Table 32.3). He also concluded that the drug was more effective in patients who had the worst symptoms. Though this is statistically significant, it does not represent a large number of patients who were actually improved to a marked degree. Moreover, patients did not act as their own controls which may have been a better approach to this study. There was no mention of side-effects and the worsening rate for the two groups was only 3 per cent. This seems unusually low since in practice there are often more problems than this, a particular complaint being weight gain. It is of course possible that the patients who dropped out were those who had significant side-effects.

Progestogens do seem to have some value as first or second line agents in the treatment of premenstrual syndrome. In practical terms they are particularly useful where other symptoms such as menorrhagia, dysmenorrhoea, prolonged or irregular cycles also need correction.

Progestogens have also been used in combination with other drugs. This is most commonly in the form of the combined oral contraceptive.

Combined oral contraception

There has been considerable interest in the use of combined oral contraceptive agents for the relief of premenstrual symptoms. There have been some well-planned studies, but the majority have looked at groups of women already taking the pill and are retrospective. The overall impression is that these women have significantly less symptoms than nonpill-takers. Herzberg & Coppen (1970) compared the symptoms of pill-users with users of other contraceptive measures; 136 oral contraceptive-users showed markedly less irritability and less depression than 27 control subjects. Moos (1969) had previously shown in a large group of 710 patients that symptoms were much less in those taking the pill. The Report of the Royal College of General Practitioners (1974) showed premenstrual syndrome to be 29 per cent less in pill-takers. It also appears that the more progestogenic pills are more effective in their relief (Culberg, 1972; Kutner & Brown, 1972). These reports seem promising, though it must be remembered that patients who choose to be on the pill were compared with those who chose alternative methods. It is possible that the women using alternative methods avoided oral contraception because it made their symptoms worse, hence, there has been a pre-selection process to transfer all the patients experiencing worsening of symptoms to the control group. The few prospective studies have not really clarified the situation. Silbergeld et al (1971) showed that in a small group of 8 patients, premenstrual anxiety was suppressed when compared with placebo. Morris & Udry (1972) showed no difference between active and placebo therapy.

It appears that the pill has a definite beneficial effect in a certain group of patients. This group is difficult to define and can only be determined empirically. In young women without contraindications and without a desire to become pregnant, this form of therapy should probably be the first line of approach. In women who are over 35, and particularly smokers, alternative methods of treatment may be preferable. Many women elect to take the pill continuously because either pre-menstrual symptoms or migraine occur during the pill-free week.

Other forms of combined therapy have been recommended in the form of hormonal implants with intermittent progestogen treatment. Studd & Nagos (1983) reported complete or almost complete relief in 84 per cent of patients using this approach.

Bromocriptine

The conflicting data on prolactin levels in the menstrual cycle and in premenstrual syndrome have been discussed. Many of these studies included the assessment of bromocriptine therapy and data are available from several other studies. Bromocriptine is a dopamine agonist and thus inhibits prolactin secretion. It is probably because this drug has been evaluated more recently that all the therapeutic studies appear to be double-blind. Benedek-Jazmann & Hearn-Sturtevant (1976) gave 5 mg of bromocriptine daily from day 10 of the menstrual cycle. This, when compared with placebo, showed a significant improvement in mood disturbance, weight increase, oedema and breast symptoms. Unfortunately, subsequent investigation has not been able to reproduce these findings (Harrison & Letchworth, 1976; Ghose & Coppen, 1977; Andersch et al,

1979). In all these studies, the drug was found to be no more effective than placebo except for the treatment of breast symptoms. Other studies have produced equivocal results except for the improvement in breast symptoms (Andersen et al, 1977; Andersch et al, 1976; Graham et al, 1978). It should be noted that in all of these protocols, treatment was not started as early in the cycle as in the work of Benedek-Jazmann & Hearn-Sturtevant (1976), and in some studies only 2.5 mg of bromocriptine daily was used. These factors may account for the difference in findings. Its value in the treatment of breast symptoms seems clear and this has been confirmed in a study looking predominantly at breast pain (Mansel et al, 1978). In this study, bromocriptine, 5 mg daily, produced a significant reduction in cyclical breast pain though it had no effect on non-cyclical breast symptoms or on the other PMS symptoms.

The drug is therefore useful, at least for the treatment of breast symptoms. However, it is often complicated by side-effects such as fainting and nausea. These problems are generally avoided by administration of therapy at night (Ch. 26)

Danazol

The anti-gonadotrophin, danazol, has now been established as a first-line treatment for endometriosis (Greenblatt et al, 1971) and a second-line drug for the treatment of menorrhagia (Chimbira et al, 1979). In doses sufficient to suppress the menses and ovulation, one would expect premenstrual syndrome symptoms to be completely suppressed. However, in the few trials performed to date, results have proved disappointing. In a study by Mansel et al (1979), looking mainly at the effects on breast pain, but also the general symptoms of premenstrual syndrome, there was little improvement apart from the breast symptoms. Another study using this drug (Day, 1979b) suggested that there was improvement in all symptoms but particularly breast symptoms. The study did not, however, include placebo therapy. The side-effects of this drug are not insignificant and in high doses hirsuitism, weight increase and deepening of the voice have been reported fairly frequently. Both this and the high price of the drug, should be considered prior to commencement of the study, particularly if long term therapy is anticipated.

Prostanoids

Prostaglandins and similar compounds are found throughout the body. They may well be related to premenstrual syndrome. They are locally acting hormones derived from various dietary essential fatty acids, and synthesis is dependent on a group of enzyme systems collectively known as prostaglandin synthetase. There is good evidence that prostaglandin synthetase inhibitors are valuable in the treatment of pain in both arthritis and in dysmenorrhoea. The role of prostaglandins is not established in premenstrual syndrome but treatment by both enhancement of prostaglandin levels and inhibition of synthesis, has been attempted. The prostaglandin synthetase inhibitor, mefenamic acid, has been evaluated in a double-blind placebo controlled trial (Wood & Jakubowicz, 1980). This study showed significant improvement in pain, headache, depression, tension and irritability. The opposite approach has been tried using dietary precursors of prostaglandins. The oil of evening primrose (Efamol) containing linoleic and dihomogammalinolenic acid, has been studied at St Thomas's Hospital, London (Brush, 1981). This study produced a reduction in all symptoms though, unfortunately, was not placebo controlled and, therefore, a valid judgement of therapy cannot yet be made. Preece & Mansel (1981) again looking at breast pain, did conduct a double-blind trial. They found a significant improvement in the treatment of cyclical breast pain but not non-cyclical pain.

This seemingly paradoxical effect of inhibitors and promoters of prostaglandin synthesis may imply that the levels of prostaglandins are less important than the balance between the various series of prostaglandins, particularly E_1 and E_2. Much more work is obviously needed on this subject before valid conclusions can be drawn.

CONCLUSIONS AND RECOMMENDATIONS

Management of the patient with premenstrual syndrome

Although a large number of studies have been performed, one might be forgiven for still being very uncertain how to treat patients presenting with premenstrual syndrome. The following is a guide to treatment, based on the better controlled trials in the literature, and the subsequent clinical experience derived from this.

History

In clinical practice, the diagnosis is entirely dependent upon the history. It is useful if the patient can complete a mood chart for 2 months prior to the first appointment in which she should also record the time of menstruation and her daily weight. This will enable the clinician to see at a glance the timing and character of the symptoms for diagnosis and enable him to calculate the timing of therapy.

Characteristics of the menstrual cycle should be ascertained, particularly with regard to duration and amount of bleeding and the length of the cycle itself. This will influence choice of therapy. A history of inter-menstrual or post-coital bleeding needs gynaecological evaluation as does any abnormal bleeding. These aspects are of primary importance and treatment of premenstrual syndrome should await their investigation. It is important to distinguish premenstrual syndrome from gynaecological disorders such as endometriosis; this may require laparoscopy. It is also important to distinguish it from psychiatric disorders; the presence of the symptom-free week following menstruation is of importance here.

By the time the patient attends the premenstrual or gynaecological clinic, she will usually have had some form of treatment. This should be recorded, together with the contraceptive method employed. The patient's attitude to treatment is important. Some women demand hormonal therapy and others refuse any type of hormone. We also need to know her sexual, family and social history, and whether she smokes.

Clinical examination

Some clinicians, particularly those running premenstrual syndrome clinics, who are not gynaecologically trained, often omit the clinical examination. This, however, is important for two reasons. Firstly, it helps to exclude the many conditions which may be confused with, or coexist with premenstrual syndrome. Secondly, the reassurance afforded to the patient is part of the treatment. This is particularly true where breast pain or pelvic pain are amongst the presenting symptoms. Many patients, not surprisingly, will have a fear of cancer of the breast or genital tract, and without gynaecological examination, we are not able to reassure them.

Further investigations

If the patient has not already presented her symptom chart, then this can be started. Some tests may be arranged for the luteal phase of the cycle. These include oestrogen, progesterone, prolactin, urea and electrolytes, which may be of some use in determining therapy and monitoring. Follicle stimulating hormone and luteinising hormone should be assayed in the older patient whose symptoms may be due to the climacteric rather than premenstrual syndrome.

Specific treatment

The treatment begins as soon as the patient is seen. The psychotherapeutic effect of discussing her symptoms must not be under-estimated. Formal psychotherapy, however, is time consuming and of doubtful value. It does help to tell the patient that the symptoms disappear with menstruation and also that many women experience similar symptoms. Advice may be given regarding diet and modification of her important activities to suit the menstrual cycle. When considering treatment, it should be remembered that one drug does not cure all symptoms or all patients and that treatment depends on the history,

Table 32.4 Drug treatment of premenstrual syndrome

Oral contraceptives
Dydrogesterone, progesterone, norethisterone
Pyridoxine
Diuretics (preferably spironolactone)
Bromocriptine
Danazol
Prostaglandin synthetase inhibitors

symptom assessment and, to some extent, the blood tests.

Drug treatment. Of the large number of drugs available for the treatment of PMS only a few have proved valuable (Table 32.4). Oral contraception is the best first line approach to treatment. Predominantly progestogenic pills or triphasic pills seem to be preferable. The pill should be prescribed in the normal cyclical way though some women find greater improvement with continuous therapy. Not all women, however, will accept missing their regular menstruation. If the woman is over 35 and smokes, the higher risk of thrombo-embolic disease should be considered. If she wishes to become pregnant, then another form of therapy will obviously be necessary.

If the patient is not suitable for oral contraception, then the character of the menstrual cycle should be studied. When dysmenorrhoea, heavy bleeding, or an irregular cycle occur, then progesterone or a progestogen should be used. Pure progesterone given as a pessary or a suppository appears to benefit certain patients, although its efficacy has not been proven in any studies. Dydrogesterone seems to be the best evaluated progestogen to date. If the plasma progesterone is low, then again progesterone or a progestogen should be prescribed.

In the patient with a normal cycle and who is not suitable for oral contraception, the specific nature of the symptoms should be assessed. The patient with cyclical breast symptoms could be treated with danazol, Bromocriptine or Efamol, though to date the best evaluated of these is Bromocriptine. This should be given in the higher dose, 5 mg from day 10 of the menstrual cycle, preferably at night.

Patients whose symptoms are predominantly psychological should be treated with vitamin B_6 and if this is ineffective, an anxiolytic or other psychoactive drug can be considered.

In patients whose symptoms are somatic and show definite increase in weight or fluid retention, a diuretic should be used and the diuretic of choice is spironolactone. Thus, the complications of rebound and secondary aldosteronism leading to cyclical oedema may be avoided. One hundred mg daily should be prescribed, commencing 3 days before the expected onset of symptoms. Serum potassium and sodium should be monitored at intervals throughout the therapy, and potassium supplements must *not* be given.

If premenstrual pelvic pain is an important symptom, then prostaglandin synthetase inhibitors, such as mefenamic acid, will be of value.

If successful treatment has not been achieved by this stage, then the initial diagnosis should be questioned since the majority of patients will have improved. If the diagnosis is re-confirmed, then the other available drugs should be tried.

Treatment should continue for 3 months and then re-assessed. If unsuccessful, then alternative measures should be taken. If successful, the treatment should be continued. The duration of therapy will vary from patient to patient but the effect of discontinuing therapy should be assessed at 6 monthly intervals.

Planning research studies in premenstrual syndrome

Until an objective means of assessing this syndrome is produced, the value of any study will be somewhat limited scientifically and our initial efforts should be aimed in this direction. Whilst menstrual charts are adequate for diagnosis, they are totally inadequate for the assessment of symptoms, particularly with regard to their severity. Presently, we can only assess mood change and weight change. Mood change should be assessed either by the Moos' Menstrual Distress Questionnaire or the more sensitive visual analogue scales. The symptoms included in the visual analogue mood chart can be adapted to suit the particular needs of each individual study. In studies which are designed to assess changes in the cycle but not the effect of the treatment, a minimum of two, and preferably three, cycles should be studied. The symptomatic and control groups should be differentiated scientifically and not on the patient's impression of her symptoms. This is probably best done again by using the Moos' technique or the visual analogue scale.

In studies to evaluate therapy, it is of paramount importance that placebo treatment is included in the study design. A minimum of five cycles should be studied. This should include a pre-treatment cycle where mood change, hormonal change and any other characteristics, can be evaluated accurately. This should be followed by two cycles of treatment and two placebo cycles in a double-blind cross-over format.

It is hoped that a more scientific approach to this syndrome will allow a more accurate assessment of symptomatology and other changes of the syndrome. We would, therefore, be in a better position to understand the aetiology and, subsequently, offer more rational treatment to the many women suffering from this syndrome.

REFERENCES

Adams P W, Rose D P, Folkard J, Wynn V, Seed M, Strong R 1973 Effect of Pyridoxine Hydrochloride (Vitamin B6) upon depression associated with oral contraception. Lancet i: 897–904

Aitken R C B 1969 Measurement of feelings using visual analogue scales. Proceedings of the Royal Society of Medicine 62: 989–993

Altman M, Knowles E, Bull H D 1941 A psychosomatic study of the sex cycle in women. Psychosomatic Medicine 3: 199–225

Andersch B, Abrahamsson L, Wendestem C, Ohman R, Hahn L 1979 Hormone profile in premenstrual tension: effects of Bromocriptine and diuretics. Clinical Endocrinology 11: 657–664

Andersch B, Hahn L, Isaksson B 1978a Body water and weight in patients with premenstrual tension. British Journal of Obstetrics and Gynaecology 85: 546–550

Andersch B, Hahn L, Wendestem C, Abrahamsson L 1978b Treatment of premenstrual syndrome with Bromocriptine. Acta Endocrinologica (Kbh) 88 (Suppl 216): 165–174

Andersen A N, Larsen J F, Steenstrup O R, Svendstrup B, Nielsen J 1977 Effect of Bromocriptine on the premenstrual syndrome. A double-blind clinical trial. British Journal of Obstetrics and Gynaecology 84(5): 370–374

Appleby B P 1960 A study of premenstrual tension in general practice. British Medical Journal 1: 391–393

Argonz J, Abinzano C 1950 Premenstrual tension treated with vitamin A. Journal of Clinical Endocrinology 10: 1579–1590

Backstrom T, Carstensen H 1974 Oestrogen and progesterone in plasma in relation to premenstrual tension. Journal of Steroid Biochemistry 5: 257–260

Backstrom T, Mattsson B 1975 Correlation of symptoms in premenstrual tension to oestrogen and progesterone concentrations in blood plasma. Neuropsychobiology 1(2): 80–86

Backstrom T, Aakvaag A 1981 Serum prolactin and testerone during the luteal phase in women with premenstrual tension syndrome. Psychoneuroendocrinology 6: 245–251

Backstrom T, Wide L, Sodergard R, Carstensen H 1976 FSH LH TeBG — capacity, oestrogen and progesterone in women with premenstrual tension during the luteal phase. Journal of Steroid Biochemistry 7: 473–476

Backstrom C T, Boyle H, Baird D T 1981 Persistence of symptoms of premenstrual tension in hysterectomized women. British Journal of Obstetrics and Gynaecology 88: 530–536

Baden W F, Lizcano H R 1963 Evaluation of a new diuretic drug (Quinethazone) in the premenstrual tension syndrome. Journal of New Drugs 3: 167–171

Belfer M L, Shader R I, Carroll M 1971 Alcoholism in women. Archives of General Psychiatry 25: 540–544

Benedek-Jaszmann L J, Hearn-Sturtevant M D 1976 Premenstrual tension and functional infertility. Aetiology and treatment. Lancet i: 1095–1098

Billig H E, Spaulding C A 1947 Hyperinsulinism of menses. Industrial Medicine 16: 336–339

Biskind M S 1943 Nutritional deficiency in the aetiology of menorrhagia, cystic mastitis and premenstrual tension; treatment with vitamin B complex. Journal of Clinical Endocrinology 3: 227–234

Block E 1960 The use of vitamin A in premenstrual tension. Acta Obstetricia et Gynaecologica Scandinavica 39: 586–592

Brahams D 1981 Premenstrual Syndrome: A disease of the mind. Lancet ii: 1238–1240

Broughton Pipkin F, Hunter J C, Turner S R, O'Brien P M S 1981 Prostaglandin E_2 attenuates the pressor response to Angiotensin II in pregnant but not in non-pregnant subjects. American Journal of Obstetrics and Gynecology 142: 168–176

Brown J J, Davies D L, Lever A F, Robertson J I S 1964 Variations in plasma renin during the menstrual cycle. British Medical Journal 2: 1114–1115

Bruce J, Russell G F M 1962 Premenstrual tension. A study of weight changes and balances of water, sodium and potassium. Lancet ii: 267–271

Brush M G 1977 The possible mechanisms causing the premenstrual syndrome. Current Medical Research and Opinion 4 (Suppl 4): 9–15

Brush M G 1981 Efamol in the treatment of premenstrual syndrome. Proceedings of first symposium on the clinical uses of Efamol and essential fatty acids. London

Carstairs M W, Talbot D J 1982 A placebo controlled trial of Tenavoid in the management of premenstrual syndrome. British Journal of Clinical Practice 35: 403–409

Charvat J, Holececk V 1966 Studies on antidiuretic hormone. Acta Medica Academica Scientia Hungarica 23: 81–93

Chesley L C, Hellman L M 1957 Variation in body weight and salivary sodium in the menstrual cycle. American Journal of Obstetrics and Gynecology 74: 46–50

Chimbira J H, Cope E, Anderson A B M, Bolton F G 1979 The effects of danazol on menorrhagia, coagulation mechanisms, haematological indices and body weight. British Journal of Obstetrics and Gynaecology 86: 46–50

Coppen A, Kessel N 1963 Menstruation and personality. British Journal of Psychiatry 109: 711–721

Coppen A J, Milne H B, Outram D H, Weber J C P 1969 Dytide, Norethisterone and Placebo in the premenstrual syndrome. Clinical Trials Journal 6: 33–35

Cullberg J 1972 Mood changes and menstrual symptoms with different gestagen/oestrogen combinations. Acta Psychiatrica Scandinavica (Suppl) 236: 1–86

Dalton K 1959 Comparative trial of new oral progestagenic compounds in treatment of premenstrual syndrome. British Medical Journal 2: 1307–1309

Dalton K 1964 The Premenstrual Syndrome. Heinemann, London

Dalton K 1977 The Premenstrual Syndrome and Progesterone Therapy. Heinemann Year Book Medical Publishers, London

Dalton M 1981 Sex hormone-binding globulin concentrations in women with severe premenstrual syndrome. Postgraduate Medical Journal 57: 560–561

Day J B 1979a Clinical trials in the premenstrual syndrome. Current Medical Research and Opinion 6 (Suppl 5): 40–45

Day J 1979b Danazol and the premenstrual syndrome. Postgraduate Medical Journal 55 (Suppl 5): 87–88

Edlundh K O, Jansson B 1966 Pelvic congestion syndrome — a preliminary psychiatric report. Journal of Psychosomatic Research 10: 221–229

Epstein M T, McNeilly A S, Murray M A F, Hockaday T D R 1975 Plasma testosterone and prolactin in the menstrual cycle. Clinical Endocrinology 4: 531–535

Fortin J N, Wittkower E D, Kalz F 1958 A psychosomatic approach to the premenstrual tension syndrome: a preliminary report. Canadian Medical Association Journal 79: 978–981

Frank R T 1931 The hormonal causes of premenstrual tension. Archives of Neurology and Psychiatry 26: 1053–1057

Friesen H G, Hwang P, Guyda H, Tolis G, Tyson J, Myers R 1972 Radioimmunoassay for human prolactin. In: Boyles A R, Griffiths K (eds) Prolactin and Carcinogenesis, p 64. Alpha Omega Alpha Publishing, Cardiff

Ghose K, Coppen A 1977 Bromocriptine and premenstrual syndrome: controlled study. British Medical Journal 1: 147–148

Gillman J 1942 The nature of subjective reactions evoked in women by progesterone with special reference to the problem of premenstrual tension. Journal of Clinical Endocrinology and Metabolism 2: 157–160

Graham J J, Harding P E, Wise P H, Berriman H 1978 Prolactin suppression in the treatment of premenstrual syndrome. Medical Journal of Australia 2(3 Suppl) 2: 18–20

Greenblatt R B, Dmowski W P, Mahesh V B, Scholer H F L 1971 Clinical studies with an antigonadotrophin — Danazol. Fertility and Sterility 22: 102–112

Green R, Dalton K 1953 The premenstrual syndrome. British Medical Journal 1: 1007–1011

Halbreich U 1981 Possible involvement of endorphin withdrawal of imbalance in specific premenstrual syndromes. Medical Hypotheses 7: 1045–1058

Halbreich U, Assael M, Ben-David M, Bornstein R 1976 Serum-prolactin in women with premenstrual syndrome. Lancet ii: 654–656

Harrison P, Letchworth A T 1976 Bromocriptine in the treatment of the premenstrual syndrome, pp 103–105. Proceedings of a symposium held at the Royal College of Physicians, London

Haspels A A 1980 A double-blind, placebo — controlled, multicentre study of the efficacy of dydrogesterone (Duphaston), pp 81–92. Proceedings of a workshop held during the Sixth International Congress of Psychosomatic Obstetrics and Gynaecology, Berlin

Herbert M, Johns M J, Dore C 1976 Factor analysis of analogue scales measuring subjective feelings before and after sleep. British Journal of Medical Psychology 49: 373–379

Herrman W M, Beach R C 1978 Experimental and clinical data indicating the psychotropic properties of progestagens. Postgraduate Medical Journal 54 (Suppl 2): 82–87

Herzberg B, Coppen A 1970 Changes in psychological symptoms in women taking oral contraceptives. British Journal of Psychiatry 116: 161–164

Hippocrates 1950 The Medical Works Of, p 267. Translated by Chadwick J & Mann W N. Blackwell Scientific Publications, Oxford

Hoffman J J 1979 A double blind crossover clinical trial of an OTC diuretic in the treatment of premenstrual tension and weight gain. Current Therapeutic Research 26(5): 575–580

Horrobin D F 1973 Prolactin: Physiology and Clinical Significance. MTP Press, Lancaster

Humke W 1968 In: Wagner K, Wagner H J (eds) Handbuch Der Verkehrs Medizin. Springerverlag, Berlin

Israel S L 1938 Premenstrual tension. Journal of the American Medical Association 110: 1721–1723

Janowsky D S, Berens D C, Davis J M 1973 Correlations between mood, weight and electrolytes during the menstrual cycle: a renin-angiotensin-aldosterone hypothesis of premenstrual tension. Psychosomatic Medicine 35(2): 143–154

Janowsky D S, Gorney R, Castelnuovo-Tedesco P, Stone C B 1969 Premenstrual — menstrual increases in psychiatric hospital admission rates. American Journal of Obstetrics and Gynecology 103: 189–191

Jenner F A, Gjessing L R, Cox J R, Davies-Jones A, Hullin R J, Hanna S M 1967 A manic depressive psychotic with a persistent 48-hour cycle. British Journal of Psychiatry 113: 895–910

Johansson E D 1971 Depression of the progesterone levels in women treated with synthetic gestagens after ovulation. Acta Endocrinologica 68: 779–792

Jones E M, Fox R H, Verow P W, Asscher A W 1966 Variations in capillary permeability to plasma proteins during the menstrual cycle. Journal of Obstetrics and Gynaecology of the British Commonwealth 73: 666–669

Jordon V C, Pokoly T B 1977 Steroid and prostaglandin relations during the menstrual cycle. Obstetrics and Gynaecology 49(4): 449–453

Jordheim O 1972 The premenstrual syndrome. Clinical trials of treatment with a progestogen combined with diuretic compared with both a progesterone alone and with a placebo. Acta Obstetricia et Gynaecologica Scandinavica 51: 77–80

Jungck E C, Barfield W E, Greenblatt R E 1959 Chlorothiazide and premenstrual tension. Journal of the American Medical Association 169(2): 112–114

Katz F H, Romfh P 1972 Plasma aldosterone and renin activity during the menstrual cycle. Journal of Clinical Endocrinology and Metabolism 34: 819–821

Kerr G D, Day J B, Munday M R, Brush M G, Watson M, Taylor R W 1980 Dydrogesterone in the treatment of the premenstrual syndrome. Practitioner 224: 852–855

Kindahl H, Granstrom E, Edquist L E et al 1976 Prostaglandin levels in peripheral plasma during the reproductive cycle. Advances in Prostaglandin and Thromboxane Research 2: 667–671

Klein L and Carey J 1957 Total exchangeable sodium in the menstrual cycle. American Journal of Obstetrics and Gynecology 74: 956–967

Kramer H 1962 A long acting diuretic suitable for outpatient treatment of fluid retention on oedema of pregnancy and the premenstrual tension syndrome. African Medical Journal 36: 4–6

Kutner S J, Brown W L 1972 Types of oral contraceptives, depression and premenstrual symptoms. Journal of Nervous and Mental Diseases 155: 153–162

Landau R L, Lugibihl K 1961 The catabolic and natriuretic effects or progesterone in man. Recent Progress in Hormone Research 17: 249–292

Landauer A A 1974 Choice decision time and the menstrual cycle. Practitioner 213: 703–706

Leader 1981 Premenstrual syndrome. Lancet ii: 1393–1394

McGiff J C, Crowshaw K, Itskovitz H D 1974 Prostaglandins and renal function. Federation Proceedings 33(1): 39–47

MacGregor G A, Roulston J E, Markandu N D, Jones J C, de Wardener H E 1979 Is 'idiopathic' oedema idopathic? Lancet i: 397–400

MacKinnon P C B and Mackinnon I L 1956 Hazards of the menstrual cycle. British Medical Journal 1: 555

McNeilly A S, Chard T 1974 Circulating levels of prolactin during the the menstrual cycle. Clinical Endocrinology 3: 105–112

Macht D I 1943 Further historical and experimental studies on menstrual toxin. American Journal of Medical Science 206: 281–305

Mansel R E, Preece P E, Hughes L E 1978 A double blind trial of the prolactin inhibitor bromocriptine in painful benign breast disease. British Journal of Surgery 65: 724–727

Mansel R E, Wisbey J R, Hughes L E 1979 The use of Danazol in the treatment of painful benign breast disease: preliminary results. Postgraduate Medical Journal 55 (Suppl 5): 61–65

Mattson B, Van Schoulz B 1974 A comparison between lithium, placebo and a diuretic in premenstrual tension. Acta Psychiatricia Scandinavica (Suppl) 255: 75–84

Michelakis A M, Yoshida H, Dormis J C 1975 Plasma renin activity and plasma aldosterone during the normal menstrual cycle. American Journal of Obstetrics and Gynecology 123: 724–726

Moos R H 1968 The development of a menstrual distress questionnaire. Psychosomatic Medicine 30: 853–867

Moos R H 1969a Menstrual distress questionnaire preliminary manual. Department of Psychiatry Stanford University School of Medicine, Stanford, California

Moos R H 1969b A typology of menstrual cycle symptoms. American Journal of Obstetrics and Gynecology 103: 390–402

Morris N M, Udry J R 1972 Contraceptive pills and the day-to-day feelings of well-being. American Journal of Obstetrics and Gynecology 113: 763–765

Morton J H 1950 Premenstrual tension. American Journal of Obstetrics and Gynecology 60: 343–352

Munday M 1977 Progesterone and aldosterone levels in the premenstrual tension syndrome. Journal of Endocrinology 73(3): 21–22

Munday M R, Brush M G, Taylor R W 1981 Correlates between progesterone, oestradiol and aldosterone levels in the premenstrual syndrome. Clinical Endocrinology 14: 1–9

O'Brien P M S 1979 Endocrine changes in premenstrual syndrome. M.D. Thesis, University of Wales

O'Brien P M S, Faratian B, Gaspar A, Johnson I, Filshie G M 1982 Quantification of premenstrual syndrome. Xth International Congress of Obstetrics and Gynaecology

O'Brien P M S, Craven D, Selby C, Symonds E M 1979 Treatment of premenstrual syndrome by spironolactone. British Journal of Obstetrics and Gynaecology 86: 142–147

O'Brien P M S, Filshie G M, Broughton Pipkin F 1977 The effect of prostaglandin E_2 on the cardiovascular response to AII in pregnant rabbits. Prostaglandins 13: 171–181

O'Brien P M S, Selby C, Symonds E M 1980 Progesterone, fluid and electrolytes in premenstrual syndrome. British Medical Journal 280: 1161–1163

O'Brien P M S, Symonds E M 1982 Prolactin levels in the premenstrual syndrome. British Journal of Obstetrics and Gynaecology 89: 306–308

Okey R, Stewart D 1933 Diet and blood cholesterol in normal women. Journal of Biological Chemistry 99: 717–727

Parker A S 1960 The premenstrual tension syndrome. Medical Clinics of North America 44: 339–348

Peninngton V M 1957 Meprobamate (Miltown) in premenstrual tension. Journal of American Medical Association 164: 638–640

Perrini A, Pilego N 1959 The increases of aldosterone in premenstrual tension. Minerva Medicine 50: 2897–2899

Piton R 1979 Evaluation of Dydrogesterone in the treatment of the premenstrual syndrome. Ars Medici 8: 1785–1794

Preece P E, Mansel R E 1981 Management of breast pain using Efamol. Proceedings of first symposium on the clinical uses of Efamol and essential fatty acids. London

Preece P E, Mansel P E, Bolton P M, Hughes L E, Baum M, Gravell I H 1976 Clinical syndromes of mastalgia. Lancet ii: 670–673

Redgrove J A 1971 In: Colquhoun W P (ed) Biological Rhythms and Human Performance. Academic Press, London

Rees L 1953a Psychosomatic aspects of the premenstrual tension syndrome. Journal of Mental Science 99: 62–73

Rees L 1953b The premenstrual syndrome and its treatment. British Medical Journal pp 1014–1016

Reeves B D, Garvin J E, McElin T W 1971 Premenstrual tension: symptoms and weight changes related to potassium therapy. American Journal of Obstetrics and Gynecology 109: 1036–1041

Reich M 1962 Variations in urinary aldosterone levels of normal females during their menstrual cycle. Annals of Medicine 1: 41–49

Reid R L, Yen S S C 1981 Premenstrual syndrome. American Journal of Obstetrics and Gynecology 139: 85–104

Robertson J I S, Weir R J, Dusterdiek G O, Fraser R, Tree M 1971 Renin, Angiotensin and Aldosterone in human pregnancy and the menstrual cycle. Scottish Medical Journal 16: 183–196

Robinson K, Huntington K, Wallace M G 1977 Treatment of the premenstrual syndrome. British Journal of Obstetrics and Gynaecology 84: 784–788

Romanini C, Liverani A, Arduini D, Lafuenti G, Manfredi L 1979 Nuove osservazioni sul trattamento di sindromi premestruali associate a dismenorrea con 6-diedro-retro-progesterone. Annali Di Ostetricia, Ginecologia Medicina Perinatale (Milano) 100: 250–265

Rosseinsky D R, Hall P G 1974 An evolutionary theory of premenstrual tension (letter). Lancet ii: 1024

Royal College of General Practitioners 1974 Oral Contraceptives and Health. Pitman Medical, London

Ruble D N 1977 Premenstrual symptoms: a reinterpretation. Science 197: 291–292

Sampson G A 1979 Premenstrual syndrome: a double-blind controlled trial of progesterone and placebo. British Journal of Psychiatry 135: 209–215

Sampson G A, Jenner F A 1977 Studies of daily recordings from the Moos' menstrual distress questionnaire. British Journal of Psychiatry 130: 265–271

Sampson G, Prescott P 1981 The assessment of the symptoms of premenstrual syndrome and their response to therapy. British Journal of Psychiatry 138: 399–405

Silbergeld S, Brast N, Noble E P 1971 The menstrual cycle: a double blind study of symptoms, mood and behaviour, and biochemical variable using enovid and placebo. Psychosomatic Medicine 33: 411–428

Simkin B, and Acre R 1963 Prolactin activity in blood during the normal human menstrual cycle. Proceedings of the Society for Experimental and Biological Medicine 113: 485–488

Singer K, Cheng R, Schou M 1974 A controlled evaluation of lithium in the premenstrual syndrome. British Journal of Psychiatry 124: 50–51

Skinner S L, Lumbers E R, Symonds E M 1969 Alteration by oral contraceptives of normal menstrual changes in plasma renin activity, concentration and subtrate. Clinical Science 36: 67–76

Slade P. Jenner F A 1980 Performance tests at different phases of the menstrual cycle. Journal of Psychosomatic Research 24: 5–8

Sletten I W and Gershon S 1966 The premenstrual syndrome: a discussion of its pathophysiology and treatment with lithium ion. Comprehensive Psychiatry 7: 197–206

Smith S L 1975 Mood and the menstrual cycle 19–58 In: Sachar E J (ed) Topics in psychoendocrinology, pp 19–58. Grune and Stratton, New York

Stieglitz M D. Kimble S T 1949 Premenstrual intoxication. American Journal of Medical Science 218: 616–623

Stokes J, Mendels J 1972 Pyridoxine and premenstrual tension. Lancet i: 1177–1178

Strecker J R 1980 An explorative study into the clinical effects of dydrogesterone in the treatment of premenstrual syndrome. In Proceedings of a workshop held during the Sixth International Congress of Psychosomatic Obstetrics and Gynaecology, Berlin, pp 71–79

Studd J W W, Nagos A L 1983 Management of the premenstrual syndrome by subcutaneous implants of oestradiol. Proceedings of 23rd British Congress of Obstetrics and Gynaecology, Birmingham

Sundsford J A, Aakvaag A 1970 Plasma angiotensin II and aldosterone excretion during the menstrual cycle. Acta Endocrinologica (Kobenhavn) 64: 452–458

Sundsford J A, Aakvaag A 1972 Plasma renin activity, plasma renin substrate and urinary aldosterone excretion in the menstrual cycle in relation to the concentration of progesterone and oestrogens in the plasma. Acta Endocrinologica 71: 519–529

Sutherland H and Stewart I 1965 A critical analysis of the premenstrual syndrome. Lancet i: 1180–1183

Sweeney J S 1934 Menstrual oedema. Journal of the American Medical Association 103: 234–236

Swyer G I M 1955 Treatment of premenstrual tension syndrome: value of ethisterone, mephenesin and a placebo compared. British Medical Journal 1: 1410–1414

Taylor R W 1977 The treatment of premenstrual syndrome with dydrogesterone ('Duphaston'). Current Medical Research and Opinion 4 (Suppl 4): 35–40

Taylor R W, James C E 1979 The clinician's view of patients with premenstrual syndrome. Current Medical Research and Opinion 6 (Suppl 5): 46–51

Thorn G W, Nelson K R, Thorn D W 1938 Study of mechanism of oedema associated with menstruation. Endocrinology 22: 155–163

Vekemans M, Delvoye P, L'Hermite M, Robyn C 1977 Serum prolactin levels during the menstrual cycle. Journal of Clinical Endocrinology and Metabolism 44: 989–993

Werch A, Kane R E 1976 Treatment of premenstrual tension with metolazone: A double blind evaluation of a new diuretic. Current Therapeutic Research 19: 565–572

Wong W H, Freedman R, Levan N E, Hyman C, Quilligan E J 1972 Changes in the capillary filtration coefficient of cutaneous vessels in women with premenstrual tension. American Journal of Obstetrics and Gynecology 114: 950–953

Wood C, Jakubowicz D 1980 The treatment of premenstrual symptoms with mefenamic acid. British Journal of Obstetrics and Gynaecology 87: 627–630

Zondek B, Bromberg Y M 1945 Endocrine allergy; allergic sensitivity to endogenous hormones. Journal of Allergy 16: 1–16

Oral contraceptives, vaginal rings and pregnancy interception

ORAL CONTRACEPTIVES

Soon after oral steroid contraceptives (OCs) became available for use by women, they rapidly became the most widely used method of contraception in developed countries among both married and unmarried women. The main reasons for the popularity of this method of contraception were ease of administration combined with an extremely high rate of effectiveness. Although accompanying side-effects which did not endanger the women's health, such as nausea, breakthrough bleeding, and breast tenderness, were not uncommon, serious side-effects, such as thromboembolism, were relatively rare. Thus, by 1965, OCs were used by an estimated 28.4 per cent of white married women in the United States practising contraception. This incidence had risen to 35.4 per cent by 1970 and remained at that level until 1975 (Westoff & Jones, 1977). In that year it was estimated that OCs were used by about 35 per cent of married women in the US utilising contraception. However, in 1975 articles began to appear in the British medical literature, linking use of OCs to an increased risk of fatal myocardial infarction and other fatal vascular diseases. In the same year the use of exogenous oestrogens was reported to be causally related to development of carcinoma of the endometrium when given in large dosages for a prolonged period of time to postmenopausal women. As women were aware that OCs also contained oestrogen, they were concerned that those formulations were also carcinogenic. Furthermore, the results of the scientific articles in the British literature, were frequently misinterpreted by lay writers who then wrote articles exaggerating the hazards of OCs which appeared in magazines read by consumers.

As a result of the risks of OCs being exaggerated to the consumer, retail sales of OCs have steadily declined in the US since 1975. Between 1975 and 1981, there was an estimated 40 per cent reduction in sales of OCs in the US.

Women have three major concerns about OCs. These are: (1) an increased risk of developing cancer; (2) problems with future childbearing and (3) an increase chance of developing heart attacks and stroke. These concerns are mostly unwarranted as the following discussion indicates.

Cancer

A thorough review of the literature reveals that there is absolutely no evidence in the 22 years of study since OCs were introduced that their use increases the risk of any type of cancer including breast cancer, cancer of the uterus, cancer of the cervix and cancer of the liver. Three large prospective studies of OC users were started in 1968, two in Great Britain — the Royal College of General Practitioners Study (RCGP) and the Oxford Family Planning Study — and one in the United States — the Walnut Creek Study. The latter was conducted under the auspices of the National Institutes of Health. Each of these studies compared large groups of women using OCs with a similar number of control women using other methods of contraception. To date, in none of these studies has there been found to be an increased risk of any type of cancer RCGP, (Vessey et al, 1976, 1974; The Walnut Creek Study, 1981).

Breast cancer. At the present time, the women using OCs in these and other studies do not have a higher incidence of breast cancer than a control group of women of similar age who are using other methods of contraception (Vessey et al 1979a; Kelsey et al, 1978).

Concern that OCs may increase the risk of breast cancer has arisen because oestrogens are known to stimulate normal breast tissue, and in women who already have cancer of the breast, oestrogens can stimulate growth of the malignant tissue. There is no evidence in humans, however, that oestrogens can initiate the development of cancer from normal breast tissue. Furthermore, OCs contain a progestogen in addition to the oestrogen, and the progestogen counteracts the stimulatory action of the oestrogen on target tissues. For this reason, women ingesting OCs have a lower incidence of non-malignant cystic disease of the breast than do controls (Ory et al, 1976; Brinton et al, 1981).

A recent multicentre epidemiological study performed

in the United States has shown there is no increased risk of breast cancer in any particular subgroup of OC users, such as those with a family histroy of breast cancer, those with and without benign breast disease, as well as those starting OCs before their first pregnancy. Furthermore, there was no change in risk of breast cancer with increasing duration of OC use of time since last OC use (Kaufman et al, 1980).

Endometrial cancer. There is no evidence that an increased incidence of carcinoma of the endometrium occurs in OC users. As a matter of fact several recently published epidemiological studies indicate that women who are using OCs are less likely to develop cancer of the endometrium than are a control group of women who do not use OCs (Kaufman et al, 1980; Weiss & Sayvetz, 1980; Hulka et al, 1982). The mistaken belief that OCs may increase the incidence of cancer of the uterus arose because of findings suggesting that postmenopausal women who were taking large doses of oestrogen without progestogen for more than 5 years had an increased incidence of cancer of the endometrium when compared to postmenopausal women who did not take oestrogen. OCs contain oestrogen, but they also contain a progestogen, and the progestogen counteracts the stimulatory effect of the oestrogen on the endometrium. For oestrogen to cause growth of the endometrium it has to react with a receptor protein in the endometrial cell. Progestogens inhibit the synthesis of these oestrogen receptors and thus, when given with an oestrogen, prevent the growth-promoting action of the oestrogen. When progestogens are given with oestrogen to postmenopausal women, they also do not have an increased incidence of endometrial cancer (Gambrell et al, 1979).

Cervical cancer. There is no evidence from any epidemiological study that users of OCs have an increased incidence of cancer of the cervix. In some studies OC users have been found to have an increased incidence of dysplasia of the cervix (including carcinoma *in situ*), compared to controls using other methods of contraception (Harris et al, 1980). Dysplasia of the cervix has also been linked with onset of sexual intercourse at a young age and with multiple sexual partners. Thus, women who began having sexual intercourse while young teenagers and have had a large number of sexual partners have a greater chance of developing dysplasia of the cervix than women with fewer sexual partners. In the studies in which OC users were found to have a higher incidence of dysplasia than the controls, it was also found that the OC users had more sexual partners and had intercourse at a younger age than did the controls who used other methods of contraception. Thus, the studies did not determine that the increased incidence of dysplasia was due to use of the OCs, but that they most likely were due to other factors, including more sexual partners, more frequent cytologic screening and increased protection by those in the control group who used diaphragms or condoms.

Liver cancer. Cancer of the liver is very uncommon in young women, and women using OCs do not have a greater chance of developing this rare cancer (Murphy, 1977). Women using OCs for more than 5 years apparently have a greater chance of developing benign liver adenomas. These benign liver tumors gradually decrease in size and eventually disappear after OCs are discontinued. Thus, these adenomas, which occur in only about one in 50 000 OC users, are temporary and do not become malignant.

Pregnancy after discontinuing use of oral contraceptives

Although the rate of return of fertility after stopping OCs in both nulligravid and nulliparous women is delayed when compared to women who stop using other methods of contraception, such as the diaphragm or IUD, eventually the percentage of women who conceive after stopping all methods is the same (Vessey et al, 1979c). Thus, although OCs produce a period of temporary infertility in some women after their discontinuation, this infertility is usually not permanent. After a 2–3 year interval, fertility rates equalise between former OC users and former users of other methods of contraception.

The spontaneous abortion rate in women who conceive in the first or subsequent months after stopping OCs is the same as the spontaneous abortion rate in the general population or that in women who stop using other contraceptive methods (Vessey et al, 1979b). There was one study which reported a high incidence of lethal chromosomal abnormalities in abortuses of women who conceived within a few months after stopping OCs. However, more recent studies have shown that abortuses of women who did not use OCs had the same incidence of these chromosomal abnormalities.

Several studies of large numbers of babies born to women who stopped using OCs have been undertaken. These studies show that these infants have no greater chance of being born with any type of birth defect (Rothman & Lovik, 1978). The incidence of congenital anomalies was the same in babies born to women who had previously used OCs as in babies born to women who had previously used other methods of contraception or women who had not used any method of contraception.

Cardiovascular disease

One of the problems with the epidemiological studies performed to determine risks of drugs producing disease is that they provide a figure called a relative risk or 'times' rate. For example, in studies of OCs it has been stated that myocardial infarction (MI) occurs three times more frequently in OC users than non-users. Nevertheless, because young women rarely develop an MI, in terms of absolute risk the chance of any one women developing the disease is extremely low. Although the relative risk figure may frighten an individual, the absolute risk figure is more important. As an example, the relative risk of dying in an airplane crash is much higher if one flies frequently. Nevertheless, many people fly frequently because the absolute risk is so low. The three prospective studies of OC users mentioned above, which have been in progress for more than 10 years, indicate that the absolute risk of any OC user developing cardiovascular disease is very low. In the United States and Britain death rates for heart attacks have decreased in women aged 20–45 during the past 15 years, years in which OC use increased dramatically. Furthermore, the decrease in heart attack death rates in these countries has been similar for men and women. If OCs, which are used by about 35 per cent of women of this age group were responsible for a great increase in the number of fatal heart attacks, one would expect that the decline in mortality rates would be different between men and women during this time period. Furthermore, analysis of the latest results from these studies indicates that a significantly increased risk of developing cardiovascular disease occurs only in current OC users over 35 years of age who smoke or those of any age who use OCs and also have some type of pre-existing vascular disease, such as hypertension, diabetes or hypercholesterolemia (Tables 33.1 and 33.2) (The Walnut Creek Study, 1981; RCGP Study, 1981). There is no reliable evidence that non-smokers under the age of 40 and smokers under 35 who use OCs have an increased chance of dying from a heart attack provided they have no other vascular disease. Thus, if a woman is under 35 and is a cigarette smoker, she can still use OCs. Likewise, a woman between 35 and 40 can continue to use OCs provided she does not smoke cigarettes or have any other type of vascular disease such as hypertension, diabetes or hypercholesterolaemia.

Data from a recent study in the US provides confirmation for these recommendations. In this study morbidity of more than 10 000 OC healthy users and 30 000 healthy controls was analysed for the 3-year period 1977–1979. During the time of study none of these women developed a heart attack. No OC user and seven controls

Table 33.1 Circulatory mortality by age and smoking

Age	Ever-users	Controls	R.R.
15–25 N.S.	0.0 (0)	0.0 (0)	—
Smok.	10.5 (1)	0.0 (0)	—
25–34 N.S.	4.4 (2)	2.7 (1)	1.6
Smok.	14.2 (6)	4.2 (1)	3.4
35–44 N.S.	21.5 (7)	6.4 (2)	3.3
Smok.	63.4 (18)	15.2 (3)	4.2*
45 N.S.	52.4 (1)	11.4 (1)	4.6
Smok.	206.7 (17)	27.9 (2)	7.4†

* Risk ~ 1/2000 year   † Risk ~ 1/500 year

From Royal College of General Practitioners' Oral Contraception Study. Further analysis of mortality in oral contraceptive users. Lancet i: 541, 1981.

Table 33.2 Walnut Creek Study — diseases of the circulatory system

	Standardised rates			R.R.	
	Never	Current	Past	Current	Past
Acute MI	0.23	0.27	0.20	1.1	0.8
Ischaemic HD	0.74	1.09	0.90	1.4	1.1
Subarachnoid hem.	0.04	0.03	0.10	2.3*	10.1
Cerebral thrombosis	0.24	0.53	0.29	2.2*	1.2
Arterial thrombosis	0.24	0.76	0.24	3.2*	1.0
Pulmonary embolism	0.38	0.22	0.29	0.6	0.0
Thrombophlebitis	0.51	0.42	0.48	0.8	1.8

* Not significant overall. RR increased only in smokers > 40.

From Ramcharan S, Pellegrin F A, Ray R M et al 1980 The Walnut Creek Contraceptive Drug Study. Journal of Reproductive Medicine 25 (Suppl): 346.

Table 33.2a Non-fatal vascular disease Group's Health Cooperative Puget Sound 1977–1979

	Non OC users	OC users	R.R.
Woman years	105 284	36 428	
Venous thrombosis	3	7	8.3
M.I.	0	0	
Stroke	7	0	
(Stroke c̄ disease)	(11)	(3)	

From Porter J B et al 1982 Obstetrics and Gynecology 59: 299

suffered a stroke (Table 33.2) (Porter et al, 1982). Among the women with medical disease such as treated hypertension or diabetes, three OC users and II non-OC users developed a stroke.

A few years ago there was concern that women should not use OCs for more than 5 years as analysis of mortality data from women enrolled in the RCGP Study suggested that there was an increased risk of dying from cardiovascular disease in women who had used OCs for more than 5 years (RCGP Study, 1977). Recent data from the same study indicate that this concern was not valid as the incidence of deaths from cardiovacular disease did not increase with increased duration of OC use (Table 33.3) (RCGP Study 1981). This information, together with data from many other epidemiological studies which show no increase in deaths from cardiovascular disease in former users of OC, indicates that the cause of myocardial infarction or stroke in OC users is due to arterial thrombosis, not

Table 33.3 Circulatory mortality by duration of OC use

Years	Rate (No)	R.R.
< 2	32.5 (5)	4.6
2–4	23.5 (4)	3.4
4–6	28.4 (5)	4.1
6–8	32.5 (5)	4.6
>8	20.1 (4)	2.9

From Royal College of General Practitioners' Oral Contraception Study. Further analysis of mortality in oral contraceptive users. Lancet i: 541, 1981.

atherosclerosis. These arterial thromboses occur mainly in women who have arterial narrowing produced by cigarette smoking or other arterial disease such as that caused by hypertension, diabetes or hypercholesterolaemia. There is no evidence that long-term use of OCs produces a permanent harmful effect on the blood vessels such as development of atherosclerosis. Thus, women can take OCs for an unlimited time period no matter how old they are when they start taking it. In addition, there is no evidence that there is need for a rest period after a few years of OC use. A rest period does not serve any value.

Other concerns

Other concerns about taking OCs that have proved to be untrue are the belief that women need to take vitamin supplements because the OCs produce vitamin deficiency. Although OCs do lower the blood levels of the B-complex vitamins and vitamin C, these low vitamin levels are not accompanied by any clinical evidence of vitamin deficiency and vitamin supplementation is not necessary. There has also been concern that OCs should not be prescribed to young teenagers as their use might cause permanent changes in their hypothalamic-pituitary-ovarian axis as well as produce premature epiphyseal closure and cause them to stop growing. Both these concerns have proved to be unfounded and OCs can be used by women of any age who have started to have regular menstrual cycles. Finally, there has been concern that OCs should not be taken by women who developed morphological alterations in their vagina and uterus due to exposure to diethylstilbestrol during fetal life. There is no evidence that when OCs are ingested by women with adenosis or other genital tract changes due to antenatal DES exposure that there is an increase in cancer or other harmful alterations. Therefore, OCs can be used safely by these women.

Adverse effects

It is important to realise that the OCs do produce certain adverse effects, although the incidence of these effects has been exaggerated. Fortunately, in most instances the more common adverse effects are relatively mild. The majority are produced by the oestrogenic component of the formulation, while the rest are produced by the progestin component alone or by a combination of the two. The most frequent symptoms produced by the oestrogenic component include nausea, breast tenderness, and fluid retention, which usually does not exceed 3–4 lb of body weight.

The synthetic oestrogen, ethinyl oestradiol, used in OCs causes an increase in hepatic production of several globulins and the amount of increase is related to the dosage of oestrogen in the OC formulation. One of the globulins, angiotensinogen, may cause an increase in hypertension. Others are involved in blood clotting and may cause an increase in venous thrombosis. Although a small percentage of women taking OCs will develop an increase in their blood pressure, this elevation is temporary and will disappear when the medication is stopped. Likewise, alterations in glucose metabolism, which are also produced by the oestrogen component, are only temporary and disappear when OC use is discontinued. There is no evidence that OC use produces diabetes mellitus or permanent hypertension.

Another adverse effect produced by the oestrogen is changes in mood and depression produced by diversion of tryptophan metabolism from its minor pathway in the brain to its major pathway in the liver. The end product of tryptophan metabolism, serotonin, is thus decreased in the central nervous system. The resultant lowering of serotonin can produce depression in some women and sleepiness and mood changes in others. This is a reversible symptom that fortunately is not too common and disappears when the OCs are stopped. The incidence of all these oestrogenic side-effects is much lower now than a decade ago because the formulations in use today contain only one-fifth as much oestrogen as the formulations that were used in the 1960s.

The progestogens, because they are structurally related to testosterone, produce certain anabolic adverse effects. These include weight gain and acne and a symptom perceived by some women as nervousness. Some women gain a considerable amount of weight when they take OCs, and this is produced by the anabolic effects of the progestin component. Although oestrogens decrease sebum production, progestins increase sebum production and can cause acne to develop and/or worsen. Thus, patients who have acne should be given a formulation with a low progestin/oestrogen ratio. The final symptom produced by the gestogenic component is failure of withdrawal bleeding or amenorrhoea. Because the progestins decrease the oestrogen receptors in the endometrium, endometrial growth is decreased, and some women have failure of withdrawal bleeding. Although this symptom is not important medically, since bleeding serves as a signal that the patient is not pregnant, it is desirable to have some amount of periodic withdrawal bleeding during the days the woman is not taking these steroids. Finally, both the oestrogen and progestin formulations can act together to produce irregular bleeding and/or chloasma. Breakthrough bleeding which is usually produced by not enough oestrogen or too much progestin or a combination of both can be alleviated by increasing the amount of oestrogen in the formulation or by switching to a more oestrogenic formulation. The symptom of chloasma, pigmentation of the malar eminences, is accentuated by sunlight and usually takes a long time to disappear after OCs are stopped.

In addition to these more common adverse effects, there is an increased risk of developing more serious problems which can lead to death or severe morbidity. The most common of these more serious adverse effects produced by OCs is cholelithiasis, which is increased about 2-fold compared to its incidence in controls. However, the absolute increased incidence is small, estimated to be about 1/1500–1/2000 women annually (RCGP Study, 1974). The risk of developing deep vein thrombophlebitis is also increased about 3–4 times, as is the risk of developing thromboembolism. However, the absolute incidence of these disorders, which are not necessarily related (i.e. patients with thromboembolism do not have to have clinical symptoms of thrombophlebitis), is of the order of about 1/10 000 users annually for thrombophlebitis and about 1/30 000 users annually for thromboembolism. OCs probably increase the incidence of thrombotic and possibly haemorrhagic stroke, although the epidemiological data are conflicting. Although the relative risk is possibly increased about three times, the actual incidence remains quite low, about 1/20 000 to 1/30 000 users/year. As mentioned above, benign liver adenomas occur very rarely in OC users, with an estimated frequency of about 1/30 000 to 1/50 000 users/year. The incidence is increased in women who have used the formulations for more than 5 years. In addition, although there is epidemiological evidence that women over 35 who smoke or have other associated risk factors, such as hypertension or hypercholesterolaemia, have an increased risk of developing myocardial infarction with OC use, the actual risk of developing myocardial infarction is very low.

Contraindications to oral contraceptive use

OCs can be prescribed for the majority of women in the reproductive age group because they are young and healthy; however, there are certain absolute contraindications for their use. These include a present and past history of vascular disease, including thromboembolism, thrombophlebitis, atherosclerosis, stroke, or systemic vascular disease, such as lupus erythematosus or haemoglobin SS disease. In addition, hypertension, diabetes mellitus, and hyperlipidaemia are contraindications to OCs, as use of these agents in women with these disorders can increase the risk of the patient developing a stroke or myocardial infarction. One of the contraindications for OC use listed by the United States Food and Drug Administration is cancer of the breast or endometrium, although there are no data indicating OCs are harmful in women with these diseases. In addition, patients who are pregnant should not ingest OCs because of the masculinising effect of the progestogens on the external genitalia of the female fetus. Patients with heart disease should use OCs with caution since the fluid retention produced by these agents could produce congestive heart failure. Finally, patients with active liver disease should not receive OCs, since the steroids are metabolised in this organ. However, patients who have had liver disease in the past but whose liver function tests have returned to normal can receive these agents. Relative contraindications

to OC use include heavy cigarette smoking, migraine headaches, amenorrhoea, and depression. Migraine headaches can be made worse by OC use, and patients who develop a stroke while taking OCs usually have an increased incidence of headaches of the migraine type, fainting, loss of vision or speech, or paraesthesias prior to development of the CVA. If any of these symptoms develop in OC users, the patient should stop ingesting these agents. Patients who are amenorrhoeic for a cause other than polycystic ovarian syndrome should probably not receive OCs, as they may have a pituitary microadenoma. OC use will mask the symptoms of both amenorrhoea and galactorrhoea, which are the symptoms produced by enlargement of the adenoma. Anyone who develops galactorrhoea while taking OCs should stop these agents, and after 2 weeks, a serum prolactin level should be measured. If the prolactin is elevated, further diagnostic evaluation, such as X-rays of the sella turcica, are indicated (Ch. 25).

Beginning oral contraceptives

Adolescents. In deciding whether the pubertal, sexually active girl should use OCs for contraception, the clinician should be more concerned about compliance in this age group than possible physiological harm. Provided the postmenarcheal girl has demonstrated maturity of the hypothalamic-pituitary-ovarian axis by having at least three regular, presumably ovulatory, cycles, it is safe to prescribe OCs without being concerned about causing permanent damage to the reproductive process. It is probably best not to prescribe OCs to women of any age with oligomenorrhoea because of the increased likelihood of their developing post-pill amenorrhoea, and oligomenorrhoea is more frequent in adolescence than later in life. One need not be concerned about accelerating epiphyseal closure in the postmenarcheal female. Their endogenous oestrogens have already initiated the process a few years prior to menarche and the contraceptive steroids will not hasten epiphyseal closure.

Following pregnancy. There is a difference in the relationship of the return of ovulation and bleeding in the postabortal woman and in the woman who has had a term delivery. The first episode of menstrual bleeding in the postabortal woman is usually preceded by ovulation. Following a term delivery, the first episode of bleeding is usually, but not always, anovulatory. Ovulation occurs sooner after an abortion, usually between 2 and 4 weeks, than after a term delivery, when ovulation is usually delayed beyond 6 weeks but may occur 4–5 weeks after delivery.

Thus after spontaneous or induced abortion of a fetus of less than 12 weeks' gestation, OCs should be started immediately to prevent conception following the first ovulation. For patients who have a delivery after 28 weeks of gestation and are not nursing, the combination pills should be initiated 2 weeks after delivery. If the termination of pregnancy occurs between 21 and 28 weeks, contraceptive steroids should be started 1 week later. The reason for delay in the latter instances is that the normally increased risk of thromboembolism occurring postpartum may be further enhanced with steroid ingestion. As the first ovulation is delayed for a period of at least 4 weeks, there is no need to expose the patient to this increased risk.

It is best for women who are nursing not to use OCs as their use diminishes the amount of milk. Women who are breast feeding every 4 hours, including the nightime, will not ovulate until at least 10 weeks after delivery and thus do not need contraception before that time.

All patients. At the initial visit, after a history and physical examination have determined that there are no medical contraindications for oral contraceptives, the patient should be informed about the benefits and risks. It is best to use a written informed consent.

Type of formulation

In determining which formulation to use, it is probably best to initially prescribe a formulation with 30 μg or 35 μg ethinyl oestradiol. A recent study from Great Britain indicated that the incidence of total deaths as well as death due to arterial causes alone was significantly decreased in patients using formulations with 30 μg ethinyl oestradiol compared with those using formulations of 50 μg ethinyl oestradiol (Table 33.4) (Mead et al, 1980). Furthermore, the incidence of ischaemic heart disease and stroke was also significantly decreased in women using the lower dose oestrogen formulations. It should be mentioned that mestranol, a component of many 50 μg formulations, is about 1.7 times less potent than ethinyl oestradiol, and there is no evidence that formulations with 50 μg mestranol are less harmful than those with a lower dose of ethinyl oestradiol. Few randomised studies have been performed comparing the different marketed formulations, and therefore the clinician has to decide which of the many formulations available is best for the majority of his

Table 33.4 Observed: expected ratios for specified events at different doses of ethinyloestradiol 1974–1977

	Ethinyloestradiol (μg)		
	30	50	X^2_1
Deaths	0.59	1.46	9.58
Non-venous	0.53	1.52	6.09
Venous	0.65	1.40	3.67
Non-venous events			
Stroke	0.82	1.20	2.64
Ischaemic heart disease	0.54	1.48	8.97

From Meade T W, Greenberg G, Thompson S G 1980 Progestogens and cardiovascular reactions associated with oral contraceptives and a comparison of the safety of 50– and 30–μg oestrogen preparations. British Medical Journal 1: 1157.

patients. Unless acne is present there is no evidence that some patients do better with formulations that are more oestrogenic while other patients do better with formulations that are more gestagenic. Until large-scale comparative studies are performed, the clinician has to decide which formulation to use based on which formulations have the least adverse effects among patients in his practice.

Follow-up

If the patient has no contraindication to OC use, the only routine laboratory tests indicated are a complete blood count, urinalysis and Pap smear. At the end of 3 months, the patient should be seen again; at this time a non-directed history should be obtained and the blood pressure measured. After this visit the patient should be seen annually, at which time a non-directed history should again be taken, blood pressure and body weight measured, and a physical examination, including a breast, abdominal, and pelvic examination (including a Pap smear), performed. The routine use of other laboratory tests is not indicated unless the patient is over 35 or has a family history of diabetes or vascular disease. For patients over 35 who wish to continue taking OCs, it is advisable to obtain a lipid panel, including HDL and LDL cholesterol, total cholesterol and triglycerides. If the lipid levels are abnormal, the OCs should be stopped. In addition, because of the increased incidence of diabetes after age 35, a 2-hour postprandial blood glucose should be obtained; if this is elevated, a full glucose tolerance test should be performed. If results of this test are abnormal, the OCs should be stopped. Routine use of these tests in women under 35 is not indicated because the incidence of positive results is extremely low. However, if the patient has a family history of vascular disease, such as myocardial infarction occurring in family members under the age of 50, it would be advisable to obtain a lipid panel before and after starting OC use, and if the patient has a family history of diabetes or evidence of diabetes during pregnancy, a 2-hour postprandial blood glucose should be obtained before and after starting OCs. If patients have a past history of liver disease, a liver panel should be obtained to make certain that the liver function is normal before starting OCs.

Drug interactions

Although synthetic sex steroids can retard the biotransformation of certain drugs, such as phenazone and meperidine, due to substrate competition, such interference is not important clinically (Hempel & Klinger, 1976). OC use has not been shown to inhibit the action of other drugs. However, some drugs can interfere clinically with the action of OCs by inducing liver enzymes that convert the steroids to more polar and less biologically active metabolites. Certain drugs have been shown to accelerate the biotransformation of steroids in the human. These include barbiturates, sulphonamides, cyclophosphamide, and rifampicin. Several investigators have reported a relatively high incidence of OC failure in women ingesting rifampicin, and these two agents should not be given concurrently. The clinical data concerning OC failure in users of other antibiotics, such as penicillin, ampicillin, and sulphonamides and analgesics, such as phenytoin, as well as barbiturates, are less clear. A few anecdotal studies have appeared in the literature, but good evidence for a clinical inhibitory effect of these drugs, such as occurs with rifampicin, is not available. Until such time as controlled studies are performed, it would appear prudent when both agents are given simultaneously to suggest use of a barrier method in addition to the OCs because of possible interference with OC action.

Non-contraceptive health benefits

In addition to being the most effective method of contraception and thus preventing the medical problems associated with both unwanted and wanted pregnancies, OCs provide several other health benefits. Some are due to the fact that the combination OCs contain a potent, orally active progestin as well as an orally active oestrogen. Since the same combination of steroids is ingested on each day of the cycle beginning on day 5, and since endogenous oestradiol secretion is markedly suppressed, there is no time when the oestrogenic target tissues are stimulated by oestrogens without a progestin (unopposed oestrogen).

It has been known for many years that both natural progesterone and the synthetic progestins inhibit the proliferative effect of oestrogen, the so-called antioestrogenic effect. Recent studies have elucidated the mechanism whereby progestins produce this effect. Oestrogens increase the synthesis of both oestrogen and progesterone receptors, while progesterone decreases their synthesis (Clark et al 1977). Thus, one mechanism whereby progesterone exerts its antioestrogenic effects is by decreasing the synthesis of oestrogen receptors. Relatively little progestin is needed to do this and the amount present in OCs is sufficient. Another way progesterone produces its antioestrogenic action is by stimulating the activity of the enzyme, oestradiol-17β dehydrogenase, within the endometrial cell. This enzyme converts the more potent oestrogen, oestradiol, to the less potent oestrone, reducing oestrogenic action within the cell (King et al, 1981).

Benefits from antioestrogenic action of progestins. As a result of the anti-oestrogenic action of the progestins in OCs, the height of the endometrium is less than in an ovulatory cycle, and there is less proliferation of the glandular epithelium. These changes produce several substantial benefits for the OC user. One is a reduction in the amount of blood loss at the time of endometrial shedding. In an ovulatory cycle the mean blood loss during menstru-

Table 33.5 Incidence of iron deficiency anaemia — RCGP study

| | Rate per 1000 woman-years | | |
	OC users	Ex-users	Controls
	5.67	5.44	9.77
RR	0.58*	0.56*	1

OC: oral contraceptive; RR: relative risk.
*P < 0.01.

From Mishell, D R Jr 1982 Noncontraceptive health benefits of oral steroidal contraceptives. American Journal of Obstetrics and Gynecology 142: 809.

ation is about 35 ml compared with 20 ml for women ingesting OCs (Hefnowi et al, 1975). This decreased blood loss makes the development of iron deficiency anaemia less likely. Data from the RCGP study (1974) showed that OC users were about half as likely to develop iron deficiency anaemia as were the controls. Moreover, the beneficial effect persisted to a similar degree in women who had previously used OCs and then stopped, probably because of an increase in the iron stores that remained for several years after the drug was discontinued (Table 33.5).

Since the OCs produce regular withdrawal bleeding, it would be expected that OC users would have fewer menstrual disorders than controls. The results of the RCGP study (1974) confirmed the fact that oral contraceptive users were significantly less likely to develop menorrhagia, irregular menstruation, or intermenstrual bleeding (Table 33.6). Since these disorders are frequently treated by curettage, OC users require this procedure less frequently.

Because progestins inhibit the proliferative effect of oestrogens on the endometrium, their constant ingestion should reduce the incidence of endometrial hyperplasia that occurs mainly in anovulatory women as a result of the unopposed action of oestrogen. Since individuals with unopposed endogenous or exogenous oestrogen also have an increased incidence of adenocarcinoma of the endometrium, it is not surprising that women who use OCs have been found to be significantly less likely to develop this oestrogen-stimulated cancer. Data from three retrospective case comparison studies indicates that the relative risk of developing endometrial cancer among OC users was only

Table 33.6 Incidence of menstrual disorders — RCGP study (numbers in parentheses)

| | Rate per 1000 woman-years | | |
	OC users	Controls	RR
Menorrhagia	12.48	23.82 (1,004)	0.52*
Irregular menses	5.19	13.08 (326)	0.65*
Intermenstrual bleeding	3.04	5.26 (178)	0.72*

OC: Oral contraceptive; RR: relative risk
*P < 0.01.

From Mishell D R Jr 1982 Noncontraceptive health benefits of oral steroidal contraceptives. American Journal of Obstetrics and Gynecology 142: 809.

Table 33.7 Incidence of endometrial cancer (CA) — Boston University Epidemiologic Survey (numbers in parentheses)

OC use	CA (152)		Controls (516)		
	No.	%	No.	%	RR*
None	136	89	411	80	1.0
<1 year	5	3	14	3	0.8
1–2 year	6	4	32	6	0.5
>3 year	5	3	53	10	0.3

OC: oral contraceptive; RR: relative risk;
* Overall RR = 0.5 (0.3 to 0.8): stopped <5 year, RR = 0.5 (0.2 to 1.0).

From Mishell D R Jr 1982 Noncontraceptive health benefits of oral steroidal contraceptives. American Journal of Obstetrics and Gynecology 142: 809.

Table 33.8 Relative risk of benign breast disease — Oxford Family Planning Associates Study (numbers in parentheses)

OC use	Fibroadenoma	Cystic disease	Breast lumps	Other
Never	1.00 (49)	1.00 (113)	1.00 (169)	1.00 (34)
Ever	0.35 (25)*	0.66 (101)*	0.58 (162)*	0.63 (36)
Current	0.16 (7)*	0.47 (41)*	0.52 (77)*	0.60 (21)

OC: oral contraceptive;
*P < 0.01.

From Mishell D R Jr 1982 Noncontraceptive health benefits of oral steroidal contraceptives. Contraception 142: 809.

half that of controls (Table 33.7) (Kaufman et al, 1980; Weiss & Sayvetz, 1980; Hulka et al, 1982). The protective effect of OCs increased the longer these agents were used and the reduced risk of endometrial cancer persisted for at least 5 years after treatment was discontinued.

Oestrogen exerts a proliferative effect on breast tissue, which also contains oestrogen receptors. Progestins probably inhibit the synthesis of oestrogen receptors in this organ as well, exerting an anti-oestrogenic action on the breast. At least ten published studies have shown that OCs reduce the incidence of benign breast disease, and two prospective studies have indicated that this reduction is directly related to the amount of progestin in the drugs (Ory et al, 1976; Brinton et al, 1981).

The data from the 1974 RCGP study revealed a significantly decreased risk of chronic cystic breast disease but not fibroadenoma among OC users (RCGP 1974). This reduced incidence became apparent after 2 years of OC use and showed a further reduction with increasing use. Ory et al (1976) in a prospective study of OC users beginning in 1970 in Boston found a significant reduction in fibrocystic disease but not fibroadenomas in OC users. The reduced risk developed after 1–2 years of OC use. Women who took OCs for more than 2 years had a 65 per cent reduction in the incidence of fibrocystic disease and a 50 per cent reduction in the incidence of fibroadenoma.

Data from the Oxford Study indicate that three types of benign breast disease were found significantly more frequently among controls than among women who had used OCs (8). The largest reduction in risk occurred for fibroadenomas where the relative risk was 0.35 — a 65 per cent protection. Low risks were also discovered for chronic cystic breast disease, 0.66 — a 34 per cent reduction, and non-biopsied breast lumps, 0.58 — a 42 per cent reduction (Table 33.8). Current users of OCs were at lowest risk of developing benign breast disease, with a significant reduction of 84 per cent for fibroadenomas, 53 per cent for chronic cycstic disease 48 per cent for non-biopsied breast lumps, and a non-significant reduction of 40 per cent for other breast disease. The first three categories showed decreasing risk with increasing duration of OC use. After

6 or more years of drug use, there was a 50 per cent reduction in these three categories of benign breast disease. This reduced risk persisted for about 1 year following discontinuation of OCs, after which no reduction was observed.

Benefits from inhibition of ovulation. Other non-contraceptive medical benefits of OCs result from their main action, inhibition of ovulation. The occurrence of ovulatory menstrual cycles throughout most of a woman's reproductive years is a relatively recent phenomenon. A few generations ago most of a woman's reproductive years were anovulatory because she was either pregnant or lactating. Thus, what has been termed 'incessant ovulation' is really a result of modern civilisation. Some disorders, such as dysmenorrhoea and premenstrual tension, occur much more frequently in ovulatory than anovulatory cycles. In fact, inhibition of ovulation by exogenous steroids has been used as therapy for severe dysmenorrhoea for decades. The 1974 report of the RCGP study showed that oral contraceptive users had 63 per cent less dysmenorrhoea and 29 per cent less premenstrual than controls.

Another serious adverse effect of ovulatory menstrual cycles is the development of functional ovarian cysts, specifically, follicular and luteal cysts, that sometimes require a laparotomy because of enlargement, rupture or haemorrhage. When ovulation is inhibited, functional cysts do not develop. The RCGP study (1974) found the incidence of benign ovarian neoplasms to be reduced by 64 per cent. In a survey performed by the Boston Collaborative Drug Surveillance Program of 25 000 patients, who were contraceptive users, admitted to hospitals in the greater Boston area, only one of 60 (1.7 per cent) women with a discharge diagnosis of functional ovarian cysts was taking OCs in contrast to 170 of 842 (20 per cent) controls (Ory,

Table 33.9 Surgically removed ovarian cysts — Boston Collaborative Drug Surveillance Program (24 hospitals)

	Controls (n = 842)	Functional cysts (n = 60)	Nonfunctional cysts (n = 70)
OC users	170 (20%)	1 (1.7%)	14 (20%)
RR	1.0	0.07*	1.0

OC: oral contraceptive; RR: relative risk;
*P < 0.02.

From Mishell D R Jr 1982 Noncontraceptive health benefits of oral steroidal contraceptives. Contraception 142: 809.

1974). The age-adjusted risk ratio was 0.07. In contrast, 14 of 70 (20 per cent) women with non-functional cysts were taking OCs, an incidence similar to that observed in the controls (Table 33.9).

Another disorder linked to incessant ovulation is ovarian cancer. Several case control studies have shown that the risk of developing ovarian cancer decreases as the number of pregnancies increases, and Beral et al (1978) reported that the incidence of ovarian cancer correlated inversely with the number of children born. The trauma to the ovarian surface epithelium produced by incessant ovulation may in some way contribute to the development of ovarian cancer. Casagrande et al (1979) reported data from a case control study which indicated that the relative risk of ovarian cancer decreased as the numbers of live births and incomplete pregnancies and OC use increased. When the anovulatory years from all three factors were added together, the decreased relative risk was statistically significant. These investigators found that the protective effect of OCs was about the same as pregnancy with 12 months of OC use, protecting to about the same degree as one live birth. Two recent case control studies reported that OC users had only about one-half the risk of developing ovarian cancer and this protection persists for at least 10 years after the OC was stopped (Table 33.10) (Kaufman et al, 1980; Rosenberg et al, 1982).

Table 33.10 Ovarian cancer and OC use

Duration	CA	Controls	R.R.
None	103	352	1.0
<1 year	11	49	0.9
1–4 year	12	76	0.6
≥5 year	6	51	0.3

Overall R.R 0.6 (0.4–0.9)
From Rosenberg et al Journal of the American Medical Association 247: 3210, 1982

Other benefits. The RCGP study (1974) showed that the risk of developing rheumatoid arthritis in OC users was only 49 per cent that of controls, 0.31 per 1 000 woman-years versus 0.63 per 1000 woman-years. Additional evidence of this protective effect was obtained from the Rochester Epidemiologic Program Project, which showed that the incidence of rheumatoid arthritis increased from 1950 to 1964 in men and women but declined in women after that date with no decline in men (Linos et al, 1978). This decline occurred during the time when OC use increased in the United States.

Another benefit produced by OC use is protection against salpingitis, commonly referred to as pelvic inflammatory disease (PID). There have been at least II published epidemiological studies estimating the relative risk of developing PID among OC users. Seven of these studies compared OC use to non-use of any other contraception. With one exception the relative risk of developing

PID among OC users compared with non-users was 0.3–0.9 (Senanayke & Kramer, 1980). In the one study that showed an increased risk of PID among OC users, the definition of this entity included non-specific nonmenstrual pelvic or abdominal pain, which probably caused a spuriously high rate. The largest study analysing data on PID in OC users was the RCGP study (1974). It is reported that the rate of PID in OC users was 0.42 per thousand woman-years and in controls 0.89, for a relative risk in oral contraceptive users of 0.47. It has been estimated that between 15 and 20 per cent of women with cervical gonorrhoeal infection will develop salpingitis. In a study from Sweden, where all cases of suspected salpingitis were confirmed by laparoscopic visualisation 1 day after admission, a total of 672 patients with culture-proved gonorrhoea were seen from 1973 to 1977 (Ryden et al, 1979). Eighty-seven, or 12.9 per cent had acute salpingitis. Of those who used contraception other than the IUD and oral steroids, 37 of 245 (15.1 per cent) developed salpingitis; about half, 30 of 342 (8.8 per cent), of those who used OCs developed salpingitis (P < 0.02). The age, marital status, and number of sexual contacts were similar in the two groups. The results of this study indicate that OCs prevent the development of salpingitis in women infected with gonorrhoea. This protection may be related to the decreased duration of menstrual flow which permits a smaller number of gonococcal organisms to ascend to the upper genital tract and allows the body's defenses to eliminate them more easily.

Westrom (1980) compared data on the use of contraceptives and the incidence of PID in 20- to 29-year-old women in Lund, Sweden, between 1970 and 1974. He found that 172 of 4032 sexually active noncontraceptive users developed PID for a rate of 3.42 per 100 woman-years, while only 148 of 16 311 OCs users developed PID for a rate of 0.91 per 100 woman years. Increased use of OCs by the population at greatest risk — sexually active women between 15 and 24 years of age — would greatly reduce this disease with its high cost of treatment and resultant infertility.

One of the sequale of PID is ectopic pregnancy, an entity that has tripled in incidence in the last decase. Oral contraceptives reduce the risk of ectopic pregnancy by more than 90 per cent.

To summarise these benefits Ory recently estimated that of 100 000 women in the United States using OCs each year, their use will prevent 320 from developing iron deficiency anaemia, 32 from developing rheumatoid arthritis and 450 from developing PID which does not require hospitalisation (Ory, 1982). In addition, there will be 150 fewer women hospitalised for PID, 235 fewer hospitalised for breast disease, 35 fewer hospitalised for ovarian tumours and 117 fewer hospitalised for tubal pregnancies (Table 33.11). Ory estimated each year about one out of every 750 women taking OCs will not develop a serious

Table 33.11 Rate and No. hospitalisations prevented yearly by OC use*

Disease	Rate (per 100 000)	No.
Benign breast	235	20 000
Ovarian cysts	35	3000
FE-def anaemia	320	27 200
PID (episodes)	600	51 000
PID (hospitalisations)	156	13 300
Ectopic pregnancy	117	9900
Rheumatoid arthritis	32	2700
Endometial CA	5	2000
Ovarian CA	4	1700

* Ory, H W Fam. Plan. Perspectives 14: 182, 1982

disease which she would have developed if she did not take this drug. He estimated that use of OCs prevents 50 000 women from being hospitalised in the United States each year. It is unfortunate that the infrequent adverse effects of OCs have received widespread publicity, while information about the more common non-contraceptive health benefits has attracted little attention.

VAGINAL RINGS

Another method of contraception that has been studied for the last 20 years is the administration of contraceptive steroids through a doughnut-shaped Silastic ring which originally was impregnated with a variety of gestagens alone and more recently has been impregnated with a combination of norgestrel and oestradiol (Fig. 33.1). These contraceptive vaginal rings (CVR) are placed in the vagina by the patient herself for a period of 3 weeks beginning on the fifth day after menses begins and than removed for a period of 1 week to allow withdrawal bleeding to occur. While the rings are in place, the steroids are released from the surface and absorbed through the vaginal mucosa into the circu-

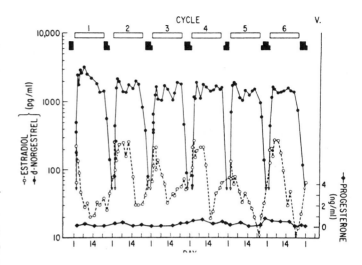

Fig. 33.2 Serum oestradiol and d-norgestrel levels on a log scale and progesterone levels during six treatment cycles. Open bars represent 3-week treatment cycles with rings in place. Black bars represent bleeding days (full height for bleeding and half height for spotting). Rings were inserted on day 1 and removed on day 21 during each cycle. From Mishell D R Jr, Moore D E, Roy S, Brenner P F, Page M A 1978 Clinical performance and endocrine profiles with contraceptive vaginal rings containing a combination of estradiol and d-norgestrel

lation at a fairly constant rate (Fig. 33.2) (Mishell et al, 1978). The serum level of steroids found in patients using the rings is sufficient to inhibit ovulation but several times less than the peak levels obtained with daily oral administration of steroids. Ovulation continues to be inhibited during the week that the rings are not in place. Sufficient steroid is present in each ring so it can be used for 6 months. Patients can insert and remove the rings without difficulty. With the use of rings containing a combination of norgestrel and oestradiol, breakthrough bleeding is minimal and similar to that occurring with the combination oral contraceptives. Withdrawal bleeding after the ring is removed occurs within a day or two, lasts for 3 to 4 days and is usually similar in amount to the normal flow. Measurement of angiotensinogen shows that levels are not increased in patients using CVRs in comparison with the several-fold increase that occurs in patients using oral contraceptive steroids (Mishell, 1979). Reasons for lack of the oestrogenic effect on hepatic globulins with CVRs may be due to three factors. Firstly, a natural oestrogen, oestradiol, is used instead of the synthetic oestrogen, ethinyl oestradiol; secondly, only a small amount of oestrogen is absorbed and, thirdly, the steroid is not absorbed through the gut into the portal system and thus bypasses the liver after it is first absorbed into the circulation. Studies have been done showing that there is no increase in weight, change in haemoglobulin or blood pressure in patients using CVRs and there are no significant alterations in tests of glucose tolerance or liver function (Sivin et al, 1981b). Because levonorgestrel is androgenic, there is a significant decrease in most circulating lipids and lipoproteins,

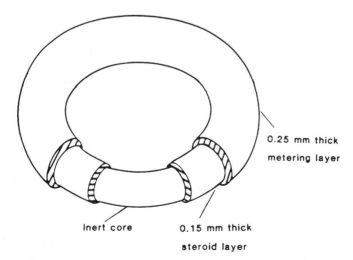

Fig. 33.1 Sectional view of a 'Shell' ring. From Jackanicz T M 1981 Levonorgestrel and estradiol release from an improved contraceptive vaginal ring. Contraception 24: 323

including cholesterol, triglycerides, HDL cholesterol and LDL cholesterol; however, the cholesterol/HDL cholesterol ratio is not significantly changed and, therefore, it is thought that these changes in lipoproteins are not clinically significant (Robertson et al, 1981). Colposcopic changes of the vagina have shown no alterations when the ring is in place and histological examination of the vaginal mucosa in patients who have worn the ring have shown no alterations in the normal histological pattern. Bacteriological studies have been performed comparing users of the rings and those using oral contraceptives with no significant differences noted between the two techniques in patients using them for a period of 6 months (Roy et al, 1981). Since preliminary studies with the ring were promising, in 1978 the Population Council initiated a multicentre international study comparing the CVR with an oral contraceptive containing levonorgestrel and ethinyl oestradiol. More than 1000 ring users were compared with more than 500 oral contraceptive users. Results of analysis of the event rates after 1 year indicated that there was no significant differences in pregnancy rates or continuation rates between the two methods but significantly more women discontinued using the ring because of vaginal problems and use-related problems (Table 33.12) (Sivin et al 1981a). However, more women discontinued using oral contraceptives for medical reasons such as headache and nausea. Patient and partner acceptance is good and the ring can be removed if desired for a few hours during the time of sexual intercourse. Ovulation occurs promptly after discontinuation of use of this method. In conclusion, the CVR provides an acceptable alternative reversible method of contraception for certain couples. It provides a convenient, once a month method that inhibits ovulation and has an acceptable rate of contraceptive effectiveness and abnormal bleeding.

PREGNANCY INTERCEPTION

Morris & van Wagenen suggested in 1966 that high doses of oestrogen given in the early post-ovulatory period will prevent implantation in women. Morris has suggested that the term 'interception' be used for what is commonly called the 'morning after pill'. The oestrogen compounds which have been utilised by various investigators for interception include diethylstilboestrol, 25–50 mg/day; diethylstilboestrol diphosphate, 50 μg/day; ethinyloestradiol, 1–5 mg/day, and conjugated oestrogens, 20–30 mg/day. Treatment is continued for 5 days and if it is begun within 72 hours after an isolated mid-cycle act of coitus, its effectiveness is very good. If more than one episode of coitus has occurred or if treatment is initiated later than 72 hours after coitus, the method if much less effective. In 1973, Morris & van Wagenen summarised the literature and found that in 9000 mid-cycle exposures treated with oestrogen, there was a total of 29 pregnancies for a pregnancy rate of approximately 0.3 per cent. Only three of these pregnancies appeared to be due to method failure for a Pearl index of 0.4/100 woman-years. Of the 20 pregnancies, three were ectopic, an incidence of approximately 10 per cent. A more recent review by Garcia et al (1977) of 4595 treatment cycles revealed a failure rate of 0.7 per cent. Side-effects associated with this therapy are, as expected, nausea and vomiting, breast soreness and menstrual irregularities. The US Center for Disease Control performed a five centre study comparing use of ethinyl oestradiol 5 μg/day with conjugated oestrogen 30 μg/day for 5 days. Treatment with ethinyl oestradiol resulted in a slightly lower pregnancy rate (0.7 per cent) compared with conjugated oestrogen (1.6 per cent). (Dixon et al, 1980). However, patients treated with ethinyl oestradiol also had a greater incidence of nausea and vomiting, indicating the potency of this dose of this oestrogen may have been greater. If treatment was begun 2 days after coitus, the pregnancy rate was 1.7-fold greater than if it was begun the day after coitus. Thus it is best to start treatment within 24 hours of coitus. As the side-effects of high dose oestrogen cause failure of some women to complete the 5-day course, a regimen of two tablets of ethinyl oestradiol 0.05 mg and dl-norgestrel 0.5 mg (Ovral) given twice with an interval of 12 hours has been tested in Canada. Effectiveness is comparable to the high dose oestrogen regime with a shorter duration of adverse symptoms. Yuzpe et al (1982) recently summarised experience with this regimen among 692 women treated in

Table 33.12 All segments. One-year termination and continuation rates per 100 acceptors by regimen and reason for termination

| Rate | Net Rates | | |
| | CVR | | |
	50 mm	58 mm	Nordette
Pregnancy	1.8	1.0	2.0
Medical termination	23.5	22.5	18.7
Use-related termination	6.6	4.4	2.0
Personal termination	8.8	9.7	11.2
Moving	2.0	2.1	2.0
Loss to Follow-Up	8.5	9.9	25.9
Continuation, LFU a termination	48.8	50.4	38.2
Continuation, LFU not a termination	54.0	56.8	55.4

Type of Termination	Events		
Pregnancy	9	5	10
Medical reasons	119	115	95
Use-related reasons	35	23	10
Personal reasons	45	47	55
Moving	10	10	10
Loss to Follow-Up	46	53	133
All	264	253	313
No. of women enrolled	547	556	553
No. of women at risk, mo. 12	239	220	193

From Sivin I, Mishell D R Jr, Victor A, Diaz S et al 1981 A multicenter study of levonorgestrel-estradiol contraceptive vaginal rings. I. Use effectiveness. Contraception 24: 341.

24 clinics. There were 11 pregnancies (1.6 per cent) but four of the subjects had unprotected intercourse more than 72 hours prior to treatment and, therefore, should not have been included in the study. Excluding those four subjects, the pregnancy rate was 1.0 per cent. About half of the subjects (42.4 per cent) had no side-effects, while nausea and/or vomiting occurred in 51.7 per cent. Other side-effects such as mastalgia and menorrhagia were infrequent, occurring in less than 1 per cent of the women. Thus the effectiveness of this method is similar to that of higher dosages of oestrogen alone and results in a lower incidence of abnormal and delayed menses. Side-effects appear to be less and, because of the 1-day treatment regimen, patient compliance may be greater with this technique. If the patient has a continuing need for contraception, after the cycle in which interception is used, one of the conventional contraceptive methods should be utilised.

REFERENCES

Beral V, Fraser P, Chilvers C 1978 Does Pregnancy protect against ovarian cancer? Lancet i: 1083

Brinton L A, Vessey M P, Flavel R et al 1981 Risk factors for benign breast disease. American Journal of Epidemiology 113: 203

Casagrande J T, Pike M D, Ross R K et al 1979 'Incessant ovulation' and ovarian cancer. Lancet ii: 170

Clark J H, Hsueh A L, Peck E J 1977 Regulation of estrogen receptor replenishment by progesterone. Annals of New York Acadamy of Science 286: 161

Dixon G W, Schlesselman J J, Ory H W, Blye R P 1980 Ethinyl estradiol and conjugated estrogens as post-coital contraceptives. Journal of American Medical Association 244: 1336

Gambrell R D Jr, Massey F M, Castaneda K A, Ugenas A J, Ricci C A 1979 Reduced incidence of endometrial cancer among post-menopausal women treated with progestogens. Journal of American Geriatric Society 27: 389

Garcia C-R, Huggins G R, Rosenfeld D L et al 1977 Postcoital contraception: Medical and social factors of the morning after pill. Contraception 15: 445

Harris R W C, Brinto L A, Cowdell R H, Skegg D C G, Smith P G, Vessey M P, Doll R 1980 Characteristics of women with dysplasia or carcinoma in situ of the cervix uteri. British Journal of Cancer 42: 359

Hefnawi F, Saleh A A, Kandil O et al 1975 Blood loss with IUDs. In: Hefnawi E, Segal S J (eds) Analysis of Intra Uterine Contraception, p 373. Elsevier, Amsterdam

Hempel E, Klinger W 1976 Drug stimulated biotransformation of hormonal steroid contraceptives: clinical implications. Drugs 12: 422

Hulka B A, Chambless L E, Kaufman D G, Fowler W C Jr, Greenberg B G 1982 Protection against endometrial carcinoma by combination-product oral contraceptives. Journal of the American Medical Association 247: 475

Kaufman D W, Shapiro S B, Slone D, Rosenberg L, Miettinen O S, Stolley P D, Knapp R C, Leavitt T Jr, Watring W G, Rosenhein N B, Lewis J L Jr, Schottenfeld D, Engle R I Jr, 1980 Decreased risk of endometrial cancer among oral contraceptive users. New England Journal of Medicine 303: 1045

Kelsey J L, Holford T R, White C, Mayer E S, Kilty S E, Acheson R M 1978 Oral contraceptives and breast diseases: An epidemiological study. American Journal of Epidemiology 107: 236

King R J B, Townsend P T, Whitehead M I 1981 The role of estradiol dehydrogenase in mediating progesterone effects on endometrium from post-menopausal women receiving estrogens and progestins. Journal of Steroid Biochemistry 14: 235

Linos A, Worthington J W, O'Fallon W M et al 1978 Rheumatoid arthritis and oral contraceptives. Lancet i: 871

Mead T W, Greenberg G, Thompson S G, 1980 Progestogens and cardio-vascular reactions associated with oral contraceptives and a comparison of the safety of 50- and 30-μg oestrogen preparations. British Medical Journal 1: 1157

Mishell D R Jr 1979 Intrauterine devices: Medicated and non-medicated. International Journal of Gynaecology and Obstetrics 16: 487

Mishell D R Jr, Moore D E, Roy S, Brenner P F, Page M A 1978 Clinical performance and endocrine profiles with contraceptive vaginal rings containing a combination of estradiol and d-norgestrel. American Journal of Obstetrics and Gynecology 130: 55

Morris J McL, Van Wagenen G 1973 Interception: The use of postovulatory estrogens to prevent implantation. American Journal of Obstetrics and Gynecology 12: 377

Murphy P G 1977 ACS commission on cancer survey supports suggested association between oral contraceptive usage and liver tumors. American College of Surgery Bulletin, p 28

Ory H W 1974 Functional ovarian cysts and oral contraceptives. Journal of the American Medical Association 228: 68

Ory H W 1982 The noncontraceptive health benefits from oral contraceptptive use. Family Planning Perspectives 14: 182

Ory H W, Cole P, MacMahon B, Hoover R 1976 Oral contraceptives and reduced risk of benign breast diseases. New England Journal of Medicine 294: 419

Porter J B, Hunter J R, Danielson D A, Jick H, Stergachis A 1982 Oral contraceptives and nonfatal vascular disease — recent experience. Obstetrics and Gynecology 59: 299

Robertson D N, Alvarez F, Sivin I, Brache V et al 1981 Lipoprotein patterns in women in Santo Domingo using a levonorgestrel/estradiol conceptive ring. Contraception 24: 469

Rosenberg L, Shapiro S, Slone D, Kaufman D W et al 1982 Epithelial ovarian cancer and combination oral contraceptives. Journal of the American Medical Association 247: 3210

Rothman K J, Louik C 1978 Oral contraceptives and birth defects. New England Journal of Medicine 299: 522

Roy S, Wilkins J, Mishell D R Jr 1981 The effect of a contraceptive vaginal ring and oral contraceptives on the vaginal flora. Contraception 24: 481

Royal College of General Practitioners 1974 Oral Contraceptives and Health: An Interim Report from the Oral Contraceptive Study of the Royal College of General Practitioners. Pitman Publishing, New York

Royal College of General Practitioners' Oral Contraceptive Study: Mortality among oral contraceptive users 1977 Lancet ii: 727

Royal College of General Practitioners' Oral Contraception Study: Further Analyses of Mortality in Oral Contraceptive Users 1981 Lancet i: 541

Ryden G, Fahraeus L, Molin L et al 1979 Do contraceptives influence the incidence of acute pelvic inflammatory disease in women with gonorrhea? Contraception 20: 149

Senanayake P, Kramer D G 1980 Contraception and the etiology of pelvic inflammatory disease: new perspectives. American Journal of Obstetrics and Gynecology 138: 852

Siven I, Mishell D R Jr, Victor A, Diaz S et al 1981a A multicenter study of levonorgestrel-estradiol contraceptive vaginal rings. I. Use effectiveness. Contraception 24: 341

Siven I, Mishell D R Jr, Victor A, Diaz S et al 1981b A multicenter study of levonorgestrel-estradiol contraceptive vaginal rings. II. Subjective and objective measures of effects. Contraception 24: 359

The Walnut Creek Contraceptive Drug Study, Volume III 1981 Center for Population Research Monograph. NIH Publication No. 81–564

Vessey M, Doll R, Peto R, Johnson B, Wiggins P 1976 A long-term follow-up study of women using different methods of contraception. An interim report. Journal of Biosocial Sciences 8: 3737

Vessey M P, Doll R, Jones K, McPherson K, Yeates D 1979a An epidemiological study of oral contraceptives and breast cancer. British Medical Journal 1: 1757

Vessey M P, Meisler L, Flavel R, Yeates D 1979b Outcome of
  pregnancy in women using different methods of contraception.
  British Journal of Obstetrics and Gynaecology 86: 348
Vessey M P, Wright N H, McPherson K, Wiggins P 1979c Fertility
  after stoppine different methods of contraception. British Medical
  Journal 1: 265
Weiss N S, Sayvetz T A 1980 Incidence of endometrial cancer in
  relation to the use of oral contraceptives. New England Journal of
  Medicine 302: 551

Westoff C F, Jones E F 1977 Contraception and sterilization in the
  United States, 1965–1975. Family Planning Perspectives 9: 153
Westrom L 1980 Incidence, prevalence and trends of acute pelvic
  inflammatory disease and it's consequences in industrialized
  countries. American Journal of Obstetrics and Gynecology 138: 880
Yuzpe A A, Smith R P, Rademaker A W 1982 A multicenter clinical
  investigation employing ethinyl estradiol combined with dl-
  norgestrel as a postcoital contraceptive agent. Fertility and Sterility
  37: 508

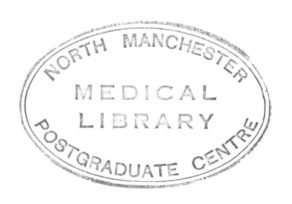

Long acting hormonal contraceptives

INTRODUCTION

Simple and convenient long acting methods of contraception have been pursued actively for at least the last 50 years. The first successful approach was the intra-uterine device although this system had a very chequered early career. Soon after the initial studies with successful oral oestrogen–progestogen contraceptives in the late 1950s it was realised that the desired temporary inhibition of ovulation could also be obtained by the infrequent injection of other related hormonal preparations. Early studies with monthly oestrogen-progestogen combinations and longer acting progestogen only formulations were encouraging and have been followed by an enormous amount of further research and development.

Apart from the obvious convenience of prolonged duration these hormonal contraceptive methods have several other advantages which are summarised in Table 34.1. On the debit side are a number of disadvantages and concerns (Table 34.2) which new methods are designed to minimise or eliminate. The range of methods currently being studied and developed is designed to appeal to a spectrum of users with differing personal and cultural preferences. However, much of the technology involved in these developments is quite complex and hence expensive.

This has severely limited the number of new approaches which have been pursued. The published literature on long acting hormonal contraception is too voluminous to be adressed thoroughly in a short review and readers are referred to several other publications for additional references (Benagiano, 1977; Fraser & Weisberg, 1981; Mishell, 1983).

HISTORY AND POLITICS OF INJECTABLE CONTRACEPTION

A review of long acting hormonal contraceptives cannot be considered complete without a careful analysis of the history of development and political involvement in the development of injectable contraceptives. Of necessity this discussion must revolve around the most widely available and longest used preparation: depot medroxy progesterone acetate (DMPA; Depo-Provera, Upjohn Company). However, many of the issues are also relevant to other long acting methods.

In 1953 it was found that esterification of a progestogen alcohol resulted in a preparation which had long lasting effects when injected (Junkmann, 1954). This was rapidly followed by the synthesis of a number of long acting progestogens including norethisterone oenanthate (Junk-

Table 34.1 Advantages of long acting progestogen-only contraceptives

Long action with one injection
Simplicity of administration
Independent of coitus
Freedom from 'fear of forgetting' daily pills
Safety margin for timing of successive injections
High method efficacy
High 'use effectiveness'
High acceptability and high continuation rates of use
No oestrogenic side-effects
Minimal gastrointestinal disturbance
Almost invariable reduction of menstrual blood loss
Amenorrhoea may be a health benefit and a convenience
Regular contact with health personnel
No suppression of lactation
Injections regarded as 'potent medicine' in many communities

Table 34.2 Concerns about long acting progestogen-only contraceptives

Method least in control of the woman herself
Cannot be rapidly reversed
Invariable change in menstrual pattern
Delay in return of fertility but no permanent sterility
Other side-effects (weight gain, headache, 'bloating')
Minor metabolic changes
Theoretical effects on fetus and on breastfed neonate
Theoretical concerns about neoplasia
Controversy about the interpretation of animal toxicology
Problems of informed consent and 'potential for abuse'
Suspicion of the integrity of the scientific community and multinational drug companies

mann & Witzel, 1958) and DMPA (Babcock et al, 1958). A large number of long acting oestrogen and progestogen formulations were prepared and tested in small clinical trials (Benagiano, 1977) but only a small number of these have reached the stage of widespread evaluation.

Schering began clinical trials on norethisterone oenanthate (NET-OEN; Norigest; Noristerat) in 1957, and Upjohn soon followed with trials of DMPA. In 1960 the United States Food and Drug Administration (USFDA) approved DMPA for marketing as a treatment for threatened or habitual abortion and endometriosis on the basis of its safety, but without good data on efficacy. The observation that women given high doses of DMPA (1–4 g) to suppress uterine activity in premature labour failed to conceive 1–1½ years postpartum lead to the first contraceptive trials in 1963 and the first reports of contraceptive efficacy in 1966 (Coutinho & De Souza; 1966; Csapo et al, 1966; Zanartu & Onetto, 1966).

Upjohn first applied to USFDA in 1967 for permission to market Depo-Provera as a contraceptive in the USA and the subsequent saga is one of the most fascinating modern tales about the emotions, distortions and lack of desire for factual accuracy which occur at the interface between science and politics (Benagiano & Fraser 1981; Fraser & Holck, 1983). The first delays occurred over questions about reversibility, the relationship to breast cancer in beagle dogs and possible cervical carcinoma *in situ*. However, in 1973 the USFDA announced its intention to approve Depo-Provera as a contraceptive, but final approval was quashed by political action. Following this the USFDA withdrew its approval for marketing of DMPA for abortion and endometriosis because of alleged ineffectiveness in these conditions and because of the observation that other progestogens administered during pregnancy might have an occasional association with congenital defects. As questions concerning the irrelevance of breast tumours in beagle dogs to risk of cancer in women were being sorted out, a further toxicological enigma appeared with the occurrence of uterine (possibly endometrial or endocervical) adenocarcinomas in two rhesus monkeys treated with very high dose DMPA for 10 years. Eventually, in 1978, following two recommendations for approval by its own Obstetrics and Gynecology Subcommittee and much antagonistic political activity, the USFDA decided to refuse marketing approval for DMPA as a contraceptive in the USA. Four years later the promised Public Board of Inquiry has only just called for submissions and is unlikely to report before 1984. Similar events have occurred in the United Kingdom where, in 1982, the Minister of Health refused to accept the recommendation for marketing approval of his own expert scientific body, the Committee for the Safety of Medicines (CSM) (Leading article 1982). He has since agreed to a public hearing on the whole question. One of the few governments of countries with a thorough drug review system which has had the courage to agree to the recommendation of its scientific advisory body for the general marketing of Depo-Provera as a contraceptive is Sweden (Swedish National Board of Health and Welfare, 1981).

It is fascinating to note that every independent scientific group which has thoroughly reviewed all the data on DMPA has recommended its wider use as a safe contraceptive. This includes the Obstetrics and Gynecology and Biostatistics Advisory Committees of the USFDA, the United Kingdom CSM, the Swedish Board of Health and Welfare, an Ad Hoc Consultative Panel on DMPA of the US Agency for International Development, the International Medical Advisory Panel of the International Planned Parenthood Federation and several groups convened by the Special Programme of Research in Human Reproduction of the World Health Organisation.

However, it must be recognised that there are legitimate concerns about injectable contraceptives (Table 34.2), many of which are not directly medical. Emphasis has often been placed on the potential for abuse of this type of contraception and the issue of informed consent. One of the major concerns has been widespread use in mentally retarded girls and underprivileged or disadvantaged groups where proper consent may not have been obtained. Injectable contraceptives may actually have major advantages in these groups, but extra care is obviously required in pretreatment counselling. A frequent criticism is that injectable contraception is the method least in the control of the women herself since the hormonal effect cannot be reversed for many weeks after administration. Although occasional individual problems have been reported this has not been a problem in practice in the major, well supervised trials (Benagiano, 1977). Good continuation rates attest to the acceptability of this type of contraception in most communities.

Part of the consumer concern about DMPA has been bound up with community suspicion of the power and profits of multinational corporations, specifically the Upjohn Company. The Company has often been accused of hiding damaging data, but thorough independent review has not revealed anything serious or unexpected.

One of the most disturbing aspects of the public forum on DMPA has been a recent trend to publication of misleading, misinformed and emotional articles in the lay press in several countries. One newspaper in Australia even refused to publish a scientifically balanced and carefully referenced letter correcting many inaccuracies in one of its articles on Depo-Provera (National Times, 1981). This type of unscientific reporting has been called 'trial by media' and does an enormous disservice to our society in the long run. One of the most widely circulated of these articles (Minkin, 1980) has been written in a superficially convincing scientific style but contains many errors, discrepancies and unjustified conclusions (Hutton, 1980; Benagiano & Fraser, 1981).

Other major concerns include the interpretation of animal toxicology, potential effects on the exposed fetus or breast fed neonate, and the other medical effects detailed in Table 34.2. These are discussed below.

It remains to be seen whether new injectables and new delivery systems will avoid these problems.

AVAILABLE APPROACHES TO PROLONGED HORMONAL CONTRACEPTIVE ACTION

Current approaches and ongoing research are geared to provide a range of choices which appeal to different women. Many international agencies and pharmaceutical companies have contributed to this field. Those public sector agencies with major ongoing development programmes are the World Health Organisation, the United States

National Institute of Child Health and Human Development, the Population Council, the United States of America Agency for International Development and the Program for Applied Research in Fertility Regulation. These programmes are independent of each other but regular coordination ensures that the research and development work is generally complementary rather than competitive.

The scope of the field is summarised in Table 34.3. This table covers methods which utilise a wide range of technologies (Fraser, 1982a). The more traditional injectable methods consist of steroid acetates or esters which have been formulated in oily solutions or microcrystalline suspensions. The steroid esters in oily solution appear to be distributed to storage sites in adipose tissue from which they are slowly released into the circulation. The active steroid moiety is then cleaved from the ester after which

Table 34.3 Current long acting hormonal contraceptives

Duration of action	Type of system	Existing systems in human use or trial	State of development	Comments
Monthly	Injectable	1. DMPA (25 mg) + EC (5 mg)	Post phase III	Dose reduction studies underway
		2. NET-OEN (50 mg) + EB (5 mg)	Phase II	
		3. NET-OEN (20 mg) alone	Phase II	
		4. DHPA (150 mg) + EOE (10 mg)	Post phase III	
		5. Others	Phase I–II	
	Oral	1. Several formulations	Phase II–III	Peoples' Republic of China only
2–3 monthly	Injectable	1. NET-OEN (200 mg)	Marketing	First order release
		2. DMPA (150 mg)	Marketing	First order release
		3. NET microcapsules (100 mg)	Phase I	Possible zero-order release
		4. Others	Pre-phase I	
	Vaginal ring (daily release rates)	1. LNG (300 μg) + E_2 (180 μg)	Phase III	Cyclical use 3 weeks out of 4; with ovulation inhibition
		2. LNG (20 μg)	Phase II	Continuous use; zero-order release; minipill effect
		3. Others	Phase I	Potential for longer duration of use
6 monthly	Injectable	1. DMPA (450 mg)	Marketing	First order release
		2. NET microcapsules (200 mg)	Phase I	Possible zero-order release
		3. Others	Pre-phase I	
	Implant -biodegradable	1. NET-cholesterol pellets	Phase I	Attenuated first order release
		2. BIDS-LNG	Pre-phase I	Single implant
	-non biodegradable	1. NET-acetate silastic (500 μg)	Phase II	Single implant
1–2 years	Implant -biodegradable (daily release rates)	1. Caprolactone LNG pellets (50 μg)	Phase I	Single implant
	-non biodegradable	1. ST1435 silastic (120 μg)	Phase I	Single implant
	Intrauterine devices	Progesterone or progestogen releasing	Phase I to marketing	Near zero-order release
5 years +	Implant -non biodegradable	1. Norplant I (30–50 μg)	Marketing	6 implants
		2. Norplant II (30–50 μg)	Phase III	2 implants

DMPA = depot medroxyprogesterone acetate; NET-OEN = norethisterone oenanthate; DHPA = dihydroxyprogesterone acetophenide; LNG = levonorgestrel; EC = oestradiol cypionate; EB = oestradiol benzoate; EOE = oestradiol oenanthate; E_2 = oestradiol 17β; BIDS = biodegradable implantable delivery system.

it is able to exert its biological effect. Microcrystalline suspensions remain as a depot at the site of injection and the active steroid or ester is slowly released from the surface of the crystals.

In recent years a concerted effort has been made to find new progestogenic steroids and to develop new progestogen esters with long acting properties. A particularly commendable effort involving several of the leading chemists in the field and a network of centres in developing countries has been supported by the World Health Organisation (Crabbe et al, 1980). This programme has sponsored the synthesis of over 200 systematically selected esters of norethisterone and levonorgestrel. Four of the esters of levonorgestrel have a duration of biological activity at least twice that of existing long acting progestogens (World Health Organisation, 1981), and at least one of these (probably the cyclobutyl carboxylate of levonorgestrel) will be developed further. During the course of this programme it has been found that the exact pharmaceutical formulation of the microcrystals or solution of the compound is critical for maximum duration of action, and the optimum formulation varies from compound to compound.

Attention is also being directed to the synthesis of novel steroids which may have advantages over existing compounds. Most of these are at an early stage of development but one new group of compounds with interesting progestogenic properties are oximes of existing progestogens (for example, levonorgestrel acetate oxime: norgestimate).

Perhaps the most exciting developments in the 'long acting' field are the delivery systems designed to release steroids systemically at a more or less constant rate (zero-order release) over a lengthy period of time. The main aims of these developments are to reduce the initial surge in blood levels seen with current injectables and to reduce the total steroid load to the body while extending the duration of action in a more predictable manner. Most of these controlled release systems have utilised either biodegradable or non-biodegradable polymers.

Non-biodegradable systems are mainly based on small poly-dimethyl siloxane (Silastic) capsules packed with the chosen progestogen. This silicon elastomer membrane permits relatively constant diffusion of the progestogen, and the rate and duration of diffusion can be widely modified by technical alterations to the size, shape and thickness of the capsule (Nash et al, 1978). These can be effective and acceptable contraceptives (Coutinho et al, 1978). The major disadvantage is that these capsules ultimately require removal. The Population Council has developed a system of six implants — 'Norplant' — which will provide contraception with levonorgestrel for over 7 years (Sivin et al, 1980).

Biodegradable capsules have been developed to avoid the necessity for removal but to permit early removal if desired or if unexpected side-effects occur. Several approaches have been tried (Benagiano & Gabelnick, 1979). One such system (Bioerodible Delivery System — levonorgestrel; BIDS-LNG; developed by the Alza Corporation with the support of WHO and the National Institutes of Health (NIH) involves small rods of a hydrophobic polyorthoester which erode slowly at the surface and steadily release the steroid which is evenly dispersed through the matrix. This is highly advanced technology and it is likely to be many years before devices of this type are widely available for clinical use. A second type of biodegradable implant has been developed by the NIH and is now in clinical trial (World Health Organisation, 1981). This is based on a polycaprolactone polymer shell which releases levonorgestrel steadily over a 1–2 year period. The polymer shell only biodegrades very slowly over a period of several years. These devices are all 2–3 mm in diameter and are implanted subcutaneously with the use of local anesthetic, a small incision and a trocar at a site chosen according to local preference (mainly upper arm, forearm, thigh or suprapubic region).

This technology has also been used to develop micro capsules based mainly on polylactide or polylactide-polyglycolide polymer formulations (Beck et al, 1981). These microcapsules can be prepared by a variety of techniques with the steroid dispersed evenly through the matrix. They can be injected intramuscularly through a large needle, where they form a depot for slow release by diffusion and surface erosion. They suffer the small disadvantage that removal is not possible after administration.

A completely different range of delivery systems has been developed for continuous local release of contraceptive steroids within the genital tract. These include intrauterine devices (IUD), intracervical devices (ICD) and vaginal rings. A progesterone-releasing IUD (Progestasert; Alza Corporation, Palo Alto) has been marketed for several years. This device releases about 65 μg of progesterone daily within the uterine cavity for up to a year. The steady release of progesterone is maintained by a specially designed controlled release membrane in the stem of the IUD. This system has one major advantage over other IUDs in that it will greatly reduce the volume of menstrual flow, but only at the expense of an increase in the number of days of spotting. More advanced hormone releasing IUDs containing potent progestogens which will last for several years are being studied at present (Luukkainen & Nilsson, 1978).

Intra-cervical devices releasing low doses of progestogens or spermicides initially appeared very attractive because they would not produce significant systemic steroid effects nor cause the same menstrual disturbances as IUDs, yet would provide prolonged duration of action (World Health Organsiation, 1979a; Kurunmäki et al, 1981). Unfortunately major difficulties have been encountered by several groups with repeated expulsions and local tissue irritation, and the ICD approach is now being pursued much less actively.

By contrast local delivery of contraceptive steroids by vaginal rings has reached the stage of large scale testing and has a great deal of promise (Mishell et al, 1970; Diczfalusy & Landgren, 1981; Population Council, 1981). These rings are very precisely manufactured from different silicon elastomers and parts of the core are filled with the active steroid. The type of silastic, surface area, thickness of the wall, loading and distribution of the steroid within the core, type of steroid and other characteristics will all influence the rate of diffusion of steroid into the vagina. The vagina is an efficient surface for absorption of steroids and has the additional benefit that absorbed steroids avoid the metabolic effect of "first pass" through the portal system of the liver. The ring can be designed to release low doses of progestogen alone which will have a "minipill" effect or higher doses of oestrogen and progestogen or progestogen alone which will inhibit ovulation. This system can be removed and reinserted at any time and is therefore in the full control of the woman herself (Ch. 33).

Types of long acting contraceptives and current world wide usage

These methods are summarised in Table 34.3, which also illustrates their stage of development. It can be seen clearly that the aim of those working in the field is to develop a full range of different long acting methods which are safe and effective, and will provide a choice with appeal to many different individuals and health care programmes.

Monthly administration

Numerous combinations of injectable oestrogens and progestogens have been studied in small clinical trials (Benagiano, 1977; Toppozada, 1977; Hall & Fraser, 1983), but only a small number of preparations are undergoing further development. None has reached the stage of general marketing. These preparations are all given by deep intramuscular injection once every 4 weeks, and are 100 per cent effective in preventing pregnancy because unnecessarily large doses were utilised in the early formulations. Dose reduction studies are underway. Another major advantage of these preparations is that they achieve more satisfactory menstrual bleeding patterns than the longer acting methods, but they suffer the inconvenience of monthly visits for the injection.

The preparation which has been most extensively studied (dihydroxyprogesterone acetophenide 150 mg plus oestradiol oenanthate 10 mg) is not being developed further because of unresolved toxicology concerns (Benagiano, 1977). Very low dose progestogens alone may have some advantages (Prema et al, 1981) but there is still uncertainty about their efficacy.

Oral long-acting oestrogen and progestogen combi-nations have been tested extensively as monthly pills in the Peoples' Republic of China (Fan, 1981). These are combinations of the long-acting oestrogen — quinestrol — with norgestrel, chlormadinone or 16-methylene chlormadinone. They are highly effective contraceptives but face major concerns about endometrial hyperplasia and metabolic effects.

Two to three monthly administration

Two preparations are already marketed widely in numerous countries and are highly effective contraceptives. DMPA is marketed for contraception in 84 countries as a microcrystalline suspension of 150 mg administered once every 90 days and there are very few countries where it is not registered for other indications. It is calculated that 12–14 million year equivalents of Depo-Provera have been used for contraception since 1963 and approximately 1.7 million year equivalents were used in 1980. Several other pharmaceutical companies apart from Upjohn make DMPA preparations of uncertain formulation and efficacy. The extent of use of these formulations is unknown. DMPA has been extensively studied with mention in over 1000 published papers, and is probably the most thoroughly investigated single hormonal contraceptive preparation in existence. Over 3.2 million woman-months of surveillance have been reported in controlled trials and approximately 20 large scale clinical studies are currently in progress.

NET-OEN is marketed as a contraceptive in over 40 countries and is administered in doses of 200 mg in oily solution every 56–84 days. World-wide usage in 1980 amounted to 100–120 000 year-equivalents. Usage is rapidly increasing and numerous large scale trials are underway at present. NET-OEN does not face the same political pressures as DMPA, but does face the same type of metabolic, clinical and toxicology issues.

DMPA and NET-OEN both exhibit first order release of steroid with high initial blood levels. Theoretically, a better approach is the use of norethisterone-releasing polymer microcapsules which are presently undergoing early clinical trails (Beck et al, 1981). These can be injected through a needle and should provide near zero-order release of NET over 3–6 months depending on the steroid-loading of the microcapsules. Modifications to the polymer and use of levonorgestrel should provide an even longer duration of action.

Vaginal rings can be designed for any duration of use from 1 month to 1 year (and probably longer), but most studies have used rings which were designed to be changed after about 3 months. None of these devices has reached the stage of general marketing but they have already demonstrated a potentially large market because of zero-order release, possible wide variations in design and generally good acceptability.

Six monthly administration

Only one preparation is marketed. This is DMPA usually given in a dosage of 450 mg every 180 days, but it is not widely used. Injectable NET or LNG microcapsules offering near zero-order release may have a small place as 6-monthly injectables although this is probably the practical limit of duration of action of a non-recoverable injection. For this prolonged duration of action implants which are potentially recoverable, at least during the first 1–2 months after administration, are psychologically more attractive to most doctors and clients. Several of these approaches are in the early stages of clinical trial (Benagiano & Gabelnick, 1979).

Duration of action greater than one year

These devices are all subcutaneous implants or IUDs and all offer the potential for early removal if the client changes her mind or experiences an untoward reaction. Most of these are based on levonorgestrel (e.g. the NIH polycaprolactone implant and the Population Council's Norplant Systems), but many other progestogens have been used in implants while have reached the stage of early clinical trial (Benagiano, 1977; Coutinho, 1978). A progestogen which has potential advantages in lactating women is ST1435 (Coutinho et al, 1976) because it has no oral activity and is unlikely to be absorbed by the neonate. The only implant system which has been very widely tested and is now being released for marketing is 'Norplant'. It is hoped to introduce a simpler two implant system (Norplant II) to replace the six implant system within a few years.

Uses of long acting progestogens other than for contraception

Long acting injectable progestogens, in particular DMPA, have been used extensively fo a wide variety of medical conditions, and are of great benefit in many of these (Fraser & Weisberg, 1981). Gynaecological conditions which may respond well include endometriosis, hirsutism, the premenstrual syndrome, dysfunctional uterine bleeding including cystic glandular hyperplasia of the endometrium, menstrual epilepsy and menstrual migraine. DMPA may be a useful chemotherapeutic adjunct in the treatment of a number of different malignant conditions. It is of particular value in the treatment of endometrial adenocarcinoma, but has been of use also in cancers of the kidney, bone, testes, cervix, ovary and breast. A miscellaneous group of conditions may also respond, including precocious puberty, acromegaly, diabetic retinopathy, recurrent aphthous ulcers, sleep apnoea, Pickwickian Syndrome and autoimmune liver disease. Progestogens may be useful for the treatment of male conditions including prostatic hypertrophy, and have been studied as possible long acting male contraceptives.

PHARMACOLOGY

Pharmacokinetics

Most injectable contraceptives exhibit first order release of the active steroid with initial high rate of release followed by an exponential decay in the circulating blood level (Fig. 34.1). The absolute levels of the peak and the rate of disappearance of the progestogen or oestrogen from the plasma depend on the dosage and formulation as well as many aspects of absorption from the injection site, blood and tissue distribution, plasma binding, metabolism and excretion. Rapid early absorption may be caused by excessive massaging of the injection site.

Depot medroxyprogesterone acetate. This represents a microcrystalline preparation and the progestogen circulates as the active free steroid. There is relatively little plasma binding and most of this is to albumin. Very little binds to sex hormone binding globulin. Plasma levels have been measured by radioimmunoassay and gas-liquid chromatography. The early assays lacked specificity and probably also measured conjugates and metabolites of MPA (Cornette et al, 1971; Mathrubutham & Fotherby, 1981). Recent assays are sensitive to <0.3 nmol/l and provide good agreement on the pattern of serum levels. However, there is still some variation in specificity and sensitivity of these assays. It is generally agreed that peak levels of 2.5–12 nmol/l are reached within 1–2 weeks following injection falling to a plateau of 2.5–4 nmol/l between 1 and 2 months later (Kaiser et al, 1974; Ortiz et al, 1977; Mathrubutham & Fotherby, 1981).Thereafter there is a gradual decline to a mean of 0.5 nmol/l during the 6 months after a single injection. It is possible that there may be ethnic differences in the pharmacokinetics (Fotherby et al, 1980). As a result of the lack of plasma binding there is rapid removal of MPA from the plasma resulting in a high metabolic clearance rate. Plasma levels between 2 and 4 nmol/l are usually present at the time of the next 90 day injection and there has been concern that accumulation of MPA may occur in the circulation with repeated injections. However two careful cross sectional studies indicate that this does not occur to any appreciable extent even after several years of continuous use (Koetsawang et al, 1979; Jeppsson et al, 1982). A careful pharmacokinetic study of different dosages of DMPA showed little difference in blood levels between doses of 100 and 150 mg in a small number of Thai women (Fotherby et al, 1980). This suggests that doses of 100 mg may provide satisfactory contraception in some ethnic groups. Such dosage reduction studies are currently underway.

Norethisterone oenanthate. This represents a preparation containing a progestogen ester in oil. A great deal of recent information has been provided on this formulation by the London group (Sang et al, 1981). Following intramuscular injection of 200 mg there is uptake of the ester into the circulation where it is distributed and stored in adipose

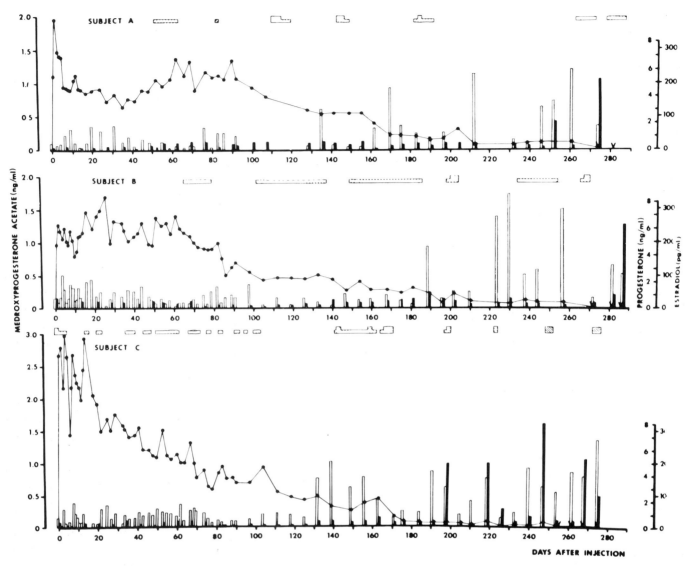

Fig. 34.1 Plasma levels of MPA (●), oestradiol (open columns) and progesterone (black columns) in three subjects following a single injection of DMPA. Episodes of vaginal bleeding are recorded as horizontal hatched bars at the top of each graph
(from Ortiz et al, 1977 with permission)

tissue. Slow release then occurs over the following weeks. Both norethisterone oenanthate and free norethisterone are detectable in the circulation although there are wide individual variations in serum levels. Norethisterone oenanthate reaches a peak of around 4 ng/ml at 1–4 days following injection with a rapid fall thereafter to <1 ng/ml by 15 days. On the other hand serum norethisterone reaches a peak of around 10 ng/ml at about 7 days and this is followed by a less rapid fall to <1 ng/ml by 35 days. It may remain detectable in serum for anything between 54 and 120 days. In humans it appears that NET-OEN is hydrolysed mainly in the liver (Back et al, 1981). The many factors which affect the duration of action of NET-OEN have been thoroughly discussed by Fotherby (1981).

Less information is available on the pharmacokinetics of monthly injectables. However, they do show first order release and there is some evidence that the dosages are

much higher than necessary with a tendency to accumulation of steroid from one injection period to the next (Gual et al, 1973; Fotherby et al, 1980). Dosage reduction studies are underway.

Several animal species have been studied as possible models for investigating the pharmacokinetics and pharmacodynamics of injectable contraceptives. There is now good evidence that rhesus monkeys (Mora & Johansson, 1976) and baboons (Fotherby & Goldzieher 1980) are adequate models for this.

Several delivery systems manage to attain near zero-order release with relatively constant serum levels over prolonged periods of time. One of the most successful approaches to this has been the development by the Population Council of a 7 year levonorgestrel releasing subcutaneous implant system — Norplant (Croxatto et al, 1980). This system achieves serum progestogen levels of

0.35 ± 0.03 ng/ml (mean ± s.e. (mean), 110 women) after 1 year. This falls to a mean of 0.29 ± 0.02 ng/ml after 5 years. This is a six implant system but a number of single implants have been tested. One of these silastic systems releases norethisterone acetate over a 6–7 month period (Laumas et al, 1981). This achieves plasma norethisterone levels of 1 ng/ml at 1 month declining to 0.5 ng/ml at 6 months. It is of some interest that this decline in plasma level appears to be due to an increase in the metabolic clearance rate of norethisterone acetate over several months of exposure, rather than a change in the rate of delivery of norethisterone acetate from the implant (Singh et al, 1982). Another very successful zero-order release system is the vaginal ring (Diczfalusy & Landgren, 1981). These systems appear to have virtually eliminated the initial high peak in serum levels following insertion and these decline at a very slow rate thereafter (Fig. 34.2). For example a norethisterone ring releasing approximately 200 µg per day produces plasma levels of 2.5 nmol/l following insertion and these decline slowly to around 2.0 nmol/l after 90 days. The equivalent values for a levonorgestrel ring releasing 20 µg

per day are 0.49 nmol/1 declining to 0.4 nmol/1 after 90 days. Characterisation of the rings has revealed that levonorgestrel and norethisterone are absorbed differently by the vagina. It appears that peak serum levels are achieved within 1 hour of insertion of a levonorgestrel releasing ring whereas peak levels are not achieved for 24 hours with norethisterone.

The other delivery system which has some promise as a near zero-order system is the injectable polylactide micro capsule system. This can be engineered to release most of the available steroids and early pharmocokinetic and clinical trials are currently underway (Beck et al, 1981).

Pharmacodynamics

There is general agreement that the classical injectables like DMPA, NET-OEN and the combined oestrogen-progestogen monthly injectables act predominantly by the effective inhibition of ovulation (Fig. 34.1). Most progestogens given in high dosage inhibit pituitary FSH and LH secretion to the low normal range (Goldzieher et al, 1970). Plasma oestradiol is also significantly suppressed into the early follicular phase range and progesterone remains very low for many months (Jeppsson et al, 1973; Ortiz et al, 1977). As progestogen levels fall there appears to be a persistent inhibition of the positive feedback response to oestradiol (Ortiz et al, 1977). This is clearly demonstrated by the reappearance of cyclic oestradiol secretion well before the occurrence of ovulation. It appears that follicle maturation resumes at MPA levels between 0.25 and 0.5 ng/ml but ovulation does not occur until the plasma levels are <0.1 ng/ml (Ortiz et al, 1977). Unlike the combined pill DMPA does not suppress the response of the pituitary to gonadotrophin releasing hormone (Toppozada et al, 1978). In general the monthly injectables produce greater suppression of pituitary ovarian function equivalent to that seen with the combined oral contraceptive pill. Norethisterone oenanthate also inhibits ovulation in a manner similar to DMPA but the effect wears off between 60 and 120 days compared with the 3–9 months following DMPA. It is possible that there are substantial ethnic differences in these responses (Benagiano et al, 1980).

All these progestogens have important effects on the function of the endometrium, Fallopian tube, cervical mucus and corpus luteum. It seems likely that these subsidiary effects are more important in the contraceptive action of NET-OEN than DMPA or the monthly injectables.

DMPA produces an endometrium with the appearance of inhibited secretion or 'suppression' and at 20–30 days following injection the endometrium becomes thin and atrophic (Lee, 1968; Khoo et al, 1971). Atrophic changes tend to become more marked with progressive injections. The ultrastructural appearances of the endometrium during one treatment cycle have been well described

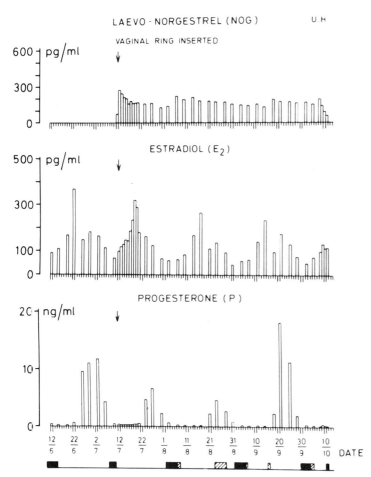

Fig. 34.2 Plasma levels of levonorgestrel, oestradiol and progesterone in a single subject using a contraceptive vaginal ring releasing approximately 20 µg of levonorgestrel daily. Episodes of vaginal bleeding are illustrated as horizontal bars at the bottom of the figure. (from Diczfalusy and Landgren 1981, with permission)

(Roberts et al, 1975). NET-OEN produces much more variable effects upon the endometrium depending on the stage of the injection cycle (Benagiano et al, 1980). Effects can also be demonstrated on the Fallopian tubes (El Mahgoub et al, 1972; Zanartu & Navarro, 1968), on cervical mucus (Kesseru-Koos, 1971) and on corpus luteum function (Weiner & Johansson, 1976). Progestogens may also suppress sex hormone binding globulin which may temporarily contribute to the changes in plasma hormone levels but this returns to normal before the next injection (Jeppsson et al, 1982). It is very encouraging to see that there is no greater suppression of any of these hormone levels after 10 years of use of DMPA than after one cycle (Jeppsson et al, 1982).

Since the low dose zero-order release systems do not act by the invariable suppression of ovulation it is likely that their effects on cervical mucus, Fallopian tube function, corpus luteum and endometrial function are extremely important for their contraceptive action as they are with the progestogen-only mini pill (Diczfalusy & Landgren, 1981; Laumas et al, 1981).

Progestogens all bind to progesterone receptors but depending on their individual structures may also bind to other receptors (e.g. androgen or cortico-steroid receptors) and may act in slightly different ways depending on their structure (Rozenbaum, 1982). MPA may act partly through androgen receptors to induce gonadotrophin suppression (Perez-Palacios et al, 1981), although it does not have an overt androgenic activity in humans. In fact in women it can be shown to have an anti androgenic action. Effects of progestogens on androgen and cortico-steroid receptors may be seen with progressively increasing doses, usually at a level well above the standard contraceptive range. The injectable progestogens produce significant suppression of oestrogen receptors in the endometrium and cervix (Tseng & Gurpide, 1975; Rall et al, 1978).

The multiple effects seen with high dose injectable contraceptives contribute to a very high efficiency of these agents. The failure of the low dose zero-order systems to inhibit ovulation does mean that they have a slightly lower contraceptive efficacy although initial trials indicate that the pregnancy rates will be quite low enough to be widely acceptable.

Clinical aspects

Contraceptive efficacy

The major injectable preparations are highly effective contraceptives. DMPA has been very extensively studied in a dosage of 150 mg every 3 months and over a dozen large scale clinical trials have been reported. The pregnancy rates have varied between 0.01 and 1.2 per 100 woman-years (Fraser & Weisberg, 1981). In the major trials the pregnancy rates have generally been less than 0.5

per 100 woman-years and this figure compares very favourably with the rates reported in combined oral contraceptive trials. The major advantage of the injectables over oral contraceptives is that the use effectiveness approaches theoretical effectiveness. Clearly factors such as disturbed absorption, missed pills and drug interactions do not contribute to the failure rate. It is possible that doses as low as 100 mg every 3 months may provide similarly effective contraception in some ethnic groups (Fotherby et al, 1980). DMPA has also been used as a 6 monthly injection, usually in a dosage of 400–500 mg. In general these 6 monthly regimens have been associated with slightly higher pregnancy rates than 150 mg every 3 months (Rall et al, 1977).

Norethisterone oenanthate is also a highly effective contraceptive but in general the pregnancy rates have been slightly higher than with DMPA. The first randomised multicentre World Health Organisation study of NET-OEN and DMPA had to be terminated prematurely because the pregnancy rate with NET-OEN 200 mg given once every 90 days (3.6 pregnancies per 100 woman-years) exceeded predetermined criteria (World Health Organisation, 1977). The second WHO multicentre comparison of these two agents studied two regimens of NET-OEN administration. Both regimens utilised 200 mg every 60 days for the first 6 months. One of these groups continued with this same schedule while the other reverted to less frequent injections of 200 mg every 84 days (World Health Organisation, 1982a). The interim report of this trial indicates that both NET-OEN regimens are more effective than the original regimen of 200 mg every 90 days. However the pregnancy rate at 18 months with the group who switched to 84 day injections was significantly higher than with DMPA users (1.6 compared with 0.2 pregnancies per 100 woman-years). The pregnancy rate with the NET-OEN 60 day regimen remained constant at 0.6 per 100 woman-years. NET-OEN has also been used successfully in the very low dosage 20 mg given as a monthly injectable (Prema et al, 1981).

Numerous small scale clinical trials of monthly injectables have been published and not a single pregnancy has been reported with any of the oestrogen-progestogen combinations (Benagiano, 1977; Toppozada, 1977; Hall & Fraser, 1983). This extraordinarily high contraceptive efficacy is in keeping with the indication from pharmacokinetic data that dosage levels are unnecessarily high (Gual et al, 1973).

Much less information is available about the zero-order release systems. Initial clinical experience with subcutaneous progestogen releasing implants was not satisfactory (Coutinho, 1978) but more recent experience, particularly with the Norplant indicates a very high efficacy for up to 5 years of use (Diaz et al, 1979; Sivin et al, 1980). It is anticipated that the vaginal ring systems will also provide good contraceptive efficacy and this should certainly be the case with those releasing a combination of an oestrogen and a progestogen (Population Council, 1981).

Acceptability and continuation rates

One of the major advantages of injectable contraceptives is their high acceptability in those communities where they are widely available. They have fairly widespread appeal to a number of couples because of the advantages outlined in Table 34.1. However, it must be acknowledged that many women find that the concerns and disadvantages summarised in Table 34.2 outweigh the potential advantages. It is probably true to say that acceptability in a particular community can only be assessed when the method is widely available and can be offered in a free choice situation or 'cafeteria' style clinic. In a country like New Zealand where DMPA has been generally marketed as a contraceptive for many years it is estimated that approximately 10 per cent of contraceptive users rely on this injectable. There is little doubt that usage would be much greater but for the emotion and controversy which have been generated by the Depo-Provera debate.

In almost all trials where continuation rates with injectables have been compared against other contraceptive methods the continuation rates have been very similar or even better for the injectables (Fraser & Weisberg, 1981). Most of the studies have involved DMPA and continuation rates with this injectable have generally been in the range of 50–80 per cent at the end of 1 year but in one exceptional study were as low as 18.3 per cent (Bloch, 1971). There are clearly many factors which affect the attitude of the patient and the physician to these contraceptives in any particular centre. In some communities continuation rates at the end of 2 years may be as high as 70 per cent (McDaniel & Pardthaisong, 1974). Continuation rates with norethisterone oenanthate (200 mg every 56 days) are of the same order with continuation of 77 per cent at 1 year, 64 per cent at 2 years and 34 per cent at 3 years (Howard et al, 1982). Similar comments apply to the oestrogen-progestogen monthly injectables (Hall & Fraser, 1983). With all of these preparations menstrual disturbances are the single major medical reason for discontinuation and the more extreme disturbances such as amenorrhoea and prolonged/heavy bleeding are responsible for the highest proportion of discontinuations. Other medical causes only account for a very small proportion of the total.

Initial indications are that subcutaneous implants and vaginal rings will also have a high acceptability in certain communities (Coutinho et al, 1978; Faundes et al, 1981).

Menstrual disturbance

Injectable contraceptives produce an almost invariable disturbance of the menstrual cycle and this may be a source of major concern to the woman especially if adequate coun-selling has not been given before treatment started. The more extreme disturbances are produced by the progestogen-only methods, especially the higher dose first-order release formulations like DMPA.

A wide range of disturbances have been reported with these contraceptives. They include frequent amenorrhoea, frequent oligomenorrhoea, less frequent irregular or prolonged bleeding or spotting and very occasional heavy bleeding. The most consistent finding is the complete unpredictability of the bleeding patterns.

DMPA causes amenorrhoea of greater than 90 days duration in up to 40 per cent of women by the end of 12 months of use (Schwallie & Assenzo, 1973; World Health Organisation, 1978a; Gray, 1980). NET-OEN causes less amenorrhoea than DMPA even with 2 monthly rather than 3 monthly administration although the incidence of other types of menstrual disturbance is similar with both these preparations (World Health Organisation, 1978a; Howard et al, 1982a).

In one DMPA trial over 70 per cent of women did not experience even one 'normal' cycle throughout 1 or more years of treatment and during any one injection interval only 7 per cent of women recorded normal cycles (World Health Organisation, 1978a). The incidence of amenorrhoea and infrequent bleeding increases with duration of treatment. Heavy bleeding in uncommon except in the puerperium (Murphy, 1979).

Monthly injectables which contain both oestrogen and progestogen give the best approximation at the present time to a normal menstrual cycle with injectable contraceptives. Although there are widespread differences between different trials, in general 75–80 per cent of women will experience cycles between 24 and 35 days (Hall & Fraser, 1983). However, it does seem that long cycles tend to increase in frequency with time and complete amenorrhoea has been reported in up to 26 per cent of patients. In a detailed study of Cycloprovera (DMPA 25 mg, oestradiol cypionate 5 mg, Upjohn Company) the incidence of amenorrhoea fluctuated around 10 per cent during the first year but gradually increased to around 25 per cent after 2 years (Koetsawang et al, 1978). Irregular bleeding, profuse and prolonged bleeding have also been reported with these preparations.

Menstrual disturbances are also seen with the lower dose zero-order release systems although these disturbances are usually of lesser degree than those recorded with DMPA and NET-OEN (Faundes et al, 1978).

It seems that the actual incidence and type of menstrual disturbances which occur in different communities treated with these contraceptive methods is similar. However, tolerance of such disturbances by individual women may vary very greatly from society to society. There is no doubt that menstrual disturbances are the commonest medical reason for discontinuation of use of these long acting methods and it seems that extreme disturbances —

including amenorrhoea and prolonged or heavy bleeding — are most likely to lead to discontinuation. However, the frequency of discontinuation is greatly influenced by physician attitude and by the extent of appropriate counselling. It seems clear nowadays that education of the women before they start use of progestogen-only contraceptives, and continuing counselling by physicians and health workers who are convinced of the value of injectables, is very important in terms of high continuation rates. There are many cultural beliefs about menstruation and in some societies any disturbance of the accepted normal pattern is seen as being undesirable. The World Health Organisation (1979b) has just completed a very detailed study in ten cultural groups in different countries. Out of that social acceptability study the women decided that they prefer the contraceptive methods which ensure that there is no amenorrhoea, that there is no increase or decrease in the regular blood loss, that they should continue to have regular, preferably short, bleeding episodes, that there should be an accurate prediction of when the next bleeding days are going to be, and that there should be no change in the blood consistency or the colour of the blood which is lost. This is an ideal which does not occur even without contraception and it is salutary to look at the very high continuation rate with injectable contraception in order to show how a woman's natural and inner feelings and her tolerance of menstrual disturbances· can be modified by appropriate counselling. There is some evidence that a contraceptive which produces predictable amenorrhoea would have a high acceptability amongst a proportion of individuals in most communities.

The development of amenorrhoea is usually clearly related to development of an atrophic endometrium. However, the mechanism behind the unpredictable bleeding episode is quite unknown. It does not appear to be related to fluctuation in circulating hormone levels but may be related in some way to the development of abnormal vessels, particularly dilated thin walled sinusoids, in the superficial endometrium. Oestrogen and progesterone receptors are greatly suppressed and there is a likelihood of abnormalities of function of lysosomes, prostaglandins and the local haemostatic system. The extent to which any of these factors contribute is unknown. These menstrual side-effects and the underlying mechanisms are considered to be of such importance that they were recently the sole topic of a 3 day World Health Organisation expert symposium (Diczfalusy et al 1980).

Management of bleeding disturbances with these agents in unsatisfactory (Koetsawang, 1980; Fraser 1981). It is widely felt that if a woman cannot tolerate amenorrhoea or irregular scanty bleeding she should not use progestogen-only methods. On the other hand it has been shown by several groups that regular cyclical administration of oestrogen will usually produce withdrawal bleeding in women who have developed amenorrhoea (El-Habashy et al, 1970; McDaniel & Pardthaisong, 1973). The type of oestrogen appears to be important and should preferably be of a short acting type. Somewhat surprisingly oestrogens do not always produce predictable withdrawal bleeding in progestogen-only users and this is probably due to the suppression of endometrial receptors preventing hormone action (Tseng & Gurpide, 1975). Regular oestrogen administration makes the method much more complicated and negates one of the major advantages of using progestogens alone.

A very wide range of oestrogen regimens have been used to treat irregular, prolonged or heavy bleeding disturbances but there is no good evidence that bleeding patterns really do improve in the long run. There is reasonable evidence that in adequate dosage oestrogens are capable of stopping an episode of bleeding but in many cases a new episode will start soon afterwards. It is encouraging that oestrogen administration only appears to be occasionally indicated and in a comparative World Health Organisation trial (Gray, 1980) oestrogen was only required in 0.5 cases per 100 woman years of use of DMPA or NET-OEN. Administration of the next DMPA or NET-OEN injection earlier than scheduled has been suggested but never adequately tested. Other agents proposed for the treatment of spontaneous dysfunctional uterine bleeding have never been tested with bleeding disturbances following progestogen contraception. Curettage is very rarely required to stop an episode of bleeding but may be indicated for diagnostic purposes, especially in older women.

In view of the high incidence and unpredictability of these menstrual disturbances urgent research is needed to establish underlying mechanisms as well as to develop new steroids and new delivery systems which may minimise the occurrence of the disturbances (Fraser & Diczfalusy, 1980). The immediate prospects for developing a progestogen only method which does not cause irregular bleeding or which produces predictable amenorrhoea are not good. Therefore pre-injection counselling remains of paramount importance.

Delay in the return of fertility

As in other areas DMPA is the preparation which has been most thoroughly studied. There is now clear evidence that this preparation causes an unpredictable delay in the return of ovulation, menstruation and fertility following discontinuation (McDaniel & Pardthaisong, 1973; Schwallie & Assenzo, 1974; Pardthaisong et al, 1980; Pardthaisong 1981 Fig. 34.3). This delay is due to the persistence of the drug in the circulation following slow removal from the depot injection site as discussed above. Once ovulation has recurred it usually continues regularly thereafter. The largest and best controlled comparative study of the return of fertility following DMPA use indicates that the conception rate curve is similar in shape to non-contraceptive

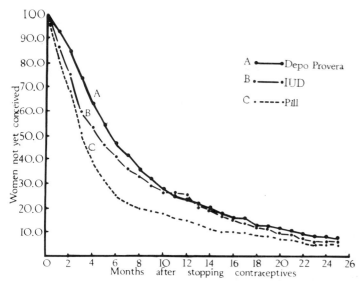

Fig. 34.3 Cumulative conception rates in women stopping Depo-Provera, oral contraceptives or an intrauterine device in order to fall pregnant. Time O for Depo Provera has been calculated from 15 weeks after the last injection
(from Pardthaisong 1981, with permission)

users and the median delay is only 5.5 months. This delay compares favourably with the 4.5 months delay following intra-uterine device use in the same populations (Pardthaisong et al, 1980). Most studies indicate a re-establishment of menstruation and ovulation in 50 per cent of subjects by 6 months after the last injection, in 75 per cent by 12 months and 85 per cent by 18 months. Equivalent conception rates are over 60 per cent by 12 months and 85 per cent by 24 months. There is no evidence whatsoever that DMPA or any other injectable causes persistent amenorrhoea or permanent infertility. Encouraging recent evidence indicates that prolonged use of DMPA does not increase the delay before conception and that nulliparous women are not at more risk of delay (Pardthaisong, 1981).

NET-OEN, the monthly injectables and the other delivery systems have not been studied nearly as extensively as DMPA but the limited data available on return of ovulation and fertility suggest that these methods are less likely to cause a delay than DMPA (Kesseru-Koos et al, 1973; Hall & Fraser, 1983).

Other side-effects and complications

Numerous reviews of injectable contraception have reaffirmed that other side-effects have never presented a problem in clinical trials and are not a common cause of discontinuation (Nash, 1975; Benagiano, 1977; Fraser & Weisberg, 1981). However, mention of side-effects during the counselling session prior to commencement of treatment appears crucial to the success of injectable contraception. Weight gain, headaches, dizziness, abdominal bloating, fatigue, nervousness and other mood changes have been reported with frequencies varying between 5 and

15 per cent of users. This frequency of complaint is not dissimilar to users of oral contraceptives and intra-uterine devices (Scutchfield et al, 1971; Schwallie & Assenzo, 1972). It is quite possible that many of these complaints may not be directly due to the exogenous hormones (Aznar-Ramos et al, 1969; Goldzieher et al, 1971). An average weight gain of 0.5–2.0 kg by the end of 1 year has been reported in most studies with the occasional patient gaining much more than this but these gains are partially offset by the 20–40 per cent of users who actually lose weight. In one trial only 0.37 per cent of participants actually complained about weight gain (World Health Organisation, 1978a).

Small mean decreases in blood pressure have frequently been reported with DMPA and NET-OEN but occasional individuals show a rise (Giwa-Osagie et al, 1978; Ojo, 1979). One investigator has reported a rise in mean diastolic blood pressure with DMPA and nearly 25 per cent of his users exhibited a significant individual rise (Leiman, 1972). This study stands out from all the others and is difficult to explain. There is no evidence that injectable progestogens adversely affect blood coagulation and the risk of venous thrombosis (Nash, 1975; Howard et al, 1981). These are probably the hormonal contraceptives of choice for women with a previous history of venous thromboembolism. Clearly it would be inadvisable to use the oestrogen containing monthly injectables in this situation. Somewhat different minor symptoms have been described with some of the monthly injectables and these include breast tenderness, dysmenorrhoea and premenstrual symptoms.

It is worth noting that progestogen-only methods may be associated with some beneficial side-effects including a significant reduction in the incidence of vaginal moniliasis (Toppozada et al, 1979) and a probable reduction in the incidence of acute pelvic inflammatory disease in women with gonorrhoea (Senanayake & Kramer, 1980).

Neoplasia

Currently all hormonal contraceptives are under the microscope of various consumer groups and the media and their theoretical potential for causing cancer is a topic of major concern. Although there is no good evidence that the combined oral contraceptives or the long acting hormonal contraceptives cause any type of cancer there are several areas of controversy (World Health Organisation, 1978b). Much of the concern arises from animal toxicity studies (see below) but the lack of well-designed studies and the potentially long latent period of neoplasms in humans ensure that the questions cannot be ignored.

The chief areas of concern are neoplasms of the breast, cervix and endometrium. Several studies have examined the relationship between DMPA and breast cancer. None of these showed any increase in the risk of breast cancer with DMPA use but only two included an appropriate comparison group (Greenspan et al, 1980). Breast cancer has been of particular concern because this is such a common cancer in many countries and only a small increase in relative risk would result in a large number of additional tumours. High doses of DMPA will actually cause breast atrophy and a proportion of patients with metastatic breast carcinoma will respond very favourably to treatment with DMPA (Cuna et al, 1978). Theoretically it is quite possible that DMPA and perhaps other progestogens may actually provide a small protective effect against the development of breast cancer.

Early clinical studies suggested that DMPA use may predispose to the development of cervical neoplasia (Powell & Seymour, 1971) but at least eight other studies have shown either no difference or a reduced incidence of cytological abnormality among DMPA users (Fraser & Weisberg, 1981). All these studies of cervical cancer among DMPA users have suffered from numerous methodological problems and in the early studies the DMPA users appeared to have numerous known risk factors for cervical neoplasia. These data are inconclusive and the results of extensive studies still in progress are awaited.

Toxicology studies in rhesus monkeys have raised the possibility of an increased risk of endometrial or possibly endocervical carcinoma with DMPA use (see below). However none of the available human data suggest such an association. In fact the paucity of cases of endometrial carcinoma among women who have used DMPA is quite remarkable. Only one case has been reported in a DMPA user and in retrospect it seems most likely that the cancer was present before DMPA use was initiated for treatment of her irregular bleeding (Stamm & De Grandi, 1981). This may represent under reporting but is remarkable considering the widespread use of the drug and the recent interest in this possible complication. In view of the recent evidence which indicates that combined oral contraceptive use is protective against the later development of endometrial carcinoma (Weiss & Sayvetz, 1980) it seems very likely that progestogen only contraceptives will also be proven to have a protective effect in due course. It must be remembered that DMPA is used with considerable success as a treatment for endometrial carcinoma in women (Rozier & Underwood, 1974; Bonte et al, 1978).

There is no evidence that DMPA, NET-OEN or the low dose delivery systems influence the risk of hepatic neoplasia or pituitary adenomas, although those agents which act by the inhibition of ovulation may help to reduce the risk of ovarian carcinoma (Casagrande et al, 1979).

Exposure of the fetus to hormonal contraceptive steroids

During the 1960s large numbers of women were treated with progestogens in high dosage in order to prevent threatened or habitual abortion. Most of the published information on fetal exposure to steroids comes from patients who were treated for pregnancy maintenance and not because of failed contraception or an inadvertently administered contraceptive dose. Some of these studies do indicate that there may be a small risk associated with exposure of the fetus to these agents. However even with the very high dosage of steroids given for pregnancy maintenance the risk to the fetus from any point of view, if any, is extremely small. The literature on the teratogenic potential of contraceptive steroids has been thoroughly reviewed on several occasions in recent years (Rothman & Louik, 1978; Benagiano & Goldzieher, 1979; Schwallie, 1981; Gray, 1983).

When given in large doses DMPA is capable of virilising rat and rabbit fetuses (Pincus, 1965) but in human studies with doses as high as 400 mg given on several occasions during the pregnancy reports of virilisation or other abnormalities are very rare. There only appear to be two reports of mild virilisation following exposure to high dose DMPA during human pregnancy (Wilkins et al, 1958; Burstein & Wasserman, 1964). On the other hand exposure to massive doses of norethisterone (10–40 mg daily) from the 4th to 35th weeks of pregnancy was associated in one study with some degree of masculinisation among 18 per cent of female infants born to 82 mothers (Jacobson, 1962). Norethisterone does appear to have a weak androgenic effect in humans but when lower doses or shorter exposure periods occur (Keith & Burger, 1977) the incidence rate appears to be generally less than 1 per cent. It is possible that progestogens increase the risk of hypospadias but the excess risk of this uncommon condition, if any, is likely to be small (Gray, 1983).

A considerable amount of information relates to malformations of the cardiovascular and central nervous systems and a small part of these data have been analysed in relation to exposure to progestogens alone. Several studies including the very large Collaborative Perinatal Project have indicated that there may be an increase in risk of congenital heart defects of up to 2-fold in fetuses exposed to high doses of progestogen (Heinonen et al, 1977; Gray, 1983). Data relating to other systems do not reach the level of statistical significance although a few individual studies show small trends. The authors of most of these studies have acknowledged the fact that an excessive number of malformations might well be expected among the babies born to mothers with a history of threatened or habitual abortion (Harlap et al, 1975). Meaningful conclusions about these very low teratogenic risks are unlikely ever to be reached because the accidental pregnancy rate with injectable contraceptives is so low. Any risk associated with the low dose zero-order release systems is also likely to be extremely low.

There is also theoretical concern that exogenous steroid hormones could affect reproductive or sexual development of the fetus if given at susceptible periods of early life

(Duncan et al, 1976; Cox, 1979). The only study of injectable contraceptives which has suggested any possible effect
on sexual behaviour involved 15 girls exposed to DMPA
in utero who appeared to have an enhanced effect on their
normal feminine behaviour compared with controls
(Ehrhardt et al, 1977). A similar study of 13 boys showed
no effects on sexual behaviour (Meyer-Bahlburg et al,
1977). A recent editorial has found little evidence to implicate prenatal progestogen use in the modification of later
sexual behaviour (Editorial, 1981).

Lactation

It is clear that one of the major benefits of established
lactation is its contraceptive action. However, it is also
clear that in most societies the long-term contraceptive
action for the individual is unreliable and effective
additional contraception is an increasing necessity
(Dobbing, 1982). There is great demand for a method
which is effective and safe for use during lactation. The
injectable progestogens have several advantages in this situation but there are also concerns about the effect of any
exogenous progestogen transferred in the milk to the
neonate.

In contrast to studies of oestrogen containing oral
contraceptives most studies of injectable progestogens
report an increase or no change in the volume of milk
produced (Hull, 1981). Most of the reported investigations
have involved DMPA but a small number have involved
NET-OEN (Karim et al, 1971). Studies of the milk content
of lactose, protein and lipids have also been reported but
the results are variable and confusing (Fraser & Weisberg,
1981; Hull, 1981). Such studies are very difficult to execute
accurately because of changes in milk composition and
volume with time and even during the course of a single
feed. It is only very recently that well-executed studies
have been initiated to look carefully at individual nutrient
compounds in the milk. At the present time it seems probable that the progestogens do not adversely influence the
volume or content of milk in women with established
lactation. A similar body of evidence suggests that DMPA
does not have any adverse effect on growth or early development of the neonate (Fraser & Weisberg, 1981).

An area of increasing scientific interest and theoretical
concern is the transfer of contraceptive steroids to the fetal
circulation through the milk. This offers the theoretical
possibility of effect on steroid receptors in the brain or
genital tract with subsequent long-term effects on reproduction or sexual behaviour.

There is now well-documented evidence that circulating
progestogens are transferred from the maternal plasma into
milk. It seems that only the non-protein bound fraction of
plasma steroids is transferred into milk. MPA has a low
protein binding in maternal plasma and is found in milk
in virtually the same concentration as in plasma (Saxena et

al, 1977). In contrast the 19-nor progestogens have a high
and specific binding in plasma and are only found in milk in
a concentration of 15–25 per cent of that in plasma.

Of critical importance is the amount of active steroid
which is absorbed by the infant. Various calculations have
been made based on the measurements of steroid transfer
into milk. These indicate that an infant would only ingest
0.08–0.25 µg/kg/day of MPA. This is a very small dose but
there is good evidence to indicate that the exposure of the
neonate is reduced even further by a relatively low efficiency of steroid absorption from the gut. Extrapolation
from adult data suggests that absorption of MPA will be
poor whereas the 19-nor progestogens are likely to be more
efficiently absorbed. Monkey studies are currently being
undertaken to look at these aspects in more detail. There
are interesting preliminary data to indicate that the novel
progestogen ST-1435 is very poorly absorbed and therefore
the subcutaneous implants which have been developed
with this progestogen may have a particular application in
lactating women.

It is interesting to note that small amounts of progesterone may be transferred to the neonate in normal human
breast milk in the early neonatal period (Kulski et al,
1977). However, these amounts are probably quite low
compared with the amounts of progesterone and oestrogen
which may be transferred to children who are bottle fed
with cow's milk. Virtually nothing is known about the
actual levels of contraceptive steroids which reach the
neonatal circulation. Only one group has reported measurement of NET in plasma samples from four breast fed
infants 2–5 days following injection of NET-OEN (Melis
et al, 1981). In these cases NET could not be detected
using an assay system with a lower limit of detection of
0.05 ng/ml. There is no evidence that these extremely small
amounts of progestogen represent a potential biological risk
to the infant (Schwallie, 1981) but there is evidence from
animals that pre-natal or early post-natal exposure to sex
steroid hormones may exert an organising effect on certain
aspects of central nervous system function and responsiveness to later hormonal stimulation (Rubin et al, 1981).
However, the importance of progestogens in this situation
is unknown. Major changes in circulating levels of LH,
FSH, oestradiol and testosterone occur in both male and
female infants in the few weeks following birth and these
probably have some importance in determining reproductive and sexual behaviour later in life. There is no evidence
that contraceptive steroids affect this process but this
clearly requires detailed and urgent investigation. Studies
are currently underway.

Metabolic effects

A wealth of metabolic data now exists from studies on
combined oral contraceptives, oestrogens and progestogens
alone and there is considerable controversy about the

extent and the importance of the individual findings (see Ch. 35). Numerous studies have looked at various metabolic aspects of long acting hormonal contraceptives, mainly DMPA and to a lesser extent NET-OEN. monthly injectables and other systems. Although variable changes have been reported with the higher dose preparations biochemical abnormalities are virtually undetectable with the low dose zero-order release systems.

Carbohydrate metabolism

Small but significant changes in carbohydrate metabolism have been reported within most studies of contraceptive doses of DMPA, NET-OEN and the monthly injectables. The most consistent finding appears to be an exaggerated insulin response to the oral or intravenous glucose tolerance test and this may be more common with higher doses. This certainly occurs with some, although not all, patients who are receiving very high doses of DMPA for the treatment of cancer (Vecchio, 1972). Even in these patients the development of clinical diabetes has been rare. A metabolic study of NET-OEN also suggests that only a small number of individual women developed a minor abnormality of response to a glucose tolerance test (Howard et al, 1982b). Some studies of DMPA have reported a small increase in fasting levels of glucose as well as insulin and an enhanced glucose and insulin response to the glucose tolerance test (Spellacy et al, 1972; Vermuelen & Thiery, 1974), but changes in plasma glucose levels have not been confirmed in all studies (Tuttle & Turkington, 1974; Tankeyoon et al, 1976; Beck et al, 1977; Dhall et al, 1977; Amatayakul, 1979). It is not clear if these changes become more prominent with very long duration of treatment with DMPA although this seems unlikely with NET-OEN (Howard et al, 1982). In one study from the USA which stands out as being different from all other investigations the response to a glucose tolerance test became borderline or abnormal in 15 per cent of 37 women (Spellacy et al, 1972) and the question has been raised whether ethnic differences or a pre-diabetic tendency may be important.

The changes in carbohydrate metabolism are of the order of changes seen with injections of natural progesterone in animals (Kalkhoff, 1982) and are equivalent to those occurring in pregnancy. It is suggested that they are due to a direct progestogenic affect. The underlying mechanism is uncertain but could also be due to the very weak corticosteroid-like effect of DMPA (Amatayakul, 1979) and perhaps of other progestogens also. Any deterioration in glucose tolerance does not appear to be due to changes in growth hormone, glucagon, thyroxin, cortisol or trytophan metabolism or secretion (Fraser & Weisberg, 1981). It seems fair to conclude that the diabetogenic effect of the injectable progestogens is definite but slight and is of the same order as that seen with combined oral contraceptives.

Lipid metabolism

Long acting hormonal contraceptives are certainly capable of modifying the circulating levels of various lipids (Fraser, 1982b; Fotherby et al, 1982). The exact nature of some of the changes is unclear but there is little doubt that progestogens and oestrogens may have substantial effects on lipid metabolism. The effects are generally dose related and are more pronounced with the 19-nor testosterone progestogens than the C-21 17-acetoxy progestogens. The major concern about changes in circulating lipids arises from the epidemiological observations that risk of coronary artery disease is inversely related to the circulating high density lipoprotein cholesterol (HDL-C) concentration and is directly related to an increase in the levels of low density lipoprotein cholesterol (LDL-C) levels and serum triglycerides (Gordon et al, 1977; Miller et al, 1977). However there are others who dispute the direct relevance of depressed levels of HDL-C (Keys, 1980; Lees & Lees, 1982) and there is at least one situation where drug related lowering of HDL-C is associated with a decrease in the subsequent incidence of myocardial infarction (Miettinen et al, 1981). Progestogens do not have any influence on fasting triglyceride levels whereas oestrogens usually elevate these. Some progestogens have been reported to produce minor changes in the composition of phospholipids but the relevance of these is quite unclear. Progestogens tend to suppress circulating levels of HDL-C and increase circulating LDL-C. Oestrogens tend to increase HDL-C (Bradley et al, 1978). With contraceptive doses of DMPA and NET-OEN fasting levels of triglycerides and total cholesterol remain unchanged (Amatayakul, 1979; Dhall et al, 1977) whereas a small reduction of 15–20 per cent is noted in HDL-C (Kremer et al, 1980; Fotherby et al, 1982). Changes with most monthly injectables can be expected to parallel those seen with combined oral contraceptives whereas no detectable change occurs with long-term low dose progestogen release from an intrauterine device, subcutaneous implant or intramuscular injection (Croxatto et al, 1978; Bamji et al, 1981; Nilsson et al, 1981).

Liver function

Injectable progestogens such as DMPA and NET-OEN do not appear to affect liver function adversely. At contraceptive doses they do not cause any clinically significant alterations in the enzymatic or excretory functions (Schwallie & Assenzo, 1973; Tankeyoon et al, 1976; Dusitsin, 1978; Amatayakul, 1979). In several of these studies bromsulphthalein retention was also measured and showed no significant alteration. No change was found in a study of 52 women with metastatic breast cancer who received extraordinarily high doses of DMPA — 1500 mg daily for 30 days (Pannuti et al, 1978). However two studies from

Egypt have indicated significantly abnormal bromsul-phthalein retention in DMPA and NET-OEN users (Saleh & Abd-el-Hay, 1977; Guirgis et al, 1980). Why these two studies are different remains unclear particularly since a study designed specifically to look at women with severe liver fluke infestation found no clinically significant alterations in liver function during treatment with DMPA (Grossman et al, 1979).

There is no evidence of any change in other aspects of liver function. In particular a group of women with a history of recurrent obstetric cholestasis did not show a recurrence of symptoms or liver function test abnormality when treated with DMPA (Kreek & Sleisenger, 1970). It is suggested that this is mainly an oestrogen related effect and therefore is more likely to be expected with the monthly injectables. Benign hepatic adenomas or focal nodular hyperplasia are a rare association with combined oestrogen-progestogen oral contraceptives but very few of the many reported cases have been associated with progestogen therapy alone (Nissen et al, 1977). It has been suggested that these tumours are mainly oestrogen induced.

Other metabolic effects

No changes have been recorded in blood coagulation or fibrinolysis with injectable progestogens (Beller & Porges, 1967; Whigham & Howie, 1979; Howard et al, 1982b). However, changes comparable to the combined oral contraceptive would be expected with the monthly injectables. There is also no evidence for any change in renal function, numerous electrolytes, standard haematological parameters, plasma proteins or vitamin status (Amatayakul, 1979). A series of careful metabolic balance studies in Thai women suggests that the small weight gain sometimes associated with DMPA use is due to deposition of fat and maybe due to an increase in appetite (Amatayakul et al, 1980). There appears to be no change in body nitrogen balance or fluid retention.

In common with progesterone and other progestogens MPA and NET can be shown to have a weak suppressive effect on wound healing, cell mediated immunity and some circulating antibody responses (Turcotte et al, 1968; Munroe, 1971; Lenco et al, 1975). In many cases these are of the same order as immunological changes seen in pregnancy and may be due to the weak glucocorticoid effect of the progestogens. However, experimental results on immunological parameters are conflicting and vary greatly depending on the animal model, the experimental design and the endpoint measured. There is no clinical evidence of immunological disturbance and since many of these minor effects are seen with progesterone itself it is unlikely that they have any serious long-term implications.

Massive doses of DMPA can cause major adrenal cortical suppression (Hellman et al, 1976) and this is clearly due to the weak glucocorticoid effect of MPA. This glucocorticoid effect ensures that there is no clinical evidence of adrenal suppression . A single contraceptive dose of DMPA causes a slight suppression of adrenocortical activity but does not interfere with the circadian rhythm or the responsiveness of the adrenal cortex (Aedo et al, 1981). DMPA may cause a small rise in basal serum prolactin levels in lactating women (Choudhury et al, 1977) but not in non-lactating women (Jeppsson et al, 1982). DMPA may also produce a slight accentuation of the prolactin response to suckling and to certain prolactin stimulating drugs (Choudhury et al, 1977; Bohnet et al, 1978).

Metabolic studies of other long acting hormonal contraceptives apart from DMPA and NET-OEN are very limited. The high dose oestrogen-progestogen monthly injectables will cause more extensive metabolic changes but the dose reduction studies which are currently underway should ensure that the metabolic changes are no greater than those seen with combined oral contraceptives. The low dose progestogen only methods should have minimal effects on all of these parameters.

The confusing role of animal toxicology

Toxicology testing in animals is a crucial part of the development of a new drug before and during the early stages of human trials. Those countries which have drug regulatory agencies have laid down regulations for this testing and in many countries these are particularly stringent for hormonal contraceptive agents (Berliner, 1974). These tough regulations have been introduced because hormonal contraceptives may be given to otherwise healthy women for prolonged periods of time for mainly social reasons.

Clinical studies of new drugs are usually carried out in three phases from short-term intensive studies in a small number (10–20) of volunteer subjects (phase I) through medium duration (e.g. three cycles) in up to 50 subjects (phase II) up to large scale full clinical trials (phase III). Prior to initiation of each phase certain animal toxicology requirements must be completed or long-term animal studies started. These require increasing durations of treatment in two or more species at different dose levels (Berliner, 1974).

The classical aim of toxicology testing is to expose the animal to progressively higher doses of a drug (up to 50 times the human dose) over most of its lifespan in order to *produce* adverse reactions and pathological conditions which may orientate clinicians and epidemiologists to *possible* side-effects in women (Benagiano & Fraser, 1981). Animal studies may provide evidence about three types of important reaction: (1) *acute toxicological reactions*; (2) *rare events*, which would be unlikely to appear in premarketing clinical trials (such as thrombo-embolic phenomena in oral contraceptive users); and (3) *induction of neoplasia* which, in humans, may have a latency period of many years.

However, many reactions will be species-specific and many will result from the desired pharmacological action of the drug. The final proof about effects, or lack of effects, in human can only come from careful clinical trials following initial reassurance that the drug is not toxic.

It is the species-specific reactions which have caused so much confusion in the unravelling of the relevance of toxicology data in the DMPA story. Before discussing these in detail it is worth highlighting the remarkable lack of side-effects and serious complications in animals treated with extremely high doses of DMPA. For example, amongst the rhesus monkeys treated with 50 times the human dose for 10 years there were more survivors than in the untreated control group. On the other hand, it is now clear that hormones behave differently at higher dosages because of the overlap in stimulating other types of cellular receptor. Therefore, it may not be appropriate to assess the toxicology of hormones by merely observing effects of very high doses.

Uncertainty and controversy have raged around two particular toxicological observations in animals treated with high dose injectable progestogens.

Mammary nodules in beagle bitches

The beagle bitch was chosen as a toxicology model to predict the breast cancer risk in women using hormonal agents, because of its high spontaneous incidence of benign and malignant breast nodules. Early toxicology trials soon indicated that the beagle was not a good animal species for testing progestogens because many of the animals developed a pyometra of severe degree. A number of these animals died. Many of the animals also developed major metabolic disturbances (including diabetes), precocious senile changes and an acromegalic syndrome. All these adverse effects are species-specific and have no parallel in primates or humans (Benagiano & Fraser, 1981). The animals which were observed for the development of breast disease required an initial hysterectomy before entry into the study. Soon after this it was reported that there was a significantly increased incidence of benign and malignant breast nodules in the progestogen treated groups. However, initially this only occurred with certain progestogens of the C-21:17acetoxy group such as MPA, chlormadinone acetate and megestrol acetate (Finkel & Berliner, 1973; Graf & El-Etreby, 1979). This did not occur initially with the 19-nor progestogens. However recent detailed investigations have thrown new light on the situation (Leading Article, 1979). It is now clear that the C-21 progestogens are especially potent in the beagle and bind well to its progestogen receptors. However, precisely the same response can be induced with other progestogens including progesterone itself provided that they are given in appropriate doses, equivalent to their binding affinity to the dog's progestogen receptor.

In addition to differences in function it is now clear that the beagle breast has a completely different structure from the human breast and, in fact, has multiple microscopic areas of neoplastic potential which contain receptors which are capable of stimulation by progestogens. It is now obvious that the development of breast nodules in the beagle is more a reflection of progestogen potency in that species than a discriminating test of carcinogenic potential in women. A substantial body of evidence has now discredited this animal as being of any value in predicting the risk of breast cancer in women and many drug regulatory agencies like the United Kingdom Committee for the Safety of Medicines and the Swedish National Board of Health and Welfare no longer require the beagle bitch for contraceptive testing. The USFDA concedes that, while evidence of tumorigenic effect in animals does not mean the drug will cause tumours in humans, evidence that it is not tumorigenic in animals allows a drug to be marketed with 'a certain measure of assurance' of its safety for humans (Berliner, 1974). It should not be forgotten that NET-OEN causes breast and pituitary nodules in rats because of a species specific oestrogenic effect. In view of this apparent inappropriateness of the rat as a test animal the USFDA has been willing to approve for human oral contraception norethisterone derivatives which have slight tumorigenic effects in rodents (Population Report, 1975).

Endometrial carcinomas in rhesus monkeys

A totally unexpected and surprising finding in the long-term DMPA rhesus monkey toxicology study was the detection of endometrial carcinomas in two out of 12 animals at terminal autopsy. One of these tumours had metastasised to the lung. These animals had been treated with 50 times the human dose for approximately 10 years. These carcinomas appeared against a histological background of endometrial atrophy with predecidual stromal changes at all dose levels. There were no malignant precursor lesions in any other animal. Recently, doubt has been cast on this histological diagnosis and the suggestion made that the tumours might be of endocervical origin. This suggestion has not received widespread support.

Very recently an endometrial or endo-cervical carcinoma has also been reported in the ongoing NET-OEN long-term rhesus monkey toxicology study. Reports have also become available recently on long term monkey toxicity studies with other contraceptive agents. In two of these studies premalignant endometrial lesions were identified in animals from control groups. However, the interpretation of the finding of uterine cancers in monkeys treated with such prolonged massive doses is unclear.

Two explanations have been advanced for the appearance of these tumours. There is evidence from other experimental situations that massive prolonged hormonal stimulation of any hormonally responsive tissue may induce neoplasia (IARC Monograph, 1974) and there can be little dispute that the treatment dosage of the affected rhesus monkeys was massive and prolonged. Contraceptive use of DMPA and NET-OEN cannot be regarded in the same manner. The second explanation is that the tumours have developed from an endometrial cell type which is not present in women. Such a cell type does indeed exist in the rhesus monkey endometrium and has been known for some time (Rossman, 1940). This cell is progestogen sensitive and under the simultaneous stimulation of implantation or local trauma it develops into an endometrial plaque at the placental site during normal pregnancy (Rossman, 1940; Wadsworth et al, 1980). There are, apparently, similarities between the histology of the endometrial plaque and cells in the reported rhesus monkey endometrial tumours but this explanation is not widely favoured. Laboratory and clinical studies in women again indicate that this animal model is probably not of any use in predicting the risk of carcinogenesis in the endometrium in women.

All progestogens face some toxicology problems but there is obviously more concern with the longer acting methods. Fortunately the possibility of any clinical risk is not substantiated by any of the rapidly accumulating human toxicology data. Extensive data are only available for DMPA but the concern should be even less for the long acting low dose zero-order systems. The only small concern with the new systems involves the effects of local release of oestrogens and progestogens by rings in the vagina. The limited available data on this issue are reassuring.

Assessment of safety of long acting contraceptives

The assessment of safety of these long acting hormones poses particular problems by the very nature of the prolonged duration of action. This aspect of long acting methods has gained increasing importance in recent years, especially as a result of political and consumer group pressure. Numerous organisations have reviewed safety aspects, and most recently the World Health Organisation has published a detailed report of an interagency meeting on the safety of injectables held in October 1981 (World Health Organisation, 1982b). As a result of requests from Governments and Health Care Programmes the World Health Organisation has also prepared a detailed and critical technical guide on injectable contraceptives for health care administrators and programme planners to permit realistic appraisal of these methods for possible national programmes (World Health Organisation, 1982c).

It is clear that long acting hormonal contraceptives rarely show any acute toxic effects and current studies are geared almost entirely to the identification and delineation of rare long-term effects such as metabolic effects, neoplasia or sequelae for the breast-fed neonate. It is apparent from the large number of studies which have already been published and from interim analyses of current studies that these risks, if present at all, must be very small. These risks are certainly no greater than those faced by long-term combined pill users, and may indeed by less especially for the new zero-order release systems. Unfortunately, pressures from politicians, the general public and the media indicate that scientists are increasingly expected to develop drugs that are 100 per cent effective and have no side-effects or long term complications. The topic 'How safe does a drug have to be?' was recently addressed in a leading article in the Lancet which reasoned that safety must always be relative (Leading article, 1981). It concluded by quoting Sir Douglas Black: 'certainly not absolutely safe, which would imply that it was totally ineffective, but as safe as reasonable precautions by all concerned can make it, consistent with appropriate therapeutic benefit'. The majority of scientists who have critically assessed the available long acting hormonal contraceptives would agree that they meet the above criteria.

Conclusions

Long acting hormonal contraceptives are probably the most controversial group of fertility regulating agents available today. However, they exhibit a wide range of potential advantages, which ensure their acceptance by many individuals in most societies. In particular, they are highly effective and convenient contraceptives.

One repeatedly voiced criticism is that these agents have been insufficiently investigated. A brief study of the published literature will reveal that this is quite untrue and that one such agent — DMPA — is probably the most extensively investigated hormonal preparation ever used as a contraceptive. It has now been in use for 20 years. Short-term safety of these contraceptives is well established and there is reasonable assurance about the longer term effects. In spite of this there is a need, as with all drugs, for continuing vigilance for possible very long-term effects. Newer developments are aimed at minimising side-effects and preventing potential long-term adverse effects.

The single major problem with these contraceptive systems is frequent disturbance of the menstrual cycle. As yet there are few good leads to the prevention and cure of this disturbance and urgent research into basic pathophysiology is necessary to understand and eliminate this frequent reason for discontinuation of method use. Some long acting agents produce an inconvenient and unpredictable delay in the return of fertility, but none cause permanent sterility. Other side-effects are generally minor. Incompletely resolved questions include inadvertent exposure of the fetus in utero, exposure of the breast fed infant, beneficial or adverse effects on neoplasia and the inherent difficulties of interpreting animal toxicology data. However, it is fair to say that these agents do not face any more unresolved problems than combined pills, intrauterine devices or surgical sterilisation.

REFERENCES

Aedo A-R, Landgren B-M, Diczfalusy E 1981 Studies on ovarian and adrenal steroids at different phases of the menstrual cycle. III. Steroid and lutropin levels before and after the administration of a single contraceptive dose of depot medroxy progesterone acetate. Contraception 24: 117–128

Amatayakul K 1979 Safety and hazards of injectable hormonal contraceptives. Singapore Journal Obstetrics and Gynecology 9: 57–67

Amatayakul K, Sivasomboon B, Thanangkul O 1980 A study of the mechanism of weight gain in medroxy progesterone acetate users. Contraception 22: 605–622

Aznar-Ramos R, Giner-Velasquez J, Lara-Ricalde R, Martinez-Manatou J 1969 Incidence of side effects with contraceptive placebo. American Journal of Obstetrics and Gynecology 105: 1144–1149

Babcock J C, Gutsell E S, Herr M E 1958 Six methyl seven hydroxprogesterone seventeen acylates: A new class of potent progestins. American Chemical Society Journal 80: 2092–2093

Back D J, Breckenridge A M, Chapman C R, Crawford F E, Olsen K A, Orme M L, Rowe P H 1981 Studies on enzymatic cleavage of norethisterone oenanthate. Contraception 23: 125–136

Bamji M S, Safaya S, Prema K 1981 Low dose injectable contraceptive, norethisterone enanthate 20 mg monthly: II Metabolic side effects. Contraception 23: 23–36

Beck P, Zimmerman D E, Eaton R P 1977 Effect of contraceptive steroids on arginine stimulated glucagon and insulin secretion in women: III Medroxyprogesterone acetate. Metabolism 26: 1193–1198

Beck L R, Ramos R A, Flowers C E, Lopez G Z, Lewis D H, Cowsar D R 1981 Clinical evaluation of injectable biodegradable contraceptive system. American Journal of Obstetrics and Gynecology 140: 799–805

Beller F K, Porges R F 1967 Blood coagulation and fibrinolytic enzyme studies during cyclic and continuous application of progestational agents. American Journal of Obstetrics and Gynecology 97: 448–452

Benagiano G 1977 Long-acting systemic contraceptives. In: Diczfalusy E (ed) Regulation of Human Fertility, pp 323–360. Scriptor, Copenhagen

Benagiano G, Gabelnick H 1979 Biodegradable systems for the sustained release of fertility regulating agents. Journal of Steroid Biochemistry 11: 449–454

Benagiano G, Goldzieher J 1979 Effects of contraception on progeny. Reviews of Perinatal Medicine 3: 115–132

Benagiano G, Fraser I S 1981 The Depo-Provera debate: Commentary on the article 'Depo-Provera, a critical analysis'. Contraception 24: 493–528

Benagiano G, Fotherby K, Coutinho E, De Souza J C, Hingorani V, Takker D, Koetsawang S, Srisupandit S 1980 Return of ovarian function and endometrial morphology in women treated with norethisterone oenanthate: a pilot study. Fertility and Sterility 34: 456–460

Berliner V R 1974 Food and drug administration requirements for toxicity testing of contraceptive products. In Briggs M H, Diczfalusy E (eds) World Health Organisation Symposium on Pharmacological Models in Contraceptive Development, Acta Endocrinologica 185 (Suppl): 240–253

Bloch B 1971 Depot medroxyprogesterone acetate (Depo-provera) as a contraceptive preparation. South African Medical Journal 45: 777–781

Bohnet H G, Naber N G, Del Pozo E, Schneider H P G 1978 Effect of synthetic gestagens on serum prolactin and growth hormone secretion in amenorrhoeic patients. Archives of Gynecology 226: 233–237

Bonte J, Decoster J M, Ide P, Billiet G 1978 Hormonoprophylaxis and hormonotherapy in the treatment of endometrial adenocarcinoma by means of medroxyprogesterone acetate. Gynecological Oncology 6: 60–68

Bradley D D, Wingerd J, Petitti D B, Krauss R M, Ramcharan S 1978 Serum high density lipoprotein cholesterol in women using oral contraceptives, estrogens and progestins. New England Journal of Medicine 299: 17–20

Burstein R, Wasserman H C 1964 The effect of provera on the fetus. Obstetrics and Gynecology 23: 931–934

Casagrande J T, Louie E W, Pike M C 1979 'Incessant ovulation' and ovarian cancer. Lancet ii: 170–173

Choudhury R R, Chompootaweep S, Dusitsin N 1977 The release of prolactin by medroxyprogesterone acetate in human subjects. British Journal of Pharmacology 59: 433–434

Cornette J C, Kirton K T, Duncan G W 1971 Measurement of medroxyprogesterone acetate by radio immunoassay. Journal of Clinical Endocrinology and Metabolism 33: 459–465

Coutinho E 1978 Clinical experience with implant contraception. Contraception 18: 411–428

Coutinho E M, De Souza J C 1966 Conception control by monthly injections of medroxyprogesterone suspension and a long-acting oestrogen. Journal of Reproduction and Fertility 15: 209–218

Coutinho E, da Silva A R, Kraft H-G 1976 Fertility control with subdermal silastic capsules containing a new progestin (ST-1435). International Journal of Fertility 21: 103–108

Coutinho E Da Silva A R, Mottos C E R, Diaz S, Croxatto H B 1978 Contraception with long acting subermal implants: 1. An effective and acceptable modality in International Clinical Trials. Contraception 18: 315–334

Cox J W 1979 Factors influencing the time of introduction of steroidal contraception in the breast feeding mother. Australian and New Zealand Journal of Obstetrics and Gynaecology 19: 7–15

Crabbè P, Diczfalusy E, Djerassi C 1980 Injectable contraceptive synthesis: an example of international cooperation. Science 209: 992–994

Croxatto H B, Diaz S, Pavez M 1978 Clinical chemistry in women treated with progestogen implants. Contraception 18: 441–450

Croxatto H B, Diaz S, Miranda P, Elamsson K, Johansson E D B 1980 Plasma levels of levonorgestrel in women during long term use of Norplant. Contraception 22: 583–592

Csapo A, De Souza-Filho M B, De Souza J C, De Souza O 1966 The effects of massive progestational hormone treatment on the human uterus. Fertility and Sterility 17: 621–626

Cuna G R, Calciati A, Strada M R 1978 High dose medroxyprogesterone acetate (MPA) treatment in metastatic carcinoma of the breast: a dose-response evaluation. Tumori 68: 143–149

Dhall K, Kumar N, Rastogi G K, Devi P K 1977 Short term effects of norethisterone oenanthate and medroxyprogesterone acetate on glucose, insulin, growth hormone and lipids. Fertility and Sterility 28: 156–158

Diaz S, Pavez M, Robertson D N, Croxatto H B 1979 A three year clinical trial with levonorgestrel silastic implants. Contraception 19: 557–569

Diczfalusy E, Fraser I S, Webb F T G (eds) 1980 Endometrial Bleeding and Steroidal Contraception. Pitman Press, Bath

Diczfalusy E, Landgren B-M 1981 New delivery systems: Vaginal rings. In: Chang C F, Griffin D, Woolman A (eds) Recent Advances in Fertility Regulation, pp 43–69. Atar S.A., Geneva

Dobbing J 1982 Maternal nutrition, breast feeding and contraception. British Medical Journal 284: 1725–1726

Duncan G W, Wyngarden L J, Cornette J C 1976 Ante and postnatal steroid environment as it affects development of mammalian reproductive mechanisms. Revue Canadienne de Biologie 26: 237–248

Dusitsin N, Tankeyoon M, Larsson-Cohn U 1978 Liver function in Thai women using different types of hormonal contraceptive agents. Journal of Medical Association of Thailand 61: 381–389

Editorial 1981 Prenatal determination of adult sexual behaviour. Lancet ii: 1149–1150

Ehrhardt A A, Grisanti G C, Meyer-Bahlburg H F 1977 Prenatal exposure to medroxyprogesterone acetate in girls. Psychoneuroendocrinology 2: 391–398

El-Habashy M A, Mishell D R, Moyer D L 1970 Effect of supplemental oral estrogen on long-acting injectable progestogen contraception. Obstetrics and Gynecology 35: 51–54

El Mahgoub S E, Karim M, Ammar R 1972 Long term effects of

injected progestogens on the morphology of human oviducts. Journal of Reproductive Medicine 8: 288–293

Fan H M 1981 Studies on long acting oral contraceptives. In: Chang C F, Griffin D, Wooman A (eds) Recent advances in Fertility Regulation, pp 378–393. Atar S.A., Geneva

Faundes A, Sivin I, Stern J 1978 Long acting contraceptive implants: An analysis of menstrual bleeding patterns. Contraception 18: 355–366

Faundes A, Hardy E, Reyes Q, Pastene L, Portes-Carrasco R Acceptability of the contraceptive vaginal ring by rural and urban populations in two Latin American countries. Contraception 24: 393–414

Finkel M G, Berliner V R 1973 The extrapolation of experimental findings (animal to man): The dilemma of systemically administered contraceptives. Bulletin of Society for Pharmacology and Environmental Pathology 1: 13–17

Fotherby K 1981 Factors affecting the duration of action of the injectable contraceptive norethisterone enanthate. Contraceptive Delivery Systems 2: 249–257

Fotherby K, Goldzieher J W 1980 Animal models for the development of long-acting injectable contraceptives. In: Phamacological Models; Serio M, Martini L (eds) pp 461–473. Raven Press, New York

Fotherby K, Koetsawang S, Mathrubutham M 1980 Pharmacokinetic study of different doses of Depo-Provera. Contraception 22: 527–536

Fotherby K, Traynes I, Howard G, Hamawi A, Elder M G 1982 Effect of injectable norethisterone oenanthate (Norigest) on blood lipid levels. Contraception 25: 435–446

Fraser I S 1981 Abnormal uterine bleeding due to hormonal steroids and intrauterine devices. In: Griffin D, Woolman A (eds) Recent Advances in Fertility Regulation, pp 265–300. Atar S.A., Geneva

Fraser I S 1982a Long acting injectable hormonal contraceptives. Clinical Reproduction and Fertility 1: 67–88

Fraser I S 1982b Lipid changes and medroxyprogesterone acetate. Contraceptive Delivery Systems 4: 1–7

Fraser I S, Diczfalusy E 1980 A perspective of steroidal contraceptives and abnormal bleeding. In: Diczfalusy E, Fraser I S, Webb F T G (eds) Endometrial Bleeding and Steroidal Contraception, pp 384–409. Pitman Press, Bath

Fraser I S, Weisberg E 1981 A comprehensive review of injectable contraception with special emphasis on Depomedroxyprogesterone acetate. Medical Journal of Australia 1 (Special Suppl): 1–19

Fraser I S, Holck S 1983 Depot medroxyprogesterone acetate. In: Mishell jr D R (ed). Vol 2. Long Acting Steroid Contraception. Advances in Human Fertility and Reproductive Endocrinology. Raven Press, New York, pp 1–30

Giwa-Osagie O F, Savage J, Newton J 1978 Norethisterone oenanthate as an injectable contraceptive: A study of patients discontinuing treatment. Contraception 18: 517–529

Goldzieher J W, Kleber J W, Moses L E, Rathmacher R P 1970 A cross-sectional study of plasma FSH and LH levels in women using sequential, combination or injectable steroid contraceptives over long periods of time. Contraception 2: 225–238

Goldzieher J W, Moses L E, Averkin E 1971 A placebo controlled double-blind crossover investigation of side effects attributed to oral contraceptives. Fertility and Sterility 22: 609–614

Gordon T, Cistelli W P, Hjortland M C, Kannel W B, Dawber T R 1977 High density lipoproteins as a protective factor against coronary heart disease. The Framingham Study. American Journal of Medicine 62: 707–714

Graf K J, El Etreby M F 1979 Endocrinology of reproduction in the female beagle dog and its significance in mammary gland tumorigenesis. Acta Endocrinologica (Suppl) 22: 1–34

Gray R H 1980 Patterns of bleeding associated with the use of steroidal contraceptives. In: Diczfalusy E, Fraser I S, Webb F T G (eds) Endometrial Bleeding and Steroid Contraception, pp 14–49. Pitman, Bath

Gray R H 1983 Teratogenesis. In: Benagiano G, Diczfalusy E, Zulli P (eds) Progestogens in Therapy. Raven Press, New York, pp 109–125

Greenspan A R, Hatcher R A, Moore M, Rosenberg M J, Ory H W 1980 The association of depot medroxyprogresterone acetate and breast cancer. Contraception 21: 563–569

Grossman R A, Assawasena V, Calpati S, Taewtong D 1979 Effects of the injectable contraceptive depot medroxyprogesterone acetate in Thai women with liver fluke infestation: final results. Bulletin of the World Health Organisation 57: 829–837

Gual C, Perez-Pelacios G, Perez A E 1973 Metabolic fate of a long acting injectable estrogenprogestogen contraceptive. Contraception 7: 271–279

Guirguis F K, El-Sowy M, Abd-el-Hay M M, Saleh F M 1980 Serum phospholipid fractionation after the use of long acting progestational contraceptives. Contraception 21: 479–489

Hall P, Fraser I S 1983 Monthly injectable contraceptives. In: Mishell jr D R (ed). Vol 2. Long Acting Steroid Contraception. Advances in Human Fertility and Reproductive Endocrinology. Raven Press, New York, pp 65–82

Harlap S, Prywes R, Davies A M 1975 Birth defects and oestrogens and progestogens in pregnancy. Lancet i: 682–684

Heinonen O P, Sloane D, Manson R R, Hook E B, Shapiro S 1977 Cardiovascular birth defects and antenatal exposure to female sex hormones. New England Journal of Medicine 296: 67–69

Hellman L, Yoshida K, Zumoff B, Levin J, Kream J, Fukushima D 1976 The effect of medroxyprogesterone acetate on the pituitary-adrenal axis. Journal of Clinical Endocrinology and Metabolism 42: 912–917

Howard G, Elder M G, Fotherby K 1981 The use of norethisterone oenanthate, an injectable contraceptive in patients at risk of venous thrombosis. In: Greenhalgh R M (ed) Hormones and Vascular Disease, pp 294–299. Pitman Medical, London

Howard G, Blair M, Chen J K, Fotherby K, Muggeridge J, Elder M G, Bye P G 1982a A clinical trial of norethisterone oenanthate (Norigest) injected every two months. Contraception 25: 333–343

Howard G, Blair M, Fotherby K, Trayner I, Hamawi A, Elder M G 1982b Some metabolic effects of long term use of the injectable contraceptive norethisterone oenanthate. Lancet i: 423–425

Hull V 1981 The effect of hormonal contraceptives on lactation: current findings, methodological considerations and future priorities. Studies in Family Planning 12: 134–163

Hutton J D 1980 Analysis of published references cited in 'Depo-Provera: a critical analysis' by S Minkin. An unpublished review

IARC 1974 Sex hormones. Monographs on the Evaluation of Carcinogenic Risk of Chemicals to Man. IARC, Lyon 6: 243

Jacobson B D 1962 Hazards of norethindrone therapy during pregnancy. American Journal of Obstetrics and Gynecology 84: 962–967

Jeppsson S, Johansson E D B, Sjoberg N O 1973 Plasma levels of oestrogens during long-term treatment with depot medroxyprogesterone acetate as a contraceptive. Contraception 8: 165–176

Jeppsson S, Gershagen S, Johansson E D B, Rannevik G 1982 Plasma levels of medroxyprogesterone acetate (MPA), sex hormone-binding globulin, gonadal steroids, gonadotrophins and prolactin in women during long term use of depo-MPA (Depo-Provera) as a contraceptive agent. Acta Endocrinologica 99: 339–343

Junkmann K 1954 Über protrahiert wirksame Gestagene (on the prolonged action of gestagens). Naunyn-Schmie deberg's Archiv Für Experimentelle Pathologie und Pharmakologie 223: 244–247

Junkmann K, Witzel H 1958 Chemie und pharmakologie von steroidhormono-estern (chemistry and pharmacology of steroidal hormone esters). Zeitschrift für Vitamin-, Hormon- und Fermentforschung 9: 97–102

Kaiser D G, Carlson R G, Kirton K T 1974 GLC determination of medroxyprogesterone acetate in plasma. Journal of Pharmaceutical Science 63: 420–425

Kalkhoff R K 1982 Metabolic effects of progesterone. American Journal of Obstetrics and Gynecology 142: 735–738

Karim M, Ammar A, El Mahgoub S 1971 Injected progestogen and lactation. British Medical Journal 1: 200–203

Keith L, Berger G 1977 The relationship between congenital defects and the use of exogenous progestational 'contraceptive' hormones during pregnancy — a 20 year review. International Journal of Gynecology and Obstetrics 15: 115–124

Kesseru-Koos E 1971 Influence of various hormonal contraceptives on sperm migration in vivo. Fertility and Sterility 22: 584–588

Kesseru-Koos E, Hurtado-Koo H, Larranaga-Leguia A, Scharff H J 1973 Fertility control with norethindrone enanthate. A long standing parenteral progestogen. Acta Europaea Fertilitas 4: 203–207

Keys A 1980 Alpha lipoprotein (HDL) cholesterol in the serum and the risk of coronary heart disease and death. Lancet ii: 603–606

Khoo S K, Mackay E V, Adam R R 1971 Contraception with a six monthly injection of progestogen: 3. Effects on the endometrium. Australian and New Zealand Journal of Obstetrics and Gynaecology 11: 226–232

Koetsawang S 1980 Management of abnormal bleeding with steroidal contraceptives. In: Diczfalusy E, Fraser I S, Webb F T G (eds) Endometrial Bleeding and Steroidal Contraception, pp 50–58. Pitman Press, Bath

Koetsawang S, Srisupandit S, Kiriwat O, Koetsawang A 1978 Monthly injectable contraceptive: a two year clinical trial. International Journal of Gynaecology and Obstetrics 16: 61–64

Koetsawang S, Shrimanker K, Fotherby K 1979 Blood levels of medroxyprogesterone acetate after multiple injections of Depo-provera or Cycloprovera. Contraception 20: 1–12

Kreek M J, Sleisenger M H 1970 Estrogen induced cholestasis due to endogenous and exogenous hormones. Scandinavian Journal of Gastroenterology (Suppl) 7: 123–131

Kremer J, De Bruijn H W, Hindricks F R 1980 Serum high density lipoprotein cholesterol levels in women using a contraceptive injection of depot medroxyprogesterone acetate. Contraception 22: 359–367

Kulski J K, Smith M, Hartman P E 1977 Perinatal concentrations of progesterone, lactose and α-lactalbumin in the mammary secretion of women. Endocrinology 74: 509–515

Kurunmäki H, Toivonen J, Lähteenmaki P, Luukkainen T 1981 Intracervical release of levonorgestrel for contraception. Contraception 23: 473–481

Laumas V, Jain A K, Jha P, Rahman S A, Kumar D, Malik B K, et al 1981 Correlation between serum norethindrone levels attained after insertion of a silastic implant releasing norethindrone acetate and the endogenous hormones. Contraception 23: 211–223

Leading Article 1979 Hounding the pill. Medical Journal of Australia 2: 406

Leading Article 1981 How safe does a drug have to be? Lancet i: 1297–1298

Leading Article 1982 Rejecting scientific advice. British Medical Journal 284: 1426

Lee R A 1968 Contraceptive and endometrial effects of medroxyprogesterone acetate. American Journal of Obstetrics and Gynecology 104: 130–134

Lees R S, Lees A M 1982 High density lipoproteins and the risk of atherosclerosis. New England Journal of Medicine 306: 1546–1548

Leiman G 1972 Depot medroxyprogesterone acetate as a contraceptive agent — effect on weight and blood pressure. American Journal of Obstetrics and Gynecology 114: 97–102

Lenco W, McNight M, McDonald A S 1975 Effects of cortisone acetate, methyl prednisone and medroxyprogesterone on wound contracture and epithelialisation in rabbits. Annals of Surgery 181: 67–73

Luukkainen T, Nilsson C H 1978 Sustained intrauterine release of d-norgestrel. Contraception 18: 451–458

Mathrubutham M, Fortherby K 1981 Medroxyprogesterone acetate in human serum. Journal of Steroid Biochemistry 14: 1–4

McDaniel E B, Pardthaisong T 1973 Depot medroxyprogesterone acetate as a contraceptive agent: Return of fertility after discontinuation of use. Contraception 8: 407–414

McDaniel E B, Pardthaisong T 1974 Use effectiveness of six-month injections of DMPA as a contraceptive. American Journal of Obstetrics and Gynecology 119: 175–180

Melis G B, Strigini F, Fruzzetti F, Paoletti A M, Rainer E, Dusterberg B et al 1981 Norethisterone oenanthate as an injectable contraceptive in puerperal and non-puerperal women. Contraception 23: 77–88

Meyer-Bahlburg H F, Grisanti G C, Ehrhardt A A 1977 Prenatal effects of sex hormones on human male behaviour: medroxyprogesterone acetate. Psychoneuroendocrinology 2: 383–390

Miettinen T A, Huttenen J K, Strandberg T, Naukkarinen V, Mattila S, Kumlin T 1981 Lowered HDL cholesterol and incidence of ischaemic heart disease. Lancet ii: 478

Miller N E, Forde O H, Taelle D S, Mijos O D 1977 The Tromso heart study. High density lippoprotein and coronary disease: a prospective case-control study. Lancet i: 965–968

Minkin S 1980 Depo-provera: a critical analysis. Women and Health 5: 49–69

Mishell D R jr (ed) 1983. Vol 2. Long Acting Steroid Contraception. Advances in Human Fertility and Reproductive Endocrinology. Raven Press, New York

Mishell D R jr, Talas M, Parlow A F, Moyer D L 1970 Contraception by means of a silastic vaginal ring impregnated with medroxyprogesterone acetate. American Journal of Obstetrics and Gynecology 107: 100–107

Mora G, Johannsson E D B 1976 Plasma levels of medroxyprogesterone acetate (MPA), estradiol and progesterone in the rhesus monkeys after intramuscular administration of Depo-provera. Contraception 14: 343–350

Munroe J S 1971 Progesteroids as immuno suppressive agents. Journal of Reticuloendothelial Society 9: 361–375

Murphy H W 1979 Effect of depot medroxyprogesterone acetate on vaginal bleeding in the puerperium. British Medical Journal 2: 1400–1401

Nash H 1975 Depo-provera: a review. Contraception 12: 377–391

Nash H A, Robertson D N, Moo Young A J, Atkinson L E 1978 Steroid release from silastic capsules and rods. Contraception 18: 367–394

National Times Aborigines given birth control drug banned in U.S. Canberra Australia 15 March 1981

Nilsson C G, Kostiainen E, Ehnholm C 1981 Serum lipids and high density lipoprotein cholesterol in women on long-term sustained low dose IUD treatment with levonorgestrel. International Journal of Fertility 26: 135–137

Nissen E D, Kent D R, Nissen S E 1977 Etiologic factors in the pathogenesis of liver tumours associated with oral contraceptives. American Journal of Obstetrics and Gynecology 127: 61–70

Ojo O A 1979 Depot medroxyprogesterone acetate for contraception. A continuing controversy. International Journal of Gynaecology and Obstetrics 16: 439–441

Ortiz A, Hiroi M, Stanczyk F Z 1977 Serum medroxy progesterone acetate concentrations and ovarian function following intramuscular injection of depot medroxyprogesterone acetate. Journal of Clinical Endocrinology and Metabolism 44: 32–38

Pannuti F, Martoni A, Lenaz G R, Piana E, Nanni P 1978 A possible new approach to the treatment of metastatic breast cancer: Massive doses of MPA. Cancer Treatment Reports 62: 499–504

Pardthaisong T 1981 Return of fertility and outcome of pregnancy after dicontinuation of the injectable contraceptive, depot medroxyprogesterone acetate. PhD Thesis University of London

Pardthaisong T, Gray R H, McDaniel E B 1980 Return of fertility after discontinuation of depot medroxyprogesterone acetate and intrauterine devices in Northern Thailand. Lancet i: 509–511

Perez-Palacios G, Fernandez-Aparicio M A, Medina M 1981 On the mechanism of action of progestins. Acta Endocrinologica 97: 320–328

Pincus G 1965 The Control of Fertility p 360. Academic Press, New York

Population Council: An International Comparative Trial 1981 A multicentre study of levonorgestrel — estradiol contraceptive vaginal rings. 1. Use-effectiveness. Contraception 24: 341–358

Population Reports: Injectables and Implants 1975 Series K. No 1, March. Population Information Program, George Washington University Medical Center, Washington, DC

Powell L C, Seymour R J 1971 Effects of depot medroxyprogesterone acetate as a contraceptive agent. American Journal of Obstetrics and Gynecology 119: 36–48

Prema K, Gayathri T L, Ramalakshmi B A, Madhavapeddi R, Phillips F S 1981 Low dose injectable contraceptive norethisterone enanthate monthly. I. Clinical trials. Contraception 23: 11

Rall H G S, Van Niekerk W A, Englebrecht B H J, Van Schalkwyk D G 1977 Comparative contraceptive experience with three months and six months medroxyprogesterone acetate regimens. Journal of Reproductive Medicine 18: 55–58

Rall M J, Soto Ferreira G, Hanssens K Y 1978 Effect of medroxyprogesterone acetate contraception on cytoplasmic estrogen receptor content of the human cervix uteri. International Journal of Fertility 23: 51–56

Roberts D K, Morbelt D V, Powell L C 1975 The ultrastructural response of human endometrium to medroxyprogesterone acetate. American Journal of Obstetrics and Gynecology 123: 811–818

Rossman I 1940 The deciduomal reaction in the rhesus monkeys (macaca mulatta). 1. The epithelial proliferation. American Journal of Anatomy 66: 277–285

Rothman K J, Louik C 1978 Oral contraceptives and birth defects. New England Journal of Medicine 299: 522–526

Rozenbaum H 1982 Relationships between chemical structure and biological properties of progestogens. American Journal of Obstetrics and Gynecology 142: 719–724

Rozier J C jr, Underwood P B jr 1974 Use of progestational agents in endometrial adenocarcinoma. Obstetrics and Gynecology 44: 60–68

Rubin R T, Reinisch J M, Haskett R F 1981 Postanatal gonadal steroid effects on human behaviour. Science 211: 1318–1324

Saleh F M, Abd-el-Hay M M 1977 Liver function tests after the use of long acting progestational contraceptives. Contraception 16: 409–417

Sang G W, Fotheby K, Howard G, Elder M, Bye P G 1981 Pharmacokinetics of norethisterone oenanthate in humans. Contraception 24: 15–27

Saxena B N, Shrimanker K, Grudzinskas J G 1977 Levels of contraceptive steroids in breast milk and plasma of lactating women. Contraception 16: 605–614

Schwallie P C 1981 Effect of depot medroxyprogesterone acetate on the fetus and nursing infant. Contraception 23: 375–386

Schwallie P C, Assenzo J R 1972 Contraceptive use-efficacy study utilizing Depo-provera adminstered as an injection once every six months. Contraception 6: 315–322

Schwallie P C, Assenzo J R 1973 Contraceptive use-efficacy study utilising Depo-Provera administered as an injection every 90 days. Fertility and Sterility 24: 331–342

Schwallie P C, Assenzo J R 1974 The effect of depot medroxyprogesterone acetate on pituitary and ovarian function and the return of fertility following discontinuation. Contraception 10: 81–89

Scutchfield F D, Long W M, Correy B, Tyler W 1971 Medroxyprogesterone acetate as an injectable female contraceptive. Contraception 3: 21–32

Senanayake P, Kramer D G 1980 Contraception and the etiology of pelvic inflammatory disease: new perspectives. American Journal of Obstetrics and Gynecology 138: 852–864

Singh H, Uniyal J P, Jha P, Takkar D, Murguesan K, Hingorani V et al 1982 Pharmacokinetics of norethindrone acetate in women after insertion of a single subdermal implant releasing norethindrone acetate. Acta Endocrinologica 99: 302–308

Sivin I, Robertson D N, Etern J, Croxatto H B, Diaz S 1980 Norplant, reversible implant contraception. Studies in Family Planning 11: 227–238

Spellacy W N, McLeod A G W, Buhi W C, Burk S A 1972 The effects of medroxyprogesterone acetate on carbohydrate metabolism. Fertility and Sterility 23: 239–246

Stamm H, De Grandi P 1981 Adenocarcinoma of the endometrium in a patient on contraceptive treatment with Depo-provera. Paper presented to the Swiss Gynecologic Society

Swedish National Board of Health and Welfare 1981 Press release following approval of Depo-provera for the new indication of contraception for women in Sweden, 11th September 1981

Tankeyoon M, Dusitsin N, Poshyachinda V, Larsson-Cohn U 1976 A study of glucose tolerance, serum transaminase and lipids in women using depot medroxyprogesterone acetate and a combination-type oral contraceptive. Contraception 15: 199–214

Toppozada M 1977 The clinical use of monthly injectable contraceptive preparations. Obstetrical and Gynecological Survey 32: 335–346

Toppozada M, Parmat C, Fotherby K 1978 Effect of injectable contraceptives Depo-provera and norethisterone oenanthate on pituitary gonadotrophin response to luteinizing hormone releasing hormone. Fertility and Sterility 30: 545–551

Toppozada M, Onsey A F, Fares E 1979 The protective influence of progestogen-only contraception against moniliasis. Contraception 20: 99–206

Tseng L, Gurpide E 1975 Effects of progestins on estradiol receptor levels in human endometrium. Journal of Clinical Endocrinology and Metabolism 41: 402–409

Turcotte J G, Haines R F, Brody G L, Meyer T J, Schwartz S A 1968 Immunosuppression with medroxyprogesterone acetate. Transplantation 6: 248–260

Tuttle S, Turkington F E 1974 Effects of medroxy-progesterone acetate on carbohydrate metabolism. Obstetrics and Gynecology 43: 685–689

Vecchio T J 1972 Injectable medroxyprogesterone acetate contraception: metabolic and endocrine effects. Journal of Reproductive Medicine 10: 193–196

Vermuelen A, Thiery M 1974 Hormonal contraceptives and carbohydrate tolerance. II. Influence of medroxyprogesterone acetate and chronic oral contraception. Diabetologia 10: 253–259

Wadsworth P F, Lewis D J, Heywood R 1980 The ultrastructural features of progestogen-induced decidual cells in the rhesus monkey (macaca mulatta). Contraception 22: 189–200

Weiner E, Johansson E D B 1976 The influence of norethisterone oenanthate on ovarian function. Acta Endocrinologica 83: 386–390

Weiss N N, Sayvetz T A 1980 Oral contraceptive use and endometrial carcinoma. New England Journal of Medicine 302: 511–514

Whigham K A, Howie P W 1979 The effect of an injectable progestogen contraceptive on blood coagulation and fibrinolysis. British Journal of Obstetrics and Gynaecology 86: 806–816

Wilkins L, Jones H W, Holman G H, Stempsel R S 1958 Masculinization in the female foetus associated with the administration of oral and intramuscular injections of progestins during gestation: Non adrenal pseudo hermaphroditism. Journal of Clinical Endocrinology and Metabolism 18: 559–568

World Health Organisation Expanded Program of Research, Development and Research Training in Human Reproduction (Task Force on long-acting systemic agents for the regulation of fertility) 1977 Multinational comparative clinical evaluation of two long acting injectable contraceptive steroids: Norethisterone enanthate and medroxyprogesterone. I. Use effectiveness. Contraception 15: 513–533

World Health Organisation Expanded Program of Research, Development and Research Training in Human Reproduction (Task Force on long acting systemic agents for the regulation of fertility) 1978a Multinational comparative clinical evaluation of two long-acting injectable contraceptive steroids: norethisterone oenanthate and medroxyprogesterone acetate: II. Bleeding patterns and side effects. Contraception 17: 395–407

World Health Organisation Technical Report 1978b Steroid contraception and the risk of neoplasia. Series No 619

World Health Organisation Special Programme of Research in Human Reproduction 1979a Intravaginal and intracervical devices for the delivery of fertility regulating agents. Journal of Steroid Biochemistry 11: 461–467

World Health Organisation Special Programme of Research in Human Reproduction 1979b 8th Annual Report

World Health Organisation Special Programme of Research in Human Reproduction 1981 10th Annual Report

World Health Organisation 1982a Multinational comparative clinical trial of long acting injectable contraceptives: norethisterone enanthate given in two dosage regimens and depot medroxyprogesterone acetate. A preliminary report. Contraception 25: 1–11

World Health Organisation 1982b Facts about injectable contraceptives. Bulletin of the World Health Organisation 60: 199–210

World Health Organisation 1982c Injectable hormonal contraceptives: technical and safety aspects. WHO Offset Publication No 65: 1–45

Zanartu J, Onetto E 1966 Long-acting injectable progestagens in fertility control. In: Proceedings of the Sixth Pan-American Congress of Endocrinology, Mexico City, October, 1965. Exerpta Medica (International Congress Series No 112), p 134. Amsterdam

Zanartu J, Navarro C 1968 Fertility inhibition by an injectable progestogen acting for 3 months — a clinical survey of 130 fertile women treated with norethisterone oenanthate. Obstetrics and Gynecology 31: 1627–1630

M. H. Briggs & Maxine Briggs

Pharmacology of hormonal contraceptives

CHEMISTRY

Molecular structures

Human contraceptives based on natural and synthetic steroid hormones are used worldwide in family planning programmes. The most frequently used preparations contain oestrogens derived from oestradiol-17β, and progestogens derived from either 17α-hydroxy-progesterone or 19-norsteroids (estranes or gonanes). Many progestogens are 17α-ethynyl compounds, though limited use has also been made of 17α-vinyl and 17α-cyanomethyl derivatives. Aside from substitution at C-17, progestogens also possess varying numbers of unsaturations and esterifications. Only one androstane has found commercial use (dimethisterone) and this is a 17α-methylethynyl derivative of testosterone with an α-methyl group at C-6. A number of pregnane derivatives are widely used. Most are 17α-acetoxy-progesterones with substituents at C-6, though other functional groups have also been used. Oestrogens may be either steroidal or non-steroidal. The principal substances used in oral contraceptives are ethynylestradiol (EE), and its 3-methyl ether, mestranol (MEE). Long acting esters of EE are effective by either the oral or intramuscular routes, but are used for contraception mainly in Eastern Europe and China. A variety of esters of oestradiol-17β have been used in experimental injectable contraceptives (17-cypionate, 3-benzoate, 17-undecylate, 17-enanthate).

Chemical and physical properties

Table 35.1 summarises available information on the major compounds used in hormonal contraceptives.

BIOLOGICAL ACTIVITIES

Animal tests

A large number of tests in laboratory animals have been used routinely to compare the relative activities of oestrogens and progestogens. The relevance of such tests to humans is highly suspect, and can, at most, offer only a very approximate guide to actions of these compounds within human tissues, or to the necessary clinical dosage regimens required to produce a particular effect. The reasons for these differences between animal findings and effects in humans are multiple, but the following are important factors:

1. different metabolism of steroids, especially those requiring metabolic activation (e.g. EE* is about 30 times more active than MEE in rats, due to poor demethylation, but the two are approximately equipotent in women);
2. pregnancy maintenance requires progesterone in all mammals, but oestrogen requirements are variable, while progesterone release by the placenta begins early in some species but late in others (e.g. early pregnancy is fully maintained in ovariectomised hamsters by LNG* or MPA alone, but not in rats or rabbits which require supplementary oestrogen);
3. species differences in receptor affinities and regulation (e.g. NET is a good progestogen in women, but weak in rodents and dogs); relative affinities for human cytosol receptors are summarised in Table 35.2.
4. routes of administration (e.g. many steroids are more active in the rabbit when given by mouth than the s.c. route; the reverse is often true of the rat);
5. maturity of the test animals (e.g. steroid hormones require adequate receptor sites in target tissues to produce optimum effects: these may be lacking in immature animals).

With these reservations, a brief description will be given of the principal animal tests routinely conducted on contraceptive steroids.

Allen-Doisy Test. Young female rats are castrated and after 14 days receive the test compound. The controls receive oestradiol. Vaginal smears are taken 2–3 days later and threshold doses (50 per cent pro-oestrus) calculated.

---

* See Table 35.1 for abbreviations used.

Table 35.1 Physico-chemical properties of contraceptive steroids

Group	Compound	Abbreviation	Molecular formula	M.Wt.	(°C)	Water	Alcohol
Oestrogens							
(a) Endogenous	Oestradiol	E2	$C_{18}H_{24}O_2$	272.4	178–9	i	s
	Oestrone	E1	$C_{18}H_{22}O_2$	270.4	260–2	i	s.s
	Oestriol	E3	$C_{18}H_{24}O_3$	288.4	288d	i	s
(b) Ethynyl	Ethynylestradiol	EE	$C_{20}H_{24}O_2$	296.4	146	s.s	s
	Mestranol	MEE	$C_{21}H_{26}O_2$	310.4	150–4	i	s
	Quinestrol	QEE	$C_{25}H_{32}O_2$	364.5	107–108	i	s
	Deposition	DEE	$C_{23}H_{30}O_5S$	413.5		s.s	
(c) E$_2$-esters	Oestradiol cypionate	ECP	$C_{25}H_{36}O_3$	396.5	149–53	i	s
	Oestradiol benzoate	EBZ	$C_{25}H_{28}O_2$	376.5	190–8	i	s.s
	Oestradiol undecylate	EUD	$C_{29}H_{44}O_3$	440.7	109–110	i	s
	Oestradiol enanthate	EDE	$C_{25}H_{36}O_3$	384.6	94–96	i	s
(d) Non steroids	Diethylstilbestrol	DES	$C_{18}H_{20}O_2$	268.4	169–72	i	s.s
	Hexestrol	HEX	$C_{18}H_{22}O_2$	290.3	145	i	s.s
	Dienestrol	DIN	$C_{13}H_{18}O_2$	266.3	230–5	i	s
Progestogens							
(a) endogenous	progesterone	PRO	$C_{21}H_{30}O_2$	314.4	127–31	i	s
	17α-hydroxyprogesterone	HPO	$C_{21}H_{30}O_3$	330.5	222–223		
	Pregnanediol	PGD	$C_{21}H_{36}O_2$	320.5	238	i	s.s
(b) Oestranes	Norethisterone	NET	$C_{20}H_{26}O_2$	298.4	203–4	i	s
	Norethisterone acetate	NEA	$C_{22}H_{28}O_3$	340.5	161–2	i	s
	Norethisterone enanthate	NEE	$C_{27}H_{39}O_3$	410.6	68–73	i	s
	Lynestrenol	LYN	$C_{20}H_{28}O$	284.4	160–4	i	s
	Ethynodiol diacetate	EDA	$C_{24}H_{32}O_4$	384.5	126–31	s.s	s
	Quingestanol acetate	QGA	$C_{27}H_{36}O_3$	408.5	182–4	i	s
	Norgestrienone	NGT	$C_{20}H_{22}O_2$	294.4	169		
	Norgesterone STS–557	NGO	$C_{19}H_{27}O_2$	287.4	142–143		
	Norethynodrel	NED	$C_{20}H_{26}O_2$	298.4	169–70	i	ss
(c) Gonanes	Norgestrel	NG	$C_{21}H_{28}O_2$	312.5	205–10	s.s	s.s
	Levonorgestrel	LNG	$C_{21}H_{28}O_2$	312.5	205–10	i	s.s
	Norgestimate	NGT	$C_{23}H_{31}O_3N$	369.6	214–216	?	?
	Desogestrel	DOG	$C_{21}H_{30}O$	298.3	110–112	?	?
	Mestrinone	MTN	$C_{21}H_{24}O_2$	308.5	148–152	?	?
	Gestodene	GON	$C_{21}H_{26}O_2$	310.5	198.3	?	?
(d) Androstanes	Dimethisterone	DMT	$C_{23}H_{32}O_2H_2O$	358.5	100°d	i	s
(e) Pregnanes	Medroxyprogesterone acetate	MPA	$C_{24}H_{34}O_4$	386.5	200–10	s.s	s.s
	Megestrol acetate	MGA	$C_{24}H_{32}O_4$	384.5	210–20	s.s	s.s
	Chlormadinone acetate	CMA	$C_{23}H_{29}O_4Cl$	404.9	210–11	i	s
	Cyprtoterone acetate	CPA	$C_{24}H_{29}O_4Cl$	416.9	200–201	i	s.s
	Superlutin	SLU	$C_{24}H_{30}O_4$	382.5	233–234	?	?
	Droxone	DPA	$C_{28}H_{35}O_4$	435.6	150–151	?	?
	16-Methylene chlormadione acetate	MCA	$C_{24}H_{29}O_4Cl$	416.9	?	?	?
(f) Others	Norgesterone	NGO	$C_{21}H_{27}O_2$	313.5	?	?	?
	STS-557	—	$C_{20}H_{25}O_2N$	311.4	?	?	?

Rubin's test. Infant female mice receive the test compound or oestradiol for 3 days, are killed on day 4 and uterine weights measured. It has been claimed that some synthetic oestrogens produce greater effects on the uterus than the vagina (e.g. EE or DES), while others act better on the vagina than the uterus (e.g. MEE or equilin).

Clauberg test. Immature female rabbits are primed with s.c. estradiol for 6 days, then receive either progesterone or test compound on days 7 to 11. After sacrifice on day 12, endometrial proliferation is estimated, usually on a scale of 1 to 4 introduced by McPhail. In this test NET and related progestogens are relatively weak, LNG is intermediate, while pregnanes like CPA and CMA are potent.

Pregnancy maintenance. Pregnant rats undergo ovariectomy on day 8 and progesterone or test compound is given from day 7 to day 20. The number of live fetuses is determined on day 21. Similar tests may also be conducted in pregnant rabbits, hamsters, or guinea-pigs, but there are major species differences (e.g. LNG or MPA without oestrogen fully maintain pregnancy in guinea-pigs and

Table 35.2 Relative affinities of some natural and synthetic steroids for human sex hormone receptors

Steroid	Receptor Affinity		
	Oestrogen receptor	Progesterone receptor	Androgen receptor
Chlormadinone acetate	W	I	W
Cortisol	W	W	W
Desogestrel	W	W	W
Dextronorgestrel	W	W	I
Oestradiol	S	W	W
Ethynodiol diacetate	W	W	W
Ethynylestradiol	S	W	W
3-Ketodesogestrel	W	S	I
Levonorgestrel	W	S	I
Lynestrenol	W	W	W
Medroxyprogesterone acetate	W	S	W
Megestrol acetate	W	I	W
Mestranol	W	W	W
Norethisterone	W	S	I
Norethynodrel	W	W	W
Progesterone	W	S	W
Testosterone	W	W	S

S = strong.
I = intermediate.
W = weak or insignificant.

hamsters, but oestrogen supplementation is required in rats and rabbits for progesterone and NET).

Inhibition of ovulation. Beginning at metoestrus, mature rats with regular cycles receive graded doses of the test compound for 4 days. Unilateral ovariectomies are conducted on days 4 and 5 and oviducts examined for ovulations. In this test EE is about twice as effective as MEE. Progesterone (alone) is also active, but a relatively high dose is needed. Compared to progesterone, LNG is at least 100 times more effective, while MPA is at least 50 times. NET and CPA rank about 30 times, while NED and EDA are about 10 times more effective.

Parabiosis test. Infant female and castrated male rats of the same litter are given a cross circulation so that the increased gonadotrophin release of the male stimulates growth of the female's ovaries. The male receives progesterone, or a test compound, for 12 days and prevention of ovarian growth is measured. Again in this test, LNG is very active, being at least 100 times as potent as progesterone. MPA, NED and LYN are about 30 times, while NET is about 10 times more potent. Surprisingly, CPA shows about the same activity as progesterone, while CMA is only half as potent as the standard.

Testicular inhibition. Infant male rats receive control treatment, progesterone, or test compound daily for 2 weeks. Weights of testes and seminal vesicles are measured on day 15. One of the most active compounds in this test

is MPA (>500 times progesterone potency), while LNG and NED are about 300 times, and CMA about 100 times as potent.

Abortion (interceptive) actions. A number of steroids will interrupt pregnancy following implantation, while even more will disrupt fertilisation, zygote transport, and/or nidation. In rats blastocysts are thought to implant on day 5. Tests are conducted on mated rats from days 7 to 12. Fetal absorptions are determined. EE is about 10 times more effective than MEE in this test. Non-steroidal compounds, including DES, are also active, though correlation between interceptive effects in rats and rhesus monkeys are poor.

Antiandrogenic effects. This is usually conducted by a modification of the standard Hershberger test. Young castrated male rats, 8 days post-operative, receive s.c. testosterone plus placebo or test compound for 2 weeks. On day 15 the seminal vesicle and prostate gland weights are determined. The antagonistic effects (if any) of the test compound on testosterone stimulated growth of the male accessory organs are calculated. The most potent antiandrogen is CPA, which has an activity about 45 times that of progesterone in this test. CMA, and to a lesser extent MPA, are also active, but LNG, NET, and related progestogens, are inactive.

Antioestrogenic effects. Activity is usually measured by a modification of Rubin's test (see above) in which a compound is given in graded doses simultaneously with estradiol for 3 days. Antagonistic action to the oestrogenic stimulation of uterine growth is determined. Most progestogens are much more active in this test when given i.m. than by mouth. Very high potency (125 × progesterone) is shown by i.m. NET, less active are pregnanes (CMA 40×, MPA 8×), with NED being inactive.

Glucocorticoid activity. A number of contraceptive steroids are associated with changes in laboratory animals similar to those following cortisone, or other glucocorticoids. In most cases it is unclear whether these are due to direct effects of the steroid, or to enhancement of endogenous corticosteroid actions. Due to the multiple sites of action of glucocorticoids in mammals, simple tests are unavailable. Practical tests include measurements of nitrogen loss, liver glycogen deposition, thymus involution, antigranuloma activity, adrenal weight suppression, induction of eosinopenia, and relative affinity for corticosteroid receptors. Most contraceptive steroids are only weakly active, if at all, in these tests, but MPA, CPA and other pregnanes have probably the greatest relative potency.

Other tests. A number of other properties can be detected in animal tests of some contraceptive steroids. These include anaesthetic actions, anti- and pro-prolactins, effects on sexual and other behaviour, mammary differentiation and development, changes in the immune response, hepatotoxicity, erythropietic actions, and interactions with the control of bone metabolism. Most of these are poorly

Table 35.3 Biological activities of contraceptive steroids in animal tests*

Oestrogens Test	Species	Route	Standard (=1)	EE	MEE	DES
Allen-Doisy	Rat	s.c.	E_2	1	0.3–0.1	?
Uterine weight	Rat	s.c	E_2	1.2	0.6	1.1
Ovulation inhibition	Rat	s.c.	E_2	1.5	0.05	?
Abortion	Rat	s.c.	E_2	1.5	0.15	?
Parabiosis	Rat	s.c.	E_2	3.0	1.0	?

Progestogens Test	Species	Route	Standard	NET	LYN	LNG	NED	CPA	CMA
Clauberg	Rabbit	s.c.	PRO	12	2.5	66	2.5	250	78
		p.o.	NET	–	0.3	5.6	0.3	10	3.3
Pregnancy maintenace	Rat	s.c.	PRO	?	?	30–100	?	2	2
	Hamster	s.c.	PRO	4.2	?	3.3	1.0	0.01	0.05
Antiovulation	Rat	s.c.	PRO	30	2	>100	2	30	4
Parabiosis	Rat	s.c.	PRO	10	30	100	30	3	0.6
Testicular inhibition	Rat	s.c.	PRO	330	?	660	300	10	100
Anti-oestrogen (uterus)	Rat	p.o.	PRO	11	9	26	0	?	3.5
Antiandrogen (prostate)	Rat	s.c.	PRO (s.c.)	0	0	0		4.5	1.5
Allen-Doisy	Rat	s.c.	E_2	.003	.02	0	0.03	0	0
Androgenicity	Rat	s.c.	testosterone	0.03	0.03	0.06	0.03	0	0

* From Briggs & Brotherton, 1970; Brotherton, 1976.

investigated and their relevance to humans is even more poorly understood than conventional tests.

The activity profiles of various oestrogens and progestogens in animal tests are shown in Table 35.3

Human tests

Delay of menstruation. There are obvious problems in assessing the relative activities of sex hormonal drugs in humans, but the postponement of menstruation test was introduced as a comparative assay of progestogens by Greenblatt et al (1958); then later refined by Swyer (1960, 1974) and others (Harkness & Charles, 1965; Østergaard, 1965). Unfortunately there are significant differences in the published results with the same progestogens evaluated at different centres.

Briggs & Briggs (1981) have compared all the major oral progestogens in commercial use by the same protocol in healthy young women with regular menstrual cycles.

Pure progestogens were micronised to <5.0 μm diameter and packed with lactose in gelatine capsules. Bioavailability from this presentation is known to be good (Fotherby & Warren, 1976). Treatment was started on day 20 of the menstrual cycle, with one capsule of progestogen taken daily, together with a 50 μg ethynyloestradiol tablet. Hormone treatment was continued until cycle day 40, or until menstrual bleeding was noticed. For all progestogens, the initial daily dose was 1.0 mg. If this was effective in delaying menstruation, the dose was halved for the subsequent cycle; if ineffective it was doubled.

The ED_{50} of twelve progestogens are listed in Table 35.4 together with the number of observations on which the calculation is based.

Biochemical parameters. An alternative approach to comparing contraceptive steroids in humans is to follow changes in biochemical parameters. It is known, for example, that dose-related changes occur in many plasma proteins in women receiving synthetic oestrogens (Briggs & Briggs, 1971). A comparison of MEE and EE for effects

Table 35.4 Delay of menstruation test (Briggs & Briggs, 1981)

Compound	No. of observations	Mean ED_{50}* (mg/day)
MPA	19	2.0
NED	22	1.6
CMA	26	1.5
EDA	31	1.5
LYN	34	1.5
MGA	15	1.5
NEA	39	1.4
CPA	13	1.3
NET	40	1.3
NG (racemate)	51	0.15
LNG	53	0.075

* Administered with 50 μg EE as a single dose.

on specific plasma proteins has been published by Briggs & Briggs (1973), who concluded that at any dose MEE produced significantly smaller changes than EE. The ratio of activity of the two oestrogens, however, was different for each protein, ranging from 1:1.5 for haptoglobin to 1:6.0 for ceruloplasmin.

The use of plasma corticosteroid-binding globulin as an assay for oestrogenicity has been investigated by Moore et al (1978) using a variety of oestrogens, alone and in combination with progestogen. Alternative oestrogen-sensitive proteins are angiotensinogen and 'pregnancy-zone protein'. Briggs (1975a) has compared antioestrogenic effects of progestogens in women by following antagonism of oestrogen-induced changes in plasma proteins. Significant reversal of changes induced by either 30 μg or 50 μg EE daily were observed with 0.25 mg LNG daily, but not with 1.0 mg NET daily.

Other. A further approach to the assessment of contraceptive steroid relative activities in humans is to determine the minimum daily dose used in successful commercial formulations. There is considerable interest within the

pharmaceutical industry to determine the lowest effective dose of contraceptive steroids, for both medical and marketing reasons. Table 35.5 lists the lowest effective dose of the various compounds as included in a number of international surveys (Briggs, 1977; Fotherby, 1977; Brotherton, 1976).

TOXICOLOGY

Acute toxicity

Hormonal steroids are of very low systemic toxicity when given to the usual laboratory animal species by the oral or intravenous routes (Table 35.6). Generally speaking, synthetic sex hormones show acute toxicities with LD_{50} in the 3 to 8+ g/kg body weight range. A review by Heywood & Wadsworth (1980) deals specifically with the toxicity of oestrogens in laboratory animals, while Heywood (1980) and Briggs (1982) have reviewed progestogen toxicity.

Acute overdosage with contraceptive steroids does not appear to be hazardous in humans. There are several reports of young children who swallowed up to 200 mg of combined oral contraceptive steroids at one time (and of adults who took up to 400 mg) with no ill effects (Picchioni, 1965). A further report on OC accidental overdosage in young children lists nausea, vomiting and drowsiness as usual symptoms, with occasional vaginal bleeding in girls (Wynne, 1968).

Chronic toxicity

Contraceptive steroids intended for human contraception are required by the US Food and Drug Administration to

Table 35.5 Lowest effective doses of of contraceptive steroids

Class	Steroid (see Table 35.1)	Route	Lowest dose	(frequency)
Oestrogens (usually + progestogen)	EE	p.o.	20–30 μg	(daily)
	MEE	p.o.	50 μg	(daily)
	QEE	p.o.	1 mg	(monthly)
	DEE	p.o.	1 mg	(weekly)
	ECP	i.m.	10 mg	(monthly)
	EBZ	i.m.	10 mg	(monthly)
	EUD	i.m.	50 mg	(monthly)
	EDE	i.m.	10 mg	(monthly)
Progestogen (+ oestrogen)	NET	p.o.	0.4 mg	(daily)
	NEA	p.o.	0.5 mg	(daily)
	LYN	p.o.	0.75 mg	(daily)
	EDA	p.o.	0.5 mg	(daily)
	QGA	p.o.	0.5 mg	(daily)
	NGT	p.o.	0.5 mg	(daily)
	NGO	p.o.	0.5 mg	(daily)
	LNG	p.o.	50–125 μg	(daily)
	NGT	p.o.	125 μg	(daily)
	DOG	p.o.	150 μg	(daily)
	MTN	p.o.	5 mg	(weekly)
	GON	p.o.	75 μg	(daily)
	CMA	p.o.	1.5 mg	(daily)
	MPA	p.o.	2 mg	(daily)
		i.m.	150 mg	(3 monthly)
	MGA	p.o.	0.1 mg	(daily)
	SLU	p.o.	5 mg	(daily)
	DMT	p.o.	25 mg	(daily)
Progestogen (alone)	NET	p.o.	300 μg	(daily)
	NEA	p.o.	300 μg	(daily)
	NEE	i.m.	200 mg	(3 monthly)
	LYN	p.o.	500 μg	(daily)
	EDA	p.o.	350 μg	(daily)
	QGA	p.o.	300 μg	(daily)
	LNG	p.o.	30 μg	(daily)
	NG	p.o.	75 μg	(daily)

Table 35.6 Acute LD_{50} of contraceptive steroids (mg/kg)*

	Rat	Mouse	Dog
CMA	>8000 p.o.	—	—
CPA	4000 s.c.	6000 s.c.	3000 s.c.
DMT	—	7600 p.o.	—
MGA	—	5000 p.o.	—
NEA	>4000 p.o.	>2500 s.c.	—
NG	—	>2500 p.o. + s.c.	—
EE	>5000 p.o.	>2500 p.o. + s.c.	—

Comparisons: Rat acute LD_{50} (mg/kg)		
	fluoracetic acid	0.05
	copper sulphate	50
	caffeine	200
	asprin	150
	carbon tetrachloride	2900
	sodium choloride	3900
	phenacetin	4100
	penicillin	6700

* Brotherton (1976).

Table 35.7 Effects of very high dose progestogens*

Expected from pharmacological properties:
Loss of condition
Reduced body weight and food intake
Redistribution of fatty tissues
Hair loss
Altered vaginal bleeding patterns
Uterine changes
Mammary nodules
Ovarian atrophy
Pituitary adenomas

Unexpected from pharmacological properties:
Liver nodules
Gall bladder hyperplasia
Retinal changes
Altered plasma proteins (fibrinogen)
Adrenal cortical degeneration

* Heywood (1980).

Table 35.8 Toxicity of high dose oestrogens in laboratory animals

Species	Compound	Effect (Reference)
Mice	EE	Mortality ↑ (1)
	Various	Scrotal hernia (2)
	Various	Decreased weight gain (1)
	EE or ME	Pituitary hypertrophy and adenomata (3)
	DES	Testicular tumours (4)
	DES, EE or MEE	Mammary tumours (2,5)
	EE	Endometrial squamous metaplasia (1)
	Various	Cervical lesions and carcinoma (6)
	Various	Testicular atrophy (1)
	Oestradiol dipropionate	Interstitial cell hypertrophy and tumors (7)
	Various	Prostate squamous metaplasia (1)
	Various	Adrenocortical hypertrophy (8)
Rats	Various	Bilateral alopecia (9)
	Various	Reduced food intake and weight gain (10)
	7α-Me-NET	Cataracts (11)
	Various	Pituitary hypertrophy and tumors (1,9)
	Various	Mammary tumours (12)
	EE	Mammary fibroadenomata (1)
	Various	Dermal and epidermal thinning (9)
	Various	Seminiferous tubular atrophy (9)
	Various	Prostate squamous metaplasia (9)
	Various	Cystic ovaries (9)
	DES	Endometrial hypertrophy, squamous metaplasia and pyometrial (13)
	Various	Adrenocortical hyperplasia (1)
	Various	Thymus involution and cysts (14)
	EE	Liver tumours (5)
Dogs	Various	Bilateral alopecia (1, 15, 16)
	DES or QEE	Inguinal hernia (16, 17)
	DES	Anaemia, thrombocytopenia, gingival bleeding and petechia (18)
	Various	Mammary hyperplasia (16, 19, 20, 21)
	DES	Ovarian tumours (22, 23)
	Various	Uterine hyperplasia, oedema necrosis and pyometra (16, 17, 19, 24)
	Various	Testicular atrophy (1)
	Various	Prostate epithelial hyperplasia and metaplasia (1, 16, 25)
	DES or QEE	Pituitary aciophils ↑ (16, 17)
	DES	Adrenocortical atrophy (26)
Non-human primates	Various	Development of sex skin (27)
	Various	Testicular atrophy (28)
	Various	Suppression of menstruation (27)
	DES or E_2B	Uterine mesothelioma (29) endometrial gland cystic dilatation (29, 30)
	Various	Mammary ductal hyperplasia (21, 30)
	Various	Prostate hyperplasia (31)
	Various	Urogenital hyperplasia and metaplasia (1, 32)
	Various	Vaginal hyperplasia and epithelial cornification (28)

(1) Heywood & Wadsworth (1981) (2) Shimkin & Grady (1941) (3) CSM (1972) (4) Andervont et al (1960) (5) IARC (1974) (6) Pan &Gardner (1948) (7) Bonser & Robson (1940) (8) Westberg et al (1957) (9) Gibson et al (1967) (10) Sullivan & Smith (1957) (11) Ray & Schut (1969) (12) McKenzie (1955) (13) Morrell & Hart (1941) (14) Geschickter & Byrnes (1942) (15) Dow (1960) (16) Schwartz et al (1969) (17) Jabara (1962b) (18) Castrodale et al (1941) (19) Mulligan (1947) (20) Finkel & Berliner (1972) (21) Geil & Lamar (1977) (22) Jabara (1962a) (23) O'Shea & Jabara (1971) (24) Dow (1959) (25) Mulligan (1944) (26) Mulligan & Becker (1947) (27) Hisaw & Hisaw (1966) (28) Hisaw & Hisaw (1961) (29) McClure & Graham (1973) (30) Geschickter & Hartman (1959) (31) Zuckerman (1938) (32) van Wagener (1935).

undergo toxicity testing for 2 years in rats, 7 years in dogs, and 10 years in monkeys (Berliner, 1974). The dosage is based on the human dose and must be up to ×100 in rats, ×50 in monkeys, and ×25 in dogs.

Growth curves of male and female rats receiving progesterone at four dose levels by two routes, have been compared with similar tests with synthetic progestogens, such as allylestrenol. The growth rate of treated female rats (at all doses) was greater than for untreated controls. Less effect was seen with the male rats, though the groups attaining the greatest final mean body weights were receiving hormones. Longer term studies with higher doses have produced somewhat different results: major findings are summarised in Table 35.7 while toxic effects of high dose oestrogens are summarised in Table 35.8. Long-term administration of NEA to rats has been studied by Schardein (1980) with the results listed in Table 35.9. Some of these changes are neoplastic, or preneoplastic; especially the increase in liver and uterine pathology seen in the high dose group.

Carcinogenicity

It has been known for many years that the administration of natural or synthetic sex hormones, for long periods, at doses several multiples of either the endogenous production rate, or of the human therapeutic dose (on a mg per kg basis), leads to the development of benign, or less frequently, malignant neoplasia. The evidence has been reviewed in IARC Monographs (1974, 1980)and a summary of selected data is given in Table 35.10. It should be noted that pathological responses vary from species to species, are markedly influenced by strain (especially in rodents), while the same hormone dose may influence neoplastic development in quite different organs of different species.

Chronic toxicity testing of contraceptive steroids in mice and rats was undertaken by the UK Committee on Safety

Table 35.9 Chronic administration NEA* (105 weeks: male and female rats)

		Untreated controls	Low dose† (× 10)	High dose‡ (× 10)
General effects				
Relative weight gain		100	70–80	50–68
Percentage survival		10	22	
Hair loss		+	+ +	+ + +
Neoplasia and related changes				
% Animals with	(M)	49	49	44
tumours	(F)	81	80	60
		7.2	7.6	6.0
Average	(M)			
tumours/animal	(F)	17.1	15.6	13.0
Liver: nodules (%)		1	2	7
cell foci (%)		2	1	21
Uterus: adenoma/polyps (%)		1	10	16
squamous metaplasia (%)		11	20	48
Mammary glands: mastopathy (%)		13	12	17
Atrophic changes				
Males: testes (%)		17	36	46
accessory organs (%)		1	4	20
Females: ovaries (%)		44	38	70

* Schardein (1980)
† 0.3–0.4 mg/kg
‡ 3.2–4.2 mg/kg
Human contraceptive dose = 0.006–0.08 mg/kg

Table 35.10 Sex hormone overdose and carcinogenesis*

Sex hormone	Dose (× human)	Species	Tumours
Testosterone	4 mg/7 day (× 170)	Mouse	Uterus/cervix
	2.5 mg/7 day (× 15)	Rat	Uterine/ovary
Testosterone +	200 mg/year (× 20) + 50 mg/year (× 10)	Hamster	Uterus/ epididymis
Stilbestrol	240 mg (× 6)	Squirrel monkey	Uterus
	50 µg/7 day (× 5)	Mouse	Breast
	0.3 mg/day (× 15)	Hamster	Kidney
Oestradiol	50 µg/7 day (× 15)	Mouse	Testis/breast
	60 µg/7 day (× 10)	Guinea-pig	Uterus
	20 mg (× 12)	Hamster	Kidney
	12 mg/month (× 200)	Rat	Breast/ pituitary
Progesterone	14 mg/month (× 17)	Mouse	Breast/ovary

* IARC Monographs Vols 6 and 21.

of Medicines following a report that MEE induced liver nodules in rats. Investigations were made of all marketed contraceptive progestogens, and progestogen-oestrogen combinations, in 80-week studies in mice, and 104-week studies in rats. Animals received the steroids mixed with their diet at three dose levels, thought to represent approximately 2–5, 50–150, and 200–400 times the human contraceptive dose, though actual doses are unstated.

NET and NED increased benign liver neoplasia in male rats (but not in females): NED also increased the incidence of malignant neoplasia in males. The only striking effect of any progestogen in females was with MGA, which increased malignant, though not benign, hepatic neoplasia. For progestogen + oestrogen combinations, male rats showed increased liver neoplasia with NED + MEE (less with higher oestrogen:progestogen ratio), NET + MEE, and MGA + EE (oestrogen: progestogen ratio without effect). The only marked change in female rats was for MGA + EE, where two dose regimens increased the incidence of both benign and malignant tumours. At least for NED (alone or in combination with MEE) there was some evidence of direct dose relationship.

In mice NED did not increase hepatic neoplasia, though some other progestogens did. Any attempt to seek some biological, biochemical, or pharmacological explanation for these findings has met with little success (Heywood, 1980; Briggs, 1982). The observed increase in liver tumours

associated with NED has been suggested to relate to its oestrogenicity, but the lack of effect of synthetic potent oestrogens make this unlikely.

Several progestogens, alone or in combination with an oestrogen, have been shown to induce mammary tumours in beagle dogs when given at up to × 25 the human dose (Geil & Lamar, 1977; Weikel & Nelson, 1977; Briggs, 1977; El Etreby & Gräf, 1979; El Etreby, 1979). Compounds in this category include progesterone itself, MPA, MGA, CMA, angestone acetate, chlorethynyl-norethisterone, chlorethynyl-norgestrel, and lynestrenol. Given alone to women, progestogens do not influence breast growth or alter pituitary secretion of growth hormone (which has mammotrophic activity). In contrast, mammary growth in the bitch is markedly stimulated by progestogens, even in ovariectomised animals, while there is massive release of growth hormone.

Benign mixed adenomata of the breast are common in old dogs, while careful examination of whole mount sections of untreated, intact, mature bitches has revealed multiple microscopic neoplasia.

If all progestogens, including progesterone itself, are tumourogenic to the dog breast, then it becomes impossible to differentiate between compounds by these tests. Paradoxically, those progestogens which have not so far been shown to be tumourogenic in the dog are most potent in women. Most authorities now believe that progestogen-induced mammary tumours in the bitch are unhelpful in predicting possible breast effects in women using oral contraceptives.

A careful examination of the literature, which has been subjected to review at frequent intervals, has revealed no spontaneous case of endometrial cancer in the rhesus monkey, though two cases in untreated control animals have been found in regulatory toxicology studies. Cancer at this site is exceptionally rare in most non-human primates. The only apparently reported case in the literature is of endometrial carcinoma *in situ* of a chimpanzee (Briggs, 1982).

With this background, the occurrence of two cases of adenocarcinoma of the uterine endometrium in 12 rhesus monkeys receiving high dose depot-MPA for up to 10 years is surprising, though there is a recent unpublished report of endometrial carcinoma in a rhesus monkey receiving high dose NET-enanthate, while two cases of endometrial cancer were found in older, though still unpublished, studies of high dose CMA in this species. The situation is very different to the rodent hepatic, or the canine mammary neoplasia, which both occur with frequency in untreated animals.

Long-term monkey studies of MGA (the molecule which differs from MPA by only two hydrogen atoms) have recently been completed, but no uterine (or other) neoplasia were found.

Mutagenicity

The development of the *Salmonella*/microsome test by Bruce Ames and associates led to its introduction as a mutagen screening procedure. The results for four progestogens in this test, and also for three oestrogens, have been recently published by Lang & Redmann (1979). Using *Salmonella* strains to detect either base-pair substitutions or frameshift mutations, no positive results were obtained with any of the progestogens or oestrogens, applied alone, or following incubation with microsomes from rat or mouse liver. Similar negative results are reported by Dayan et al (1980). Paradi (1981) failed to find any X-linked recessive lethal mutations above the control value in larval *Drosophila melanogaster* fed EDA, NED, or NG, in combination with EE or MEE.

Teratology

Effects of progestogens on rodent development depend largely on pharmacological properties. MPA in the rat induces virilisation of female fetuses (Lyster et al, 1959; Suchowsky & Junkmann, 1961).Progesterone at approximately the same dose is devoid of this masculinising effect (Revesz et al, 1970), and so is gestonerone caproate (Mey, 1967). CPA, a progestogen with anti-androgenic activity, induces virilisation in female offspring, and feminisation of males, when administered during pregnancy in a variety of laboratory species (Neumann et al, 1974). High doses of many commonly used progestogens have been studied by Andrew et al (1973), who found one strain of mice which appeared particularly susceptible. Malformations reported include cleft palate, club foot, exencephaly, hydroencephaly, abdominal haemorrhage, retardation of fetal growth, multiple uro-genital defects, abnormal ossification of ribs and/or skull, cranioschisis and partial duplication of the kidney. In fetal rats, cleft palate and

exencephaly were not found at comparable doses, but some cases of cleft palate were seen in rabbits exposed *in utero* to MPA. Full reproduction studies with CMA in pregnant mice and rabbits have been reported by Takano et al (1966). High doses were teratogenic in both species, with cleft palate being one of the more common malformations.

Studies on progestogen/oestrogen combinations have been reported (Saunders & Elton, 1967; Saunders, 1967). NED + MEE induced malformations in rats and rabbits, but EDA + MEE was without significant effect. As both progestogens require metabolism to NET in humans before they become progestationally active, the difference between these compounds in laboratory species may be due to the metabolic products.

Steroid hormone transfer from mother to fetus is based largely on biological evidence rather than published investigation of labelled compounds. Transplacental passage in a number of species has been demonstrated, particularly for corticosteroids, by Bashore et al (1970) and Migeon et al (1961). The first demonstration for transplacental transfer of sex hormones was by Courrier (1924) who gave oestrogen to pregnant guinea-pigs and observed stimulation of the vagina and breasts of female fetuses. Numerous publications describe effects of maternal oestrogens or androgens on genital tract development in fetal rodents (see Green et al, 1939; Raynaud, 1942). Toxic effects of the synthetic non-steroidal oestrogen, DES, by the transplacental route are more dramatic and are listed in Table 35.11.

Some of the effects of pre-natal exposure to sex

Table 35.11 Transplacental transfer effects of DES

Species	Sex of offspring	Effects (Reference)
Human	Female	Cervical and vaginal clear-cell adenocarcinoma (1) Vaginal adenosis (1) Cervical erosions (1) Irregular cycles (1)
	Male	Epididymal cysts (1) Lypotrophic testes (1) Capsular induration (1)
Mice	Female	Reduced fertility or infertility (2) Persistent urogenital sinus (3) Portio vaginalis hypertrophy (3)
	Male	Reduced fertility or infertility (2) Undescended testes (3) Testicular hypogenesis (3)
Hamsters	Female	Reproductive tract hypertrophy and neoplasia (4)
	Male	Testicular and epididymal spermatic granuloma (4)
Monkeys	Female	Cervical hooding (5) Vaginal ridging and adenosis (5)
	Male	Undescended testes (5) Preputial adhesions (5)

(1) Bibbo et al (1977) (2 McLachlan et al (1975) (3) Nomura & Kanzaki (1977) (4) Rustia & Shubik (1976) (5) Hendricks et al (1978).

hormones on later behaviour are known. Androgen exposure of female fetuses can lead to masculine-type behaviour in later adulthood (Pheonix et al, 1959). Pre-natal exposure to oestrogens and/or progestogens may change behaviour (Reinisch & Karow, 1977). A review of sex hormonal actions on human fetal development, and the incidence of malformations, has been published by Briggs & Briggs (1979a). While there is no doubt that fetal damage can be induced in some laboratory animals given large amount of sex hormones, the doses required are very much larger than those used in human obstetrics and gynaecology. When the evidence for each type of malformation allegedly associated with sex hormone use is examined critically, it becomes very insubstantial. That masculinised female infants have been born to mothers exposed during pregnancy to sex hormones is unquestionable, but the vast majority of pregnant women receiving similar treatments have not produced abnormal offspring (there are several countries in which obstetric support therapy with sex hormones is given routinely for early pregnancy). Masculinisation of female infants also occurs in untreated women. The risk of masculinisation during pregnancy from sex hormone treatment cannot be estimated reliably; if it exists at all it is very small.

It seems at least possible that the tenuous association between sex hormone exposure and malformations reported by some, but no means all, surveys is fortuitous, and that reported malformations are due to some other, unrelated, factor or factors (WHO Scientific Group, 1981).

Conclusion

The purpose of animal toxicology is to predict adverse effects in humans at the usual therapeutic doses, not to investigate bizarre effects occurring at astronomically high dose levels in species with poorly understood physiology and pathology. The guidelines for toxicity studies of contraceptive steroids laid down by regulatory agencies are now widely acknowledged to be of little relevance to human safety.

FORMULATION AND ADMINISTRATION

Formulation effects

Most progestogens and oestrogens are well absorbed when taken by mouth in either capsule, tablet or pill form. There is some evidence that micronisation of progestogens increases biological activity (Gibian et al, 1968), though the basis for this effect is uncertain. The bioavailability of oestrogens, such as EE, is only about 40–50 per cent, due to metabolic inactivation during intestinal absorption, and first pass through the liver (Speck et al, 1976; Goldzieher et al, 1980a, b).

Table 35.12   Bioavailability of progestogens (percentage of oral dose)

Compound	Species			
	Rat	Beagle bitch	Rhesus monkey	Woman
LNG	9	22	9	100
GON	13	36	9	100
NET	31	44	17	60
CPA	100	75	91	100

Bioavailability for progestogens varies with the individual substance, but is generally higher than for oestrogens (Table 35.12).

Depot contraceptives take the form of solutions in oil (e.g. NEE) or microcrystalline suspensions in an aqueous base (e.g. MPA). Following intramuscular injection, the steroid is gradually released into the circulation. For compounds like MPA, which are intrinsically active, contraceptive effects are direct. For many esters, however, enzymic hydrolysis is required. In particular, NEE enters the circulation and is de-esterified, primarily in the liver. The same is probably true of long acting oestradiol esters, also sometimes given by the i.m. route in long acting injected contraceptives.

Other delivery systems are less well known. Commercial progestogen-releasing IUDS have undergone systematic engineering studies to provide optimum constant release rates (Pharris, 1974). Despite this their performance has not been much better than traditional non-medicated devices, though menstrual blood loss is reduced (Wagatsuma, 1981). Similarly, there has been considerable interest is progestogen implants, of both the biodegradable and silastic types, but again no commercially viable product has yet appeared.

Experimental use of intranasally sprayed contraceptive steroids has failed to demonstrate any particular advantage for this route and the dose required is close to that for oral administration.

Absorption and bioavailability

The bioavailability and terminal half-lives in plasma for various progestogens in several species have been studied by Düsterberg et al (1981). Their results are summarised in Tables 35.12 and 35.13. There are obvious major differences between compounds and between species. Three of the four progestogens examined had high bioavailability in women, but were poor in the other three species. There were also major differences in the plasma terminal half-lives of the compounds.

Comment has been made previously on the bioavailability and absorption of EE in humans. About 50–60 per cent of an oral dose undergoes sulphation during first pass through the intestines and liver, reducing bioavailability to 40–50 per cent. There appear to be major individual differ-

Table 35.13 Terminal half-lives of progestogens (hours) (based on plasma values following oral administration

Compound	Species			
	Rat	Beagle bitch	Rhesus monkey	Woman
LNG	0.5	1.2	4.4	26.4
GON	0.4	4.6	4.0	14.6
NET	3.7	6.3	109	16.6
CPA	26.3	1.9	25.3	48.0

Table 35.14 Human pharmacokinetics of oral MEE and EE*

	MEE	EE
Plasma peak (h)	2–4	1–2
Plasma $T_\frac{1}{2}$ distribution (h)	1–4	1–3
Plasma $T_\frac{1}{2}$ elimination (h)	8–16	6–14
Urinary $T_\frac{1}{2}$ (h)	27–42	24–29
MCR (l/day)	1740	1345
Total body clearance (l/h)	60–282	27–76
Urinary excretion (%)	30–60	42–60
Urinary metabolites conjugated (%)	85–90	85–90
Faecal excretion (%)	40–70	40–58

* Goldzieher et al (1980a,b); other major studies are by Speck et al (1976) Warren & Fotherby (1973), Kaul et al (1981), Kaufman et al (1981) and Longcope & Williams (1977).

ences between women. Mestranol and EE have similar bioavailabilities in the human, but are significantly different in other species — such as the rat — due to poor demethylation systems.

PHARMACOKINETICS AND METABOLISM

Plasma concentration profiles

While several major research groups have published papers on the pharmacokinetics of contraceptive steroids in humans, comparison of their results is difficult due to use of both male and female subjects, and the administration of either pure steroids or commercial preparations. It is also apparent that the number of subjects in each study has been small, while other confounding factors include differences in methods for calculating volumes of distribution, clearance rates, and the various kinetic models used, together with the precision of different analytical methods. There are several recent reviews (e.g. Briggs, 1981).

The most commonly used contraceptive oestrogen is ethynyloestradiol (EE). When administered in tablet or solution form EE is absorbed in humans with great rapidity, with a half-life of absorption of 12–20 min. There is, however, significant metabolism (mainly to the 3-sulphate) during absorption through the intestinal wall and during the first liver pass (Speck et al, 1976; Goldzieher et al, 1980a, b). This reduces the amount of biologically active steroid available for contraception to only 40–50 per cent of the oral dose. Due to the rapid absorption, peak plasma concentration is attained within 2 hours after ingestion of the compound, though there are very large individual variations in the concentration found. The major pharmacokinetic parameters of EE are listed in Table 35.14 and compared with mestranol (MEE) a second commonly used oestrogen which undergoes rapid and extensive metabolism to EE in humans.

A study by Goldzieher et al (1980a) has compared plasma concentrations and pharmacokinetics of EE in women resident in a variety of different countries. In these investigations single oral doses of EE ranging from 35 to 100 µg were given to a total of 98 women resident in Nigeria, Singapore, Sri Lanka, Thailand, and the USA.

Using a highly specific radioimmunoassay, plasma levels of free EE were determined and appropriate pharmacokinetic parameters calculated. With doses of 50–80 µg EE, two-thirds of North American women showed detectable plasma EE concentrations at 24 hours. All parameters of the tri-exponential kinetic curve were calculated for women in the Sri Lankian study and for one of the USA investigations, while partial kinetic data were obtained for other countries. Strikingly lower plasma EE levels were consistently observed in Nigerian women, while Thai women showed highest concentrations, even when corrected for differences in body surface area.

In these investigations, the half-life of the absorption phase ranged from 4 to 22 min, while the half-life of the distribution phase was from 1–3 hours; half-life of the elimination phase was 6–14 hours. The apparent volume of the distribution was around 200 l/m², while the total body clearance was between 38 and 60 l/m²/h.

A high degree of correlation ($r = 0.95$) was reported between the peak plasma EE concentration and area under the curve of plasma EE values. The origin of these substantial differences in the kinetics of EE between women located in various countries remains to be identified, but could be of considerable clinical significance.

For MEE the ratio of plasma EE (following oral EE) to plasma MEE (following oral MEE) ranged from about one in Sri Lankan women to four in Thai women. As the groups were small it is not yet known whether these represent true biological differences between the various populations. The total body clearance of MEE ranged from 60 to 282 l/h, while that of EE derived from MEE ranged from 27 to 76 l/h. A comparison of areas under the plasma response curves showed no significant difference between EE derived from MEE and EE given as such. This is further confirmation that EE and MEE are bioequivalent over the usual dose range used in oral contraceptives.

For oestradiol esters (i.m.), lower plasma oestrogen levels have been found with the cypionate than with either the valerate or benzoate used at the same dose (Oriowo et al, 1980).

The pharmacokinetics of NET have been compared at

14 different international centres by Fotherby et al (1979). Plasma concentrations were measured at various times following a standard dose (1 mg). Inter-centre differences were of the same order as intra-centre differences and body size did not appear to influence the rate of NET disappearance from blood. A summary of the mean ranges found in this study is presented in Table 35.15. Results on plasma peak concentrations, plasma half-life, and metabolic clearance rate from other published studies of NET are reviewed in Table 35.16 which also provides information on the dose and route, sex of the subjects investigated, and whether or not estrogen was simultaneously administered. Both NET and LNG show significant affinity for human plasma sex hormone-blinding globulin, which increases markedly following oestrogen administration. The plasma concentration profile of these progestogens is therefore

Table 35.15 Plasma profile of NET (1 mg p.o.)*

Time (h)	Range	Extremes (nmol/l) Mean
0.5	4.5–13.1	8.8
1.0	8.9–18.8	13.8
2.0	8.7–20.0	14.3
4.0	7.5–16.1	12.8
8.0	3.8–9.2	6.5
12.0	2.7–6.3	4.5
24.0	1.1–3.1	2.2

* Fotherby et al (1979).

significantly influenced by concurrent use of oestrogen.

Using specific radioimmunoassays, Mishell et al (1977) have measured serum levels of LNG at intervals after the ingestion of various NG + EE tablets (0.5 mg NG + 50 μg

Table 35.16 Human pharmacokinetics of NET

Parameter	Results	Dose	Conditions Oestrogen	Sex	Reference
Plasma peak concentration	141 ± 23 nmol/l (42 ± 6.8 μg/l)	5 mg NET	—	F	Okerholm et al (1978)
	68 ± 6 nmol/l (20 ± 1.7 μg/l)	5 mg NET	—	M	Okerholm et al (1978)
	24 ± 4 nmol/l (7.2 μg/l)	1 mg NET	50 μg EE	F	Pasqualini et al (1977)
	19 nmol/l (5.7 μg/l)	1 mg NET	50 μg EE	F	Stanczyk et al (1978)
	14 ± 4 nmol/l (4.2 μg/l)	1 mg NET	—	F	Fotherby et al (1979)
	20 nmol/l (5.9 μg/l)	1 mg NEA	50 μg EE	F	Back et al (1978)
	28 nmol/l (8.3 μg/l)	1 mg NEA	50 μg EE	F	Back et al (1978)
	16 nmol/l (4.8 μg/l)	1 mg NEA	20 μg EE	F	Back et al (1978)
	24–52 nmol/l (7.2–15.3 μg/l)	1 mg EDA	50 μg EE	F	Walls et al (1977)
	22–29 nmol/l (6.5–8.7 μg/l)	1 mg EDA	50 μg EE	F	Vose et al (1979)
	21 nmol/l (6.2 μg/l)	0.5 mg NET	35 μg EE	F	Stanczyk et al (1978)
	11 nmol/l (3.2 μg/l)	0.35 mg NET	—	F	Stanczyk et al (1978)
	26–41 nmol/l (7.7–12.3 μg/l)	0.35 mgNET	—	F	Prasad et al (1979)
	16–50 nmol/l (4.7–14.8 μg/l)	0.35 mg NET	—	F	Prasad et al (1979)
Plasma half-life (elimination)	4.6 ± 0.5 h	10 mg NET	—	M	Okerholm et al (1978)
	7.0 h	1 mg NET	50 μg EE	F	Pasquelini et al (1977)
	1.0 ± 0.4 h	0.35 mg NET	—	F	Prasad et al (1979)
	1.5 ± 0.3 h	0.35 mg NET	50 μg EE	F	Prasad et al (1979)
	4.0–6.9 h	1 mg EDA	50 μg EE	F	Vose et al (1979)
	34.8 h	^{3}H-NEA(i.v.)	—	F	Singh et al (1979)
Metabolic clearance rate (MCR)	531 ± 56 l/day	NET (i.v.)	—	F	Mahesh et al (1977)
	495 l/day	NEA (i.v.)	—	F	Singh et al (1979)

Table 35.17 Pharmacokinetics of LNG (results of studies in women)

Parameter	Results (nmol/l)	Dose (μg)	Oestrogen	Reference
Plasma peak	0.68 (0.6–0.8)	30	—	Spona et al (1980)
	1.5 (1.3–1.8)	50	—	
	1.6 (1.2–2.0)	100	—	
	3.2 (2.3–4.2)	150	—	
	5. (3–7)	150	30	Laehteenmaeki & Nilsson
	(13–26)	250	50	(1978)
	19.5	150	30	Brenner et al (1977)
	(4.8–6.4)	37.5		Elstein et al (1976)
	(2.9–6.4)	30	—	Stanczyk et al (1975)
				Weiner et al (1976)

EE, 0.3 mg NG + 50 ;μg EE, 0.075 mg NG + 30 μg EE. Inhibition of ovulation appears to require a peak concentration in serum of 3μg/l LNG (10.1 nmol/l) and /or a minimum level of 1 μg/l LNG (3.4 nmol/l) when the oral contraceptive is taken orally once daily. A summary on the major pharmacokinetic parameters of LNG is given in Table 35.17.

Less well studied are the pregnane progestogens. Humpel et al (1977) found a plasma peak at 4 hours for cyproterone acetate (CPA) in women taking 2 mg CPA + 50 μg EE. The mean value was 18 ± 3.4 nmol/l (7.2 ± 1.4 μg/l). The major metabolite was 15β-hydroxy-CPA and this also showed maximum concentrations in plasma at 4 hours (31 ± 9.6 nmol/l, or 11.8 ± 3.7 μg/l). Oral progesterone (100 mg) gives a plasma peak of 22–34 nmol/l at 4 hours (Whitehead et al, 1980). A 50 mg oral dose of MGA gave a plasma peak of 182–263 nmol/l at 3–4 hours, while a 10 mg oral dose of MPA gave a plasma peak of 3.1 nmol/l at 3 hours (Martin & Adlercreutz, 1977). Following i.m. 150 mg MPA the plasma peak is reached within 24 hours and ranges from 2.6 to 7.8 nmol/l (Ortiz et al 1977). The peak of plasma NET following 200 mg i.m. NEE is not reached for about 7 days, and averages 40 to 57 nmol/l (Goebelsmann et al, 1979). Lower levels of unchanged NEE can also be detected in plasma.

Contraceptive steroid metabolism

Oestrogens. Irrespective of the route of administration, contraceptive steroids are generally efficiently absorbed and enter the circulation to be widely distributed to most tissues and organs. Little free steroids are excreted; the major end-products being conjugates (principally glucuronides and sulphates). These are excreted in both urine and bile, with some of the biliary metabolites undergoing enterohepatic recycling.

The metabolism of contraceptive steroids has been the subject of a number of previous reviews (James, 1972; Fotherby, 1974; Breuer, 1977; Ranney, 1977; Briggs, 1981; Bolt, 1979). It is apparent that there are major species differences in metabolic pathways for many steroids, while there may be significant differences between individuals for reasons that are not yet clear.

In most species MEE is efficiently demethylated to yield EE; following this conversion the subsequent metabolism of MEE is the same as that of EE in all species studied. Unique metabolites of MEE are the 17-glucuronide and 2-hydroxy-MEE (Williams M.C. et al, 1975a, b), though these are minor metabolites in women. The two principal excretion products of either MEE or EE are EE-3-sulphate and EE-3-glucuronides.

MEE and EE also undergo D-homoannulation to yield D-homoestrone and D-homoestradiol-17αβ. This reaction occurs extensively in the rabbit, but is a very minor pathway in humans and the rat (Abdel-Aziz & Williams, 1969, 1970).

The extent of de-ethynylation of EE and MEE is controversial. According to Kulkarni & Goldzieher (1970) and Williams et al (1975b) between 15 and 20 per cent of human urinary glucuronide metabolites of EE were de-ethynylated (oestrone, oestradiol, oestriol and 2-methoxy-oestradiol), however, Williams et al (1975a) found only 1 to 2 per cent de-ethynylation in women given labelled EE or MEE. It is recognised that there is prompt partial conversion by intestine and liver of EE to its sulphate (Bird & Clarke, 1975), which is known to have a relatively long biological half-life.

The 3-methoxy group of MEE renders the compound more lipophilic than EE, so that the tissue pool of MEE is larger than for the same dose of EE, due to storage in fats (Appelgren & Karlsson, 1971; Bold & Remmer, 1972; Bolt & Bolt, 1974). An even more lipophilic compound is quinestrol (QEE), which is the 3-cyclopentylether of EE. Dealkylation of QEE to release EE occurs to varying degrees in different species. It is a minor pathway in the rabbit (Layne & Williams, 1967), but the principal pathway in humans (Williams et al, 1967) and the rat (Meli et al, 1968), though the ratio of excretion in bile and in urine varies significantly with species. In humans, biliary excretion is important, with about 40 per cent of an oral dose of EE being recoverable from faeces (via biliary excretion) compared to 60 per cent in urine (Cargill et al,

Table 35.18 Contraceptive steroid metabolites

Class	Compound	Principal metabolites identified*
Oestrogens	EE	2-OH-EE
		2-OH, 3-MeO-EE
		2-MeO-EE
		4-OH-EE
		6α-OH-EE
		16α-OH-EE
		D-homo-E_2
		E_2
		E_1
	MEE	EE
		As for EE
	QEE	6α-OH-QEE
		EE
		As for EE
	E_2-esters	E_2
Progestogens	NET	4,5-epoxy-NET
		1β-OH-NET
		EE(?)
		de-ethynyl-NET
		3α-dihydro-NET
		5α-dihydro-NET
		3α,5α-tetrahydro-NET
		3β-dihydro-NET
		5β-dihydro-NET
		3β,5β-tetrahydro-NET
		3α,5β-tetrahydro-NET
		3β,5α-tetrahydro-NET
	NEE	NET
		As for NET
	LYN	EDO
		NET
		As for NET
	EDA	EDO
		NET
		As for NET
	LNG	2α-OH-LNG
		6β-OH-LNG
		16β-OH-LNG
		3α-dihydro-LNG
		5β-dihydro-LNG
		3α,5β-tetrahydro-LNG
		Hydroxy-dihydro-LNG
		Hydroxy-tetrahydro-LNG
	DNG	1β-OH-DNG
		16α-OH-DNG
		16β-OH-DNG
		D-homo-DNG
	DOG	3α-OH-DOG(?)
		3β-OH-DOG
		11-methylene-LNG
	NGM	LNG-3-oxime
		LNG
		As for LNG
	MPA	6-OH-MPA
		21-OH-MPA
		17-deacetyl-MPA
	MGA	6-OH-MGA
		Dihydroxy-MGA
		Deacetyl-MGA
	CPA	15β-OH-CPA

Table 35.18 (contd)

Class	Compound	Principal metabolites identified*
	CMA	1β-OH-CMA
		2α-OH-CMA
		2β-OH-CMA
		2-OH-△¹-CMA
		5-OH-CMA
		3α-dihydro-CMA
		3β-dihydro-CMA
		5α-dihydro-CMA
		5β-dihydro-CMA
		2α-OH-3α-dihydro-CMA
		2α-OH-3β-dihydro-CMA
		2β-OH-3β-dihydro-CMA
		3α,5β-tetrahydro-CMA
		3β,5β-tetrahydro-CMA

* Often as conjugates (glucuronidates, sulphates, glutathionates): there are significant individual and species differences.

1969; Reed et al, 1972; Fotherby, 1973). Biliary excretion is also important in the rat and guinea-pig (Reed & Fotherby, 1975), but in baboons urinary excretion of EE metabolites greatly predominates (Kulkarni, 1970).

There appear to be major individual, as well as species differences, in the metabolism of contraceptive oestrogens (De la Pena et al, 1975; Ranney, 1977; Helton & Goldzieher, 1977; Nilsson & Nygren, 1978; Bolt, 1979).

Oestradiol esters undergo hydrolysis to yield free E_2, which is then metabolised by the same pathways as endogenous E_2. There are significant differences in the rates of hydrolysis of these esters between organs, species and individuals (Oriowo et al, 1980).

Oestranes. Structurally related progestogens include norethisterone (NET), norethynodrel (NED), lynestrenol (LYN), and ethynodiol diacetate (EDA), together with the esters norethisterone acetate (NEA) and norethisterone enanthate (NEE) (Table 35.18). There is conclusive evidence that these compounds are all metabolised to NET, which is the active substance producing hormonal effects. For the oral progestogens in this series, the metabolism in humans is rapid and efficient, occurring partly during first passage through the intestines and liver.

Unlike the rabbit, where excretion occurs in urine, the principal route of excretion of NET in the rat is via bile. Hanasono & Fischer (1974) reported recovery of 80 per cent of the label within 8 hours from bile duct-cannulated rats given [³H]-NET. Metabolites in bile were conjugates that participated in an enterohepatic circulation. Kappus & Remmer (1975) have shown that rat liver microsomes convert NET *in vitro* to a compound (believed to be NET-4,5-epoxide) that binds covalently to tissue proteins. The gut wall of the rat also metabolises NET (Back et al, 1978).

Mahesh et al (1977) present studies on the human metabolism, metabolic clearance rate, blood metabolites and blood half-life of NET. Investigations were made following a single i.v. injection. NET disappeared rapidly from the circulation, but metabolites appeared to persist. Administration of [³H]-NET for 6 days at 24 hour intervals revealed a 'staircase' effect on blood radioactivity, with no indication of a plateau, though on discontinuation the metabolites slowly cleared with a half-life of about 70 hours. The major metabolites were all ring A-reduced compounds, including the 3α, 5α-, 3α, 5β-, and 5α, 3β derivatives. In blood an additional metabolite was identified as 5β-dihydro-NET.

Early studies on the metabolism of NET in humans followed the excretion of the radioactive label. Layne et al (1963) gave oral doses of [³H]-NET and measured urinary excretion. In 7 days after oral administration of the compound 50–70 per cent of ³H appeared in the urine, and the major fraction of the label was conjugated as glucuronides. Fotherby et al (1966) did a similar study using [¹⁴C]-NET. More than 90 per cent of the urinary metabolites were found still to possess the 17-ethynyl group. Fotherby & Klopper (1968a) also reported studies on the metabolism of [¹⁴C]-NET in women. In seven subjects given ¹⁴C-NET intravenously, 40–80 per cent of the ¹⁴C appeared in the urine in 5 days. Only 3 per cent of the radioactivity was free steroid. Fifteen per cent was present as sulphate conjugates, and about 50 per cent was present as glucuronides. There was little or no de-ethynylation.

Detailed identification of norethisterone metabolites was provided by Murata (1968), who gave [³H]-NET orally and analysed urine for metabolites. About 9 per cent of urinary ³H was free. Twenty-five per cent was conjugated as glucuronides, and 40 per cent was present as sulphates. In general, the metabolic transformations were saturation of the double bond and reduction of 3-keto to a hydroxyl group.

Gerhards et al (1971) gave [³H]-or [¹⁴C]-NET orally to three women and identified plasma and urinary metabolites. Plasma radioactivity reached a peak 2 hours after administration of the labelled drug. The disappearance of plasma radioactivity showed a half-life of 9 hours while the half-life of NET was 2 hours. Sulphates composed 80–90 per cent of the conjugates, and of these 3β, 5β-tetrahydro-NET was the major metabolite. Urinary radioactivity amounted to 40–50 per cent of the dose, and 50–65 per cent of urinary ³H or ¹⁴C was present as sulphate conjugates.

Arai et al (1962), studied [³H]-NED in rabbits, some of which had bile duct cannulas. Mean recovery of radioactivity was 21 per cent in urine, 17 per cent in faeces, and 33 per cent in bile, compared with 50 per cent in urine and 16 per cent in faeces of intact rabbits. The principal metabolite in bile was 3β-dihydro-NED, together with NET and 10β-hydroxylated derivatives. Urine also contained these same compounds as conjugates, together with what were thought to be de-ethynylated metabolites. In bile duct-cannulated rats, Hanasono & Fischer (1974) found 70 per cent of the label from [³H]-NED appeared in the bile

within 7 hours and also demonstrated enterohepatic circulation.

EDA is rapidly deacetylated and oxidised to NET following administration to humans. Walls et al (1977) have measured plasma NET following oral tablets of 1 mg EDA + 50 μg EE taken by four normal women. Comparison of mean areas under the plasma concentration-time curves indicated that the absorption of EDA could be monitored by measurements of plasma NET.

A further study on bioavailability and pharmacokinetics of NET in women receiving oral EDA, has been published by Vose et al (1979). Results are presented on plasma NET responses in healthy women who received either oral contraceptives containing 1 mg EDA + 50 μg EE, or a solution containing EDA + EE in ethanol.

The pharmacokinetics of NEA in women has been studied by Singh et al (1979). Previously untreated healthy female volunteers received a single i.v. injection of tritiated NEA dissolved in 10 per cent alcoholic saline. Blood specimens were collected at intervals up to 72 hours. Following intravenous injection, NEA is rapidly metabolised to NET, which then disappears from the plasma with an average half-life of 34.8 hours. Unidentified tritiated metabolites persisted in the free steroid fraction of plasma in significant amounts for as long as 72 hours after the injection.

An interesting comparative pharmacokinetic study of three progestogens (LYN, CPA, LNG) has been published by Humpel et al (1977). The micronised compounds, labelled with either ¹⁴C or ³H, were administered orally combined with 50 μg EE to six women. Plasma progestogen concentration and total radioactivity were recorded up to 5 and 8 days after ingestion. All progestogens were completely absorbed at comparable rates. Post-maximum courses of disposition were characterised by two phases, the first of which had a half-life of about 3 hours and was not substance specific. The half-life of the second phase was about the same for LNG and CPA (1.5 and 1.7 hours respectively), but was significantly higher for LYN (2.5 hours). Percentages of doses recovered in urine and faeces respectively were: LNG 48, 46; LYN 50, 39; CPA 30, 58. There was a marked discrepancy between plasma radioactivity and NET concentration following LYN. This was not due to unconverted LYN and presumably related to some other metabolite.

LYN is converted to NET via ethynodiol (3β-dihydro-NET) in humans, but 3α-dihydro-NET has been detected in vitro in rabbit liver homogenates incubated with LYN (Fotherby, 1974b). The efficiency of conversion of 3-deoxysteroids to the active 3-keto metabolites presumably depends on the amount lost along competing pathways, such as formation of 3-conjugates from the 3-hydroxy precursors.

NET-enanthate (NEE) has been widely used as a long acting depot contraceptive. It is thought to act as a depot progestogen from which NET is gradually released by hydrolysis. The conversion of NEE to NET has been studied by Back et al (1981). When incubated with blood plasma from rabbits, rats, or guinea pigs there was extensive hydrolysis within 90 min. In contrast, blood plasma from dogs, goats and humans showed negligible hydrolysis (less than 2.5 per cent). Good hydrolytic activity *in vitro* was also demonstrated for liver, kidney, gut wall, stomach, heart and skeletal muscle of rabbits, but incubation with human muscle or fat showed little hydrolysis. It would appear that this ester is rapidly hydrolysed following intramuscular injection in the rabbit, whereas in humans the liver is probably the main site of hydrolysis and the ester is largely unaffected by blood enzymes.

The conversion of NET (and related progestogens) to oestrogens, such as EE, has been the subject of some controversy. Labelled EE has been recovered unequivocally from the urine of women receiving labelled NET (see Breuer, 1977), but a principal intermediate is 1β-hydroxy-NET. This compound is readily aromatised by acid or alkali and EE extracted from urine of women receiving NET was probably formed during the analytical procedure, rather than by human metabolism.

Gonanes. It is of considerable interest to know if the metabolism of active LNG is the same or different to that of DNG. This problem has been investigated by Sisenwine et al (1975) who administered 1.5 mg of ^{14}C-labelled compound (either $(+)-$, $(-)-$, or $(\pm)$-NG) to women. Mean percentage recovery of radioactivities was as follows (in 7 days): LNG — urine 45, faeces 32; DNG — urine 64, faeces 25; NG — urine 58, faeces 23. No significant oestrogen formation was observed with metabolism of LNG, though minor amounts of phenols were seen with DNG. Other metabolic pathways may be summarised as follows: LNG — 2α-hydroxylation, 3α, 5β-reduction, 16β-hydroxylation; DNG-1β-hydroxylation, 16β-hydroxylation, 16β-hydroxylation, D-hommannulation.

Metabolism of NG by the female baboon has been investigated by Sisenwine et al (1978). Using ^{14}C-NG, following a single administration, unchanged drug was absent from the urine, but metabolites noted in other primates, including 3α, 5β-tetrahydro NG, 2α-hydroxy NG, 16β-hydroxy NG, and 13-ethyl-D-homogon-4-ene-3, 17α-dione were detected in both unconjugated and conjugated fractions. The sulphated metabolites of NG detected in human urine were not evident, and 3α, 5β-tetrahydro NG was the major metabolite in one baboon. The metabolite pattern seen in the African green monkey is closer to that in women where 16β-hydroxy NG (as sulphate) appears to constitute about one-third of the total urinary activity following oral labelled-NG.

Sisenwine et al (1977) used [^{14}C]-norgestimate in rhesus monkeys, given as a single intragastric dose (0.5 mg/kg). There was rapid absorption into blood and two major metabolites were detected (LNG and LNG-3-oxime). The authors suggest that norgestimate is rapidly converted to LNG-3-oxime, which is then more slowly converted to LNG. The principal metabolite of the latter is probably a glucuronide conjugate of 13β-ethyl-17α-ethynyl-5β-gona-3α, 17β-diol (3, 5 -tetrahydro-LNG).

Human pharmacokinetics of norgestimate in the presence and absence of EE has been studied by Weintraub et al (1978). Investigations were made on seven healthy women who received a single capsule of ^{14}C-labelled norgestimate either alone or in combination with [^{3}H]-EE. The dose of norgestimate was 0.49 or 0.50 mg, while the EE dose was 140 μg. The mean elimination of ^{14}C following oral [^{14}C]-norgestimate over the 2 week collection period was 83.5 per cent with a range of 64–94 per cent. Urinary radioactivity accounted for a mean 46.8 per cent, while a mean 36.8 per cent was recovered in the faeces. EE appeared to have little effect on the routes or amounts of elimination.

The active metabolite of DOG appears to be 3-keto-DOG (which is 11-methylene-LNG). The latter shows high binding affinity for progesterone receptors, which DOG lacks (Viinikka et al, 1979). An intermediate is presumably 3α-hydroxy-DOG or 3β-hydroxy-DOG (or both), by analogy with the metabolic activation of LYN. The efficiency of conversion of DOG to its active metabolite is uncertain. Viinikka et al (1980) have studied plasma distribution and elimination in volunteers, together with recovery from urine and faeces. In single dose studies, 83 per cent of DOG radioactivity was recovered over a 8 day period from urine and faeces (48 per cent from urine, 35 per cent from faeces). The corresponding recoveries in the volunteers pretreated with DOG plus EE were 76 per cent total recovery, with 45 per cent in urine and 31 per cent in faeces.

Pregnanes. MPA and CMA have found use both as oral and injectable contraceptives, while MGA has been used in oral contraceptives and in implants. Reviews on the metabolism of these compounds have been published by Fotherby & James (1972) and Fotherby (1974a).

Much of the label from progestogens in this group is excreted primarily via the urine in primates, though the dog favours biliary (and faecal) excretion (Hill, 1972). Slaunwhite & Sandberg (1961) recovered in humans up to 42 per cent of label from i.v. [^{14}C]-MPA in urine compared with up to 13 per cent in faeces. The biological half-life appeared to be about 14.5 hours (about half that of NET). Similarly for labelled-MGA, Cooper & Kellie (1968) recovered up to 78 per cent in urine and up to 30 per cent in faeces. The values for CMA were up to 43 per cent in urine and up to 28 per cent in faeces (Dorfman, 1971).

Hydroxylation of the 17-acetoxyprogestogens occurs at C-6 with MPA (Helmreich & Huseby, 1962: Castegnaro & Sala, 1962), MGA (Cooper & Kellie. 1968), and melengestrol acetate (Cooper et al, 1967) and at C-21 with MPA (Helmreich & Huseby, 1962).

Martin & Adlercreutz (1977) have measured the concentration of these two progestogens in human plasma following oral administration. At the same dose there was much higher plasma concentration of MGA than MPA. Metabolites of MGA in human bile were almost exclusively glucuronide conjugated, whereas in urine both sulphate and glucuronide conjugated metabolites were found. Monohydroxylated metabolites predominated, though evidence of MGA reduction was also apparent. In dogs metabolites were similar to those found in humans.

A comparison of CMA metabolism in the rat, rabbit, dog and human is discussed by Honma et al (1977). Fourteen unconjugated metabolites and three conjugated metabolites were isolated from urine, faeces and bile following oral administration. A marked species difference in metabolic pattern was established. The major urinary metabolite in man was the 2-hydroxy CMA, with significant amounts of 3-hydroxy and 5β-metabolites. The occurrence of 1-hydroxylation and 5-hydroxylation reactions, which are new metabolic pathways, is described for both the rat and human. One of the main metabolites in humans and rats is 3-β-hydroxy CMA.

The metabolic fate of MAP was studied in intact baboons and in those with bile fistulas by Ishihara et al (1976). Following i.v. administration of labelled MAP only a small percentage (less than 15 per cent) of the administered dose was recovered in the urine in 7 hours in intact baboons, as well as in the urine of baboons with biliary fistulas. Higher amounts of radioactivity were excreted in the bile (approximately 25 per cent), amounting to almost double the percentage excreted in the urine. The similarity in the urinary excretion of radioactivity intact and biliary fistula animals indicates that, even though a substantial biliary excretion of the labelled MAP occurred, the amount involved in an enterohepatic circulation is probably small. Glucuronates were the predominant conjugates, both in the urine and bile. The loss of the 17α-acetate group appeared to be rather extensive, ranging from 30 to 70 per cent, among different conjugated and unconjugated metabolites of MAP. The deacetylation of the 17α-acetate in MAP was similar to that observed in humans given the drug. Oxygenation of MAP at position 1 and/or 2 appeared to be minimal (<5 per cent). The major metabolic conversions of contraceptive steroids are summarised in Table 35.18

MODE OF ACTION

Combined OCs, when taken correctly, and in the absence of confounding factors (poor gastrointestinal absorption, interference by other drugs, etc.), appear to be highly efficient inhibitors of ovulation in the majority of women. This appears to be largely independent of either the particular oestrogen or progestogen used in the combination, or of the type of formulation (high or low dose fixed combination, sequential, biphasic, or triphasic). The actions on various target organs are summarised in Table 35.19.

Inhibition of ovulation is produced by the elimination of the mid-cycle surge in plasma gonadotrophin concentration. Basal gonadotrophin secretion is less affected, though there is some suppression, especially with higher dose combinations.

Plasma gonadotrophin response to a bolus of GnRH, given into a peripheral vein, is moderately suppressed in some, but not all, users of combined OC. Response is greater with lower dose combinations, but appears unrelated to duration of OC use. In contrast, plasma prolactin in basal concentration is often raised in OC users and prolactin response to a peripheral bolus of TRH is enhanced.

Contraceptive steroids alter activity of the higher brain centre — hypothalamus-anterior-pituitary axis in many ways in animal models, but effects in women are uncertain. It is likely that contraceptive steroids (oestrogens and progestogens) interact with target cell receptors in many brain areas, aside from the hypothalamus and pituitary (though direct effects on these latter organs also occur).

Prolonged use of combined OCs probably alters concentrations and tissue distribution of sex hormone receptors, and also of GnRH secretion and its receptors in the anterior pituitary. Short feedback effects on gonadotrophins may also change. Production of brain neurotransmitter substances, and prostaglandins, are difficult to investigate, but are likely to be altered by contraceptive steroids.

Combined OCs have secondary contraceptive effects, mediated via sex hormone receptors, on the uterine endometrium, cervical mucus, oviducts, and may also interfere with spermatozoan transport and capacitation in the female tract.

The mode of action of contraceptive steroids administered by routes other than oral is less well investigated, especially for newer products. A summary of published data is given in Table 35.20.

METABOLIC AND ENDOCRINE EFFECTS

Contraceptive steroids induce major changes in a wide range of metabolic processes of women (Table 35.21). While the majority of these metabolic changes appear to be due to the estrogen components of many preparations, there is also good evidence that progestogens alone induce significant changes in a number of important metabolic parameters. There is evidence for an interaction between oestrogens and progestogens when administered together. Amongst the changes that have been reported are a deterioration of glucose tolerances tests, accompanied by an increase in plasma insulin response. In the fasting state plasma triglyceride and cholesterol tends to be elevated, largely due to alterations in the pattern of lipoproteins.

Table 35.19 Mode of action of OC*

Target organ	Criterion	Effect of OC
Ovary	Luteal phase increase in plasma progesterone, 17α-hydroxyprogesterone and oestradiol concentrations	Often eliminated (Diczfalusy, 1968)
	Peri-ovulatory increase in plasma oestradiol and 17α-hydroxyprogesterone	Often eliminated (Diczfalusy, 1968)
	Direct ovarian examination (laparoscopy or culdoscopy)	General absence of corpora lutea; cystic and atretic follicles (Ryan et al, 1964; Diddle et al, 1967; Zussman et al, 1967; Sanchez-Rivers et al, 1968)
	Ovarian response to exogenous hCG	Reduced (Lunenfeld et al, 1963; Hecht-Lucari, 1964)
	Steroidal sex hormone biosynthesis	Inhibited (Appelgren, 1969; Fotherby, 1977; Saure et al, 1977; Schürenkämper & Lisse, 1978; Shinada et al, 1978)
	Gonadotrophin receptor concentrations	Reduced (Wardlow et al, 1975)
Pituitary gland	Peri-ovulatory surge of gonadotrophins in plasma	Absent or reduced (Briggs et al, 1970; Briggs, 1975a; Johansson, 1976; Goldzieher et al, 1975a)
	Basal gonadotrophin concentrations in plasma	Moderately suppressed (Cohen & Katz, 1981)
	Cytosol receptor concentration (oestrogen and progestogen receptors)	Altered (Naess & Attramadal, 1978; Moguilewsky & Raynaud, 1979)
	Gonadotrophin responses to i.v. bolus of GnRh	Moderately suppressed (Mischell et al, 1977; Rubinstein et al, 1978; Scott et al, 1978b; Wan et al, 1981)
	Concentration of GnRH receptors in pituitary	Reduced (Spona, 1975)
Hypothalamus	Concentration of sex hormone receptors	Altered (MacLuskey & McEwan, 1978)
	GnRH secretion	Reduced
Higher brain centres	Neurotransmitter concentrations (noradrenaline, dopamine, serotonin, 5-HIAA)	Altered (Bernasconi et al, 1976; Algeri et al, 1977)
	Prostaglandin effects on GnRH	Altered (Craig, 1976; Roberts et al, 1976)
Uterine endometrium	Usual cyclic changes	Eliminated (Ober, 1977)
	Glandular proliferation	Diminished or abolished (Magnco-Topele et al, 1963)
	Spiral arterioles	Fail to develop (Ober, 1977)
	Intimal layers of uterine arterial branches	Cellular proliferation (Osterholzer et al, 1977)
	Cytosol receptors for oestrogens	Reduced (Sanborn et al, 1978; Pollow et al, 1978)
	Cytosol receptors for progesterone	Reduced (Sanborn et al 1978; Pollow et al, 1978)
	Enzyme histochemistry	Altered (Connell et al, 1967)
Uterine cervix	Sperm penetration of cervical mucus (*in vitro* or *in vivo*)	Reduced by progestogens (Elstein et al, 1973)
	Viscosity of cervical mucus	Increased by progestogens (Odeblad, 1968; Kesserü, 1971; Cohen, 1978)
	Mucoprotein content of mucus	Altered (Elstein et al, 1973)
	Oestrogen-receptors and progesterone-receptors in cervical cytosols	Reduced (Sanborn et al, 1978)
Oviducts	Contractions in tubal musculature	Altered (Coutinho, 1973)
	Spontaneous motility	Reduced (Elder et al, 1978)
	Cilial action	Altered (Aksu, 1979)
	Ovum transport	Altered (Harper et al, 1976)
Spermatozoa	Motility and viability	Reduced
	Capacitation	Inhibited (Gwatkin & Williams, 1970; Briggs, 1973a)

* Effects are modified by the presence or absence of oestrogen, the soe and regimen of contraceptive steroid(s) used, and the individual compounds present.

Table 35.20 Mode of action of contraceptive steroids administered by routes other than oral

Steroid	Dose	Route	Principal contraceptive effects	Reference
NEA	40 μg/day	Intranasal	Mid-cycle LH ↓ Luteal progesterone ↓	Carol et al (1980)
PRO	60 μg/day	IUD	Endometrium	Newton et al (1979)
LNG	?/day	IUD	Endometrium	El-Magoub (1981)
MPA	150 mg/3 month	i.m.	Mid-cycle LH + FSH ↓ Luteal progesterone ↓	Vecchio (1976)
NEE	200 mg/3 months	i.m.		
LNG	6 × 35 mg	Silastic implant	Endometrium Other?	Sivin et al (1980)
NGT	6 × 35 mg	Silastic implant	Endometrium Other?	Sivin et al (1980)
E_2	4 × 25 mg (reducing)	Pellet Implant	Endometrium Other?	Nezhat et al (1980)
NET	200 μg	Silastic Vaginal ring	Ovulation Endometrium	
LNG +	290 μg +	Silastic	Ovulation Endometrium	Mishell et al (1978)
E_2	180 μg/day	Vaginal ring	Other?	

This alteration with many commonly used oral contraceptives may favour enhanced atherosclerotic changes. There is increased input of triglycerides into the plasma pool, and while triglyceride removal is also increased, it does not balance the increased input.

Aside from changes in the lipoproteins there are also significant alterations in many other plasma proteins of hepatic origin. These include important carrier proteins for many hormones, trace elements, and vitamins. There are also major changes in the concentration of the renin substrate that may contribute to significant alterations in blood pressure in oral contraceptive users.

Many steroidal contraceptives act by inhibiting the mid-cycle surge of the pituitary gonadotrophins associated with ovulation. They generally have little effect on basal secretion of gonadotrophins, though basal prolactin secretion is somewhat enhanced. There are also increases in plasma growth hormone; thyrotrophin concentration is largely unchanged, but adrenocorticotrophin is suppressed. Marked alterations are seen in many plasma steroidal hormones, often due to alterations in their binding protein. The characteristic changes in oestradiol and progesterone seen in an untreated menstrual cycle are eliminated, while the pattern of plasma androgens is markedly altered. Plasma cortisol and, to a lesser extent aldosterone, are increased.

Most users of contraceptive steroids show no alterations in plasma marker enzymes for organ damage, but there is often an increase in enzymes associated with hepatic microsomal activity. Alterations have also been reported in red cell enzymes requiring B vitamins for their coenzymes, while blood platelet enzymes associated with lysosome activity tend to be enhanced. Changes have been reported in steroid metabolising enzymes of the uterus during the use of contraceptive steroids.

There are many methodological problems facing the

Table 35.21 Metabolic and endocrine effects of combined OC*

Group	Test	Effects
Carbohydrates (and insulin) (Adams & Oakley, 1972; Beck, 1973; Spellacy 1969, 1976, 1978)	Fasting blood glucose concentration	Sometimes increased
	Oral glucose tolerance test	Often deteriorates
	Intravenous glucose tolerance test	Sometimes deteriorates
	Glucose tolerance test with corticosteroid pretreatment	Often deteriorates
	Insulin response during glucose tolerance test	Usually increased
	Proinsulin	Small increase (Haussman et al, 1975)
	Peripheral cell insulin-receptors	Altered concentration and affinities (Gambhir et al, 1978; Tsibris et al, 1980; Di Pirro et al, 1981)
Lipids and lipoproteins (Basdevant et al, 1976; Beck, 1975; Lederer & Vastesaeger, 1977)	Fasting triglycerides in blood plasma/serum	Often increased, especially by E.
	Fasting total cholesterol in blood plasma/serum	Usually small increase
	Post-heparin lipolytic activity	Decreased (influenced by P:E balance)

* For further information see reviews by Corfman, 1969; Salhanick et al, 1969; Briggs et al, 1970; Bingel & Benoit, 1973; Warren, 1973; Miale & Kent, 1974; Weindling & Henry, 1974; Briggs, 1976; Spellacy, 1978; Briggs & Briggs, 1981)

Table 35.21 (contd)

Group	Test	Effects
	Lipoprotein fractions: HDL (α-LP) VLDL (β-LP) LDL (pre-β-LP)	Increase and/or decreases depending upon P:E balance (Rössner et al, 1971; Ravens & Jipp, 1976; Van der Steeg & Pronk, 1977; Bradley et al, 1978; Briggs & Briggs, 1979b).
	Lipoprotein cholesterol: HDL-cholesterol VLDL-cholesterol LDL-cholesterol	Increase and/or decreases depending upon P:E balnce (Rössner et al, 1971; Ravens & Jipp, 1976; Van der Steeg & Pronk, 1977; Bradley et al, 1978; Briggs & Briggs, 1979b).
	Fasting non-esterified Fatty acids (NEFA): Free fatty acids (FFA)	Decreased by E
Proteins and enzymes (Ambrus et al, 1976; Meade et al, 1976; Poller, 1978; Briggs & Briggs, 1979c)	Metallo-proteins: transferrin ceruloplasmin	Some increase Increased
	Hormone-binders: Transcortin (TC) Sex hormone-binding globulin (SHBG) Thyroxine-binding globulin (TBG) Thyroxine-binding prealbumin (PBPA) Aldosterone-binding globulin (ABG)	Increased Increased Increased Increased Increased
	Vitamin-binders: Transcobalamins (TCOB) Retinol-binding protein (RBP) Folate-binding protein (FBP)	Increased Increased Increased
	Blood coagulation and fibrinolytic factors: Prothrombin Fibrinogen Factor VI Factor VII Factor VIII Factor IX Factor X Antifactor Xa Factor XI Factor XII Factor XIII Antithrombin III α₂-macroglobulin Fibrinolytic activator	No change Increased No change Increased Increased No change ? Increased Decreased No change Increased Small decrease Decreased Increased Decreased

Table 35.21 (contd)

Group	Test	Effects
	Miscellaneous: Albumin Haptoglobulin Orosomucoid	Reduced Reduced Reduced
Amino acids (free) (Craft & Peters, 1971; Briggs, 1978a, Oepen et al, 1978)	Serine Histidine Phenylalanine Ornithine Tryptophan Asparagine Glutamine Glycine Valine Isoleucine Tyrosine Aspartate Methionine α-aminobutyrate Proline Leucine Threonine Arginine Citrulline	Decreased Decreased Decreased Decreased Decreased Decreased Reduced Reduced Reduced Reduced Reduced Reduced Reduced Reduced Increased Increased Increased Increased Increased
Protein hormones	Basal gonadotrophins Mid-cycle gonadotrophins Prolactin Thyroid-stimulating hormone (TSH) Adrenocrorticotrophin (ACTH) Insulin (during GTT) Glucagon (arginine-stimulated) Growth hormone Angiotensin I and II	Some reduction Eliminated Some increase No change Some reduction Increased Decreased Increased Increased
Non-protein hormones	Cyclic changes in oestradiol, progesterone, and metabolites Basal oestradiol, progesterone, and metabolites Dehydroepiandrosterone (sulphate) Androsterone (sulphate) Total testosterone + 5α-dihydrotestosterone Free testosterone + 5α-dihydrotestosterone Total cortisol Free cortisol Total thyroxine (T₄) Total triiodothyroxine (T₃)	Eliminated Unchanged ? Reduced Reduced Increased No change Increased Small increase ? Increased Increased
Mineral elements (Smith & Brown, 1976)	Na, K, Cl Cu Fe I	No change Increased by E Increased by E Increased by E

Table 35.21 (contd)

Group	Test	Effects
	Zn	Decreased by depot-P and by oral E/P
	Mn	Decreased by E
Vitamin status (Larsson-Cohn, 1975; Wynn, 1975; Bamji, 1978; Tonkin, 1981)	A	Increased by E
	B_1	Decreased (?)
	B_2	Decreased by E
	B_6	Decreased
	B_{12}	Decreased
	C	Decreased
	D	Decreased (?)
	E	Decreased (?)
	Niacin	Increased
	Folate	Decreased (?)

Table 35.22 Methods of investigating biochemical effects of pharmaceuticals

		Problems
Cross-sectional:	Compare biochemistry of those taking drugs with controls not taking drug (or taking alternative drug)	Do reasons for taking (or not taking) drug influence biochemistry (e.g. disease, social status, race, nutrition, genetics)?
		Are groups closely matched on confounding factors (e.g. age, sex, menstrual status, weight, duration of treatment, smoking)?
Prospective:	Compare biochemistry pretreatment and at intervals during treatment (a control group receiving no treatment, or an alternative drug, may or may not be added)	Are any changes due to drug, or to alterations in confounding factors (e.g. weather, diet, weight, occupation, disease)?
		If controls were used, are they closely matched to test group (see above)?

study of metabolic changes related to the use of any pharmaceutical agent. Aside from individual and temporal factors, there are fundamental difficulties related to usual study designs (Table 35.22). These are often very difficult to standardise in studies with contraceptive steroids.

The clinical significance of these numerous biochemical alterations has been the subject of considerable discussion and debate, and it is generally believed that many of the alterations are undesirable. The present trend in the development of new steroidal contraceptives has been to formulate products in which these metabolic changes are minimised or eliminated entirely (Briggs, 1979).

DRUG INTERACTIONS

Interactions reported

Several reviewers have published lists of interactions between contraceptive steroids and other pharmaceutical agents (see Stockley, 1976; Robertson & Johnson, 1976; Breckenridge, 1977; Breckenridge et al, 1979, 1980; Editorial, 1980). A compilation of these, together with some more recent reports is provided in Table 35.23. The references are incomplete as interaction reports are now extensive.

Interactions between two pharmaceutical agents are usually complex and involve a variety of biochemical mechanisms. The usual clinical consequence is a change in the biological effects of one or both drugs. Where interaction primarily changes efficacy of a steroidal contraceptive, a usual sign is increased spotting and BTB suggesting inadequate steroid hormone supply to the uterine endometrium so that contraceptive efficacy may be in doubt. There are far more accounts of irregular bleeding than of unwanted pregnancies in contraceptive users taking interacting drugs.

The opposite interaction is where a second agent increases efficacy. This appears to occur with large doses of vitamin C (Back et al, 1981; Briggs, 1981), which by competitive blocking of intestinal sulphatases, increases the amount of non-sulphated EE (the biologically active fraction) entering the circulation from an OC (enhanced bioavailability).

A different type of interaction is where the steroid contraceptive shows no apparent change in efficacy, but a second drug taken simultaneously shows a marked change. This occurs, for example, with troleandomycin, which produces jaundice in many women using OCs but rarely in non-users (Miguet et al, 1980). Similar increased toxicity in OC users appears to occur with a number of other drugs, including imipramine, acenocoumarol, and vincristine.

Mechanisms of interactions

The various possible ways in which steroid contraceptive–drug interactions may occur have been reviewed by Robertson & Johnson (1976). The include:

1. a direct physical or chemical combination influencing absorption;
2. displacement from binding sites;
3. activation or inhibition of hepatic enzymes affecting biodegradation;
4. competition for a common receptor site;
5. interactions through opposing physiological mechanisms;
6. interference with urinary excretion.

Interactions involving changes in absorption may presumably occur with various antacids, while liquid paraffin is another possibility (Swyer, 1979). More subtle absorption changes include the ascorbic acid-EE effect

Table 35.23   Pharmacological interactions with contraceptive steroids

Group	Substance	Effects	Reference
Anticonvulsants	Phenytoin	BTB; pregnancy	(1) (2)
	Phenobarbitone	BTB; pregnancy	(2) (3)
	Phenytoin/pehenobarbitone	BTB; pregnancy	(2) (3)
Antibiotics (anti-infectives)	Ampicillin	Pregnancy	(4) (12)
	Chloramphenicol	Pregnancy	(3)
	Troleandomycin	Jaundice	(5)
	Metronidazole	Ovulation	(6)
	Rifampicin	BTB; pregnancy	(10)
	Tetracycline	Pregnancy	(11)
Anti-inflammatory	Phenylbutazone	BTB	(7)
Analgesics	Amidopyrine	BTB; impaired clearance	(8) (9)
	Noramidopyrinemethyl-sulphonate	BTB; impaired clearance	(20)
	Phenacetin	BTB	(3)
Antacids	Kaolin	Reduced availability	(13)
	Aluminium hydroxide	Reduced availability	(13)
	Magnesium trisilicate	Reduced availability	(13) (21)
	Activated charcoal	Reduced availability	(13)
Tranquilisers/antidepressants	Chlordiazepoxide	Impaired clearance	(14)
	Meprobamate	BTB	(3)
	Imipramine	Reduced antidepressant effect: increased toxicity	(25)
Miscellaneous	Caffeine	Impaired clearance	(15)
	Polybrominated biphenyls	Enhanced steroid clearance	(16)
	Dihydroergotamine	Preganancy	(3)
Anticoagulants	Dicoumarol	Reduced effect	(22)
	Acenocoumarol	Enhanced effect	(19)
Anticancer agents	Vincristine	Enhanced cytotoxicity	(17)
		Augmented thrombocytosis	(18)
Vitamins	Ascorbic acid	Enhanced steroid absorption	(23)
	Cholecalciferol	Impaired clearance	(24)
	B-vitamins	Reduced absorption: altered carrier proteins	(26)

(1) Nenyon (1972) (2) Janz & Schmidt (1974) (3) Von Hempel et al (1973) (4) Dossetor (1975) (5) Miguet et al (1980) (6) Joshi et al (1980) (7) Böhm (1980) (8) Sonnenberg et al (1980) (9) Abernethy & Greenblatt (1981) (10) Reimers & Jezek (1971) (11) Bacon & Shenfield (1980) (12) Friedman et al (1980) (13) Fadel et al (1979) (14) Roberts et al (1979) (15) Patwardhan et al (1980) (16) McCormack et al (1979) (17) Rosner et al (1978) (18) Cantwell et al (1979) (19) de Teresa et al (1979) (20) Voigt et al (1977) (21) Khalil & Invagnu (1976) (22) Schrogie et al (1967) (23) Briggs (1981) (24) Carter et al (1975) (25) Prang et al (1972) (26) Tonkin (1981).

described above, or antibiotic induced changes in intestinal flora altering enterohepatic cycling of contraceptive steroids.

Changes in binding-sites on plasma carrier proteins have been inadequately investigated, but there is evidence that they may be important. Administration of EE, for example, greatly increases the binding-site concentration of plasma sex hormone-binding globulin (SHBG), which is a carrier protein not only for endogenous testosterone and estoestradiol, but also for many progestogens, including LNG, NET and 3-keto-DOG. These progestogens also antagonise the EE-induced increase in SHBG, so that available binding-sites are determined by a complex interaction of both EE and progestogen dose. For other drugs, there is evidence that anticonvulsants increase the binding of progestogens to SHBG, and so reduce the free plasma pool (Backstrom & Sodergard, 1977).

It is well known that many drugs — such as barbiturates, anticonvulsants, and rifampicin — are potent inducers of hepatic microsomal enzymes responsible for their own oxidative metabolism, but which also act on many other pharmaceutical agents. There is convincing evidence (Breckenridge et al, 1980) that the simultaneous administration of contraceptive oestrogen plus progestogen with another drug which induces microsomal oxidases leads to significantly lower plasma levels of both steroids. This is probably sufficient to explain the increased risk of BTB and pregnancy in OC users also receiving microsomal oxidase inducers.

The reverse effect — blocking of hepatic enzymes by steroids — appears to occur with amidopyrine, imipramine, and possibly also troleandomycin. These drugs are poor inducers, so that their simultaneous use with contraceptive steroids leads to competition for the same limited number of microsomal oxidases.

The clinical significance of drug interactions with contraceptive steroids is still being debated, but clearly any steroid user who is prescribed another drug requires extra surveillance. Pregnancies are relatively rare, and most are due to rifampicin. Women at particular risk of contraceptive failure from interactions are likely to be unreliable users, or those with intrinsically high rates of contraceptive steroid metabolic turnover. Presumably, users of low dose contraceptives will be at greater risk than those treated with larger doses. Toxic effects from the second drug may also depend largely on intrinsic metabolic differences and steroid doses, so that titration of the doses of both steroid and second drug may be required to reduce risks.

REFERENCES

Aakvaag A 1969 Formation of steroid hormones in the porcine ovary in vitro. Journal of Endocrinology 43: 25–26

Abdel-Aziz M T, Williams K I H 1969 Metabolism of 17x-ethynylestradiol and its 3-methyl ether by the rabbit: an in vivo D-homoannulation. Steroids 13: 809–820

Abernethy D R, Greenblatt D J 1981 Impairment of antipyrine metabolism by low-dose oral contraceptive steroids. Clinical Pharmacology and Therapeutics 29: 106–110

Abu-Fadil S, DeVane G, Siler T M, Yen S S C 1976 Effects of oral contraceptive steroids on pituitary prolactin secretion. Contraception 13: 79–85

Adams P W, Oakley N W 1972 Oral contraceptives and carbohydrate metabolism. Clinics in Endocrinology and Metabolism 1: 697–720

Adams P W, Wynn V, Folkard J, Seed M 1976 Influence of oral contraceptives, pyridoxine, and tryptophan on carbohydrate metabolism. Lancet 1: 759

Adlercreutz H, Eisalo A, Heino A, Luukainen T, Penttila I, Saukkonen T 1968 Investigations on the effect of an oral contraceptive and its compounds on liver function, serum proteins, copper, ceruloplasmin and gamma glutamyl peptidase in post menopausal women. Scandinavian Journal of Gastroenterology 18: 273

Ahren T, Lithell H, Victor A, Vessby B, Johnsson E D B 1981 Comparison of the metabolic effects of two hormonal contraceptive methods: an oral formulation and a vaginal ring II. Contraception 24: 451–468

Alberga A, Ferrez M, Baulieu E E 1976 Estradiol-receptor DNA interaction: liquid polymer phase partition. FEBS Letters 61: 223–226

Algeri, Bonati M, Curcio M, Jori A, Ladinsky H, Pouzio F, Garattini S 1977 Biochemical effects of steroid contraceptive drugs on some neurotransmitters in the central nervous system. In: Garattini S, Berendes H W (eds) Pharmacology of Steroid Contraceptive Drugs, pp 53–71. Raven Press, New York

Amatayakul K, Sivasomboon B, Thanangkul O 1978 Vitamin and trace mineral in medroxyprogesterone acetate users. Contraception 18: 253–269

Ambrus J L, Mink I B, Courney N G, Niswander K, Moore R H, Ambrus C M, Lillie M A 1976 Progestational agents and blood coagulation. American Journal of Obstetrics and Gynecology 125: 1957

Andervont H B, Shimkin M B, Canter H Y 1960 Susceptibility of 7 inbred strains and the F_1 hybrids to estrogen-induced testicular tumors in strain BALB/C mice. Journal of the National Cancer Institute 25: 1069–1081

Andrew F D, Christensen H D, Williams T L, Thompson M G, Wall M E 1973 Comparative teratogenicity of contraceptive steroids in mice and rats. Teratology 7: A11–A12

Appelgren L E 1969 Interference with progesterone synthesis of some antifertility compounds as shown by histochemistry. European Congress on Sterility 2, 6

Appelgren I E, Karlsson R 1971 The distribution of [14C]-4-mestranol in mice. Acta Pharmacologica et Toxicologica 29: 65–74

Arai K, Golab T, Layne D S, Pincus G 1962 Metabolic fate of orally administered [3H]-norethynodrel in rabbits. Endocrinology 71: 639–648

Areekul S, Pantampon P, Doungbarn J, Yamarat P, Vongyathithum M 1977 Serum vitamin B_{12}, serum and red cell folates, vitamin B_{12}, and folic acid-binding proteins in women taking oral contraceptives. Southeast Asian Journal of Tropical Medicine and Public Health 81: 480–485

Asku M F 1979 Histo-morphologic and histochemical evaluation of tubal epithelium in oral contraceptive users. Proceedings World Congress of Obstetrics and Gynecology, Tokyo, Abstract 337

Atger M, Baulieu E E, Milgrom E 1974 Investigation of progesterone receptors in guinea-pig vagina, uterine cervix, mammary glands, pituitary and hypothalamus. Endocrinology 94: 161

Back D J, Breckenridge A M, Crawford F E, MacIver M, Orme M L, Rowe P H, Smith E 1978 Kinetics of norethindrone in women. II. Single-dose kinetics. Clinical Pharmacology and Therapeutics 24: 448–453

Back D J, Breckenridge A M, Crawford F E, MacIver M, Orme M L, Rowe P H 1981 Interindividual variation and drug interactions with hormonal steroid contraceptives. Drugs 21: 46–61

Backstrom T, Sodergard R 1977 The influence of antiepileptic drugs on steroid plasma levels and binding during the menstrual cycle. Acta Endocrinologica 85 (Suppl 212): 42

Bacon J F, Shenfield G M 1980 Pregnancy attributable to interaction between tetracycline and oral contraceptives. British Medical Journal 280: 293

Bamji M S 1978 Implications of oral contraceptive use on vitamin nutritional status. Indian Journal of Medical Research 68: 80–87

Bamji M S, Ahmed F 1978 Effects of oral contraceptive steroids on vitamin A status of women and female rats. World Review of Nutrition and Dietetics 31: 135–140

Barbosa J, Seal U S, Doe R P 1973 Anti-estrogens and plasma proteins. II. Contraceptive drugs and gestagens. Journal of Clinical Endocrinology and Metabolism 36: 706–714

Basdevant A, deLignieres B, Mauvais-Jarvis P 1976 Lipid disorders and increased vascular risk due to contraceptive steroids. Nouvelle Presse Medicale 6: 1496–1472

Bashore R A, Smith F, Gold E M 1970 Placental transfer and metabolism of 4-14C-cortisol in the pregnant monkey. Nature 228: 774–775

Bates G W, Edman C D, Porter J C, MacDonald P C 1979 Catechol-O-methyl transferase activity in erythrocytes of women using oral contraceptive steroids. American Journal of Obstetrics and Gynecology 133: 691–593

Baulieu E E 1978 Mechanism of action of estrogens. Klinische Wochenschrift 56: 685–695

Baulieu E E, Godeau F, Schorderet M, Schorderet-Slatkine S 1978 Steroid-induced meiotic division in Xenopus laevis oocytes: surface and calcium. Nature 275: 593–598

Baxter J D, Funder J W 1979 Hormone receptors. New England Journal of Medicine 301: 1149–1161

Beck K J, Leyendecker G, Nocke W 1972 Comparison of estradiol-17β and progesterone concentrations in cervical mucus and serum. European Congress on Sterility, Abstracts, 3: 104

Beck P 1973 Contraceptive steroids: modifications of carbohydrate and lipid metabolism. Metabolism 22: 841–855

Beck P J 1975 Alterations of lipid metabolism by contraceptive steroids. Journal of Steroid Biochemistry 6: 957–959

Beck P J, Eaton R P, Arnett D M, Alsever R N 1976 Effects of contraceptive steroids on arginine-stimulated glucagon and insulin secretion in women. Metabolism 25: 23

Beckerhoff R, Vetter W, Armbruster H, Luetscher J A, Siegenthaler W 1973 Plasma aldosterone during oral contraceptive therapy. Lancet 1: 1218

Bergink E W, Holma P, Pyörälä T 1981 Effects of oral contraceptive combinations containing levonorgestrel on serum proteins and androgen binding. Scandinavian Journal of Clinical and Laboratory Investigations 41: 663–568

Berliner V R 1974 Food and Drug Administration requirements for toxicity testing of contraceptive products. In: Briggs M H,

Diczfalusy E (eds) Pharmacological Models in Contraceptive Development, pp 240–265. W H O, Geneva

Bernasconi S, Garattini S, Samanin R 1976 Effect of steroid contraceptives on the concentrations of brain monoamines in rats and mice. Archives Internationale Pharmacodynamics 222: 272–281

Bibbo M, Gill W B, Azizi F, Blough R, Fang V S, Rosenfield R L et al 1977 Follow-up study of male and female offspring of DES-exposed mothers. Journal of Obstetrics and Gynecology 49: 1–8

Boettcher B 1974 Molecular nature of sperm agglutinins and sperm antibodies in human sera. Journal of Reproduction and Fertility Supplement 21: 151

Böhm S 1980 Medicamentous enzyme induction and hormonal contraception: effects of phenobarbital and phenybutazone on hormonal contraception. Zentralblatt für Gynäkologie 102: 966–973

Bohnet H G, Mühlenstedt D, Hanker J P F, Schneider H P G 1977 Prolactin oversuppression. Archiv Gynäkologie 223: 173–178

Bolt H M 1979 Metabolism of estrogens — natural and synthetic. Journal of Pharmacology and Therapeutics 4: 155–181

Bolt H M, Bolt W H 1974 Pharmacokinetics of mestranol in man in relation to its oestrogenic activity. European Journal of Clinical Pharmacology 7: 295–305

Bolt H M, Bolt M, Kappus H 1977 Interaction of rifampicin treatment with pharmacokinetics and metabolism of ethynyloestradiol in man. Acta Endocrinologica 85: 189–197

Bolt H M, Remmer H 1972 The accumulation of mestranol and ethynyloestradiol metabolites in the organism. Xenobiotica 2: 489–498

Bonser G M, Robson J M 1940 The effects of prolonged oestrogen administration upon male mice of various strains: development of testicular tumours in the Strong A strain. Journal of Pathology and Bacteriology 51: 9–22

Bradley D D, Wingerd J, Petitti D B, Krauss R M, Ramcharan S 1978 Serum high-density lipoprotein cholesterol in women using oral contraceptives. New England Journal of Medicine 299: 17–20

Bradwell A R, Brunett D, Ramsden D B, Burr W A, Prince H P, Hoffenberg R 1976 Preparation of a monospecific antiserum to thyroxine-binding globulin for its quantitation by rocket immunoelectrophorisis. Clinica Chemica Acta 71: 501–510

Braselton W E, Lin T J, Mills T M, Ellegood J O, Mahesh V B 1977 Identification and measurement by gas chromatography-mass spectrometry of norethindrone and metabolites in human urine and blood. Journal of Steroid Biochemistry 8: 9–18

Braselton W E, Lin T J, Ellegood J O, Mills T M, Mahesh V B 1979 Accumulation of norethindrone and individual metabolites in human plasma during short and long term administration of a contraceptive dosage. American Journal of Obstetrics and Gynecology 133: 154–160

Breckenridge A 1977 Drug interactions with oral contraceptives: an overview. In: Garattini S, Berendes H W (eds) Pharmacology of Steroid Contraceptive Drugs, pp 307–311. Raven Press, New York

Breckenridge A M, Back D J, Orme M 1979 Interactions between oral contraceptives and other drugs. Journal of Pharmacology and Therapeutics 7: 617–626

Breckenridge A M, Back D J, Crawford F E, MacIver M, Orme M, Rowe P H 1980 Drug interactions with oral contraceptives: clinical and experimental studies. In: Newton J R, Jacobs H S, Caldwell A D S (eds) Workshop on Fertility Control: Royal Society of Medicine International Congress and Symposium, Series 31, pp 1–11. Academic Press, London

Bregulla K, Frölich M 1977 Results of in vitro sperm penetration tests in cervical mucus during the use of sequential oral contraceptives. Archives fur Gynäkologie 233: 187–193

Bregulla K, Hausser H 1975 In vitro sperm penetration of cervical mucus during the normal cycle and under the influence of combined or sequential oral contraceptives. Archives fur Gynäkologie 218: 227

Brenner R M 1973 Hormonal regulation of oviductal epithelium. In: Segal S J et al (eds) Regulation of Mammalian Reproduction, C C Thomas, Springfield, pp 337–351

Breuer H 1977 Metabolic pathways of steroid contraceptives drugs. In: Garattini S, Berendes H W (eds), pp 73–88. Raven Press, New York

Briggs M H 1973a Blood platelet biochemistry in women receiving steroid contraceptives. Haematologia 7: 347–367

Briggs M H 1973b Lysosomal enzyme activation by steroid hormones in vivo. Journal of Steroid Biochemistry 4: 341–347

Briggs M H 1973c Steroid hormones and the fertilizing capacity of spermatozoa. Steroids 22: 547

Briggs M H 1975a Effects of oral progestogens on estrogen-induced changes in plasma proteins. Journal of Reproductive Medicine 15: 100–103

Briggs M H 1975b Contraceptive steroid binding to the human uterine progesterone-receptor. Current Medical Research and Opinion 3: 95–98

Briggs M H 1975c Biochemical effects of oral contraceptives. Advances in Steroid Biochemistry and Pharmacology 5: 65–160

Briggs M H 1975d Hormonal contraceptives and plasma sex hormone binding globulin. Contraception 12: 149–153

Briggs M H 1975e Effects of oral progestogens on estrogen induced changes in plasma proteins. Journal of Reproductive Medicine 15: 100

Briggs M H 1975f Minimizing the metabolic effects of oral contraceptives. Bulletin of the Post-Graduate Committee in Medicine (University of Sydney) 31: 175–181

Briggs M H 1977 Combined oral contraceptives. In: Diczfalusy E (ed) Regulation of Human Fertility, pp 253–282. Scriptor, Copenhagen

Briggs M H 1978a Steroid contraception: metabolic and endocrine effects. In: Sciarra J J et al (eds) Risks, Benefits and Controversies in Fertility Control, pp 214–229. Harper and Row, New York

Briggs M H 1978b Effects of oral contraceptives on amino acid, protein and vitamin metabolism. Proceedings of the 6th Asia and Oceania Congress of Endocrinology 1: 114–118

Briggs M H 1979 Biochemical basis for the selection of oral contraceptives. International Journal of Gynaecology and Obstetrics 16: 509–516

Briggs M H 1980 Endocrine effects of oral contraceptives. Proceedings of the 28th International Congress of Physiological Sciences, Hungarian Academic and Scientific Publishing House, Budapest

Briggs M H 1981 Megadose vitamin C and metabolic effects of the pill. British Medical Journal 283: 1547

Briggs M H 1982 Comparative investigation of oral contraceptives using randomized, prospective protocol. In: Haspels A (ed) Benefits and Risks of Hormonal Contraception, pp 115–130. M T P Press, Lancaster

Briggs M H, Briggs M 1971 Effects of oral ethinylestradiol on serum proteins. Contraception 3: 381

Briggs M H, Briggs M 1972a Plasma hormone concentrations in women receiving steroid contraceptives. Journal of Obstetrics and Gynaecology of the British Commonwealth 79: 946–950

Briggs M H, Briggs M 1972b Relationship between plasma monoamine oxidase activity and sex hormone concentration. Journal of Reproduction and Fertility 29: 447–449

Briggs M H, Briggs M 1973a Hormonal influences on erythrocyte catechol-O-methyl transferase activity in humans. Experientia 29: 278–279

Briggs M H, Briggs M 1973b Effects of some contraceptive steroids on serum proteins of women. Biochemical Pharmacology 22: 2277–2281

Briggs M H, Briggs M 1975 Biochemical Contraception. Academic Press, New York

Briggs M H, Briggs M 1977 Oral Contraceptives — 1, pp 67–68 Eden Press, Montreal

Briggs M H Briggs M 1979a Oral Contraceptives — 3, pp 231–249. Eden Press, Montreal

Briggs M H, Briggs M 1979b Plasma lipoprotein changes during oral contraception. Current Medical Research and Opinion 6: 249–253

Briggs M H, Briggs M 1979c Oral contraceptives and plasma protein metabolism. Journal of Steroid Biochemistry 11: 425–428

Briggs M H, Briggs M 1981 Relative activity of commonly used oral progestogens in the delay of menstruation test in normal women. Gine Dips 10: 538–542

Briggs M H, Briggs M 1982 Randomized prospective studies on metabolic effects of oral contraceptives. Acta Obstetrica Gynecologica Scandinavica, Suppl 105: 25–32

Briggs M H, Briggs M, Austin J 1971 Effects of steroid pharmaceuticals on plasma zinc. Nature 232: 480

Briggs M H, Brotherton J 1970 Steroid Biochemistry and Pharmacology, p 424. Academic Press, New York

Briggs M H, Pitchford A G, Staniford M, Barker H M, Taylor D 1970 Metabolic effects of steroid contraceptives. Advances in Steroid Biochemistry and Pharmacology 2: 111–222

Brody S, Kerstall J, Nilsson L, Suanborg A 1968 The effect of some ovulation inhibitors on the different plasma lipid fractions. Acta Medica Scandinavica 183: 1–7

Brosens I, Van Assche A, Koninckx P, Heyns W, De Hertogh R 1976 New combined oral contraceptive with incremental progestogen dosage regimen. European Journal of Obstetrics and Gynaecology and Reproductive Biology 6: 315–318

Brotherton J 1976 Sex Hormone Pharmacology, pp 198–222. Academic Press, London

Bulbrook R D, Herian M, Tong D, Hayward J L, Swain M C, Wang D Y 1973 Effects of steroidal contraceptives on levels of plasma androgen sulphates and cortisol. Lancet 1: 628–630

Buller R E, O'Malley B W 1976 Biology and mechanism of steroid hormone receptor interaction with the eukaryotic nucleus. Biochemical Pharmacology 25: 1–12

Bullock L P, Bardin C W 1977 Androgenic, synadrogenic, and antiandrogenic actions of progestins. Annals of the New York Academy of Sciences 286: 321–330

Cain M D, Walters W A, Catt K J 1971 Effects of oral contraceptive therapy on the renin-angiotensin system. Journal of Clinical Endocrinology and Metabolism 33: 671–676

Cantwell B M, Begent R H, Rubens R D 1979 Augmentation of vincristine-induced thrombocytosis by norethisterone. European Journal of Cancer 15: 1065–1069

Cargill D J, Steinetz B G, Gosnell E, Beach V L, Meli A, Fujimoto G J, Raynolds B M 1969 Fate of ingested radiolabelled ethynylestradiol and its 3-cyclopentyl ether in patients with bile fistulas. Journal of Clinical Endocrinology and Metabolism 29: 1051–1061

Carol W, Borner A, Lauterbach H, Klinger G, Bohm W, Greinke C 1980 Effects of intranasally administered low dose progesterone on the pituitary and gonadal functions. Endokrinologie 75: 159–166

Carr B R, Parker C R, Madden J D, MacDonald P C, Porter J C 1979 Plasma levels of adreno corticotropin and cortisol in women receiving oral contraceptive steroid treatment. Journal of Clinical Endocrinology and Metabolism 49: 346–349

Carter D E, Goldman J M, Bressler R, Huxtable R J, Christian C D, Heine M W 1974 Effect of oral contraceptives on drug metabolism. Journal of Clinical Pharmacology and Therapeutics 15: 22

Castegnaro E, Sala G 1962 Isolation and identification of 6β, 17α 21-trihydroxy-6α-methyl- $\triangle^4$pregnene-3, 20-dione (21-acetate) from the urine of human subjects treated with MGA. Journal of Endocrinology 24: 445–452

Castrodale D, Bierbaum O, Helwig E B, MacBryde C M 1941 Comparative studies of the effects of estradiol and stilbestrol upon the blood, liver and bone marrow. Endocrinology 29: 363–373

Chamness G C, Jennings A W, McGuire W L 1974 Estrogen receptor binding to isolated nuclei: a nonsaturable process. Biochemistry 13: 327–331

Chan L, O'Malley B W 1978 Steroid hormone action: recent advances. Annals of Internal Medicine 89: 694–701

Chayen J. Bitensky L, Butcher R G, Altman F P 1974 Cellular biochemical assessment of steroid activity. Advances in Steroid Biochemistry and Pharmacology 4: 1–60

Cheng Y-G, Karavolas H J 1975 Subcellular distribution and properties of progesterone ($\triangle^4$-steroid) 5α-reductase in rat medial basal hypothalamus. Journal of Biological Chemistry 250: 7997–8003

Cohen B L, Katz M 1981 Further studies on pituitary and ovarian function in women receiving hormonal contraception. Centraception 24: 159–175

Cohen M R 1968 Cervical mucorrhea and spinnbarkeit in patients taking norethindrone plus mestranol. Fertility and Sterility 19: 405

Cole F E, Weed J C, Schneider G T, Holland J B, Geary W L, Rice B F 1973 The gonadotropin receptor of the human corpus luteum. American Journal of Obstetrics and Gynecology 117: 87–95

Committee on Safety of Medicines 1972 Carcinogenicity Tests of Oral Contraceptives, p 23. Her Majesty's Stationery Office, London

Connell E B, Senia A, Stone M L 1967 Endometrial enzymes histochemistry in oral contraceptive therapy. Fertility and Sterility 18: 35–45

Connell E B 1972 Endometrial histochemistry. In: Balin H, Glasser S (eds) Reproductive Biology, Excerpta Medica, Amsterdam, pp 727–747

Cooper J M, Elce J S, Kellie A E 1967 Metabolism of melengestrol acetate. Journal of Biochemistry 104: 57

Cooper J M, Kellie A E 1968 Metabolism of megestrol acetate in women. Steroids 11: 133–149

Costanzi J J, Young B K, Carmel R 1978 Serum vitamin B_{12} and B_{12}-binding protein levels associated with oral contraceptives. Texas Reports on Biology and Medicine 36: 69–77

Courrier R 1945 Endocrinologie de la Gestation, Masson, Paris

Coutinho E M 1973 Hormonal control of tubal musculature. In: Segal S J et al (eds) Regulation of Mammalian Reproduction, pp 385–399. C C Thomas, Springfield

Craft I L, Peters I J 1971 Quantitative changes in plasma amino acids induced by oral contraceptives. Clinical Science 41: 301–307

Craig G M 1976 Prostaglandins, possible mediators of the effects of oestrogens on luteinizing hormone output. Medical Hypothesis 2: 116

Crowell E B, Clatenoff D V, Kiekhofer W 1971 Factor VIII changes with oral contraceptives. Journal of Laboratory and Clinical Medicine 77: 551

Davies I J, Naftolin F, Ryan K J, Siu J 1975 Specific, high-affinity, limited-capacity estrogen binding component in the cytosol of human fetal pituitary and brain tissues. Journal of Clinical Endocrinology and Metabolism 40: 909–912

Dayan J, Crajer M C, Bertozzi S, Lefrancois S 1980 Application of the salmonella typhimurium microsome test to the study of 25 drugs belonging to 5 chemical series. Mutation Research 77: 301–306

De Pirro R, Forte F, Bertoli A 1981 Changes in insulin receptors during oral contraception. Journal of Clinical Endocrinology and Metabolism 52: 29–35

De Teresa E, Vera A, Ortigosa J, Alonso Pulpon L, Peunte Arus A, De Artaza M 1979 Interaction between anticoagulants and contraceptives: an unsuspected finding. British Medical Journal 2: 1260–1261

Diczfalusy E 1968 Mode of action of contraceptive drugs. American Journal of Obstetrics and Gynecology 100: 136–163

Diddle A W. Watts G F, Gardner W H, Williamson P J 1967 Oral contraceptive medication: a prolonged experience. American Journal of Obstetrics and Gynecology 95: 489–495

DiSorbo D, Rosen F, McPartland R P, Milholland R J 1977 Glucocorticoid activity of various progesterone analogs: correlation between specific binding in thymus and liver and biologic activity. Annals of the New York Academy of Sciences 286: 355–368

Doar J W H, Wynn V, Cramp D G 1969 Studies on venous blood pyruvate and lactate levels during oral and intravenous glucose tolerance tests in women receiving oral contraceptives. In: Shalhanick H A et al (eds) Metabolic Effects of Gonadal Hormones and Contraceptive Steroids, pp 178–192. Plenum Press, New York

Dorfman R 1971 In: Kewitz H (ed) Nebenwirkungen Contraceptiver Steroide, p. 139. Westkreuz-Verlag, Berlin

Dossetor J 1975 Drug interactions with oral contraceptives. British Medical Journal 4: 467–468

Dow C 1959 Experimental reproduction of the cystic hyperplasia-pyometra complex in the bitch. Journal of Pathology and Bacteriology 78: 267–278

Dow C 1960 Oestrogen induced atrophy of the skin in dogs. Journal of Pathology and Bacteriology 80: 434–435

Dugwekar Y G, Narula R K, Laumas K R 1973 Distribution of a 1-^{3}H-Chlormadinone acetate in the reproductive tract of women. Contraception 7: 313

Dunn F G, Jones J V, Fife R 1975 Malignant hypertension associated with use of oral contraceptives. British Heart Journal 37: 336

Editorial 1980 Drug interaction with oral contraceptive steroids. British Medical Journal 2: 93–94

Elder M G, Myatt L, Chaudhuri G 1978 Effect of norgestrel and clogestone on the spontaneous motility of the human fallopian tube. International Journal of Fertility 23: 61–64

El Etreby M F, Gräf K J 1979 Effect of contraceptive steroids on mammary gland of the beagle dog and its relevance to human carcinogenicity. Pharmacology and Therapeutics 5: 369–402

El Etreby M F, Gräf K J, Beir S, Elger W, Günzel P, Neumann F

1979 Suitability of the beagle dog as a test model for the tumorogenic potential of contraceptive steroids. Contraception 20: 237–256

El-Magoub S 1981 The norgestrel-T IUD. Abstract in III World Congress of Human Reproduction, Berlin

Elstein M, Moghissi K S, Borth R 1973 Cervical Mucus in Human Reproduction, p. 163. Scriptor, Copenhagen

Fadel H, Abd Elbary A, Nour El-Din E, Kassem A A 1980 Availability of norethisterone acetate from combined oral contraceptive tablets. Pharmazie 34: 49–50

Fern M, Rose D P, Fern E B 1978 Effect of oral contraceptives on plasma androgenic steroids and their precursors. Obstetrics and Gynecology 51: 541–544

Fink G 1979 Feedback actions of target hormones on hypothalamus and pituitary with special reference to gonadal steroids. Annual Review of Physiology 41: 571–585

Finkel M J, Berliner V R 1973 The extrapolation of experimental findings (animal to man): The dilemma of the systemically administered contraceptives. Bulletin of the Society for Pharmacological and Environmental Pathology 4: 13–18

Fisch I R, Frank J 1977 Oral contraceptives and blood pressure. Journal of the American Medical Association 237: 2499–2503

Fotherby K 1973 Pharmacokinetics of contraceptive steroids in humans. Proceedings of the 5th International Congress on Pharmacology 1: 230–239

Fotherby K 1974a Metabolism of contraceptive steroids. In: Briggs M H, Diczfalusy E (eds) Pharmacological Models in Contraceptive Development. W H O, Geneva

Fotherby K 1974b Metabolism of synthetic steroids by animals and man. In: Briggs M H, Diczfalusy E (eds) Pharmacological Models in Contraceptive Development: Animal Toxicity and Side Effects, pp 119–147. W H O, Geneva

Fotherby K 1977 Low doses of gestagens as fertility regulating agents. In: Diczfalusy E (ed) Regulation of Human Fertility, pp 283–322. Scriptor, Copenhagen

Fotherby K, Abdel-Rahman N A, De Souza J C, Coutinho E M, Koetsawang S, Nukulkarn P et al 1979 Rate of metabolism of norethisterone in women from different populations. Contraception 19: 39–45

Fotherby K, James F 1972 Metabolism of synethetic steroids. Advances in Steroid Biochemistry and Pharmacology 3: 67–165

Fotherby K. Kamjab S, Littleton P, Klopper A 1966 Metabolism of 17α-ethynyl steroids. Journal of Biochemistry 99: 14p

Fotherby K Warren R J 1976 Bioavailability of contraceptive steroids from capsules. Contraception 14: 261

Fowler R E, Chan S T H, Walters D E, Edwards R G, Steptoe P C 1977 Steroidogenesis in human follicles approaching ovulation as judged from assays of follicular fluid. Journal of Endocrinology, 72: 259–271

Fregly M J, Fregly M S (eds) 1974 Oral Contraceptives and High Blood Pressure. Dolphin Press, Gainesville

Friedman C I, Huneke A L, Moon H K, Powell J 1980 The effect of ampicillin on oral contraceptive effectiveness. Journal of Obstetrics and Gynecology 55: 33–37

Funckes C G, Chvapil M, Carrol R W, Bressler R 1976 Effect of a long-acting contraceptive drug, norethindrone enanthate, on serum zinc and copper in human volunteers. Contraception 14: 291–295

Gallagher T F, Mueller M N, Kappas A 1966 Estrogen pharmacology IV. Studies on the structural basis for estrogen-induced impairment of liver function. Medicine, Baltimore 45: 471–479

Gambhir K K, Turner V, Archer J A, Carter L, Robinson T J, Hollis V 1978 Chronic oral contraceptive therapy in man: decrease of insulin binding. Journal of Steroid Biochemistry 9: 859

Geil R G, Lamar J K 1977 F D A studies of estrogen, progestogens and estrogen/progestogen combinations in the dog and monkey. Journal of Toxicology and Environmental Health 3: 179–193

Geschikter C F, Byrnes E W 1942 Factors influencing the development and time of appearance of mammary cancer in the rat in response to estrogen. Archives of Pathology 33: 334–356

Geschickter C F, Hartman C G 1959 Mammary response to prolonged estrogenic stimulation in the monkey. Cancer 12: 767–781

Ghezzo F, Mele A, Pegoraro L 1980 Effects of oestro-progestogenic oral contraceptives on blood coagulation, fibrinolysis, and platelet aggregation. Haematologica 65: 738–745

Ghoneim S M, Toppozada H K, El-Heneidy A R, Taha M M 1975 Effect of an oral contraceptive on acid-base balance, blood gases and electrolytes. Contraception 12: 395–405

Gibian H, Kopp R, Kramer M, Neumann F, Richter H 1968 Effect of particle size on biological activity of norethisterone acetate. Acta Physiologica Latinoamericano 18: 323

Gibson J P, Newberne J W, Kuhn W L, Elsea J R 1967 Comparative chronic toxicity of three oral estrogens in rats. Toxicology and Applied Pharmacology 11: 489–510

Glueck C J, Scheel D, Fishback J, Steiner P 1971 Progestogens, anabolic-androgenic compounds, estrogens: effects on triglycerides and post-heparin lipolytic enzymes. Lipids 7: 110

Goebelsmann U, Stanczyk F Z, Brenner P, Goebelsmann A, Gentzchein E, Mishell D R 1979 Serum norethindrone (NET) concentrations following intramuscular NET enanthate injection. Effect upon serum LH, FSH estradiol and progesterone. Contraception 19: 283–313

Goldzieher J W, Chenault C B, de la Pena A, Dozier T S, Kraemer D C 1978a Comparative studies of the ethynyl estrogens used in oral contraceptives: effects with and without progestational agents on plasma androstenedione, testosterone, and the testosterone binding in humans, baboons and and beagles. Fertility and Sterility 29: 388–396

Goldzieher J W, Chenault C B, de la Pena A, Dozier T S, Kraemer D C 1978b Comparative effects of the ethynyl estrogens used in oral contraceptives. VI Effects with and without progestational agents on carbohydrate metabolism in humans, baboons, and beagles. Fertility and Sterility 30: 146–153

Goldzieher J W, de la Pena A, Chenault C B, Woutersz T B 1975 Comparative studies of ethynyl estrogens used in oral contraceptives. II. Antiovulatory potency. American Journal of Obstetrics & Gynecology 122: 619–624

Goldzieher J W, Dozier T S, de la Pena A, Ojo O A, Lean T S, Chinnatamby S, Basnayake S, Koetsawang S 1980a Plasma levels and pharmacokinetics of ethinyl estrogens in various populations. Contraception 21: 1–16

Goldzieher J W, Dozier T S, de la Pena A, Ojo O A, Lean T S, Chinnatamby S, Basnayake S, Koetsawang S 1980b Plasma levels and pharmacokinetics of ethinyl estrogens in various populations. Contraception 21: 17–27

Gordon D B, Sachin I N 1977 Chromatographic separation of multiple renin substrates in women: effect of pregnancy and oral contraceptives. Proceedings of the Society for Experimental Biology and Medicine 156: 461–464

Gordon D B, Sachin I N, Dodd V N 1976 Heterogeneity of renin substrate in human plasma: effect of pregnancy and oral contraceptives. Proceedings of the Society for Experimental Biology and Medicine 153: 314–318

Gordon R, Castelli W P, Hjortland M C, Kannel W B, Dawber T R 1977 High density lipoprotein as a protective factor against coronary heart disease. American Journal of Medicine 62: 707–711

Gorski J, Gannon F 1976 Current models of steroid hormone action: a critique. Annual Review of Physiology 38: 425–450

Goulding A, McChesney R 1977 Oestrogen-progestogen oral contraceptives and urinary calcium excretion. Clinical Endocrinology 6: 449–454

Green R R, Burrill M W, Ivy A C 1939 Experimental intersexuality: effect of antenatal androgens on sexual development of female rats. American Journal of Anatomy 65: 415–421

Greenblatt R B, Jungck E C, Barfield W E 1958 A new test of efficacy of progestational compounds. Annals of the New York Academy of Sciences 71: 717

Griffiths J, Linklater H 1972 Radioisotope method for catechol-O-methyltransferase in blood. Clinica Chimia Acta 39: 383–386

Gwatkin R B L, Williams D T 1970 Inhibition of sperm capacitation in vitro by contraceptive steroids. Nature 227: 182

Hafs H D, Haynes N B 1977 Prostaglandins and pituitary hormone secretion. In: Silver D K (ed) Prostaglandins and Therapeutics, Upjohn, Kalamazoo, 3: 3–4

Hagenfeldt L. Hagenfeldt R, Wahren J 1977 Influence of contraceptive steroids on the turnover of plasma free arachidonic and oleic acids. Hormone and Metabolic Research 9: 66–69

Hähn N, Paschen K, Haller J 1972 Variations in copper, iron, magnesium, calcium, and zinc in women with normal menstrual cycles, under treatment with ovulation inhibitors, and during pregnancy. Archives Gynäkologie 213: 176–186

Haller J 1970 Direct effect of medroxyprogesterone acetate on the intrasplenic ovarian graft in guinea pigs. Hormonal Steroids 3: 215. New York: Excerpta Medica

Halstead J A, Hackley B H, Smith J C 1968 Plasma zinc and copper in pregnancy and after oral contraceptives. Lancet 2: 278

Hanasono G K, Fischer L J 1974 The excretion of tritium-labelled chlormadinone acetate, mestranol, norethindrone and norechynodrel in rats and the enterohepatic circulation of metabolites. Drug Metabolism and Disposition 2: 159–168

Harkness R A, Charles D 1965 Studies on the biological activity and metabolism of the cyclopentyl-3-enol ether of progesterone. American Journal of Obstetrics and Gynecology 93: 1005

Harper M K J, Pauerstein C J, Adams C E, Coutinho E M, Croxatto H B, Paton D M 1976 Ovum Transport and Fertility Regulation, p. 568. Scriptor, Copenhagen

Harrison R F, Walker E, Youssefnejadian E, Craft I 1975 Comparison of serial $PGF_{2\alpha}$ concentrations in serum of normal women and in those receiving oral contraceptives. Prostaglandins 10: 729–732

Haussman L, Goebel K M, Klahn D, Kaffarnik H 1975 Insulin and proinsulin: secretion under the influence of contraceptive steroids. Klinische Wochenschrift 53: 853

Hecht-Lucari G 1964 Central and peripheral action of fertility-inhibiting progestogens. International Journal of Fertility 9: 205–216

Helmreich M L, Huseby R A 1962 Disposition of radioactive 17α-hydroxyprogesterone, 6α-methyl-17α-acetoxyprogesterone and 6α-methyl prednisolone in human subjects. Journal of Clinical Endocrinology 22: 1018

Hendricks A G, Benirschke K, Thompson R S, Ahern J, Lucas W E, Oi R 1978 The effects of prenatal diethylstilbestrol (DES) exposure on the genitalia of pubertal Macaca mulatta. Teratology 17: 23A

Hery M, Laplante E, Kordon C 1976 Participation of serotonin in the phasic release of LH. I. Evidence from pharmacological experiments. Endocrinology 99: 496–503

Heywood R 1980 The experimental toxicity of systemic fertility regulating agents in laboratory animals. In: Serio M, Martini L (eds) Animal Models in Human Reproduction, pp 433–442. Raven Press, New York

Heywood R, Wadsworth P F 1981 The experimental toxicology of estrogens. In: Chaudbury R R (ed) Pharmacology of Estrogens, pp 63–80. Pergamon Press, Oxford

Hill R 1972 Pre-clinical toxicity of steroid hormones: recent experiences with estrogens and progestogens in the dog. In: Briggs M H, Christie G A (eds) Advances in Steroid Biochemistry and Pharmacology, Vol 3, pp 29–38. Academic Press, New York

Hisaw F L, Hisaw F L 1961 Action of estrogen and progesterone on the reproductive tract of lower primates. In: Young W C (ed) Sex and Internal Secretions, 3rd edn, Vol 1, pp 556–589. Bailliere Tindal, London

Hisaw F L, Hisaw F L 1966 Edema of the skin and menstruation in monkeys (Macaca mulatta) on repeated estrogen treatments. Proceedings of the Society for Experimental Biology and Medicine 122: 66–70

Honma S, Iwamura S, Iizuka K, Kambegawa A, Shida K 1977 Identification and antiandrogenic activity of the metabolites of 17α-acetoxy-6-chloropregna-4, 6-diene-3, 20-dione (chlormadinone acetate) in the rat, rabbit, dog and man. Chemical and Pharmacological Bulletin 25: 2019–2031

Hooker C W, Gardner W U, Pfeiffer C A 1940 Testicular tumors in mice receiving estrogens. Journal of the American Medical Association 115: 443–445

Horrobin D F 1979 Prolactin: role in health and disease. Current Therapeutics, April, 97–108

Howard G, Blair M, Fotherby K, Trayner I, Hamawi A, Elder M G 1982 Some metabolic effects of long term use of the injectable contraceptive norethisterone oenanthate. Lancet 1: 423–425

Humpel M, Wendt H, Dogs G, Weiss C H R, Rietz S, Speck U 1977 Intraindividual comparison of pharmacokinetic parameters of d-norgestrel, lynestrerol and cyproterone acetate in six women. Contraception 16: 199–215

Hyne R V, Boettcher B 1978 Binding of steroids to human spermatozoa and its possible role in contraception. Fertility and Sterility 30: 322–328

Illingworth D V, Wood G P, Flinckinger G L, Mikhail G 1975 Progesterone receptor of the human myometrium. Journal of Clinical Endocrinology and Metabolism 40: 1001–1008

International Agency for Research in Cancer 1974 Monographs on the Evaluation of Carcinogenic Risk of Chemicals to Man, Vol 6, p 243. Lyon

International Agency for Research in Cancer 1980 Monographs on the Evaluation of Carcinogenic Risk of Chemicals to Man, Vol 2, p 583. Lyon

Ishihara M, Kirdani R Y, Osawa Y, Sandberg A A 1976 The metabolic fate of medroxyprogesterone acetate in the baboon. Journal of Steroid Biochemistry 7: 65–70

Jabara A G 1962a Induction of canine ovarian tumours by diethylstilboestrol and progesterone. Australian Journal of Experimental Biology 40: 139–152

Jabara A G 1962b Some tissue changes in the dog following stilboestrol administration. Australian Journal of Experimental Biology 40: 293–308

Jackson M H 1961 Observations on the use of certain orally active progestogens for the control of fertility in women. Proceedings of the Royal Society of Medicine 54: 984

Jacobi J M, Powell L W, Gaffney T J 1969 Immunological quantitation of human transferin in pregnancy and during the administration of oral contraceptives. British Journal of Haematology 17: 503–509

Jänne O, Hemminki S, Isomaa V, Kokko E, Torkkeli H, Torkkeli T, Vierikko P 1978A Progestational activity of natural and synthetic androgens. International Journal of Andrology, Supplement 2, 162–174

Jänne O, Kontula K, Luukkainen T, Vihkor J 1975 Oestrogen-induced progesterone receptor in human uterus. Journal of Steroid Biochemistry 6: 501

Janz D, Schmidt D 1974 Anti-epileptic drugs and failure of oral contraceptives. Lancet i: 1113

Johansson E D B 1972 Plasma levels of progesterone achieved by different routes of administration. Acta Obstetricia et Gynecologicia Scandinavia Supplement 19: 17

Johansson E D B 1976 Effects of exogenous steroids on gonadotrophin secretion. Clinics in Obstetrics and Gynaecology 3: 579–590

Jost A 1950 Malformation of the extremities of rat fetus by pituitary extracts. Gynecologie et Obstetrique (Paris) 49: 44

Justo G, Motta M, Martini L 1975 In vivo effects of acetylcholine on LH secretion. Experientia 31: 598–600

Kalkhoff R K 1972 Review of oral contraceptive agents and sex steroids on carbohydrate metabolism. Annual Review of Medicine 23: 429–438

Kalkhoff R K 1975 Effects of oral contraceptive agents on carbohydrate metabolism. Journal of Steroid Biochemistry 6: 949–956

Kamyab S, Baghdiantz A, Hadj Mohammadi M R 1978 Serum level and 24-hour urinary excretion pattern of potassium following intake of combined oral contraceptives. Acta Medica Iran 21: 87–94

Kaplay S S, Ramanadham M 1978 Erythrocyte membrane adenosine-triphosphatases in women using oral contraceptives. Contraception 18: 287–293

Kappus H, Bolt H M, Remmer H 1973 Affinity of ethynylestradiol and mestranol for the uterine estrogen receptor and for the microsomal mixed function oxidase of the liver. Journal of Steroid Biochemistry 4: 121

Kappus H, Remmer H 1975 Metabolic activation and disposition: the biological fate of chemicals. Drug Metabolism and Disposition 3: 338

Kasid A, Buckshee K, Hingorani V, Laumas K R 1978 Interaction of progestins with steroid receptors in human uterus. Biochemical Journal 176: 531–539

Katz F H, Romfh P, Smith J A, Roper E F, Barnes J S 1975 Combination contraceptive effects on monthly cycle of plasma aldosterone, renin activity and renin substrate. Acta Endocrinologica 79: 295–300

Kekki M, Nikkila E A 1971 Plasma triglyceride turnover during use of oral contraceptives. Metabolism 20: 878

Kenyon I E 1972 Unplanned pregnancy in an epileptic. British Medical Journal 1: 686–687

Kesserü E 1971 Influence of various hormonal contraceptives on sperm migration in vivo. Fertility and Sterility 22: 9

Khalil S A H, Iwuagwu M 1976 The in-vitro uptake of some oral contraceptive steroids by magnesium trisilicate. Journal of Pharmacy and Pharmacology 28: 47P

Khomasuridze A G, Volcheck A G, Spastnykh E I 1976 Effect of synthetic progestins on the glucocorticoid and androgenic function of the adrenal cortex. Akush Ginekologie 9: 7–10

King R J B, Mainwaring W I P 1974 Steroid Cell Interactions, p 440. Butterworths, London

Kissebah A H, Harrigan P, Wynn V 1973 Mechanism of hypertriglyceridaemia associated with contraceptive steroids. Hormone and Metabolic Research 5: 184

Kjeld J M, Puah C M Joplin G F 1976 Changed levels of endogenous sex steroids in women on oral contraceptives. British Medical Journal 2: 1354–1356

Klumpp F, Klaus D 1978 Effect of oral contraceptives on the capacity to stimulate plasma renin activity and plasma aldosterone. Medizinische Welt 29: 228–231

Kontula K, Jänne T, Luukkainen T, Vihko R 1973 Progesterone binding protein in human myometrium. Ligand specificity and some physicochemical characteristics. Biochimica et Biophysica Acta 328: 145

Kotake Y, Murakami E 1971 Possible diabetogenic role for tryptophan metabolites and effects of xanthurenic acid on insulin. American Journal of Clinical Nutrition 24: 826

Krulich L 1979 Central neurotransmitters and the secretion of prolactin, GH, LH, and TSH. Annual Review of Physiology 41: 603–615

Kudzma D J, Bradley E M, Goldzieher J W 1972 Metabolic balance study of the effects of an oral steroid contraceptive on weight and body composition. Contraception 6: 31–37

Kulkarni B D 1970 Metabolism of ^{14}C-ethynyloestradiol in the baboon. Journal of Endocrinology 48: 91–98

Kulkarni B D 1976 Steroid contraceptives in non-human primates. I. Metabolic fate of synthetic estrogens in the baboon before exposure to oral contraceptives. Contraception 14: 611–623

Kulkarni B D, Avila T D, O'Leary J A 1977 Steroid contraceptives in non-human primates. II. Metabolic fate of synthetic estrogens in the baboon after exposure to oral contraceptives. Contraception 15: 307–317

Kunin C M, McCormack R C, Abernathy J R 1969 Oral contraceptives and blood pressure. Archives of Internal Medicine 123: 362

Lang R, Redmann A 1979 Non-mutagenicity of some sex hormones in the Ames salmonella/microsome mutagenicity test. Mutation Research 67: 361–365

Laragh J H 1976 Oral contraceptive-induced hypertension: nine years later. American Journal of Obstetrics and Gynecology 126: 141–147

Larsson-Cohn U 1965 Oral contraception and serum protein-bound iodine. Lancet i: 317

Larsson-Cohn U 1975 Oral contraceptives and vitamins: a review. American Journal of Obstetrics and Gynecology 121: 84

Larsson-Cohn U, Berlin R, Vikrot O 1970 Effects of combined and low-dose gestagen oral contraceptives on plasma lipids. Acta Endocrinologica 63: 717–735

Lauweryns J, Ferin J 1964 Effects on the ovary of prolonged administration of lynestrenol: a histological study. International Journal of Fertility 9: 35–39

Layne D S, Golab T, Arai K, Pincus G 1963 The metabolic fate of orally administered [^{3}]-norethynodrel and [^{3}H]-norethindrone in humans. Biochemical Pharmacology 13: 905–911

Layne D S, Williams K I H 1967 Urinary metabolites of radioactive quinestrol in rabbits. International Journal of Fertiligy 12: 158–163

Lederer J, Vastesaeger M 1977 Contraceptive pills: their effects on lipid and carbohydrate metabolism and on the cardiocirculatory system. Bruxelles Medicine 57: 199–214

Lee D L, Kollman P A, Marsh F J, Wolff M E 1979 Quantitative relationships between steroid structure and binding to putative progesterone receptors. Journal of Medicinal Chemistry 20: 1139–1145

Lei H P, Hu Z-Y 1981 The mechanisms of action of vacation pills. In: Symposium on Recent Advances in Fertility Regulation, Beijing, September 1980

L'Hermite M, Delvoye P, Nokin T, Vekemans M, Robyn C 1972 Human prolactin secretion as studied by radioimmunoassay: some aspects of its regulation. In: Boyns A R, Griffiths K (eds) Prolactin and Carcinogenesis, p 91. Alpha-Omega Press, Cardiff

Lindholm J, Schultz-Möller N 1973 Plasma and urinary cortisol in pregnancy and during estrogen-gestagen treatment. Scandinavian Journal of Clinical and Laboratory Investigation 31: 119

Linthorst C 1966 A new progestogen-estrogen combination for gynaecologic therapy and contraception. International Journal of Fertility 11: 35–45

Littleton P, Fotherby K, Dennis K J 1968 Metabolism of [^{14}C]-norgestrel in man. Journal of Endocrinology 42: 591–598

Longcope C, Williams K I H 1977 Ethynylestradiol and mestranol: their pharmacodynamics and effects on natural estrogens. In: Garattini S (ed) Pharmacology of Steroid Contraceptive Drugs, pp 89–98. Raven Press, New York

Loraine J A, Bell E T, Harkness R A, Mears E, Jackson M C N 1965 Hormone excretion patterns during and after long-term administration of oral contraceptives. Acta Endocrinologica 59: 15–24

Lunenfeld B, Sulimovici S, Rabau E 1963 Mechanism of action of antiovulatory compounds. Journal of Clinical Endocrinology and Metabolism 23: 391–395

Lyster S C, Lund G H, Dulin W E 1959 Ability of some progestational steroids to stimulate male accessory glands to reproduction in the rat. Experimental Biology and Medicine 100: 540–543

MacLusky N J, McEwen B S 1978 Oestrogen modulates progestin receptor concentrations in some rat brain regions but not in others. Nature 274: 276–278

McCann S M, Moss R L 1975 Putative neurotransmitters involved in discharging gonadotropin-releasing neurohormones and the action of LH-releasing hormone on the CNS. Life Sciences 16: 833–852

McClure H M, Graham C E 1973 Malignant uterine mesotheliomas in squirrel monkeys following diethylstilbestrol administration. Laboratory Animal Science 23: 493–498

McCormack K M, Arneric S P, Hook J B 1979 Action of exogenously administered steroid hormones following perinatal exposure to polybraminated biphenyls. Journal of Toxicology and Environmental Health 5: 1085–1094

McGuire J L, Lisk R D 1968 Estrogen receptors in the intact rat. Proceedings of the National Academy of Sciences, U.S. 61: 497–

McKenzie I 1955 The production of mammary cancer in rats using oestrogens. British Journal of Cancer 9: 284–299

McLachlan J A, Shah H C, Newbold R R, Bullock B C 1975 The effect of prenatal exposure of mice to diethylstilbestrol on reproductive tract function in the offspring. Toxicology and Applied Pharmacology 33: Abstract 173

Maathuis J B, Kelly R W 1978 Ovarian steroids and the synthesis or catabolism of prostaglandins. Journal of Endocrinology 77: 361–371

Madden J D, Milewich L, Parker C R, Carr B R, Boyar R M, MacDonald P C 1978 Effect of oral contraceptive treatment on the serum concentration of dehydroiso androsterone sulfate. American Journal of Obstetrics and Gynecology 132: 380–384

Madjerek Z, DeVisser J, Vandervies J, Overbeek G A 1960 Allylestrenol, a pregnancy maintaining oral gestagen. Acta Endocrinologica 35: 8–19

Magneo-Topete M, Perez-Vega E, Goldzieher J W, Martinez-Manautou J, Rudel H W 1963 Comparison of the endometrial activity of three synthetic progestins used in fertility control. American Journal of Obstetrics and Gynecology 85: 427–432

Maheh V B, Mills T M, Lin T J, Ellegood J O, Braselton E W 1977 Metabolism, metabolic clearance rate, blood metabolites, and blood half-life of norethindrone and mestranol. In: Gerattini S, Berendes H W (eds) Pharmacology of Steroid Contraceptive Drugs, pp 117–130. Raven Press, New York

Mammem E F 1982 Oral contraceptives and blood coagulation: a critical review. American Journal of Obstetrics and Gynecology 142: 781–790

Martin F, Adlercreutz H 1977 Aspects of megestrol acetate and medroxyprogesterone acetate metabolism. In: Garattini S, Berendes H W (eds) Pharmacology of Steroid Contraceptive Drugs, pp 99–115. Raven Press, New York

Martin J V, Martin P J, Goldberg D M 1976 Enzyme induction as a possible cause of increased serum triglycerides after oral contraceptives. Lancet 1: 1107–1109

Maw D S J, Wynn V 1972 Relation of growth hormone to altered carbohydrate metabolism in women taking oral contraceptives. Journal of Clinical Pathology 25: 354–358

Meade T W 1980 Oral contraceptives: progestagens and thrombosis. In: Newton J R, Jacobs H S, Caldwell A D S (eds) Workshop on Fertility Control, Royal Society of Medicine International Congress and Symposium, Series 31, Academic Press/Royal Society of Medicine, London, pp 39–48

Meade T W 1982 Oral contraceptives, clotting factors and thrombosis. American Journal of Obstetrics and Gynecology 142: 758–761

Meade T W, Brozovic M, Chakrabarti R, Howarth D J, North W R S, Stirling Y 1976 An epidemiological study of the haemostatic and other effects of oral contraceptives. British Journal of Haematology 34: 353

Means A R, Vaitukaitis J 1972 Peptide hormone "receptors": specific binding of ^{3}H-FSH to testes. Endocrinology 90: 39–46

Meikle A W, Jubiz S, Matsukura G, Harade G, West C D, Tyler F H 1970 Effect of estrogen on the metabolism of metyrapone and release of ACTH. Journal of Clinical Endocrinology and Metabolism 30: 259–263

Meli A, Steinetz B G, Giannina T, Cargill D J, Manning J P 1968 Fat storage, de-etherification and elimination of quinestrol in the rat. Proceedings of the Society for Experimental Biology and Medicine 127: 1042–1048

Mey R 1967 Masculinization of the fetus by 19-norhydroxyprogesterone cuproate. Arzneimittel-Forschung 17: 439–440

Miale J B, Kent J W 1974 Effects of oral contraceptives on the results of laboratory tests. American Journal of Obstetrics and Gynecology 120: 264–272

Migeon C J, Bertrand J, Gemzell C A 1961 Transplacental passage of various steroid hormones in mid-pregnancy. Progress in Hormone Research 17: 207–243

Miguet J P, Vuitton D, Allemand H, Pessayre D, Monange C, Hirsch J P, Metreau J M et al 1980 An outbreak of jaundice due to the combination troleandomycin — oral contraceptives. Journal of Gastroenterology and Clinical Biology 4: 420–424

Miller N E 1978 Evidence for the antiatherogenicity of high density lipoprotein in man. Lipids 13: 914–921

Mills T M, Lin T J, Braselton W E, Ellegood J O, Mahesh V B 1976 Metabolism of oral contraceptive drugs. The formation and disappearance of metabolites of norethindrone and mestranol after intravenous and oral administration. American Journal of Obstetrics and Gynecology 126: 987–922

Mishell D R, Kletzky O A, Brenner P F 1977a Effect of contraceptive steroids on hypothalamic-pituitary function. American Journal of Obstetrics and Gynecology 128: 60–74

Mishell D R, Roy S, Moore D E, Brenner P F, Page M A 1977b Clinical performance and endocrine profiles with contraceptive vaginal rings containing d-norgestrel. Contraception 16: 625–636

Mishell D R, Moore D E, Roy S, Brenner P F, Page M A 1978 Clinical performance and endocrine profiles with contraceptive vaginal rings containing a combination of estradiol and di-norgestrel. American Journal of Obstetrics and Gynecology 130: 55–62

Miyamoto J 1978 Sex steroids and thyroid function tests. International Journal of Gynaecology and Obstetrics 16: 28–33

Moguilewsky M, Raynaud J P 1979 Estrogen-sensitive, progestin-binding sites in the female rat brain and pituitary. Brain Research 164: 165–175

Møller S E 1981 Effect of oral contraceptives on tryptophan and tyrosine availability: evidence for a possible contribution to mental depression. Neuropsychobiology 7: 192–200

Moore D E, Kawagoe S, Davajan V, Nakamura R M, Mishell D R 1978 An in vivo system in man for quantitation of estrogenicity. II. Pharmacologic changes in binding capacity of serum corticosteroid-binding globulin induced by conjugated estrogens, mestranol and ethinyl estradiol. American Journal of Obstetrics and Gynecology 130: 482–486

Morrell J A, Hart G W 1941 Studies on stilbestrol. I. Some effects of continuous injections of stilbestrol in the adult female rat. Endocrinology 29: 796–816

Muldoon T G 1977 Pituitary estrogen receptors. In: Allen M B, Mahesh V B (eds) The Pituitary: A Current Review, pp 295–329. Academic Press, New York

Mulligan R M 1944 Feminization in male dogs: A syndrome associated with carcinoma of the testis and mimicked by the administration of estrogens. American Journal of Pathology 20: 865–873

Mulligan R M 1947 Some effects of chronic doses of stilbestrol in female dogs. Exploratory Medicine and Surgery 5: 196–205

Mulligan R M, Becker D L 1947 Residual tissue changes in male dogs following cessation of orally administered stilbestrol. American Journal of Pathology 23: 299–310

Murata S 1968 Study of estrane strain progestins metabolism in human body. Nihon Naubumpitsu Shi 43: 1083–1096

Musa B U, Doe R P, Seal U S 1967 Serum protein alterations produced in women by synthetic estrogens. Journal of Clinical Endocrinology and Metabolism 27: 1463–1469

Mützel W, El Mahgoub S 1977 Studies with d-norgestrel-^{3}H in lactating women. In: Garattini S, Berendes H W (eds) Pharmacology of Steroid Contraceptive Drugs, pp 137–144. Raven Press, New York

Naess O, Attramadal A 1978 Progestin receptors in the anterior pituitary and hypothalamus of male rats. International Journal of Andrology Supplement 2, Pt 1: 175–183

Nallar R, Biscardi A M 1973 Hypophysial feed-back in the hypothalamic regulation of luteinizing hormone secretion. Experientia 29: 878–879

Neumann F, von Berswordt-Wallrabe R, Elger W, Steinbeck H, Hahn J D, Kramer M 1970 Aspects of androgen-dependent events as studied by antiandrogens. Recent Progress in Hormone Research 26: 337–410

Newton J, Szantagh F, Lebech P, Rowe P 1979 A collaborative study of the progesterone intrauterine device (Progestasert). Contraception 19: 575–589

Nezhat C, Karpas A E, Greenblatt R B, Mahesh V B 1980 Estradiol implants for conception control. American Journal of Obstetrics and Gynecology 138: 1151–1156

Nilsson C G, Lähteenmäki P 1978 Plasma prolactin concentrations in women treated with low dose combination type oral contraceptives and in women using a D-norgestrel releasing intrauterine device. Annals of Clinical Research 10: 242–245

Nilsson S, Nygren K-G 1978 Ethinyl estradiol in peripheral plasma after oral administration of 30 μg and 50 μg to women. Contraception 18: 469–475

Nilsson S, Victor A, Nygren K-G 1977 Plasma levels of d-norgestrel and sex hormone binding globulin during oral d-norgestrel medication immediately after delivery and legal abortion. Contraception 15: 87–92

Nitowsky H M, Davis J, Nakagawa S, Fox D 1979 Human hexosaminidase isozymes. IV. Effects of oral contraceptive steroids on serum hexosaminidase activity. American Journal of Obstetrics and Gynecology 134: 642–647

Nomura T, Kanzaki T 1977 Induction of urogenital anomalies and some tumors in the progeny of mice receiving diethylstilbestrol during pregnancy. Cancer Research 37: 1099–1104

Notelovitz M, Kitchens C S, Coone L, McKenzie L, Carter R 1981 Low-dose oral contraceptive usage and coagulation. American Journal of Obstetrics and Gynecology 141: 71–75

Nowaczynski W, Murakami T, Richardson K, Genest J 1978 Increased aldosterone plasma protein binding in women on combined oral contraceptives throughout the menstrual cycle. Journal of Clinical Endocrinology and Metabolism 47: 193–199

Ober W B 1977 Effects of oral and intrauterine administration of contraceptives on the uterus. Human Pathology 8: 513–527

Odeblad E 1971 Cervical factors. In: Diczfalusy E, Borell U (eds) Control of Human Fertility, pp 89–96. Wiley, New York

Oepen J, Oepen I, Fuchs C 1969 Influence of contraceptive pills on serum amino acids in comparison with results typical for sex,

menstrual cycle and pregnancy. Archives Gynakologie 208: 33
Oliveira H S, Oliveira C F, Abraul E 1979 Influence of the vitamin B_6 on the alterations of the glucose and insulin levels in normal women receiving oral contraceptive drugs. Abstracts 11th World Congress of Gynecology and Obstetrics, Tokyo, pp 151–152
Okerholm R A, Peterson F E, Keeley F J, Smith T C, Glazko A J 1978 Bioavailability of norethindrone in human subjects. European Journal of Clinical Pharmacology 13: 35–39
Oriowo M A, Landgren B M, Stenstrom B, Diszfalusy E 1980 A comparison of the pharmacokinetic properties of three estradiol esters. Contraception 21: 415–424
Ortiz A, Hiroi M, Stanczyk F Z, Goebelsmann U, Mishell D R 1977 Serum medroxyprogesterone acetate (MPA) concentrations and ovarian function following intramuscular injection of Depo-MPA. Journal of Clinical Endocrinology and Metabolism 44: 32–38
Osawa Y 1981 Norethisterone, a major ingredient of contraceptive pills, is a suicide inhibitor of estrogen biosynthesis. Science 215:
O'Shea J D, Jabara A G 1971 Proliferative lesions of serous membranes in ovariectomised female and entire male dogs after stilboestrol administration. Veterinary Pathology 8: 81–90
Østergaard E 1965 The oral progestational and antiovulatory properties of megestrol acetate and its therapeutic use in gynaecological disorders. Journal of Obstetrics and Gynaecology of the British Commonwealth 72: 45
Oster P, Arab L, Kohlmeier M, Mordasini R, Schellenberg B, Schlierf G 1982 Effects of estrogens and progestogens on lipid metabolism. American Journal of Obstetrics and Gynecology 142: 773–775
Osterholzer H O, Grillo D, Kruger P S, Dunnihoo D R 1977 Effect of oral contraceptive steroids on branches of the uterine artery. Obstetrics and Gynecology 49: 227–232
Palmer K, Feierabend J F, Baggett B, Wall M E 1969 Metabolic removal of a 17α-ethynyl group from the antifertility steroid norethindrone. Journal of Pharmacology and Experimental Therapeutics 167: 217–222
Pan M B, Gardner W U 1948 Carcinomas of the uterine cervix and vagina in estrogen and androgen-treated hybrid mice. Cancer Research 8: 337–341
Paradi E 1981 Mutagenicity of some contraceptive drugs in Drosophila melanogaster. Mutation Research 88: 175–178
Parke D V 1978 Pharmacology of mucus. British Medical Medical Bulletin 34: 89–94
Pasqualini J R, Castellet R, Portois M C, Hill J L, Kinel F A 1977 Plasma concentrations of ethynyloestradiol and norethindrone after oral administration to women. Journal of Reproduction and Fertility 49: 189–193
Patwardhan R V, Desmond P V, Johnson R F, Schenker S 1980 Impaired elimination of caffeine by oral contraceptive steroids. Journal of Laboratory and Clinical Medicine 95: 603–608
Perkins C M, Hancock K W, Cope G F, Lee M R 1981 Urine free dopamine in normal primigravid pregnancy and women taking oral contraceptives. Clinical Science 61: 423–428
Peters J R, Elliott J M, Grahame-Smith D G 1979 Effect or oral contraceptives on platelet noradrenaline and 5-hydroxy-tryptamine receptors and aggregation. Lancet: 933–936
Phoenix C H, Goy R W, Gerall A A 1959 Organizing action of prenatally administered testosterone propionate on the tissues mediating mating behavior of female guinea pig. Endocrinology 65: 369–382
Picchioni A L 1965 Control of poisoning. American Journal of Hospital Pharmacy 22: 486–487
Pincus G 1965 The Control of Fertility, p. 231. Academic Press, New York
Plate W P 1968 Ovarian changes after long-term contraception. In: Meglor L, Peck H M (eds) Drug-Induced Diseases, 3: 235–238
Platt D, Eimer H 1973 Lysosomal enzyme activity in human serum during use of hormonal contraceptives. Klinische Wochenschrift 51: 91–92
Poller L 1978 Oral contraceptives, blood clotting and thrombosis. British Medical Bulletin 34: 151–156
Pollow K. Geilfuss J, Boquoi E, Pollow B 1978 Estrogen and progesterone binding proteins in normal human myometrium and leiomyoma tissue. Journal of Clinical Chemistry and Clinical Biochemistry 16: 503–511
Prange A J, Wilson I C, Alltop L B 1972 Journal of the American Medical Association 219: 143
Prasad K V S, Narasingarad B S, Sivakumar B, Prema K 1979 Pharmacokinetics or norethindrone in Indian women. Contraception 20: 77–90
Prasad K V S, Sivakumar B, Narasinga Rao B S 1979 The rabbit as an animal model to study pharmacokinetics of norethindrone in women. Contraception 20: 619–632
Purvis K, Landgren B M, Cekan Z, Diczfalusy E 1975 Indices of gonadal function in the human male. II. Seminal plasma levels of steroids in normal and pathological conditions. Clinical Endocrinology 4: 247–258
Rannevik G, Jeppsson S, Kullander S 1972 Effect or oral contraceptives on the liver in women with recurrent cholestasis (hepatosis) during previous pregnancies. Journal of Obstetrics and Gynaecology of the British Commonwealth 79: 1128–1136
Ranney R E 1977 Comparative metabolism of 17α-ethynyl steroids used in oral contraceptives. Journal of Toxicology and Environmental Health 3: 139
Rao P N, Zuspan F P 1970 Urinary catecholamines excretion and basal body temperature alterations with oral contraceptives. Surgical Forum 21: 412–413
Ravens K G, Jipp P 1976 Lipoprotein changes with oral contraceptives and in pregnancy. Verhandlungen Der Deutschen Gesellschaft für Innere Medizin 82: 839
Ray J A, Schut A L 1969 Cataracts and other lesions in rats receiving a synthetic progestin-estrogen. Journal of Toxicology and Applied Pharmacology 14: 634
Raynaud A 1942 Inhibition of eyelid development in mouse embryos. Comptes Rendus Societie de Biologie 136: 337–338
Reed M J, Fotherby K 1975 Metabolism of ethynyloestradiol and oestradiol in the guinea pig. Journal of Steroid Biochemistry 6: 121–125
Reed M J, Fotherby K, Steele S J 1972 Metabolism of ethynyloestradiol in man. Journal of Endocrinology 55: 351–361
Reimers D, Jezek A 1971 Rifampicin und andere antituberkulotika bei gleichzeitiger oraler kontrazeption. Praxis und Klinik der Pneumologie 25: 255–262
Reinische J M, Karow W G 1977 Prenatal exposure to synthetic progestin and estrogen. Archives of Sexual Behavior 6: 257–263
Revesz C, Chappel C I, Gaudry R 1960 Masculinization of female fetuses in the rat by progestational compunds. Endocrinology 66: 140–144
Reymond M, Lemarchand-Beraud T 1976 Effects of oestrogens on prolactin and throtrophin responses to TRH in women during the menstrual cycle and under oral contraceptive treatment. Clinical Endocrinology 5: 429–437
Roberton Y R, Johnson E S 1976 Interactions between OC and other drugs: a review. Current Medical Research and Opinion 3: 647–661
Roberts J S, Carlson J G, McCracken J A 1976 Prostaglandin $F_{2\alpha}$ production by the brain and its role in LH secretion. Advances in Prostaglandin and Thromboxane Research 2: 609–619
Roberts R K, Desmond P V, Wilkinson G R, Schenker S 1979 Disposition of chlordiazepoxide: sex differences and effects of OC. Clinical Pharmacology and Therapeutics 25: 826–831
Robertson D M, Landgren B M, Guerrero R 1975 Oestradiol receptor levels in the human fallopian tube during the menstrual cycle. Acta Endocrinologica 80: 705–718
Rose D P, Brown R R, Price J M 1968 Metabolism of tryptophan to nicotinic acid derivatives by women taking oestrogen/progestogen preparations. Nature 219: 1259–1260
Rosner F, Hirshaut Y, Grünwald H W, Deutsch S 1978 Potentiation of vincristine cytotoxicity by hormones: corticosteroids, androgens, estrogens and progestins. American Journal of Haematology 5: 305–314
Rosner J M, Martinez I M, Mendizabal A F, Spaltro N A 1971 In vivo and in vitro uptake of labelled estradiol by different segments of the human uterus. Steroidologia 2: 283–288
Rössner S, Larsson-Cohn U, Carlson L A, Boberg J 1971 Effect of an oral contraceptive agent on plasma lipids, plasma lipoproteins, intravenous fat tolerance, and the post-heparin lipoprotein lipase activity. Acta Medica Scandinavia 190: 301
Rubinfeld Y, Maor Y, Simon D, Modai D 1979 Progressive rise in

serum copper levels in women taking oral contraceptives. Fertility and Sterility 32: 599–601

Rubinstein L, Moguilevsky J, Leiderman S 1978 The effect of oral contraceptives on the gonadotrophin response to LHRH. Obstetrics and Gynecology 52: 571–574

Rudel H W, Kincl F A 1972 Oral contraceptives. Human fertility studies and side effects. In: Tausk M (ed) Pharmacology of the Endocrine System and Related Drugs: Progesterone, Progestational Drugs and Antifertility Agents, Pergamon, Oxford, 2: 385–469

Rudel H W, Martinez-Manautou J, Maqueo-Topete M 1965 Role of progestogens in the hormonal control of fertility. Fertility and Sterility 16: 158–169

Rudorff K H, Herrmann J, Dieterich T, Kruskemper H C 1978 Effect of estrogen upon thyroid metabolism. Medizinische Klinik 73: 1109–1113

Rustia M, Shubik P 1976 Transplacental effects of diethylstilboestrol on the genital tract of hamster offspring. Cancer Letters 1: 139–146

Ryan G M, Graig J, Reid D E 1964 Histology of the uterus and ovaries after long-term cyclic norethynodrel therapy. American Journal of Obstetrics and Gynecology 90: 715–725

Salhanick H A, Kipnis D M, Van de Wiele R L 1969 Metabolic Effects of Gonadal Hormones and Contraceptive Steroids, Plenum Press, New York

Sanborn B M, Kuo H S, Held B 1978 Estrogen and progestogen binding site concentrations in human endometrium and cervix throughout the menstrual cycle and in tissue from women taking oral contraceptives. Journal of Steroid Biochemistry 9: 951–955

Sanchez-Rivera G, Merlo J G, Escudero M, Botella-Llusia J 1968 Action of several synthetic steroids on the human ovary. American Journal of Obstetrics and Gynecology 101: 665–671

Sar M, Stumpf W E 1973 Neurons of the hypothalamus concentrate ^{3}H-progesterone or its metabolites. Science 182: 1266–1268

Sar M, Stumpf W E 1975a Distribution of androgen-concentrating neurones in the rat brain. In: Stumpf W E, Grant L D (eds) Anatomical Neuroendocrinology, pp 120–133. Karger, Basel

Sar M, Stumpf W E 1975b Cellular localization of progestin and estrogen in guinea pig hypothalamus by autoradiogrphy. In: Stumpf W E, Grant L D (eds) Anatomical Neuroendocrinology, pp 142–152. Karger, Basel

Saruta T, Saade G A, Kaplan N M 1970 Possible mechanism for hypertension induced by oral contraceptives. Diminished feedback suppression of renin release. Archives of internal Medicine 126: 621–626

Sato K, Ogino M, Nakabayashi M, Sakamoto S 1978 Oral contraceptives and thromboembolism. Kokyo to Junkan 26: 212–220

Saunders F J 1967 Effects of norethynodrel combined with mestranol administered to rats during early pregnancy. Endocrinology 80: 447–452

Saunders F J, Elton R L 1967 Effects of ethynodiol diacetate and mestranol in rats and rabbits, on conception, on the outcome of pregnancy, and on the offspring. Toxicology and Applied Pharmacology 11: 229–244

Saure A, Karjalainen O, Teravaeinen T 1977 Effect of synthetic gestagens on oestrogen formation in vitro by human corpus luteum. Acta Endocrinologica Supplement 212: 70

Schally A, Kastin A J 1970 The role of sex steroids, hypothalamic LH-releasing hormone in the regulation of gonadotropin secretion from the anterior pituitary gland. In: Briggs M H (ed) Advances in Steroid Biochemistry and Pharmacology, pp 41–69. Academic Press, New York

Schardein J L 1980 Studies on the components of an oral contraceptive agent in albino rats. Journal of Toxicology and Environmental Health 6: 885–906

Schenker J G, Ben-Yoseph Y, Shapira E 1972 Erythrocyte carbonic anhydrase B levels during pregnancy and use of oral contraceptives. Obstetrics and Gynecology 39: 237

Schenker J G, Hellerstein S, Jungreis E, Polishuk W Z 1971 Serum copper and zinc levels in patients taking oral contraceptives. Fertility and Sterility 22: 229

Schneider H P G, Leyendecker G 1979 The normal and dysregulated human menstrual cycle. Advances in Steroid Biochemistry and Pharmacology 7: 23–50

Schrogie J J, Solomon H M, Zieve P D 1967 Clinical Pharmacology and Therapeutics 8 670

Schürenkämper P, Lisse K 1978 In vitro studies on the effect of d-norgestrel and norethisterone acetate on the synthesis of sex hormones by the human ovary. Endokrinologie 71: 25–34

Schwartz N B, McCormack C E 1972 Gonadal function and its regulation. Annual Review of Physiology 34: 435

Schwartz E, Tornaben J A, Boxill G C 1969 Effects of chronic oral administration of a long-acting estrogen, quinestrol, to dogs. Toxicology and Applied Pharmacology 14: 487–494

Scott J A, Brenner P F, Kletzky O A, Mishell D R 1978a Factors affecting pituitary gonadotropin function in users of oral contraceptive steroids. American Journal of Obstetrics and Gynecology 130: 817–821

Scott J Z, Kletzky O A, Brenner P F, Mishell D R 1978b Comparison of the effectos of contraceptive steroid formulations containing two doses of estrogen on pituitary function. Fertility and Sterility 30: 141–145

Seiki K, Hattori M 1973 In vivo uptake of progesterone by the hypothalamus and pituitary of the female ovariectomized rat and its relationship to cytoplasmic progesterone-binding protein. Endocrinology Japonica 20: 111–119

Segre A, Citti U, Bertaglia A, Prampolini P 1978 Plasma levels of the gonadotropins in patients taking estrogen/progestogens. Minerva Ginecologia 30: 157–165

Sepsenwol S, Hechter O 1976 Failure to observe testosterone-induced nucleus-lysosome interaction in rat ventral prostate. Molecular and Cellular Endocrinology 4: 115–129

Shaala S, Khowessah M, El-Damarawy H, El-Sahwi S, Osman M, Toppozada M 1977 Reduced uterine response to $PGF_{2\alpha}$ under oral contraceptives. Prostaglandins 14: 523–533

Shapiro S S, Dyer R D, Colas A E 1978 Synthetic progestins: in vitro potency on human endometrium and specific binding to cytosol receptor. American Journal of Obstetrics and Gynecology 132: 549–554

Shaw J E, Tillson S A 1974 Interactions between the prostaglandins and steroid hormaones. Advances in Steroid Biochemistry and Pharmacology 4: 189–207

Sheridan P J, Buchanan J M, Anselmo V C, Martin P M 1979 Equilibrium: the intracellular distribution of steroid receptors. Nature 282: 579–582

Shimkin M B, Grady H G 1941 Toxic and carcinogenic effects of stilbestrol in strain C3H male mice. Journal of the National Cancer Institute 2: 55–60

Shinada T, Tokota Y, Igarashi M 1978 Inhibitory effect of various gestagens upon the pregnenolone 3β-ol-dehydrogenase-Δ^5-isomerase system in human corpora lutea of menstrual cycles. Fertility and Sterility 29: 84–87

Shojania A M, Wylie B 1979 Effect of oral contraceptives on vitamin B_{12} metabolism. American Journal of Obstetrics and Gynecology 135: 129–134

Sidell F R, Kaminskis A 1975 Influence of age, sex and oral contraceptives on human blood cholinesterase activity. Clinical Chemistry 21: 1393–1395

Singh H, Unival J P, Murugesan K, Takkar D, Hingorani V, Laumas K R 1979 Pharmacokinetics of norethindrone acetate in women. American Journal of Obstetrics and Gynecology 135: 409–414

Sisenwine S F, Kimmel H B, Liu A L, Ruelius H W 1975 Excretion and stereo-selective biotransformations of dl- and d- and L-norgestrel in women. Drug Metabolism and Disposition 3: 180–188

Sisenwine S F, Kimmel H B, Liu A L, Ruelius H W 1977 The conversion of d-norgestrel-3-oxime-17-acetate to d-norgestrel in female rhesus monkeys. Contraception 15: 25–37

Sisenwine S F, Kimmel H B, Liu A L, Ruelius H W 1978 Urinary metabolites of norgestrel in female baboons. Federal Proceedings of the American Society for Experimental Biology 37: 813

Sivin I, Robertson D N, Stern J, Croxatto H B, Diaz S, Coutinho E et al 1980 Norplant: reversible implant contraception. Studies in Family Planning 11: 227–235

Skouby S O, Mølsted-Pedersen L, Kühl C 1982 Low dosage oral contraception in women with previous gestational diabetes. Obstetrics and Gynecology 59: 325–328

Slaunwhite W R, Sandberg A A 1961 Identification of a 6.21-

dihydroxylated metabolite of medroxyprogresterone acetate in human urine. Journal of Clinical Endocrinology and Metabolism 21: 753–764

Smith J C, Brown E D 1976 Effects of oral contraceptive agents on trace element metabolism: a review. In: Prasad A S, Oberleas D (eds) Trace Elements in Human Health and Disease, Vol 2, pp 315–346. Academic Press, New York

Sonnenberg A, Koelz R, Herz I, Benes I, Blum A L 1980 Limited usefulness of the breath test in evaluation of drug metabolism: a study in human oral contraceptive users treated with dimethylaminoantipyrine and diazepam. Hepato-Gastroenterology 27: 104–108

Southgate J, Collin G G S, Prys-Davies J, Sandler M 1970 Effect of contraceptive steroids on monamine oxidase activity. Journal of Clinical Pathology 23: Supplement 3, 43–48

Soveri P, Fyrquist F 1977 Plasma renin activity and angiotensis II during oral contraception. Annals of Clinical Research 9: 346–349

Speck U, Wendt H, Schultze P E, Jentsch D 1976 Bioavailability and pharmacokinetics of cyproterone acetate-^{14}C and ethinyloestradiol-^{3}H after oral administration as a coated tablet. Contraception 14: 151–163

Spellacy W N 1969 Review of carbohydrate metabolism and the oral contraceptive. American Journal of Obstetrics and Gynecology 104: 448–460

Spellacy W N 1976 Carbohydrate metabolism in male infertility and female fertility-control patients. Fertility and Sterility 27: 1132–1141

Spellacy W N 1978 Oral contraceptives: metabolic aspects. In: Arce B, Pujol-Amat P (eds) Human Reproduction and Fertility Regulation, pp 157–164. Espaxs, Barcelona

Spellacy W N 1982 Carbohydrate metabolism during treatment with estrogen, progestogen, and low-dose oral contraceptives. American Journal of Obstetrics and Gynecology 142: 732–734

Spellacy W N, Buhi W C, Bendel R P 1969 Insulin and glucose determination after one year of treatment with sequential type oral contraceptive. Obstetrics and Gynecology 33: 800

Spellacy W N, Buhi W C, Birk S A 1972a Effects of vitamin B$_6$ on carbohydrate metabolism in women taking steroid contraceptives. Contraception 6: 265

Spellacy W N, Buhi W C, Birk S A 1972b Effects of estrogens on carbohydrate metabolism: glucose, insulin, and growth hormone studies on 171 women ingesting premarin, mestranol, and ethinyl estradiol for six months. American Journal of Obstetrics and Gynecology 114: 378

Spellacy W N, Carlson K L, Schade S L 1967 Human growth hormone levels in normal subjects receiving oral contraceptives. Journal of the American Medical Association 202: 451–456

Speroff L 1976 Which birth control pill should be prescribed? Fertility and Sterility 27: 997–1008

Spona J 1973 LHRH stimulated gonadotropin release mediated by two distinct pituitary receptors. FEBS Letters 35: 59–62

Spona J 1975 LHRH interactions with pituitary receptors: properties and characterization. Endocrinologia Experimentalis 9: 127–134

Staemmler H J 1964 Die Gestörte Regelung der Ovarialfunktion, pp 184–189. Springer, Berlin

Stanczyk F Z, Brenner P F, Mishell D R, Ortiz A, Genzchein E K E, Boebelsmann U 1978 A radioimmunoassy for norethindrone (NET): measurement of serum NET concentrations following ingestion of NET-containing oral contraceptive steroids. Contraception 18: 615–633

Steinetz B G, Meli A, Giannina T, Beach V L 1967 Studies on bibliary metabolism of orally administered ethynylestradiol and quinestrol. Proceedings of the Society for Experimental Biology and Medicine 124: 1283–1289

Stockley I 1976 Interactions with oral contraceptives. The Pharmaceutical Journal 140–143

Suchowsky G K, Junkmann K 1961 A study of the virilizing effect of progestogens on the female rat fetus. Endocrinology 68: 341–349

Sullivan L W, Smith T C 1957 Influence of estrogens on body growth and food intake. Proceedings of the Society for Experimental Biology and Medicine 96: 60–64

Swyer G I M 1960 Problems der klinischen Beurteilung gestagener steroide. In: Nowakowski (ed) Moderne Entwicklungen auf dem Gestenge Biet, p. 100. Springer-Verlag, Berlin

Swyer G I M 1969 Liquid paraffin and oral contraceptives. Practitioner 202: 592

Swyer G I M 1974 Potency and selectivity of action of progestogens. In: Fairweather D V J (ed) Second International Norgestrel Symposium, Excerpta Medica International Congress Series, 344: 43–46

Szego C M, Seeler B J, Steadman R A, Hill D F, Kimura A K, Roberts J A 1971 The lysosomal membrane complex: focal point of primary steroid hormone action. Biochemical Journal 123: 523–538

Szego C M, Seller B J 1973 Hormone-induced activation of target-specific lysosomes: acute translocation to the nucleus after administration of gonadal hormones in vivo. Journal of Endocrinology 56: 347–360

Szontagh F E 1973 Short-loop "Internal" pituitary-hypothalamus gonadotropin feedback in the human. Endocrinologica Experimentalis 7: 65–67

Takano K, Yamamura H, Suzuki M, Nishimura H 1966 Teratogenic effects of chlormadinone acetate in mice and rabbits. Proceedings of the Society for Experimental Biology and Medicine 121: 455–457

Talley D J, Li J J, Villee C A 1975 Biochemical comparison of estrogen receptors of the hamster hypothalamus and uterus. Endocrinology 96: 1135–1144

Tonkin S Y 1981 Oral contraceptives and vitamin status. In: Briggs M H (ed) Vitamins in Human Biology and Medicine, pp 29–64. C R C Press, Florida

Tryding N, Nilsson S E, Tufuesson G, Berg G, Carlstrom S, Elmfors B, Nilsson J E 1969 Physiological and pathological influences on serum monamine oxidase level. Scandinavian Journal of Clinical and Laboratory Investigations 23: 79–84

Tseng L, Gurpide E 1972 Changes in the in vitro metabolism of estradiol by human endometrium during the menstrual cycle. American Journal of Obstetrics and Gynecology 114: 1002

Tseng L, Gurpide E 1975 Induction of human endometrial estradiol dehydrogenase by progestins. Endocrinology 97: 825

Tseng L, Gurpide E 1979 Stimulation of various 17β and 20α-hydroxysteroid dehydrogenase activities by progestins in human endometrium. Endocrinoloty 104: 1745–1748

Tsibris J C M, Raynor L O, Buhi W C 1980 Insulin receptors in circulating erythrocytes and monocytes from women on oral contraceptives or pregnant women near term. Journal of Clinical Endocrinology and Metabolism 51: 711–719

Van der Steeg H Y, Pronk J C 1977 Effect of an oral contraceptive on serum lipoproteins and skinfold thickness. Contraception 16: 29

Van Wagenen G 1935 The effects of oestrin on the urogenital tract of the male monkey. Anatomical Record 63: 387–403

Vecchio T J 1976 Long-acting injectable contraceptives. Advances in Steroid Biochemistry and Pharmacology 5: 1–65

Vertes M, King R J B 1971 Mechanism of oestradiol binding in rat hypothalamus: effect of androgenisation. Journal of Endocrinology 51: 271

Vessey M P, Mann J I 1978 Female sex hormones and thrombosis: Epidemiological aspects. British Medical Bulletin 34: 157–162

Viajayan E, McCann S M 1978 Re-evaluation of the role of catecholamines in control of gonadotropin and prolactin release. Neuroendocrinology 25: 150–165

Victor A, Johansson E D N 1977 Effects of d-norgestrel induced decreases in sex hormone binding globulin capacity on the d-norgestrel levels in plasma. Contraception 16: 115–123

Victor A, Weiner E, Johansson E D B 1976 Sex hormone binding globulin: the carrier protein for d-norgestrel. Journal of Clinical Endocrinology and Metabolism 43: 244–247

Viinikka L, Ylikorkala O, Vihko R, Masenack H G, Nieuwenhuyse H 1980 Metabolism of a new synthetic progestage, Org 2969, in female volunteers. The distribution and excretion of radioactivity after an oral dose of the labelled drug. Acta Endocrinologica 93: 375–379

Voigt R, Nöschel H, Müller B 1977 Klinische untersuchungen über den einfluss langdauernder progestageneinnahme auf den Abbau von Noramidopyrinmethansulfonatnatrium (Analgin). Zentralblatt für Gynäkologie 99: 161–164

Von Hempel E, Bohm W, Carol W, Klinger G 1973 Medicinal enzyme induction and hormonal contraception. Zentralblatt für Gynäkologie 95: 1451–1455

Vose C W, Butler J K, Williams B M, Stafford J E H, Shelton J R,

Rose D A et al 1979 Bioavailability and pharmacokinetics of norethisterone in women after oral doses of ethynodiol diacetate. Contraception 19: 119–127

Walls C, Vose C W, Horth C E, Palmer R F 1977 Radioimmunoassay of plasma norethisterone after ethynodiol diacetate administration. Journal of Steroid Biochemistry 8: 167–171

Wan L S, Ganguly M, Weiss G 1981 Pituitary response to LHRH stimulation in women on oral contraceptives: a follow-up dose response study. Contraception 24: 229–234

Wardlaw S, Lauersen N H, Saxena B B 1975 The LH-hCG receptor of human ovary at various stages of the menstrual cycle. Acta Endocrinologica 79: 568–576

Warren M P 1973 Metabolic effects of contraceptive steroids. American Journal of Medical Science 265: 4–21

Warren R J, Fotherby K 1973 Plasma levels of ethynyloestradiol after administration of ethynyloestradiol or mestranol to human subjects. Journal of Endocrinology 59: 369–370

Webster R A, Pikler G M, Spelsberg T C 1976 Nuclear binding of progesterone in hen oviduct. Biochemical Journal 156: 409–418

Weikel J H, Nelson L W 1977 Problems in evaluating chronic toxicity of contraceptive steroids in dogs. Journal of Toxicology and Environmental Health 3: 167–177

Weinberger M H, Collins R D, Dowd A J, Nokes G W, Luetscher J A 1969 Hypertension induced by oral contraceptives containing estrogen and progestogen. Effects on plasma renin-activity and aldosterone excretion. Annals of Internal Medicine 71: 891–902

Weindling H, Henry J B 1974 Laboratory test results altered by the pill. Journal of the American Medical Association 229: 1762–1768

Weintraub H S, Abrams L S, Patrick J W, McGuire J L 1978 Disposition of norgestimate in the presence and absence of ethinyl estradiol after oral administration to humans. Journal of Pharmacological Science 67: 1406–1408

Weir R J, Tree M, Fraser R 1970 Effects of oral contraceptives on blood pressure and on plasma renin, renin substrate, and corticosteroids. Journal of Clinical Pathology 23: Suppl 3, 49–53

Weir R J, Davies D L, Fraser R, Morton J J, Tree M, Wilson A 1975 Contraceptive steroids and hypertension. Journal of Steroid Biochemistry 6: 961–964

Weiss G 1970 Effects of steroid hormones on cervical mucus. Advances in Steroid Biochemistry and Pharmacology 1: 137–

Westberg J A, Bern H A, Barnawell E B 1957 Strain differences in the response of the mouse adrenal to oestrogen. Acta Endocrinologica 25: 70–82

Westphal U 1971 Steroid-protein interactions. Monographs on Endocrinology 4: Springer-Verlag, Berlin

Whitehead M I, Townsend P T, Gill D K, Collins W P, Campbell S 1980 Adsorption and metabolism of oral progesterone. British Medical Journal 280: 825–827

World Health Organization 1981 The effect of female sex hormones on fetal development and infant health. W H O Technical Report Series 657

Williams K I H, Layne D S, Hobkirk R, Nilsen M, Blahey P R 1967 Metabolism of doubly labelled ethynylestradiol-3-methyl ether in women. Steroids 9: 275–187

Williams M C, Helton F D, Goldzieher J W 1975a The urinary metabolites of 17α-ethynylestradiol 9α11ε-³H in women. Steroids 25: 229–241

Williams J G, Longcope C, Williams K I H 1975b Metabolism of 4-³H and 4-¹⁴C-17α ethynylestradiol-3-methyl ether (mestranol) by women. Steroids 25: 343–354

Winikoff D 1971 Oral contraceptives and thyroid function tests. Medical Journal of Australia 1: 1059

Wolfe L S, Coceani F 1979 Role of prostaglandins in the central nervous system. Annual Review of Physiology 41: 669–684

Wynn V 1975 Vitamins and oral contraceptive use. Lancet 1: 561

Wynn V, Godsland I, Niththyananthan R, Adams P W, Melrose J, Oakley N W, Seed M 1979 Comparison of effects of different combined oral contraceptive formulations on carbohydrate and lipid metabolism. Lancet i: 1045–1049

Wynn V 1982 Effect of duration of low-dose oral contraceptive administration on carbohydrate metabolism. American Journal of Obstetrics and Gynecology 142: 739–746

Wynn V, Niththyananthan R 1982 The effect of progestins in combined oral contraceptives on serum lipids with special reference to high-density lipoproteins. American Journal of Obstetrics and Gynecology 142: 766–772

Wynne N A 1968 Oral contraceptives. Pharmaceutical Journal II: 447

Zacherle B J, Richardson J A 1972 Irreversible renal failure secondary to hypertension induced by oral contraceptives. Annals of Internal Medicine 77: 83–85

Zakheim R M, Molteni A, Mattioli L, Mullis K B 1976 Angiotensin I converting enzyme and angiotensin II levels in women receiving an oral contraceptive. Journal of Clinical Endocrinology and Metabolism 42: 588–589

Zech P, Rifle G, Linder A 1975 Malignant hypertension with irreversible renal failure due to oral contraceptives. British Medical Journal 4: 326–327

Zuckerman S 1938 The effects of prolonged oestrogenic-stimulation on the prostate of the rhesus monkey. Journal of Anatomy 72: 264–276

Zuleski F, Loh A, Dicarlo F J 1978 Determination of ethinyl estradiol in human urine by radio chemical GLC. Journal of Pharmaceutical Science 67: 1138–1141

Zussman W V, Forbes D A, Carpenter R J 1967 Ovarian morphology following cyclic northindrone-mestranol therapy. American Journal of Obstetrics and Gynecology 99: 100–105

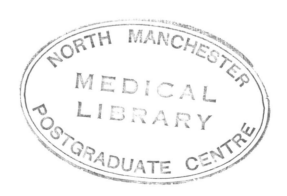

Endocrine aspects of malignancy of the breast

INTRODUCTION

The role of steroid hormones in adenocarcinoma of the breast is imperfectly understood. That these hormones play an important part in the genesis of this cancer seems clear, yet the mechanism of this malignant interaction remains muddled. Once initiated, many breast tumours remain under hormonal control. We have little idea why only a portion of tumours are hormonally regulated, and only glimmerings of how the regulation is enforced. Though we can use steroid hormones both in an adjuvant setting and in metastatic breast carcinoma, and with relative specificity, many important questions remain unanswered regarding the proper place and type of hormonal therapy. Despite the many deficiencies in our understanding of steroid hormones in breast cancer, the subject has been one of real progress and fascination. The past decade has witnessed an explosion in our understanding of breast cancer. This chapter will identify the strides made in the epidemiology, biology, and treatment of breast cancer, inasmuch as they relate to steroid hormones.

STEROID HORMONES IN THE EPIDEMIOLOGY AND AETIOLOGY OF BREAST CANCER

The epidemiological observation linking the female genital organs with breast cancer is an old one. One of the fathers of epidemiology, Bernardino Ramazzini, remarked on the relationship in his *De Morbis Artificium* in 1713: 'Experience proves that as a consequence of disturbances in the uterus, cancerous tumours are very often generated in women's breasts, and tumours of this sort are found in nuns more than in any other women. Now these are not caused by suppression of the menses but rather, in my opinion, by their celibate life. . . . Every city in Italy has several religious communities of nuns, and you can seldom find a convent that does not harbor this accursed pest, cancer, within its walls. Now why is it that the breasts suffer for the derangements of the womb, whereas other parts of the body do not suffer in this way or not so frequently? It is certainly because there is between them a mysterious sympathy that so far has escaped the researches of prosectors, though perhaps the course of time will reveal it, since the whole domain of Truth has not yet been conquered.'

More than two and a half centuries later, Ramazzini's basic insight — the 'mysterious sympathy' between the breast and the reproductive organs — remains sound, and is increasingly well-documented. The 'whole domain of Truth' also remains unconquered — a matter of fascination and frustration for investigators concerned with the problem of breast cancer.

Endogenous hormones and breast cancer

It now seems clear, a decade after the pioneering epidemiological investigations of MacMahon et al (1970), that endogenous hormonal factors affect the risk of developing breast cancer. Some of the hormonally-related factors now thought to alter a woman's risk of developing breast cancer are listed in Table 36.1.

Reproductive history is certainly important. MacMahon et al (1970), and several subsequent authors, have shown that early childbirth seems to protect a woman from breast malignancy, and that late childbirth seems to increase the risk of developing breast cancer. The difference in breast cancer incidence related to childbirth can be profound; women having a first child under the age of 18 may have only one-third the incidence of breast cancer of women having their first childbirth after age 35 (Kelsey, 1979).

Table 36.1 Hormonally-related factors affecting risk of developing breast cancer

Factors Increasing Risk	Factors Decreasing Risk
First childbirth after age 30	First childbirth at age < 20
Early menarche	
Late menopause	? High parity
Progesterone deficit	Ovariectomy at age < 35

The protective effect of first childbirth may be extended with subsequent childbirths (Lilrenfeld et al, 1975; Tulinius et al, 1978; Thien-Hlang & Thien-Maung, 1978; Adami et al, 1978), though this has not been a consistent finding in all studies.

The risk of developing breast cancer may be increased by prolonged exposure to endogenous oestrogens. Women with an early age of menarche, and women with a late age of menopause, appear to be at increased risk for developing breast cancer (reviewed by Kelsey, 1979). Ovariectomy at a young age (less than 35) appears to offer relative protection against breast cancer.

Sherman & Korenman (1974) have suggested that breast cancer risk may be elevated in patients with inadequate corpus luteum function. The 'unopposed' (by progesterone) oestrogen in these women may promote development of breast cancer.

A study from the Johns Hopkins University Obstetrical clinics has shown that progesterone-deficient premenopausal women with fertility difficulties have 5.4 times the risk of breast cancer when compared to women with non-hormonal fertility problems (Cowan et al, 1981). This study lends credence to the idea that progesterone has a protective effect in breast cancer. The argument for corpus luteum dysfunction as a risk factor in breast cancer has been discussed in detail by Sherman et al (1982).

Exogenous oestrogens and breast cancer

If variations in the hormonal environment affect risk of developing breast cancer, one must ask whether exogenous hormones alter breast cancer incidence. The question is of fairly obvious importance, given both the high incidence of breast cancer in Western societies and the number of women receiving oestrogen-containing medications. If exogenous hormones do increase breast cancer incidence in a significant way, then they represent a serious public health problem.

Exogenous oestrogens, for purposes of discussion, may be conveniently divided into two classes: those used in birth control, and those used for replacement therapy in women with natural or surgical menopause.

Interpretation of studies relating breast cancer to oral contraceptive use in necessarily fraught with hazard. Most reported investigations are case-control studies, with their attendant special qualifications. Oral contraceptives are frequently combinations of oestrogens and progestins, with potentially offsetting effects. Finally, if exogenous oestrogens do bear a causal relation to breast cancer, the relation might only manifest itself in select sub-populations, and might only be visible after a long latency period.

Oral contraceptive use and breast cancer risk have recently been reviewed (Kelsey, 1981). The majority of case-control studies to date do not implicate oral contraceptives as a causative agent in breast cancer, at least in the general population Two population-based studies (Royal College of General Practitioners, 1981; Vessey et al, 1981), showed no significant trend towards increased breast cancer risk in large groups of women receiving oral contraceptives.

Intriguingly, some case control studies (reviewed by Kelsey, 1981) have pointed out two sub-populations that may be at increased risk: firstly, women taking oral contraceptives for relatively long duration; and secondly, women taking oral contraceptives prior to their first childbirth. These two groups will require special consideration in future studies. At present, however, no special recommendations can be made to either group, given the lack of conclusive data.

The role of replacement oestrogens is controversial even if one excludes the question of breast cancer risk. The relative risks of uterine cancer (probably increased by replacement oestrogens) and bone and vascular degenerative disorders (probably decreased by replacement oestrogens) are hotly debated (see Ch. 7). The risk of developing breast cancer with replacement oestrogens may be modestly increased in the general population (reviewed by Kelsey, 1981). Breast malignancy incidence may be significantly increased in women receiving replacement oestrogens following a surgical menopause (Hoover et al, 1981; Brinto et al, 1981), and in postmenopausal nulliparous women receiving replacement oestrogens. These subpopulation deserve special attention.

Theories explaining the steroid hormone–breast cancer link

Numerous models for the association between oestrogens and breast cancer have been proposed over the years, some based on epidemiological observation and some based on laboratory investigation. They have foundered, by and large, on the conflicting laboratory data available from multiple endocrinological studies (reviewed by Korenman, 1980). Suffice it to say that current evidence does not convict the oestrogens of being tumour inducers, at least in the classic sense of tumour-inducing carcinogens. Circulating and excreted oestrogens, of any type, are not consistently elevated in breast cancer patients. Two proposed models (Korenman, 1980; Drife, 1981) view oestrogens as tumour promoters (agents that increase the risk of cancer in patients previously exposed to an inducing agent). Korenman's 'Oestrogen Window' hypothesis proposes that during certain time periods in the female reproductive life, there is increased risk ('open windows') of carcinogenesis, and that these 'windows' are periods of unopposed oestrogenic stimulation of the breast. The hypothesis is summarised in Table 36.2.

A variation on Korenman's theme is offered by Drife (1981), who suggests that pregnancy irreversibly alters the breast, making its lobules responsive to circulating progesterone present during the menstrual cycle. This proges-

Table 36.2 Estrogen window hypothesis

1. Human breast cancer is induced by carcinogens in a susceptible mammary gland.
2. Unopposed estrogenic stimulation is the most favorable state for induction.
3. There is a long latency between induction of tumor and clinical expression.
4. The duration of the estrogen window determines risk.
5. Inducibility declines with establishment of normal ovulatory menses and becomes very low during pregnancy.

(Reproduced with permission from Pike et al 1981 Hormones and Breast Cancer. Cold Spring Harbor Laboratory).

terone responsiveness would decrease or oppose the increased risk of developing breast cancer associated with endogenous or exogenous oestrogens.

STEROID HORMONE RECEPTORS IN HUMAN BREAST CANCER

Introduction

While the exact role of steroids in the aetiology of breast cancer remains uncertain, their actions in established breast cancer are better known. This is due largely to the discovery and exploitation of breast tumour steroid receptors, particularly oestrogen receptor (ER) and progesterone receptor (PgR).

Steroid receptor analysis has been a powerful tool for the researcher and a potent aid for the clinician. Our knowledge of the inner workings of the breast cancer cell has increased enormously over the past two decades. Steroid receptor determinations have altered our views of breast cancer biology, pathology, prognosis, and treatment. In this section we shall review the revolution brought about by steroid receptor investigations.

Steroid receptor measurements

While steroid receptor determinations have been performed on all the general steroid classes, interest has centred on oestrogen and progesterone receptors. Steroid receptor assays commonly measure binding of a radiolabelled steroid either to tissue slices or to soluble cytosol proteins. Oestrogen receptor may be measured by a multitude of techniques (reviewed by Chamness & McGuire, 1979), but are most commonly determined by either sucrose density gradient centrifugaion or the dextran-coated charcoal technique. Both methods are in widespread use, and provide readily reproducible results in trained hands. Oestrogen receptor assays may report either qualitative (positive versus negative) or quantitative results, and may be used to measure cytoplasmic receptor or receptor translocated to the nucleus. At present several groups are actively investigating the use of monoclonal antibodies to steroid receptors; their eventual widespread use may make present methods obsolete.

Progesterone receptor assays currently employed measure cytoplasmic receptor; measures of the nuclear form has not been reproducibly documented to date. Sucrose density gradients are the present method of choice for PgR determinations.

Steroid receptor physiology in breast cancer

Unlike polypeptide hormones, the classic steroid hormone interaction is intracytoplasmic rather than at the cell membrane. Steroids freely cross the cell membrane and enter the tumour cytoplasm. In breast cancer patients with low circulating 17β-oestradiol (E_2) levels, the tumour itself may synthesise the steroid by aromatisation of testosterone and androstenedione (Adams & Li, 1975; Varela & Dao, 1978) or by conversion from oestrone (Wilking et al, 1980). The significance of such intratumor synthesis is uncertain, though recent evidence suggests a relation between the ability to transform precursors and steroid receptor levels (Wilkins et al, 1980; Miller, et al, 1981).

Steroid hormone actions are mediated through cytoplasmic steroid receptors. One of these receptors — that for oestrogen — has become the centre piece of efforts to understand steroid actions in breast cancer. ER is a cytosolic protein with high affinity for 17β-oestradiol and lesser affinity for other steroid hormones and for nonsteroidal anti-oestrogens. Cytoplasmic ER levels may be regulated by testosterone (Zava & McGuire, 1977), progesterone (Hsueh et al, 1976), insulin (Butler et al, 1981), and cyclic adenosine 3', 5'-monophosphate (cAMP) (Cho-Chung et al, 1981). Furthermore, oestradiol may influence the levels of its own receptor (Edery et al, 1981).

Upon binding E_2, cytoplasmic ER undergoes significant changes. These changes have been characterised (Jungblut et al, 1979) as an increase in 'nucleotropy' (the ability of receptor to translocate to the nucleus) and an ability to 'activate' the receptor, i.e. an enhanced ability to induce DNA transcription in the nucleus. Neither nucleotropy nor activation are well understood. It has been suggested that the steroid–steroid receptor interaction produces a specific allosteric confirmational change (Bullock et al, 1978), and that differences in response to E_2, other steroids, and anti-oestrogens is due to differing allosteric changes (Rochefort & Borgna, 1981). Translocated ER's interaction with the

Table 36.3

Oestrogen-regulated proteins	Reference
DNA polymerase α	Edwards et al, (1980)
Thymidine kinase	Bronzert et al, (1981)
Progesterone receptor	Horwitz et al, (1975)
24 K	Edwards et al, (1980)
54 K	Adams et al, (1980)
Oestrogen-induced protein	Kaye et al, (1980)
Endogenous peroxidase	Anderson et al, (1979)
Lactalbumin	Woods et al, (1977)
Plasminogen activator	Butler et al, (1979)

DNA-histone complex awaits elucidation. The results of the interaction are several, and have been listed in Table 36.3. As a brief perusal of this list suggests, E_2 influences or is related to an astonishing range of cell functions, including cell proliferation, nucleotide salvage pathways, other steroid receptors, and fibrinolytic activity. Some oestrogen-regulated proteins (24K, 54K, oestrogen-Induced Protein) are unknown quantities at present, and the subject of much active research.

Steroid receptors, tumour pathology, and natural history

There are fundamental pathological differences between ER-positive and ER-negative tumours. These differences are reflected not in histological type (see Rosen et al, 1975) but in more sophisticated determinations of cell morphology and in cell kinetics, and in the biology of the tumours.

A consistent finding in cell morphology studies has been that ER-negative tumours tend to be less well-differentiated than ER-positive tumours, and that other negative prognostic characteristics tend to clump in ER-negative tumour populations. ER-negative tumours have greater nuclear and cellular atypia, higher number of mitoses, less tumour elastica, greater tumour necrosis, greater lymphoid infiltration of tumour, and less tubule formation (Antoniades & Specter, 1979; Rolland et al, 1980; Fisher et al, 1981). Few studies have considered cell morphology in light of steroid receptors other than ER. One study that did (Wurz et al, 1980) found that only 8 per cent of ER-negative tumours were well or moderately differentiated, as opposed to 59 per cent of tumours with multiple assayable steroid receptors.

Flow cytometry and cell kinetic studies have added to this light microscopic picture. ER-negative tumours are more aneuploid than ER-positive tumours (Muss et al, 1980), and have higher thymidine labeling indices (TLI) (Meyer et al, 1977). Of biological import is the recent observation that TLI in breast tumours is related not only to ER status but also to menopausal status: ER-negative, premenopausal patients have the highest proliferative activity (Bertuzzi et al, 1981).

The differences seen between ER-negative and ER-positive patients at a cellular level have functional correlates in the natural history of the disease. ER-negative tumours are more likely to metastasise to visceral organs than ER-positive tumours; ER-positive tumours more commonly spread to bone (Stewart et al, 1981). ER-positive patients have a longer disease-free interval (Knight et al, 1977) and better overall survival (Bishop et al, 1979) than ER-negative patients. PgR-positive patients also appear to have longer disease-free interval after surgery, and improved overall survival (Saez et al, 1981).

Summarising the pathology and natural history of breast cancer, we can state that steroid receptor status defines (albeit broadly) two major biological subsets of the disease. ER-negative tumours are characterised by aggressive, malignant features. ER-positive tumours appear to the laboratory investigator, the pathologist, and the clinician, to pursue a more benign and gradual course.

ENDOCRINE THERAPY OF BREAST CANCER

Principles of endocrine therapy of breast cancer

The endocrine manipulability of breast cancer is an old observation. The English surgeon Beatson produced remission of metastatic breast cancer in the 1890s with ovariectomy. Systematic exploitation of this effect occured in the 1950s with Huggins & Dao's (1954) experience with ovariectomy and Huggins & Bergenstal's (1951) experience with adrenalectomy.

Successes (and failures) with surgical ablation in disseminated breast cancer led to attempts at predicting who might respond best to therapy. Surgical ablation of endocrine organs produced (and produces) clinical responses in less than a third of patients ,more commonly in postmenopausal women and in women with a longer disease-free interval between primary surgery and diagnosis of metastasis. The development of oestrogen receptor analysis in the late 1960s and early 1970s provided a useful framework for earlier clinical observations. An international symposium held in 1974 (McGuire et al, 1975) summarised the basic findings relating ER and response to therapy in metastatic breast cancer. These findings have been amplified and extended in subsequent years, and collectively emphasise the need for steroid receptor analysis in all cases of breast cancer.

ER is positive in about two-thirds of sampled breast cancers. Women with ER-positive tumours respond to hormonal manipulation in 50–60 per cent of cases. ER-negative tumours respond to hormonal manipulation in less than 10 per cent of cases. There is a good correlation between ER values of primary and metastatic tumours in cases where there has been no hormonal therapy between the times of the two biopsies. ER determinations on the primary tumour accurately predict both the ER status and endocrine responsiveness of metastatic tumour. ER values tend to increase with age, ER-negative tumours being more common in premenopausal and less common in postmenopausal women. ER-negative is strong evidence against the likelihood of responding to a hormonal manipulation. ER-positivity by itself is less selective in determining response. One method of improving the predictability of response, originally proposed at the 1974 symposium, is to perform a quantitative ER on the tumour specimen. Response to hormonal manipulation increases directly with quantitative ER value.

Increasing knowledge of the cell physiology of ER has added to our ability to predict endocrine responsiveness in breast cancer. ER is translocated to the nucleus by E_2, where it interacts with nuclear DNA. One of the products of this interaction is PgR. Both nuclear ER (Fazekas & MacFarlane, 1981) and PgR (Horwitz et al, 1975) have been measured in breast cancer, and offer some measure of the completeness of the ER pathway in the tumour. Patients with measurable nuclear ER and PgR have higher response rates than patients having only cytoplasmic ER. In one combined series, 77 per cent of ER-positive, PgR-positive patients responded to endocrine manipulation, versus only 27 per cent of ER-positive, PgR-negative patients (Osborne et al, 1980). These data suggest the need for a biologically intact oestrogen receptor pathway if an endocrine manipulation of metastatic breast cancer is to succeed.

Although no single test offers complete sensitivity and specificity in predicting endocrine responsiveness, the following recommendations provide a basic framework for hormonal manipulation of metastatic breast cancer. Firstly, samples of primary breast cancer should be submitted for steroid receptor analysis on all patients. Secondly, steroid receptor analysis should include, in addition to qualitative ER, either quantitative ER, PgR determination, or (if available) both. Thirdly, ER-negative patients with metastatic breast cancer should not receive endocrine manipulation as initial therapy of their disease. Hormonal manipulation should be offered only to those patients with steroid receptor-positive tumours. Patients with unknown or borderline steroid receptor values may receive hormonal manipulation.

Treatment modalities in hormone-responsive breast tumours

Steroid receptor analysis has pinpointed a group of patients likely to benefit from endocrine manipulation. It does not spacify which treatment modality is best for the individual patient. Since the pioneering surgical manipulations of the 1950s, a host of new endocrine therapies for breast cancer has sprung up. A bewildering array of options is now available to the physician treating metastatic breast cancer. We will not examine exhaustively each of these treatments;

Table 36.4 Endocrine therapy of metastatic breast cancer — treatment options

Ablative	Additive
Surgical	Oestrogens (Diethylstilboestrol)
Ovariectomy	Progestins (Medroxyprogesterone acetate)
Adrenalectomy	Androgens
Hypophysectomy	Antiestrogens (Tamoxifen)
	Glucocorticoids
Medical	
Aminoglutethimide	
Radiotherapy	
Ovarian irradiation	

interested readers are referred to a review by Osborne & McGuire (1982) and to the standard oncology textbooks. Instead we will discuss the modalities available in a brief and general sense.

The hormonal therapy of metastatic breast cancer is conveniently divided into ablative and additive. These are listed in Table 36.4.

Ablative therapy

The classic endocrine treatments of disseminated breast cancer, developed in the 1950s, were ablative and surgical. These modalities have provided the standard against which all subsequent treatments have been measured. All three surgical ablative therapies (ovariectomy, adrenalectomy, and hypophysectomy) have similar response rates, with between 30 and 40 per cent of previously untreated patients having objective tumour responses. Between 50 and 60 per cent of ER-positive, previously untreated patients will respond to surgical ablative therapy. Duration of response to ablative therapy varies, but averages between 1 and 2 years, with some patients having a prolonged response. Soft tissue, bony, and solitary lung metastases respond more frequently than visceral metastases, though this may in part be a function of the ER-negative predominance seen in visceral metastases. Patients responding to one surgical manipulation have a good chance of responding to a second surgical (or other hormonal) manipulation. After failure of an initially successful hormonal manipulation as many as one-half of patients will respond to a second type of hormonal therapy.

Ablative surgical manipulation presumably acts through removal of the hormones stimulating breast tumours. Ovariectomy (surgical castration) in the premenopausal and perimenopausal women drastically decreases circulating oestradiol. Adrenalectomy removes steroid precursors of oestradiol that may be converted either in the adrenal gland, in peripheral fat, or in the tumour itself. Hypophysectomy depresses steroid synthesis by removal of trophic hormones. Another mechanism by which hypophysectomy might act — removal of prolactin — has not been borne out in clinical observations: patients may actually have elevated prolactin levels after hypophysectomy. As surgical ablative therapies are successful primarily with ER-positive tumours, a major (and unproven) assumption has been that the ER apparatus is somehow involved in tumour regression.

If surgical ablative therapies have similar actions and results, how then to prefer the use of one over another? The answer to this question lies primarily in the relative risks of the various procedures. The risks of ovariectomy are those involved with the operation itself, making it the endocrine modality of choice in the premenopausal women. Ovarian ablation by radiation is not to be preferred to surgical therapy: treatment is prolonged and tumour response delayed. Radiation castration should be limited to those patients unable to undergo surgical castration.

Though adrenalectomy, unlike ovariectomy, is useful in the postmenopausal patient, it is a more hazardous operation. In addition to the usual surgical complications, adrenalectomised patients are at permanent risk for adrenal insufficiency, and must receive both glucocorticoid and mineralocorticoid therapy for life (Kennedy, 1974).

Both the risk and the permanency of surgical adrenalectomy may be avoided by the use of aminoglutethimide (reviewed by Santen, 1981). Aminoglutethemide, an oral anticonvulsant, blocks cytochrome p-450-mediated steroid hydroxylation at two important steps. The conversion of cholesterol to pregnenolone is blocked, creating a 'medical adrenalectomy.' Furthermore, the drug inhibits aromitisation of androgens to oestrogens. This latter action may be of importance in patients in whom aromitisation to E_2 occurs in fat or tumour. Though the drug is not without toxicity (lethargy, ataxia, weight gain, and a morbiliform skin rash may be seen), its efficacy in breast cancer clearly is equal to that of surgical adrenalectomy.

As with surgical adrenalectomy, the medically adrenalectomized patient should receive replacement glucocorticoids (usually hydrocortisone 40–60 mg daily). Hydrococortisone has the added benefit of preventing a rise in ACTH, which might otherwise overcome the aminoglutethimide-induced block in steroid synthesis. Medical adrenalectomy undoubtedly should replace surgical adrenalectomy in the years ahead.

Hypophysectomy, though similar to other surgical manipulations for tumour response, is considerably more dangerous. Endocrine deficits such as diabetes insipides, hypoadrenalism, and hypothyroidism, necessitate replacement therapy. Meningitis, rhinorrhoea, haemorrhage, loss of vision, and impairment of taste, may be seen following surgery, and a rare patient may die as a direct result of the operation. Pituitary ablation should be considered only as a third-line therapy (at best) in patients previously responding to hormonal manipulation.

Additive therapy

Additive hormonal therapy for metastatic breast cancer has been used throughout the twentieth century. Recent years have seen the addition of both new forms of additive therapy and new ways of using old forms. Types of additive therapy include oestrogens, antioestrogens, progestins, androgens, and glucocoticoids.

The method of action of all additive therapies is uncertain. As with ablative therapies, additive therapies are successful in a significant proportion of ER-positive cases and useless for most ER-negative tumours. An assumption derived in part from this observation is that additive therapies must interact — directly or indirectly — with the oestrogen receptor apparatus.

Oestrogens are the oldest form of additive therapy for metastatic breast cancer. As with most additive therapies, the method of action for oestrogens is uncertain. Administered in vitro, E_2 will suppress DNA synthesis in pharmacological doses and stimulate it at physiological concentrations (Lippman & Bolan, 1975). One suggested mechanism for this dose-response effect involves decreased nuclear binding of steroid receptor when exposed to pharmacological E_2 concentrations (Kiang & Kennedy, 1976), though this mechanism has not been demonstrated convincingly in breast tumours.

Diethylstilboestrol (DES) has been the most frequently used oestrogen for additive therapy. In unselected postmenopausal women it produces responses in about one-third of cases, a percentage increased with ER-positivity. 'Tumour flare,' with hypercalcaemia, bone pain, and transient tumour growth, may be seen initially after beginning therapy. Tumour flare — which may be seen with all additive therapy — is not a reason to stop treatment, as patients with it frequently respond to hormonal therapy. Tumour response, when seen, is usually in the form of a partial remission. Its onset may be slow, with maximum anti-tumour effect sometimes taking several months to occur.

Patients receiving additive oestrogen may suffer from a number of side-effects, including gastrointestinal upset, skin hyperpigmentation, breast enlargement, vaginal discharge, stress incontinence, and cardiovascular side-effects. Gastrointestinal side-effects in particular are a frequent cause for drug withdrawal.

Anti-oestrogens have gradually supplanted oestrogens in the management of postmenopausal women with ER-positive metastatic tumours. Tamoxifen — the prototype drug in this class — has been compared with DES in a randomised, prospective trial (Ingle et al, 1981). This drug is of equal efficacy to DES, and on the whole is better tolerated. Tamoxifen has seen limited use in premenopausal women with ER-positive tumours. Early reports in small numbers of patients suggest that it has similar effectiveness to ovariectomy (Mourisden et al, 1978). Such comparisons require extensive confirmation in randomised prospective trials before tamoxifen can be recommended for routine use in premenopausal women. Recent crossover trials comparing anti-oestrogen therapy and medical adrenalectomy suggest that some patients failing tamoxifen will subsequently respond to aminoglutethimide. The converse does not appear to occur, leading to the recommendation that anti-oestrogen therapy should precede medical adrenalectomy in the postmenopausal women (Smith et al, 1981).

Anti-oestrogens may have several methods of action. Tamoxifen competes with E_2 for binding to ER and can induce PgR in vitro (Horwitz & McGuire, 1979). Tamoxifen, like additive oestrogens in high concentration, may interfere with nuclear processing of the ER complex, a function perhaps related to differences in salt extractability seen with the anti-oestrogen receptor complex (Katzenellenbogen et al, 1980). Tamoxifen also decreases intracellular thymidine pools (Lippman & Aitken, 1980) and cytoplasmic ER levels (Katzenellenhogen et al, 1979). An unconfirmed report suggests that there may be a high-affinity binding site for anti-oestrogens separate from ER (Sutherland et al, 1980).

Less commonly used as additive therapies are progestins and androgens. The mechanism of action of the former is unknown; the latter may act by depleting cytosolic ER (Zava & McGuire, 197). Progestins (the common preparation being medroxyprogesterone acetate — MPA) in high doses have enjoyed recent popularity in clinical trials (DeLana et al, 1979), with response rates equal to the best of other hormonal manipulations. Large multi-institutional trials are now underway in several countries testing the efficacy of MPA. Androgens are beneficial in a smaller fraction of patients than the other additive (or ablative) therapies, and in addition have the unpleasant side-effect of virilisation. Only about 20 per cent of unselected patients respond to androgen therapy.

One final additive therapy deserves brief mention. Glucocorticoids such as prednisone produce an objective tumour response in 5–10 per cent of patients. Their routine use cannot be recommended: several better endocrine manipulations are available, and the toxicity of long-term steroid therapy is unacceptable. Use of these agents ahould be limited to those specific instances (brain metastasis and hypercalcaemia) where maximum benefit may be derived.

General recommendations

Endocrine therapy, whether additive or ablative, should be limited to those patients most likely to respond; i.e. to steroid receptor-positive patients. ER-negative patients with metastatic disease are best served with chemotherapy rather than hormonal therapy. After institution of endocrine therapy, it may be necessary to observe the patient for as long as 3 months for a beneficial response. Patients failing initial endocrine therapy should proceed to chemotherapy; patients failing hormonal therapy after an initial beneficial reponse may benefit from a second hormonal intervention, and should receive a second-line endocrine therapy.

Adjuvant endocrine therapy

Two recent trials have included hormonal manipulation in adjuvant treatment following primary surgery. The National Surgical Adjuvant Breast Project (Fisher et al, 1981) compared L-phenylalanine mustard and 5-fluorouracil with and without tamoxifen; Hubay et al used cyclophosphamide, methotrexate, and 5-fluorouracil with and without tamoxifen. The results from both groups suggest that combined hormonal and chemotherapy is superior to chemotherapy. As one might expect, the benefit of tamoxifen in both groups was confined to ER-positive (particularly menopausal) patients. It remains to be shown that the short-term benefit demonstrated in both trials can be translated into long-term survival advantages or cures.

A somewhat older trial coming to similar conclusions is of historical and conceptual interest, though perhaps not of practical clinical use. In a large group of women randomised to either receive or not receive adjuvant ovarian irradiation, the postmenopausal treatment group fared significantly better in terms of survival than the postmenopausal control group. The effect of radiotherapy on survival, it should be noted, was not measurable until 3 to 5 years of follow-up, emphasising the importance of study duration in reporting treatment results (Meakin et al, 1977).

CONCLUSION

Recent years have been a time of great progress and promise in the understanding of breast cancer. Our knowledge of the underlying causes of the disease, of the tumour itself, and of its treatment, is measurably greater than it was even 15 years ago. That steroid hormones are inextricably linked to the genesis and progress of the disease now seems undeniable, and might even be said to constitute the central thesis of breast cancer research. And if, as Ramazzini stated so long ago, the whole domain of truth has not yet been conquered, then at least some preminary forays have been crowned with victory.

REFERENCES

Adami H O, Rimsten A, Stenkvist B et al 1978 Reproductive history and breast cancer. Cancer 41: 747–757
Adams J B, Li K 1979 Biosynthesis of 17β-oestrodiol in human breast carcinoma tissue and a novel method for its characterization. British Journal of Cancer 31: 420–433
Bertuzzi A, Daidone M G, DiFronzo G, Silvestrini R 1981 Relationship among estrogen receptors, proliferative activity and menopausal status in breast cancer. Breast Cancer Research and Treatment 1: 253–262
Bishop H M, Elston C W, Blamey R W, Haybittle J L, Nicholson R I, Griffiths K 1979 Relationship of oestrogen-receptor status to survival in breast cancer. Lancet ii: 283–284
Bullock L P, Bardin C W, Sherman M R 1978 Androgenic, antiandrogenic, and synandrogenic actions of progestins: role of

steric and allosteric interactions with androgen receptors. Endocrinology 103: 1768–1782

Butler W B, Kelsey W H, Goran N 1981 Effects of serum and insulin on the sensitivity of the human breast cancer cell line MCF-7 to estrogen and antiestrogen. Cancer Research 41: 82–88

Chamness G C, McGuire W L 1979 Methods for analyzing steroid receptors in human breast cancer. In: McGuire W L (ed) Breast Cancer: Advances in Research and Treatment, Vol III, pp 149–197. Plenum Press, New York

Cho-Chung Y S, Clair T, Bodwin J S, Berghoffer B 1981 Growth arrest and morphologic changes of human breast cancer cells by dibutyryl (?) cyclic AMP and 1-arginine. Science 214: 77–79

DeLena M, Brembilla C, Valagussa P et al 1979 High-dose medroxprogesterone acetate in breast cancer resistant to endocrine and cytotoxic herapy. Cancer Chemotherapy and Pharmacology 2: 175–180

Drife J O 1981 Breast cancer, pregnancy, and the pill. British Medical Journal 283: 778–779

Edery M, Goussard J, Dehinnin L, Scholler R, Reiffsteck J, Drosdowsky M A 1981 Endogenous oestradiol-17β concentration in breast tumors determined by mass fragmentography and by radioimmunoassay: Relationship to receptor content. European Journal of Cancer 17: 115–120

Fazekas A G, MacFarlane J K 1981 Nuclear estradiol receptors and regression in human breast cancer. Proceedings AACR/ASCO 22: 13

Horwitz K B, McGuire W L 1979 Estrogen control of progesterone receptor induction in human breast cancer: role of nuclear estrogen receptor. Advances in Experimental Medicine and Biology 117: 95–110

Horwitz K B, McGuire W L, Pearson O H, Segeloff A 1975 Predicting response to endocrine therapy in human breast cancer: a hypothesis. Science 189: 726–727

Hsueh A J W, Peck E J, Clark J H 1976 Control of uterine estrogen receptor levels by progestrone. Endocrinology 98: 438–444

Huggins C, Bergenstal D M 1951 Inhibition of human mammary and prostatic cancers by adrenalectomy. Cancer Research 12 :134–141

Huggins C, Dao T L 1954 Characteristics of adrenal-dependent mammary cancer. Annals of Surgery 140: 497–501

Ingle J N, Ahmann D L, Green S J et al 1981 Randomized clinical trial of diethylstilbestrol versus tamoxifen in postmenopausal women with advanced breast cancer. New England Journal of Medicine 304: 16–21

Jungblut P W, Hughes H, Ganes J et al 1979 Mechanisms involved in the regulation of steroid receptor levels. Journal of Steroid Biochemistry 11: 273–278

Katzenellenbogen B S, Tsai T S, Tateo T, Katzenellenhogen J A 1979 Estrogen and antiestrogen action: studies in reproductive target tissue and tumors. Advances in Experimental Medicine and Biology 117: 111–132

Katzenellenbogen B S, Katzenellenbogen J A, Eckert R L et al 1980 Antiestrogen action in estrogen target tissues: receptor interactions and antiestrogen metabolism. Progress in Cancer Research and Therapy 14: 309–320

Kelsey J L 1979 A review of the epidemiology of human breast cancer. Epidemiologic Reviews 1: 74–109

Kelsey J L 1981 Epidemiological studies of the role of exogenous estrogens in the etiology of breast cancer. In: Pike M C , Siiteri P K, Welsch C W (eds) Banbury Report 8 pp 215–225. Hormones and Breast Cancer, Cold Spring Harbor Laboratory

Kennedy B J 1974 Hormonal therapies in breast cancer. Seminars in Oncology 1: 119–130

Kiang D T, Kennedy B J 1976 'Intranuclear' castration effect of high dose estrogens. Proceedings of AACR/ASCO 17: 194

Knight W A III, Livingston R B , Gregory E J, McGuire W L 1977 Estrogen receptor is an independent prognostic factor for early recurrence in breast cancer. Cancer Research 37: 4669–4671

Korenman S G 1980 The endocrinology of breast cancer. Cancer 46: 874–882

Korenman S G 1981 Reproductive endocrinology and breast cancer in women. In: Pike M C, Siiteri P K, Welsch C W, (eds) Banbury Report 8 pp 71–82. Hormones and Breast Cancer, Cold Spring Harbor Laboratory

Lilrenfeld A M, Coombs J, Bross I D J, et al 1975 Marital and

reproductive experince in a community-wide epidemiologic study of breast cancer. Johns Hopkins Medical Journal 136: 157–162

Lippman M E, Aitken S C 1980 Estrogen and antiestrogen effects on thymidine utilization by MCF-7 human breat cancer cells in tissue culture. Progress in Cancer Research and Therapy 14: 3–19

Lippman M E, 8olan G 1975 Oestrogen-responsive human breast cancer in long-term tissue culture. Nature 256: 592–595

MacMahon B, Cole P, Lin T M, et al 1970 Age at first birth and Breast cancer risk. Bulletin World Health Organization 43: 209–221

McGuire W L, Vollmer E P, Corbone P P 1975 Estrogen Receptors in Human Breast Cancer. Raven Press, New York

Meakin J W, Allt W E C, Beale G A et al 1977 Ovarian irradiation and prednisone following surgery for carcinoma of the breast. In: Salmon S E, Jones S E (eds) Adjuvant Therapy of Cancer. Elsevier, Amsterdam

Miller W R, Hawkins R A, Forrest A P M 1981 Steroid metabolism and oestrogen receptors in human breast carcinomas. European Journal of Cancer and Clinical Oncology 17: 913–917

Mouridsen H, Palshof T, Patterson J, Battersby L 1978 Tamoxifen in advanced breast cancer. Cancer Treatment Review 5: 131–141

Muss H B, Kute T R, Cooper M R, Marshall R C 1980 The correlation of estrogen and progesterone receptors with DNA histograms in patients with advanced breast cancer. Proceedings AACR/ASCO 21: 172

Meyer J S, Rao B R, Stevens S C, White W L 1977 Low incidence of estrogen receptor in breast carcinomas with rapid rates of cellular replication. Cancer 40: 2290–2298

Osborne C K, McGuire W L 1982 Endocrine therapy of breast cancer. In: Bardin C W (ed) Current Endocrinologic Therapy.

Obsborne C K, Yochmowitz M D, Knight W E III, McGuire W L 1980 The value of estrogen and progesterone receptors in the treatment of breast cancer. Cancer 46: 2884–2888

Ramazzini B 1964 Diseases of Workers. Translated by W C Wright, Hafner Publishing Co, NY

Rochefort H, Borgna J L 1981 Differences between oestrogen receptor activition by oestrogen and antioestrogen. Nature 292: 257–259

Rosen P P, Menedez-Botet C J, Nisselbaum J S, Urgen J A, Mike V, Fracchia A, Schweltz M K 1975 Pathological review of breast lesions analyzed for estrogen receptor protein. Cancer Research 35: 3187–3194

Royal College of General Practitioners 1981 Breast cancer and oral contraceptives: findings in Royal College of General Practioners' Study. British Medical Journal, 282: 2089–2093

Saez S, Chouvet C, Mayer M, Cheix F 1981 Estradiol and progesterone receptor (ER, PgR) as prognostic factors in human primary breast tumors. Proceedings AACR/ASCO 21: 139

Santen R J 1981 Suppression of estrogen with aminoglutethimide and hydrocortisone (Medical adrenalectomy) as treatment of breast carcinoma: a review. Breast Cancer Research and Treatment 1: 183–202

Smith T E, Harris A L, Morgen M et al 1981 Tamoxifen versus aminoglutethimide in advanced breast carcinoma: a randomized cross-over trial. British Medical Journal 283: 1432–1434

Sherman B M, Korenman S G 1974 Inadequate corpus luteum function: pathopysiological interpretation of human breast cancer epidemiology. Cancer 33: 1306–1312

Sherman B M, Wallace R B, Korenman S G 1982 Corpus luteum dysfunction and the epidemiology of breast cancer: a reconsideration. Breast Cancer Research and Treatment 1: 287–296

Stewart J F, King R J B, Sexton S A, Millis R R, Rubens R D, Hayward J L 1981 Oestrogen receptors, sites of metastatic disease and survival in recurrent breast cancer. European Journal of Cancer 17: 449–453

Sutherland R L, Murphy L C, Foo M S, Green M D, Whybourne A M 1980 High-affinity anti-oestrogen binding site distrinct from the oestrogen receptor. Nature 228: 273–275

Thein-Hlang, Thein-Maung Myint 1978 Risk factors of breast cancer in Burma. International Journal Cancer 21: 432–437

Tulinius H, Day N E, Johannisson G, et al 1978 Reproductive factors and risk for breast cancer in Iceland. International Journal Cancer 21: 742–730

Varela R M and Dao T L 1978 Estrogen synthesis and estradiol binding by human mammary tumors. Cancer Research 38: 2429–2433

Vessey M P, McPherson K, Doll R 1981 Breast cancer and oral contraceptives: findings in Oxford-Family Planning Association Contraceptive Study. British Medical Journal 282: 2093–2094

Wilkins N, Carlstrom K, Gustaffsson S A, Skodefors H, Tollbom O 1980 Oestrogen receptors and metabolism of oestrone sulphate in human mammary carcinomas. European Journal od Cancer 16: 1339–1344

Wurz H et al 1980 Correlation of steroid hormone receptor levels with histologic grading in human breast cancer. Klin Wochenschr 58: 643

Zava D T, McGuire W L 1977 Estrogen receptors in adrogen-induced breast tumor regression. Cancer Reseaech 37: 1608–1610

Endocrine consequences of female genital tract neoplasia

The four main groups of genital tract neoplasms that produce hormones are (1) the steroid-secreting tumours of the ovaries (which need to be distinguished clinically from benign ovarian hyperplasias and from adrenal tumours); (2) the chorionic gonadotrophin-secreting trophoblastic tumours; (3) the rare ovarian tumours, chiefly teratomas, that produce other hormones; and (4) a varied group of common tumours that rarely display paraneoplastic endocrine effects.

Introduction: ovarian steroid compartments affected by neoplasia

Ovarian and adrenal steroidogenesis

The ovary and the adrenal gland produce the steroid hormones important in gynaecological oncology. Their principal products (oestradiol and progesterone; cortisol and aldosterone) are unique, but generally their steroid pathways have more in common than different (Fig. 37.1). Moreover the minor steroids produced by the ovaries and the adrenals (androstenedione, oestrone and dehydroepiandrosterone) are of particular importance as indicators (and determinants — see Ch. 5) of cancer.

Androgen production can be predominantly along the $\triangle 5$ pathway through dehydroepiandrosterone or along the $\triangle 4$ pathway through androstenedione. Testosterone is the most potent androgen. Androstenedione is weaker, and dehydroepiandrosterone (DHA) and its sulphate have only very mild androgenic activity. Androgens in females are important when produced in excess or when production of oestrogens is compromised; androgens are also the essential precursors of oestrogens.

Production of an *oestrogen* depends on the loss of the 19-carbon residue and on desaturation or aromatisation of the A-ring. These steps yield the weak oestrogen oestrone from androstenedione, and the powerful oestrogen oestradiol from testosterone; oestradiol may also be produced from oestrone by its own 17β-oxidoreductase. The weakest oestrogen, oestriol, is mainly a metabolic product of oestrone and oestradiol.

The adrenal and ovarian steroids that circulate in the highest plasma concentrations are the sulphate conjugates dehydroepiandrosterone sulphate (DHAS) and oestrone sulphate. Tight binding to plasma albumin confers on them a long plasma half-life; glucuronide conjugates of the same steroids are more loosely bound and more readily excreted. DHA and its conjugates constitute the bulk of the urinary 17-ketosteroids; androstenedione and its metabolites also contribute.

Adrenal sex steroid production is influenced mainly by ACTH. Ovarian steroid production is dependent on gonadotrophin stimulation.

Normal ovarian endocrine function

The ovary has three steroidogenic compartments: developing follicles, which produce the oestrogen that dominates the follicular phase; the corpus luteum, which produces the progesterone and oestrogen of the luteal phase; and interstitial stromal cells, which produce androgens. Though compartmentalisation of steroid production, particularly when neoplasia occurs, is not absolute (Batta et al, 1980; Dennefors et al, 1980), the following generalisations form a framework for understanding the endocrine behaviour of most ovarian tumours.

The *follicle* consists of the granulosa cells around the oocyte and the immediately adjacent stroma, as it differentiates with follicle growth into the theca interna (Fig. 37.2a). Follicle growth depends on FSH and the oestrogen that the follicle produces in response to FSH. Follicles contain membrane FSH-receptors (FSH–R) on the granulosa cells and membrane LH-receptors (LH–R) on the theca interna cells. The weight of evidence favours the general concept that in the developing tertiary follicle androgen is produced by the theca interna through the $\triangle 5$ pathway to DHA and from there to androstenedione under the stimulus of LH; the granulosa cells aromatise androstenedione to oestrone, and testosterone to oestradiol,

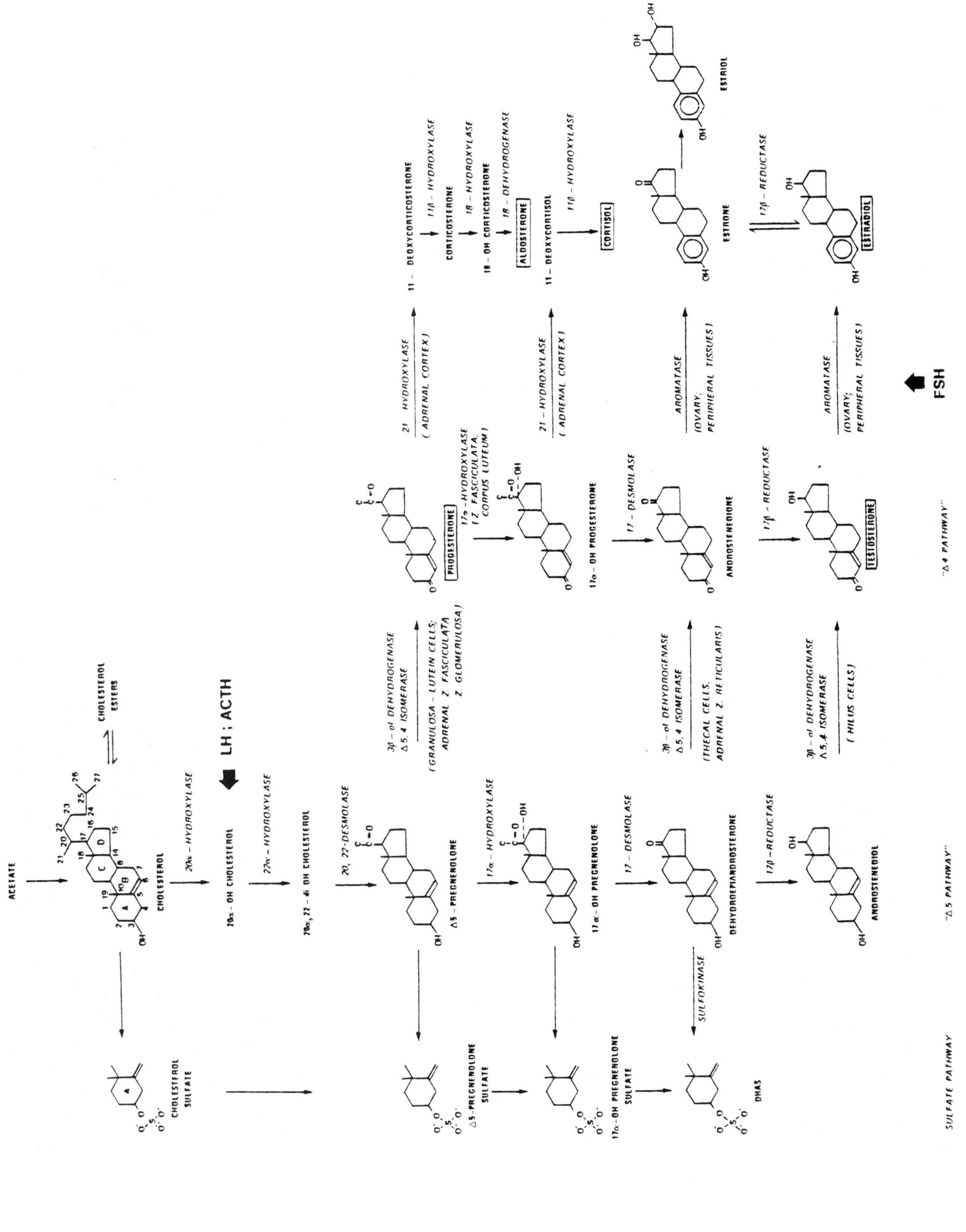
ACETATE
CHOLESTEROL
CHOLESTEROL ESTERS
20α - HYDROXYLASE
LH ; ACTH
20α - OH CHOLESTEROL
22α - HYDROXYLASE
20α, 22 - di OH CHOLESTEROL
20, 22-DESMOLASE
Δ5 - PREGNENOLONE
3β - ol DEHYDROGENASE
Δ 5, 4 ISOMERASE
(GRANULOSA - LUTEIN CELLS; ADRENAL Z. FASCICULATA Z. GLOMERULOSA)
PROGESTERONE
21 HYDROXYLASE
(ADRENAL CORTEX)
11 - DEOXYCORTICOSTERONE
11β - HYDROXYLASE
CORTICOSTERONE
18 - HYDROXYLASE
18 - OH CORTICOSTERONE
18 - DEHYDROGENASE
ALDOSTERONE
17α - HYDROXYLASE
17α - OH PREGNENOLONE
17α - HYDROXYLASE
(Z. FASCICULATA, CORPUS LUTEUM)
17α - OH PROGESTERONE
21 - HYDROXYLASE
(ADRENAL CORTEX)
11 - DEOXYCORTISOL
11β - HYDROXYLASE
CORTISOL
17 - DESMOLASE
DEHYDROEPIANDROSTERONE
3β - ol DEHYDROGENASE
Δ 5, 4 ISOMERASE
(THECAL CELLS, ADRENAL Z. RETICULARIS)
17 - DESMOLASE
ANDROSTENEDIONE
AROMATASE
(OVARY; PERIPHERAL TISSUES)
ESTRONE
ESTRIOL
17β - REDUCTASE
ANDROSTENEDIOL
3β - ol DEHYDROGENASE
Δ 5, 4 ISOMERASE
(HILUS CELLS)
17β - REDUCTASE
TESTOSTERONE
AROMATASE
(OVARY; PERIPHERAL TISSUES)
ESTRADIOL
17β - REDUCTASE
FSH
CHOLESTEROL SULFATE
Δ5 - PREGNENOLONE SULFATE
17α - OH PREGNENOLONE SULFATE
SULFOKINASE
DHAS
SULFATE PATHWAY
"Δ 5 PATHWAY"
"Δ 4 PATHWAY"

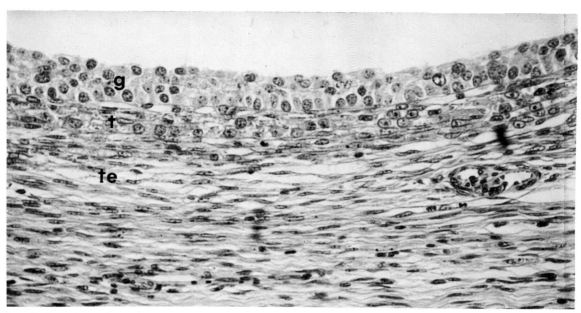

Fig. 37.2a Normal pre-ovulatory follicle. Cells of the theca interna (t) are engaged in active steroid synthesis, particularly androgens, and have plumper cytoplasm than the inactive stromal cells of the theca externa (te). The granulosa (g) layer is avascular; granulosa cells show nuclear crowding characteristic of preluteal architecture and are chiefly concerned with aromatization of thecal androgens to oestrogens (×200)

under the stimulus of FSH (Dorrington et al, 1975; Moon et al, 1978; Hillier et al, 1981). Recent evidence has made it clear that compartmentalisation of steroid production in the follicle is not quite as rigid as this scheme suggests (McNatty et al, 1979; Batta et al, 1980) and that other factors may contribute to the cooperation shown by the theca and the granulosa in oestradiol production (McNatty et al, 1980).

Androgens are deleterious to follicle growth, and promote atresia (Louvet et al, 1975). It seems, therefore, that the local ratio of oestrogen to androgen governs whether a follicle will grow or become atretic (Ross, 1976; Armstrong & Dorrington, 1977) and this in turn depends on the activity of granulosa cell FSH-dependent aromatase.

The larger follicles are capable of sequestering FSH in their antral fluid (McNatty et al, 1975) and, as well, antral fluid oestradiol concentrations reach up to 40 000 times plasma levels, both of which may enable continuing FSH action to take place as plasma FSH falls, and fewer and fewer follicles maintain a high oestrogen:androgen ratio. This sequestration of gonadotrophins and steroids in ovarian follicles may explain the occurrence of theca lutein cysts some time after evacuation of a hydatidiform mole (see below). Finally, in the normal menstrual cycle, one follicle outstrips the others in oestradiol production and growth and becomes the follicle destined to ovulate. Prolonged oestrogen action on the granulosa cells eventually induces the formation of granulosa cell LH–R in the pre ovulatory

Fig. 37.1 Steroid synthesis pathways. Acetate and cholesterol are substrates for steroid synthesis, which proceeds under the stimulus of LH in the ovaries and ACTH in the adrenal glands. Trophoblast requires cholesterol or its derivatives as substrate for steroid synthesis, which is not known to be under a tropic stimulus. The essential steps in the formation of pregnane (C–21), androstane (C–19), and oestrane (C–18) derivatives are each mediated by specific desmolases, which remove parts of the side chain progressively. The C–21 steroid △5-pregnenolone is a common precursor: its metabolism proceeds through other △5 steroids (the '△5 pathway') or through △4 steroids (the '△4 pathway'). △5 steroids are direct precursors of corresponding △4 steroids through at least three rather specific 3β-ol dehydrogenase/△5,4 isomerase enzyme systems, the tissue distribution of which is indicated. The adrenal glands, and perhaps also the ovaries, release steroid sulphates after conjugation of various precusors by sulphokinase; sulphated steroids in the adrenal glands are direct but inefficient substrates for △5 pathway enzymes (the 'sulphate pathway'). Important end products specific to ovary, adrenal or placenta are indicated in boxes. A very small amount of progesterone is released by the adrenal glands as well as by the ovaries; trophoblast lacks 17-hydroxylase and so produces progesterone as an end-product. Because 21-hydroxylase is normally confined to the adrenal glands, so too is production of aldosterone and cortisol. Aromatase is necessary for oestrogen production: it is FSH-dependent in the developing follicle, but not in peripheral adipose tissue or in trophoblast. Not shown is 16-hydroxylation of DHAS in the fetal liver: 16-OH DHAS (and probably DHAS, see text) is aromatizable substrate for trophoblast oestrogen synthesis (from Jansen & Shearman, 1981)

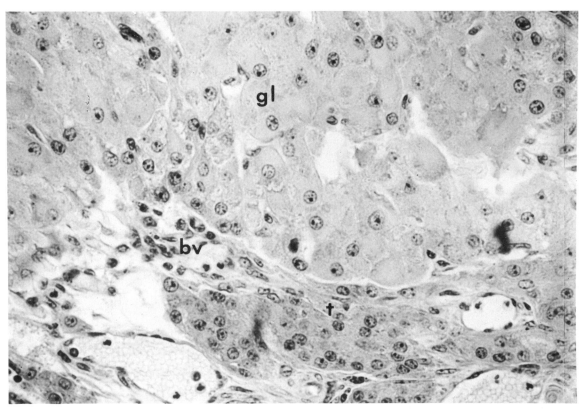

Fig. 37.2b Corpus luteum. Luteinised granulosa cells (gl) are now actively engaged in progesterone and 17α-hydroxyprogesterone synthesis. Blood vessels (bv) enter the tissue from the luteinised theca(t) (× 200)

follicle (Richards et al, 1976) and, with oestradiol production from the follicle now maximal, the midcycle LH surge begins.

The midcycle LH surge starts the luteinisation of, and the de novo steroid synthesis in, the granulosa cells (Richards, 1975; Rao et al, 1977). The granulosa cells exhibit 3β-ol dehydrogenase-△5,4 isomerase activity that differs from that of the theca (but resembles that of the adrenal gland) (Jones et al, 1968), in that it converts pregnenolone preferentially to progesterone. The switch from the △5 to the △4 pathway for steroid synthesis is also reflected by an increased output of 17α-hydroxprogesterone from the ovary.

Ovulation is followed by collapse of the follicle and further luteinisation of the granulosa as it becomes vascularised to form the *corpus luteum* (Fig. 37.2b). A whole new sequence of hormone-receptor interactions comes into play to cause the progesterone and 17α-hydroxprogesterone production that characterises the luteal phase.

The *ovarian interstitial stroma* provides the theca interna for the developing follicle, and in this respect the propensity of the interstitial cells to produce androgens through the △5 pathway under the influence of LH (Rice & Savard, 1966; Marsh et al, 1976) has already been described. During the menstrual cycle circulating androstenedione and testosterone derive about equally from the adrenals and from the interstitium of the ovaries (Mikhail,

1970; Abraham, 1974); the ovarian interstitial contribution to testosterone, androstenedione, and even DHAS, can be demonstrated by a slight mid cycle rise that accompanies the LH surge. However, it is during pregnancy (particularly molar pregnancy), after the menopause, in the polycystic ovary syndrome, and with ovarian tumours that the interstitium becomes most important endocrinologically.

In the midst of the interstitium, close to the hilus of the ovary, there are distinct cells that resemble the Leydig cells of the testis. These *hilus cells* share with Leydig cells a unique steroid 3β-ol dehydrogenase-△5,4 isomerase that appears to be capable of producing testosterone from △5 androstenediol (Jones et al, 1968).

Ovarian function in pregnancy

Pregnancy, with its chronically elevated levels of circulating hCG, has a powerful luteinising effect on the ovaries. Prolongation of the life of the corpus luteum is the first consequence of this (and a normal corpus luteum may simulate an ovarian tumour in the first trimester by becoming cystic) (Novak et al, 1975), but luteinisation also takes place in the theca surrounding atretic follicles and in the interstitial stroma (Nelson & Greene, 1958). When the luteinising stimulus is exceptionally severe, or the stromal compartment is unusually sensitive to normal amounts of hCG, thecal hyperplasia with luteinisation can occur. The

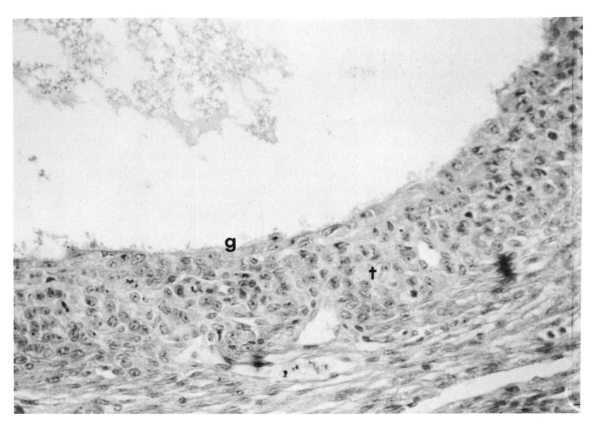

Fig. 37.2c Atretic follicle with prominent luteinised theca (t) and regression of the granulosa (g); androgen synthesis predominates (×200)

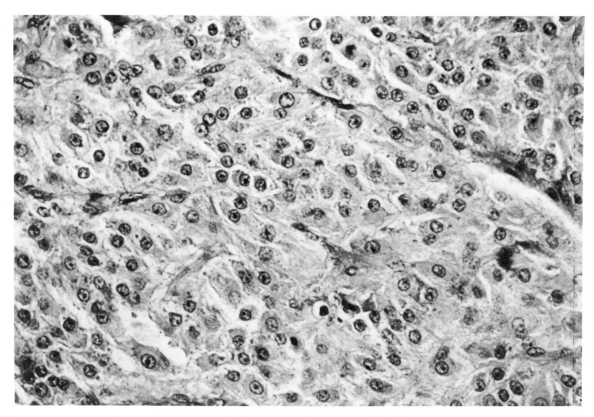

Fig. 37.2d Pregnancy luteoma with luteinized stromal cells; the tissue is well vascularised (×200)

resulting hyperthecosis can be predominantly around cystic atretic follicles (theca lutein cysts, or hyperreactio luteinialis — Fig. 37.2c), interstitial and focal (pregnancy luteoma — Fig. 37.2d), or may occur in relation to a functioning or nonfunctioning tumour in the ovary — a histological spectrum qualitatively similar, though quantitatively greater, than that found in the ovary in the non pregnant state.

Plasma free testosterone is normally unchanged in pregnancy (Rivarola et al, 1968), despite the considerable impact that hCG has on the ovarian stroma. Plasma total testosterone rises considerably, but this is accounted for by greatly increased sex hormone binding globulin (SHBG) production. Moreover, the normal placenta is thought to protect both the mother and a female fetus from possible virilisation, if for some reason testosterone production is abnormally high, by its efficient aromatising system, which converts testosterone to oestradiol (Hensleigh et al, 1975; Hensleigh & Woodruff, 1978).

Hyperplasia and luteinisation of interstitial thecal tissue in pregnancy (see above) occasionally produces a discreet ovarian tumour — a *pregnancy luteoma* — which may be palpable but which usually presents incidentally at Caesarean section or postpartum tubal ligation (Wagstaff, 1973; Garcia-Bunuel et al, 1975; Hensleigh & Woodruff, 1978). Histologically it is designated a stromal luteoma (Scully, 1977; Fig. 37.2d and also see below); its increased androgen secretion is indicated by occasional production of maternal virilisation and, less commonly, virilisation of a female fetus (Garcia-Bunuel et al, 1975; Scully, 1977; Hensleigh & Woodruff, 1978).

Pregnancy luteomas are multiple in at least half the cases (Scully, 1977). Even when only a single nodule is present, it is usual for the stroma of the same or the contralateral ovary to contain luteinised stromal cells or prominent theca-lutein cysts (Wagstaff, 1973). Spontaneous regression after pregnancy is invariable. Few patients give a history suggestive of previous endocrinopathy (Hensleigh & Woodruff, 1978). Only one case has been reported in association with trophoblastic disease: the luteoma was bilateral and was diagnosed at the time of hysterectomy (Garcia-Bunuel et al, 1975).

Theca-lutein cysts (hyperreactio luteinalis) occur commonly in molar pregnancy, but may occasionally also develop in association with multiple pregnancy (Caspi et al, 1973; Judd et al, 1973; Hensleigh & Woodruff, 1978) or rarely with normal pregnancy (Caspi et al, 1973; Hensleigh & Woodruff, 1978). Theca lutein cysts are considered further below.

Oocyte depletion and postmenopausal ovarian function

Attenuation of primordial follicle numbers through follicle growth and subsequent atresia or ovulation eventually depletes the ovary of responsive oocytes; oestrogen production fails, and menses cease — the menopause. Primordial follicles are still present at the onset of the menopause (Block, 1952), and as a group these follicles presumably represent the tail end of the distribution of gonadotrophin sensitivity. Longitudinal studies after the menopause (Brown, 1981) indicate that fluctuating ovarian steroid production, which apparently represents episodes of follicle development, can continue for months or years without producing menses. Indeed, under the stimulus of postmenopausal levels of gonadotrophins, such follicle development occasionally produces ovulation and uterine bleeding; but generally collective response of the follicles is insufficient, and their fate is atresia (Costoff & Mahesh, 1975).

With removal of oestradiol's negative feedback effects, large increases in FSH and LH production follow. The tonically elevated plasma gonadotrophins, particularly LH, constitute a striking stimulus to the remaining ovarian endocrine compartment — the interstitium — to produce androgens.

Compared with the premenopausal ovary, the postmenopausal ovary produces considerably less androstenedione — which indicates that the likely major premenopausal ovarian source of this hormone is from interstitium condensed around the follicles, the theca interna. Postmenopausally, adrenal androgen secretion is reduced, apparently due to a loss of an oestrogen trophic action (Abraham & Maroulis, 1975; Lobo et al, 1982), but nevertheless accounts for 70–85 per cent of circulating androstenedione levels (Judd et al, 1974; Vermeulen, 1976).

The position with testosterone is more complicated. Overall, plasma testosterone after the menopause is lowered only minimally (Judd, 1976); but ovarian testosterone production is increased (Judd et al, 1974; Judd, 1976, Greenblatt et al, 1976) — probably indicating the unprecedented LH stimulus to the hilus cells. Nevertheless the relative contribution of the adrenals and the ovaries to circulating testosterone remains 50 per cent for each, before and after the menopause (Judd, 1976; Vermeulen, 1976). The reason for this paradox is that plasma androstenedione is a major testosterone precursor, and the decrease in ovarian androstenedione production after the menopause is compensated for by an increase in direct ovarian testosterone production; only a small amount of direct adrenal testosterone secretion takes place (Baird et al, 1969).

The postmenopausal ovary produces minimal amounts of oestrone, and negligible amounts of oestradiol and progesterone (Judd et al, 1974; Vermeulen, 1976), although occasional exceptions are encountered (Longcope et al, 1980). Plasma oestrone, however, is only slightly lower postmenopausally than in the early follicular phase; it becomes the major circulating oestrogen. The main origin of this oestrogen is unique and important: the peripheral conversion, by adipose tissue aromatase, of androstenedione to oestrone.

Steroid production by dysgenetic gonads

The fibrous tissue of a streak gonad as classically found in ovarian dysgenesis (whether associated with short stature, Turner's Syndrome, or with normal or eunuchoid stature, 'pure gonadal dysgenesis') may be morphologically indistinguishable from normal ovarian stroma. Endocrinologically, however, the stroma differs subtly by not having been provided with the large number of theca interna cells with which many years of follicular activity and interstitial differentiation endow the stroma of normal postmenopausal ovaries; as a consequence the dysgenetic gonad's stroma may not have quite the propensity for androstenedione production that the postmenopausal ovary has (Hughesdon, 1978).

Hilus cells, though, are recognisable in the stroma of streaks both at birth and after puberty, and their androgen production may contribute at puberty to some sexual hair growth (Jones & Scott, 1971). In response to the high gonadotrophin levels of primary ovarian failure, hilus cell hyperplasia may take place (sometimes to the point of adenoma formation) and may cause clitoromegaly and hirsutism (Jones & Scott, 1971); the androgen produced is testosterone (Judd et al, 1970). The absence of germ cells and follicles from streak ovaries — a phenomenon that is not primary but occurs through total follicle atresia after birth (Jones & Scott, 1971) — means that ovarian oestrogen production is non existent. Occasional patients (usually with chromosomal mosaicism) retain a reduced complement of follicles to the time of menarche and so may present after this with a premature menopause rather than with primary amenorrhoea and infantilism.

Oestrogen production, with spontaneous breast development, has rarely been reported in patients with streak gonads and primary amenorrhoea (Saunders et al, 1975; Jones, 1976). One patient with 46,XX pure gonadal dysgenesis had a small number of follicles with presumably sufficient oestrogen to initiate thelarche but insufficient for menstruation (Jones, 1976), whereas three, all 46,XY, have had gonadoblastomas.

Testosterone production and virilisation can occur in phenotypic females who carry Y-chromosome material. Leydig cells are likely to be present in the gonads, either as hilus cells in streaks or in functioning testicular tissue, and respond to rising LH levels during late childhood. Leydig cells or luteinised stromal cells that produce testosterone (Rose et al, 1974) are a frequent component of gonadoblastomas (Scully, 1970), to which patients with Y-chromosomal material are highly predisposed (Manuel et al, 1976).

Extraglandular oestrogen production

The principal source of oestrogen after the menopause is aromatisation of circulating androstenedione to oestrone, and to a much lesser extent aromatisation of testosterone to oestradiol, in the adipocyte-supporting stroma of fat tissue (Nimrod & Ryan, 1975; MacDonald et al, 1978; Ackerman et al, 1981). Peripheral aromatisation is independent of FSH action (Folkerd et al, 1982).

The percentage of androstenedione converted to oestrone depends, firstly, on the quantity of adipose tissue available — that is, obesity (Rizkallah et al, 1975; MacDonald et al, 1978) — and, secondly, age (Grodin et al, 1973; Hemsell et al, 1974). So whereas about 1.3 per cent of androstenedione entering the circulation is converted to oestrone in young women (MacDonald et al, 1967), this rises to 2.7 per cent in postmenopausal women (Grodin et al, 1973) and continues to rise with advancing age (Hemsell et al, 1974). Recent evidence also indicates that overt diabetes mellitus is associated with increased levels of plasma oestrone independent of obesity and age (Deutsch & Benjamin, 1978). Oestrone derived by these means constitutes the major source of circulating oestradiol in postmenopausal women (Judd et al, 1982).

These causes of increased extraglandular oestrogen production are well known clinical associations of endometrial hyperplasia and adenocarcinoma. Of relevance here, though, is that this mechanism, extraglandular conversion of androgens to oestrogens, can substantially modify the biochemical and clinical expression of ovarian androgen-secreting tumours.

Sex steroid-producing ovarian and adrenal tumours

Stromal hyperplasia and hilus cell hyperplasia

After the menopause, depletion of responsive follicular units leaves the ovarian stroma as the receptive tissue on which elevated levels of pituitary gonadotrophins act (Fig. 37.3a); the physiological consequences of this have been described. Whereas it is clear that androstenedione and testosterone continue to be produced by stromal cells and hilus cells after the menopause, it is also established that normally the major tissue of origin of circulating androgens (and therefore their oestrogen metabolites) is the adrenal. Because of the LH-stimulus of the postmenopause, it is not surprising that cortical stromal hyperplasia (Fig. 37.3b), sometimes with luteinisation (Fig. 37.3c), is a common incidental pathological finding in the ovary (Yin & Sommers, 1961).

When cortical stromal hyperplasia with luteinisation is extensive (hyperthecosis), excessive ovarian steroid production is a logical consequence; but on the other hand much has been made of the difficulty in correlating clinical

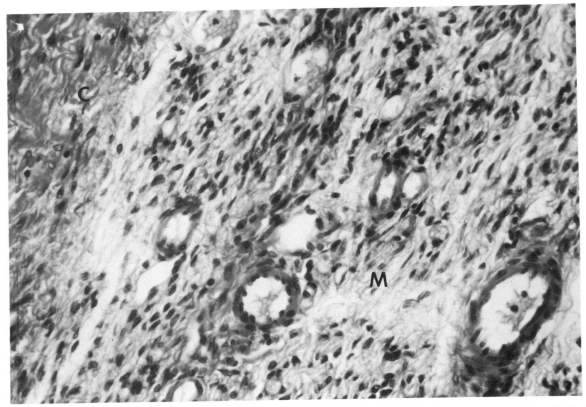

Fig. 37.3a Normal postmenopausal cortical (C) and medullary (M) stroma showing inactive stromal cells with small spindled nuclei (× 200)

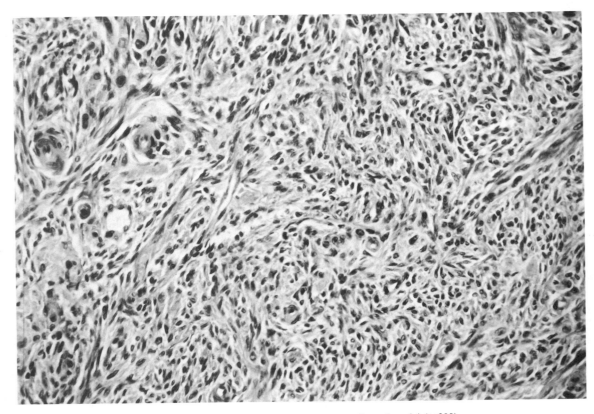

Fig. 37.3b Stromal hyperplasia showing accentuated whorled pattern and some rounding of nuclei (× 200)

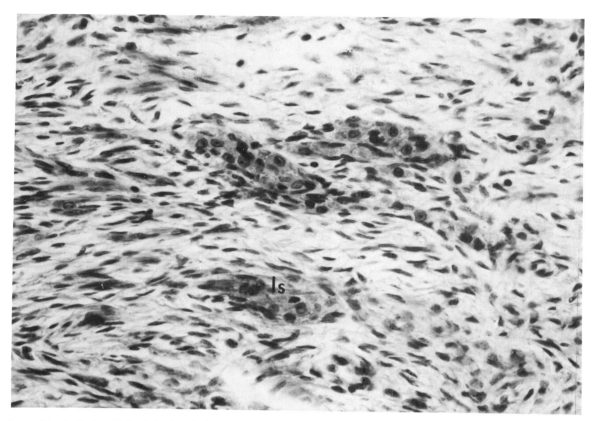

Fig. 37.3c Stromal hyperplasia with luteinization (ls) indicative of steroid synthesis (×200)

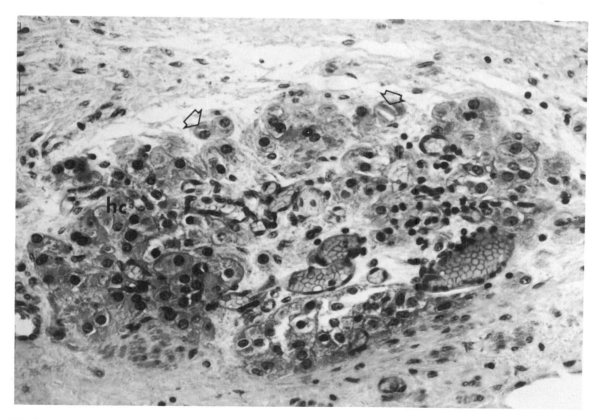

Fig. 37.3d Hilus cells (hc) are a normal constituent of the ovarian hilus, are identical to Leydig cells of the testis, synthesise testosterone, and occasionally have intracytoplasmic Reinke crystals (arrows). The same cells can differentiate elsewhere in the stroma in hyperplastic and neoplastic conditions (×200)

and biochemical evidence of steroid production with histological and histochemical observations on the ovarian stroma. Clearly, clinical expression will depend on the nature of the steroid or steroids produced (whether relatively impotent, like androstenedione, or potent, like testosterone), the production rate (governed by the size of the tumour and, in the case of feminising stromal tumours, the relationship between theca cells and granulosa cells), the availability of substrate (e.g. progesterone in pregnancy — Forest et al, 1978), the extent of peripheral steroid conversion (such as androstenedione to oestrone), and the level of tissue sensitivity to the circulating steroid. To this could be added the possibility that cortical stromal hyperplasia may merely be the result of particularly high LH levels, themselves perhaps caused by abnormal feedback by steroids not directly of ovarian origin.

Nevertheless a relationship between ovarian cortical stromal hyperplasia and postmenopausal endometrial hyperplasia and carcinoma is well established, and postmenopausal virilisation from stromal hyperthecosis is well described (Braithwaite et al, 1978). The predominant steroids produced are androgens: testosterone and, especially, androstenedione (Rice & Savard, 1966). In virilised patients urinary 17-ketosteroids are variably elevated.

Hilus cell (Leydig cell) hyperplasia (Fig. 37.3d) is distinctly less common than stromal hyperthecosis, but, because testosterone is produced preferentially, it is more likely to present clinically — both with virilisation and with endometrial hyperplasia (Taylor, 1966). Hilus cell hyperplasia is also dependent on high postmenopausal LH levels and may coexist with stromal hyperthecosis. Furthermore,

typical Leydig cells with Reinke crystals may occur in stroma well away from the hilus, presumably representing non-neoplastic transformation of stromal cells to Leydig cells (Sternberg & Roth, 1973).

Pure stromal tumours of the ovary

The close relationship of pure stromal neoplasms (fibromas, thecomas, so-called stromal luteomas and lipoid tumours, and Leydig-cell tumours) with their hyperplastic counterparts is illustrated by their benign nature, by their similar relatively high incidence in postmenopausal women (Fig. 37.4), and by their frequent bilaterality, multinodularity, and coexistence with non-neoplastic stromal or hilus cell hyperplasia (Scully, 1977; Sternberg & Dhurander, 1977). These obesrvations suggest strongly than an LH stimulus is important in their aetiology.

Pure *thecomas* (Fig. 37.5a) are commonly considered to be oestrogenic rather than androgenic (Sternberg & Dhurander, 1977). That this is normally due to direct oestrogen production has not often been shown for thecomas devoid of granulosa cell elements, and theoretical considerations make it likely that oestrogenic effects of pure thecomas are usually at least partly secondary to peripheral conversion of androstenedione to oestrone.

Androstenedione has been shown to be produced by those stromal tumours that have attained sufficient morphological evidence of steroid production to warrant the terms *stromal luteoma* or *lipoid tumour* (Fig. 37.5b) (Bonaventura et al, 1978); but such tumours may certainly sometimes also produce important quantities of other

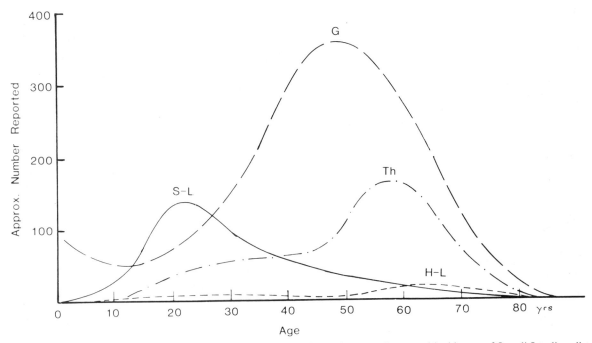

Fig. 37.4 Relative age-incidence of sex-cord stromal tumours of the ovary. Approximate total reported incidences of Sertoli-Leydig cell tumours (S-L), granulosa cell tumours (G), thecomas (Th) and hilus or Leydig cell tumours (H-L) derived from published series

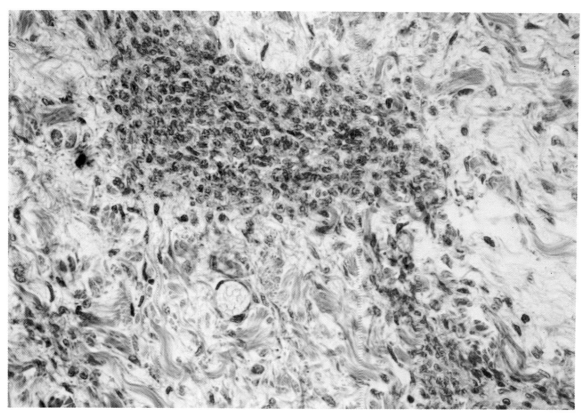

Fig. 37.5a Thecoma. Ovarian stromal neoplasia characterized by variable luteinisation of spindle-shaped cells. Androgen and/or oestrogen synthesis may occur, but cannot be predicted from the histological features (×200)

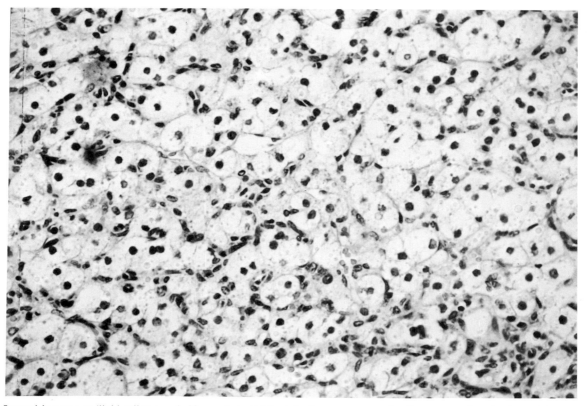

Fig. 37.5b Stromal luteoma or 'lipid cell tumour'. More substantial luteinisation causes stromal cells to accumulate fat, but, although often classified separately, there is no clear distinction between these and other stromal tumours; androgens most commonly predominate (×200)

androgens (Imperato-McGinley et al, 1981), oestrogens, (Reed et al, 1979) and even progestogens (Bonaventura et al, 1978; Weiland et al, 1978).

Because androstenedione is the predominant steroid, these tumours usually do not suppress plasma gonadotrophins. Urinary 17-ketosteroids are often elevated. Perhaps because they tend to occur in older women — in whom peripheral aromatisation of androgens to oestrogens could be expected to be efficient — most theca cell tumours, especially in older patients, are clinically oestrogenic rather than androgenic.

Leydig cell tumours, whether derived from hilus cells (*hilus cell tumours*) or from stromal cells (Sternberg & Roth, 1973; Roth & Sternberg, 1973) and irrespective of whether or not differentiation has proceeded to the point where Reinke crystals are found, typically have testosterone as their main steroid product (Rivarola et al, 1968; Casthely et al, 1977; Bonaventura et al, 1978; Weiland et al, 1978). Consequently, virilisation manifests clinically; but paradoxical uterine bleeding may occur (Novak & Mattingly, 1960; Dunnihoo et al, 1966; Mandel et al, 1981), either because of extraglandular conversion of androgens to oestrogens or because of direct oestradiol secretion (Weiland et al, 1978; Davidson et al, 1981).

Hilus cell tumours have been reported to suppress plasma gonadotrophins (Katz et al, 1977; Casthely et al, 1977), presumably because testosterone and oestradiol predominate over androstenediol and oestrone. Urinary 17-ketosteroids are usually normal. Hilus cells are stimulated by LH, and the vast majority of hilus cell tumours occur after the menopause (Fig. 37.4; Dunnihoo et al, 1966), when LH levels are elevated. Hilus cell tumours are extremely rare in women of reproductive age who do not give a history of primary ovarian failure (Lyons et al, 1980) or long-standing ovarian hyperandrogenism (Goldberg & Woodruff, 1977; Katz et al, 1977), in both of which LH levels are elevated; however, a recently reported case occurred in a 21-year-old with normal menses before and after oral contraception, the use of which immediately preceded presentation and diagnosis (Sutton et al, 1981).

Corticosteroid production from an ovarian tumour is a theoretical possibility in only two situations: acquisition of the hydroxylases needed for this route of progesterone metabolism by a functioning ovarian stromal neoplasm ('ectopic' corticosteroid synthesis); and neoplastic transformation of ectopic adrenal tissue.

Small nodules of accessory adrenal cortical tissue are identifiable in perhaps 25 per cent of total hysterectomy and bilateral salpingo-ovariectomy specimens (Falls, 1955), but their location is invariably along the infundibulopelvic fold of the broad ligament; adrenal rests are not found within the ovarian stroma. Hyperplasia or neoplasia of broad ligament adrenal rests has been reported in association with prolonged ACTH stimulation in Nelson's syndrome (Baranetsky et al, 1979; Verdonk et al, 1982).

One reported ovarian stromal tumour has been shown to have produced an elevated plasma cortisol and urinary free cortisol (Marieb et al, 1983); the patient manifested a florid Cushing's syndrome, ovarian vein plasma cortisol (but not ACTH) was high, and histologically the ovarian tumour recapitulated adrenal cortex in architecture. There are also two reports of virilising ovarian stromal tumours with *in vitro* evidence for cortisol and corticosterone production (Motlik & Starka, 1973; Imperato-McGinley et al, 1981).

Ovarian sex cord tumours

Granulosa cell tumours that do not contain theca cells (pure granulosa cell tumours; Fig. 37.6a) are less likely to be oestrogen-producing than granulosa cell tumours that do (Fig. 37.6b). Histochemical reactions typical of steroid production are usually confined to the theca cell component (Scully, 1977), but on the other hand immunohistochemical studies show oestradiol to be localised in the granulosa (Gaffney et al, 1983): the situation seems to be remarkably parallel to that of the normal developing follicle, in which granulosa cells, under the stimulus of FSH, aromatise thecal androgens. Similarly also to the developing follicle, the oestrogen produced by granulosa cell tumours with thecal elements is oestradiol (Wentz & McCranie, 1976), so endogenous gonadotrophins are usually suppressed. The tumours' efficiency in synthesising and secreting oestradiol, however, is generally much less than that of normal follicular tissue — approximately 80 per cent of the tumours being easily palpable as pelvic or abdominal masses by the time of diagnosis (Goldston et al, 1972; Lack et al, 1981).

Premenopausal patients with granulosa cell tumours continue to menstruate regularly until enough theca-initiated oestrogen production takes place to disturb ovulation, after which there is dysfunctional uterine bleeding or, less commonly, amenorrhoea (Novak et al, 1971; Fox et al, 1975; Evans et al, 1980). Young girls with granulosa cell tumours before the age of puberty may present with isosexual precocious puberty (Novak et al, 1971; Roth et al, 1979; Evans et al, 1980; Lack et al, 1981) or, occasionally, with virilisation (Lack et al, 1981). Postmenopausal patients usually present with postmenopausal bleeding (Taylor, 1966), and the association between granulosa-thecal cell tumours and endometrial hyperplasia and carcinoma is well recognised (Novak et al, 1971; Goldston et al, 1972).

There are suggestive, but not conclusive, indications that granulosa cell tumours are FSH-dependent. Though granulosa cell tumours, unlike pure theca cell tumours, may occur at any age, they are commonest after the menopause (Taylor, 1966; Novak et al, 1971; Scully, 1977; and see Fig. 37.4); their prognosis then is worse than before the menopause.

Demonstration of FSH-receptors in a granulosa cell

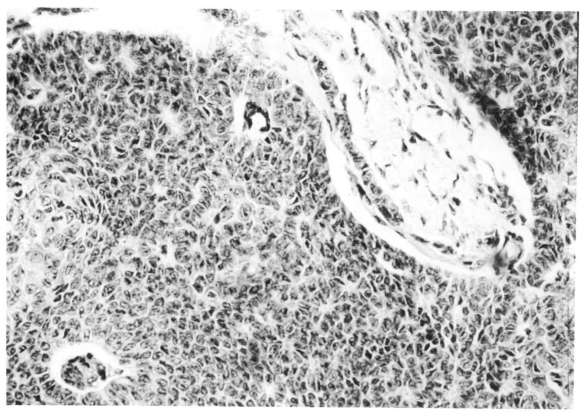

Fig. 37.6a Granulosa cell tumour. Sex-cord tumour recapitulating follicular structure (×200)

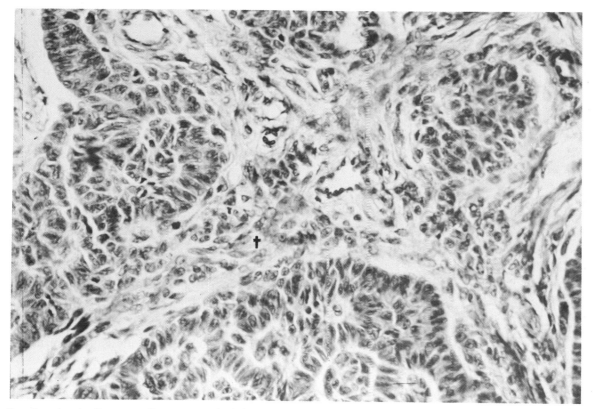

Fig. 37.6b Granulosa-thecal cell tumour. Oestrogen synthesis is most likely when thecal components (·) are present to provide aromatisable androgen substrate to the granulosa cells, but the arrangement between the two components is significantly less efficient for oestradiol synthesis than is the case in a developing follicle (×200)

tumour (Davy et al, 1977) constitutes more direct evidence of gonadotrophin sensitivity. Consequently, FSH supression with exogenous oestrogen has been suggested for the long-term management of granulosa cell tumours (Goldston et al, 1972); this seems to make sense endocrinologically, particularly for tumours after the menopause or with the advent of the menopause in younger women with previously diagnosed tumours.

Some granulosa cell tumours display granulosa cell luteinisation and at least a proportion of these show evidence of progesterone action on the endometrium — a further parallel with normal follicle cell physiology. Raised plasma progesterone levels have been reported with a metastatic granulosa cell tumour in a postmenopausal patient (Lomax et al, 1977).

Granulosa cell tumours may virilise — particularly a special group of cystic granulosa cell tumours that occur in young women and produce testosterone with normal urinary 17-ketosteroids (Norris & Taylor, 1969; Giuntoli et al, 1976). Virilisation is also occasionally found with granulosa cell tumours under the hCG stimulus of pregnancy, so that whereas granulosa cell tumours normally constitute only 2 per cent of virilising tumours (Ireland & Woodruff, 1976) in pregnancy the proportion is over 10 per cent (Verhoeven et al, 1973). The source of the androgen is considered to be the reactive thecal cells.

The classic testosterone-producing sex cord tumour is the *Sertoli-Leydig cell tumour*, androblastoma or arrhenoblastoma (Fig. 37.7a, b), in which sex cord cells instead of forming follicular structures recapitulate testicular development as tubules, cords or islands of Sertoli cells. These tumours are rare, but occur in a younger age group than granulosa cell tumours do (Taylor, 1966; and see Fig. 37.4).

Luteinised stroma and Leydig cells are more plentiful in intermediate and poorly differentiated Sertoli-Leydig cell tumours than in well-differentiated tumours (Pedowitz & O'Brien, 1960; O'Hern & Neubecker, 1962; Novak & Long, 1965; Roth et al, 1981); symptoms of defeminisation (breast atrophy and amenorrhoea) and virilisation are correspondingly more common, implying that the luteinised stroma and Leydig cells are the source of the androgen. The main steroid synthesised and secreted is testosterone (Savard et al, 1961), so plasma DHAS and urinary 17-ketosteroids are either normal or only moderately raised despite clinical virilisation, and in postmenopausal women plasma gonadotrophins are likely to be suppressed (Meldrum & Abraham, 1979). Nevertheless the tissue these tumours contain does not produce androgens particularly efficiently: almost all the tumours are well over 5 cm in diameter by the time of diagnosis. The Leydig or luteinised stromal cells almost never contain Reinke crystals (O'Hern & Neubecker, 1962; Roth et al, 1981) and, at least according to fat stains and testosterone immunofluorescence, may not have a monopoly on androgen synthesis

but may share this ability with the Sertoli cells (O'Hern & Neubecker, 1962; Kurman et al, 1978).

Clinical virilisation, though, is uncommon in well-differentiated tumours composed only of mature Sertoli cell elements (Taylor, 1966; Tavassoli & Norris, 1980; Roth et al, 1981). Pure Sertoli cell tumours may, however, manifest clinically with isosexual precocious puberty, dysfunctional uterine bleeding or postmenopausal bleeding, all of which imply oestrogen excess (Pedowitz & O'Brien, 1960; Tavassoli & Norris, 1980; Roth et al, 1981).

Aldosterone production, with severe hypertension and hypokalaemia, has been associated with an ovarian Sertoli cell tumour on at least two occasions. In the first patient described, a 9-year-old girl with precocious puberty, clinical abnormalities resolved after the tumour was excised; conversion of progesterone to mineralocorticoids was inferred from *in vitro* studies (Ehrlich et al, 1963). In the second patient, a 31-year-old with hypertension and hypokalaemic alkalosis, death occurred from the metabolic effects of primary hyperaldosteronism before an ovarian Sertoli cell tumour was diagnosed; plasma steroid levels and tissue culture studies indicated aldosterone, testosterone and oestradiol production by the tumour (Todesco et al, 1975).

Gynandroblastomas are rare sex cord-stromal tumours in which follicular structures with Call-Exner vacuoles and Sertoli cell tubules coexist and intermingle. Few tumours have been studied endocrinologically, but it seems that the tumours may virilise, feminise, or do both (Emig et al, 1959; Taylor, 1966). Testosterone was elevated and the endometrium was proliferative in a recently reported case (Anderson & Rees, 1975).

Germ cell tumours

Leydig cells or luteinized stromal cells that produce testosterone (Rose et al, 1974) and so cause virilisation are a frequent component of the *gonadoblastomas* (Scully, 1970), to which patients with Y-chromosomal material are highly predisposed (Manuel et al, 1976). This Y-chromosomal material may be impossible to detect karyotypically — even with multiple banding studies — and its inferred presence may depend on demonstrating its sensitive phenotypic sequel, the H-Y antigen (Wachtel et al, 1976). It is of correlative interest that those patients who have virilising male intersex, usually the result of partial androgen synthesis failure, have, in the gonadoblastomas that occur, significantly fewer identifiable androgen synthesising cells than is usual in gonadoblastomas in other patients (Scully, 1970).

In testicular feminisation the incidence of germ cell tumour is the least of all XY females and the incidence of dysgerminomas seems to be comparable with that in phenotypic males with undescended testes (Morris, 1953). Clinical manifestation of any endocrine disturbance is

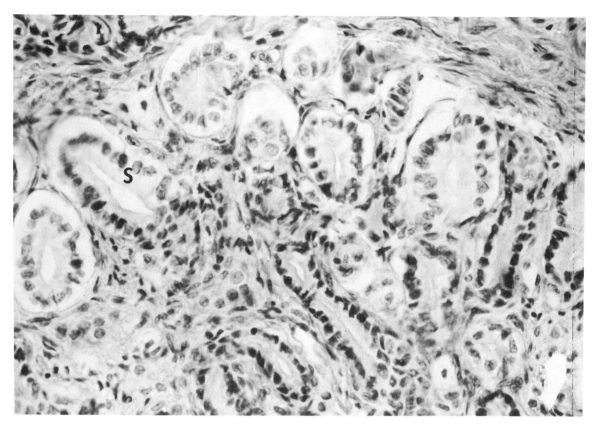

Fig. 37.7a Sertoli cell tumour, well-differentiated. Ovarian sex-cord tumour composed of Sertoli cells (S) recapitulating testicular tubular structure. In the absence of a differentiated stromal Leydig cell component these tumours are often endocrinologically inactive (×200)

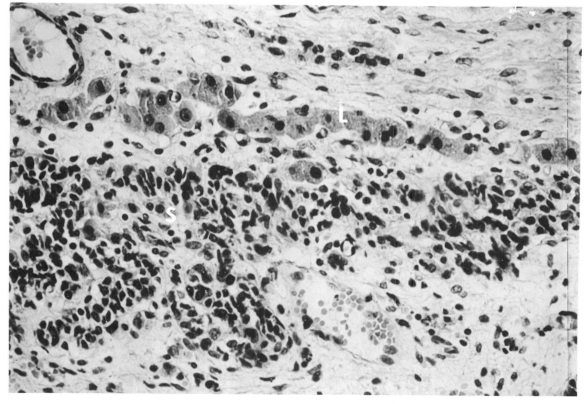

Fig. 37.7b Sertoli-Leydig cell tumour. The Sertoli cell (S) component is poorly differentiated, but the prominent Leydig cells (L) are likely to be accompanied by testosterone secretion (×200)

unlikely, because such patients already have plasma testos-terones in the normal male range but with peripheral androgen insensitivity, and because there is no uterus to disclose oestrogen over-production.

Ovarian germ cell tumours that contain trophoblastic elements (Braunstein et al, 1978) may produce hCG, which then stimulates steroid production from either the normal or the neoplastic elements, or both, of that ovary. Pre-cocious puberty or disturbance of cyclical ovarian func-tion is likely if hGC is produced in sufficient quantity (approaching that of pregnancy or trophoblastic disease) to provoke abnormal androgen synthesis from the ovarian stroma. The hCG-producing properties of germ cell tumour trophoblast are discussed more fully below. The presence of trophoblast, however, in a dysgerminoma has, in several reported cases (Castleman et al, 1972; Ueda et al, 1972), apparently also endowed the tumour with the ability to aromatise androgens to oestrogens — a property that such trophoblast therefore shares with normal gesta-tional trophoblast. The androgens that are converted to oestrogens are not necessarily of gonadal origin: males with trophoblast-containing testicular tumours have been shown to have 5- to 10-fold increases in oestrogen production rates largely accounted for by tumour metabolism of DHAS (Kirschner et al, 1970) — a direct parallel with normal trophoblastic aromatisation of fetal adrenal androgens in pregnancy.

Oestrogen production and spontaneous breast develop-ment, as mentioned earlier, has also been reported in patients with streak gonads and primary amenorrhoea (Saunders et al, 1975; Jones, 1976). It is sometimes the result of a small number of persistent follicles, presumably producing enough oestrogen to initiate thelarche but not enough to cause menstruation (Jones, 1976), but at least three patients, all 46,XY, have had gonadoblastomas (Saunders et al, 1975; Jones, 1976), which presumably contained follicle type cells capable of aromatising androgens.

Steroid production with 'non-functioning' ovarian tumours

Brenner tumours, Krukenberg tumours, mucinous and endometrioid epithelial tumours and, rarely, dermoids and germ cell tumours (none of which are usually steroid-secreting) can produce virilisation (Hughesdon, 1958; Taylor, 1966; Scott et al, 1967; Woodruff et al, 1968; Verhoeven et al, 1973; Ireland & Woodruff, 1976; Stewart et al, 1981) owing to the stimulatory effect that an expanding ovarian mass can have on surrounding stroma — an effect that seems comparable with the stromal differ-entiation of theca interna by a normal developing follicle (Hughesdon, 1958). The reactive stroma tends to produce androstenedione as well as other androgens (Rivarola et al, 1968; MacDonald et al, 1976) and urinary 17-ketosteroids are often high (Scott et al, 1967; Woodruff et al, 1968).

Extraglandular conversion of androstenedione to oestrone has been shown to occur and may account for biochemical, histological and clinical oestrogen effects (MacDonald et al, 1976; Rome et al, 1981), although direct production of oestradiol has also been documented (Quinn et al, 1983).

The common denominator in the tumours likely to produce stromal hyperplasia has been suggested to be the relatively large surface area these tumours display to the stroma (Scott et al, 1967). It is likely that more subtle mechanisms are involved, but these have not been defined. The luteinisation that takes place in the reactive stroma and the virilisation evident clinically are much enhanced both by the hCG stimulus of pregnancy and by high LH levels after the menopause. Therefore, whereas in the non-preg-nant state intrinsically non-functioning tumours constitute 21 per cent of virilising tumours (Ireland & Woodruff, 1976), in pregnancy the proportion is 45–50 per cent (Novak et al, 1970; Verhoeven et al, 1973), and after the menopause the proportion may be greater than 50 per cent (Woodruff et al, 1963).

Virilising adrenal tumours

The diagnosis of a steroid-secreting ovarian tumour is reasonably straightforward when an adnexal mass is palp-able, as it is in the majority of cases both before and after the menopause. However, hilus cell tumours — which occur mostly in postmenopausal women but can complicate pre-existing androgenic ovarian pathology in younger women — are often too small to be obvious clinically or laparoscopically (Dunnihoo et al, 1966; Casthely et al, 1977). Difficulties may therefore arise in distinguishing ovarian and adrenal virilising tumours.

Virilising adrenal tumours fall into three groups endo-crinologically. Firstly, there are those adenomas and carcinomas that increase both androgen and corticosteroid output, causing virilisation with, usually, a florid Cushing's syndrome; urinary 17-ketosteroids are markedly elevated and so is urinary free cortisol (or 17-ketogenic steroids, or 17-hydroxycorticosteroids).

The second group are those adenomas that release DHA and DHAS as well as androstenedione and testosterone, but without a detectable increase in corticosteroid production (Mahesh et al, 1968; Blichert-Toft et al, 1975; Bertagna & Orth, 1981; Gabrilove et al, 1981; Fuller et al, 1983); urinary 17-ketosteroids are high, plasma gonado-trophins are often not suppressed, and the differential di-agnosis includes an ovarian stromal tumour.

Thirdly, there are those adenomas that presumably take origin from subcapsular ovarian stromal rests (Wong & Warner, 1971) or from Leydig cell differentiation of adrenal mesenchyme (Horvath et al, 1980) and produce testosterone with relatively little androstenedione (Werk et al, 1973; Givens et al, 1974; Larson et al, 1976; Smith et al, 1978; Kable & Yussman, 1979; Spaulding et al, 1980;

Gabrilove et al, 1981); urinary 17-ketosteroids are normal. These adenomas occur mainly in postmenopausal women; plasma gonadotrophins may be suppressed, either from concomitant oestradiol production or through extraglandular conversion of testosterone to oestradiol. The differential diagnosis is an ovarian hilus cell or Leydig cell tumour.

Differential diagnosis in the second and third groups cannot be achieved with differential suppression or stimulation of the ovaries and adrenals, because these adrenal adenomas are often responsive to LH and hCG. The adenomas may be quite small — they can elude detection by adrenal scanning or computed tomography — and preoperative diagnosis may only be possible by selective catheterisation and sampling of adrenal and ovarian veins. Selective venous sampling is attended by well known problems and pitfalls (technical and anatomical difficulty with accurate selective catheterisation; adrenal steroid secretion is both episodic and increased by stress; and in women of reproductive age ovarian oestrogen secretion and androgen secretion is unilateral) and is only of clinical use when androgen production is autonomous and there is high suspicion of tumour (Wentz et al, 1976).

Feminising adrenal tumours

Adrenal carcinomas can occasionally secrete oestrogens as well as androgens and corticosteroids. Most case reports of feminising adrenal carcinomas refer to men with gynaecomastia (Wallach et al, 1957), but at least 11 cases have been reported of adrenal carcinoma in prepubertal girls being associated with isosexual precocious puberty without virilisation or obvious features of Cushing's syndrome (Drop et al, 1981).

Chorionic gonadotrophin production in trophoblastic disease

Normal trophoblast endocrinology

After the ovary, the most important source of hormones in the normal female genital tract is the trophoblast (Fig. 37.8a), from its earliest differentiation in the embryo to its fully developed form, the placenta (Villee, 1969). Detectable levels of its most prominent product — chorionic gonadotrophin (hCG) — are found in maternal plasma from the time the blastocyst hatches from the zona pellucida and implants in the endometrium, on the seventh day after ovulation and fertilisation, 1 week before the next expected menstrual period. Circulating levels then increase logarithmically over the next few weeks of early pregnancy.

Chorionic gonadotrophin is a glycoprotein of molecular weight 39 000 — a glycosylated polypeptide dimer

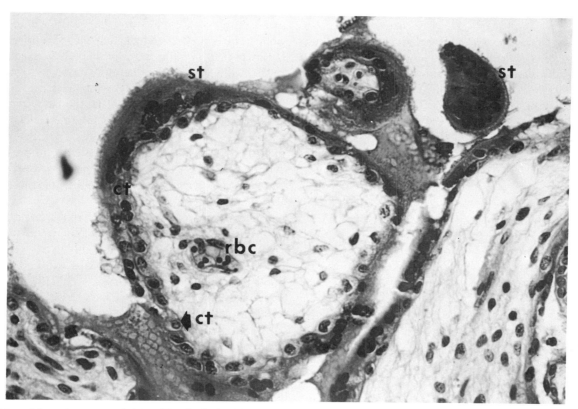

Fig. 37.8a Normal first-trimester trophoblast. The chorionic villus contains blood vessels with fetal (nucleated) red blood cells (rbc), a continuous layer of cytotrophoblast (ct) and, in contact with maternal blood, the syncytiotrophoblast (st), which is the site of production of chorionic gonadotrophin. Progesterone synthesis and aromatisation of △5-androgens to oestrogens also take place in the syncytiotrophoblast (× 200)

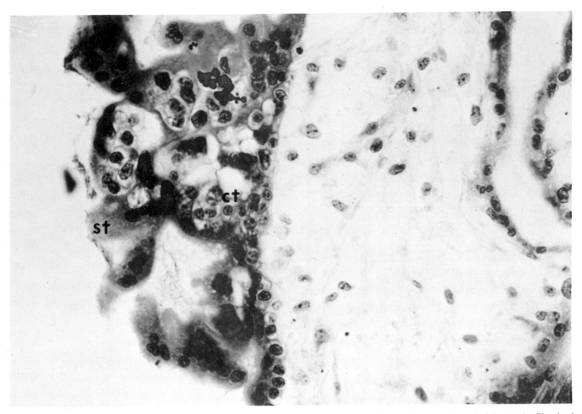

Fig. 37.8b Hydatidiform mole. The cytotrophoblast (ct) is proliferating under the peripheral rim of syncytiotrophoblast (st). Chorionic gonadotrophin production is invariable. The chorionic villi are devoid of fetal blood vessels and have become hydropic (× 200)

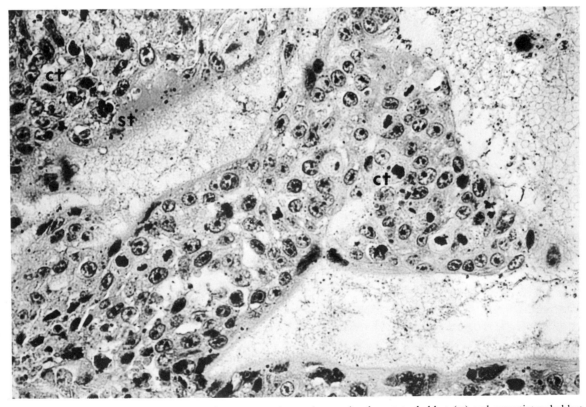

Fig. 37.8c Choriocarcinoma. Nuclear pleomorphism and numerous mitoses characterise the cytotophoblast (ct) and syncytiotrophoblast (st) (× 200)

composed of an alpha and beta subunit, with the negatively-charged sugar, sialic acid, constituting 12 per cent of the molecule's mass (Vaitukaitis et al, 1976). Synthesis of hCG occurs in the syncytiotrophoblast, perhaps at least partly under the influence of the polypeptide luteinising hormone releasing hormone (LRH), whose presence has been demonstrated in cytotrophoblast (Khodr & Siler-Khodr, 1978). Alpha-subunits are synthesised in excess and significant levels are found in the circulation; it is the rate of beta-subunit synthesis that determines the production rate of the complete molecule.

Biological activity of hCG depends not only on release of the hormone into the circulation in dimer form; it is also necessary for the molecule to be glycosylated, the abundant sialic acid of the carbohydrate portion of the molecule serving to prevent binding to receptors in the liver that otherwise clear the circulation before biological activity can be manifested. The degree to which hCG is sialylated therefore is critically important in determining plasma concentration and *in vivo* biological activity, though it affects neither immunological reactivity in assay systems nor receptor binding *in vitro*. The degree to which hCG is sialylated is variable through pregnancy, the highest ratio of biological:immunological activity being found in the first trimester; different clones of cultured trophoblast cells produce hCG of different degrees of sialylation (Vaitukaitis et al, 1976).

The morphology of immature syncytiotrophoblast reflects the commitment this tissue has to hCG production. Ultrastructurally there is an abundance of rough endoplasmic reticulum that is usually dilated to give an overall vacuolated appearance, between which the cytoplasm appears very dense; glycogen is abundant and histologically the synctium stains strongly for carbohydrates. Separate differentiation of the inner cell mass, which gives rise to the embryo itself, and the extraembryonic trophoblast is accomplished by the 64-cell blastocyst stage (Gardner & Rossant, 1976).

Chorionic gonadotrophin shares with luteinising hormone the ability to stimulate progesterone production from the corpus luteum by binding to specific receptors on the membrane of the luteal cells. Progesterone from the corpus luteum is accompanied by 17α-hydroxyprogesterone, and the pregnant state is maintained this way until progesterone of trophoblastic origin is abundant.

Steroid production — progesterone and oestrogens — takes place in the syncytiotrophoblast. Progesterone synthesis does not seem to be under gonadotrophic control, its principal requirement being availability of progesterone's immediate precursor in the steroid synthesis pathway, pregnenolone (Paul et al, 1981); provision of neither cholesterol nor hCG affects the rate of progesterone synthesis by syncytiotrophoblast *in vitro*. The placenta also cannot 17-hydroxylate progesterone or pregnenolone, so its efficient synthesis of oestrogens depends on aromatisation

of androgens, especially DHAS and its 16α-hydroxylated derivative.

Hydatidiform mole and choriocarcinoma

Fertilisation of an ovum can sometimes lead to sperm-derived male pronuclei providing the entire chromosome complement for the resultant zygote — usually because the female pronucleus has been lost or somehow prevented from undergoing syngamy with the male pronucleus, which itself undergoes duplication to produce a diploid chromosome complement (Kajii & Ohama, 1977). Cleavage divisions follow, but the inner cell mass fails to develop and trophoblast alone is left to grow into an entity, well-known as a hydatidiform mole (Fig. 37.8b), that has a propensity for malignant behaviour in the maternal host tissues, perhaps because of its solely paternal genetic origins. The malignant sequelae of hydatidiform mole include invasive mole and choriocarcinoma (Fig. 37.8c).

The endocrine properties that have been described for normal syncytiotrophoblast also characterise the abnormal syncytiotrophoblast of hydatidiform mole and choriocarcinoma (Bahn et al, 1981). Progesterone is synthesised and androgens are aromatised to oestrogens (Bahn et al, 1981). Moles and their malignant derivatives secrete high levels of hCG and precursor alpha-and beta-subunits into the circulation, quantification of which can be used to follow the clinical course of trophoblastic disease. Measurement of hCG and its subunits as tumour markers, however, is beyond this chapter's scope: it is well-described elsewhere (Bagshawe & Begent, 1981; Mackay et al, 1981). Although the secreted hCG is heterogeneous in molecular structure, a substantial proportion is present in dimeric and glycosylated form, thus constituting a marked gonadotrophic stimulus to the ovaries.

The trophoblast, whether normal or neoplastic, also produces other polypeptide hormones, notably placental lactogen (hPL), but neither have these proved particularly useful so far as tumour markers nor are there specific endocrine effects associated with these substances when produced by genital tract tumours in women, over and above those that occur with normal pregnancy.

Ovarian and other endocrine responses to trophoblast neoplasia

Theca-lutein cysts ('hyperreactio luteinalis') occur commonly in molar pregnancy. The microscopic structure of theca lutein cysts is identical to that of the cysts in the polycystic ovary syndrome (PCOS) (Fig. 37.2c), in which the LH-stimulus to the ovaries closely resembles that of hCG. The granulosa is often rather poorly developed and there is marked thecal luteinisation; only the presence of corpora albicantia and the absence of a thickened capsule, which point to previously normal cyclical ovarian function, may distinguish the ovary of hyperreactio luteinalis from that of PCOS histologically.

Evidence is strong, though, that hCG also has intrinsic FSH-like activity (Louvet et al, 1976; Siris et al, 1978; Bluestein & Vaitukaitis, 1981), which may explain the similarity that theca lutein cysts can also show to ovaries overstimulated with exogenous gonadotrophins. Sequestration of gonadotrophins within the theca lutein cysts presumably underlies the very variable time sequence of ovarian enlargement with hydatidiform mole, which often occurs weeks after evacuation of the mole, when hCG levels in the peripheral circulation are continuing to fall; the development of theca lutein cysts, however, increases to about 50 per cent the chance of persistent trophoblastic disease manifesting (Morrow et al, 1977). Ovarian enlargement can be massive, with all the coagulation. changes, ascites and haemoconcentration that can accompany hyperstimulation of the ovaries with exogenous gonadotrophins (Planner et al, 1982).

Testosterone production is increased in trophoblastic disease (Samaan et al, 1972) because of hCG's stimulatory effects on the ovarian stroma, but virilisation has not been described — presumably because the abnormal trophoblast is able to aromatise the androgens produced. Although one might consider measuring plasma androgen levels to detect the presence or to monitor the progress of theca lutein cysts, a better indicator is provided by measuring plasma 17α-hydroxyprogesterone levels (Osathanondh et al, 1973; Forest et al, 1978), which parallel corpus luteum function in the normal menstrual cycle and in pregnancy. Because it lacks 17-hydroxylase, 17α-hydroxyprogesterone is not produced by the trophoblast.

Hydatidiform moles cause abnormal thyroid function tests indicative of *hyperthyroidism* in over 50 per cent of cases (Higgins et al, 1975); clinical thyrotoxicosis is much less common (Hershman, 1972), but can be severe, and cases of high-output cardiac failure and thyroid crisis have been reported with choriocarcinoma (Soutter et al, 1981).

The mechanism by which thyrotoxicosis is produced is now clear. Commercially available hCG has TSH-like actions *in vitro* (Silverberg et al, 1978) and *in vivo* (Sowers et al, 1978), and it is well established that hCG alone is sufficient to account for thyrotrophin activity derived both from normal (Harada & Hershman, 1978) and from neoplastic (Kenimer et al, 1975) trophoblast. In one study of patients with hydatidiform mole and choriocarcinoma, biochemical hyperthyroidism was likely with serum hCG levels greater than 0.1×10^6 iu/l and clinical thyrotoxicosis occurred in most patients when levels exceeded 0.3×10^6 iu/l (Norman et al, 1981).

Other-hormone-secreting genital tract tumours

Just as the predominant, and classical, sites of hormone production in the genital tract comprise the ovary (sex ster-

oids) and the normal trophoblast (polypeptide hormones, particularly chorionic gonadotrophin), so the chief hormonally-active neoplasms in the genital tract are derived from them. But in special circumstances tumours from other tissues in the genital tract can produce clinically important hormones, and the ovary itself can produce hormones not classically associated with an ovarian source. The ovary has this ability to produce non sex steroid hormones through a unique mechanism: the ability of neoplastic germ cells to differentiate into any tissue normally found in fetal or mature life. Furthermore, the other genital tract tissues, and also the ovary, can occasionally become endocrinologically important through the mechanism widely known as ectopic hormone production.

Mature teratomas

Teratomas are germ cell tumours in which there is differentiation into tissues or even organs that normally would come from more than one germinal layer in the embryo. The frequency with which skin and its appendages are found in these tumours has led to the name *dermoid cyst* being used for them. In mature teratomas all the constituent tissues are differentiated to a degree found in mature or adult life; these tissues may then share with their conventionally located counterparts the physiological properties those tissues normally display — which, in the case of endocrine tissues, can lead to clinically important phenomena outside the ovary that contains the teratoma.

Thyrotoxicosis occurs with rather fewer than half of the patients with identifiable thyroid tissue (Fig. 37.9) in an ovarian teratoma (Kempers et al, 1970; Pantoja et al, 1975). The mechanism of the thyrotoxicosis, however, is not nearly as simple as the histological similarity between the ovarian tissue and normal thyroid would suggest. Normally, quiescence of the thyroid would be expected in the presence of autonomous thyroid activity elsewhere; but many patients with an apparently functioning ovarian stroma have a toxic goitre — which is usually adenomatous, occasionally it is Grave's disease (Woodruff & Markley, 1957; Kempers et al, 1970) — either coincidentally or sequentially. Accurate management of these patients therefore demands careful endocrine work-up and follow-up, including nuclear studies of the neck and lower abdomen to delineate areas of thyroid activity.

Chromaffin cell tumours of the ovary — *carcinoids* — may arise in pre-existing teratomas or may be seen in the absence of other recognisable teratomatous tissue; in the latter case their origin from germ cells must be in doubt, because similar primary carcinoids can be found in a variety of non-enteric tissues in which teratomas do not occur, but which, like the ovaries (Hidvegi et al, 1982), may contain argentaffin cells. Occasionally ovarian carcinoid represents metastasis from a bowel primary (Haines, 1971).

Primary ovarian carcinoids, unlike bowel carcinoids,

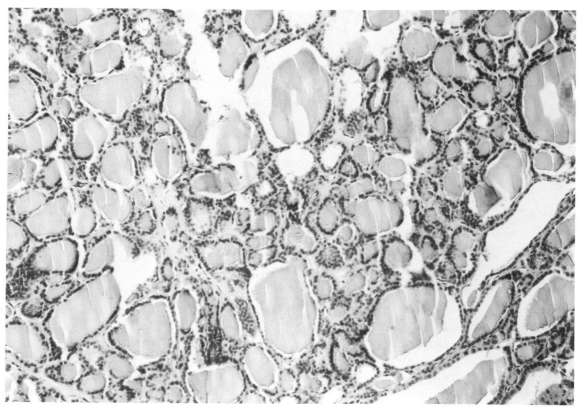

Fig. 37.9 Struma ovarii. Recapitulation of thyroid histology by an ovarian teratoma.

secrete their serotonin and other vasoactive substances directly into the systemic circulation rather than into the portal circulation, from which serotonin is quickly cleared by the liver. Ovarian carcinoids may therefore produce postprandial flushing and other manifestations of the carcinoid syndrome in the absence of hepatic metastases (Climie & Heath, 1968; Haines, 1971). About 50 per cent of ovarian carcinoid tumours produce symptoms (Haines, 1971). The carcinoid syndrome is found with carcinoids that have an insular (midgut) histologic pattern, but not with those that have a trabecular (foregut and hindgut) pattern (Robboy et al, 1975). Preoperative diagnosis is possible by demonstrating increased urinary excretion of 5-hydroxyindolacetic acid.

Malignant change in a tissue component of a mature dermoid can, especially in the presence of metastases, be accompanied by paraneoplastic phenomena, which are discussed in detail below. In a recently reported case of epidermoid carcinoma complicating a mature teratoma, hypercalcaemia and metastatic calcification followed production and secretion by the tumour of large amounts of prostaglandin E_2 (Kim et al, 1981). In at least one reported case (Peterson, 1957) a primary choriocarcinoma, probably accompanied by hCG production, has complicated an otherwise histologically benign ovarian teratoma.

Immature teratomas

Immature teratomas are almost always hormonally inactive.

Rarely syncytiotrophoblastic elements may be present and hCG may be secreted (Kurman & Norris, 1978).

Other germ cell tumours

Chorionic gonadotrophin production and secretion occurs with those malignant germ cell tumours in which there has been a histogenic attempt to recapitulate extraembryonic tissues that include trophoblast — just as α-fetoprotein (AFP) secretion occurs from those germ cell tumours that differentiate embryonic yolk-sac elements (Baylin & Mendelsohn, 1980). So hCG secretion is universal in non-gestational *choriocarcinomas*, which contain both cytotrophoblast and syncytiotrophoblast in intimate association (Fig. 37.10a); hCG production and secretion is common in *embryonal carcinomas* (Fig. 37.10b), which contain syncytiotrophoblast-like cells that are positive for hCG on immunohistochemical staining (Kurman & Norris, 1976); but hCG production does not occur in endodermal sinus tumours (Kurman & Norris, 1978), which show differentiation of primitive embryonic but not extraembryonic tissues. The commonest malignant germ cell tumours, *dysgerminomas* (Fig. 37.10c), only rarely contain syncytiotrophoblast cells, so significant levels of hCG are also rare (Kurman & Norris, 1978).

Clinical manifestations result either from hCG stimulation of the ovarian stroma outside the tumour to secrete steroids or from conversion by the abnormal trophoblast of circulating DHAS to oestrogen, and include precocious

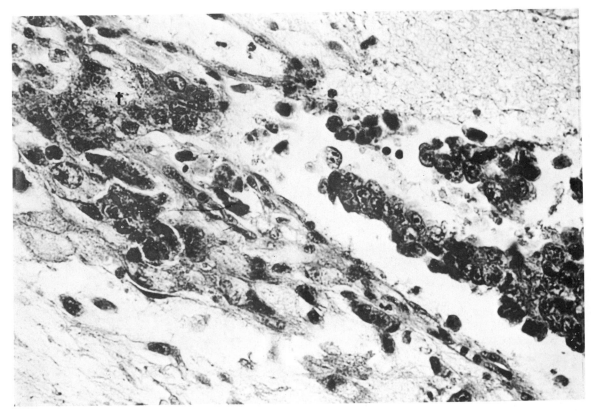

Fig. 37.10a Primary choriocarcinoma of the ovary. Malignant germ cell tumour of the ovary with discernible trophoblast (t). Chorionic gonadotrophin is produced by giant cells (syncytiotrophoblast), but feminising precocious puberty is likely to be the result of syncytiotrophoblastic aromatisation of circulating DHAS to oestrogens (see text) (×200)

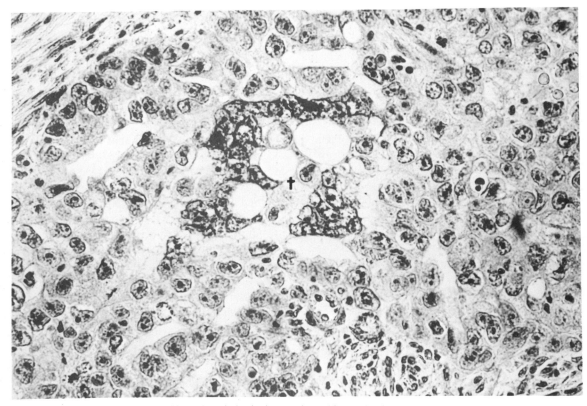

Fig. 37.10b Embryonal carcinoma with trophoblast (t) and chorionic gonadotrophin production (×200)

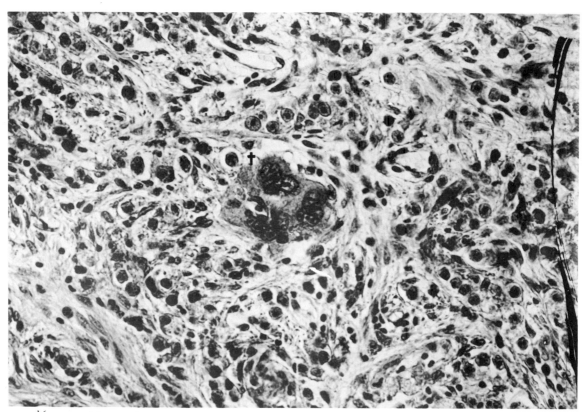

Fig. 37.10c Dysgerminoma with syncytiotrophoblast-like giant cells (t) and chorionic gonadotrophin production — a rare event with this type of tumour (×200)

puberty in girls before menarche, abnormal bleeding or amenorrhoea in women of reproductive age, and hirsutism and virilisation at any age. In 117 cases of dysgerminoma, five patients (4.3 per cent) had secondary amenorrhoea, or had oligomenorrhoea and hirsutism (Asadourian & Taylor, 1969), whereas among 15 patients with embryonal carcinoma these hormonal manifestations were present in nine (60 per cent) (Kurman & Norris, 1976). Half the prepubertal patients who develop primary choriocarcinoma of the ovary show signs of precocious puberty (Norris & Adam, 1981).

These tumours are highly malignant. Treatment is directed towards achieving survival and includes surgical excision of the tumour together with combination chemotherapy. The chief clinical importance of hCG is then its role as a tumour marker in following progress of the disease.

Phylogeny and ontogeny of ectopic hormone production

Most of the hormones of man and other vertebrates are phylogenetically ancient (Roth et al, 1982). This is especially true of the polypeptide hormones: for example, ACTH, β-endorphins, somatostatin and insulin have been found in protozoa, and insulin and hCG occur in bacteria.

These primitive synthetic capabilities are thought to have been conserved in a wide variety of human tissues:

normal tissues other than conventional endocrine tissues are known to contain, and are thought to produce, ACTH, hCG and insulin, or at least their precursor molecules, in small but measurable quantities (Ratcliff et al, 1972 — ACTH; Yoshimoto et al, 1979 — hCG; Roth et al, 1982 — insulin). Conventional endocrine and neuroendocrine phenomenology of glands and nerves compared with other tissues is therefore more a series of spectacular quantitative differences than a set of qualitatively unique attributes. The cells in normal tissues that display these abilities seem to be the partially differentiated and dividing stem cells of the tissue, and any condition (benign or malignant) that increases the number of dividing cells may increase the amount of elaborated protein (Odell et al, 1977).

The biogenic amines, prostaglandins and steroid hormones also have a substantial ancestry. Adrenalin activates adenylate cyclase in protozoa, and prostaglandins are widespread among the invertebrates. However, although various sterols are encountered in invertebrates, consistent ability to synthesise cholesterol and its steroid hormone derivatives appears to be restricted to the vertebrates.

Peptide hormones, biogenic amines, prostaglandins and steroid hormones could all be candidates for ectopic production by neoplastic cells. Indeed, it is likely that virtually all neoplasms elaborate ectopic proteins (Odell et al, 1977; Odell & Wolfsen, 1980). However, only a minority of cancers secrete hormones that are biologically active — and, qualitatively, secretion of hormones by neoplasms is far from being a random tumour feature (Baylin & Mendelsohn, 1980). Furthermore, the more complicated the enzyme systems normal tissues require for secretion of hormones in active form, the more likely it is that the neoplastic cell will need differentiation of a special sort to produce that active hormone ectopically. For example, the large precursor molecule for ACTH is of extraordinarily wide occurrence in neoplastic cells (Odell & Wolfsen, 1980), but only those neoplastic cells that acquire amine precursor uptake and decarboxylation (APUD) ability are able to convert the biologically inactive precursor polypeptide into the small polypeptides that have biological activity — and so produce an ectopic hormone syndrome.

Similarly, a degree of tumour differentiation is needed to assemble the subunits of chorionic gonadotrophin and glycosylate the molecule, giving it the resistance to metabolism and long plasma half-life it needs for biological activity. The neoplastic tissues most likely to do this are those that differentiate like trophoblast — a phenomenon so well known among germ cell tumours that the question of what constitutes 'ectopic' production becomes quite cloudy. Most gonadal or extragonadal tumours that produce hCG from trophoblastic components also produce placental lactogen (Baylin & Mendelsohn, 1980), illustrating again that hormone production by tumours is not random or chaotic but is a logical consequence of the tumour's differentiation. Immunologically detectable hCG is found with a wide range of genital (Rutamen & Seppala, 1978) and non-genital (Braunstein et al, 1978) neoplasms, but glycosylated and biologically active hCG is rarely secreted by ovarian and other tumours unless those tumours contain giant cells and have some histological resemblance to syncytiotrophoblast (Civantos & Rywlin, 1972; Skrabanek et al, 1979).

Steroid synthesis requires much specialisation, so it is not surprising that *ectopic* steroid secretion as a paraneoplastic phenomenon has not been encountered: the tumours that produce steroids occur in tissues that produce steroids — the main subject of this chapter. Again, the type of cell that is actually proliferating in a steroid-producing ovarian tumour is likely to be a relatively undifferentiated stem cell (Kurman et al, 1978) and steroid synthesis by that tumour should be seen as a sign of tissue differentiation, just as the morphological features of the tumour that allow it to be named imply differentiation. As is the case with polypeptide-producing tumours, it is more than just coincidence that morphological and functional differentiation occur in parallel more often than not, so granulosa cell tumours generally produce oestradiol and Sertoli-Leydig cell tumours generally produce testosterone.

However, we have already seen that even in normal ovarian tissues compartmentalisation of steroid synthesis is not absolute, so it should cause no surprise that with

hyperplasias (Dennefors et al, 1980), and particularly with neoplasias, divergence from conventional structure-function relationships is possible. In this sense if, say, a Sertoli cell tumour acquires the hydroxylases needed for mineralocorticoid synthesis, or even if it just acquires large amounts of aromatase and secretes oestradiol instead of testosterone, then that tumour's steroid production can arguably be considered 'ectopic'. Nothing is probably gained by extending the concept of ectopic hormone production so far as this except in drawing attention to the point that 'ectopic' is more a quantitative than a sharp qualitative distinction.

On the other hand, prostaglandin production by tissues is universal from the invertebrates through to mammalian tissues, and prostaglandin production by tumours is probably equally ubiquitous. The paraneoplastic consequences of tumour prostaglandin production are considered below.

Ectopic polypeptide hormone syndromes

Cells with APUD characteristics are rare in normal genital tract tissues (Fox et al, 1964; Hidvegi et al, 1982), so this range of ectopic hormone syndromes — Cushing's Syndrome from ectopic ACTH, water intoxication from inappropriate vasopressin, hypoglycaemia from ectopic insulin, peptic ulceration and watery diarrhoea from gut polypeptides — would not be expected to occur among genital tract tumours with the frequency they occur elsewhere. Isolated cases exist in the literature.

Cushing's syndrome with hypokalaemia from ectopic ACTH secretion has been reported with a variety of ovarian tumours, including a number of Sertoli-Leydig cell tumours, and from a small cell squamous carcinoma of the cervix (Berthelot et al, 1961; Nichols et al, 1962; Jones et al, 1976; Lojek et al, 1980). In at least one instance an ovarian tumour, of indeterminate histological type, has produced the ectopic ACTH syndrome and carcinoid syndrome together (Brown & Lane, 1965) — a classic consequence of an APUD neoplasm.

An insulin-producing ovarian neurosarcoma (Shetty et al, 1982) and an insulin-producing squamous carcinoma of the cervix (Kiang et al, 1973) have been described. Several ovarian mucinous cystadenomas have caused the Zollinger-Ellison Syndrome from ectopic gastrin production (Cocco & Conway, 1975; Long et al, 1980; Bollen et al, 1981). Malignant melanomas in the genital tract may also have the potential for producing syndromes in this category.

Hypercalcaemia

In 1956 three women with genital malignancy and hypercalcaemia were reported (Plimpton & Gellhorn, 1956); the serum calcium returned to normal after operative excision of the tumour in those cases in whom this was possible. One had a 'papillary' adenocarcinoma of the ovary; two had endometrial carcinomas. None of the patients had evidence of bony metastases or the bony changes that accompany hyperparathyroidism. Since then many other genital malignancies have been accompanied by hypercalcaemia as a paraneoplastic phenomenon and it is clear that this is the commonest clinical 'ectopic hormone' complication produced by genital cancers — just as it is the commonest endocrine complication of malignant disease in general (Blackman et al, 1978). The clinical manifestations are physical weakness and clouded consciousness.

Some tumours produce hypercalcaemia through secretion of the polypeptide hormone parathormone or a polypeptide very much like it (Hamilton et al, 1977). Parathormone-like substances have been assayed in association with large ovarian tumours, including clear cell carcinoma, granulosa cell tumour and stromal sarcoma (Holtz, 1980). However, most gynaecological and other malignancies associated with hypercalcaemia have no biochemical or radiological evidence of hyperparathyroidism (Sherwood, 1980; Stewart et al, 1982). At least some gynaecological tumours seem to produce hypercalcaemia by releasing prostaglandins into the circulation (Sherwood, 1980; Josse et al, 1981).

Gynaecological malignancies with paraneoplastic hypercalcaemia have been reviewed recently in two series (Holtz, 1980; Stewart et al, 1982): there were 19 ovarian tumours (with a distinct prevalence of clear cell tumours), eight squamous carcinomas of the vulva, eight endometrial adenocarcinomas (with a predominance of tumours with squamous components), two uterine sarcomas, one carcinoma of the cervix and one squamous carcinoma of the vagina. In a separate series, eight of 698 patients with squamous carcinoma of the cervix had clinically and biochemically apparent hypercalcaemia (Lacey & Morrow, 1979). The tumours reported have almost all been large and clinically obvious by the time hypercalcaemia was diagnosed; most of the patients, except those with cervical cancer, have been elderly. Younger patients with particularly aggressive small cell carcinomas of the ovary and hypercalcaemia have recently been described (Dickersin et al, 1982).

Erythrocytosis

Neoplasms derived from mesothelial tissues (Frohman, 1981) can produce humorally active substances different to the polypeptide-amine-prostaglandin group described above for APUD tumours and to the fetoplacental hormones described elsewhere in this chapter. Very large uterine myomas are occasionally associated with haemoglobin levels in the range 18–22 g/dl (Tumen, 1930; Nedwich et al, 1962; Shane & Naftolin, 1975); the erythrocytosis usually abates after hysterectomy. Virilising tumours in women may be accompanied by polycythaemia, but not to this degree. Although ectopic erythropoietin secretion by the myoma has been inferred, there is no direct evidence that this is the case and less direct mechanisms may operate (Lipsett et al, 1964; Hammond & Winnick, 1974).

Acknowledgments

Histological sections courtesy of Dr Peter Russell, King George V Memorial Hospital, Sydney.

REFERENCES

Abraham G E 1974 Ovarian and adrenal contribution to peripheral androgens during the menstrual cycle. Journal of Clinical Endocrinology and Metabolism 39: 340–346
Abraham G E, Chakmakjian Z H 1973 Serum steroid levels during the menstrual cycle in a bilaterally adrenalectomized woman. Journal of Clinical Endocrinology and Metabolism 37: 581–587
Abraham G E, Maroulis G B 1975 Effect of exogenous estrogen on serum pregnenolone, cortisol, and androgens in postmenopausal women. Obstetrics and Gynecology 45: 271–274
Ackerman G E, Smith M E, Mendelson C R, MacDonald P C, Simson E R 1981 Aromatization of androstenedione by human adipose tissue stromal cells in monolayer culture. Journal of Clinical Endocrinology and Metabolism 53: 412–417
Anderson M C, Rees D A 1975 Gynandroblastoma of the ovary. British Journal of Obstetrics and Gynaecology 82: 63–73
Armstrong D T, Dorrington J H 1977 Estrogen biosynthesis in the ovaries and testes. Advances in Sex Hormone Research 3: 217–258
Asadourian L A, Taylor H B 1969 Dysgerminoma. An analysis of 105 cases. Obstetrics and Gynecology 33: 370–379
Bagshaw K D, Begent R H J 1981 Trophoblastic tumors: clinical features and management. In: Coppleson M (ed) Gynecologic Oncology, pp 757–773. Churchill Livingstone, Edinburgh
Bahn R S, Worsham A, Speeg K V Jr, Ascoli M, Rabin D 1981 Characterization of steroid production in cultured human choriocarcinoma cells. Journal of Clinical Endocrinology and Metabolism 52: 447–450

Baird D T, Uno A, Melby J C 1969 Adrenal secretion of androgens and oestrogens. Journal of Endocrinology 45: 135–136
Baranetsky N G, Zipser R D, Goebelsmann U, Kurman R J, March C M, Morimoto I, Stanczyk F Z 1979 Adrenocroticotropin-dependent virilizing paraovarian tumours in Nelson's syndrome. Journal of Clinical Endocrinology and Metabolism 49: 381–386
Batta S K, Wentz A C, Channing C P 1980 Steroidogenesis by human ovarian cell types in culture: influence of mixing cell types and effect of added testosterone. Journal of Clinical Endocrinology and Metabolism 50: 274–279
Baylin S B, Mendelsohn G 1980 Ectopic (inappropriate) hormone production by tumors mechanisms involved and the biological and clinical implications. Endocrine Reviews 1: 45–77
Bertagna C, Orth D N 1981 Clinical and laboratory findings and results of therapy in 58 patients with adrenocrotical tumors admitted to a single medical center (1951 to 1978). American Journal of Medicine 71: 855–875
Berthelot P, Benhamou J P, Fauvert R 1961 Hypercortisome et cancer de L'uterus. Etude d'un cas et revue de la litterature. Presse Medicale 59: 1899–1902
Blackman M R, Rosen S W, Weintraub B D 1978 Ectopic homones. Advances in Internal Medicine 23: 85–113
Blichert-Toft M, Vejlsted H, Kehler H albrechtson R 1975 Virilizing adrenocrotical adenoma responsive to gonadrotrophin. Acta Endocrinologica 78: 77–85

Block E 1952 Quantitative morphological investigations of the follicular system in women. Variations at different ages. Acta Anatomica 14: 108–123

Bluestein B I, Vaitukaitis J L 1981 Affinity chromatography purification of solubilized FSH testicular membrane receptor. Biology of Reproduction 24: 661–669

Bollen E C M, Lamers C B H W, Jansen J B M J, Larsson L I, Joosten H J M 1981 Zollinger-Ellison syndrome due to a gastrin-producing ovarian cystadenocarcinoma. British Journal of Surgery 68: 776–777

Bonaventura L M, Judd H, Roth L M, Clearly R E 1978 Androgen, estrogen, and progestagen production by a lipid cell tumor of the ovary. American Journal of Obstetrics and Gynecology 131: 403–409

Braithwaite S E, Erkman-Balis B, Avila T D 1978 Postmenopausal virilization due to stromal hyperthecosis. Journal of Clinical Endocrinology and Metabolism 46: 295–299

Braunstein G D, Kamdar V V, Kanabus J, Rasor J 1978 Properties of human chorionic gonadotropin produced in vitro by ovarian carcinoma cells. Journal of Clinical Endocrinology and Metabolism 47: 326–332

Brown H, Lane M 1965 Cushing's and malignant carcinoid syndromes from ovarian neoplasm. Archives of Internal Medicine 115: 490–494

Brown J B 1981 Hormone profiles in young women at risk of breast cancer; a study of ovarian function during theelarche (sic), menarche, and menopause and after childbirth. In: Pike M C, Siiteri P K, Welsch C W (eds) The Banbury Report. Vol 8. Hormones and Breast Cancer, pp 33–56. Coldspring Harbor Laboratory, Coldspring Harbor, N.Y.

Caspi E, Schreyer P, Bukovsky J 1973 Ovarian lutein cysts in pregnancy. Obstetrics and Gynecology 42: 388–398

Casthely S, Diamandis H P, Pierre-Louis R 1977 Hilar cell tumor of the ovary: diagnostic value of plasma testosterone by selective ovarian vein catheterization. American Journal of Obstetrics and Gynecology 129: 108–110

Castleman B, Scully R E, McNeely B U 1972 Case records of the Massachusetts General Hospital. Case 11–1972. New England Journal of Medicine 286: 594–600

Civantos F, Rywlin A M 1972 Carcinomas with trophoblastic differentiation and secretion of gonadotrophins. Cancer 29: 789–798

Climie A R W, Heath L P 1968 Malignant degeneration of benign cystic teratomas of the ovary. Cancer 22: 824–832

Cocco A E, Conway S J 1975 Zollinger-Ellison syndrome associated with ovarian mucinous cystadenocarcinoma. New England Journal of Medicine 293: 485–486

Costoff A, Mahesh V B 1975 Primordial follicles with normal oocytes in the ovaries of postmenopausal women. Journal of the American Geriatrics Society 23: 193–196

Davidson B J, Waisman J, Judd H L 1981 Long-standing virilism in a woman with hyperplasia and neoplasia of ovarian lipidic cells. Obstetrics and Gynecology 58: 753–759

Davy M, Torjesen P A, Aakvaag A 1977 Demonstration of an FSH receptor in a functioning granulosa cell tumor. Acta Endocrinologica 85: 615–623

Dennefors B L, Janson P O, Knutson F, Hamberger L 1980 Steroid production and responsiveness to gonadotropin in isolated stromal tissue of human postmenopausal ovaries. American Journal of Obstetrics and Gynecology 136: 997–1002

Deutsch S, Benjamin F 1978 Effect of diabetic status on fractionated estrogen levels in postmenopausal women. American Journal of Obstetrics and Gynecology 130: 105–106

Dickersin G R, Kline I W, Scully R E 1982 Small cell carcinoma of the ovary. Cancer 49: 188–197

Dorrington J H, Moon Y S, Armstrong D T 1975 Estradiol-17β biosynthesis in cultured granulosa cells from hypophysectomized immature rats; stimulation by follicle-stimulating hormone. Endocrinology 97: 1328–1331

Drop S L S, Bruining G J, Visser H K A, Sippell W G 1981 Prolonged galactorrhoea in a 6-year-old girl with isosexual precocious puberty due to a feminizing adrenal tumour. Clinical Endocrinology 15: 37–43

Dunnihoo D R, Grieme D L, Woolf R B 1966 Hilar-cell tumors of the ovary. Report of 2 new cases and a review of the world literature. Obstetrics and Gynecology 27: 703–713

Ehrlich E N, Dominguez O V, Samuels L T, Lynch D, Oberhelman H, Warner N E 1963 Aldosteronism and precocious puberty due to an ovarian and androblastoma (Sertoli cell tumor). Journal of Clinical Endocrinology and Metabolism 23: 358–367

Emig O R, Hertig A T, Rowe F J 1959 Gynandroblastoma of the ovary. Review and report of a case. Obstetrics and Gynecology 13: 135–151

Evans A T III, Gaffey T A, Malkasian G D Jr, Annegers J F 1980 Clinicopathologic review of 118 granulosa and 82 theca cell tumors. Obstetrics and Gynecology 55: 231–238

Falls J L 1955 Accessory adrenal cortex in the broad ligament. Incidence and functional significance. Cancer 8: 143–150

Folkerd E J, Jacobs H S, van der Spuy Z, James V H T 1982 Failure of FSH to influence aromatization in human adipose tissue. Clinical Endocrinology 16: 621–625

Forest M G, Orgiazzi J, Tranchant D, et al 1978 Approach to the mechanism of androgen overproduction in a case of Krukenberg tumor responsible for virilization during pregnancy. Journal of Clinical Endocrinology and Metabolism 47: 428–434

Fox H, Kazzaz B, Langley F A 1964 Argyrophil and argentaffin cells in the female genital tract and in ovarian mucinous cycts. Journal of Pathology and Bacteriology 88: 479–488

Fox H, Agrawal K, Langley F A 1975 A clinicopathologic study of 92 cases of granulosa cell tumor of the ovary with special reference to the factors influencing prognosis. Cancer 35: 231–241

Frohman L A 1981 Ectopic hormone production. American Journal of Medicine 70: 995–997

Fuller P J, Pettigrew I G, Pike J W, Stockigt J R 1983 An adrenal adenoma causing virilization of mother and infant. Clinical Endocrinology 18: 143–153

Gabrilove J L, Seman A T, Sabet R, Mitty H A, Nicolis G L 1981 Virilizing adrenal adenoma with studies on the steroid content of the adrenal venous effluent and a review of the literature. Endocrine Reviews 2: 462–470

Gaffney E F, Majmudar B, Hertzler G L, Zane R, Furlong B, Breding E 1983 Ovarian granulosa cell tumors — immunohistochemical localization of estradiol and ultrastructure, with functional correlations. Obstetrics and Gynecology 61: 311–319

Garcia-Bunuel R, Berek J S, Woodruff J D 1975 Luteomas of pregnancy. Obstetrics and Gynecology 45: 407–414

Gardner R L, Rossant J 1976 Determination during embryogenesis. In: Ciba Foundation Symposium 40 (new series). Embryogenesis in Mammals, pp 5–25. Elsevier, Amsterdam

Giuntoli R L, Celebre J A, Wu C H, et al 1976 Androgenic function of a granulosa cell tumor. Obstetrics and Gynecology 47: 77–79

Givens J R, Anderson R N, Wiser W L, et al 1974 A gonadotropin-response adrenocrotical adenoma. Journal of Clinical Endocrinology and Metabolism 38: 126–133

Goldberg B, Woodruff J D 1977 Enzyme histochemistry of ovarian lipoid cell hyperplasia in a masculinized patient. Obstetrics and Gynecology 49: 69–76

Goldston W R, Johnston W W, Fetter B F, Parker R T, Wilbanks G D 1972 Clinicopathologic studies in feminizing tumors of the ovary. I. Some aspects of the pathology and therapy of granulosa cell tumors. American Journal of Obstetrics and Gynecology 112: 422–429

Greenblatt R B, Colle M L, Mahesh V B 1976 Ovarian and adrenal steroid production in the postmenopausal woman. Obstetrics and Gynecology 47: 383–387

Grodin J M, Siiteri P K, MacDonald P C 1973 Source of estrogen production in postmenopausal women. Journal of Clinical Endocrinology and Metabolism 36: 207–214

Haines M 1971 Carcinoid tumors of the ovary. Journal of Obstetrics and Gynaecology of the British Commonwealth 78: 1123–1127

Hamilton J W, Hartman C R, McGregor D H, Cohn D V 1977 Synthesis of parathyroid hormone-like peptides by a human squamous cell carcinoma. Journal of Clinical Endocrinology and Metabolism 45: 1023–1030

Hammond D, Winnick S 1974 Paraneoplastic erythrocytosis and ectopic erythroproteins. Annals of the New York Academy of Sciences 230: 219–227

Harada A, Hershman J M 1978 Extraction of human chorionic thyrotropin (hCT) from term placentas: failure to recover throtropic activity. Journal of Clinical Endocrinology and Metabolism 47: 681–685

Hemsell D L, Grodin J M, Brenner P F, Siiteri P K, MacDonald P C 1974 Plasma precursors of estrogen. II. Correlation of the extent of conversion of plasma androstenedione to estrone with age. Journal of Clinical Endocrinology and Metabolism 38: 476–479

Hensleigh P A, Woodruff J D 1978 Differential maternal-fetal response to androgenizing luteoma or hyperreactio luteinalis. Obstetrical and Gynecological Survey 33: 262–271

Hensleigh P A, Carter R P, Grotjan H E, Jr 1975 Fetal protection against masculinization with hyperreactio luteinalis and virilization. Journal of Clinical Endocrinology and Metabolism 40: 816–823

Hershman J M 1972 Hyperthyroidism induced by trophoblastic thyrotropin. Mayo Clinic Proceedings 47: 913–918

Hidvegi D, Cibils L A, Sorenson K, Hidvegi I 1982 Ultrastructural and histochemical observations of neuroendocrine granules in nonneoplastic ovaries. American Journal of Obstetrics and Gynecology 143: 590–594

Hillier S G, Reichert L E Jr, Van Hall E V 1981 Control of preovulatory follicular estrogen biosynthesis in the human ovary. Journal of Clinical Endocrinology and Metabolism 52: 847–856

Holtz G 1980 Paraneoplastic hypercalcemia in gynecologic malignancy. Obstetrical and Gynecological Survey 35: 129–136

Horvath E, Chalvardjian A, Kovacs K, Singer W 1980 Leydig-like cells in the adrenals of a woman with ectopic ACTH syndrome. Human Pathology 11: 284–287

Hughesdon P E 1958 Thecal and allied reactions in epithelial ovarian tumors. Journal of Obstetrics and Gynaecology of the British Empire 65: 702–709

Hughesdon P E 1978 Postnatal formation of ovarian stroma and its relation to ovarian pathology. International Journal of Gynaecology and Obstetrics 16: 8–19

Imperato-McGinley J, Peterson R E, Dawood M Y, Zullo M, Kramer E, Saxena B B, Arthur A, Huang T 1981 Steroid hormone secretion from a virilizing lipoid cell tumor of the ovary. Obstetrics and Gynecology 57: 525–531

Ireland K, Woodruff J D 1976 Masculinizing ovarian tumors. Obstetrical and Gynecological Survey 31: 83–111

Jones H W Jr 1976 Editorial comment. Obstetrical and Gynecological Survey 31: 217

Jones G E S, Goldberg B, Woodruff J D 1968 Histochemistry as a guide for interpretation of cell function. American Journal of Obstetrics and Gynecology 100: 76–83

Jones H W III, Plymate S, Gluck F B, Miles P A, Greene J F Jr 1976 Small cell nonkeratinizing carcinoma of the cervix associated with ACTH production. Cancer 38: 1629–1635

Josse R G, Wilson D R, Heersche J N M, Mills J R, Murray T M 1981 Hypercalcemia with ovarian carcinoma: evidence of a pathogenetic role for prostaglnadins. Cancer 48: 1233–1241

Judd H L, Scully R E, Atkins L, et al 1970 Pure gonadal dysgenesis with progressive hirsutism. New England Journal of Medicine 282: 881–885

Judd H L 1976 Hormonal dynamics associated with the menopause. Clinical Obstetrics and Gynecology 19: 775–788

Judd H L, Benirschke K, De Vane G, Reuter S R, Yen S S C 1973 Maternal virilization developing in a twin pregnancy. New England Journal of Medicine 288: 118–122

Judd H L, Judd G E, Lucas W E, Yen S S C 1974 Endocrine function of the postmenopausal ovary: concentration of androgens and estrogens in ovarian and peripheral vein blood. Journal of Clinical Endocrinology and Metabolism 39: 1020–1024

Judd H L, Shamonki I M, Frumar A M, Lagasse L D 1982 Origin of serum estradiol in postmenopausal women. Obstetrics and Gynecology 59: 680–686

Kable W T, Yussman M A 1979 Testosterone-secreting adrenal adenoma. Fertility and Sterility 32: 610–611

Kajii T, Omaha K 1977 Androgenetic origin of hydatidiform mole. Nature 268: 633–634

Katz M, Hamilton S M, Albertyn L, et al 1977 Virilization with diffuse involvement of ovarian androgen secreting cells. Obstetrics and Gynecology 50: 623–627

Kempers R D, Dockerty M B, Hoffman D L, Bartholomew L G 1970 Struma ovarii — ascitic, hyperthyroid, and asymptomatic

syndromes. Annals of Internal Medicine 72: 883–893

Kenimer J G, Hershman J M, Higgins H P 1975 The thyrotropin in hydatidiform moles is human chorionic gonadotropin. Journal of Clinical Endocrinology and Metabolism 40: 482–491

Khodr G S, Siler-Khocr T 1978 Localization of luteinizing hormone-releasing factor in the human placenta. Fertility and Sterility 29: 523–526

Kiang D T, Bauer G E, Kennedy B T 1973 Immunoassayable insulin in carcinoma of the cervix associated with hypoglycemia. Cancer 31: 801–805

Kim W, Bockman R, Lemos L, Lewis J L Jr 1981 Hypercalcemia associated with epidermoid carcinoma in ovarian cystic teratoma. Obstetrics and Gynecology 57: 81s–85s

Kirschner M A, Wider J A, Ross G T 1970 Leydig cell function in men with gonadotrophin-producing testicular tumors. Journal of Clinical Endocrinology and Metabolism 30: 504–511

Kurman R J, Andrade D, Goebelsmann U, Taylor C R 1978 An immunohistological study of steroid localization in Sertoli-Leydig tumors of the ovary and testis. Cancer 42: 1772–1783

Kurman R J, Norris H J 1976 Embryonal carcinoma of the ovary. A clinicopathological entity distinct from endodermal sinus tumor resembling embryonal carcinoma of the adult testis. Cancer 38: 2420–2433

Kurman R J, Norris H J 1978 Germ cell tumors of the ovary. Pathology Annual 13 Pt 1: 291–325

Lacey C G, Morrow C P 1979 Hypercalcemia in patients with squamous cell carcinoma of the cervix. Gynecologic Oncology 7: 215–222

Lack E E, Perez-Atayde A R, Murthy A S K, Goldstein D P, Crigler J F Jr, Vawter G F 1981 Granulosa theca cell tumors in premenarchal girls: a clinical and pathologic study of ten cases. Cancer 48: 1846–1854

Larson B A, Vanderlaan W P, Judd H L, McCullough D L 1976 A testosterone-producing adrenal cortical adenoma in an elderly woman. Journal of Clinical Endocrinology and Metabolism 42: 882–887

Lipsett M B, Odell W D, Rosenberg L E, Waldmann T A 1964 Humoral syndromes associated with nonendocrine tumors. Annals of Internal Medicine 61 733–756

Lobo R A, March C M, Goebelsmann U, Mishell D R Jr 1982 The modulating role of obesity and 17β-estradiol (E₂) on bound and unbound E₂ and adrenal androgens in oophorectomized women. Journal of Clinical Endocrinology and Metabolism 54: 320–324

Lojek M A, Fer M F, Kasselberg A G, Glick A D, Burnett L S, Julian C G, Greco F A, Oldham R K 1980 Cushing's syndrome with small cell carcinoma of the uterine cervix. American Journal of Medicine 69: 140–144

Lomax C W, May H V Jr, Panko W B, Thornton W N Jr 1977 Progesterone production by an ovarian granulosa cell carcinoma. Obstetrics and Gynecology 50 Suppl: 39s

Long T T III, Barton T K, Draffin R, Reeves W J, McCarty K S Jr 1980 Conservative management of the Zollinger-Ellison syndrome. Ectopic gastrin production by an ovarian cystadenoma. Journal of the American Medical Association 243: 1837–1839

Longcope C, Layne D S, Tait J F 1968 Metabolic clearance rate and interconversions of estrone and 17β-estradiol in normal males and females. Journal of Clinical Investigation 47: 93–105

Longcope C, Hunter R, Franz C 1980 Steroid secretion by the postmenopausal ovary. American Journal of Obstetrics and Gynecology 138: 564–568

Louvet J-P, Harman S M, Schreiber J R, Ross G T 1975 Evidence for a role of androgens in follicular maturation. Endocrinology 97: 366–372

Louvet J-P, Harman S M, Nisula B C, Ross G T, Birken S, Canfield R 1976 Follicle stimulating activity of human chorionic gonadotropin: effect of dissociation and recombination of subunits. Endocrinology 99: 1126–1128

Lyon F A 1975 The development of adenocarcinoma of the endometrium in young women receiving long term sequential oral contraception. American Journal of Obstetrics and Gynecology 123: 299–301

Lyons N F, Wilson P C, Connolly M C, Crane W A J, 1980 A virilizing hilus-cell tumour in an African patient with Turner's syndrome. British Journal of Obstetrics and Gynaecology 87: 169–173

MacDonald P C, Rombaut R P, Siiteri P K 1967 Plasma precursors of estrogen. I. Extent of conversion of plasma androstenedione to estrone in normal male and nonpregnant normal, castrate and adrenalectomized females. Journal of Clinical Endocrinology and Metabolism 27: 1103–1111

MacDonald P C, Grodin J M, Edman C D, Vellios F, Siiteri P K 1976 Origin of estrogen in a postmenopausal woman with a nonendocrine tumor of the ovary and endometrial hyperplasia. Obstetrics and Gynecology 47: 644–650

MacDonald P C, Edman C D, Hemsell D L, Porter J C, Siiteri P K 1978 Effect of obesity on conversion of plasma androstenedione to estrone in postmenopausal women with and without endometrial cancer. American Journal of Obstetrics and Gynecology 130: 448–455

Mackay E V, Khoo S K, Daunter B 1981 Tumor markers. In: Coppleson M (ed) Gynecologic Oncology pp 270–282. Churchill-Livingstone, Edinburgh

Mahesh V B, Greenblatt R B, Coniff R F 1968 Urinary steroid excretion before and after dexamethasone administration and steroid content of adrenal tissue and venous blood in virilizing adrenal tumors. American Journal of Obstetrics and Gynecology 100: 1043–1054

Mandel F P, Voet R L, Weiland A J, Judd H L 1981 Steroid secretion by masculinizing and 'feminizing' hilus cell tumors. Journal of Clinical Endocrinology and Metabolism 52: 779–784

Manuel M, Katayama K P, Jones H W Jr 1976 The age of occurrence of gonadal tumors in intersex patients with a Y chromosome. American Journal of Obstetrics and Gynecology 124: 293–300

McNatty K P, Hunter W M, McNeilly A S, Sawers R S 1975 Changes in the concentration of pituitary and steroid hormones in the follicular fluid of human Graafian follicles throughout the menstrual cycle. Journal of Endocrinology 64: 555–571

McNatty K P, Makris A, De Grazia C, Osathanondh R, Ryan K J 1979 The production of progesterone, androgens and oestrogens by human granulosa cells in vitro and in vivo. Journal of Steroid Biochemistry 11: 775–779

McNatty K P, Makris A, De Grazia C, Osathanondh R, Ryan K J 1980 Steroidogenesis by recombined follicular cells from the human ovary in vitro. Journal of Clinical Endocrinology and Metabolism 51: 1286–1292

Marieb N J, Spangler S, Kashgarian M et al 1983 Cushing's syndrome secondary to ectopic cortisol production by an ovarian carcinoma. Journal of Clinical Endocrinology and Metabolism 57: 737–740

Meldrum D R, Abraham G E 1979 Peripheral and ovarian venous concentrations of various steroid hormones in virilizing ovarian tumors. Obstetrics and Gynecology 53: 36–43

Mikhail G 1970 Hormone secretion by the human ovaries. Gynecologic Investigation 1: 5–20

Moon Y S, Tsang B K, Simpson C, Armstrong D T 1978 17β-estradiol biosynthesis in cultured granulosa and thecal cells of human ovarian follicles: stimulation by follicle-stimulating hormone. Journal of Clinical Endocrinology and Metabolism 47: 263–267

Morris J McL 1953 The syndrome of testicular feminization in male pseudohermaphrodites. American Journal of Obstetrics and Gynecology 65: 1192–1211

Morrow C P, Kletzky O A, Disaia P J, Townsend D E, Mishell D R, Nakamura R M 1977 Clinical and laboratory correlates of molar pregnancy and trophoblastic disease. American Journal of Obstetrics and Gynecology 128: 424–429

Motlik K, Starka L 1973 Adrenocortical tumour of the ovary. Neoplasia 20: 97–110

Nedwich A, Frumin A, Meranze D R 1962 Erythrocytosis associated with uterine myomas. American Journal of Obstetrics and Gynecology 84: 174–178

Nelson W W, Green R R 1958 Histology of human ovary during pregnancy. American Journal of Obstetrics and Gynecology 76: 66–90

Nichols J, Warren J C, Mantz F A 1962 ACTH-like excretion from carcinoma of the ovary. The clinical effect of m,p'-DDD. Journal of the American Medical Association 182: 713–718

Nimrod A, Ryan K J 1975 Aromatization of androgens by human abdominal and breast fat tissue. Journal of Clinical Endocrinology and Metabolism 40: 367–372

Norman R J, Green-Thopson R W, Jialal I, Soutter W P, Pillay N L, Joubert S M 1981 Hyperthyroidism in gestational trophoblastic neoplasia. Clinical Endocrinology 15: 395–401

Norris H J, Adam A E 1981 Malignant germ cell tumours of ovary. In: Coppleson M (ed) Gynecologic Oncology, pp 680–696. Churchill Livingstone, Edinburgh

Norris H J, Taylor H B 1969 Virilization associated with cystic granulosa tumors. Obstetrics and Gynecology 34: 629–635

Novak E R, Long J H 1965 Arrhenoblastoma of the ovary. A review of the Ovarian Tumor Registry. American Journal of Obstetrics and Gynecology 92: 1082–1093

Novak E R, Mattingly R F 1960 Hilus cell tumor of the ovary. Obstetrics and Gynecology 15: 425–432

Novak D J, Lauchlan S C, McCawley A C, Faiman C 1970 Virilization during pregnancy. American Journal of Medicine 49: 281–290

Novak E R, Kutchmeshgi J, Mupas R S, Woodruff J D 1971 Feminizing gonadal stromal tumors. Analysis of the granulosa-theca cell tumors of the ovarian tumor registry. Obstetrics and Gynecology 38: 701–713

Novak E R, Lambrou C D, Woodruff J D 1975 Ovarian tumors in pregnancy. An ovarian tumor registry review. Obstetrics and Gynecology 46: 401–406

O'Hern T M, Neubecker R D 1962 Arrhenoblastoma. Obstetrics and Gynecology 19: 758–770

Odell W D, Wolfsen A R 1980 Hormones from tumours: are they ubiquitous? American Journal of Medicine 68: 317–318

Odell W, Wolfsen A, Yoshimoto Y, Weitzman R, Fisher D, Hirose F 1977 Ectopic peptide synthesis: a universal concomitant of neoplasia. Transactions of the Association of American Physicians 90: 204–227

Osathanondh R, Goldstein D R, Tulchinsky D, Finn A E 1977 Serum 17-α hydroxyprogesterone in patients with gestational trophoblastic neoplasms. Obstetrics and Gynecology 49: 77–79

Pantoja E, Noy M A, Axtmayer R W, et al 1975 Ovarian dermoids and their complications. Comprehensive historical review. Obstetrical and Gynecological Survey 30: 1–20

Paul S, Das C, Jailkhani B L, Talwar G P 1981 Progesterone synthesis by human placental syncytiotrophoblast in vitro. Preferred precursor and effect of human chorionic gonadotrophin. Journal of Steroid Biochemistry 14: 311–313

Pedowitz P, O'Brien F B 1960 Arrhenoblastoma of the ovary. Review of the literature and report of 2 cases. Obstetrics and Gynecology 16: 62–77

Peterson W F 1957 Malignant degeneration of benign cystic teratomas of the ovary. A collective review of the literature. Obstetrical and Gynecological Survey 12: 793–830

Planner R S, Abell D A, Barbaro C A, Beischer N A 1982 Massive enlargement of the ovaries after evacuation of hydatidiform moles. Australian and New Zealand Journal of Obstetrics and Gynaecology 22: 96–102

Plimpton C H, Gellhorn A 1956 Hypercalcemia in malignant disease without evidence of bone destruction. American Journal of Medicine 21: 750–759

Quinn M A, Baker H W G, Rome R, Fortune D, Brown J B 1983 Response of a mucinous ovarian tumor of borderline malignancy to human chorionic gonadotropin. Obstetrics and Gynecology 61: 121–126

Rao M C, Richards J S, Midgley A R Jr, Reichert L E Jr 1977 Regulation of gonadotropin receptors by luteinizing hormone in granulosa cells. Endocrinology 101: 512–523

Ratcliffe J G, Knight R A, Besser G M et al 1972 Tumor and plasma ACTH concentrations in patients with and without the ectopic ACTH syndrome. Clinical Endocrinology 1: 27–44

Reed M J, Hutton J D, Beard R W, Jacobs H S, James V H T 1979 Plasma hormone levels and oestrogen production in a postmenopausal woman with endometrial carcinoma and an ovarian thecoma. Clinical Endocrinology 11: 141–150

Rice B F, Savard K 1966 Steroid hormone formation in the human ovary: IV. Ovarian stromal compartments; formation of radioactive steroids from aurate-1-^{14}C and action of gonadotropins. Journal of Clinical Endocrinology and Metabolism 26: 593–609

Richards J S 1975 Estradiol receptor content in rat granulosa cells during follicular development: modification by estradiol and gonadotropins. Endocrinology 97: 1174–1184

Richards J S, Ireland J J, Rao M C, Bernath G A, et al 1976 Ovarian follicular development in the rat: hormone receptor regulation by estradiol, follicle stimulating hormone and luteinizing hormone. Endocrinology 99: 1562–1570

Rivarola M A, Forest M G, Migeon C J 1968 Testosterone, androstenedione and dehydroepiandrosterone in plasma during pregnancy and at delivery: concentration and protein binding. Journal of Clinical Endocrinology and Metabolism 28: 34–40

Rizkallah T H, Tovell H M, Kelly W G 1975 Production of estrone and fractional conversion of circulating androstenedione to estrone in women with endometrial carcinoma. Journal of Clinical Endocrinology and Metabolism 40: 1045–1056

Robboy S J, Norris H J, Scully R E 1975 Insular carcinoid primary in the ovary. A clinicopathologic analysis of 48 cases. Cancer 36: 404–418

Rome R M, Fortune D W, Quinn M A, Brown J B 1981 Functioning ovarian tumors in postmenopausal women. Obstetrics and Gynecology 57: 705–710

Rose L I, Underwood R H, Williams G H, Pinkus G S 1974 Pure gonadal gysgenesis. Studies of in vitro androgen metabolism. American Journal of Medicine 57: 957–961

Ross G T 1978 Disordered follicular maturation and atresia. In: Givens J R (ed) Endocrine Causes of Menstrual Disorders, pp 223–236. Year Book Medical Publishers, Chicago

Roth L M, Sternberg W H 1973 Ovarian stromal tumors. II. Pure Leydig cell tumor, non-hilar type. Cancer 32: 952–960

Roth L M, Nicholas T R, Ehrlich C E 1979 Juvenile granulosa cell tumor. A clinicopathologic study of three cases with ultrastructural observations. Cancer 44: 2194–2205

Roth L M, Anderson M C, Govan A D T, Langley F A, Gowing N F C, and Woodcock A S 1981 Sertoli-Leydig cell tumors: a clinicopathologic study of 34 cases. Cancer 48: 187–197

Roth J, LeRoith D, Shiloach J, Rosenzweig J L, Lesniak M A, Havrankova J 1982 The evolutionary origins of hormones, neurotransmitters, and other extracellular chemical messengers. Implications for mammalian biology. New England Journal of Medicine 306: 523–527

Rutamen E-M, Seppala M 1978 The HCG-beta subunit radioimmunoassay in nontrophoblastic gynecologic tumors. Cancer 41: 692–696

Ryan K J, Petro Z, Kaiser J 1968 Steroid formation by isolated and recombined ovarian granulosa and thecal cells. Journal of Clinical Endocrinology and Metabolism 28: 355–358

Samaan N A, Smith J P, Rutledge F N, Barcellona J M 1972 Plasma testosterone levels in trophoblastic disease and the effects of oophorectomy and chemotherapy. Journal of Clinical Endocrinology and Metabolism 34: 558–561

Saunders D M, Barratt J, Grudzinskas G 1975 Feminization in gonadal dysgenesis associated with ovarian gonadoblastoma. Obstetrics and Gynecology 46: 93–97

Savard K, Gut M, Dorfman R I, Gabrilove JL, Soffer L J 1961 Formation of androgens by human arrhenoblastoma tissue in vitro. Journal of Clinical Endocrinology and Metabolism 21: 165–174

Scott J S, Lumsden C E, Levell M J 1967 Ovarian endocrine activity in association with hormonally inactive neoplasia. American Journal of Obstetrics and Gynecology 97: 161–170

Scully R E 1970 Gonadoblastoma. A review of 74 cases. Cancer 25: 1340–1356

Scully R E 1977 Ovarian Tumors. A review. American Journal of Pathology 87: 686–720

Shane J M, Naftolin F 1975 Aberrant hormone activity by tumors of gynecologic importance. American Journal of Obstetrics and Gynecology 121: 133–147

Sherwood L M 1980 The multiple causes of hypercalcemia in malignant disease. New England Journal of Medicine 303: 1412–1413

Shetty M R, Boghossian H M, Duffell D, Freel R, Gonzales J C 1982 Tumor-induced hypoglycemia. A result of ectopic insulin production. Cancer 49: 1920–1923

Silverberg J, O'Donnell J, Sugenoya A, Row V V, Volpe R 1978 Effect of human chorionic gonadotropin on human thyroid tissue in vitro. Journal of Clinical Endocrinology and Metabolism 46: 420–424

Siris E S, Nisula B C, Catt K J, Horner K, Birken S, Canfield R E, Ross G T 1978 New evidence for intrisic follicle-stimulating

hormone-like activity in human chorionic gonadotropin and luteinizing hormone. Endocrinology 102: 1356–1361

Skrabanek P, Kirrane J, Powell D 1979 A unifying concept of chorionic gonadotrophin production in malignancy. Investigations in Cell Pathology 2: 75–85

Smith H C, Posen S, Clifton-Bligh P, Casey J 1978 A testoterone-secreting adrenal cortical adenoma. Australian and New Zealand Journal of Medicine 8: 171–175

Soutter W P, Norman R, Green-Thopson R W 1981 The management of choriocarcinoma causing severe thyrotoxicosis. Two case reports. British Journal of Obstetrics and Gynaecology 88: 938–943

Sowers J R, Hershman J M, Carlson H E, Pekary A E 1978 Effect of human chorionic gonadotropin on thyroid function in euthyroid men. Journal of Clinical Endocrinology and Metabolism 47: 898–901

Spaulding S W, Masuda T, Osawa Y 1980 Increased 17β-hydroxysteroid dehydrogenase activity in a masculinizing adrenal adenoma in a patient with isolated testosterone overproduction. Journal of Clinical Endocrinology and Metabolism 50: 537–540

Sternberg W H, Dhurander H N 1977 Functional ovarian tumors of stromal and sex cord origin. Human Pathology 8: 565–582

Sternberg W H, Roth L M 1973 Ovarian stromal tumors containing Leydig cells. I. Stromal-Leydig cell tumor and non-neoplastic transformation of ovarian stroma to Leydig cells. Cancer 32: 940–951

Stewart K R, Casey M J, Gondos B 1981 Endodermal sinus tumor of the ovary with virilization. Light- and electron-microscope study. American Journal of Surgical Pathology 5: 385–391

Stewart A F, Romero R, Schwartz P E, Kohorn E I, Broadus A E 1982 Hypercalcemia associated witwh gynecologic malignancies. Biochemical characterization. Cancer 49: 2389–2394

Sutton G P, Lyles K W, Wiebe R H 1981 Steroid secretion and testosterone binding in a woman with an ovarian hilus cell tumor and thyrotoxicosis. American Journal of Obstetrics and Gynecology 141: 535–538

Tavassoli F A, Norris H J 1980 Sertoli cell tumors of the ovary. A clinicopathological study of 28 cases with ultrastructural observations. Cancer 46: 2281–2297

Taylor H B 1966 Functioning ovarian tumors and related conditions. Pathology Annual 1: 127–147

Todesco S, Terribile V, Borsatti A, Mantero F 1975 Primary aldosteronism due to a malignant ovarian tumor. Journal of Clinical Endocrinology and Metabolism 41: 809–819

Tumen H J 1930 The association of polycythemia with occlusion of the inferior vena cava. American Journal of Obstetrics and Gynecology 20: 417–420

Ueda G, Hamanaka N, Hayakawa K, et al 1972 Clinical, histochemical, and biochemical studies of an ovarian dysgerminoma with trophoblasts and leydig cells. American Journal of Obstetrics and Gynecology 114: 748–754

Vaitukaitis J L, Ross G T, Braunstein G D, Rayford P L 1976 Gonadotropins and their subunits: basic and clinical studies. Recent Prigress in Hormone Research 32: 289–331

Verdonk C, Guerin C, Lufkin E, Hodgson S F 1982 Activation of virilizing adrenal rest tissues by excessive ACTH production. An unusual presentation of Nelson's syndrome. American Journal of Medicine 73: 455–459

Verhoeven A T M, Mastboom J L, Van Leusden H A I M, Van der Velden W H M 1973 Virilization in pregnancy coexisting with an (ovarian) mucinous cystadenoma. A case report and review of virilizing ovarian tumors in pregnancy. Obstetrical and Gynecological Survey 28: 597–622

Vermeulen A 1976 The hormonal activity of the postmenopausal ovary. Journal of Clinical Endocrinology and Metabolism 42: 247–253

Villee D B 1969 Development of endocrine function in the human placenta and fetus. New England Journal of Medicine 281: 473–484

Wachtel S S, Koo G C, Breg W R, et al 1976 Serologic detection of a Y-linked gene in XX males and XX true hermaphrodites. New England Journal of Medicine 295: 750–754

Wagstaff T I 1973 Luteoma in pregnancy. Australian and New Zealand Journal of Obstetrics and Gynaecology 13: 232–235

Wallach S, Brown H, Englert E Jr, Eik-Nes K 1957 Adrenocortical carcinoma with gynecomastia: a case report and review of the literature. Journal of Clinical Endocrinology and Metabolism 17: 945–958

Weiland A J Bookstein J J, Clearly R E, Judd H L 1978 Preoperative localization of virilizing tumors by selective venous sampling. American Journal of Obstetrics and Gynecology 131: 797–802

Wentz A C, McCranie W M 1976 Circulating hormone levels in a case of granulosa cell tumor. Fertility and Sterility 27: 167–170

Wentz A C, White R I Jr, Migeon C J et al 1976 Differential ovarian and adrenal vein catheterization. American Journal of Obstetrics and Gynecology 125: 1000–1007

Werk E E, Sholiton L J, Kalejs L 1973 Testosterone-secreting adrenal adenoma under gonadotropin control. New England Journal of Medicine 289: 767–770

Wong T-W, Warner N E 1971 Ovarian thecal metaplasia in the adrenal gland. Archives of Pathology 92: 319–328

Woodruff J D, Markley R L 1957 Struma ovarii. Demonstration of both pathologic change and physiologic activity; report of four cases. Obstetrics and Gynecology 9: 707–719

Woodruff J D, Williams T J, Goldberg B 1963 Hormone activity of the common ovarian neoplasm. American Journal of Obstetrics and Gynecology 87: 679–698

Woodruff J K, Goldberg B, Jones G S 1968 Enzymic histochemical reations in two Krukenberg tumors associated with clinically different endocrine patterns. American Journal of Obstetrics and Gynecology 100: 405–417

Yin P-H, Sommers S C 1961 Some pathologic correlations of ovarian stromal hyperplasia. Journal of Clinical Endocrinology and Metabolism 21: 472–477

Yoshimoto Y, Wolfsen A R, Hirose F, Odell W D 1979 Human chorionic gonadotropin-like material: presence in normal human tissues. American Journal of Obstetrics and Gynecology 134: 729–733

Endocrine aspects of genito-urinary neoplasia

INTRODUCTION

The association between hormonal factors and tumours of the genito-urinary tract was first documented more than two centuries ago (Pott, 1779; Hunter, 1786). Experimental and epidemiological data link the hormonal milieu and the genesis of cancer of the testis, kidney and prostate gland, and there is evidence to suggest that the growth of these tumours is hormonally dependent.

In this chapter, we review the aetiological, clinical and therapeutic associations between hormones and neoplasia of the genito-urinary tract.

TESTICULAR CANCER

Although uncommon in the general community, testicular malignancy represents a major cause of neoplastic morbidity and mortality in young males. The annual incidence in the male community is 3–6/100 000 (Mostofi & Price, 1973; Pugh, 1976), with a peak in the 15–35 age group. Moreover, it has been suggested that the incidence of the disease is rising (Clemmeson 1968).

The majority of testicular tumours (including seminomas and teratomas, or non-seminomatous germ cell tumours) have been shown to be of germinal origin, arising from germ cells that have migrated from the yolk sac to the genital ridges during fetal life (Dixon & Moore, 1952; Mostofi & Price, 1973; Teilum, 1976), as reviewed elsewhere (Raghavan & Neville, 1983). In addition to these tumours, malignant lymphomas, Leydig cell and Sertoli cell tumours, gonadoblastomas and metastatic tumours may be found less frequently in the testicles — these uncommon tumours will not be discussed here in detail.

The aetiology of germ cell tumours is unknown, although associated factors have been defined, including testicular maldescent, congenital abnormalities of the urogenital tract, trauma, mumps, sporadic familial associations and chromosomal abnormalities (Mostofi & Price, 1973; Raghavan & Neville, 1983).

A large body of circumstantial and experimental evidence suggests a close association between hormonal factors and the genesis of testicular germ cell tumours. The physiology of testicular function, with the complex interactions of the hypothalamic-pituitary-end organ axis, has already been reviewed (Ch. 3) and will not be repeated here. Nevertheless, major abnormalities of endocrine function have been demonstrated in patients with germ cell tumours (*vide infra*), and it is uncertain whether they represent the causes or effects of these tumours.

Experimental models

The intra-testicular injection of metallic salts in cockerels frequently induces the development of testicular teratomas. Of considerable interest has been the demonstration that this phenomenon is seasonally dependent, the most frequent production of testicular teratomas occurring when the experiments are carried out in spring, the time of maximum gonadotrophin secretion (Michalowsky, 1926; Carleton et al, 1953; Guthrie, 1964). It has also been claimed that the growth rate of cells derived from testicular tumours in tissue culture is modified by the addition of androgenic steroids to the culture medium, in some cases being enhanced and in others suppressed (Kallen & Rohl, 1962). However, these data are difficult to evaluate because of the lack of characterisation of the cells in culture (whether these populations represent tumour tissue or fibroblast outgrowths).

In a study in male rats, Dmitriev (1977) has shown that the growth of experimentally induced testicular tumours can be arrested by treatment with parenteral oestrogens, and has postulated the suppression of circulating follicle stimulating hormone (FSH) as the major determinant of tumour regression. In another study with rats, Prudencio et al (1973) have demonstrated regression of induced testicular tumours in response to hypophysectomy. More recently, Damjanov & Solter (1981) have demonstrated that maternal factors influence the development of testicular tumours in mice of the 129 strain. This strain has previously been shown to be susceptible to testicular tumours (Stevens, 1962) and has provided an important model of testicular malignancy and of the interactions between the factors governing normal organ development (ontogenesis) and the initiation of malignant change (oncogenesis). Certain strains of the these mice, so-called 'permissive' strains, are associated with a greater prevalence of tumours. The mating of reciprocal F_1 hybrids of 'permissive' and 'non-permissive' strains has shown that maternal factors determine the eventual prevalence of tumours in the offspring.

The use of immunosuppressed animals, including cortisone-treated hamsters, congenitally athymic (T-cell deficient) 'nude' mice and thymectomised and irradiated mice, as hosts for fragments of implanted tumours has provided another experimental model for the study of the endocrinology of testicular cancer. These 'xenografted' tumours have been used, in particular, to characterise the production of hormones and of tumour marker substances (for example, human chorionic gonadotrophin and alpha-foetoprotein) as discussed elsewhere (Pierce et al, 1959; Selby et al, 1979; Raghavan et al, 1980, 1981a; Raghavan & Selby, 1981). Another animal model that links the hormonal environment and the genesis of testicular tumours is the initiation of Leydig cell tumours in mice by the repeated administration of oestrogens (Bonser & Robson, 1940; Hooker et al, 1940); these effects are accelerated by chorionic gonadotrophin and anterior pituitary hormones. Subsequent serial transplantation is dependent upon the administration of oestrogens; however, once initiated, the transplant becomes hormone-independent.

Epidemiology and natural history

In man, the maximum incidence of germ cell tumours is found in late adolescence and in the third decade (Mostofi & Price, 1973; Pugh, 1976), corresponding to a period of maximum reproductive activity and possibly of peak circulating blood androgen levels. The tumours found in these age groups are mainly seminomas, embryonal cell carcinomas and teratocarcinomas. The majority of seminomas, in fact, occur in somewhat older patients and only rarely are seen in children. They are associated with a better prognosis than are maliganant teratomas (non-seminomatous germ cell tumours or NSGCT) which occur in the younger age groups. Seminomas appear to be characterised by slower growth rates, later metastasis and greater radiosensitivity — whether these features reflect the endocrine environment is not known.

The spectrum of testicular germ cell tumours in pre-pubertal males is quite different. The majority of testicular neoplasms in this age group are yolk sac tumours (50–75 per cent) or differentiated teratomas (25 per cent) (Brown, 1976; Brosman, 1979). Although the yolk sac tumours are highly malignant whatever the age of the patient, the other germ cell tumours that occur in pre-pubertal males tend to be more differentiated, with a concomitantly more benign behaviour. Similarly, in females, excluding yolk sac tumours, NSGCT tend to be more differentiated, with a better prognosis (Caruso, 1971). In fact, the majority of the ovarian germ cell tumours are dysgerminomas, with similar behaviour patterns to seminoma, their male equivalent (Kurman & Norris, 1976).

There is marked variation in the natural history of sacrococcygeal germ cell tumours — they have an excellent prognosis if treated surgically at birth, but can be highly malignant if left untreated for a few months (Donellan & Swenson, 1968). Paradoxically, these tumours are characteristically benign if they first present in older patients, perhaps representing a selection process or an altered natural history in a different hormonal environment.

The ingestion of stilboestrol during pregnancy has been shown to be associated with the subsequent development of vaginal adenocarcinoma in female offspring (Herbst et al, 1971). Similar correlations for genital tract cancer have been sought in male offspring. Although early reports have not shown an increased incidence of testicular cancer in this setting (Henderson et al, 1973; Bibbo et al, 1975; Loughlin et al, 1980), an increased prevalence of urogenital tract anomalies, including testicular hypoplasia has been noted in males exposed to diethylstilboestrol in utero (Gill et al, 1977; Cosgrove et al, 1977) and, more recently, Henderson et al (1979) have demonstrated an increased prevalence of oestrogen ingestion in the mothers of 131 patients with testicular cancer, as compared to matched controls, although the statistical significance of the study was limited by the numbers of patients. The association of testicular maldescent and subsequent testicular cancer has been extensively documented (Pott, 1779; Gilbert & Hamilton, 1940; Blandy et al, 1970). Whether this represents oncogenesis due to trauma, the hormonal milieu or other factors is not known. Nevertheless, a 20- to 30-fold increase in prevalence of these tumours is found in patients with a history of testicular maldescent. In some instances, the testicular tumour occurs on the contralateral side from the maldescended testis. Of possible relevance to this phenomenon is the demonstration in rats that ischaemia induced in one testicle is associated with subsequent damage to the contralateral testis if the originally injured testicle is not removed — this may represent an immunological phenomenon, and is associated with disruption of spermatogenesis (Harrison et al, 1981).

Further evidence on this subject is provided by the description of carcinoma in situ of the testis (Skakkebaek, 1975), characterised by the presence of pre-invasive intratubular 'atypical' germ cells with increased size, irregular chromatin patterns, increased DNA content and a raised mitotic index. These cells have been described in infertile males (Nuesch-Bachman & Hedinger, 1977; Skakkebaek, 1978), in the contralateral testes of patients with germ cell tumours (Berthelsen et al, 1979), in cryptorchid and ectopic testicles (Waxman, 1976; Krabbe et al, 1979) and in 'normal' tissue adjacent to germ cell tumours (Skakkebaek, 1975). Further support for the association of infertility and testicular cancer is provided by the reports of testicular tumours that have occurred in males treated for infertility with clomiphene, human chorionic gonadotrophin and mesterolone (Reyes & Faiman, 1973; Rubin, 1973; Neoptolemos et al, 1981). The occurrence of carcinoma in situ in a variety of conditions associated with testicular cancer and with hormonal abnormalities suggests an interaction of endocrine factors in the genesis of germ cell tumours, although it remains difficult to separate the components of cause and effect.

The majority of patients with testicular tumours do not have cryptorchidism or infertility. Nevertheless, endocrinological abnormalities have been reported in such patients; for example, before treatment, low circulating FSH levels have been demonstrated (Reiter & Kulin, 1971), as well as decreased testosterone levels (Fossa et al, 1980). In addition, the testes of patients with testicular tumours do not respond to markedly elevated circulating levels of hCG that may be present, although they may respond to injections of luteinising hormone (Kirschner et al, 1970). Before orchidectomy, or immediately thereafter, these patients often have markedly depressed sperm counts (Thachil et al, 1981; Bracken & Smith, 1980).

At issue is the significance of these observations: Is the observed infertility related to the aetiology of the cancer or merely an effect of it? Previously there was little information to resolve this issue because the treatment itself was considered to cause infertility. For example, retroperitoneal lymph node dissection damages the autonomic nerves that control the emission of semen, causing the patient to have a 'dry ejaculate' (Kom et al, 1971). Furthermore, cytotoxic chemotherapy was thought to cause permanent loss of spermatogenesis (Thachil et al, 1981). However, it has now been demonstrated that effective lymphadenectomy can be accomplished in many patients without permanent loss of ejaculation (Narayan et al, 1982), and that spermatogenesis will often return after the use of standard chemotherapy regimens such as cis-platinum, vinblastine and bleomycin (Drasga et al, 1982; Lange et al, 1983). In many of the patients who have undergone one or both of these treatments, sperm analysis returns to normal (Lange et al, 1983). These data, as well as the evidence that patients with other malignancies (such as Hodgkin's disease) have abnormal semen (Chapman et al, 1981), suggest that infertility in patients with testicular cancer may be a direct effect of the disease itself.

Endocrinological aspects of diagnosis

Clinical Presentation

Testicular cancers are frequently associated with endocrine manifestations, both clinically and in the laboratory. Gynaecomastia is seen in approximately 5 per cent of patients with Sertoli or Leydig cell tumours. This may be accompanied by galactorrhoea. The basis of gynaecomastia in germinal malignancy is not fully understood. Conflicting data have resulted from the available studies, which relate this feature to increased circulating levels of prolactin, human chorionic gonadotrophin, oestrone, oestradiol and to low levels of testosterone (Stepanas et al, 1978) or to an altered oestrogen: testosterone ratio (Lindenmeyer et al, 1973; Siiteri & MacDonald, 1973). In addition, immunocytochemical studies have demonstrated human chorionic gonadotrophin and human placental lactogen (hPL) to be produced by tumours in patients with gynaecomastia (Heyderman, 1979). However, the numbers of patients studied have been small, and no data have been included to specify other possible causes of gynaecomastia (such as drug use — for example, metoclopamide, which stimulates prolactin secretion).

In children with Leydig cell tumours, precocious puberty may occur, with hypertrophy of genitalia, precocious skeletal and muscular growth.

Laboratory investigation

The inadequacy of conventional imaging techniques (Husband, 1980) has stimulated the search for more sensitive and specific indices of viable tumour tissue. One probe that has offered such a potential is the monitoring of tumour markers, substances regularly and reliably produced by viable tumour tissue. The 'ideal' tumour marker, produced by only one type of tumour cell, would be truly monoclonal in origin and should be readily and reproducibly measured when present in only minute amounts in the tissues, body fluids or excreta, and should correlate directly with viable tumour mass.

In testicular cancer, most of the known tumour markers are 'onco-developmental' antigens, expressed both by tumour cells and by cells of the developing embryo. As these substances are normally found during development, their presence in tumour tissue is probably not the result of mutation, but rather the re-expression of genes that have been repressed at some stage during development. This phenomenon may reflect an inter-relationship between normal organ development and the mechanisms of malignant transformation (Abelev, 1974). The onco-developmental proteins, human chorionic gonadotrophin and alphafoetoprotein (AFP) are the two most useful tumour markers in clinical practice today, although they do not fulfil the 'ideal' criteria.

Human chorionic gonadotrophin (hCG). hCG is a glycoprotein with a molecular weight of about 38 000, normally produced by placental trophoblastic tissue. It is composed of two dissimilar polypeptide chains, α and β, the former subunit being common to luteinising hormone (LH), thyroid stimulating hormone (TSH) and FSH, and the latter conferring immunological and biological specificity (Vaitukaitis, 1979). Antisera raised against the whole hCG molecule cross react with LH, whereas antibodies raised against the β subunit of hCG cross react to only a small degree with LH in physiological concentrations and are thus a more specific marker of vital tumour.

Zondek (1929, 1930) first demonstrated the production of large quantities of gonadotrophic hormones by males with testicular tumours, using bioassay techniques. Hamburger et al (1936) characterised the hormones and attempted to correlate their production with tumour histology and response to treatment, but without great success. Several workers were able to demonstrate histological evidence that a variety of tumour types were associated with the production of FSH and chorionic gonadotrophin (Hamburger et al, 1936; Furuhjelm, 1941; Twombley, 1947) prior to the introduction of immunocytochemical localising techniques.

With the use of more sensitive assay procedures, the prevalence of detectable hCG in patients with NSGCT has risen to about 50 per cent and it appears that this proportion may be even higher if immunocytochemical procedures are used to demonstrate hCG in fixed tumour tissues (Raghavan et al, 1982a). These procedures also allow the sites of production of hCG to be demonstrated — the marker is elaborated by trophoblastic tissue, by syncytial giant cells and by undifferentiated cells found singly or in clusters (Heyderman & Neville, 1976; Kurman et al, 1977; Heyderman et al, 1981). These cells may be present in NSGCT or in seminoma, explaining the association of hCG with both tumour types. The prevalence of increased levels of hCG in patients with seminoma and no histological evidence of NSGCT elements is between 10 and 30 per cent (Lange et al, 1980; Kohn & Raghavan, 1981).

hCG is not completely specific to the placenta and testicular tumours — 'ectopic' hCG production may be found in association with other malignancies (including carcinoma of the liver, lung, ovary, breast, kidney, bladder and gastrointestinal tract) and in some non-malignant conditions (Table 38.1).

The metabolic half-life of the whole hCG molecule in the human circulation is between 24 and 36 hours (Vaitukaitis, 1979), although its component sub-units have much shorter half-life values. Tumours do not always produce whole hCG molecules; some produce only α-hCG or β-hCG fragments. Nevertheless, the metabolic clearance characteristics of hCG can be of considerable importance in patient management, as discussed below. Lectin binding assays have demonstrated micro-heterogeneity of hCG production — i.e. different molecular structures, with different binding characteristics (Yoshimoto et al, 1977). A detailed review of the physiology of hCG production is beyond the scope of this chapter, and has been covered elsewhere (Vaitukaitis, 1979; Kohn & Raghavan, 1981;

Norgaard-Pedersen et al, 1981; Lange & Raghavan, 1983).

Alphafetoprotein (AFP). AFP, a glycoprotein of molecular weight 70 000, is a single chain molecule produced by the fetal yolk sac, liver and gastrointestinal tract in many species. In the human fetus, it reaches a peak at about the third month of gestation and then gradually declines. In normal children older than one year and in adults, levels as high as 14 to 16 μg/l may be detected. Its function is unknown, but it appears to act as an albumin-like protein in the fetus, and may have an immuno-regulatory function (Ruoslahti & Hirai, 1978). This protein was first detected 25 years ago in the sera of animals with chemically induced hepatomas, and has been demonstrated in up to 70 per cent of patients with hepatomas, 70 per cent of patients with germ cell tumours, in association with liver metastases and occasionally in other tumour types (Table 38.1).

Its metabolic clearance half life is about 4–6 days in man.

Table 38.1 Causes of raised AFP or HCG levels

Condition	AFP	hCG	Comments
Pregnancy	+ + +	+ + +	
Early infancy	+ + +	+ + +	Persistent decline
Cross reaction with LH	–	±	Resolve with testosterone stimulation
Marijuana	–	± ?	?LH effect?
Benign liver	± ±	–	Note liver function tests
Ataxia telangiectasia	± ±	–	
Neural tube defects	± ±	–	
Hereditary tyrosinaemia	± ±	–	
Malignancy			
Hepatoma	± → + + +	+/–	70% of Pts with AFP
Germ cell tumours	± → + + +	± → + + +	80% of Pts with AFP and/or hCG
Gestational neoplasia	–	+ + +	
Lung	–	±	hCG usually <50 miu/l
Breast	–	±	hCG usually <50 miu/l
Kidney	–	±	hCG usually <50 miu/l
Bladder	–	±	hCG usually <50 miu/l
Ovary	–	±	hCG usually <50 miu/l
Cervix	–	±	hCG usually <50 miu/l
Gastrointestinal	± ±	±	hCG usually <50 miu/l

Key: ± range of values from 'normal' to small elevation; + + + range of values up to markedly elevated; LH luteinising hormone; AFP alphafetoprotein; hCG human chorionic gonadotrophin.

The use of lectin binding studies (for example, with con-canavalin-A) has demonstrated heterogeneity of these pro-teins — for example, in man, two types of AFP have been demonstrated: concanavalin-A 'binding' and 'non-binding' fractions. Fetal liver tissue and hepatomas are associated with 'bound' fractions of approximately 95 per cent, where-as AFP from amniotic fluid or germ cell tumours only has a 50 per cent binding ratio — this forms the basis of a useful test to determine the nature of the tumour associated with AFP production in clinical practice (Vessella et al, 1983).

Immunocytochemical studies have localised the produc-tion of AFP to classical hepatoma, yolk sac carcinoma, undif-ferentiated cells within germ cell tumours and, more recently, to a solid variant of yolk sac tumour that resem-bles seminoma morphologically (Kurman et al, 1977; Heyderman, 1979; Raghavan et al, 1980b; Heyderman et al, 1981). However, raised levels of AFP in patients with apparently 'pure' seminoma imply the presence of occult foci of NSGCT and that the patient should be treated as if NSGCT had been demonstrated (Lange et al, 1980; Raghavan et al, 1982b).

Other tumour markers. Several potential tumour markers have been described in association with testicular tumours, including carcinoembryonic antigen (CEA), fibronectin, lactic acid dehydrogenase (LDH), placental alkaline phos-phatase, human placental lactogen, prolactin, SP-1, oestrone and oestradiol (Table 38.2). A thorough review of the physiology and applications of these substances to the management of testicular cancer has been rpovided else-where (Lange & Raghavan, 1983; Norgaard-Pedersen et al, 1981).

Although a variety of cell surface antigens have been described in murine testicular cancer (Artzt et al, 1973) and in human studies (Holden et al, 1977; Hogan et al, 1977; McIlhinney, 1981), there are no published data on the presence or absence of steroid receptors on the surface of testicular tumours. Although steroid receptors have been demonstrated in normal testicular tissue, and the phenom-enon of negative or 'down' regulation of receptors by LH,

prolactin and hCG in mice and rats has been described (Klemcke & Bartke, 1981; Chan et al, 1981), no analogous studies have yet been reported in patients with testicular cancer.

Clinical applications of tumour markers

Monitoring of treatment. To be of maximum clinical value, both AFP and hCG should be measured because of the large percentage of patients with raised circulating levels of only one marker. In a review of more than 400 patients with metastatic NSGCT, 25 per cent had raised levels of only AFP and 15 per cent had raised hCG as the only detectable marker (Kohn & Raghavan, 1981). In addition, discordance may occur — when one marker level falls and the other rises or remains unchanged in response to therapy (Braunstein et al, 1973; Lange et al, 1977; Raghavan et al, 1980).

For practical purposes, persistently elevated circulating marker levels in patients with germ cell tumours equate with the presence of active neoplastic disease. However, the monitoring of serial samples is of the greatest import-ance to ensure the following:

1. that a random laboratory error has not occurred;
2. that the increased level is not merely a reflection of metabolic decay of a high initial level — for example, a patient with an initial AFP level of 2000 μg/l at the time of orchidectomy would normally have an AFP level of 250 μg/l 2 weeks after the operation in accordance with a metabolic half-life of 5 days (*vide supra*);
3. that the diagnosis of recurrent tumour is made as early as possible — detectable elevations of tumour marker levels in the blood may be found several weeks before recurrent tumour can be detected with imaging techniques, such as X-rays, CT scans and radionucleide scans.

It should be noted that many commercially available radioimmunoassays for the β-subunit of hCG cross react with LH, yielding low positive values in the absence of active tumour, an important consideration in patients with

Table 38.2 Other markers of testicular cancer

Marker	Localised in tumour tissue	Present in blood	Radioimmunoassay	Clinical uses or comments
CEA	Yes	Yes	Yes	Poor correlation with course of disease
LDH	No	Yes	No	Correlates with bulky tumour Unstable antigen for measurement
PlAP	Yes	Yes	Yes	Monitor for some seminomas
SP–1	Yes	Yes	Yes	Marked overlap with hCG
AAT	Yes	Yes	No	Marked overlap with AFP
Ferritin	Yes	Yes	No	Poor correlation with course of tumour
HPL	Yes	Yes	Yes	? Poor correlation with course of tumour
Fibronectin	Yes	Yes	No	? Unknown

Key: CEA carcinoembryonic antigen; LDH lactic acid dehydrogenase; PlAP placental alkaline phosphatase; AAT α₁ antitrypsin; HPL human placental lactogen; SP–1 Schwangerschafte protein–1.

only one or no testicles and who may also have been rendered hypogonadal (with grossly elevated LH) by chemotherapy. In this situation, retesting of hCG after the patient has received a short course of testosterone (to suppress LH production) may help to resolve the issue (Catalona et al, 1979).

It should be emphasised that the absence of detectable markers does not equate with the absence of tumour — up to 30 per cent of patients with metastatic NSGCT have no detectable levels of AFP or hCG (Kohn & Raghavan, 1981; Raghavan et al, 1980), and metastatic seminomas are usually not associated with these tumour markers. In the latter context, placental alkaline phosphatase appears to be useful in monitoring the progress of these patients (Wahren et al, 1979; Lange et al, 1982a). Furthermore, in some patients with raised circulating marker levels at presentation, the levels will fall in response to treatment, although persistent tumour tissue can be demonstrated, representing residual non-marker-producing 'clones' of cells, a function of the cellular heterogeneity of these tumours (Raghavan et al, 1980).

With the awareness of these potential pitfalls, AFP and hCG together provide a major clinical aid in monitoring of response to treatment and as a harbinger of recurrence, as they can be detected as an index of viable cell masses 100 times smaller than can be seen with conventional imaging techniques. Furthermore, detection of prolonged metabolic clearance times of tumour markers correlates with persistent tumour or resistance of the tumour cells to treatment — this reflects the balance of metabolic clearance rate versus continued production of markers by viable cells (Kohn, 1978; Lange et al, 1982b).

Prognostic implications. One issue that remains to be resolved is whether AFP or hCG, in themselves, have prognostic significance — i.e. is marker elevation merely a reflection of tumour mass or does the production of markers indicate an inherent aggressiveness, metastatic potential or resistance to treatment? When data are not corrected for tumour bulk or histology, high marker levels appear to be an adverse prognostic sign (Scardino et al 1977; Bagshawe, 1980; Newlands et al, 1980; Friedman et al, 1980; Peckham et al, 1981). However, when the cases are separated into subgroups on the basis of histology and tumour mass (bulk), raised levels of hCG do not appear to be an independent prognostic variable (Scardino & Skinner, 1979; Peckham et al, 1981; Raghavan et al, 1982a). The situation regarding AFP is less certain, and further studies will be required. In patients with seminoma, AFP is of adverse progostic significance because it implies the presence of NSGCT.

However, in this setting, the significance of hCG is uncertain, with conflicting data (Wilson & Woodhead, 1972; Maier & Sulak, 1973; Mauch et al, 1979; Lange et al, 1980). Finally, as previously discussed, the presence of a prolonged metabolic clearance time (half-life) appears to

be an adverse prognostic factor, as it implies the continued presence of viable tumour despite treatment.

Tumour localisation techniques. In addition to the conventional assay techniques which demonstrate raised blood marker levels, two methods have been developed that may reveal the site of marker production in an individual patient:

1. Selective venous catheterisation: Percutaneous catheterisation of the veins that drain the groin and retroperitoneum allows sampling of venous blood at intervals for the assay of α-hCG. Because of the short halving time of this subunit (20 min), there is little accumulation in the peripheral circulation and marked local increases in concentration can sometimes be detected; however, the technique is complicated and of limited practical use (Javadpour, 1980).

2. Radio-immuno-localisation: radiolabelled anti-CEA antibodies can be used to locate deposits of CEA-producing tumours in animals and in humans (Goldenberg et al, 1978). The technique involves the labelling of specific antibodies with a radio-isotope, such as [123]iodine, and the use of [131]iodine and subtraction imaging techniques to eliminate the blood pool background (that would be caused by circulating levels of CEA) on a computer print-out or screen. More recently, antibodies raised against hCG and AFP have been radiolabelled and used to localise deposits of germ cell tumours with some early successes (Goldenberg et al, 1980a,b) and antibodies raised against cell surface antigens that are expressed by germ cell tumours have been used in experimental models (Moshakis et al, 1981). These techniques have not yet been proved in routine clinical practice and it remains uncertain whether the resolution is greater than for conventional imaging procedures. One important theoretical benefit is the requirement for viable tumour to produce tumour markers — thus the demonstration of a true positive radio-immuno-localisation scan may be a useful method of detecting live tumour deposits, thus distinguishing benign masses, fibrosis or necrosis.

Endocrine therapy of testicular cancer

The role of hormonal manipulation in the treatment of germ cell testicular cancer has not been proven, although a series of anecdotal reports suggest that some tumours may respond to such treatment. Regression of metastases from germ cell tumours has been reported in response to bilateral orchidectomy (McClelland, 1943; Saleeby, 1944), treatment with testosterone (Davis & Shumway 1958), diethylstilboestrol (Shivers & Axilrod, 1952) and progestational agents (Coutts & Vargas-Zalazar, 1945; Bloom & Hendry, 1973; Klepp et al, 1977).

However, in most instances, the numbers of patients studied have been small, the follow-up details scanty, and in some cases patients have been treated with other modalities concurrently (Coutts & Vargas-Zalazar, 1945; Bloom & Hendry, 1973; Klepp et al, 1977), thus making the evaluation of these data extremely difficult.

Another approach reported has been the treatment of patients with hCG-producing tumours by the injection of antisera raised against gonadotrophic hormones; however, no clinical responses were noted and, in fact, the levels of gonadotrophins (as measured in urinary excretion) increased (Twombley, 1947), which probably represented increased clearance due to antigen-antibody binding.

Although endocrine manipulation may provide another useful treatment option for patients with drug-resistant germ cell tumours, the available data are conflicting and represent studies that were initiated without acceptable trial design criteria.

Endocrine therapy may also have a place in the treatment of the infertility caused by cytotoxic chemotherapy. Experiments in rats have suggested that analogues of luteinising hormone release factor can protect germ cells from the detrimental effects of chemotherapy, possibly by retarding the metabolic rate of the cells (Glode et al, 1981). In humans, progestational agents appear to protect against chemotherapy-induced amenorrhoea (Chapman & Sutcliffe, 1981), and studies in males with Hodgkin's disease or testicular cancer are in progress, using a variety of agents that lower serum FSH levels.

RENAL CELL CARCINOMA

Tumours of the kidney constitute approximately 3 per cent of malignancies in Caucasian populations, with an annual incidence of 5.6/100 000 males and 2.8/100 000 females. The male:female ratio ranges from 2:1 to 3.8:1 (Mostofi, 1967; Matsuda et al, 1976), rising after the age of 30 years. The sex incidence in children is equal (Shellhammer & Smith, 1973). Unlike testicular tumours, the predominant age group for renal carcinomas is 60 to 80 years, with the exception of Wilms' tumour (nephroblastoma) which occurs predominantly in the paediatric population. Eighty per cent of renal malignancies are renal cell carcinomas (Grawitz tumours) — there are experimental links between the hormonal environment and the initiation of these tumours, and it has been suggested that some renal cell carcinomas are responsive to changes in this environment.

Experimental data

Renal structure and function in laboratory animals are influenced by sex hormones, as measured by growth and development of renal tissue and by the concentration and distribution of enzymes in the kidney (Koronchevsky &

Ross, 1940; Selye 1941; Ludden et al, 1941; Lattimer, 1942). In the frog, a circadian rhythm has been demonstrated for the mitotic index of normal and malignant cells in the renal tubules (Marlow & Mizel, 1976).

Labelled diethylstilboestrol (DES) is taken up by renal tubular epithelium in hamsters, to a greater extent in males than in females (Ghaleb, 1961). Oestrogen binding proteins or oestrogen receptor sites have been demonstrated in normal rodent renal tissue (King, 1967; de Vries et al, 1972; Li et al, 1974). In addition, androgen receptors (Bullock & Bardin, 1974) and progesterone receptors (Li et al, 1977) have been demonstrated. Although the exact function of those receptors in the normal kidney of rodents has not been ascertained, it has been shown that protein synthesis is stimulated by the interaction of androgens and their receptors in the kidney (Gehring et al, 1971; Bullock & Bardin, 1974; Noronha, 1975).

The endocrine function of renal tumours has been studied in several animal models. In the dog, there is a marked male sex predominance in the occurrence of spontaneous renal cancers (Lucke & Kelly, 1976). However, it is the Syrian hamster that has offered a model of renal carcinoma that has been most extensively studied. Histologically, these tumours appear to be of proximal tubular origin, although interstitial elements are also present (Kirkman, 1959). Renal tumours can be induced in these animals by the administration of oestrogens (Kirkman & Bacon, 1952; Bloom et al, 1963a; Bloom, 1972). The induction of these tumours is prevented by the administration of exogenous progestagens (Bloom et al, 1963a,b) and by the natural progesterone production of the hamsters (Kirkman, 1959, 1974). Similarly, it has been demonstrated that the growth of these tumours is inhibited by the administration of progestagens (Bloom et al, 1963a,b), a paradoxical finding as the administration of progestagens induces hypertrophy of the kidney in the rat and mouse (Bloom et al, 1963a). Receptor activity for oestrogens, progesterone and androgens has been demonstrated in normal and malignant renal tissue in the Syrian hamster (Li et al, 1979). However, it has also been suggested that the correlation between hormone dependency and oestrogen receptor status in these tumours is not proven (Steggles & King, 1968, 1972). Furthermore, doubts have been raised as to the adequacy of this model as a reflection of human renal cell carcinoma, the suggestion having been made that it more accurately represents interstitial carcinoma of the kidney (Llombart-Bosch & Peydra, 1975). Nevertheless, these tumours remain sensitive to oestrogens (which stimulate their growth) and to oestrogen antagonists, such as tamoxifen (which slows the growth rates), after several years of serial transplantation. Tumours also regress in response to bilateral adrenalectomy and bilateral orchidectomy, an effect that is neutralised by the administration of oestrogens or androgens (Bloom et al, 1963a,b). It is of interest to note, however, that other tissues in the

Syrian hamster have demonstrable oestrogen receptor activity, but do not undergo malignant change in response to treatment with oestrogens (Li et al, 1976).

Although the mechanisms of carcinogenesis are not known, it has been demonstrated that oestrogen treatment appears to induce the development of progesterone receptors in the hamster kidney before the onset of any obvious malignancy (Li et al, 1977). In summary, histological studies and analyses of lipid content (Li, personal communication) suggest similarities between the Syrian hamster model and human renal cell carcinoma. However, the relevance of the hormone-dependence characteristic of this model to the human disease state remains unclear.

Renal carcinoma has also been studied in spontaneous mouse tumours (Murphy & Hreshesky 1973; Soloway & Myers, 1973). In these models, treatment with progestagens has not influenced tumour growth rates, although decreased take rates have been demonstrated in oestrogen pre-treated mice, and growth retardation in established tumours treated with testosterone or oestrogens (Soloway & Myers, 1973).

The data available from *in vitro* preparations of renal cell carcinoma are conflicting — androgens and progestagens have been incubated with cultures of these tumours, but without consistent patterns of growth stimulation or inhibition (Tchao et al, 1968; Card et al, 1970).

Clinical studies

Receptors

As an extension of the studies described above, specimens of human kidney and renal carcinoma have been analysed for evidence of hormonal sensitivity. Receptor activity for aldosterone, testosterone and progesterone has been found in the nuclei and cytosol of both normal and malignant renal tissue (Fanestil et al, 1974), greater testosterone and progesterone uptake being demonstrated in the malignant tissue. Oestrogen receptor activity has been revealed in normal renal tissue (more pronounced in the medulla than in the cortex) and in renal carcinoma (Bojar et al, 1975). In a detailed study of 20 patients, Concolino (1979) demonstrated oestrogen receptors in 12, progesterone receptors in 14, both receptors in nine and no receptors in three patients. In this study, there was no correlation between receptor activity and histological differentiation. The progesterone receptors were characterized in greater detail and were shown to have a higher binding capacity but lower receptor affinity for progesterone than the receptors in normal kidney tissue.

Treatment

Building on the results of the experimental and clinical studies detailed above, attempts have been made to treat patients with renal cell carcinoma with a variety of hormonal manipulations to induce tumour regression (Bloom, 1971, 1973). Despite initial enthusiasm for this management approach, supported by a plethora of anecdotal reports, the objective response rates using currently acceptable criteria have been quite disappointing, as summarised in Tables 38.3 to 38.5. An important problem

Table 38.3 Progestagens and renal cancer

Reference	Response rate	Comments
Samuels et al (1968)	3/22	PRs/?survival
Paine et al (1970)	1/15	PR/2 excluded*
Bloom (1971)	8/79	PR/4 excluded*
Wagle & Murphy (1971)	6/37	PR/? 3–31/12
Talley (1973)	7/61	CR & PR/?criteria
Alberto & Senn (1974)	0/20	—
Morales et al (1975)	0/18	—
Stolbach et al (1981)	1/22	—
Total	26/274 (9.5%)	

* Exclusions because of unacceptable citeria of response.

Table 38.4 Androgens and renal cancer

Reference	Response rate	Comments
Jenkin (1967)	1/15	PR
Samuels et al (1968)	1/11	PR
Wagle & Murphy (1971)	2/27	CR, PR
Talley (1973)	0/37	—
Alberto & Senn (1974)	0/23	—
Morales et al 1975)	1/20	PR
Lokich & Harrison (1975)	0/37	—
Papec et al (1977)	1/16	PR
Total	6/186 (3.2%)	

Table 38.5 Other hormonal agents and renal cell carcinoma

Drug	Response rate	Reference	Comments*
Corticosteroids	0/13	Lokich (1975)	—
	0/38	Talley (1973)	—
Tamoxifen	0/15	Glick (1980)	—
	5/79	Al Sarraff (1981)	2 CR; 3 PR
Nafoxidine	3/20	Legha (1976)	2 CR; 1 PR
	1/21	Feun (1979)	1 PR
	3/19	Stolbach (1981)	2 CR; 1 PR
Estracyt	0/16	Swanson (1981)	—

* CR: complete remission;   PR: partial remission

in evaluating the published data has been to distinguish between true tumour responses and the phenomena of 'spontaneous regression' (Robinson, 1969; Fairlamb, 1981; Katz & Shapiro, 1982) and slow natural progression of disease. 'Spontaneous regression' — a clinical situation in which measurable tumour deposits decrease in size without overt therapeutic intervention — has been reported in several tumour types, but most commonly in renal cell carcinoma. Although it occurs more frequently in male patients (Bloom, 1973), it is not common; it was recorded in less than 1 per cent of cases in a series of 571 unselected patients (deKernion & Berry, 1980) and the very existence of such a phenomenon is controversial. Alternatively these observations may be explained by the concept of the 'self-healing' hypernephroma — this attributes the areas of cortical renal scarring that are commonly found in these tumours to regression caused by the 'intrinsic frailty' of the tumour (Zak, 1957).

Renal cell carcinomas are characterised by Gompertzian growth kinetics, the growth rates decreasing with increasing tumour mass (Steel, 1977); hence, in the clinical setting of metastatic disease, their growth rates are often slow, creating a difficult distinction between 'stable' disease and 'slowly progressive' disease. A further complicating feature is the well documented observation of tumour regression after nephrectomy, in which metastases decrease in size in the months following surgical removal of the primary tumour. Although these features are not unique to renal cell carcinoma, they occur with greater frequency than in many other tumours and thus introduce substantial doubt as to the accuracy and relevance of many of the early reports of successful hormonal treatment of renal cancer (Robinson, 1969; Katz & Shapiro, 1982).

Progestagens. Much of the published data has been devoted to reports of progesterone therapy of these tumours. As shown in Table 38.3, the overall response rate, summarising some of the larger series of cases, is less than 10 per cent, the majority of responses being incomplete or partial responses of relatively short duration. The response rates range from 0 to 17 per cent, the variation being due to different criteria of response and perhaps to different dose schedules.

The physiological effects of treatment with high dose progestagens include glucocorticoid side-effects, including steroid euphoria (Samuels et al, 1968) and suppression of the pituitary-adrenal axis (Hellman et al, 1976), with decreased growth hormone response to stimulation and decreased circulating corticosteroid levels (Sadoff & Lusk, 1974). However, these effects are difficult to distinguish from abnormalities found in patients with disseminated cancer on no treatment. Concolino (1979) has reported that measurement of progesterone receptors in tumour specimens is a useful predictor of response to hormonal manipulation; however, this series reflected only small numbers

of patients with short follow up periods, and will require corroboration.

Androgens. As with progestagen treatment, the response rate to androgen therapy from accumulated series is less than 5 per cent, the majority being only partial responses (Table 38.4). Similarly, difficulties in evaluating the different criteria of response and short follow up periods apply.

Oestrogens and corticosteroids. The use of oestrogens in the management of advanced renal cell carcinoma has been less extensively characterised. However, there have been several recent reports of the use of oestrogen antagonists in this situation (Table 38.5), with low but apparently reproducible response rates.

By contrast, no responses have been reported in two series with a total of 51 patients treated with glucocorticoids (Talley, 1973; Lokich & Harrison, 1975).

In summary, despite the obvious interest generated from the animal models, hormonal treatment, as currently applied, does not appear to offer a solution to the problems posed by the patient with disseminated renal cell carcinoma. In order to evaluate accurately the place of hormonal manipulation, it will be necessary for prospective, randomised trials to be initiated, with rigid response criteria, documentation of pre-treatment tumour growth rates, histological review and the testing of hormonal receptor status. In addition, further exploitation of the animal models may yield insights into more appropriate doses and schedules for the hormones to be used.

PROSTATIC CANCER

Although the prostate gland has been studied extensively, its physiological function remains a mystery. It contributes to the fluid of the ejaculate, but the role of its secretions in a biological or functional sense is unknown. With increased age, the gland is associated with benign and malignant hyperplasias that appear to be related to the hormonal environment, an association first documented two centuries ago in a report that castration was followed by a decrease in the size of the prostate gland (Hunter, 1786).

The normal prostate gland

The prostate develops in embryonic life as an outgrowth of the urogenital sinus, a series of tubules developing and then fusing to form the gland. In the female, the prostate remains vestigial, corresponding to the lateral and middle lobes of the male gland, and lacking a posterior lobe (Mostofi & Price, 1973). It weighs approximately 1 g at birth, grows to about 4 g before puberty and weighs about

20 g at the start of the third decade, usually remaining stable for many years until a second growth phase commences in the fifth to seventh decades (Swyer, 1944).

On cross section, four regions can be identified — central, peripheral, mucosal and an anterior fibromuscular stroma. It has been suggested that there is no embryological distinction between these regions (Scott, 1963). However, data have also been presented to show that prostatic hyperplasia always arises from the preprostatic region, an area adjacent to the central zone and derived from the Wolffian duct, as distinct from the remainder of the gland, which is derived from the urogenital sinus (McNeal, 1981), implying a monoclonal origin for benign prostatic hyperplasia (BPH). In addition, the stroma of the prostate is essential for the response of the glandular elements to the stimulus (testosterone) that induces hyperplasia (Cunha & Lung, 1979).

The growth and development of the prostate are under hormonal control, primarily by androgens (Huggins et al, 1941; Huggins & Hodges, 1941). The current concepts of the physiology of the prostate are summarised in Fig. 38.1. In the normal male, the major circulating androgen is testosterone, of which 95 per cent is of testicular origin, being produced predominantly by the Leydig cells. These cells are stimulated by the gonadotrophins, primarily luteinising hormone (LH), to synthesise testosterone from cholesterol and acetate. The average testosterone concentration in the blood is 6000 μg/l in males aged 25 to 70 years, but may decline subsequently (Stearns et al, 1974; Vermeulen, 1976). Recent data suggest that there is,

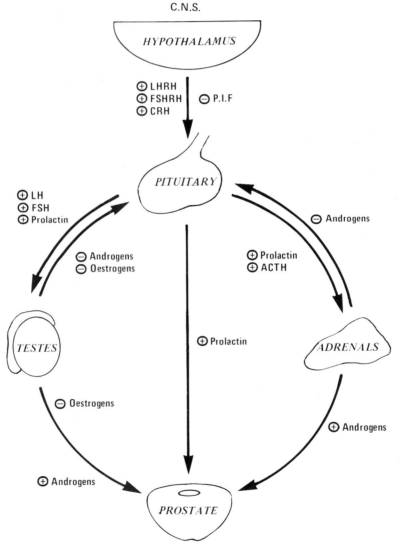

Fig. 38.1 Physiological interactions in prostatic cancer. + represents a factor likely to stimulate tumour growth; − represents a factor likely to inhibit tumour growth; C.N.S.: central nervous system; LHRH: luteinising hormone releasing hormone; FSHRH: follicle stimulating hormone releasing hormone; CRH: corticotrophin releasing hormone; P.I.F.: prolactin inhibiting factor; LH: luteinising hormone; FSH: follicle stimulating hormone; ACTH: adrenal corticotrophic hormone

in fact, no true decline in circulating levels with increasing age if healthy male volunteers are sampled, and that the predominant change is a decrease in Leydig cell reserve (when stressed with gonadotrophins) (Harman & Tsitouras, 1980 and see Ch 3).

Testosterone is bound to two major proteins in the blood — sex hormone binding globulin (SHBG) and albumin — and is in dynamic equilibrium with the unbound or 'free' fraction. This latter component enters the cells, is converted to the active form in the prostate, dihydrotestosterone (DHT), by a reductase enzyme (Bruchovsky & Wilson, 1968a, b), and is then transported to the nucleus, where it interacts with chromosomes, initiating gene transcription and protein synthesis (Higgins & Gehring, 1978).

It appears that the levels of SHBG alter with increasing age, which may explain the apparent decline in total testosterone observed (Vermeulen et al, 1972, 1976). The levels of SHBG in the blood are increased by the administration of exogenous oestrogens and decreased by testosterone (Burton & Westphal, 1972).

In addition to the effects of testosterone in the prostate, oestrogens and progestagens interact with this gland. Approximately 75 to 90 per cent of the circulating oestrogens of young, healthy males are derived from the peripheral conversion of androgens (Siiteri & MacDonald, 1973). Oestrogens and androgens compete for SHBG binding sites, although testosterone has a greater avidity for the protein. Because of these interactions, there is a 40 per cent rise in the ratio of free oestradiol/free testosterone in males over 50 years of age. The major effect of oestrogens on the prostate gland appears to be mediated via the hypothalamo-pituitary-gonodal axis, with inhibition of testicular synthesis of testosterone. If oestrogens and testosterone are administered jointly to castrate animals, normal growth of the prostate gland occurs — oestrogens do not appear to block the replacement effect of the administered testosterone.

C_{19}-androgenic steroids are also produced by the adrenal gland, and may stimulate prostatic growth and metabolism (Harper et al, 1974). In the normal male, with high circulating levels of testicular androgens, the adrenal steroids are unlikely to have a major physiological role in prostate metabolism; however, in the eunuch, this balance may be altered (*vide infra*).

Prolactin also has a function in the growth and metabolism of the prostate gland. In hypophysectomised rats, exogenous androgens are unable to restore full prostatic growth unless supplemented by prolactin (Grayhack et al, 1955). Similarly the interaction of testosterone and prolactin has been confirmed *in vitro* in fragments of human prostatic tissue (Farnsworth et al, 1981). In addition, prolactin has been reported to stimulate production of adrenal androgenic steroids (Millington et al, 1976).

Specific receptor sites for the hormones discussed above

have been sought in prostatic tissue. In the dog and the human prostate, oestrogen receptor activity has been demonstrated in some, but not all, studies (Hawkins et al, 1975; Ekman et al, 1979a, b). Androgen receptors have been demonstrated in prostatic cytoplasm (Mobbs et al, 1975) and nuclei (Mainwaring & Milroy, 1973; Lieskovsky & Bruchovsky, 1979). An important problem in the determination of putative 'androgen receptor activity' is the risk of contamination of tissue specimens by even small amounts of SHBG, which mimics the cytoplasmic androgen receptor in its binding and avidity for dihydrotestosterone (DHT). This problem is compounded by the minute amounts of receptor present, and its lability even at low temperatures. To circumvent these problems, a synthetic androgen, methyltrienolone (R1881) has been used in receptor assays as it binds to the cytoplasmic receptors but not to SHBG (Bonne & Raynaud, 1975; Menon et al, 1978). However, a limitation of this technique is the progestational activity of R1881, with consequent binding to progesterone receptors (Dube et al, 1976). This problem can be avoided by the use of triamcinolone acetonide, in excess concentrations, to saturate the progesterone receptors before using R1881 in the androgen receptor assay. Despite these measures, there is persistent concern that the steroid specificity of R1881 binding to human prostatic tissue differs from that demonstrated in the studies of rat ventral prostate, for which the assay was originally used (Asselin et al, 1976). Furthermore, there is uncertainty regarding the relative components of androgen and progesterone receptor binding with R1881 (Shain & Boesel, 1978). However, on the basis of competitive binding studies with testosterone and DHT, it appears that R1881 functions as a measure of androgen receptor activity at least in nuclear extracts.

Prolactin receptors have been demonstrated in the prostate gland and testis (Aragona & Friesen, 1975) — presumably, these mediate the interaction of prolactin in testosterone uptake and metabolism by the prostate, as discussed below.

Another factor that may interact in the physiology of the prostate gland is a steroid binding protein that has been described in rat prostatic secretions (Heynes et al, 1977). Its production is stimulated by androgenic steroids (Parker & Scrace, 1979), but its function is as yet unknown. A marked deoxyribonucleic acid sequence homology exists between the polypeptides that form its two component subunits, suggesting that duplication of an ancestral gene has occurred with subsequent genetic divergence yielding the capacity to bind steroids (Parker et al, 1982).

Benign prostatic hyperplasia (BPH)

Benign hyperplasia of the prostate gland is a concomitant of ageing in most dogs and in man (Moore, 1943). An absolute requirement is the presence of functioning testicles. However, the aetiology of this condition is not known, although postulated factors abound, including infection, neoplastic change, race, venereal transmission, frequency of sexual activity, religion and occupation.

Histologically, the glands in BPH show marked variation in structure, as compared to the uniformity of the normal prostate (Moore, 1943; Mostofi & Price, 1973). Varying degrees of hyperplasia of the constituents of the prostate — fibrous, muscle and glandular tissue — are present, the acini usually being enlarged with papillary processes encroaching on the lumina. Acid phosphatase activity is prominent in the lumina of the glandular structures. Adjacent to foci of BPH, areas of atrophy or epithelial metaplasia may be seen (Moore, 1943; Mostofi & Price, 1973).

Experimental models

Several models of BPH have been studied in an effort to duplicate the human disease state. For example, Fingerhut & Veenema (1966) have been able to induce prostatic hypertrophy in mice by the administration of oestrogens — however, the histological patterns obtained differ markedly from their human counterparts.

Castro and his group have used the technique of xenografting to grow explants of BPH tissue in immunosuppressed animals (Castro, 1973). Although in these studies the xenografted tissues did not greatly increase in size, they remained viable for up to 12 weeks and showed maintenance of histology and acid phosphatase production. In addition, the tumours took up ³H-testosterone and were able to be serially transplanted (Williams et al, 1978).

Perhaps the most 'physiological' model of BPH is found in aged dogs, the only other major species in which the disorder is found without artificial stimuli. However, histological differences from the human disease are pronounced, and there are doubts as to the adequacy of canine BPH as a model of human disease. For example, dogs tend to develop enlargement of the posterior prostate, with consequent rectal, rather than urinary, obstruction. In the dog, BPH is associated with a predominantly glandular proliferation of a diffuse nature, rather than disease arising in the periurethral area.

Physiology of benign prostatic hyperplasia

As noted above, the effects of ageing on male endocrine function have been studied in detail, providing as a corollary information regarding the hormonal concomitants of BPH. Although testosterone levels may fall after the age of 60 years (Vermeulen, 1976), there is no significant difference between control populations and patients with BPH. In fact, the onset of BPH occurs up to 20 years before the testosterone levels are thought to decline (Vermeulen et al, 1972). There is disagreement as to

whether DHT levels alter in patients with BPH (Ghanadian et al, 1977; Hammond et al, 1978). It has, however, been shown that DHT does not increase with age (Lewis et al, 1976). DHT has been measured in normal and hyperplastic prostate tissue (Meikle et al, 1980) and has been found to be greatly increased in the latter. Furthermore, it has been measured in normal prostatic tissue with histological evidence of early hyperplasia — markedly raised levels were found in the hyperplastic regions only (Siiteri & Wilson, 1970). Thus, DHT is associated with the development of BPH, but it is not known whether this represents cause or effect.

This association has been studied more extensively in the dog. Raised levels of DHT have been demonstrated in hyperplastic zones of canine prostates (Gloyna et al, 1970). The administration of 3α-androstenediol to castrated dogs causes an accumulation of DHT in the prostate which is greater than if DHT itself is administered directly to these animals; the administration of 3α-androstenediol causes the development of BPH, which does not occur in animals treated with conventional doses of DHT (Moore et al, 1979a; De Klerk et al, 1979). In fact, if pharmacological doses of DHT are used, BPH can be induced in dogs. Hence the intracellular mediator of BPH is, in fact, DHT, although the mechanisms of its action are unknown; earlier experiments to the contrary probably reflected the use of inadequate doses.

Despite the increased formation of oestrogens from androgenic precursors with increasing age, there appears to be no difference between plasma oestrogen levels in patients with BPH versus age-matched controls without prostatic disease (Bartsch et al, 1979). The decrease in the testosterone: oestrogen ratio with increased age may facilitate a second growth spurt in the prostate, but may not be an important causative factor. However, it appears that 17β-oestradiol has a synergistic promoting effect on the development of BPH (De Klerk et al, 1979), which may be due, in part, to the enhancing effect of oestrogens on cytoplasmic androgen receptor content in prostatic tissue (Moore et al, 1979b). However, this increased androgen receptor activity could represent contamination by increased levels of SHBG (secondary to the increased levels of oestrogens in the blood) in the cytosol preparations.

Nevertheless, it has also been shown that the mean concentration of androgen receptor activity in the nuclei of hyperplastic human prostate tissue is 1.4 times greater than that of normal prostate (Lieskovsky & Bruchovsky, 1979), with an assay that is not contaminated by SHBG. These data are not supported by all studies (Trachtenberg et al, 1982). Although oestrogen receptors have been demonstrated in the prostate, there is controversy as to whether they are present in hyperplastic tissue (Ekman et al, 1979a, b) and thus the mechanism of interaction of oestrogens and androgens in human BPH is not yet fully resolved. It has been shown that androgen receptor activity increases in response to the administration of oestrogens, but the significance of this finding is not known (Mobbs et al, 1975).

Carcinoma of the prostate gland

The incidence of carcinoma of the prostate (CAP) also rises with age, with a prevalence of about 80 per cent in males older than 80 years (Hirst & Bergman, 1954), and it is often found as an incidental feature at autopsy (Mostofi & Price, 1973). The aetiology of CAP is unknown, although an increased prevalence has been documented in workers exposed to cadmium (Kipling & Waterhouse, 1967). The role of sex hormones in the genesis of CAP has been investigated because of the observation that eunuchs do not develop this disease (Moore, 1947) and the fact that many prostatic cancers regress in response to a decrease in circulating androgens (Huggins & Hodges, 1941); however, no clear aetiological relationship has been demonstrated in man. It has recently been suggested that familial factors influence the incidence of prostate cancer — in a study in Utah, it was shown that there was a significantly higher incidence among the brothers of patients with the disease than in control groups (Meikle & Stanish, 1982). Paradoxically, the probands, their sons and brothers had lower circulating testosterone levels than controls of comparable age. However, an important limitation is that the population in Utah, which has an unusually high proportion of Mormons, may not be representative of 'average' males with prostatic cancer. Furthermore, probands were selected on the basis of disease diagnosed before the age of 62 years, which could have selected a subgroup of 'juvenile'-onset prostatic cancer. The epidemiological and aetiological data and hypotheses regarding this disease have been reviewed in detail elsewhere (Hutchison, 1981).

This tumour occurs naturally in man and in dogs (as is seen with BPH), but also in horses, bulls and monkeys. The histological features of human CAP often show only a subtle difference from BPH, and the diagnosis sometimes is made on the basis of metastatic disease. However, other features include increased anaplasia, architectural changes, invasion and alterations in the histochemical staining patterns and reactions (Mostofi & Price, 1973). An added factor in the diagnosis of CAP may be the demonstration of ultrastructural pleomorphism, with changes in the distribution of organelles in the cytoplasm. The diagnosis is often made more difficult by the spectrum of differentiation present, with regions of normal prostate and hyperplastic zones abutting areas of frank carcinoma which also manifest considerable histological heterogeneity. This heterogeneity is reflected functionally by the variation in patterns of acid phosphatase production and in the spectrum of sensitivity of CAP to hormonal therapy.

Experimental models

Prostatic tumours have been artificially induced in rodents by the injection into the prostate of benzpyrene (Moore & Melchionna, 1937) and methylcholanthrene (Dunning et al, 1946), and by the subcutaeous implantation of fragments of prostatic epithelium with methylcholanthrene crystals (Horning, 1946). The histological patterns demonstrated in these tumours include squamous cell carcinoma, leiomyosarcoma and adenocarcinoma, and variable hormonal sensitivity has been documented in treated animals.

A hormonally sensitive adenocarcinoma of the prostate has been discovered in an aged male Copenhagen rat and has been serially transplanted in syngeneic animals. The hormonal responsiveness of this R3327H tumour has been demonstrated as a function of its growth properties in intact and castrated male rats and in female rats (Voigt & Dunning, 1974; Smolev et al, 1977) and it has been shown to be composed of two populations of cells: hormone-sensitive and hormone-resistant. Receptors for androgens, oestrogens and progestagens have been demonstrated and characterised in this tumour (Voigt et al, 1975; Heston et al, 1979; Lea & French, 1981).

Similar studies have been performed in carcinoma of the dorsal prostate in Nb mice (Noble, 1980a, b) with distinct oestrogen- and androgen-dependent cell lines.

Malignant transformation has been induced in cultures of hamster prostate cells by the injection of Simian virus 40 (Paulson et al, 1968), when the tranformed cells are injected into syngeneic animals, acid phosphatase-producing malignant tumours result.

Fragments of CAP have been cultured in vitro and have shown a response to incubation with testosterone, manifested as increased differentiation in some cases, and an increased mitotic index in one anaplastic tumour (McMahon et al, 1972). In addition to the xenografting of BPH tissue, fragments of CAP have been implanted into immunosuppressed mice (Mickey et al, 1977; Williams et al, 1978) and have been shown to maintain characteristics such as histology, ultrastructure and acid phosphatase production. In the studies reported to date, metastases of CAP to bones or other sites have not been documented, a feature shared by most xenografted tumours (Raghavan & Selby, 1981).

In addition to their use as models of the endocrine physiology of CAP, some of these animal tumours have been applied to the testing of potential new therapies for CAP, including new drugs and schedules. In these studies, tumour growth inhibition or regression has been compared in treated and untreated tumours, including the effects of Flutamide, a non-steroidal anti-androgen (Smolev et al, 1977); tamoxifen, an anti-oestrogen (Noble, 1980a, b); and estramustine phosphate, a combination of an alkylating agent conjugated to a steroid nucleus (Catane et al, 1980).

Physiology

No consistent data have been produced to show a persistent endocrine abnormality associated with CAP — most studies have failed to reveal any difference between healthy controls and patients with CAP in the levels of plasma LH, FSH, prolactin, SHBG, oestrogens or androgens. However, there have been sporadic reports that alterations in testosterone/oestrogen ratios correlate with the presence of CAP, although these remain to be substantiated (Rannikko et al, 1981). A major difficulty is to distinguish between the hormonal effects related directly to the presence of disseminated carcinoma or to the stress associated with it, as distinct from factors that are associated with the genesis of the tumour. For example, the demonstration of a lack of ACTH-cortisol response to insulin-induced hypoglycaemia in patients with CAP (Madajewicz et al, 1980) could be explained on the basis of underlying stress or metabolic changes due to the cancer. Similarly, decreased levels of binding proteins could be part of a more generalised hypoproteinaemic state.

The exact role of prolactin in the physiology of CAP is not clear. It enhances the uptake, metabolism and function of testosterone in prostatic cancer cells, as well as in BPH (Farnsworth et al, 1981). As previously noted, prolactin stimulates the production of androgenic steroids by the adrenal gland (Millington et al, 1976). It has also been shown that oestrogen administration causes sustained hyperprolactinaemia (Harper et al, 1976) which, in theory, could cause a growth increase resulting in 'oestrogen resistance'.

Ekman et al (1979a, b, 1980) have demonstrated receptor activity for androgens, progestagens and gluco-corticoids in specimens from five patients with CAP, but no oestrogen receptors (although several of their patients had previously been treated with oestrogens or estramus-tine phosphate, thus potentially interfering with the assay). A correlation of strongly postive receptor assays with subsequent response to hormonal treatment has been demonstrated (Ekman et al, 1980; Ghanadian et al, 1981) and it has been suggested that the nuclear androgen receptor is a more useful predictor than the cytoplasmic assay (Ghanadain et al, 1981).

Diagnosis

Carcinoma of the prostate, like the germ cell tumours, is a neoplasm characterised by tumour markers which reflect, to some extent, viable tumour mass; however, as with germ cell tumours, CAP is a heterogeneous tumour, composed of marker-producing and non marker-producing elements, thus limiting the effectiveness of the tumour markers in clinical practice.

Acid phosphatase. To date, the most useful tumour marker for CAP has been serum acid phosphatase. This protein, consisting of isoenzymes with a molecular weight of approximately 100 000, is found in prostate, red blood cells, bone, liver and the kidney. The specificity of each isoenzyme appears to be determined by sialic acid residues (Chu et al, 1975). The available assays include biochemical methods, counter-immuno-electrophoresis (CIEP) and radioimmunoassays (RIA), the latter being the most sensitive. In an effort to increase the sensitivity of the assays, acid phosphatase has been measured in bone marrow aspirates, following reports of an earlier detectable elevation of the protein in that site than in the blood (Gursel et al, 1974). However, doubts have been cast on the true utility of the bone marrow assay (Reynolds et al, 1973). Whether acid phosphatase accurately reflects tumour mass, stage or potential response to treatment remains controversial, with conflicting data. Between 10 and 80 per cent of patients with CAP have been reported to have detectably raised serum levels of acid phosphatase, depending on the stage of the disease and the sensitivity of the asay used. There appears to be little doubt that this protein has no value as a screening test for CAP, even in high-risk population groups, in view of the proportion of false positive and false negative assays (Watson & Tang, 1980).

Specific antigens. More recently, Chu and his group have characterised a 'specific' prostatic cancer antigen, which was originally detected by immunodiffusion assays and immunoelectrophoresis (Papsidero et al, 1980). They have subsequently developed an enzyme immunoassay to facilitate quantitation of this prostate-specific antigen, and are able to detect blood levels as low as 0.1 μg/l. To date, this antigen has only been found in human prostate tissue and in blood samples from males, the levels being higher in patients with BPH and CAP than in healthy controls (Kuriyama et al, 1980).

A monoclonal antibody, aPro3, has been described which recognizes an antigen from prostate tissue (Ware et al 1982). This antigen has a molecular weight of 175 000 and is composed of subunits of molecular weight 54 000. It appears to be present on the surface of cultured prostatic cancer cells. However, its specificity for prostatic tissue will require further study and its relevance *in vivo* has not yet been reported. Whether aPro3 recognises the antigen described by Chu has not yet been reported.

Several non-specific tumour markers of CAP have been described, including alkaline phosphatase, carcinoembryonic antigen, ribonuclease, polyamines, creatine phosphokinase isoenzyme BB and lactic acid dehydrogenase. However, a review of the physiology and applications of these antigens is beyond the scope of this chapter, and has been provided elsewhere (Catalona & Menon, 1981; Harper et al, 1981).

Hormonal therapy of carcinoma of the prostate

Since John Hunter's report of a decrease in prostatic size

following castration (Hunter, 1786), prostatic symptoms have been treated by castration, initially on an empirical basis without histological proof of the nature of the prostatic disorder (White, 1895; Cabot, 1896). It was not until the series of clinical and experimental studies of the Nobel laureate, Charles Huggins, and his collaborators were reported that a physiological basis for this practice was defined (Huggins & Hodges, 1941; Huggins et al, 1941). These workers showed that histological and functional prostatic atrophy followed castration, that replacement of testosterone reversed these changes, and that the atrophy could be re-induced by the addition of stilboestrol to the drug regimen. In fact, Huggins & Hodges (1941) showed that acid and alkaline phosphatase estimation could be used to monitor the course of patients after castration or the initiation of oestrogen therapy for CAP.

An important limitation to the 'hormonal' approach to the treatment of CAP is the heterogeneity of the tumour cells, with populations of cells that are sensitive to hormonal manipulations and others that are resistant or hormonally independent. However, as noted previously, it may be that a prediction of hormonal sensitivity can be made on the basis of androgen receptor activity of resected prostatic cancer tissue (Ekman et al, 1980; Ghanadian et al, 1977, 1981).

An ancillary determinant of prognosis following hormonal therapy is the measurement of tumour ploidy or DNA profiles with flow cytometric techniques (Tavares et al, 1966; Zetterberg & Esposti, 1980). In these studies, poor response to endocrine therapy and short subsequent survival correlate with increased heteroploidy (and, in turn, decreased differentiation); whereas a diploid DNA content reflects greater differentiation and improved survival. Such a technique appears to have most value in the analysis of moderately differentiated tumours, particularly because of the subjective variation in classifying 'differentiation' with the light microscope. Furthermore, flow cytometry provides a tool for monitoring the efficacy of hormonal treatment, based on alterations in the ploidy of tumours during treatment (Leistenschneider & Nagel, 1980).

From a clinical standpoint, prostatic carcinoma is a difficult tumour to evaluate prospectively. For example, a high proportion of patients have mixed lytic and sclerotic bone metastases and occult lymph node deposits — with non-invasive techniques, it is often difficult to distinguish progression and regression. The more easily evaluable visceral metastases are uncommon in this disease. Furthermore, the advanced age group of the patients, with their propensity for non-cancerous musculo-skeletal disorders, and the long natural history of prostatic cancer make morbidity and survival statistics difficult to interpret.

In an effort to rationalise the monitoring of treatment and the accurate determination of objective response rates, the United States National Prostatic Cancer Project has

Table 38.6 NPCP criteria of response

Complete regression:
  Tumour masses, if present, totally disappeared and no new lesions appeared
  Elevated acid phosphatase, if present, returned to normal
  Osteolytic lesions, if present, recalcified
  Osteoblastic lesions, if present, disappeared
  If hepatomegaly is significant, there must be complete return to normal size and return of liver function tests to normal

Partial regression:
  At least one tumour mass, if present, is reduced by $\geq$ 50% in cross-sectional area
  Elevated acid phosphatase, if present, returned to normal
  Osteolytic lesions, if present, undergo recalcification in one or more, but not necessarily all
  Osteoblastic lesions, if present, do not progress
  If hepatomegaly is a significant indicator, there must be at least a 30% reduction in liver size and at least a 30% improvement in all pretreatment abnormalities of liver function
  No increase in other lesions
  No new lesions
  No significant cancer-related deterioration in weight (>10%), symptoms or performance status

established criteria of response, which have been widely accepted, as summarised in Table 38.6 (Murphy et al, 1976). However, many of the studies of hormonal treatment for CAP have not adhered to well-defined criteria of response and it is often difficult to evaluate the available data regarding 'objective' versus 'subjective' response and the significance of 'stable disease'. Despite these problems, certain features have emerged among the more extensive studies of hormone therapy, as discussed below.

The major options available for such treatment are: removal of the source of circulating androgens; inhibition of the stimulus to androgen production; the use of androgen antagonists or blockers; the use of hormone-cytotoxic compounds.

Removal of the source of circulating androgens

Orchidectomy. As discussed above, the rationale for bilateral orchidectomy in the management of prostatic carcinoma was determined by Huggins et al (1941). This procedure results in a substantial decrease in plasma testosterone, mean levels falling from 5000–6500 μg/l before castration to 400–500 μg/l (Young & Kent, 1968; Shearer et al, 1973; Clark & Houghton, 1977; Bracci et al, 1977) and often remaining low for several years.

Subcapsular orchidectomy was introduced in an effort to provide a more cosmetically and psychologically acceptable operation (Riba, 1942); but subsequently Leydig cells demonstrated in the tunica vaginalis (McDonald & Calams, 1959) were shown to be responsive to gonadotrophic stimulation on the basis of measured urinary androgen excretion (O'Conor et al, 1963). However, more recent data have shown no significant increase in plasma testosterone after subcapsular orchidectomy in patients stimulated with gonadotrophins (Burge et al, 1976; Clark & Houghton, 1977). Several studies have documented that suppression of testosterone production persist for several years after orchidectomy (Shearer et al, 1973; Clark & Houghton, 1977; Bracci et al, 1977) and that androgen levels often remain suppressed in the presence of reactivation of the disease (Walsh & Siiteri, 1975; Bracci et al, 1977), implying that androgens have not caused the relapse.

Another role for orchidectomy that has been proposed is its use in the management of patients who have relapsed after oestrogen treatment. An important potential limitation to this approach is the probability that the relapse may be a function of 'hormonally resistant' clones of cells that would be resistant to orchidectomy. A recent study has addressed this issue and showed a 5 per cent objective response rate and a 15 per cent subjective response rate to secondary orchidectomy (Stone et al, 1980), although others have reported an objective response rate of 17 per cent (Bjorn et al, 1979); different criteria of 'oestrogen escape' and 'objective response' explain these differences.

Medical and surgical adrenalectomy. It has been postulated that the efficacy of castration is limited by the production of androgens from sources other than the testicles — for example, the adrenal glands, as previously discussed. In castrated men, adrenal testosterone production is less than 3 per cent of the output of testosterone in the intact male (Sanford et al, 1977). Furthermore, adult pre-pubertal castrates have atrophic prostates with no prostatic secretion. Despite the lack of objective evidence to date to support the adrenal glands as sites of significant androgen production with respect to CAP, subjective and objective response rates of 20 to 30 per cent have been recorded following surgical adrenalectomy (Reynoso & Murphy, 1972; Mahoney & Harrison, 1972) or after medical adrenalectomy with aminoglutethimide (Robinson et al, 1974; Walsh & Siiteri, 1975; Santen et al, 1976; Robinson, 1980; Worgul et al, 1981). In addition, many of the responses to adrenalectomy have been of several months' duration.

Inhibition of the stimulus to androgen production

Oestrogens. In males who have not been castrated, the primary effect of oestrogens is suppression of LH secretion with a consequent decrease in testosterone production. In addition, oestrogens may directly inhibit the function of Leydig cells (Jones et al, 1978). The nature of any direct effect of oestrogens on prostate cancer cells is uncertain — it has been reported that in castrated animals, oestrogens synergise with androgens to stimulate prostatic growth (Tesar & Scott, 1964); however, Symes & Milroy (1978) were unable to demonstrate any *in vitro* effect of a range of doses of diethylstilboestrol incubated with human prostatic cancer cells on either nuclear uptake of DHT or on 5α-reductase activity. Further data will be required to resolve this issue.

Veterans Administration Cooperative Urological Research Group (VACURG) studies. The most extensive appraisal of the use of oestrogens in the management of prostatic cancer was undertaken by the VACURG, a multi-centre collaborative group based in American Veterans Administration Hospitals, between 1960 and 1975 (VACURG 1967, 1968; Byar, 1973, 1980a, b). In their first study, patients with stage I (no palpable tumour) and stage II (palpable tumour not extending beyond the prostate) disease were treated with radical prostatectomy and were then randomised to receive either placebo or 5 mg of diethylstilboestrol daily by mouth. In both stages, there were more cancer deaths in the placebo group than in the oestrogen-treated group, but the differences were not significant. However, stage I patients receiving oestrogens had a higher mortality rate which was related to an increased risk of cardiovascular death. There was no difference in survival in the two groups of stage II patients. Lower tumour progression rates were observed in the oestrogen-treated patients with stage I and II disease. An important drawback to this study is that patients in the 'placebo group' were frequently treated with oestrogens upon relapse, thus altering the survival figures at the time of analysis.

Patients with stage III and IV disease (local and distant metastases, respectively) were randomised at presentation to receive with placebo only, placebo plus orchidectomy, diethylstilboestrol (5 mg daily) plus orchidectomy, or diethystilboestrol alone. Although oestrogen was effective in reducing the number of cancer deaths and retarding the progression of the disease, this treatment was associated with an excess of cardiovascular deaths, particularly in stage III patients. A second important result was that orchidectomy did not appear to be superior to oestrogens, and the combination of the two treatments did not confer a survival benefit over either treatment used alone. Once again, important limitations of trial design were incorporated into the study (including 'cross-over' from placebo to treatment groups, inadequate staging procedures, and uncertainty regarding patient compliance in taking oral medications) and may have caused major errors of interpretation of the data (Coune, 1978).

A second study was commenced in 1967. Patients with stage III and IV disease were randomised at presentation to receive one of the following treatments: placebo; diethylstilboestrol (DES), 0.2 mg daily; DES, 1 mg daily; DES, 5 mg daily. Patients treated with the two highest DES dose schedules had fewer cancer deaths than those receiving placebo or 0.2 mg of DES. However, the 5 mg dose was associated with a greater cardiovascular mortality rate than the lower doses or placebo. Again the survival of patients treated initially with placebo for stage III disease exceeded that among the patients treated with 5 mg of DES. However, in stage IV disease, treatment with 1 or 5 mg of DES conferred a survival benefit over treatment with placebo or 0.2 mg DES.

A third study has suggested that there is no benefit in treating patients with 2.5 mg of Premarin or 30 mg of Provera (a synthetic progestagen) daily, rather than with 1 mg of DES daily.

Notwithstanding the important errors of trial design in the VACURG studies, they have had a strong influence on the timing and use of oestrogens in clinical practice. Since the completion of these studies, it has been demonstrated that, in most patients, the optimal dose of stilboestrol is 3 mg per day, a schedule that yields a more effective suppression of circulating androgen levels than 1 mg daily, but without an increased cardiovascular mortality rate (Shearer et al, 1973). It has also been shown that oestrogen treatment of castrated males does not suppress testosterone to levels lower than for orchidectomy or oestrogens used alone (Shearer et al, 1973). Similar dose-response data have been reported for other oestrogens, including Premarin and ethinyl oestradiol. However, chlorotrianisene (TACE), which has been used widely in clinical practice, has little demonstrable effect on the production of testosterone, LH or FSH (Shearer et al, 1973; Baker et al, 1973).

Anti-oestrogens

In addition to the inhibitory effects of oestrogens on the growth of CAP, it has been reported that the anti-oestrogen tamoxifen has activity against refractory prostatic carcinoma, with responses noted in two of 29 patients treated (Glick et al, 1980b). The mechanism of its action is unknown. However, rapid deteriorations ('flare' reactions) have also been reported in such patients, and further assessment will be required before the introduction of tamoxifen into routine management of prostatic cancer (Patterson, 1980).

Pituitary ablation

After castration, LH and FSH levels rise to a plateau level which has been shown to persist for as long as five years (Bracci et al, 1977). Adopting the hypothesis that these levels may stimulate tumour growth, pituitary ablation by surgery or irradiation has been studied in patients with relapsed prostatic cancer and preliminary data have shown symptomatic responses (Reynoso & Murphy, 1972). However responses are often of short duration. An added theoretical benefit of hypophysectomy is the associated decrease in production of prolactin (a stimulator of prostatic growth).

Prolactin inhibitors

As an alternative to hypophysectomy, prolactin inhibitors have been evaluated in the management of metastatic CAP. In theory, such inhibitors could interfere with the direct and indirect effects of prolactin on the prostate and testis discussed previously. L-Dopa (Farnsworth & Gonder, 1977) and bromocriptine (Jacobi et al, 1980) have yielded response rates as high as 70 per cent in series of untreated and pre-treated patients, although these are usually of only short duration. The major responses reported have been amelioration of bony pain.

Danazol

Danazol, a 2,3-isoxazol of 17α-ethynyl testosterone, has been used predominantly for the treatment of endometriosis (Greenblatt et al, 1971) and benign cystic disease of the breast (Madanes & Farber, 1982). The exact mechanism of its action remains controversial, but it appears to inhibit directly sex steroid synthesis and may competitively inhibit the binding of sex steroids to their cytoplasmic receptors in target tissues (Madanes & Farber, 1982), and has been reported to inhibit gonadotrophin production (Potts et al, 1974).

In a current study, Danazol has been used in 14 patients with hormonally-resistent metastatic CAP who have undergone bilateral orchidectomy and, in some cases, treatment with oestrogens (Raghavan et al, unpublished). To date, three patients have experienced complete pain relief of up to 3 months duration, but have not fulfilled the NPCP criteria for objective remission, and the drug will require further evaluation.

Analogues of luteinising hormone releasing hormone

The acute administration of 'superactive' analogues of luteinising hormone releasing hormone (LHRH) causes a prolonged release of pituitary gonadotrophins with consequent increased Leydig cell function and increased plasma testosterone levels (Schally et al, 1980). Paradoxically, the chronic administration of large doses of LHRH analogues causes suppression of pituitary and Leydig cell function (Schally et al, 1980) and induces regression of prostatic tumours in experimental animals (deSombre et al, 1976). Tolis et al (1982) have reported responses in nine of ten patients with advanced carcinoma of prostate treated with LHRH analogues for periods ranging from 6 weeks to 12 months. One attraction of this therapeutic approach is the lack of associated gynaecomastia.

Antagonists of androgen function

An alternative approach for the control of CAP is the use of anti-androgens, agents that compete directly with circulating androgens at their target organs and inhibit the nuclear uptake of DHT. The first generation drugs are structural analogues of testosterone — for example, cyproterone acetate, the most extensively characterised anti-androgen. Cyproterone is a progestational drug that inhibits the release of gonadotrophins (thus lowering testosterone levels) and also blocks the formation of the DHT-receptor complex in prostatic nuclei (Walsh 7 Korenman, 1971). Remissions have been reported in up to 70 per cent of patients (Scott & Schirmer, 1966; Geller et al, 1968), with decreased pain and reduced acid phosphatase levels, although doubts have been raised about the real significance of these 'responses' (Tveter et al, 1978).

Flutamide (Sch 13521) is a non-steroidal pure anti-androgen that is not a progestagen. It is structurally an anilide derivative that does not inhibit gonadotropins, has no adrenocortical function and does not suppress androgen synthesis. It has been reported to cause decreased pain and/or obstructive symptoms in 20 to 30 per cent of previously treated patients (Stoliar & Albert, 1974; Sogani & Whitmore, 1979), although lower response rates of only short duration have been reported by others (Narayana et al, 1981).

Many progestagens are structural analogues of the androgens and react with both androgen and progesterone receptor sites, thus functioning as competitive inhibitors of androgens. For example, megestrol acetate, a synthetic progestagen, blocks the intracellular effects of the androgens, including binding of DHT to the cytoplasmic receptor and the 5α-reductase enzyme, in addition to suppressing plasma testosterone levels by inhibiting gonadotrophins (Geller et al, 1981). This drug has yielded response rates in 40 to 90 per cent of previously treated and untreated patients (Johnson et al, 1975; Geller et al, 1978), although, once again, most of these responses have lasted less than 6 months. More recently, Geller et al (1981) have re-induced responses of longer duration in a small number of patients with the combination of megestrol acetate and low dose (0.1 mg) diethylstilboestrol.

Hormone-cytotoxic compounds

As noted previously, prostatic cancer is characterised by the presence of mixed populations of tumour cells, including those that are sensitive to hormonal manipulations and others that show no response to such treatment. To date, the results of treatment with conventional cytotoxic agents, such as cyclophosphamide, adriamycin, the nitrosoureas, and cisplatinum, have been disappointing in patients with CAP, whether or not their tumours have been shown to be hormone-sensitive (Murphy, 1980). One line of investigation has been to apply hormone-cyctotoxic compounds, conjugates of a steroid nucleus with a cytotoxic agent, to the management of patients with disseminated prostatic cancer (Jonsson & Hogberg, 1971; Fossa & Miller, 1976; Mittelmann et al, 1976; Nagel & Kolln, 1977). The rationale of such an approach is that the steroid nucleus may 'home in' on receptor sites, carrying the cytotoxic drug with it; in addition, the steroid may exert its own tumoricidal effect (Muntzing et al, 1974).

Estramustine phosphate. Estramustine phosphate (Estracyt), a nor-nitrogen mustard bound to oestradiol-17-phosphate, is the most extensively investigated of the hormone-cytotoxic compounds. During the first nine years of its clinical use, encouraging response rates were reported from several centres (Jonsson & Hogberg, 1971; Fossa & Miller, 1976; Mittelmann et al. 1976; Nagel & Kolln, 1977; Edsmyr et al, 1980). with as many as 60 per cent of patients showing 'objective' responses. The enthusiasm for this drug was such that it was introduced into combination chemotherapy regimens for patients with hormonally-insensitive prostatic carcinoma (Soloway et al, 1981). However, serious doubts have been raised as to the adequacy of reporting criteria used in the early studies of this drug (Chisholm et al, 1977). Furthermore, in a preliminary report of a randomised trial of estramustine phosphate versus conventional oestrogens in the initial treatment of well or moderately differentiated prostatic carcinoma, no difference was noted between the two arms with respect to frequency or duration of remission or in adverse side-effects. Nevertheless, there may be a limited role for this drug in the management of patients who have already failed conventional hormonal therapy (Edsmyr et al, 1980; Chisholm et al, 1977).

Prednimustine. Prednimustine is a combination of an alkylating agent (chlorambucil) and a corticosteroid (prednisolone) linked by an ester bond. Because of the apparent response rates reported with estramustine phosphate in patients with CAP, trials have been initiated to assess the efficacy of this drug against prostatic cancer. Catane et al (1978) have reported a 35 per cent objective response rate to this drug, using NPCP criteria; however, the length of follow-up was inadequate to allow a realistic evaluation of the drug.

From the same centre, Beckley et al (1981) assessed the efficacy of chlorambucil plus prednisolone administered to a series of 11 patients with CAP, and compared their results with the earlier data — because of the small number of patients studied in each report, no useful conclusion can be drawn, although there were no gross differences in therapeutic responsiveness.

Nevertheless, in both studies, patients experienced useful pain relief of several months duration, and thus the drug will require further evaluation.

SUMMARY

There are extensive experimental and clinical links between the hormonal milieu and cancer of the testis, prostate and kidney, both with respect to the initiation of malignancy and its subsequent treatment. Although hormonal factors may be involved in the genesis of testicular cancer, the major clinical association is in the production of marker substances by these tumours. By contrast, renal cell carcinoma has been shown to be hormone dependent in a series of experimental models, both with respect to the induction of malignant change and treatment, but there is little objective evidence to support significant clinical applications at present. Prostatic cancer, however, is uneqivocally sensitive to hormonal treatment in clinical practice, and is characterised by its elaboration of relatively sensitive and specific tumour markers. Although it is an age-dependent tumour, the mechanisms of tumour induction demonstrated in animal models have not yet been extrapolated to the human situation.

The management of testicular cancer has now been rationalised with the judicious use of staging procedures, surgery and chemotherapy, augmented by tumour marker monitoring. However, the management of hormone-resistant prostatic cancer remains a significant problem,

which will require the development of new drugs and schedules and greater understanding of the heterogeneity of the tumour. In order for progress to be made, rigid criteria of response and adequate sampling of tumour tissue (for histological and receptor analysis) will be essential. To date, clinical progress in the management of metastatic renal cell carcinoma has been very limited. Extensive experimental and clinical investigation, using the available animal models, receptor assays and drug development programmes will be required if further progress is to be made. As with carcinoma of the prostate, there remains a great need to adopt strenuous and detailed criteria of response, augmented by thorough follow-up data, in order to avoid the indefinite propagation of useless therapeutic programmes.

REFERENCES

Abelev G I 1974 Alpha-fetoprotein as a marker of embryo-specific differentiations in normal and tumor tissue. Transplantation Reviews 20: 3–37

Al Sarraff M, Eyre H, Bonnet J, et al 1981 Study of tamoxifen in metastatic renal cell carcinoma and the influence of certain prognostic factors: a SWOG study. Cancer Treatment Reports 65: 447–451

Alberto P, Senn H J 1974 Hormonal therapy of renal carcinoma alone and in association with cytostatic drugs. Cancer 33: 1226–1229

Aragona C, Friesen H 1975 Specific prolactin binding sites in the prostate and testis of rats. Endocrinology 97: 677–684

Artzt K, Dubois P, Bennett D, Condamine H, Babinet C, Jacob F 1973 Surface antigens common to mouse cleavage embryos and primitive mouse teratocarcinoma cells in culture. Proceedings of the National Academy of Science (USA) 70: 2988–2992

Asselin J, Labrie F, Gourdeau Y, Bonne C, Raynaud J P 1976 Binding of ^{3}H-methyltrienolone (R 1881) in rat prostate and human benign prostatic hypertrophy (BPH). Steroids 28: 449–453

Baker H W G, Burger H G, de Kretser D M, Hudson B, Straffon W G 1973 Effects of synthetic oral oestrogens in normal men and patients with prostatic carcinoma. Lack of gonadotropin suppression by chlorotrianisene. Clinical Endocrinology 2: 297–306

Bagshawe K D 1980 Marker proteins as indicators of tumour response to therapy. British Journal of Cancer 41 (Suppl IV): 186–190

Bartsch W, Becker H, Pinkenburg F A, Krieg M 1979 Hormone blood levels and their inter-relationships in normal men and men with benign prostatic hyperplasia. Acta Endocrinologica 90: 727–736

Beckley S, Wajsman L Z, Slack N H, Murphy G P 1981 Chemotherapy in metastatic hormone refractory prostatic cancer using chlorambucil in combination with prednisolone versus conjugate, prednimustine (Leo 1031). Urology 17: 446–448

Berthelsen J G, Skakkebaek N E, Morgensen P, Sorensen B L 1979 Incidence of carcinoma in situ of germ cells in contralateral testis of men with testicular tumours. British Medical Journal 2: 363–364

Bibbo M, Al-Naqueeb M, Baccarini I, et al 1975 Follow-up study of male and female offspring of DES treated mothers. A preliminary report. Journal of Reproductive Medicine 15: 29

Bjorn G L, Gray C P, Strauss E 1979 Orchidectomy after presumed oestrogen failure in treatment of carcinoma of the prostate. Western Journal of Medicine 130: 363–364

Blandy J P, Hope-Stone H F, Dayan A D 1970 Tumours of the Testicle pp 12–30. William Heinemann Medical Books Limited, London

Bloom H J G 1971 Medroxyprogesterone acetate (Provera) in the treatment of metastatic renal cancer. British Journal of Cancer 25: 250–265

Bloom H J G 1972 Renal cancer. In Stoll B A (ed) Endocrine Therapy in Malignant Disease, pp 339–349. W B Saunders, London

Bloom H J G 1973 Hormone-induced and spontaneous regression of metastatic renal cancer. Cancer 32: 1066–1071

Bloom H J G, Hendry W F 1973 Possible role of hormones in treatment of metastatic testicular teratomas: Tumour regression with medroxyprogesterone acetate. British Medical Journal 3: 563–567

Bloom H J G, Wallace 1964 Hormones and the kidney: Possible therapeutic role of testosterone in a patient with regression of metastases from renal adenocarcinoma. British Medical Journal 2: 476–430

Bloom H J G, Dukes C E, Mitchley B C V 1963a The oestrogen-induced renal tumour of the Syrian hamster. Hormone treatment and possible relationship to carcinoma of the kidney in man. British Journal of Cancer 17: 611–645

Bloom H J G, Baker W H, Dukes C E, Mitchley B C V 1963b Hormone dependent tumours of the kidney: II. Effect of endocrine ablation procedures on the transplanted oestrogen-induced renal tumour of the Syrian hamster. British Journal of Cancer 17: 646–656

Bojar H, Wittliff J L, Balzer K, Dreyfurst R, Boeminghaus F, Staib W 1975 Properties of specific estrogen-binding components in human kidney and renal carcinoma. Acta Endocrinologica (Suppl) 193: 51–60

Bonne C, Raynaud J P 1975 Methyltrienolone, a specific ligand for cellular androgen receptors. Steroids 26: 227–232

Bonser G M, Robson J M 1940 The effects of prolonged oestrogen administration upon male mice of various strains: Development of testicular tumours in Strong A strain. Journal of Pathology and Bacteriology 51: 9–22

Bracci U, DiSilverio F, Sciarra F, Sorcini G, Piro C, Santoro F 1977 Hormonal pattern in prostatic carcinoma following orchidectomy: 5-year follow-up. British Journal of Urology 49: 161–166

Bracken R B, Smith K B 1980 Is semen cryopreservation helpful in testicular cancer? Urology 15: 581–583

Braunstein G D, McIntire K R, Waldmann T A 1973 Discordance of human chorionic gonadotropin and alpha-fetoprotein in testicular teratocarcinomas. Cancer 31: 1065–1068

Brown N J 1976 Yolk-sac tumour (orchioblastoma) and other testicular tumours of childhood. In Pugh R C B (ed) Pathology of the Testis, pp 356–70. Blackwell Scientific Publications, Oxford

Brosman S A 1979 Testicular tumors in pre-pubertal children. Urology 13: 581–588

Bruchovsky N, Wilson J D 1968a The conversion of testosterone to 5a-androstan-17B-ol-3-one by rat prostate in vivo and in vitro. Journal of Biological Chemistry 243: 2012–2021

Bruchovsky N, Wilson J D 1968b The intranuclear binding of testosterone and 5a-androstan-17B-ol-3-one by rat prostate. Journal of Biological Chemistry 243: 5953–5960

Burge P D, Harper M, Hartog M, Gingell J C 1976 Subcapsular

orchidectomy — an effective operation? Proceedings of the Royal Society of Medicine 69: 663–664

Bullock L P, Bardin W C 1974 Androgen receptors in mouse kidney: A study of male, female and androgen insensitive (tfm/y) mice. Endocriniology 94: 746–756

Burton R M, Westphal U 1972 Steroid hormone binding proteins in blood plasma. Metabolism 21: 253–260

Byar D P 1973 The Veterans' Administration Cooperative Urological Research Group's studies of cancer of the prostate. Cancer 32: 1126–1130

Byar D P 1980a VACURG studies of conservative treatment. Scanianavian Journal of Urology and Nephrology supplement 55: 99–102

Byar D P 1980b VACURG studies of post-prostatectomy survival. Scandinavian Journal of Urology and Nephrology supplement 55: 113–116

Cabot A T 1896 The question of castration for enlarged prostate. Annals of Surgery 24: 265–309

Card D J, Kohorn E I, Lyttun B 1970 Effects of hormones on whole organ cultures of renal cell carcinoma. Surgical Forum 21: 532–540

Carleton R L, Friedman N B, Bomze E J 1953 Experimental teratomas of the testis. Cancer 6: 464–473

Caruso P A, Marsh M R, Minkowitz S, Karten G 1971 An intense clinico-pathologic study of 305 teratomas of the ovary. Cancer 27: 343–348

Castro J E 1973 A method of in vivo maintenance of human prostatic tissue in immunosuppressed mice. British Journal of Urology 45: 163–168

Catalona W J, Menon M 1981 New screening and diagnostic tests for prostate canncer and immunologic assessment. Urology (Suppl) 17: 61–65

Catalona W J, Vaitukaitis J L, Fair W R 1979 Falsely positive specific human chorionic gonadotropin assays in patients with testicular tumors: Conversion to negative with testosterone administration. Journal of Urology 122: 126–128

Catane R, Kaufman J H, Madajewicz S, Mittelman A, Murphy G P 1978 Prednimustine therapy for advanced prostatic cancer. British Journal of Urology 50: 29–32

Catane R, Mittelman A, Murphy G P, Sandberg A A 1980 Effects of testosterone on estracyt localisation in rat prostate. Oncology 37: 357–359

Chan V, Katikineni M, Davies T F, Catt K J 1981 Hormonal regulation of testicular luteinizing hormone and prolactin receptors. Endocrinology 108: 1607–1612

Chapman R N, Sutcliffe S B 1981 Protection of ovarian function by oral contraceptives in women receiving chemotherapy for Hodgkin's disease. Blood 58: 849–851

Chapman R N, Sutcliffe S M, Malpas J S 1981 Male gonadal dysfunction in Hodgkin's disease. Journal of the American Medical Association 245: 1323–1328

Chisholm G D, O'Donoghue E P N, Kennedy C L 1977 The treatment of oestrogen-escaped carcinoma of the prostate with estramustine phosphate. British Journal of Urology 49: 717–720

Chiu C L, Weber J 1974 Prostatic carcinoma in young adults. Journal of the American Medical Association 230: 724–730

Chu T M, Bhargava A, Barnard E A et al 1975 Tumor antigen and acid phosphatase isoenzyme in prostatic cancer. Cancer Chemotherapy Reports 59: 97–101

Clark P, Houghton L 1977 Subcapsular orchidectomy for carcinoma of the prostate. British Journal of Urology 49: 419–425

Clemmesen J 1968 A doubling of morbidity from testis carcinoma in Copenhagen. Acta Pathologica Microbiologica Scandanavica 72 (Section A): 348–349

Concolino G 1979 Renal cancer: Steroid receptors as a biochemical basis for endocrine therapy. In: Thompson E B and Lippman M E (eds) Steroid Receptors and the Management of Cancer, Vol I, pp 173–196. CRC Press Inc, Boca Raton, Florida

Cosgrove M D, Benton B, Henderon B I 1977 Male genitourinary abnormalities and maternal diethylstilboestrol. Journal of Urology 117: 220–222

Coune A 1978 Carcinoma of the prostate. In Staquet M (ed) Radnomized Trials in Cancer: A Critical Review by Sites, pp 389–409. Raven Press, New York

Coutts W E, Vagas-Zalazar R 1945 Rev chilena de hig y med prev 7: 57–61 quoted Shivers C H, Axilrod H D p 538

Cunha G R, Lung B 1979 The importance of stroma in morphogenesis and function activity of urogenital epithelium. In Vitro 15: 50–71

Davis P L, Shumway M H 1958 Tumors of the testicle: Temporary suppression of pulmonary metastases with testosterone. Journal of Urology 80: 62–64

Damjanov I, Solter D 1982 Maternally transmitted factors modify development and malignancy of teratomas in mice. Nature 296: 95–96

deKernion J B, Berry D 1980 The diagnosis and treatment of renal cell carcinoma. Cancer 45: 1947–1956

deKlerk D P, Coffey D S, Ewing L L et al 1979 Comparison of spontaneous and experimentally induced canine prostatic hyperplasia. Journal of Clinical Investigation 64: 842–849

Dixon F J, Moore R A 1952 Tumors of the Male Sex Organs. Atlas of Tumor Pathology, Fascicles 31b and 32, Armed Forces Institute of Pathology, Washington

Dmitriev V N 1977 Hormonal treatment of precancerous diseases of the testis in rats. Bulletin of Experimental Biology and Medicine (USSR) 83: 540–542

Donnellan W A, Swenson O 1968 Benign and malignant sacrococcygeal teratomas. Surgery 64: 834–836

Dodge A M 1974 Fine structural, Hal Vgas antigen, and reverse tanscriptase study of the Syrian hamster stilbestrol-induced renal carcinoma. Laboratory Investigation 31: 250–253

Drago J R, Gershwin M E, Maurer R E, Ikeda R M, Eckless D D 1979 Immunobiology and therapeutic manipulation of heterotransplanted Nb rat prostate adenocarcinoma into congenitally athmic (nude) mice. I. Hormone dependency and histopathology. Journal of the National Cancer Institute 62: 1057–1066

Drasga R E, Williams S D, Stevens E E et al 1982 Gonadal function after plantinum, vinblastine, bleomycin +/− adriamycin in testicular cancer. Proceedings of the American Society of Clinical Oncology 1: 105(abst)

Dube J Y, Chapdelaine P, Tremblay R R, Bonne C, Raynaud J P 1976 Comparative binding specificity of methyltrienolone in human and rat prostate. Hormone Research 7: 341–352

Dunning W F, Curtis M R, Segaloff A 1946 Methylcholanthrene squamous cell carcinoma of rat prostate with skeletal metastases, and failure of rat liver to respond to the same carcinogen. Cancer Research 6: 256–262

Edsmyr F, Esposti P L, Andersson L 1980 Estramustine phosphate therapy in poorly differentiated carcinoma of the prostate. Scandinavian Journal of Urology and Nephrology (Suppl) 55: 139–142

Ekman P, Snowchowski M, Dahlberg E, Bressian D, Hogberg B, Gustafsson J A 1979a Steroid receptor content in cytosol from normal and hyperplastic human prostates. Journal of Clinical Endocrinology and Metabolism 49: 205–215

Ekman P, Snowchowski M, Dahlberg E, Gustafsson J A 1979b Steroid receptors in metastatic carcinoma of the human prostate. European Journal of Cancer 15: 257–262

Ekman P, Gustafsson J A, Hogberg B, Pousette A, Snochoswski M 1980 Prediction of tumor response to endocrine therapy in prostatic carcinoma based on steroid receptor assay. Scandinavian Journal of Urology and Nephrology (Suppl) 55: 83–89

Fairlamb D J 1981 Spontaneous regression of metastases of renal cancer. Cancer 47: 2102–2106

Fanestil D D, Vaughn D A, Ludens J H 1974 Steroid hormone receptors in human renal carcinoma. Journal of Steroid Biochemistry 5: 338(abst)

Farnsworth W E, Gonder M J 1977 Prolactin and prostate cancer. Urology 10: 33–40

Farnsworth W E, Slaunwhite W R Jr, Sharma M, et al 1981 Interaction of prolactin and testosterone in the human prostate. Urological Research 9: 79–88

Feun L G, Drelichman A, Singhakowinta A, et al 1979 Phase II study of nafoxidine in the therapy for advanced renal carcinoma. Cancer Treatment Reports 63: 149–150

Fingerhut B, Veenema R J 1966 Histology and radioautography of induced benign enlargement of the mouse prostate. Investigative Urology 4: 112–124

Forbes A P 1978 Chemotherapy, testicular damage and gynaecomastia: an endocrine 'black hole' (editorial) New England Journal of Medicine 299: 42–43

Fossa S D, Miller A 1976 Treatment of advanced carcinoma of the prostate with estramustine phosphate. Journal of Urology 115: 406–408

Fossa S D, Klepp O, Aakvaag A 1980 Serum hormone levels in patients with malignant testicular germ cell tumours without clinical and/or radiological signs of tumour. British Journal of Urology 52: 151–157

Friedman A, Vugrin D, Golbey R B 1980 Prognostic significance of serum tumor biomarkers (TM), alpha-fetoprotein (AFP), beta subunit of human chorionic gonadotrophin (bHCG), and lactate dehydrogenase (LDH) in nonseminomatous germ cell tumors. Proceedings of the American Society of Clinical Oncology 21: 323(abst)

Furuhjelm L 1941 Excretion of gonadotropic hormones in urine in cases of tumor of testis. Nordiske Medizin 11: 2603–2609

Geller J, Vazakas G, Fruchtman B, et al 1968 The effect of cyproterone acetate on advanced carcinoma of prostate. Surgery, Gynecology and Obstetrics 127: 748–758

Geller J, Albert J, Yen S S C 1978 Treatment of advanced cancer of the prostate with megestrol acetate. Urology 12: 537–541

Geller J, Albert J, Yen S S C, Geller S, Loza D 1981 Medical castration with megestrol acetate and minidose of diethylstilbestrol. Urology 17 (supplement): 27–33

Gehring U, Tomkins G M, Ohno S 1971 Effect of the androgen-insensitivity mutation on a cytoplasmic receptor for dihydrotestosterone. Nature, New Biology 232: 106

Ghaleb H A 1961 The metabolism of stilboestrol and the diphosphate ester in relation to treatment of carcinoma of the prostate. PhD thesis, University of London, quoted by Bloom H J G 1964 Hormone treatment of renal tumours: Experimental and clinical observations. In: Riches E (ed) Tumours of the Kidney and Ureter vol 5, p 311. E and S Livingstone Ltd, Edinburgh

Ghanadian R, Lewis J G, Chisholm G D, O'Donoghue E P N 1977 Serum dihydrotestosterone in patients with benign prostatic hypertrophy. British Journal of Urology 49: 541

Ghanadian R, Auf G, Williams G, Davis A, Richards B 1981 Predicting the response of prostatic carcinoma to endocrine therapy. Lancet ii: 1418

Gilbert J B, Hamilton J B 1940 Studies in malignant testis tumors: Incidence and nature of tumors in ectopic testes. Surgery, Gynecology and Obstetrics 71: 731–743

Gill W B, Schumacher G F B, Bibbo M 1977 Pathological semen and anatomical abnormalities of the genital tract in human male subjects exposed to diethylstilboestrol in utero. Journal of Urology 117: 477–480

Glick J H, Wein A, Torri S, et al 1980a Phase II study of Tamoxifen in patients with advanced renal cell carcinoma. Cancer Treatment Reports 64: 343–344

Glick J H, Wein A, Padavic K, et al 1980b Tamoxifen in refractory metastatic carcinoma of the prostate. Cancer Treatment Reports 64: 813–818

Glode L N, Robinson G A, Gould S F 1981 Protection from cyclophosphamide-induced testicular damage with an analog of gonadotropin-releasing hormone. Lancet i: 1132–1134

Gloyna R E, Siiteri P K, Wilson J D 1970 Dihydrotestosterone in prostatic hypertrophy. II. The formation and content of dihydrotestosterone in the hypertrophic canine prostate and the effect of dihydrotestosterone on prostate growth in the dog. Journal of Clinical Investigation 49: 1746–1753

Goldenberg D M, de Land F, Kim E et al 1978 Use of radiolabelled antibodies to carcinoembryonic antigen for the detection and localization of diverse cancers by external photscanning. New England Journal of Medicine 298: 1384–1388

Goldenberg D M, Kim E E, de Land F H, vanNagell J R, Javadpour N 1980a Clinical radioimmunodetection of cancer with radioactive antibodies to human chorionic gonadotropin. Science 207: 1284–1286

Goldenberg D M, Kim E E, deLand F, et al 1980b Clinical studies on the radioimmunodetection of tumors containing alpha-fetoprotein. Cancer 45: 2500–2505

Grayhack J T, Bunce F L, Kearns J W, Scott W W 1955 Influence of the pituitary on prostatic response to androgen in the rat. Bulletin of the Johns Hopkins Hospital 96: 154–163

Greenblatt R B, Dmowski W P, Mahesh V B, Scholer H F L 1971 Clinical studies with an antigonadotropin — Danazol. Fertility and Sterility 22: 102–112

Gursel E O, Rezvan M, Sy F A, Veenema R 1974 Comparative evaluation of bone marrow acid phosphatase and bone scanning in staging of prostatic cancer. Journal of Urology 111: 53–57

Guhthrie J 1964 Observations on the zinc induced testicular teratomas of fowl. British Journal of Cancer 18: 130–142

Hamburger C, Bang F, Nielson J 1936 Studies on gonadotropic hormones in cases of testicular tumors: Attempt at classification of testicular tumors on the basis of their hormonal, histological and clinico-radiological properties. Acta Pathologica Microbiologica Scandanavica 13: 75–102

Hammond G L, Kontturi M, Vihko P, Vihko R 1978 Serum steroids in normal males and patients with prostatic disease. Clinical Endocrinology 9: 113

Harman S M, Tsitouras P D 1980 Reproductive hormones in aging men. I. Measurement of sex steroids, basal luteinizing hormone and Leydig cell response to human chorionic gonadotropin. Journal of Clinical Endocrinology and Metabolism 51: 35–40

Harper M E, Pike A, Peeling W B, Griffiths K 1974 Steroids of adrenal origin metabolised by human prostatic tissue in vivo and in vitro. Journal of Endocrinology 60: 117–125

Harper M E, Peeling W B, Cowley T, et al 1976 Plasma steroid and protein hormone concentrations in patients with prostatic carcinoma before and during oestrogen therapy. Acta Endocrinologica 81: 409–426

Harper M E, Chaisiri P, Slade J, Peeling W B, Griffiths K 1981 Hormonal relationships, receptors and tumour markers. In Duncan W (ed.) Prostate Cancer (Recent Results in Cancer Research) Vol. 78, pp 44–59. Springer Verlag, Berlin

Harrison R G, Lewis Jones D I, de Marvel M J M, Connolly R C 1981 Mechanism of damage to the contralateral testis in rats with an ischaemic testis. Lancet 2: 723–725

Hawkins E F, Nijs M, Brassinne C, Tagnon H J 1975 Steroid receptors in the human prostate. 1. Estradiol -17B binding in benign prostatic hypertrophy. Steroids 26: 458–469

Henderson B E, Benton B D A, Weaver P T, Linden G, Nolan J F 1973 Stilbestrol and uro-genital tract cancer in adolescents and young adults. New England Journal of Medicine 288: 354

Henderson B E, Benton B, Jing J, Yu M C, Pike M C 1979 Risk factors for cancer of the testis in young men. International Journal of Cancer 23: 598–609

Hellman L, Yoshida K, Zumoff B, Levin J, Kream J, Fukushima D K 1976 The effect of medroxyprogesterone acetate on the pituitary-adrenal axis. Journal of Clinical Endocrinology and Metabolism 42: 912–917

Herbst A L, Ulfelder H, Poskanzer D C 1971 Adenocarcinoma of the vagina. Association of maternal stilbestrol therapy with tumor appearance in young women. New England Journal of Medicine 284: 878

Heston W D W, Menon M, Tanaris C, Walsh P C 1979 Androgen, estrogen and progesterone receptors of the R3327H Copenhagen rat prostatic tumor. Cancer Letters 6: 45–50

Heyderman E 1978 Multiple tissue markers in human malignant testicular tumours. Scandinavian Journal of Immunology 8 supplement 8: 119–123

Heyderman E, Neville A M 1976 Syncytiotrophoblasts in malignant tumours. Lancet ii: 103

Heyderman E, Raghavan D, Neville A M 1981 Functional pathology of testicular tumours. In Peckham M J (ed) The Management of Testicular Tumours, pp 42–49. Edward Arnold, London

Heynes W, Peeters B, Mous J 1977 Influence of androgens on the concentration of prostatic binding protein (PBP) and its m-RNA in rat prostate. Biochemical and Biophysics Research Communications 77: 1492–1499

Higgins S J, Gehring U 1978 Molecular mechanisms of steroid hormone action. Advances in Cancer Research 28: 313–326

Hirst A E Jr, Bergman R T 1954 Carcinoma of the prostate in men 80 or more years old. Cancer 7: 136–141

Hogan B, Fellous M, Avner P, Jacob F 1977 Isolation of a human teratoma cell line, which expresses F9 antigen. Nature 270: 515–518

Holden S, Bernard O, Artzt K, Whitmore W F Jr, Bennett D 1977 Human and mouse embryonal carcinoma cells in culture share an embryonic antigen (F9). Nature 270: 518–520

Hooker C W, Gardner W U, Pfeiffer C A 1940 Testicular tumors in mice receiving estrogens. Journal of the American Medical Association 115: 443–445

Horning E S 1946 Induction of glandular carcinomas of prostate in mouse. A preliminary communication. Lancet ii: 829–830

Huggins C, Hodges C V 1941 Studies on prostatic cancer. I. The effect of castration, of estrogen, and of androgen injection on serum phosphatases in metastatic carcinoma of the prostate. Cancer Research 1: 293–297

Huggins C, Stevens R A, Hodges C V 1941 Studies on prostatic cancer. II. Effects of castration on advanced carcinoma of the prostate gland. Archives of Surgery 43: 209–223

Hunter J 1786 Observations on Certain Parts of the Animal Oeconomy, p 39. Bibliotheca Osteriana, London

Husband J 1980 Diagnostic techniques: Their strengths and weaknesses. British Journal of Cancer 41(suppl iv): 21–29

Hutchison G B 1981 Incidence and etiology of prostate cancer. Urology (Suppl) 17: 4–10

Jacobi G H, Altwein J E, Hohenfellner R 1980 Adjunct bromocriptine treatment as palliation for prostate cancer: Experimental and clinical evaluation. Scandinavian Journal of Urology and Nephrology supplement 55: 107–112

Javadpour N 1980 The role of biologic tumor markers in testicular cancer. Cancer 45: 1755–1761

Jenkin R D 1967 Androgens in metastatic renal adenocarcinoma. British Medical Journal 1: 361

Johnson D E, Kaesler K E, Ayala A C 1975 Megestrol acetate for treatment of advanced carcinoma of the prostate. Journal of Surgical Oncology 7: 9–15

Jones T M, Fang V S, Landau R L, Rosenfield R 1978 Direct inhibition of Leydig cell function by estradiol. Journal of Clinical Endocrinology and Metabolism 47: 1368–1373

Jonsson G, Hogberg B 1971 Treatment of advanced prostatic carcinoma with Estracyt: A preliminary report. Scandinavian Journal of Urology and Nephrology 5: 103–107

Kallen B, Rohl L 1962 Steroid influence of testicular tumor growth, studied in tissue culture. Journal of Urology 87: 906–913

Katz S E, Shapiro H E 1982 Spontaneous regression of genitourinary cancer — an update. Journal of Urology 128: 1–4

King R J B 1967 Fixation of steroids to receptors. Archives of Anatomy, Microscopy, Morphology and Experimentation 56 supplement 3–4: 570–580

Kipling M D, Waterhouse J A H 1967 Cadmium and prostatic carcinoma. Lancet i: 730–731

Kirkman H 1959 Oestrogen-induced tumors of the kidney in the Syrian hamster. III and IV. National Cancer Institute Monograph 1: 1–59

Kirkman H 1974 Autonomous derivatives of estrogen-induced renal carcinomas and spontaneous renal tumours in the Syrian hamster. Cancer Research 34: 2728–2744

Kirkman H, Bacon R L 1952 Oestrogen induced tumours of the kidney. Journal of the Ntional Cancer Institute 13: 743–755

Kirscher M A, Cohen F B, Jespersen D 1974 Estrogen production and its origin in men with gonadotrophin-producing neoplasm. Journal of Clinical Endocrinology and Metabolism 39: 112–118

Kirschner M A, Wider J A, Ross G T 1970 Leydig cell function in men with gonadotrophin producing testicular tumors. Journal of Clinical Endocinology and Metabolism 30: 504–511

Klemcke H G, Burtke A 1981 Effects of chronic hyperprolactinaemia in mice on plasma gonadotrophin concentrations and testicular human chorionic gonadotropin binding sites. Endocrinology 108: 1763–1768

Klepp O, Klepp R, Host H, Asbjornsen G, Talle K, Stenwig A E 1977 Combination chemotherapy of germ cell tumors of testis with vincristine, adriamycin, cyclophosphamide, actinomycin-D and medroxyprogesterone acetate. Cancer 40: 638–646

Kohn J 1978 The dynamics of serum alpha-fetoprotein in the course of testicular teratoma. Scandinavian Journal of Immunology 8 (Suppl 8): 103–107

Kohn J, Raghavan D 1981 Tumour markers in malignant germ cell tumours. In; Peckham M J (ed) The Management of Testicular Tumours, pp 50–69. Edward Arnold, London

Kom C, Mulholland S G, Edson M 1971 Etiology of infertility after retroperitoneal lymphadenectomy. Journal of Urology 105: 528–530

Koronchevsky V M, Rose M A 1940 Kidney and the sex hormones. British Medical Journal 1: 645–647

Krabbe S, Skakkebaek N E, Berthelsen J G, et al 1979 High incidence of undetected neoplasia in maldescended testes. Lancet i: 999–1000

Kuriyama M, Wang M C, Papsidero L D et al 1980 Quantitation of prostate-specific antigen in serum by a sensitive enzyme immunoassay. Cancer Research 40: 4658–4662

Kurman R J, Norris H J 1976 Malignant mixed germ cell tumors of the ovary: A clinical and pathologic analysis of 30 cases. Obstetrics and Gynecology 48: 579–589

Kurman R J, Scardino P T, McIntire K R, Waldmann T A, Javadpour N 1977 Cellular localisation of alpha-fetoprotein and human chorionic gonadotrophin using an indirect immunoperoxidase technique. Cancer 40: 2136–2151

Lange P H, Raghavan D (1983) Clinical applications of tumor markers in testicular cancer. In: Donohue J P (ed) Management of Testicular Cancer. Williams and Wilkins, Baltimore, pp 111–130.

Lange P H, McIntire K R, Waldmann T A, Hakala T R, Fraley E E 1977 Alpha-fetoprotein and human chorionic gonadotropin in the management of testicular tumors. Journal of Urology 118: 593–596

Lange P H, Nochomovitz L E, Rosai J, et al 1980 Serum alpha-fetoprotein and human chorionic gonadotropin in patients with seminoma. Journal of Urology 124: 472–478

Lange P H, Millan J L, Stigbrand T, Vessella R L, Ruoslahti E, Fishman W H 1982a Placental alkaline phosphatase as a tumor marker for seminoma. Cancer Research 42: 3244–3247

Lange P H, Bosl G J, Kennedy B J, Fraley E E 1982b Marker half-life analysis as a prognostic tool in testicular cancer. Journal of Urology

Lange P H, Narayan P, Vogelzang N J, Shafer R P, Kennedy B J, Fraley E E (1983) Changing concepts about infertility after treatment for testicular tumors. Journal of Urology

Lattimer J K 1942 The action of testosterone proprionate upon the kidneys of rats, dogs and men. Journal of Urology 48: 778–784

Lea O A, French F S 1981 Androgen receptor protein in the androgen-dependent Dunning R-3327 prostate carcinoma. Cancer Research 41: 619–623

Legha S, Muggia F 1976 Antiestrogens in the treatment of cancer. Annals of Internal Medicine 84: 751

Leistenscheider W, Nagel R 1980 Cytological and DNA-cytometric monitoring of the effect of therapy in conservatively treated prostatic carcinomas. Scandinavian Journal of Urology and Nephrology supplement 55: 197–204

Lewis J G, Ghanadian R, Chisholm G D 1976 Serum 5a-dihydrotestosterone and testosterone changes with age in man. Acta Endocrinologica 82: 444–451

Li J J, Talley D J, Li S A, Villee C A 1974 An estrogen binding protein in the renal cytosol of intact, castrated and estrogenized golden hamster. Endocrinology 96: 1106–1113

Li J J, Talley D J, Li S A, Villee C A 1976 Receptor characteristics of specific estrogen binding in the renal adenocarcinoma of the golden hamster. Cancer Research 36: 1127–1132

Li J J, Li S A, Cuthbertson T L 1979 Nuclear retention of all steroid hormone receptor classes in the hamster renal carcinoma. Cancer Research 39: 2647–2651

Li S A, Li J J, Villee C A 1977 Significance of the progesterone receptor in the estrogen-induced and –dependent renal tumor of the Syrian golden hamster. Annals of the New York Academy of Sciences 286: 369–383

Lieskovsky G, Bruchovsky N 1979 Assay of nuclear androgen receptor in human prostate. Journal of Urology 121: 54–58

Lindenmeyer D, Hornung D, Korner F 1973 Hormonal changes in urine and plasma in patients with various testicular tumors before and after treatment. Urology International 28: 127–144

Llombart-Bosch A, Peydra A 1975 Morphologic, histochemical and ultrastructural observations of diethylstilbestrol-induced kidney tumors in the Syrian golden hamster. European Journal of Cancer 2: 403

Lokich J J, Harrison J H 1975 Renal cell carcinoma: Natural history and chemotherapeutic experience Journal of Urology 114: 371–374

Loughlin J E, Robboy S J, Morrison A S 1980 Risk factors for cancer of the testis. New England Journal of Medicine 303: 112–113

Lucke W M, Kelly D F 1976 Renal carcinoma in the dog. Veterinary Pathology 13: 264–269

Ludden J B, Kreuzer E, Wright I S 1941 Effect of testosterone proprionate, estradiol benzoate and deoxycorticosterone acetate on kidneys of adult rats. Endocrinology 28: 619–623

Madajewicz S, Bhargava A, Wajsman Z, Mittelman A, Fitzpatrick J, Murphy G P 1980 Hypothalamopituitary-adrenal axis in patients with prostatic carcinoma. Oncology 37: 373–375

Madanes A E, Farber M 1982 Danazol. Annals of Internal Medicine 96: 625–630

Mahoney E M, Harrison J H 1972 Bilateral adrenalectomy for palliative treatment of prostatic carcinoma. Journal of Urology 108: 936–938

Maier J G, Sulak M H 1973 Radiation therapy in malignant testis tumors. Cancer 32: 1212–1216

Mainwaring W I, Milroy E J 1973 Characterisation of the specific androgen receptors in the human prostate gland. Journal of Endocrinology 57: 371–377

Marlow P B, Mizel S 1976 Evidence for rhythm of mitotic activity in normal and adenocarcinoma cells of the renal tubules of Rana pipiens. Journal of the National Cancer Institute 57: 1069–1076

Matsuda M, Osafure M, Kotake K, Sonoda T 1976 A clinical study on renal cell carcinoma. Japanese Journal of Urology 67: 635–641

Mauch P, Weichselbaum R, Botnick L 1979 The significance of positive chorionic gonadotropins in apparently pure seminoma of the testis. International Journal of Radiation Oncology, Biology and Physics 5: 887–889

McClelland J C 1943 Discussion of article by Davis E, Journal of Urology 49: 31

McDonald J H, Calams J A 1959 Extra-parenchymal Leydig-like cells; observations following subcapsular orchidectomy. Journal of Urology 82: 145–147

McIlhinney R A J 1981 Cell surface molecules of human teratoma cell lines. International Journal of Andrology supplement 4: 93–110

McMahon M J, Butler A V J, Thomas G H 1972 Morphological responses of prostatic carcinoma to testosterone in organ culture. British Journal of Cancer 26: 388–394

McNeal J E 1981 Normal and pathologic anatomy of prostate. Urology 17 (Suppl): 11–16

Meikle A W, Stanish W M 1982 Familial prostatic cancer risk and low testosterone. Journal of Clinical endocrinology and Metabolism 54: 1104–1108

Meikle A W, Collier E S, Middleton R G, Fang S-M 1980 Supranormal nuclear content of 5a-dihydro-testosterone in benign hyperplastic prostate of humans. Journal of Clinical Endocrinology and Metabolism 51: 945–947

Menon M, Tananis C E, Hicks L L, Hawkins E F, McLoughlin M G, Walsh P C 1978 Characterisation of the binding of a potent synthetic androgen, methyltrienolone, to human tissues. Journal of Clinical Investigation 61: 150–162

Michalowsky J 1926 Die experimentelle erzeugung einer teratoiden neubildung beim hoden beim hahn. Cbl. Allg. Pathologie Pathologische Anatomie 38: 585–587

Mickey D D, Stone K R, Wunderli H, Mickey G H, Vollmer R T, Paulson D F 1977 Heterotransplantation of a human prostatic adenocarcinoma cell line in nude mice. Cancer Research 37: 4049–4058

Millington D S, Golder M P, Crowley T H, et al 1976 In vitro synthesis of steroids by a feminising adrenocortical carcinoma: Effect of prolactin and other protein hormones. Acta Endocrinologica 82: 561–569

Mittelman A, Shukla S K, Murphy G P 1976 Extended therapy of stage D carcinoma of the prostate with oral estramustine phosphate. Journal of Urology 115: 409–412

Mobbs B G, Johnson I E, Connolly J G 1975 In vitro assay of androgen binding by human prostate. Journal of Steroid Biochemistry 6: 453–458

Montie J E, Stewart B H, Straffon R A et al 1977 The role of adjunctive nephrectomy in patients with metastatic renal cell carcinoma. Journal of Urology 117: 272–275

Monaghan P, Raghavan D, Neville A M 1982 Ultrastructural studies of xenografted human germ cell tumors. Cancer 49: 683–697

Moore R A 1943 Benign hypertrophy of the prostate. A morphologic study. Journal of Urology 50: 680–710

Moore R A 1947 Endocrinology of Neoplastic Disease p 147. Oxford University Press, New York

Moore R A, Melchionna R H 1937 Production of tumors of the prostate of the white rat with 1: 2-benzpyrene. American Journal of Cancer 30: 731–74

Moore R J, Grazak J M, Wilson J D 1978a Regulation of cytoplasmic dihydrotestosterone binding in dog prostate by 17 B-estradiol. Journal of Clinical Investigation 63: 351–357

Moore R J, Razak J M, Quebbeman J F, Wilson J D 1979b Concentration of dihydrotestosterone and 3a-androstanediol in naturally occuring and androgen-induced prostatic hyperplasia in the dog. Journal of Clinical Investigation 64: 1003–1010

Morales A, Kiruluta G, Lotts J 1975 Hormones in the treatment of metastatic renal cancer. Journal of Urology 114: 692–693

Moshakis V, McIlhinney R A J, Raghavan D, Neville A M 1981 Radioimmunodetecion of a human testicular teratoma using anti-teratoma monoclonal antibodies. British Journal of Cancer 44: 91–99

Mostofi F K 1967 Pathology and spread of renal cell carcinoma. In: King J S (ed) Renal Neoplasia, pp 41–85. Little & Brown, Boston

Mostofi F K, Price E B 1973 Tumors of the male genital system. A.F.I.P. Atlas of Tumor Pathology, Armed Forces Institute of Pathology, Washington D.C., Fascicle 8

Muntzing J, Shukla S K, Chu T M, Mittelmann A, Murphy G P 1974 Pharmacoclinical study of oral estramustine phosphate (Estracyt) in advanced carcinoma of the prostate. Investigative Urology 12: 65–68

Murphy G P 1979 Cancer of the prostate. In: Javadpour N, (ed) Prinicples and Management of Urolgic Cancer, pp 403–418 Williams and Wilkins Company, Baltimore

Murphy G P, Hresheský W J 1973 A murine renal cell carcinoma. Journal of the National Cancer Institute 50: 1013–1025

Murphy G P, Saroff J, Joiner J R, et al 1976 Chemotherapy of advanced prostatic cancer by the National Prostatic Cancer Project. Seminars in Oncology 3: 103–106

Nagel R, Kolln C-P 1977 Treatment of advanced carcinoma of the prostate with estramustine phosphate. British Journal of Urology 49: 73–79

Narayan P, Lange P H, Fraley E E 1982 Ejaculation and fertility after extended retroperitoneal lymph node dissection for testicular cancer. Journal of Urology 127: 685–688

Narayana A S, Loening S A, Culp D A 1981 Flutamide in the treatment of metastatic carcinoma of the prostate. British Journal of Urology 53: 152–153

Neoptolemos J P, Locke T J, Fossard D P 1981 Testicular tumour associated with hormonal treatment for oligospermia. Lancet ii: 754

Newlands E S, Begent R H J, Kaye S B, Rustin G J S, Bagshawe K D 1980 Chemotherapy of advanced malignant teratomas. British Journal of Cancer 42: 378–384

Noble R L 1980a Production of NB rat carcinoma of the dorsal prostate and response of estrogen-dependent transplants to sex-hormones and tamoxifen. Cancer Research 40: 3547–3550

Noble R L 1980b Development of androgen-stimulated transplants of NB rat carcinoma of the dorsal prostate and their response to sex hormones and tamoxifen. Cancer Research 40: 3551–3554

Norgaard-Federsen B, Raghavan D (eds) et al 1981 Germ cell tumours: A collaborative review. Onco-Developmental Biology and Medicine 1: 327–347

Noronha R F X 1975 The inhibition of dimethylnitrosamine induced renal tumorigenesis in NZO/B1 mice by orchidectomy. Investigative Urology 13: 136

Nuesch-Bachmann I H, Hedinger C 1977 Atypische spermatogonien also prakanzerose. Schweizerische Medizin Wochenschrift 107: 795–801

O'Conor J, Chiang S P, Grayhack J T 1963 Is supcapsular orchidectomy a definitive procedure? Studies of hormone excretion before and after orchidectomy. Journal of Urology 89: 236–240

Paine C H, Wright F W, Ellis F 1970 The use of progesterone in the treatment of metastatic carcinoma of the kidney and uterine body. British Journal of Cancer 24: 277–282

Papec R J, Ross S A, Levy A 1977 Renal cell carcinoma: Analysis of

31 cases with assessment of endocrine therapy. American Journal of Medical Sciences 274: 281–285

Papsidero L D, Wang W C, Valenzuela L A, Murphy G P, Chu T M 1980 A prostate antigen in sera of prostatic cancer patients. Cancer Research 40: 2428–2432

Parker M G, Needham M, White R 1982 Prostatic steroid binding protein: Gene duplication and steroid binding. Nature 298: 92–94

Parker M G, Scrace G T 1979 Regulation of protein synthesis in rat ventral prostate — cell free translation of mRNA. Proceedings of the National Academy of Science (USA) 76: 1580–1584

Patterson J S 1980 Use of antioestrogens in prostatic carcinoma. Scottish Medical Journal 25: 162

Paulson D F, Rabson A S, Faley E E 1968 Vital neoplastic transformation of hamster prostate tissue in vitro. Science 159: 200–201

Pierce G B, Dixon F J Jr, Verney E 1959 Endocrine function of a heterotransplantable human embryonal carcinoma. Archives of Pathology 67: 204–210

Peckham M J, Barrett A, McElwain T J, Hendry W, Raghavan D 1981 Non-seminoma germ cell tumours of the testis: Results of treatment and an analysis of prognostic factors. British Journal of Urology 53: 162–172

Pott P 1779 The Chirurgical Works of Percivall Pott, cited by Blandy et al 1970, p 4

Potts G O, Beyler A L, Shane H P 1974 Pituitary gonadotrophin inhibitory activity of danazol. Fertility and Sterility 25: 367–372

Prudencio R F, Clark S S, Das Gupta T K 1973 Effect of hypophysectomy on an experimental testicular tumor. Surgical Forum 24: 547–548

Pugh R C B 1976 Testicular tumours: Introduction. In: Pugh R C B (ed) Pathology of the Testis, pp 139–159. Blackwell Scientific Publications, Oxford

Raghavan D, Neville A M (1983) The biology of testicular tumours. In: Innes-Williams D and Chisholm G (eds) Scientific Foundations of Urology, 2nd ed, pp 785–796. William Heinemann Medical Books, London

Raghavan D, Selby P J 1981 Testicular tumour xenografts and other experimental models. In: Peckham M J (ed) The Management of Testicular Tumours, pp 70–82. Edward Arnold, London

Raghavan D, Gibbs J, Nogueira-Costa R, et al 1980 The interpretation of marker protein assays: A critical appraisal in clinical studies and a xenograft model. British Journal of Cancer 41 supplement IV: 191–194

Raghavan D, Heyderman E, Monaghan P, et al 1981a When is a seminoma not a seminoma? Journal of Clinical Pathology 34: 123–128

Raghavan D, Gibbs J, Heyderman E, et al 1981b Functional and morphological aspects of human teratoma xenografts. In: Bastert G B A, Fortmeyer H, and Schmidt-Matthiesson, H (eds) Thymusaplastic Nude Mice and Rats in Clinical Oncology, pp 439–445Gustav Fischer Verlag, Stuttgart

Raghavan D, Peckham M J, Heyderman E, Tobias J S, Austin D E 1982a Prognostic factors in clinical stage I non-seminomatous germ-cell tumours of the testis. British Journal of Cancer 45: 167–173

Raghavan D, Sullivan A L, Peckham M J, Neville A M i982b Elevated serum alphafetoprotein and seminoma: Clinical evidence for a histologic continuum? Cancer 50: 982–989

Rannikko S, Kairento A-L, Karonen S-L, Adlercreutz H 1981 Hormonal patterns in prostatic cancer. Acta Endocrinologica 98: 625–633

Reiter E O, Kulin H E 1971 Suppressed FSH in men with chorionic gonadotrophin secreting testicular tumors. Journal of Clinical Endocrinology and Metabolism 33: 957–961

Reyes F I, Faiman C 1973 Development of a testicular tumour during cisclomiphene therapy. Canadian Medical Association Journal 109: 502–506

Reynolds R D, Greenberg B R, Martin N D, et al 1973 Usefulness of bone marrow acid phosphatase in staging carcinoma of the prostate. Cancer 32: 181–184

Reynoso G, Murphy G P 1972 Adrenalectomy and hypophysectomy in advanced prostatic carcinoma. Cancer 29: 941–945

Riba L W 1942 Subcapsular castration for carcinoma of prostate. Journal of Urology 48: 384–387

Robinson C E 1969 Spontaneous regression of renal carcinoma. Canadian Medical Association Journal 100: 297

Robinson M R G 1980 Aminoglutethimide: Medical adrenalectomy in the management of carcinoma of the prostate. A review after 6 years. British Journal of Urology 52: 328–329

Robinson M R G, Shearer R J, Fergusson J D 1974 Adrenal suppression in the treatment of carcinoma of the prostate. British Journal of Urology 46: 555–559

Rubin S-O 1973 Malignant teratoma of testis in a subfertile man treated with HCG and HMG. Scandinavian Journal of Urology and Nephrology 7: 81–84

Ruoslahti E, Hirai H 1978 Alpha-fetoprotein. Scandinavian Journal of Immunology (Suppl) 8: 3–26

Sadoff L, Lusk W 1974 The effect of large doses of medroxyprogesterone acetate (MPA) on urinary estrogen levels and serum levels of cortisol, T4, LH and testosterone in patients with advanced cancer. Obstetrics and Gynecology 43: 262–267

Saleeby E R 1944 Teratoma of the testicle: Metastasis to the epigastrium treated by bilateral orchidectomy — recovery. Annals of Surgery 119: 262–265

Samuels M L, Sullivan P, Howe C D 1968 Medroxyprogesterone acetate in the treatment of renal cell carcinoma (hypernephroma). Cancer 22: 525–532

Sanford E J, Drago J R, Thomas J R, Santen R, Lipton A 1976 Aminoglutethimide medical adrenalectomy for advanced prostatic carcinoma. Journal of Urology 115: 170–174

Sanford E J, Paulson D F, Rohner T J, et al 1977 The effects of castration on adrenal testosterone secretion in men with prostatic carcinoma. Journal of Urology 118: 1019–1021

Santen R J, Lipton A, Kendall K 1974 Successful medical adrenalectomy with aminoglutethimide. Journal of the American Medical Association 230: 1661–1664

Schally A V, Arimura A, Coy D H 1980 Recent approaches to fertility control based on derivatives of LH-RH. Vitamins & Hormones (N.Y.) 38: 257–323

Scardino P T, Skinner D G 1979 Germ cell tumors of the testis: Improved results in a prospective study using combined modality therapy and biochemical tumor markers. Surgery 86: 86–94

Scardino P T, Cox H D, Waldmann T A, et al 1977 The value of serum tumor markers in the staging and prognosis of germ cell tumors of the testis. Journal of Urology 118: 994–999

Scott W W 1963 Growth and development of the human prostate gland. National Cancer Institute Monograph 12: 111–130

Scott W W, Schirmer H K A 1966 A new oral progestational steroid effective in treating prostatic cancer. Transactions of the American Association of Genitourinary Surgeons 58: 54–60

Selby P J, Heyderman E, Gibbs J, Peckham M J 1979 A human testicular teratoma serially transplanted in immune-deprived mice. British Journal of Cancer 39: 578–583

Selye A 1941 Effect of hypophysectomy on morphological appearance of kidney and on renotropic action of steroid hormones. Journal of Urology 46: 110–115

Shain S A, Boesel R W 1978 Human prostate steroid hormone receptor quantitation. Investigative Urology 16: 169–174

Shearer R J, Hendry W F, Sommerville I F, Fergusson J D 1973 Plasma testosterone: An Accurate monitor of hormone treatment in prostate cancer. British Journal of Urology 45: 668–677

Shellhammer P F, Smith M J V 1973 Renal cell carcinoma in children. Southern Medical Journal 66: 1345–1350

Shivers C H, Axilrod H D 1952 Clinical Effect of estrogen therapy on metastatic lesions from carcinoma of testis. Journal of Urology 67: 537–542

Siiteri P K, MacDonald P C 1973 Role of extraglandular estrogen in human endocrinology. In: Greep R O and Astwood E B (eds) Handbook of Physiology section VII, Endocrinology, Vol II, pp 615–629. Williams and Wilkins, Balti more

Siiteri P K, Wilson J D 1970 Dihydrotestosterone in prostatic hypertrophy I. The information and content of dihydrotestosterone in the hypertrophic prostate of man. Journal of Clinical Investigation 49: 1737–1745

Skakkebaek N E 1975 Atypical germ cells in the adjacent 'normal' tissue of testicular tumours. Acta Pathologica et Microbiologica Scandinavica 83: section A: 127–130

Skakkebaek N E 1978 Carcinoma-in-situ of the testis: Frequency and relationship to invasive germ cell tumours in infertile men. Histopathology 2: 157–170

Smolev J K, Heston W D W, Scott W W, Coffey D S 1977 Characterisation of the Dunning R3327H prostatic adenocarcinoma: An apppropriate animal model for prostatic cancer. Cancer Treatment Reports 61: 273–287

Sogani P C, Whitmore W F Jr 1979 Experience with flutamide in prveiously untreated patients with advanced prostatic cancer. Journal of Urology 122: 640–643

Soloway M S, Myers G H Jr 1973 The effect of hormonal therapy on a transplantable renal cortical adenocarcinoma in syngeneic mice. Journal of Urology 109: 356–361

Soloway M S, deKernion J B, Gibbons R P, et al 1981 Comparison of estramustine phosphate and vincristine alone or in combination for patients with advanced, hormone refractory, preveiously irradiated carcinoma of the prostate. Journal of Urology 125: 664–667

deSombre E R, Johnson E S, White W F 1976 Regression of rat mammary tumors effected by a gonadoliberin analog. Cancer Research 36: 3830–3833

Steggles A W, King R J 1968 The uptake of 16,7-3H-oestradiol by oestrogen dependent and independent hamster kidney tumours. European Journal of Cancer 4: 395–400

Steggles A W, King R J 1972 Oestrogen receptors in hamster tumours. European Journal of Cancer 8: 323–334

Steel G G 1977 Growth Kinetics of Tumours, pp 5–55. Clarendon Press, Oxford

Stepanas A V, Samaan N A, Schultz P N, Holoye P Y 1978 Endocrine studies in testicular tumor patients with and without gynecomastia. Cancer 41: 369–376

Stevens L C 1962 Testicular teratomas in fetal mice. Journal of the National Cancer Institute 28: 247–268

Stearns E L, MacDonald J A, Kaufman B J, Lucman T S, Winter J S, Faiman L 1974 Declining testicular function with age; hormonal and clinical correlates. American Journal of Medicine 57: 761–766

Stolbach L L, Begg C B, Hall T, Horton T 1981 Treatment of renal carcinoma: A phase III randomized trial of oral medroxyprogesterone (Provera), hydroxyurea and nafoxidine. Cancer Treatment Reports 65: 689–692

Stoliar B, Albert D J 1974 Sch 13521 in the treatment of advanced carcinoma of the prostate. Journal of Urology 111: 803–807

Stone A R, Hargreave T B, Chisholm G D 1980 The diagnosis of oestrogen escape and the role of secondary orchiectomy in prostatic cancer. British Journal of Urology 52: 535–538

Swanson D A, Johnson D E 1981 Estramustine phosphate (Emcyte) as treatment for metastatic renal carcinoma. Urology 17: 344–346

Swyer G I M 1944 Postnatal growth changes in human prostate. Journal of Anatomy 78: 130–145

Symes E K, Milroy E 1978 An experimental approach to the optimum oestrogen dosage in prostatic carcinoma. British Journal of Urology 50: 562–566

Talley R W 1973 Chemotherapy of adenocarcinoma of the kidney. Cancer 32: 1062–1065

Tavares A S, Costa J, deCarvalho A, Reis M 1966 Tumour ploidy and prognosis in carcinoma of the bladder and prostate. British Journal of Cancer 20: 438–443

Tchao R, Easty G C, Ambrose E A, Raven R W, Bloom H J 1968 Effect of chemotherapeutic agents and hormones on organ cultures of human tumours. European Journal of Cancer 4: 39–44

Teilum G 1971 Special Tumors of Ovary and Testis and Related Extragonadal Lesions, pp 31–78, 327–372. Munksgaard, Copenhagen

Tesar C, Scott W W 1964 A search for inhibitors of prostatic growth stimulators. Investigative Urology 1: 482–498

Thachill M V, Jewett M A S, Rider W D 1981 The effects of cancer and cancer therapy on male infertility. Journal of Urology 126: 141–145

Tolis G, Ackman D, Stellos A 1982 Tumor growth inhibition in patients with prostatic carcinoma treated with luteinizing hormone-releasing agonists. Proceedings of the National Academy of Sciences (USA) 79: 1658–1662

Trachtenberg J, Bujnovsky T, Walsh P C 1982 Androgen receptor content of normal and hyperplastic human prostate. Journal of Clinical Endocrinology and Metabolism 54: 17–21

Tveter K J, Otnes B, Hannestad R 1978 Treatment of prostatic carcinoma with cyproterone acetate. Scandinavian Journal of Urology and Nephrology 12: 115–118

Twombley G H 1947 The relationship of hormones to testicular tumors. In: Twombley G H and Pack G T (eds) Endocrinology of Neoplastic Disease, pp 228–244. Oxford University Press, Oxford

Vaituakaitis J L 1979 Human chorionic gonadotropin: A hormone secreted for many reasons. New England Journal of Medicine 301: 324–326

Van der Werf Messing B, van Gilse H A 1971 Hormonal treatment of metastases of renal cell carcinoma. British Journal of Cancer 25: 423–427

Vermeulen A 1976 Testicular hormonal secretion in ageing in males. In: Grayhack J T, Wilson J D, Scherbenske M J (eds) Benign Prostatic Hyperplasia, NIAMDD Workshop Proceedings, pp 177–182. Government Printing Office, Department of Health Education and Welfare, Washington

Vermeulen A, Reubens R, Verdonck L 1972. Testosterone secretion and metabolism in male senescence. Journal of Clinical Endocrinology 34: 730–735

Vermeulen A, De Sy W 1976 Androgens in patients with benign prostatic hyperplasia before and after prostatectomy. Journal of Clinical Endocrinology and Metabolism 43: 1250–1254

Vessella R L, Santrach M, Lange P H 1983 Concanavalin-A affinity molecular variance of human alpha-fetoprotein in testicular tumor. Journal of Urology

Voigt W, Dunning W F 1974 In vivo metabolism of testosterone-3H in R3327, and androgen-sensitive rat prostatic adenocarcinoma. Cancer Research 34: 1447–1450

Voigt W, Feldman M, Dunning W F 1975 5α-dihydrotestosterone-binding proteins and androgen sensitivity in prostatic cancers of Copenhagen rats. Cancer Research 35: 1840–1845

de Vries J R, Ludens J H, Fanestil D D 1972 Estradiol renal receptor molecules and estradiol-dependent an anti-naturesis. Kidney International 2: 95–101

Veterans Administration Cooperative Urological Research Group 1967 Carcinoma of the prostate: Treatement comparisons. Journal of Urology 98: 516–522

Veterans Administration Cooperative Urological Research Group 1967 Factors in the prognosis of carcinoma of the prostate: A cooperative study. Journal of Urology 100: 59–65

Wagle D G, Murphy G P 1971 Hormonal therapy in advanced renal cell carcinoma. Cancer 28: 318–321

Wahren B, Holmgren P A, Stigbrand T 1979 Placental alkaline phosphatase, alphafetoprotein and carcinoembryonic antigen in testicular tumors: tissue typing by means of cytologic smears. International Journal of Cancer 24: 749–753

Walsh P C, Korenman S G 1971 Mechanism of androgenic action: Effect of specific intracellular inhibitors. Journal of Urology 105: 850–857

Walsh P C, Siiteri P K 1975 Suppression of plasma androgens by spironolactone in castrated males with carcinoma of the prostate. Journal of Urology 114: 254–255

Ware J L, Paulson D F, Parks S F, Webb K S 1982 Production of monoclonal antibody aPro3 recognizing a human prostatic carcinoma antigen. Cancer Research 42: 1215–1222

Watson R A, Tang D B 1980 The predictive value of prostatic acid phosphatase as a screening test for prostate cancer. New England Journal of Medicine 303: 497–499

Waxman M 1976 Malignant germ cell tumor in situ in a cryptorchid testis. Cancer 38: 1452–1456

White J W 1895 The results of double castration in hypertrophy of the prostate. Annals of Surgery 22: 1–80

Williams G, Ghanadian R, Castro J E 1978 The growth and viability of human prostatic tissue maintained in immunosuppressed mice. Clinical Oncology 4: 347–351

Wilson J M, Woodhead D M 1972 Prognostic and therapeutic implications of urinary gonadotropin levels in the management of testicular neoplasia. Journal of Urology 108: 754–756

Worgul T J, Santen R J, Samajlik A, et al 1981 Clinical and biochemical effect of aminoglutethimide in the treatment of advanced prostatic carcinoma. Proceedings of the American Society of Clinical Oncology 22: 471 (abstract)

Yoshimoto Y, Wolfsen A R, Odell W D 1977 Human chorionic gonadotrophin-like substance in neuro-endocrine tissues of normal subjects. Science 197: 575–577

Young H H II, Kent J R 1968 Plasma testosterone levels in patients with prostatic carcinoma before and after treatment. Journal of Urology 99: 788–792

Zak F G 1957 Self healing hypernephromas. Journal of the Mount Sinai Hospital 24:1352–1353

Zetterberg A, Esposti P L 1980 Prognostic significance of nuclear DNA levels in prostatic carcinoma. Scandinavian Journal of Urology and Nephrology supplement 55: 53–58

Zondek B 1929 Versuch einer biologischen (hormonalen) Diagnostik bein malignen Hoden tumor. Chirurgerie 2: 1072–1073

Zondek B 1930 Ueber die Hormone des Hypophysenvorderlappens. III. Follikelreifungshormon (Prolan A) und Tumoren. Klinische Wochenschrift 9: 679–682

Zondek B 1935 Hormones des Ovariums und des Hypophysenvorderlappens, pp 459–475. Julius Springer, Vienna

Index